Women in Medicine

A Bibliography
of the Literature on Women Physicians

compiled and
edited by

SANDRA L. CHAFF

RUTH HAIMBACH

CAROL FENICHEL

NINA B. WOODSIDE

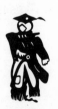

The Scarecrow Press, Inc.
Metuchen, N.J. & London
1977

This project was supported in part by NIH Grant LM 02332 from the National Library of Medicine.

Library of Congress Cataloging in Publication Data

Main entry under title:

Women in medicine.

    Includes indexes.
    1.   Women physicians--Bibliography.   I.   Chaff, Sandra L.
Z7963.M43W65[R692]   016.61069'52   77-24914
ISBN 0-8108-1056-5

TABLE OF CONTENTS

INTRODUCTION
vii

EXPLANATORY NOTES
x

HISTORY OF WOMEN IN MEDICINE
1
In addition to biographies of pre-19th century personalities, the literature cited here gives historical context to the status, education, and practice patterns of healers and physicians. (Histories of specific institutions are located under MEDICAL INSTITUTIONS, SOCIETIES, AND THEIR JOURNALS)

BIOGRAPHIES
75
Specific physicians of the 19th and 20th centuries are the subjects of this section. Comprehensive life histories are included, as well as articles which list educational and career data, and material which consists of biographical segments about travel and other experiences. (Material focusing only on one aspect of a physician's life, i.e., missionary activity or war work, can be found in the classification which relates to that activity.) Fictionalized accounts of the lives of historical figures are also included in this section

RECRUITMENT
385

MEDICAL EDUCATION
393
Included are statistical articles on medical education, general discussions about how women should acquire that education, and material relating in a general manner to medical students, faculty, administration, and educational trends. Undergraduate and premedical education articles are cited as well. (Discussions about women's motivations for entering medicine can be found under PSYCHO-SOCIAL FACTORS. General histories of medical education are located in HISTORY OF WOMEN IN MEDICINE)

GRADUATE MEDICAL EDUCATION
442
Material concentrates on internships, residencies, fellowships, retraining programs, and continuing education programs

MEDICAL ACTIVITY 460
Statistical and narrative material covers practice patterns, specialties, teaching, and administration. (Material discussing societal attitudes or cultural patterns which ultimately affect medical activity is cited in PSYCHOSOCIAL FACTORS)

SPECIALTIES 543
Articles discuss specific specialties--careers in, difficulties encountered, dangers, rewards, and opportunities, as well as historical aspects of women's involvement in specific specialties

MISSIONARY ACTIVITY 581
Along with material on missionary organizations, this section contains material which focuses on the missionary work of individual physicians

WARTIME ACTIVITY 610
Covered are the activities of specific organizations during times of war, which directly relate to war. Material on specific women emphasizes work in war situations or in the military service

PSYCHOSOCIAL FACTORS 648
Literature cited in this section examines social and cultural attitudes affecting women in medicine: the suitability of women for medical study and practice, motivations for entering medicine, the need for women's influence in health care, the problems faced by women physicians, and the attitudes they hold. (Attitudinal material on medical students will be found in MEDICAL EDUCATION. Reports of the debates over women physicians by specific medical institutions or societies are listed under MEDICAL INSTITUTIONS, SOCIETIES, AND THEIR JOURNALS. Material discussing psychosocial factors from a historical perspective are located in HISTORY OF WOMEN IN MEDICINE)

MEDICAL INSTITUTIONS, SOCIETIES, AND THEIR JOURNALS 761
Included: general discussions and statistical data primarily relevant to specific medical schools; the experience of women in medical societies or organizations; and the history and policies of medical journals. (For information about medical education not focusing on specific schools, see MEDICAL EDUCATION)

GENERAL 894
The literature cited here mentions multiple aspects of women in medicine, and gives overviews of the situation for women physicians

FICTION 952
References appear for literature which deals with non-historical figures

iv

NONMEDICAL ACTIVITY   958

APPENDICES   963
   Directories   966
   Collections

INDEXES   969
   Author   995
   Subject   1075
   Personal Name

INTRODUCTION

This bibliography brings together and provides reference to the published literature about women physicians. Such a resource comes not only at a time of increasing interest in women's lives, but also in a period when many basic assumptions about the health care delivery system are being questioned. With the recent rapid rise in the numbers of women in medical school in countries such as the United States, it has become obvious that women will play an increasing role in health care. This work provides citations to literature which documents this increasing involvement of women in medicine, and examines the causes and future course of this trend. It includes, also, material about the lives of specific women physicians and groups of women physicians and helps provide insight into how the careers of most women physicians have differed from those of their male colleagues. The history of women physicians and healers, as well as institutions and issues related to this history, are also represented in the literature cited. We sincerely hope the bibliography will be used by persons representing a wide range of interests and information needs: by researchers, guidance counselors, and people and agencies in general who wish to know woman's heritage.

Our goal was to provide a comprehensive coverage of the literature about women physicians in all parts of the world. We have examined over 95 per cent of the more than 4000 items cited herein, and have indicated those items which we were unable to secure for examination. Of the total number of entries, approximately nine per cent are from non-English-language literature. For these items, English title translations and English annotations are provided. The bibliography represents literature from the 18th century through December 1975 (our earliest cited piece is a 16-page German work by F. Boerner entitled, in translation, Should Women Practice Medicine?, published in Leipzig in 1750). Within this time span, the lives of women physicians and healers from the beginnings of recorded history are discussed. Only published material has been cited: included are books, medical and non-medical journal articles, alumnae and alumni magazine articles, and doctoral theses. Biographical dictionaries and newspaper articles have not been included; nor have sections on women physicians from history of medicine textbooks, or letters-to-the-editor which appeared in medical journals, unless new or unusual information was presented. As in most bibliographic projects with finite resources and a time constraint, it proved impossible to locate everything, especially in relation to the non-English-language material. We are confident that this resource does provide a comprehensive view of what has been written about women physicians, that very few United States publications have been missed, and that the international literature has received a substantial representation.

This bibliography was developed at the Medical College of Pennsylvania as a special project of the Florence A. Moore Library of Medicine in cooperation with the Center for Women in Medicine. In order to collect the material, the unique Women in Medicine Collection of the College's library was tapped, and provided a solid foundation from which to proceed. In addition, letters soliciting information were sent to women's organizations, medical schools, medical societies, state and other geographically-oriented historical archives, and individuals throughout the world. Subject bibliographies provided yet another resource used in collecting material. The annotations were written to assist in deciding whether or not a particular item is one which the user would wish to secure and peruse further. They were written to convey the flavor as well as the content of the items. We have attempted to avoid the use of evaluative words in description and where such words and phrases do occur, they reflect the tone and phrasing of the original material. A few items were felt to have titles sufficient to indicate the content of the material and were not annotated at all.

Most of the publications cited in this bibliography have been collected and are housed in the Florence A. Moore Library of Medicine at the Medical College of Pennsylvania. As the Female Medical College of Pennsylvania (1850-1866) and Woman's Medical College of Pennsylvania (1867-1969), this institution has been the leader in the education of women physicians for over 125 years. The College's collection, as well as other U.S. collections which have substantial holdings relating to women physicians, are described in the Collections Appendix.

ACKNOWLEDGMENTS

A bibliography of this magnitude would not have been possible without the cooperation and assistance of many women. Our appreciation to Janet Cooper who worked on the project in its beginning phases; Ruth Bornholdt who labored with us during the last half of the effort; and Nancy Harper, the medical student who devoted a goodly portion of her spare time for several months. We should also like to acknowledge the translators who provided annotations for the non-English-language material: The Medical Documentation Service at the College of Physicians of Philadelphia, and Ursula Lieber, who annotated most of the German material. And finally, our special gratitude goes to the women who make up the staff of the Florence A. Moore Library of Medicine where this bibliography was produced--especially Margaret Jerrido, who worked dauntlessly for many months to see that the manuscript was produced in readable form for the publisher; Lillian Cannon, whose conscientious effort in the final stages was invaluable; and Claire Schultz, the library director, who gave continual support to the project. Truly, without these women our task would have been impossible.

EXPLANATORY NOTES

In dealing with a bibliography of this size, one question which compilers must face is how best to arrange the material and index it to provide simple yet maximum access. Our approach has been to provide four modes of access to the material: 1) each citation appears alphabetically under a broad classification heading (and more specific geographical designation) which best reflects the primary concern of the material: each item is listed under only one classification; 2) index terms have been assigned to each citation which reflect important concerns of that item; 3) when women physicians are mentioned in any substantial way in the material, these women are indexed as well, and appear in the Personal Name Index; and 4) each item is indexed by author. These access modes may be used separately or in conjunction with one another. The simplest searching may require only one approach; more complex research needs may demand a more active use of the four modes. There is, in short, a constant interaction among the classifications, the Subject Index, and the Personal Name Index, of which the researcher must be aware to use this bibliography effectively. Following are examples designed to illustrate how one might approach the bibliography.

EXAMPLE 1: If a user is interested in securing material relating to missionary activity among women physicians, the approach would be as follows:

A. Scan the citations and annotations in the classification section which pertains to one's interest. In this case, the classification MISSIONARY ACTIVITY would be scanned. The user should notice the names which appear frequently in the annotations under this classification, such as Clara Swain and Anna Dengel.

B. Turn to the Subject Index and check under the index term which is most nearly synonymous with the classification term (i.e., Missionaries and Missionary Activity). These terms will contain citation numbers to all references which deal in some way with missionary activity of women physicians but which do not appear under the MISSIONARY ACTIVITY classification for one reason or another: for example, an article which treats the entire life of a particular woman whose career included a brief period of missionary activity will be cited under the BIOGRA-PHIES classification but indexed under Missionary Activity.

C. Finally, check the Personal Name Index for citations to the names of women which have been noted as appearing frequently in the annotations under the classification MISSIONARY ACTIVITY (e.g., Clara Swain and Anna Dengel).

EXAMPLE 2: If a user is interested in researching Marie Zakrzewska, an early and prominent woman physician in America, the approach would be as follows:

A. Check for Zakrzewska's name in the Author Index. This will lead to citations of articles written by Zakrzewska which deal with the subject of women physicians. Scan the annotations for these articles, noting the names of people and places that occur frequently.

B. Check the Personal Name Index for Zakrzewska's name. Scan the citations and annotations thus found, noting again the names of people and places that occur frequently in the annotations. The user will observe, for example, that Zakrzewska's name appears frequently in association with the name of Emily Blackwell and the New England Hospital for Women and Children.

C. Turn to the Subject Index and proceed to the citations listed under the term New England Hospital for Women and Children. Here the user will find not only more material on Zakrzewska, but also leads to additional subject terms to check.

D. Turn to the Personal Name Index for citations listed under Emily Blackwell's name.

HISTORY OF
WOMEN IN MEDICINE

In addition to biographies of pre-19th century personalities, the literature cited here gives historical
context to the status, education, and practice patterns
of healers and physicians. (Histories of specific institutions are located under MEDICAL INSTITUTIONS,
SOCIETIES, AND THEIR JOURNALS.)

AFRICA

1. Kuhnke, Laverne. "The 'Doctoress' on a Donkey: Women Health Officers in Nineteenth Century Egypt." Clio Medica, 9:3 (September 1974) 193-205.

   Most other studies refer to the 19th-century Egyptian school described in this paper as a midwifery school because it emphasized obstetrics. However, this author distinguishes between untrained folk midwives--dayas--and hakimas--a term for "doctoresses." The School for Hakimas required six years of training and at least rudimentary theoretical science--a prodigious amount of instruction for women in the Middle East at that time. Detailed are the development of a women's auxiliary health corps in Egypt, recruitment, the professional activities of the Egyptian "doctoress," and the sociological factors which contributed to the decline in numbers of medical women in the early 20th century.

2. Stephens, Nannie A. "Woman in Gynecology and Obstetrics." American Journal of Surgery and Gynecology, 12 (January 1899) 144-145.

   Dr. Stephens presents a history of women in gynecology and obstetrics which concentrates on women of ancient Egypt. She concludes her article with examples of her own experiences as a specialist in the field.

ASIA

3. Jhirad, J. "Pioneer Work by and for Medical Women." Journal of the Association of Medical Women in India, 39:2 (May 1951) 29-34.

   This article opens with the mention of the first medical women in the U.S. and Great Britain. In 1869 Clara Swain of America became India's first woman physician. The accomplishments of several other women, many of them medical missionaries, are also cited, along with those of women's medical schools and associations. In conclusion, the author urges medical women to rise to India's pressing problem of preventive medicine, and to prepare themselves for teaching posts and for research.

4. Wong, K. Chimin and Wu, Lien-Teh. History of Chinese Medicine: Being a Chronicle of Medical Happenings in China from Ancient Times to the Present Period. Tientsin Press, Ltd., Tientsin, China, 1932, xviii, 706 pp. figs., illus., photos., ports.

   Scattered information on women healers and physicians is found throughout this history, which traces the Chinese medical evolution from an indigenous and mysterious art form in 2697 B.C. to the widespread assimilation of "Western" medicine in the 1930s. The authors note that Ch'un Yü-yen, an obstetrician of the Han dynasty, is the first woman doctor mentioned in Chinese medical history. Not until the 19th century, however, do women begin to emerge in the profession. This book brief-ly profiles several distinguished women, including Hü King-eng, Ida Kahn, Mary Stone (Shih Mei-yu), and Yamei Kin (Y. May King). Foreign women physicians, many of them missionaries, are also mentioned. Medical education of women, and hos-pitals staffed and founded by women are described as well. Appendixes include chronological tables of events, geographical, name, and subject indexes, and an extensive bibliography.

AUSTRALIA & NEW ZEALAND

5. Morgan, Elma Sandford. A Short History of Medical Women in Australia. Burroughs Wellcome and Company (Austra-lia), Ltd., Australia, 1970.
    This history was produced for the Australian Federation of Medical Women on the occasion of the 12th Congress of the Medical Women's International Association, Melbourne, Aus-tralia. [Item not examined by editors.]

6. "Women in Medicine." Medical Journal of Australia, 1:2 (9 January 1971) 54-56. (Comments.)
    A discussion of the opening of medical schools and hospital posts to women includes profiles of Australia's first women physicians. While contrasting early opposition to medical wo-men with the present situations in Australia, the author points out that women still face medical school quota systems, un-equal pay, and inflexible employment conditions that force wo-men with multiple responsibilities to become part of the pro-fession's "wastage" statistics.

7. Younger Ross, Isabella. "The Advent of Women into Medicine." Medical Journal of Australia, (30 May 1953) 777-779. (Presentation, Australasian Medical Congress, 22-29 Au-gust 1952.)
    On June 2, 1865, Dr. Wilhelmina Ferguson, a graduate of the Woman's Medical College of Pennsylvania, became the first woman to apply for medical registration in Victoria. The opinion of the medical community regarding a woman's registra-tion ran so negative that Dr. Ferguson never approached the Medical Board again. It was not until 20 years later that an-other woman (Dr. Laura Morgan, a graduate of New York Med-ical Woman's College) applied for registration. Her application also was unsuccessful and she returned to America. The first woman to practice in Victoria was Dr. Constance Stone, an Australian-born, American and Canadian-educated physician. Sydney was the first university to admit women to medical studies, but the University of Melbourne was the first school

to actually grant medical degrees to women. The story of the seven women who opened the doors of the University of Melbourne and the problems they faced follows.

CANADA

8. Abbott, Maude E. History of Medicine in the Province of Quebec. McGill University, Montreal, Canada, 1931, 97 pp. facsim., figs., photos., ports.
This regional history covers Quebec medicine from the mid-16th century to the 1920s. Although written by a woman physician, there is little mention of the role of women doctors, with the exception of an account of the admission of women to the Bishop's College Medical School in 1890. Ten women were graduated from that institution from 1893 to 1905, when it merged with the McGill Faculty of Medicine. This book, however, details the known facts of Dr. James Miranda Stuart Barry, the British army officer who, upon an autopsy in 1865, was found to have been a woman. Dr. Barry, a graduate of Edinburgh, entered military service in 1813 and was made a staff surgeon in military hospitals of Canada. Dr. Barry was later made inspector general of all British hospitals. Her true sex was apparently successfully concealed throughout her entire career. Sources for this data are documented in the bibliography, and a picture of Dr. Barry has been included in the text.

9. Bean, E. S. "Pioneer Women in Medicine." Nova Scotia Medical Bulletin, 21 (April 1942) 113-123.
[Article not examined by editors.]

10. Beaton-Mamak, Mary. "Women Doctors: Ruffles in the Profession." Dimensions in Health Service, 52:1 (January 1975) 38. port. (Profiles.)
An overview of the history of Canadian women in medicine, this article mentions the accomplishments of several distinguished women physicians.

11. Godfrey, C. M. "The Origins of Medical Education of Women in Ontario." Medical History (London), 17:1 (January 1973) 89-94. tables.
This article traces the development of medical education for women in Ontario, Canada. The first women medical students were recruited for a special course at the Royal Medical College in Kingston in 1880. Protests of male students in 1882-1883 forced the organization of a separate school for women in Kingston in 1883. In 1895 this institution merged with the Ontario Medical College for Women in Toronto. In 1905 the Ontario Medical College for Women became part of the University of Toronto. Concurrent with the growth of this school was the Women's College Hospital, established in 1910. Tables showing the percentage of women matriculates to graduate from

both the Kingston and Toronto institutions during the 1880s are
included.

12. Hacker, Carlotta. The Indomitable Lady Doctors. Clarke,
    Irwin & Company Limited, Toronto, Canada, 1974, 259 pp.
    photos. , ports. , table.
    The publication of this volume marks the golden jubilee of the
    Federation of Medical Women of Canada. As a memorial to
    women who pioneered in Canadian medicine, whole chapters
    are devoted to biographical sketches of such physicians as
    James Barry, Emily Stowe, Augusta Stowe-Gullen, Jennie
    Trout, the first graduates of the Queen's University medical
    course for women (Elizabeth Beatty, Elizabeth Smith-Shortt,
    and Alice McGillivray), Maria Anguin, Charlotte Ross, vari-
    ous medical missionaries, Elizabeth Scott Matheson, Helen
    MacMurchy, and Maude Abbott. Brief notes on other women
    physicians follow most chapters. Included is a section of
    notes, four statistical appendices, a selected bibliography, and
    an index. There are photographs of many of the physicians
    discussed.

EUROPE, EASTERN

13. Belicza, B[iserka]. ["The First Croatian Women Physicians"].
    Liječnički Vjesnik, 92:10 (1970) 1187-1197. (Cro)
    This article traces the general history of women of Slavic ori-
    gin who practiced medicine in Croatia from the 13th century to
    the first decade of the 20th century when the first women phy-
    sicians graduated from medical schools abroad. Draga Slava
    is the first woman physician whose name is recorded as being
    conferred with the right to practice medicine (in 1330) "be-
    cause of successful cures and the good result she had achieved
    in treating podagric and eye diseases." After women were al-
    lowed to attend the School of Medicine at Zürich, Ljočić-Milo-
    šević of Šabac, Serbia, was, in 1879, the first woman physician
    of the Slavic south who graduated at Zürich. Dr. Milica Švig-
    lin-Čavov was the first Croatian woman to become a qualified
    physician by graduating from Zürich in 1893. In 1898 a
    Health Service Organization Act of Croatia prohibited women
    physicians from practicing medicine there. Dr. Karola Milo-
    bar was the first woman physician to practice in Zagreb by
    obtaining a special work permit. Becoming an expert in gastro-
    enterology, she started a practice "for diseases of the diges-
    tive system and women's diseases." Another pioneer, Augusta
    Buček, obtained her degree in 1903 and specialized in derma-
    tology. Ema Pavlekovič also earned her medical degree in
    1903 but did not practice medicine in Croatia until 1920, hav-
    ing practiced abroad until then. Milana Gavrančic-Novak, Van-
    da Betlheim, and Emilia Lazič also received their medical de-
    grees in Switzerland. According to the available data, Zlata
    Havliček was the first Croatian woman to graduate from the
    School of Medicine in Vienna (in 1911). [The journal includes
    an English translation of this article, pp. 68-78.]

14. Chojna, J. W. ["Participation of the First Women-Physicians in Warsaw Medical Society and the Attitude of the Society Towards the Problem of Women in Health Care"]. Archiwum Historii Medycyny (Warszawa), 36 (1973) 177-185. (Russian and English Abstracts.) (Pol)
[Article not examined by editors.]

15. Huppert, M. P. "Women Doctors in the Middle Ages." History of Medicine, 5:3 (Autumn 1973) 25-26.
While women in Italy during the Middle Ages were legally entitled to medical school education, women's social position made it difficult for them to utilize the privilege. Therefore, most women doctors obtained "licences to practice," which were granted after a demonstration of medical knowledge.
This article mentions many women doctors, from the first recorded to have practiced in Southern Italy (Federica Vitali of the School of Salerno), to Alessandra Giliani of Bologna. The era came to an end with the expansion of universities in the middle of the 15th century; women were barred from obtaining the now-essential academic qualifications, and could no longer acquire the non-academic practicing licences.

16. Kempler, K. ["Fight for the Admission of Women to Universities in Hungary at the End of the 19th Century"]. Orvosi Hetilap, 115:30 (28 July 1974) 1775-1777. (Hun)
In the 19th century, Hungarian medical schools were closed to women and they were particularly denied the right to dispense drugs. A Union for the Rights of Women was led particularly by Countess Anna Bolza. Nevertheless, it was not until 1895 that she and several of her associates were granted the Diploma in Medicine by a decree of the legislature. The National Congress of Dispensers had been strongly opposed to the admission of women in their August 1874 meeting, but several prominent medical men enthusiastically supported the admission of women. The minister of culture decreed in 1888 that women could practice medicine if associated with male physicians. At that time there were 14 women in Budapest who had medical diplomas from the University of Paris and one who had received her diploma from Zurich in 1879. The latter, Vilma Hugonnay, was the first woman admitted to practice in Budapest. The decrees in question are quoted in full. The government decree was fully effective in June 1895, but the full equality of women physicians did not come until 1913. Matild Schorr, Ida Szendeffy, and Lea Koenigsberger received their diplomas in 1897; all previously had been midwives. By 1913, of a class of 113 graduates admitted to practice, 10 were women. One of these, Ilonka Szoradi, practiced for 25 years.

17. Lazarewitch, Radmilla. "Women Physicians in Serbia." Woman's Medical Journal, 29[19]:12 (December 1919) 256.
Draga Ljotchitch-Miloshevitch became the first woman physician in Serbia after graduating from the University of Zurich in 1878. Despite early opposition to medical women, there is

now no difference in their privileges and those of male physicians.

EUROPE, WESTERN

18. Alvarez Ricart, Maria Del Carmen. ["Women in 19th Century Spanish Medicine: the First Women to Obtain Medical Degrees"]. Asclepio, 21 (1969) 43-48. (Spa)
The entrance of women into the medical sciences and medicine in Spain in the 19th century precipitated a deluge of polemic in contemporary journals by the women's male colleagues, who questioned not their qualifications and training so much as the appropriateness of women's desire to enter the world of academic life and the medical societies. The first of these women was Dolores Aleu, who passed the examinations of the anatomy and dissection groups in 1875 with high honors and was awarded the Premio Extraordinario by these organizations. Shortly thereafter, she was enrolled by the therapeutics group and was appointed an assistant in the department of Sr. Carbo at Barcelona. An article published by Aleu in 1878 on rheumatism and reprinted under the title of "Feminine First Steps" set off a series of articles in several of the journals, apparently because she had disagreed with some opinions of a male colleague. The first woman to be invested with the doctorate was another Barcelonan, Martina Castells. The male reaction was apparently summed up in one comment: "Our sincere congratulations--but don't let it happen again!" Castells died early in the year 1884, less than a year and a half after receiving her degree. In 1886, Dolores Lleonart y Casanovas became a Licenciate in Medicine from the University of Barcelona at the age of 19, and in the same year Luisa Dominga became a Licenciate of the University of Valladolid. In 1889 the Faculty of Medicine of Valencia awarded the Licenciate in Medicine and Surgery to Maria Concepcion Aleixandre y Ballestar. Two years later her application for membership in the Spanish gynecological society was rejected after heated discussion by the (male) members.

19. Baudouin, Marcel. ["Female Doctors in France during the 13th and 14th Century"]. Gazette Medicale de Paris, 22 (1 June 1901) 169-172. (Fre)
The author briefly discusses several women of the period who were honored for their medical skills: Saint Jutta, practicing about 1252; Mistress Hersend, who accompanied St. Louis on the Seventh Crusade in the mid-13th century as a physician, perhaps to Louis' queen Marguerite; Isabel (Elizabeth) queen of Portugal, later beatified by Urban VII; and Sarah, wife of Abraham, a Jewess known to have been practicing and teaching in 1326. He presents a list of eight women who were practicing medicine illegally, i.e. without proper studies or diplomas, at the end of the 13th and beginning of the 14th century. A part of the article is devoted to consideration of two lists found

by earlier researchers of women accused of, or excommunicated for, practicing medicine illegally in the first half of the 14th century, with a discussion of sources of confusion in names: in addition to differences in spelling, this includes such questions as whether several listings of the name Clarisse may refer to individuals or simply to members of the religious order of Clarisses (names for St. Claire of Assisi). The author selects five from these lists for brief discussion: Clarice of Rouen, wife of Pierre, excommunicated in 1311 or 1312; Jehanne (Jeanne) Converse of Salins, brought to court with her husband by the Medical Faculty of Paris and excommunicated in 1322; Laurence, wife of Jehan de Gaillon, 1327; Jehanne Clarisse, 1331; and Jacobe Félicie, fined and excommunicated in 1322.

20.   Baudouin, Marcel. ["Female Physicians of Ancient Greece (Biographical Notes). (First Century B.C.--First Century A.D.)"]. Gazette Medicale de Paris, 12th Series, 1:7 (16 February 1901) 49-51. illus. (Fre)
Among women healers mentioned in ancient writings are Artemisia II, queen of Carie (a midwife, according to Pliny), Anyte of Epidaurus, Lais of Athens, Olympias of Thebes, Salpe, Sotira, and Agnodice of Athens. Most are mentioned by Pliny; all were probably midwives, if they existed at all.

21.   Baudouin, Marcel. ["Female Physicians of Ancient Greece (First Century B.C.--First Century A.D.). (Biographical Notes)"]. Gazette Medicale de Paris, 12th Series, 1:8 (23 February 1901) 57-59. (Fre)
The author has found evidence, in a collection of Greek inscriptions from tombstones, that the Greeks had women doctors whom they called Elatreiua or latriue. One inscription mentions Empiria, wife of Vettianus, as a woman doctor. Two other names have recently been discovered--Basila (or Basilla) of Corycos and Thecla of Seleucia, both buried in Christian cemeteries. Nothing else is known about them.

22.   Baudouin, Marcel. ["Women Surgeons in the School of Salerno"]. Archives Provinciales de Chirurgie, 9 (1900) 202-205. port. (Fre)
Brief biographies are presented of three distinguished women from the famous school of Salerno, who could be considered to be surgeon specialists. The first, Trotula (Trota, Trocta, Trottola), lived and practiced in the 11th century. There has been considerable controversy over exactly who she was and whether she actually wrote the major work attributed to her (De Passionibus Mulierum), but current opinion is that Trotula is more than a legend. Her works have survived only as fragments quoted by later authors. The second, Mercuriade, is known for four works in surgical pathology, all of which have been lost. The third, Francoise, wife of Mathieu de Romana, passed an examination before a committee of physicians and surgeons and was granted "doctoral permission in surgery" in 1321 by the Duke of Calabria.

23. Bayon, H. P. "Trotula and the Ladies of Salerno: A Contribution to the Knowledge of the Transition between Ancient and Mediaeval Physick." Proceedings of the Royal Society of Medicine, 33 (10 January 1940) 471-475. photo.
The author traces the perpetuation of the belief that Trotula of Salerno was a legend, from Charles Singer in 1924 through Thorndike (1929) and Powicke and Emden (1936). In 1930 and 1938, however, Kate Hurd Mead challenged these opinions. The author finds investigation into the truth of Trotula's existence too "invidious" a task to undertake, but does try to present an "unambiguous conception of the importance and significance of De Passionibus against the background of medical knowledge and practice of the 12th to 13th centuries in Southern Italy, and its consequent influence across time and land in relation to medicine."

24. Beckh, H. ["Centenary of Women in Medicine"]. Bayer Aerztebl., 26 (January 1971) 42-46.
[Article not examined by editors.]

25. Caldwell, Ruth. "Women in Medicine: Chapter I. The First Women in Medicine." Medical Woman's Journal, 37:2 (February 1930) 40-42.
Women have acted as physicians as long as there has been a history of medicine. Women were the first nurses and practitioners of the healing art. Ancient Greek epics, mythology, and history mention a variety of women healers: Hygea, goddess of health; the daughter of Augea; the Egyptian Polydamna; Cleopatra's sister, Arsenoe; Pythagoras' wife, Theano; Antiochus; Victoria; and Leoparda. Greek history also records the life of Agnodice, a woman who disguised herself as a man in order to study under the great male physicians of her day. She wished to care for women whose modesty would not allow them to be helped by male physicians during childbirth and other "private diseases." When it became known that Agnodice was a woman, she was condemned to death. The noble women she had helped, which included most of the women of the city, surrounded her house and "before the judges ... told them they would no longer account them for husbands and friends, but for cruel enemies that condemned her to death who restored to them their health, protesting they would all die with her if she were put to death." As a result, the magistrates annulled the law forbidding gentlewomen the right to study medicine.

26. Caldwell, Ruth. "Women in Medicine: Chapter II. Medieval Women Physicians." Medical Woman's Journal, 37:3 (March 1930) 72-75.
During the early Christian period (the fourth and fifth centuries) many female converts became physicians. Indeed, before 500 A.D. there were four women saints who were physicians: Saint Zenais, Saint Philomela, Saint Theodosia, and Saint Nicerata. Fabiola founded the first hospital of Rome. During

the Middle Ages, nunneries and monasteries became centers for healing the sick and the wounded in battle. "The healing art" became part of the curriculum in convent schools. Frequently, women characters in Medieval epics were prepared to give first aid. Saint Hildegarde wrote medical treatises and nearly all of the methods of diagnosis now used are to be found or at least hinted at in her work. At Salerno, Trotula headed a department of medicine on women's diseases which was entirely under the supervision of women professors. North of the Alps women were active in medicine, but in 1292 the Faculty of Paris passed an edict "which forbade the practice of medicine to all who were not members of that body, to which only unmarried men were admitted." In England, women were able to practice medicine, but not for long "because the male competitors became jealous."

27. Caldwell, Ruth. "Women in Medicine: Chapter III. Women in Medicine--'Modern History.'" Medical Woman's Journal, 37:4 (April 1930) 96-98.
After the "Dark Ages," as more men were educated, the place that women had held in medicine was usurped "by the jealous males"--especially in northern Europe. The women of Italy and southern Europe were able to retain their positions in medicine longer, not only as midwives but also as highly regarded medical experts in other fields such as anatomy, dissection, and the physical education of children. At one time, women exclusively were midwives and as such were as highly regarded as magistrates, physicians, and surgeons, "but they lost their respectable position because they were denied the opportunities of needful study and careful instruction." Queen Victoria also contributed to the decline of women as midwives when she employed "men-midwives" during her confinement. At that time women midwives believed the use of chloroform was wrong and would not use it. In Russia, because of the customs of the Graeco-Russian Church, midwives still flourished and medical men were rarely consulted. The mortality rate was far lower in Russia than in England.

28. Chéreau, A. ["Proceeding Instituted, in 1322, by the Faculty of Medicine, Against a Woman Illegally Practicing Medicine"]. L'Union Médicale, 31:93 (7 August 1866) 241-248. (Fre)
A list of taxpayers in Paris in the year 1292 includes (in addition to 151 barbers, male and female) 29 "mires" or male doctors and eight "meiresses" or female doctors. The author of this paper found a list of 24 individuals practicing medicine illegally in Paris in 1322; the city at that time had an estimated population of 275,000. The list includes two women. The Faculty of Medicine of Paris took action against these illegal practitioners; earlier it had obtained a sentence of excommunication against a Clarice of Rouen and successfully brought suit against Jehanne Converse and her husband, and the Faculty was awaiting a promised papal bull threatening excommunication of

anyone practicing medicine without proper certification in Paris
or its suburbs. This article quotes the complaints against one
Jacobea Felicie in August 1322 and the testimony of eight witnesses who had been treated by her. In spite of their reports
of apparent cures, Jacobea Felicie was fined and excommunicated.

29. Coues, William Pearce. "Women Physicians in Medieval
Times." Boston Medical and Surgical Journal, 172:3 (21
January 1915) 119. (Letters to the Editor.)
Dr. Coues offers a prose translation of "Erec and Enide" by
Chrétien de Troyes, a French poet of the 12th century. The
poem describes women's skill in healing a wounded soldier.

30. Coury, C. and Pecker, A. ["Notes on the Teaching of Obstetrics in France in the Eighteenth Century--Angelique du
Coudray at Grenoble"]. In: [20th International Congress
of the History of Medicine, Berlin, Germany, 22-27 August 1966.] Edited by Heinz Goerke and Heinz Müller-
Dietz. George Olms, Hildesheim, Germany, 1968, pp.
671-678. (Fre)
It was only in the 18th century that men began to carry out
increasingly the duties of an accoucheur; prior to that they
had been called in only when serious difficulties occurred during delivery. Most women in labor were attended by poorly
educated older women. In 1780 a royal edict set up a refresher course in practical obstetrics at the veterinary school at
Alfort under the direction of Angelique Marguerite Le Boursier
du Coudray (also spelled Ducoudrai or Du Coudrai). She had
been born in Paris, practiced there and in Auvergne as a midwife, and had invented a "machine" for demonstrating obstetric
maneuvers. In 1767 she was given a yearly salary by Louis
XV to teach in all the provinces. Jealous surgeons were
strongly opposed to her teaching.

31. Creutz, Rudolf. ["Women of Salerno in the Service of Aesculapius from the 11th to the 15th Century"]. Die Frau,
(1932) 110-115. (Ger)
The "high period" of the medical school at Salerno was remarkable, among other things, for the appearance of a number
of women medical students. Unfortunately, it is hard to separate legend and history, although there is no doubt that the
women existed and contributed to the care of women and children. Most of their published works are known only as names
in the works of later authors, and there is controversy over
whether they actually wrote the books attributed to them. The
author describes what little is known about six of these women
who practiced in the 11th through 15th centuries: Trotula,
Abella, Mercuriadis, Rebecca Guarna, Francesca de Roma,
and Constantia Calenda. In addition, he mentions the unnamed
and unnumbered women healers who practiced a kind of folk
medicine among the general population, and cites a number of
remedies popular in that period for the care of the skin and
hair.

32.   Damour, Felix.   [Louise Bourgeois: Her Life, Her Work].
         Jouve & Boyer, Paris, France, 1900, 110 pp.   illus.
         (M. D. thesis.   No. 603.)   (Fre)
This thesis was presented to the faculty of medicine of the
University of Paris.   After an introductory survey of midwifery
of the 16th century, the author summarizes the life of Louise
Bourgeois, taken from portions of her writings including her
books.   Louise Bourgeois was born in 1563 in the Faubourg
St. -Germain, and married Martin Boursier, a surgeon in the
royal army.   During the civil war, she and her three children
had to flee Paris, and during their period of exile, she studied
midwifery with her husband.   After their return to Paris, she
took the examinations for accreditation as a midwife and soon
became as popular with court society as she had previously
been with the common people.   She presided at the births of
the six royal infants, starting with Louis XIII in 1601.   Her
writings consist of three books of instruction and observations
on diseases of pregnancy and abnormal deliveries, a collection
of "secrets, " and a defense against doctors.   The first to describe the treatment of chlorosis with iron, to advocate induced
delivery in cases of severe hemorrhage, and to enumerate the
different fetal presentations, Louise Bourgeois was the first
woman to write in France on the obstetric arts.

33.   Darcanne-Mouroux.   "History of French Medical Women. "
         Medical Woman's Journal, 29:10 (October 1922) 238-240.
This brief summary of French women who opened the medical
profession to women begins with the request of Madeline Bres
for the right to matriculate at the Medical Faculty of Paris
(1866).   In 1881 Mlle. Edwards was instrumental in obtaining
permission for women to compete for the "externat, " and later,
the "internat. "   In 1889 Mlle. Wilbouchewitch became the second woman to receive "interne titulaire. "   Because of the success of these women, 34 women were received as interns from
1887 to 1922, and there are now 357 French women matriculated at the Faculty of Paris.   There are 160 women doctors
practicing in Paris, and many women have distinguished themselves during the war.   Several contemporary physicians are
mentioned.

34.   Fichna, Margarete.   ["Pioneers for Women in Medical Studies
         in Austria"].   Zeitschrift d. Bauvereines der d. Akademi-
         kerinnen Österreichs, 12:2 (1959) 13 passim.   (Ger)
This article concentrates on the pioneers for women's medical
studies and practice in Austria.   Dr. Rosa Kerschbaumer was
the first woman to obtain licensure in Austria.   Dr. Anna
Bayer practiced as the first public health physician in Bosnia.
After studying in Switzerland, Gabriele Possaner von Ehrenthal
obtained the doctorate in Austria after a long, drawn-out fight
ended by an imperial decree that allowed all women who had
studied abroad to obtain an M. D. degree in Austria.   And finally, the first woman to study in Austria and to obtain her M. D.
from an Austrian university was Margarete Hoenigsberg-Hil-

ferding. All these women fought against severe prejudice in the scientific community and in the public.

35. Fischer, J. ["Women in the Service of Aesculapius"]. _Wiener Medizinische Presse_, 42 (1900) 1913-1917. (Ger)
In the controversy over women's admission to medical studies, the author reviews the book by H. Schelenz, _Women in Esculapius' Realm_, an essay on the history of women in medicine. It contains a brief overview of women practicing or promoting medicine in antiquity and the Middle Ages, of midwifery, and of the influence of rich noblewomen, who furthered science and pharmacology for humanitarian reasons. Schelenz is accused of prejudiced reporting, especially on female pharmacists, whom he accuses of having a passion for poison and of misusing their knowledge to satisfy their vices. The author praises the historic research of Schelenz's book but cannot agree with his conclusion that "women are born to be a man's companion."

36. Flatow, F. ["Outstanding Women in Medicine during the Past"]. _Die Medizinische Welt_, 52 (24 December 1932) 1879-1884. ports. (Ger)
In this article the author concentrates on the writings of women in medicine during the 17th and 18th centuries. He gives a short biography and then underlines the publications of these midwives and physicians. The longest passage is devoted to Dorothea Christiana [Erxleben] Leporin--in particular, to the controversy between her and three male physicians accusing her of quackery. The author stresses the important contributions women made to obstetrics before the field was taken over by their male colleagues.

37. Friedenwald, H. "Jewish Doctoresses in the Middle Ages." _Medical Pickwick_, 6 (1920) 283.
[Article not examined by editors.]

38. Goodell, William. _A Sketch of the Life and Writings of Louyse Bourgeois, Midwife to Marie De' Medici, the Queen of Henry IV. of France. The Annual Address of the Retiring President Before the Philadelphia County Medical Society._ Published by the Society, Philadelphia, Pennsylvania, 1876, 52 pp. port.

39. Gordon, Charles Alexander. "Medical Women." _Medical Press and Circular_, 117 (10 August 1898) 131-133.
[Article not examined by editors.]

40. Gordon, J. Elise. "Some Women Practitioners of Past Centuries." _Practitioner_, 208 (April 1972) 561-567. facsim.
There were women doctors called medicae in ancient Rome, as well as highly regarded and respected women healers who functioned as doctors during medieval times and into the 17th century.

41. Grangée, F. M. ["The Woman Physician: Reflections on a Study Written Over 50 Years"]. Vie Méd., 4 (1923) 1417-1420. (Fre)
[Article not examined by editors.]

42. Guardia, J. M. ["Spanish Philosophers: Oliva Sabuco"]. Revue Philosophique, (1886) 42-60; 272-292. (Fre)
Oliva Sabuco des Nantes Barrera--the exact name is uncertain --published in 1587 a book entitled A New Philosophy of the Nature of Man, Not Known or Achieved by the Ancient Philosophers, Which Will Improve Human Life and Health..., and dedicated to Phillip II of Spain. The author, although not a physician, pointed out the causes of error which have misled both ancient and "modern" physicians. This paper presents the little that is known about her and the times in which she wrote, the circumstances in which the book was republished in 1728 and, at some length, the theories of medicine contained in it. The "passions" are considered the cause of all disease and death. Fear, anger, despair, love (unrequited or deprived), shame, anxiety, compassion, etc., all greatly influence the secretions of the brain which in turn control the health of the body. Advice is given by this "doctor without diploma" on proper diet and habits, including the effects of taste, color, odor, heat, and cold. The sources of all actions, sentiments, movements, all vital phenomena, resides in the head, through which they are influenced by external events.

43. Hamilton, George L. "Trotula." Modern Philology, 4 (October 1906) 377-380.
Hamilton offers a heavily documented explanation of why the name of Trotula should appear as the author of one of the books in the Vade Mecum of Jankin in the Wife of Bath's Prologue: "Trotula was the first and most distinguished of the female representatives of the medical school of Salerno," and as such her name was very well known.

44. Hedvall, Gunnel. ["On Our First Women Doctors"]. Nordisk Medicinskhistorisk Årsbok, (1974) 167-172. facsim., photo. (Swe)
At a lecture at the Medical Assembly in December 1973, the speaker reviewed the gradual development of the idea of medical careers for women, starting in the early 1800s with the need for parish doctors for women and infants, through the lengthy deliberations of the Medical Council, the medical academic establishment and the Riksdag (the legislature), to the admission of women to the medical schools in the early 1870s and the first woman to receive an M.D. degree from a Swedish school (Karolina Widerström in 1888). By 1900 there were 14 women doctors of a total of 1300 physicians; in 1910 there were 31, and in 1970, 31 per cent of the doctors in Sweden were women. Most of the early women doctors were also active in social reform movements, women's rights, universal

education, and the early radical political movements. Widerström, especially, was a leader in the demand for equality for
women physicians.

45.   Heise, Agnete.   "The First Women Doctors of Denmark."
           Journal of the American Medical Women's Association, 4:
           2 (February 1949) 70-72.   port.
        Nielsine Mathilde Nielsen was the first woman physician of
        Denmark, receiving her degree from the University of Copen-
        hagen in 1885 after a struggle to have the University open its
        door to women, which it ultimately did in 1875.   The work of
        Drs. Eli Moeller and Alvilda Harbou Hoff is also mentioned.

46.   Hovorka, Ostar.   ["Female Physician in Ancient Rome"].
           Klinish-Therapeutische Wochenschriften, 21:1 (1914) 6-8.
           (Ger)
        In this article the author attempts to illustrate the important
        role female medical doctors played in ancient Rome.   He bases
        his study on epitaphs from Roman monuments and tombstones
        from which he quotes liberally.   He concludes that contrary to
        popular belief the "medicae" were trained and practicing phy-
        sicians who worked mainly, though by no means exclusively,
        for female patients.   They practiced obstetrics, but their role
        was not restricted to that of a midwife.   They were well read
        and enjoyed considerable esteem in the community, as indi-
        cated by their financial success and the grateful epitaphs on
        their tombstones.

47.   Hurd-Mead, Kate Campbell.   "Concerning Certain Medical Wo-
           men of the Late Middle Ages."   Medical Life, 42:3 (March
           1935) 110-128.   port.
        "Women doctors of the late Middle Ages were very much like
        the women of today, pacifists, sympathetic with the sick, gentle,
        and unobtrusive wherever they were obliged to compete with
        men, grateful for small favors, and asking in those days only
        for the opportunity to study and to be let alone in their work....
        [The] attitude of masculine bravado and feminine subservience
        lasted until the middle of the nineteenth century when women
        took the matter into their own hands...."   Dr. Hurd-Mead
        provides information on several outstanding personalities, the
        hospitals they built, and the contributions they made during the
        medieval period.

48.   Hurd-Mead, Kate Campbell.   "Trotula."   Isis, 25 (1930) 349-
           367.
        Dr. Hurd-Mead reviews the evidence of manuscripts and printed
        books of several centuries to prove that "Trotula was a woman
        doctor of Salerno of the eleventh century who wrote a famous
        gynecology which was used for hundreds of years as a text book
        and work of reference by students and doctors."

49.   Hurd-Mead, Kate Campbell.   "Trotula's Gynecology and Ob-
           stetrics."   Women in Medicine, 72 (April 1941) 20-21.

The then current president of the American Women's Medical Association, Elizabeth Mason-Hohl, translated Trotula's Passionibus Mulierum Curandorum from the Aldine Press edition published in Venice in 1547; Aldine was the second firm to publish it by machinery. The Diseases of Women remained in print for many centuries wherever there were students of medicine. It is interesting to find that purified preparations of the drugs in use in old Salerno are still prepared and advertised by pharmacists today. [This selection by Dr. Hurd-Mead is included as part of an obituary to Mary McKibben-Harper. This obituary, entitled "Kate Campbell Hurd-Mead: 1876-1941," appears in the BIOGRAPHIES section of this bibliography.]

50. ["It's Coming!"]. El Siglo Medico, 17:856 (5 June 1870) 463. (Spa)

This is a very brief notice of Elizabeth Garrett-Anderson's graduation from the Medical Faculty of Paris.

51. Jantsch, Marlene. ["The Development of Medicine as a Profession for Women: On the 100th Birthday of Dr. Gabriele Possanner-von Ehrenthal"]. Mitteilungs-blatt d. Ärztekanammer f. Wien, 12:6 (1960) 6-15. (Ger)

In commemoration of the 100th birthday of Dr. Gabriele Possaner-von Ehrenthal, the nineteenth century Austrian physician, this article surveys the history of women in medicine in her country. Dr. Possaner-von Ehrenthal's pioneer work as the first woman to obtain a medical doctorate in Austria is underlined. Although she had previously obtained her M.D. in Switzerland, Austrian authorities forced her to retake her exams in Austria in order to practice medicine. The article also mentions a number of other Austrian women physicians who did important pioneer work in the universities and in various medical specialties.

52. Jougla, G. ["Medical Women in History"]. Monaco-méd., 5: 76 (1901) 7. (Fre)

[Article not examined by editors.]

53. Kitchin, Kathleen F. "The Study of Anatomy by Women." Medical Women's Federation News-Letter, (March 1927) 38-44.

The achievements of specific women healers and scholars are mentioned in this article, which discusses five groups of female anatomical students: surgeons, midwives, philosophers, dilettanti ("ladies of fashion who flocked to public dissections as to-day they might go to the theatre"), and professional anatomists.

54. Kull-Schaffner, R. ["Barbara von Roll, A Great Doctor in Her Time"]. Zeitschrift Krankenpfl, 64 (October 1971) 356-357. photo. (Ger)

On the 400th anniversary of her death in 1571, it seems fit-ting to remember this woman of the 16th century. She was born in the canton of Solothurn in Switzerland in 1502, into a family which is still important in industry and trade. As a girl she studied Latin texts in philosophy and medicine and became interested in botany, especially medicinal plants. At age 17 she married Hieronymus von Luternau. After she became a wealthy widow at 47, Barbara devoted herself to medicine and the use of plant materials in medications. In her time she was considered a learned and scientific physician and was consulted often by the doctors in the town hospital. To the poor she gave not only medicine but the food and drink they needed to return to health. She was well aware of the interrelation of body and mind and pioneered the humane treatment of mental illness. She corresponded with a number of learned men in Switzerland and in foreign countries. Barbara von Roll died in 1571, mourned by the whole city.

55.　Lesky, Erna.　["The First Generation of Austrian Women Physicians"].　Österreichische Arztezeitung, 5 (10 March 1975) (unpaged).　(Ger)

Women were admitted to the professions in Austria relatively late, compared to the U.S., because they could not obtain the type of secondary education necessary for admission to the university until nearly 1900. The first woman doctor to settle in Austria was Gabriele Possaner, who obtained her medical education in Switzerland and was finally given an M.D. in Vienna in 1897. Because of the cost in time and money, the first women doctors were daughters of upper middle class or noble families. Several of them served in military hospitals and as hospital directors during World War I. Some specialized in such fields as dentistry, pediatrics, or gynecology, but most chose general practice (83 per cent of 387 women practicing in 1926). By the third decade of the 20th century women were occupying high-level positions and had organized their own medical society. In the thirties they began to be researchers, and Anna Dengel had founded the Medical Mission Sisters for work in foreign countries.

56.　Lipinska, Melanie.　["Women Physicians of Rome"].　Le Progres Medical, 9 (3rd series) (29 April 1899) 276-279.　(Fre)

In the early years of Rome, there were no practitioners with special titles or functions as doctors; and, as in most primitive societies, medicine was closely tied to religion. During the first century A.D., Greek medical practitioners were permitted to settle in Rome; women were probably among them. In later years there was a distinction between obstetrices (midwives) and medicae (practitioners of all forms of medicine). The third book of Octavius Horatianus (4th century) is dedicated to a Victoria who was learned in diseases of women. Numerous funerary inscriptions have been found in various parts of the Roman world honoring medicae, both slave and free women. Several Christian women are mentioned by early authors as versed in medicine, but very little is known about them.

57. Lipinska, Melanie and Mackenzie, (Lady) Muir. "Women Doctors: A Historic Retrospect." Contemporary Review, 108 (October 1915) 504-510.
   This article also appeared in Littell's Living Age, 287 (13 November 1915) 419-424. [Article not examined by editors.]

58. Mason-Hohl, Elizabeth. "Trotula: Eleventh Century Gynecologist." Medical Woman's Journal, 47:12 (December 1940) 349-356. facsims. (Inaugural Address, Annual Meeting, American Medical Women's Association, New York, June 10, 1940.)
   This article includes informative data on Trotula, her writings and her times, taken from the author's experiences in researching this 11th century physician. Concluding the article are portions taken from the author's translation (into English) of Trotula's treatise, Passionibus Muliebrium Curandarum Aegritu. Reproductions of early texts are included.

59. Münster, Ladislao. [Italian Female Doctors from the 13th to the 15th Century]. Editrice Sigurtà Farmacentici, Milan, Italy, 1952, 11 pp. (Lo Smeraldo, No. 6.) (Ita)
   From the middle of the 12th century to the end of the 13th century, Italy had a surprisingly high number of female physicians. Most were wives, widows, or daughters of physicians. The practice of medicine, made possible after passing an examination before a commission, did not require academic studies. When (towards the end of the 13th century) public school training and university studies became prerequisites for practicing medicine in Italy, the number of women doctors declined rapidly, as the social barriers to women in universities remained. The author mentions female physicians in different areas of Italy, underlining that there were no legal barriers to their professional endeavor. They were particularly numerous in Tuscany. Little biographical data is given. The article contains a bibliography.

60. Münster, L[adislao]. "Women Doctors in Medieval Italy." Ciba Foundation Symposium, 10 (1962) 136-140.
   In addition to providing biographies of several notable Italian women healers, the author sets forth reasons for the prominence of women doctors in medieval times and the disappearance of women practitioners in the Renaissance period.

61. "'Old Dame Trot,' Magistra Medicinae." New York State Journal of Medicine, 38:5 (1 March 1938) 397-398. (Across the Desk.)
   A few facts about Trotula of Salerno are extracted primarily from K. C. Hurd-Mead's History of Women in Medicine.

62. Papara, Dora. "Medical Women in Greece." Journal of the American Medical Women's Association, 7:7 (July 1952) 265-267.
   The author is associate director of a mental hospital in the

Greek Ministry of Health. She has been studying in the United States on international fellowships. This article reviews a variety of women who practiced medicine in Greece and traces them in their contexts up to the article's present. Women were healers in Greece until the Golden Age ended with wars and invasions and the Turkish occupation, which left behind a tradition against women. This state, woman as man's chattel, continued until after the liberation of northern Greece in 1896 when Dr. Panagrotatu [sic], the first woman doctor from Greek territory proper, studied in the Greek University. Acknowledgment is made to Dr. Pournaropoulos, assistant professor of the history of medicine in the University of Athens, for the information used in this article.

63. Petrén, Gustaf. ["From the Discussion on Increasing Women's Civil Rights in the 1860s and Their Admission to Medical Careers and the University in the Early 1870s"]. Medicinska Föreningens Tidskrift, 25:2 (1947) 41-46. port. (Swe)
The author reviews the discussions in the Riksdag (the legislature) on the demands of the women's rights movement and the demands for equal educational opportunities beginning about 1860 until about 1873, and quotes some of the royal decrees on the subject. It was in 1870 that the medical-philosophical examination was opened to women, and in 1873 the king ordered that they should be admitted to the licenciate examination which would allow them to practice. The first woman doctor educated in Sweden, Karolina Widerström, took the medical-philosophical examination at Uppsala and was admitted to the Karolinska Institute in 1880. She completed her medical education there and was licensed in 1888. In 1885, Nielsine Nielsen became the first woman doctor in Denmark.

64. "A Pioneer of Modern Medical Women and Her Predecessors of the Middle Ages." Lancet, 1 (18 January 1908) 173-174.
In this article, the Lancet editors take issue with another journal's claim that Nadezhda Prokoffievna Susslova-Golubeva was the first woman doctor in all Europe. Although "Madame Susslova-Golubeva" was Russia's first female physician, the first famous European woman physician was Trotula of Salerno. And, although no women have been granted medical degrees in England in the past century, Henry VIII granted medical licenses "to certain women to attend the sick poor who could not afford to pay the fees of regular practitioners yet did not wish to depend entirely on charity."

65. Pirami, Edmea. ["The Woman Physician Throughout the Centuries"]. Bull. Sci. Med. (Bologna), 138:2 (April-June 1966) 205-213. (Ita)
The author traces the history of women in medicine from the herb experts of ancient Greece to the present, with principle emphasis on Italy. During the early Christian times and the Middle Ages, women continued to treat the sick and wounded

in Italy. The medical school at Salerno trained several notable women, such as Trotula and Costanza Calenda. Others
were taught by and carried on the practices of husbands and
families, often after passing examinations at the medical
schools. France did not allow women to study medicine until
the end of the 19th century, but several countries accepted
them earlier: examples given are Catharina Schrader, who
first described placenta previa in 1700 in Holland, and Dorothea Leporin [Erxleben], who graduated in Germany in 1754.
These women often did research along with their practices
and published and defended their results. By the early 20th
century most Western countries accepted women doctors, although there were still obstacles placed in their paths. Today,
especially since World War II, women practice on a par with
men and occupy positions once reserved solely for men.

66. Potter, Ada. "The History of Dutch Medical Women." Medical Woman's Journal, 30:1 (January 1923) 5-6. (Presentation, Convention, Medical Women's International Association, Geneva, Switzerland, 6 September 1922.)
Dr. Potter's speech opens with brief biographies of Alletta
Jacobs (Holland's first woman physician) and Catharina Van
Tuschenbroek (Holland's second woman physician and the first
woman medical student at the University of Utrecht). Dr. Potter's description of the present status of Dutch medical women
includes statistics on the enrollment of women in medical
schools. Because of strong cooperation between men and women physicians, Dutch women have no need for separate medical societies. In view of women's equality Dr. Potter tells
her audience that she cannot agree with the conference's wish
to form a National Medical Woman's Board in Holland.

67. Raulin, Louis. ["Notes on Prehistoric Medicine: Midwives
and Medical Women in Ancient Rome"]. Gazette Hebdomadaire des Sciences Médicales, 41:36 (5 September 1920)
425-426. (Fre)
In ancient Egypt and Greece there were myths of goddesses acting as midwives or as protectors of women in labor. The
Greek cults survived, with changes of names, in Italy, but human midwives also began to appear--some of them highly
skilled. Many of these women also cared for infants and children, and some became competent general practitioners. We
know of these women generally only through inscriptions on
tombstones or (in the case of a few) through mentions by ancient authors. Although they were probably poorly educated,
at least some of them were called physicians during the period
of the Republic. The women practitioners disappeared after
the fall of the empire and did not reappear until the tenth century when Italy became a center for medical education.

68. Salzi, Francesco. [Medical Women]. Tipografia Romana,
Rome, Italy, 1877, 31 pp. (Ita)
Dedicated to Her Excellency Princess Elena Borghese, this

booklet contains brief biographical notes on 50 women said to
be versed in the healing arts, from pre-Christian Greeks and
Romans to Florence Nightingale. Many of the women included
are probably mythical and very few of them were doctors in
the modern sense; the very sketchy notes contain dates for
only about 15 of the subjects.

69.   Schelenz, Hermann. [Women in the Realm of Esculapius, a
       Study for a History of Women in Medicine and Pharmacy;
       With Consideration of the Future of the Modern Woman Doc-
       tor and Pharmacist]. Ernst Guenther, Leipzig, Germany,
       1900, iv, 74 pp. (Ger)
The book contains material found by the author during research
for a large work on the history of pharmacy. Much of it is
devoted to women healers in ancient times and of the Germanic
tribes. The Middle Ages, especially at the Salerno School,
saw the first educated women physicians, although many of
them were as famous for their secret remedies as for their
knowledge of medical science. The last 20 pages are given
over to the development of freedom for women in pharmacy
and medicine in the 19th century and to related philosophical
discussion. The work does contain a name index, but no
table of contents or bibliography.

70.   Segre, Marcello. ["Jewish Female Doctors in the Middle
       Ages"]. Pagina di Storia della Medicina, 14:5 (1970) 98-
       106. (Ita)
Despite rulings by the church that Jewish doctors should not
be allowed to treat Christian patients, Jews dominated the medical profession in the 12th to 15th centuries and occupied high
positions in the papal courts. During this period, women had
free access to the universities in several countries. In the
13th and 14th centuries, the doctorate became less important
as many cities set up their own examinations for approving the
qualifications of physicians trained in private schools, encouraging women in particular to study near their homes. After
1400 the doctoral degree again became necessary for medical
practice, and the number of women entering practice decreased.
The author lists and briefly discusses a number of women doctors, mostly Jews, in Italy and in the German states. In
Salerno: Rebecca Guarna, Costantia Calenda, Federica Vitale,
Francesca Romana, Venturela Cisinato, Maria Incarnata, Abella, and of special note, Trotula (Dame Trot, in English writings, who was probably a highly skilled midwife early in the
11th century). Many of the Jewish women doctors were wives,
widows, or daughters of well-known physicians, like the Sicilian
Virdimura, wife of Pasquale, physician of Catania. In the late
15th century, rumors of ritual murders led to denunciation,
trial, and execution of a number of Jews at Trento, including
the physician Brunetta, accused of providing the instruments
used. In France, a Jewish woman named Sarah practiced in
Paris at the end of the 12th century, and Sara de Saint Gilles,
widow of Abraham, practiced in Marseilles in the early 1300s.

Many Jewish women practiced in the German states, often as eye doctors.

71.   "Some Pioneer Scandinavian Women Doctors. " World Medical
          Journal, 11:1 (January 1964) 34.
        The first woman to become a doctor in Denmark (1885), Niel-
        sine Nielsen had to go abroad to study gynecology because of
        male physicians' resistance in her own country. In Sweden, the
        first woman physician (1888), Karolina Widerstrom, also spe-
        cialized in gynecology, and later, obstetrics. Both women
        practiced successfully.

72.   Steudel, J[ohannes]. "Medical Women of the Occident. " Jour-
          nal of the American Medical Women's Association, 17:1
          (January 1962) 52-55. (Lecture, University of Kiel, 1958.)
        This article, the first of a two-part article which first appeared
        in Zentralblatt für Gynäkologie, 81:8 (February 21, 1959) 284-
        295, was translated by Catharine Macfarlane. In it, the au-
        thor reviews incidents in the European struggle of women to
        enter medical schools. Switzerland first permitted women to
        study medicine at the University of Zürich in 1864, Bern and
        Geneva in 1872, and Basel in 1890. Only 50 years prior to
        this article were they permitted to study in Austria and Ger-
        many. Prior to the turn of the century, women could occa-
        sionally be permitted to attend a lecture or clinical course,
        but if they chose to do so, they were exposed to curiosity and
        rudeness. In England, the London School of Medicine for Wo-
        men, founded in 1874, played an important role in the admis-
        sion of women students to medical facilities. Elizabeth Black-
        well was the first American woman physician; Marie Heim
        Vögtlin was the first Swiss woman physician (she passed the
        State examination in 1872 with distinction). Madeleine Brés
        was, in 1875, the first French woman to receive the title of
        Doctor of Medicine. Franziska Tiburtius and Emilie Lehmus
        were, for fifteen years, the only women physicians in Berlin.
        Midwifery, as a forerunner of medical practice for women, is
        traced with emphasis on the work of Louise Bourgeois in the
        late 16th and early 17th century in Paris (Bourgeois, in 1601,
        became midwife to the Queen Marie de Medici), and Justine
        Siegemund who practiced midwifery in 17th century Germany.
        Siegemund was the first in Germany to teach the correct treat-
        ment of head and face presentations.

73.   Steudel, J[ohannes]. "Medical Women of the Occident. " Jour-
          nal of the American Medical Women's Association, 17:2
          (February 1962) 139-142.
        The conclusion of a two-part article which first appeared in
        Zentralblatt für Gynäkologie, 81:8 (February 21, 1959) 284-
        295, is here translated by Catharine Macfarlane. The enroll-
        ment of women in medical colleges since the beginning of the
        century has substantially increased, but prior to the second
        half of the nineteenth century the difficulties for women in
        medicine were nearly insurmountable. The first woman to be

granted a degree and thus admitted to the practice of medicine was Dorothea Christiane Erxleben of Quedlinburg in the 18th century. At about the same time in Italy, several women achieved academic degrees: Maria delle Donne in 1799 received the degree of Doctor of Medicine and permission to practice medicine. Anna Morandi-Manzolini in 1756 was appointed Professor of Anatomy at the University of Bologna. Trotula of Salerno is also discussed in the context of her 12th century life, along with Hildegarde von Bingen, the healer and mystic whose medical and scientific writings as well as the record of her political influence have survived the ages. "From the activities of women of past centuries in the healing art," writes the author, "this conclusion may be drawn: Medical thinking and medical treatment must not be the exclusive privilege of men."

74. Strassmann, P. ["Louise Bourgeois as Midwife (1601-1610) to Queen Marie de Medici, Wife of Henry IV of France"]. Allgemeine Deutsche Hebammen-Zeitung, 19:13 (19 June 1904) 203-207; 226-229. port. (Ger) Louise Bourgeois--also called Boursier--born in 1564, came to the palace in 1601, at the age of 37, as midwife to the French queen. In those times physicians attended deliveries only occasionally. Although many midwives were poorly educated, some, like Mme. Bourgeois, had studied from texts by such authorities as Ambroise Paré, and even wrote books themselves. Part 1 describes how Bourgeois became a midwife, how she secured the position as royal midwife, the delivery of the dauphin, the deliveries of the other two sons and three daughters of the royal couple, and her retirement with a life pension. Part 2 reviews her books as a source of information about Bourgeois herself and about the status of midwifery at that time. The books contain advice on diet for new mothers and various remedies for mother and baby, as well as more clinical subjects such as the management of abnormal presentations.

75. Stuard, Susan Mosher. "Dame Trot." Signs: Journal of Women in Culture and Society, 1:2 (Winter 1975) 537-542. This article reviews and comments on the centuries-old debate among historians about Trotula of Salerno. "Could eleventh-century Salerno accommodate a woman as a professor and physician? [and] If [Trotula] did exist, could she have composed the manuscripts ascribed to her by tradition?" Among the medical historians mentioned are Elizabeth Mason-Hohl and Kate Campbell Hurd-Mead, both of whom defended Trotula's existence.

76. Walsh, James Joseph. Medieval Medicine. A. & C. Black, Ltd., London, England, 1920, xii, 221 pp. illus., photos. Walsh devotes one chapter (pages 154-168) in this book to the situation of medical women during the Middle Ages. According to Walsh, women were encouraged to study medicine in the

Italian universities in the 12th century. Records of the history of Salerno show that women physicians staffed the entire department of female diseases. Outstanding among these women was Trotula, to whom many books are attributed. Another significant medical woman of the 12th century was the Benedictine Abbess Hildegarde who wrote two texts on medicine. Thirteenth century records at Bologna show women as students and faculty members in that medical school. One of these, Alessandra Giliani, was a prosector in anatomy at Mondino. Although it was believed that women physicians practiced in France in the Middle Ages, no records of distinguished contributions among them exists. It was hypothesized that the Heloise-Abelard incident at the University of Paris led to the exclusion of women from higher education. As Paris served as the model for Oxford and Cambridge, this might account for the absence of women in the histories of these English universities. The situation in Italy was apparently unique. By the 16th century, the role of women in medicine had diminished.

77.   Winckel, Franz von. ["The Woman as Physician: A Lecture in the Gynecological Clinic on 5 March 1898"]. In: Franz von Winckel: Eighteen Lectures from His Estate. Edited by Max Stumpf. J. F. Bergmann, Wiesbaden, Germany, 1914, 126-141. (Ger)
This lecture, given by the famous gynecologist to his students and colleagues in Munich, briefly reviews some mentions of women healers by the ancient Greek and Roman writers. Most of the text is devoted to the writings of the 17th-century midwives Marguerite de la Marche (née Tertre) in France and Justina Siegmundin in Germany. The speaker apparently intended to continue the historical review but never did so, according to the editor.

78.   "Women Doctors in the Viking Age." British Medical Journal, (20 January 1917) 95.
Information about women healers of the Viking Age (eighth, ninth, and tenth centuries) can be gleaned from Norse sagas. A discussion of this subject was held at a meeting of the Viking Society for Northern Research. [This article also appears in the Boston Medical and Surgical Journal, 176 (24 May 1917) 746-747.]

GERMANY

79.   Becker, W. ["The First Female Doctor in the Middle Ages"]. Die Medizinische Welt, 9 (4 March 1939) 307-308. (Ger)
This article is a brief biography of Dorothea Christiane Erxleben. In response to a similar claim made for Dorothea von Schloezer of Goettingen University, the author stresses Erxleben's outstanding position as the first woman ever to obtain a doctorate from a German university.

80.   Beiswenger, Immanuel.   [A Contribution to the History of Ob-
          stetrics: Justine Siegemundin and Her Achievements].
          Munich, Germany, 1899.   (M.D. thesis.)   (Ger)
      This medical thesis deals with the achievements of Justine
      Siegemundin, a 17th-century German midwife.   Her outstanding
      contribution was a book on difficult deliveries in which she de-
      scribes various techniques for repositioning and delivering the
      infant.   The thesis contains a short biography and then analyzes
      the various techniques and maneuvers outlined in Justine Siege-
      mundin's book on obstetrics.

81.   Berger, E.   [The Development of Women's Medical Education].
          Marburg, Germany, 1947.   (Ph.D. Thesis.)   (Ger)
      [Thesis not examined by editors.]

82.   Billig, Anton Hermann.   [Dorothea Christiana Erxleben: the
          First German Woman Physician.]   München University,
          München, Germany, 1966, 72 pp.   (Ph.D. Thesis.) (Ger)
      In his Ph.D. thesis on the first German woman physician, the
      author analyzes and describes the development of women's edu-
      cation from Luther's to Gottsched's times, emphasizing the
      writers and philosophers who favored better possibilities for
      female education.   He then gives a biography of Dorothea
      Erxleben, which concentrates on the events surrounding her
      doctorate examination.   The main section is devoted to her
      publications, especially her first book (which deals with the
      reasons why women do not study), and her thesis presented
      during her doctorate examination.   The author emphasizes Dr.
      Erxleben's influence as a pioneer of women's education and
      liberation.

83.   Blumenthal, Annemarie.   [Discussions on Women in Higher
          Education in Berlin].   University of Berlin, Berlin, Ger-
          many, 1965.   (Medical Thesis.)
      This medical thesis discusses the controversial issue of wo-
      men in medicine during the second half of the 19th century in
      Germany.   After an introduction to the history of women in
      medicine, the author describes the evolution of women's ad-
      mission to medical studies and quotes contemporaries on the
      issue.   The thesis contains a bibliography.

84.   Brohl, Ilse.   [The Struggle for Women in Medicine in the 19th
          Century].   University of Berlin, Berlin, Germany, 1943.
          (Medical Dissertation.)   (Ger)
      [Article not examined by editors.]

85.   Buchheim, Liselotte.   ["When the First Woman Doctors Gradu-
          ated in Leipzig"].   Wissenschaftliche Zeitschrift Der Karl-
          Marx-Universität Leipzig, 6:3 (1956-1957) 365-381.
          tables.   (Ger)
      In this study of the history of women medical students at Leip-
      zig University, two periods are reviewed: the time before wo-
      men were admitted to medical studies and participated as au-

ditors and the period after 1906 when they became regular students and could obtain their medical degrees. Permission for women to attend lectures was dependent on the arbitrary decision of the individual teacher and the University. The requirements were strict, especially for Russians and other foreigners but also for German women. The number of German women attending these lectures was small and fairly constant between 1900 and 1906. After 1906 women could register for courses, but only in 1911 were regular female students more numerous than auditors. One of the problems was the insufficient training of women, who had to fulfill the same requirements for admission as men without having free access to all high schools Female auditors could obtain a Ph.D. after 1902, but until 1906 few utilized this option, and between 1906 and 1914, 40 women obtained their doctor's degree in Leipzig. They were on the average older than their male counterparts, and most had obtained their high school training in private courses and schools. Their theses included independent research work. Eight of them married, all practiced. Though increasing numbers of women study medicine, only nine have become university professors since 1900.

86.   Burger, Elisabeth. [Development of Medical Education for Women]. University of Marburg, Marburg, Germany, 1947. (Medical Dissertation.) (Ger)
[Article not examined by editors.]

87.   Creutz, Rudolf. ["Marie-Louise Lachapelle and Marie-Anne Victorine Boivin, M.D., h.c., two Representatives of Obstetrics at the Turn of the 19th Century."] Die Medizinische Welt, 15 (10 April 1937) 520-524. port. (Ger)
After a short introduction on the influence of women on obstetrical practice, the author gives biographies of Marie Louise Lachapelle and Marie Anne Victorine Boivin. He underlines their respective merits and publications. He also describes their roles as teachers and practicing midwives in the 18th century. Boivin obtained an honorary doctorate at the University of Marburg in Germany in 1827. On this occasion she dedicated a book to the university: the book contains a widely praised chapter on internal pelvimetry, showing her interest in research and science.

88.   ["Curiosa from Old Medical Writings. 16. The Study of Medicine by Women"]. Hippokrates, 33 (15 September 1962) 728. (Ger)
[Article not examined by editors.]

89.   Engbring, Gertrude M. "Saint Hildegard, Twelfth Century Physician." Bulletin of the History of Medicine, 8:6 (June 1940) 770-784. (Presentation, Medical History Club, Loyola University Medical School, February 1940.)

90.   Field, G. W. "The First Woman Doctor of Medicine in Ger-

many. " <u>Woman's Medical Journal</u>, 10:11 (November 1900)
468-473. (Biographical.)
Dorothea Christian Erxleben in 1754 had conferred upon her
(at the age of 39) the degree of Doctor of Medicine from the
Friedrichs Academia in Halle.

91.   Fisher-DeFoy, Werner. ["The Story of the Graduation of Doro-
      thea Christiana Erxleben, the First German Female Phy-
      sician"]. <u>Archiv Fuer. Geschichte der Medizin</u>, 4:6 (1911)
      440-461. (Ger)
In this article on the first woman to obtain a medical doctorate
at a German university, the author contends that Dorothea
Erxleben did not apply for the examination of her own free
will, but was forced into it. In fact, three Quedlinburg physicians had accused her of unlawful medical practice and Dorothea Erxleben was therefore ordered to take the medical doctorate examination for which she had obtained the royal consent
13 years previously (in 1741). The exchange of letters between
the three physicians, the governor, and Dorothea Erxleben is
reproduced in its entirety. The article also contains the letters concerning her graduation in Halle in 1754. It concludes
with a quote from her obituary deploring her death in 1762 at
the age of 47 years.

92.   Frank, Julia Bess. "The Surgeon and the Surgeon's Wife: En-
      graving by Martin Engelbrecht (1684-1756), Augsburg. "
      <u>Journal of the History of Medicine and Allied Sciences</u>,
      30:2 (April 1975) 164-165. facsims.
In two illustrations from the early 18th century portraying a
male surgeon and his wife, the male surgeon is the one who
holds the instruments of tonsure and surgery, while the woman
carries the barber's tools. While women, with few exceptions,
did not attend German universities at this time, not many of
the men practitioners did either. "Many women of the seventeenth and eighteenth centuries actively assisted fathers, husbands, or brothers in the practice of medicine or surgery, and
after such an apprenticeship, soon became independent practitioners. Even though she ranks beneath her husband, this
surgeon's wife represents a link in the chain of women in medicine that stretches, thin at times, but never broken, into the
furthest reaches of antiquity. "

93.   Heischkel, Edith. ["Dorothea Christine Erxleben, a Pioneer
      for Women's Admission to University Studies in the 18th
      Century"]. <u>Die Aerztin</u>, 11 (1940) 329+ . (Ger)

94.   Horwitz, L. ["Frederic the Great and the First Female Gen-
      eral Practitioner in Prussia"]. <u>Muenchner Medizinische
      Wochenschrift</u>, 79 (1932) 1367. (Ger)
This article contains a brief historical survey of the events
leading to the granting of a medical doctor title to Dorothea
Christiane Erxleben (née Leporin), the 17th-century German
physician. The article underlines the intervention of Frederic

the Great, who had to grant a special dispensation for this
first woman physician to be admitted to the doctorate examination.

95. Kaiser, [Professor]. ["When the First Woman Graduated as
     a Doctor"]. Daheim (1914) 25. (Ger)
     This short article describes the examination to obtain a med-
     ical doctorate taken by Dorothea Christiane Leporin [Erxleben]
     in June 1754. Dr. Leporin was the first German woman phy-
     sician.

96. Knabe, Lotte. ["The First Graduation of a Woman in Germany
     as a Doctor of Medicine at the University of Halle, 1754"].
     In: [450 Years of the Martin Luther University at Halle-
     Wittenberg. Vol 2]. Halle University, Halle, Germany,
     1952, 109-124. port. (Ger)
     If it is hard to believe in 1952 that only about 50 years ago
     there was serious protest against women in the professions and
     major obstacles were still placed in the way of their obtaining
     general or technical education, it is even harder to realize that
     the first German woman to obtain an M.D. and start practice
     did so nearly 200 years ago. She was able to do so only
     through the intervention of the king of Prussia, who permitted
     her to take the necessary examinations. Dorothea Leporin was
     born in 1715 in Quedlinberg, the daughter of a physician. A
     frail, often sickly child, she became interested in books at an
     early age; her father later educated her and her brother to-
     gether in Latin, basic sciences, and medicine. The brother
     entered the University of Halle in 1740 but fled with his father
     when called up for military duty. Dorothea petitioned the king
     to allow her brother to return and to permit them both to study
     at Halle. A royal rescript granting her request was issued in
     April 1741. Instead of entering the university, however, Doro-
     thea married and continued to study medicine while raising her
     family. A complaint filed in 1753 by three local doctors
     against her and "other Feldschers, bathers, barbers and mid-
     wives" for soliciting patients and illegally practicing medicine
     inspired her to again seek official approval. In June 1754 she
     presented and defended a thesis, and received a doctor of medi-
     cine degree. Dorothea Leporin Erxleben, by her actions, an-
     swered many of the questions which would be raised 150 years
     later about whether women were capable of learning the sci-
     ence of medicine and physically able to carry on a practice,
     and whether they could cope simultaneously with home and ca-
     reer.

97. Koenig-Warthausen, G. von. ["On the Medical Studies of Wo-
     men 70 Years Ago ('Good Old Days')"]. Medizinische Welt
     (Stuttgart), 3 (19 January 1963) 171-173. (Ger)
     [Article not examined by editors.]

98. Kraetke-Rumpf, Emmy. [The Physician of Quedlinburg: A
     Biography of Germany's First Female Medical Doctor].

Hase and Koehler, Leipzig, Germany, 1939, 252 pp. plates. (Ger)

This book is a dramatized biography of Dorothea [Christiana Erxleben] Leporin, the first German woman to obtain a medical degree. It concentrates on her social environment and on her family background. The problems of her pioneer position are dealt with mainly as expressed in the prejudice of her male colleagues and stressed in scenes from her medical doctorate examination in Halle in 1754. The book is written as a novel. It contains no index and no bibliography. It includes 11 illustrations showing Quedlinburg and personages that were important in her life and career.

99.   Nauck, E. th. [Women Studying at the University of Freiburg in Breisgau]. University of Freiburg in Breisgau, Freiburg, Germany, 1953, 80 pp. tables. (Contributions to the History of Freiburg Research and University, No. 3.) (Ger)

This book on the history of the education of women in Freiburg consists of five chapters: the early history of the movement for education of women; negotiations concerning the introduction of women's education in Freiburg (1873-1900); the early years of women at Freiburg (1899-1911); numbers of female students and their courses of study; and the contributions of women students to the intellectual and social life of the university. As late as 1884 the medical faculty rejected a 100,000-mark endowment for scholarships for needy women students in medicine, pharmacy, and chemistry, but by 1895 women were auditing courses and in 1900 they were officially permitted to matriculate. Five women who had been auditing were listed as having started their studies in the previous year, making Freiburg the first German university to admit women. Appendix IX gives the numbers of women matriculated in each of the faculties each year from 1900 to 1952; until 1909 medical students made up more than half of the total, and they continued to be the biggest group (except for 1927-30) until 1945, when the opportunities for medical students decreased markedly. Appendix XI gives the number of doctoral degrees awarded to women by the various faculties in the years 1895 to 1952; the M.D. degrees total 1039, compared to 380 for the combined philosophy/natural philosophy faculties. Eighteen appendices, a bibliography, and person/place and subject indexes are included.

100.   Quentin, E. ["Hildegard von Bingen: a Modern Woman Physician--800 Years Ago"]. Munchener Medizinische Wochenschrift, 109:47 (24 November 1967) 2509-2510. (Ger)

"Hildegard von Bingen was born around 1098 and died in 1179 as Abbess of Ruppertsberg Abbey, near Bingen, founded by herself. Her works provide a lively impression of her comprehensive knowledge and her unique personality. Her spiritual and medical assistance was requested by many men, even by princes. For the physician the two chapters of her work 'Causae et Curae' and 'Physika' might be particularly interesting. " [Article English summary.]

101.　Rall, Jutta. ["The Female Doctor in German Medical History"]. Deutsche Aerzteblatt-Aerztliche Mitteilung, 64: 42 (21 October 1967) 1-12. (Ger)
As stated in this lecture, given to the German Women Physician's Association on an unspecified date, the first German woman physician was probably Hildegard, Abbess of the Benedictines at Bingen. She was interested in natural science as well as medicine and published a number of theological and medical works, said to have been dictated in German and later translated into Latin. In the 15th century there were said to be 15 women doctors in Frankfurt, mostly surgeons and eye doctors. During the 17th and 18th centuries there were a number of well-known and respected midwives. The first German woman to receive the doctor's degree was Dorothea Erxleben, who defended her thesis in 1754 at Giessen. Regina von Siebold and her daughter Charlotte Heidenreich received degrees at Giessen in 1819 and 1817 respectively. In the 1870s Franziska Tiburtius and Emilie Lehmus were the first women physicians to settle in Berlin, where they established a clinic for women. They were followed by Agnes Bluhm in 1884 and an increasing number of others. After 1900, women were accepted at most of the German universities, although they still had many difficulties to overcome. At the time this article was written, about 20 per cent of the doctors in West Germany were women.

102.　Reimerdes, Ernst Edgar. ["Dorothea Christiane Erxleben, the First German Female Physician. (1715-1915)"]. Deutsche Medizinische Wochenschrift, 45 (4 November 1915) 1343-1344. (History of Medicine.) (Ger)
This brief biography of Dorothea (Leporin) Erxleben is published in honor of the 200th anniversary of her birth on November 13, 1715. In her early years she became so interested in science and medicine that her father, a physician, had her educated with her brother in the theoretical and practical bases of medicine, as well as in languages and in household arts. In spite of poor health, she made great progress in her studies and in 1741 was granted royal permission to take the examinations of the medical faculty at Halle. She did not take advantage of this permission until 1754, when, after 12 years of marriage and four children, she presented and defended a thesis and received a doctoral degree in medicine at Halle. She returned to her native town of Quedlinburg, where she died in June 1762, after eight years of successful practice.

103.　Runge, Hans. ["Contemporary Reports on Germany's First Woman Physician, Dorothea Christ. Leporin of Quedlinburg"]. Münchener Medizinische Wochenschrift, 87:51

(20 December 1940) 1435.   (Ger)
The author gives biographical data on Dorothea Christ. Erxleben, née Leporin, which he found in the Hannoverischen
Beyträgen zum Nützen und Vergnügen, no. 41, May 21, 1762,
in an article titled "Information on Some Learned Members
of the Fair Sex." The information on Leporin was taken
from a biographical sketch attached to her doctoral dissertation, entitled in Latin, "Medica exponens quod nimis cito ac
jucunde curare saepius fiat causa minus rutae curationis."
Leporin was born in 1715, the daughter of a well-known physician, who taught her Latin and other foreign languages in
her early youth; from him she learned the love of medicine
that sustained her during her struggle for education. She
married in 1742. Friends, husband, and relatives considered
her desire to study medicine unsuitable or even indecent, and
in 1749 she wrote a justification which was published anonymously in several German magazines and literary journals
under the title "Rational Thoughts on Education of the Fair
Sex." Leporin finally received her doctoral degree in June
1754, when she was a 40-year-old housewife and mother of
several children. Emperor Frederick the Great informed
her that he would "raise no objection" if she were to join the
faculty at the University at Halle. However, she returned to
her home town of Quedlinburg in the Hartz Mountains where
she carried on a large and successful practice.

104.   Singer, Charles. "The Scientific Views and Visions of Saint
        Hildegard (1098-1180)." In: Studies in the History and
        Method of Science, edited by Charles Singer. Oxford
        University Press, London, England, 1917, 1-55. figs.,
        plates.
        This analysis of the life and thought of Hildegard of Bingen
        details her visionary scientific and philosophic thought, her
        ideas on the structure of the material universe, and her de-
        scription of anatomy and physiology according to a macro-
        cosmic scheme (she insisted on a relationship among the
        qualities of the soul, the constitution of the external cosmos,
        and the structure of the body). The monk Theodoric credits
        her with miraculous powers of healing in the treatment of
        the sick, and she has been called a pioneer of the hospital
        system. However, there is no real evidence that her treat-
        ment went beyond exorcism and prayer, regardless of her un-
        disputed acquaintance with the science of her day.

105.   Strecker, Gabriele. "Medical Women in Germany." Journal
        of the American Medical Women's Association, 2:11 (No-
        vember 1947) 506-508.
        Dorothea Erxleben, having obtained a special license from
        Frederic II to study medicine, received her degree in 1784
        from a Prussian university and became the first woman phy-
        sician in Germany. While it was not until 1908 that the Ger-
        man Reich allowed women to attend classes at its universi-
        ties, in 1876 two German medical women returned from

Zurich with medical degrees and founded the Clinic of Women Doctors in Berlin in the midst of great intolerance. The first German Association of Medical Women was founded in 1923. Issues it identified as important were women's sports from the point of view of a woman doctor, and social welfare for women under arrest. It dissolved itself in May 1933 when Hitler came to power. In 1945 a similar group was founded and licensed by the military government in 1947. Issues this group identified as important were the maintenance of economic interests of medical women, representation on medical boards, and an adequate number of women on committees in charge of the distribution of jobs in the medical field. The Nazis issued restrictions against women working when the husband should be the one earning the living for the family. Barbara von Renthe, vice-president of the Board of Medical Affairs for the Soviet Zone, reported that the Russian occupied zone had 35 to 40 per cent women doctors. Directly after the war, there was an abundance of doctors (especially when the army doctors returned), and it was felt in the Western sector that "we cannot take the responsibility of permitting a married woman to practice when there are innumerable men who cannot make a living as resident doctors or as free practitioners."

106. Stricker, W. ["The Treatment of Syphilis in the Male by a Woman Physician"]. Janus, 11 (1847) 196. (Ger)
An advertisement appeared in a Frankfurt newspaper in 1746. In it, Maria Franziska Charlotte Geringin announces her treatment of a variety of physical diseases, including blindness (even if it was congenital). She also claims a secret venereal disease cure which is less disagreeable for the patient than the current treatments. Patients can send their maids or servants, should they be embarrassed to come themselves.

107. Van Der Velden, Friedrich. [The History of Female Medical Practitioners]. Tuebingen, Germany, 1892. (Thesis.) (Ger)
[Thesis not examined by editors.]

108. Zaunick, Rudolph. ["Dorothea Erxleben, nee Leporin (1715-1762): Germany's First Woman Physician: On the 200th Anniversary of the Conferring of Her Degree in the University of Halle"]. Zeitschrift fuer Aerztl. Fortbildung, 48:22 (1954) 780-786. facsim., port. (Ger)
The official disapproval and public scorn that met Franziska Tiburtius and Emilie Lehmus when, after receiving their medical degrees at Zurich, they set up the first polyclinic for women in Berlin in 1878, makes all the more remarkable the achievement of Dorothea (Leporin) Erxleben. Born on 13 November 1715, she was tutored along with her older brother by their doctor father. He introduced both of them to the theory and practice of medicine, including bedside teaching.

In about 1740 the father and two brothers fled to evade military service; Dorothea managed to obtain from the royal court forgiveness for them and permission for the older brother and herself to study at the university. She did not attend, however, but in 1742 married Johann Christian Erxleben, deacon of St. Nicholas in Quedlinburg, a widower with four children. The same year she published a book on education for women, with a foreword by her father, which was later reprinted anonymously. Over the next 12 years she studied, wrote, bore four children, and helped the sick poor to the extent that three local doctors accused her in 1753 of illegal practice of medicine. In her reply, Erxleben demanded that she be allowed to take the doctoral examination or be examined by her accusers. A royal decree forced the university to permit her to take the examinations, which she passed with great ease. With faculty and Court approval, the doctoral diploma was awarded to her on 12 June 1754. She returned to Quedlinburg, where she died in June 1762 of a hemorrhage, probably tubercular.

GREAT BRITAIN

109.   Bell, E. Moberly.   Storming the Citadel: The Rise of the Woman Doctor.   Constable & Co. Ltd., London, England, 1953, 200 pp.   illus., ports.
This book chronicles in historical perspective the movement of English medical women for education and professional recognition. It begins with Elizabeth Blackwell and Elizabeth Garrett and moves through the Edinburgh struggle led by Sophia Jex-Blake, the founding of the London School of Medicine for Women, the work of women physicians in India, the First World War, World War II, and ends with the Goodenough Report which established coeducation in English medical schools. It is extensively indexed and includes pictures of Elizabeth Garrett Anderson, Elizabeth Blackwell, Sophia Jex-Blake, Isabel Thorne, and Mary Scharlieb.

110.   Burstyn, Joan N.   "Education and Sex: The Medical Case Against Higher Education for Women in England, 1870-1900."   Proceedings of the American Philosophical Society, 117:2 (April 1973) 79-89.
In this essay the author covers the ferment in Victorian England dealing with male intellectuals' objections to the higher education of women. Many of these objections had "medical basis," such as the "effect" mental strain had on reproductive function. A portion of the article deals with objections to women in the medical curriculum. Gynecologists and obstetricians, the first to be affected by competition from women physicians, were prominent in the attack. Reference is made to Elizabeth Garrett Anderson, whose life as a wife, mother, and practicing physician challenged the arguments against educating women, and whose writings refute the "medical" bases of the popular objections.

111.   Cockram, E. Joyce. "Tribute to Sabine." Journal of the
            Medical Women's Federation, 43:3 (July 1961) 86-89.
            (Address, 44th Annual General Meeting, Medical Wo-
            men's Federation, Plymouth, Mass., 4 May, 1961.)
        This address is an account of Sabine Saunders, a Tudor
        Englishwoman born in 1520, who, like all wives of her day,
        also acted as "physician" to her family. The article lists
        many Tudor women well-known for their medical knowledge,
        and quotes from diaries, poems, plays, and contemporary
        herbals to illustrate women's role in medicine and the pre-
        scriptions they might make.

112.   Dopson, Laurence. "Pioneer Women Doctors of Hastings."
            Sussex County Magazine, (September 1950).
        [Article not examined by editors.]

113.   Franz, Nellie Alden. English Women Enter the Professions.
            Printed by Columbia University Press for the author,
            Cincinnati, Ohio, 1965, 317 pp.   photo., port.
        The author devotes a chapter each to the entrance of English
        women to several professions. The chapter on medicine be-
        gins at the very beginning--with Aesculapius, Hippocrates,
        and Galen--and discusses early fragmentary information on
        women healers, herb-doctors, and midwives. Two 18th-cen-
        tury practitioners, Crazy Sally and Ellen Haythornethwaite,
        are mentioned. Then the author discusses those 19th-century
        English women whose efforts served to open the way for med-
        ical women: Elizabeth Blackwell ("the first English-born wo-
        man to receive a degree in medicine"), Elizabeth Garrett-
        Anderson, and Sophia Jex-Blake (who, with four other women,
        succeeded in gaining admission to the University of Edinburgh).
        There is a section on the Woman's Hospital Corps and other
        war work by women, and socialized medicine is briefly dis-
        cussed. Lastly, results of the Goodenough Report are given;
        the report covered abuses having to do with the higher educa-
        tion of women doctors and recommended coeducation for
        every medical school in the United Kingdom.

114.   Garrett-Anderson, E. "The History of a Movement." Fort-
            nightly Review, 59 (March 1893) 404-417.
        The history and development of the movement (in Great Brit-
        ain and Ireland) to admit women to the medical profession,
        including the part played by Garrett-Anderson in this move-
        ment, are outlined. The author describes how she tried to
        do in England what Elizabeth Blackwell had done in America
        for medical women. She describes the struggles of Mary
        Putnam Jacobi and Sophia Jex-Blake to obtain a medical de-
        gree. There are now six examining bodies prepared to give
        women diplomas, and these schools, including their require-
        ments and tuition, are described. The struggle to become
        legally qualified practitioners has been won, but women now
        want the best possible education so that they can become first-
        rate doctors. There are many encouraging signs that the

position of women, after they get their medical degrees, is improving. The New Hospital in the Euston Road, run entirely by women, has done much to improve the image of women physicians. Women are also doing impressive work at Clapham Maternity Charity, Notting Hill Dispensary, a small North London hospital, and in private practice and at official posts. Many have become medical missionaries. It is hoped that women, in recognition of their great contributions, will soon be admitted to all medical societies.

115. Jex-Blake, Sophia. "Medical Women." Nineteenth Century, 22 (November 1887) 692-707.
    Dr. Jex-Blake reviews events over the last ten years (in England and abroad) relating to medical education and acceptance of women. The difficulties are summed up by Dr. Jex-Blake as: (1) remaining jealousy and ill-will towards medical women by a portion of the medical profession itself; (2) the exclusion of women students from medical schools; and (3) financial difficulties.

116. Jex-Blake, Sophia. Medical Women: A Thesis and a History. Oliphant, Anderson, & Ferrier, Edinburgh, Scotland; Hamilton, Adams, & Co., London, England, 1886, 256, 100 pp.
    This work is a presentation of Dr. Jex-Blake's original two essays on women physicians (Medical Women: Two Essays, 1872). For this edition, the author rewrote the essays, hoping "to give as complete and comprehensive a view as brevity would allow of the whole question of medical practice by women."

117. Jex-Blake, Sophia. Medical Women: Two Essays. William Oliphant & Co., Edinburgh, Scotland, Hamilton, Adams, & Co., London, England, 1872, 162 pp.
    This book's first essay, "Medicine as a Profession for Women," was reprinted ("with large additions") from Woman's Work and Woman's Culture. To counter opposition to women in medicine in England, Jex-Blake summarizes medical history, showing how the practice of medicine was exclusively appropriated by men only recently, while women had been practitioners since antiquity. The second essay, "Medical Education of Women," is the substance of a lecture delivered in St. George's Hall, London, on 26 April 1872. The essay is primarily a recounting of Jex-Blake's battle in Edinburgh, during which she and four other women braved riots to win the right to matriculate and be awarded medical degrees. She recalls the founding of the London and Edinburgh medical schools for women (the Edinburgh school continued until women were finally admitted to degrees at the University of Edinburgh in 1894). An appendix includes summaries of the Edinburgh legal actions, and extensive notes quote opinions, correspondence, petitions, and rebuttals from all sides of the controversy. ["Medical Education of Women" subsequently

appeared in a number of journals which include Transactions of the National Association for the Promotion of Social Science, 1873, London, (1874) 385-393; Medical Magazine, London, 1 (1892-1893) 1138-1149.]

118. Lloyd, Hilda. "Looking Back." Journal of the Medical Women's Federation, 40:3 (July 1958) 180-181.
Dame Hilda Lloyd, ex-president of the Royal College of Obstetricians and Gynaecologists and emeritus professor of obstetrics and gynaecology at the University of Birmingham and United Hospitals, briefly reviews the past forty years over which she had been in the medical profession, pointing out history and trends related to that profession.

119. Lutzker, Edythe. Women Gain a Place in Medicine. McGraw-Hill Book Company, New York, New York, 1969, 160 pp. illus., photos., ports.
Written for "the young people of this generation and those to follow," this book tells the story of five British women who sought, in the second half of the 19th century, to enter the medical profession. Sophia Jex-Blake became interested in a medical career while visiting the United States in 1866, tried and failed to gain admittance to a medical school in England, and finally attended the University of Edinburgh-- but not without a fight. She led a group of five women determined to be admitted to the medical school, and on October 29, 1869 her petition for admission was approved. She wrote in her diary: " 'If I can be the first woman to open a British University then surely I ... shall have served, my heart and I--even if I die straightway....' " Her comrades in this venture were Edith Pechey, Isabel Thorne, Matilda Chaplin, and Helen Evans. The " 'gallant little band,' " as bona fide matriculated students of Edinburgh University, then faced the problem of how to gain admission to the Royal Infirmary for training in the wards. That won, the university continued to raise obstacles in the women's path, finally refusing to graduate them. This led to the founding of the tremendously successful London School of Medicine for Women. "Not only had the women won the right to a medical education, to hospital training, and to inclusion in the Medical Register, but they had also brought the entire subject of education to the fore; they had involved Parliament itself in the question." The book contains both a bibliography and an index. The text is liberally illustrated with photographs.

120. McKibben-Harper, Mary. "English Women in Medicine." Medical Woman's Journal, 32:9 (September 1925) 247-250. photos.
In England, women physicians have been members of the British Medical Association since 1895 when the male membership rescinded the vote of 1878 refusing membership to women. American women physicians would do well to be as organized as the English. English medical women were first

educated at the London School of Medicine for Women founded
by Dr. Jex-Blake and then received their practical training
at the Royal Free Hospital.

121.   "Medical Women. 'The History of a Movement.'" Woman's
            Medical Journal, 1:3 (March 1893) 54-55.
        Mrs. Garrett Anderson's paper, "The History of a Movement,"
        published in Fortnightly Review, inspired this sketchy review
        of English medical women's advances over the past few dec-
        ades.

122.   Sandes, Gladys M. "Women Medical Students in Britain."
            Women in Medicine, 88 (April 1945) 8-10. photos.
        A history is given of the struggle of women physicians in
        Britain which began after the second woman physician (Eliza-
        beth Garrett Anderson) was admitted to the list of the Med-
        ical Register (Elizabeth Blackwell being the first woman ad-
        mitted). The Society of Apothecaries, the only British insti-
        tution at the time which permitted the admission of women,
        was determined that no more women should be admitted.
        This struggle spawned the incipient Elizabeth Garrett Ander-
        son Hospital, the London School of Medicine for Women
        (1874), and the cooperation between this school and the Royal
        Free Hospital. Just prior to and during World War I, wo-
        men were beginning to be admitted to London hospitals and
        their medical schools. Admission of women to the London
        School of Medicine is discussed. Although many positions in
        medicine are theoretically open to both men and women, no
        women are ever appointed to leading posts.

123.   Thorne, May. "The Romance of the Medical Education of
            Women in England." Medical Woman's Journal, 32:8
            (August 1925) 207-209. (Address, Meeting, Medical Wo-
            men of Chicago, April 15, 1925.)
        The history of women in medicine in England began when
        Elizabeth Blackwell, a native of England, was accepted at
        Geneva College in New York State in 1847. When Dr. Black-
        well returned to England with her medical degree, she quali-
        fied on the first register of duly qualified medical practition-
        ers. Elizabeth Garrett Anderson, after having been refused
        admittance to medical schools, qualified herself for, and
        passed, the examinations in medicine of the Society of Apothe-
        caries in London. As a result, this Society created a rule
        that only certificates of instruction from qualified medical
        schools (none of which would accept women) would be accep-
        table. This "effectively blocked the way for any other wo-
        man to qualify in medicine." Sophia Jex Blake led a group
        of five women who applied at the University of Edinburgh;
        after much energy and expense were expended, they were
        admitted to the examinations. After these women took honors,
        the Senate refused other women students admittance. In
        1874, the Royal Free Hospital founded the London School of
        Medicine for Women. In 1877, the Royal Free Hospital in

London and the King and Queen's College of Physicians in
Ireland opened its professional examinations facilities to women. In 1906, women held staff positions as physicians and
surgeons at the Royal Free Hospital. While women have
been accepted in many medical schools around England, they
have not been allowed positions of responsibility as staff:
therefore, women's medical schools and hospitals are needed.

124.   Thorne, May. "Women in Medicine: The Early Years."
          Postgraduate Medical Journal, 27 (July 1951) 355-357.
        In 1869 five women, led by Sophia Jex-Blake, made applica-
        tion to the medical school at the University of Edinburgh,
        and their battle with school authorities contributed to the
        opening of the medical profession to women. The author's
        mother was one of the five women students.

125.   Webb-Johnson, Alfred. "Mainly About Women." British
          Medical Journal, 2 (8 August 1942) 165-166. (Address.
          London School of Medicine for Women, London, England,
          24 July 1942.)
        Following a discussion of the "seeds sown in the 18th cen-
        tury" for women's entrance into the professions, Sir Webb-
        Johnson focuses on two pioneer medical women: Elizabeth
        Garrett and Sophia Jex-Blake. Garrett, who "used her fem-
        inine arts to get her way," serves as an example of individual
        success. Jex-Blake, who attained her goal through "strife,
        riot, and public protests," fought for others as well as her-
        self. The speaker (president of the Royal College of Sur-
        geons) then gives a history of women and the College. He
        concludes with brief speculations concerning the future of
        medical women.

126.   "Women in Medicine." Nursing Mirror and Midwives Journal,
          140:10 (6 March 1975) 41. ports.
        In a speech before the Royal Society of Arts in London, Dame
        Albertine Winner traced the history of women in medicine
        from ancient Egypt to the present. The talk, summarized in
        this article, concentrated on the advancements made by Brit-
        ish women physicians.

INTERNATIONAL

127.   Ackerman, Emma M. "Progress of Women in Medicine."
          Journal of Iowa State Medical Society, 23:7 (July 1933)
          361-362. (Address, State Society of Iowa Medical Wo-
          men, Thirty-sixth Annual Meeting, Des Moines, Iowa,
          10 May 1933.)
        A historical summary of the gradually improving position of
        women in the field of medicine is presented by Dr. Acker-
        man, who touches briefly upon the accomplishments of ma-
        jor women in the struggle--from such ancient pioneers as
        Fabiola of Rome and Trotula of Salerno, to 19th-century

leaders such as Elizabeth Garrett and Mary Putnam Jacobi, and on to more recent trailblazers such as Estelle Ford Warner, Rosalie Morton, and Bertha Van Hoosen.

128. Aitken, Janet. "Women in Medicine in the Ages." Journal of the Medical Women's Federation, 46:3 (July 1964) 175-179. (Presentation, Osler Club of London, London, England, 30 October 1963.)
Beginning with the fact that there have been both men and women doctors from about 6000 B.C., Dr. Aitken sketches an outline of women in medicine up to the present.

129. Angwin, Maria L. "Woman in Medicine." Woman's Medical Journal, 6:8 (August 1897) 241-249.
A brief summary of the success of two ancient female practitioners (Agnodice and Marie Zega) serves as the springboard for a defense of the presence of women in the field of medicine. Universities and medical schools now open to women are listed, and the accomplishments of more contemporary women physicians (Jex-Blake, Garrett-Anderson, Blackwell, Cushier, Prideau, et al.) are related. Angwin hopes to put to rest "senseless twaddle about 'woman's sphere' and trying to keep her in paths whose sole recommendation is their sanction by long ages of custom."

130. Austin, Margaret. "History of Women in Medicine; A Symposium: Early Period." Bulletin of the Medical Library Association, 44:1 (January 1956) 12-15. (Presentation, Midwinter meeting, Midwest Regional Group, Medical Library Association, Chicago, Illinois, February 1955.)
This article discusses women in medicine from the first woman physician who practiced in Egypt c. 2730 B.C. through Sophia Jex-Blake, who was educated at the University of Edinburgh in Scotland.

131. Bass, Elizabeth. "The March of Women in Medicine: A Collection of Medical Literature." Women in Medicine, 83 (April 1944) 16-17.
This article [a reprint from The Mississippi Doctor (August 1943) 83-84] is a brief overview of the evolution of woman's place in medicine as gleaned from the Elizabeth Bass Collection of Women in Medicine at Tulane University. It is also a celebration of the day a law was passed "for the appointment of female physicians and surgeons in the Medical Corps of the Army and Navy" (17 April 1943).

132. Baudouin, Marcel. [Female Physicians: Study of International Social Psychology. Portraits and Biographies. History. Statistics. Special and Practical Medical Teachings. Volume I: Female Physicians of the Past]. Institut International de Bibliographie, Paris, France, 1901, 263 pp. illus. (Fre)

The work consists of short biographies arranged chronolog-
ically in six chapters: 1) the Greek Period, 2) the Roman
Period, 3) the School of Salerne, 4) Middle Ages and Modern
Times, 5) Modern Military Women Physicians, and 6) Women
Writers and Practitioners (not physicians). The author attempts to account for all women physicians mentioned by earlier writers, notably P. A. Delacoux in Bibliographie des
Sages-femmes célèbres, anciennes, modernes, et contem-
poraines (Paris, 1834), and Melanie Lipinska in Historie des
Femmes-Médecines (Paris, C. Jacques et cie, 1900). The
work is of particular interest due to the author's emphasis
on primary documents and variant meanings in translation of
words. The author cites the identifying epitaph or text as it
appeared on a woman physician's monument, gravestone,
statue, or written record, and discusses various translations.
For example, "Maia," cited as a woman physician by several authors, is discounted here, "Maia being a term which
designates a profession, rather than a feminine proper name."
Care is taken to compare the primary document with published literature to clarify and correct any distortions or
errors. Many women previously identified as physicians are
here described as wise women, midwives, or legend. An
alphabetical name index is appended.

133. Beaugrand, A. ["Female Physicians: Part I"]. Gazette
Hebdomadaire de Médecine et de Chirurgie, 9 (2nd series): 34 (23 August 1872) 545-549. (Fre)
This first part of a three-part historical survey of women
physicians covers the classical period of Egypt, Greece, and
Rome. The author notes that he is concerned only with physicians, not with midwives, although in some periods the latter were considered the equivalent of doctors in some medical fields. Aside from female deities and legendary human
females, the Greek practitioners were probably primarily
midwives. Women had much more freedom in Rome and
there were apparently a number who were called medicae and
treated a range of ailments beyond those of women and infants. [This article was to appear in the next volume of the
Encyclopedic Dictionary of Medical Sciences.]

134. Beaugrand, A. ["Female Physicians: Part II"]. Gazette
Hebdomadaire de Médecine et de Chirurgie, 9 (2nd series): 35 (30 August 1872) 561-567. (Fre)
Part 2 of Beaugrand's historical review covers the time from
about the beginning of the Christian Era through the 15th century. In spite of the uncertainty about the writings of the
women doctors of antiquity, it is certain that the practice of
medicine was open to both sexes. During the Middle Ages
in the Arab countries, women "learned in medicine" were
the only practitioners allowed to treat women patients, and
the same situation prevailed in the Orient, although these
educated women were rare in both areas. At the medical
school in Salerno a number of women graduates became well

known for their teachings and writings and for their knowledge of medicines; very little, however, is known about the lives of these women. Medically trained women were rare in other countries in this period. Although royal decrees in the 14th century permitted women to practice surgery in Paris, by the 16th century medical and surgical practice by women had almost entirely disappeared.

135. Beaugrand, A. ["Female Physicians: Part III"]. Gazette Hebdomadaire de Médecine et de Chirurgie, 9 (2nd series): 38 (20 September 1872) 609-621. (Fre)
Part 3 of Beaugrand's historical survey covers the period from the 16th century to the mid-19th century. It starts with Oliva Sabuco de Nantes Barrera, author of a Spanish book, A New Philosophy of the Nature of Man. That the author was a woman is about all that is known about her, and there is some doubt about that. Several women who wrote medical books in the 17th century are briefly mentioned. By the end of the 18th century, women doctors had become uncommon, especially in France. The greater part of the article is a review of the arguments presented by various medical men for and against the idea of allowing women to become doctors of medicine. This fight is related to the general struggle for the emancipation and rights of women and, like it, is further advanced in America and England. The author quotes at length from a commentary by Montanier which concludes that a woman would have to give up every feminine characteristic to become a doctor--sensitivity, modesty, tenderness, etc.--as well as sacrifice marriage and maternity to the demands of a medical career. He is shocked at the idea of male and female students sharing dissections and instruction in physiology, medicine, and especially surgery, citing unspecified "scandals" in Edinburgh and Philadelphia. Because of his belief in freedom, he must agree that women should have access to all facilities, but only under the same rigorous academic requirements applied to men.

136. Bochalli, R. ["Famous Medical Women of the Past and the First Noted Women-Physicians of Our Time"]. Medizinische Monatsschrift (Stuttgart), 17 (June 1963) 383-385. (Ger)
[Article not examined by editors.]

137. Bolton, H. Carrington. "The Early Practice of Medicine by Women." Popular Science Monthly, 18 (December 1880) 191-202. (Address, Commencement Exercises, Woman's Medical College of the New York Infirmary, New York, 27 May 1880.)
Women healers in mythology and of ancient and medieval times are the subject of the major portion of this article. Also mentioned are women practitioners of 18th-century Europe and colonial America. The author concludes by contrasting today's much improved educational opportunities for

medical women with the "formerly well-nigh insurmountable impediments and obstacles."

138. Brunton, Lauder. "Some Women in Medicine." Canadian Medical Association Journal, 48:1 (January 1943) 60-65. (Men and Books.) (Presentation, 3rd Annual Memorial Meeting, Osler Society of McGill University, 27 March 1942.)

After a review of the beginnings of medical education for women, Brunton traces the history of women in medicine through the lives of outstanding medical women: Louise Bourgeois, a 17th-century French midwife; Hildegarde of Bingen, a 12th-century nun who was a physician and "notable seer of visions"; Trotula of Salerno; James Barry; Elizabeth Blackwell; Lucy Wanzer, the first woman doctor to graduate in the state of California; Elizabeth Garrett-Anderson; Christine Murrell; and Maude Abbott.

139. Caldwell, Ruth. "Women in Medicine: Chapter IV. The Pioneer Medical Women." Medical Woman's Journal, 37:5 (May 1930) 129-131.

Before the American Revolution, only men practiced medicine; women were midwives. "During this colonial period the medical profession in the United States was not organized in any way, and the type of medicine practiced was deplorable." After the Revolution, medicine improved when doctors started going to Europe; but women remained excluded and midwives were suppressed. Six women in the United States pioneered in medicine in the 1840s. Harriot Hunt of Boston practiced without a diploma. Harvard refused to accept her for fear that all their male students would go to Yale. "At the same time three colored students were refused." Mary Putnam Jacobi responded to this incident by writing, "whenever a woman proves herself capable of an intellectual achievement, this latter ceases to constitute an honour for the men who had previously prized it. Hence the urgent necessity of excluding women from all opportunity of trying." Elizabeth Blackwell was awarded her degree in 1849 and Emily Blackwell was awarded hers in 1852. Together they founded the New York Infirmary so that women physicians could have medical companionship and access to dispensary practice, and so that women medical students would have a place to train. Marie Zakrzewska, Ann Preston, and Emmeline Cleveland were also pioneer medical women at this time. In 1867, Nadejda Suslawa, a Russian, was the first woman to obtain a degree from the University of St. Petersburg and in 1870 Elizabeth Garrett of England received her degree from the Sorbonne. In 1878, Sophia Jex-Blake became the first medical woman to receive a medical degree in England.

140. Chadwick, James R. "The Study and Practice of Medicine by Women." International Review, (October 1879) 444-471.

The article presents a historical summary of women in medicine, from antiquity (including mythology) to the 1878 admission of three women to the American Medical Association. Virtually every "pioneer," every major controversy, and every major advance in the progress towards opening the medical field to women is covered. Conclusions affirm that the movement to admit women to medical careers is worldwide, that many existing medical schools are opening their doors to women without calamitous results, and that the scope of the demand for the medical education for women is in direct ratio to the enlightenment of the country. The question is no longer whether to allow women to practice medicine, but whether to give women the best possible instruction in order to protect the community from imperfectly trained practitioners.

141. Cordell, Eugene F. "Woman as a Physician. Illustrious Examples Drawn from History. --The Advantages of the Female Medical Students of To-Day Compared with Those of Her Predecessors, with Suggestions as to Their Proper Utilization." Maryland Medical Journal, 10 (6 October 1883) 353-356. (Introductory Lecture, Woman's Medical College of Baltimore, 1 October 1883.)
This lecture abstract surveys the progress made by women medical students since Old Testament times, when the midwife held a distinct office, as she did for centuries. The author mentions Agnodice, obstetrician in ancient Athens; Aspasia, a gynecologist; Fabiola, a Roman woman who had charge of a hospital; the School of Salerno, which had women professors in the Middle Ages; Louyse Bourgeois, midwife to Marie de Medicis and writer of a book on obstetrics; Marie Louise Lachapelle, first director of La Maternité in Paris; and Marie Boivin, prolific obstetrical writer in eighteenth-century France. He discusses medical colleges now open to women, and concludes by telling the students that nowadays women have "the freest privileges," and that his discussion should "not merely lead you to strive to equal those who have preceded you, but to surpass them. "

142. Cuthbert, Sister M. "Women in Medicine." Medical Missionary, 32:1 (January-February 1958) 7-9. photos, port.
Sister Cuthbert gives a historical overview of women in medicine. When the College of Physicians in London was founded in 1811, 66 women were licensed, half of them in surgery. This situation changed, however, at the time of the Protestant Reformation, when the Guild of Surgeons was founded in England under Henry VIII, and deliberately excluded women from practice. Education of women sharply declined from that time on, until in the 19th century lay women broke through the barrier and began making the medical field "respectable" for women. The work of Dr. Agnes McLaren, a Scottish missionary who converted to Catholicism, is reviewed in conclusion.

143. Drinkwater, H. "Woman's Place in Medicine: Historical Sketch. " Liverpool M. -Chir. J. , 32 (1912) 19-38. [Article not examined by editors.]

144. Ehrenreich, Barbara and English, Deirdre. Witches, Midwives, and Nurses: A History of Women Healers. Feminist Press, Old Westbury, New York, 1973, 45 pp. illus. , photos. (Glass Mountain Pamphlet No. 1.)
"To know our history is to begin to see how to take up the struggle again, " state the authors, who assert that women have always been healers. In this pamphlet, Ehrenreich and English concentrate on two phases in the suppression of women health workers and the male professional takeover: the persecution of witches in medieval Europe, and the rise of the male medical profession in 19th-century America. The oppression of women medical workers is shown to be a political struggle--a part of the history of sex struggle, and a part of class struggle. The publication is liberally illustrated and contains an annotated bibliography.

145. Ghrist, Jennie. "President's Address. Women in Medicine. " Woman's Medical Journal, 22:7 (July 1912) 147-149. (Original.) (Presentation, Fifteenth Annual Meeting, State Society of Iowa Medical Women, Burlington, Iowa, 7 May 1912.)
Upon the occasion of her election to the presidency of the State Society of Iowa Medical Women, Dr. Ghrist discoursed on three periods in the development of the science of medicine as it relates to women: (1) the accidental discovery of a few remedies which happened to work (women healers were often thought to possess powers of witchcraft), (2) the establishment of facts making medicine a science (women were then barred from educational and professional privileges), and (3) the "germ era" (Elizabeth Blackwell and other pioneers began to unbar doors once shut to women). Women physicians have contributed much, but they are advised to "do more of [their] own thinking on the unknown problems of medicine and surgery. " More women should specialize.

146. Glasgow, Maude. "Women in the Medical Profession. " Medical Record, 88 (4 December 1915) 951-955.
Dr. Glasgow discusses women in medicine throughout history --in Greek literature, as witches in the Middle Ages, and up through the present.

147. Glasgow, Maude. "Women Physicians. " Journal of the American Medical Women's Association, 9:1 (January 1954) 24-25.
"Caring for the sick was woman's job, even before human history began, " writes Dr. Glasgow who sketches the history of women in prominent positions relating to medicine, from Sumeria, through ancient Egypt and Greece, to Rome and up through medieval, Renaissance, and 18th-century Europe, to

1847 and Elizabeth Blackwell's historic opening of the door "for the re-entrance of women into their old profession."

148. Harding, Frances Keller. "Women Doctors: Past, Present and Future." Ohio State Medical Journal, 68 (December 1972) 1082-1085.
Dr. Harding, "a member of a three-generations-of-women-doctors sequence," briefly reviews some of the historical references to women physicians: their early modern struggles to obtain recognition as a professional class; the statistics of women vs. men who are active in medicine; women physicians' geographical distribution patterns in the United States; and their changing professional opportunities.

149. Hughes, Muriel Joy. Women Healers in Medieval Life and Literature. King's Crown Press, Morningside Heights, New York, 1943, 180 pp. illus.
Women in medieval times held much of the responsibility for the administration of medical aid. Since healing fell so obviously within the sphere of women, they were naturally accepted in contemporary writing. Hughes's first chapter deals with some famous women healers in literature: Morgan le Fay, Queen Isolt of Ireland, Arnine, Nicolette, Amable, and Pertelote. "The Layman's Medicine" is followed by a chapter on "Lay Women Healers." Hughes's "Academic Medicine begins with the schools of the 12th century, mainly Salerno in Italy and its rival school, Montpellier in France. Women practitioners and medieval midwives and nurses each receive their own discussion. The work is footnoted and an appendix lists women practitioners of the later Middle Ages by type of practice (i.e., barbers, doctors, surgeons, empirics, midwives, and nurses), by their country, and by their century. A glossary of herbs, a bibliography, and an index conclude the work.

150. Hurd-Mead, Kate Campbell. "A Contribution to the Study of Women in Medicine. Were There Qualified Women Doctors Before the Nineteenth Century?" New England Journal of Medicine, 199:11 (13 September 1928) 527-534.
"There are many proofs that from the beginning of time women were quietly and efficiently tending the sick...." Dr. Hurd-Mead recites the evidence for this claim, from monuments, tombstones, and writings of other physicians. Specific women healers are discussed.

151. Hurd-Mead, Kate Campbell. "History of Medicine." Women in Medicine, 72 (April 1941) 21-22.
Kate Mead's Volume II of the History of Women in Medicine, which includes the eastern hemisphere, Australia to Ireland, South Africa to China, was ready for a publisher. Dr. Mead was still working on Volume III which will include the western hemisphere from the Arctic to the Antarctic, from the Hawaiian Islands to the northeastern tip of Canada. "Several

universities are including medical history in the curriculum and yet they skate glibly over the part played by women. At the recent convention of the Association of the History of Medicine, no women were on the program ... it is very difficult to get photographs of medical women in their prime, or of those who have died. Men's portraits are evidently forthcoming with alacrity. Not so of these women." [This selection by Dr. Hurd-Mead is included as part of an obituary by Mary McKibben-Harper. This obituary, entitled "Kate Campbell Hurd-Mead: 1876-1941," appears in the BIOGRAPHIES section of this bibliography.]

152.   Hurd-Mead, Kate Campbell. A History of Women in Medicine: From the Earliest Times to the Beginning of the Nineteenth Century. The Haddam Press, Haddam, Connecticut, 1938, xvi, 569 pp. illus., photos., ports.
One of the first histories of women in medicine, Dr. Hurd-Mead's comprehensive work begins with medical women in ancient times and progresses through the 18th century. There are ten main chapters which divide the work chronologically by century (with the exception of Chapter II which discusses Trotula and the School of Salerno). Within each of these chapters, Dr. Hurd-Mead covers such aspects of women in medicine as the cultural milieu in which they practiced, social conditions, legal considerations, medical concerns, and medical institutions of the period. Dr. Hurd-Mead began collecting material for this history in 1890. It was at the historical club of Johns Hopkins Hospital, in that year, that Drs. Osler, Welch, and Kelly inspired her to search for the story of women's place in the development of medicine. Dr. Howard A. Kelly of Johns Hopkins University wrote the introduction for the book. Many illustrations illuminate Dr. Hurd-Mead's text, and a 42-page index concludes the work.

153.   Hurd-Mead, Kate Campbell. "The Seven Ages of Women in Medicine." Bulletin of the Medical Women's National Association, 35 (January 1932) 11-15.
The author reflects on the paucity of information about great women in general and women physicians in particular. She asks, "Are we now a professional equality with the best medical men so that our followers will ever continue to progress? Or is there likely to occur another subsidence of women, as in the past, and again a super abundance of the obnoxious feminine inferiority complex?" The seven times in history when women "threw off their dependence" and several rose to prominence are recounted.

154.   Hurd-Mead, Kate Campbell. "A Study of the Medical Education of Women." Journal of the American Medical Association, 116:4 (25 January 1941) 339-347. (American Medical Association Student Section.)
In her "tightly compressed article," Dr. Hurd-Mead gives a century-by-century account of medical women, showing how

"there has been no age in which the two sexes have not worked side by side in order to improve the health and the happiness of the people around them as well as to augment their own fortunes." Outstanding personalities from the first century A.D. to the present are noted. Dr. Hurd-Mead also quotes statistics relevant to the medical education and practice of women.

155. Landau, Richard. [History of Jewish Physicians: A Contribution to the History of Medicine]. S. Karger, Berlin, Germany, 1895, [144 pp.?]. (Ger)
In the belief that one cannot completely understand the present unless one knows what has gone before, the author traces the history of Jewish doctors and their contributions to knowledge from Old Testament times through the 19th century. During the Dark Ages, the Jews, along with the Arabs, kept scientific and medical knowledge alive, and were instrumental in spreading that knowledge to the awakening West at the end of that period. A few women physicians are mentioned: Rebecca, who taught at Salerno during the high period of that school's life; Sarah, who practiced medicine in Paris in the 13th century; another Sarah, who in 1419 was given permission to practice in the diocese of Wuerzburg on payment of an annual tax of ten "gulden"; and a Jewish woman named Zerlin who practiced in Frankfurt at about the same time. These women enjoyed a large clientele and a high reputation; Zerlin was even permitted to live outside the ghetto. Jewish women doctors were listed on the rolls of Frankfurt throughout the 15th century.

156. Latham, Vida A. "Early Women Physicians." Journal of the American Medical Women's Association, 10:8 (August 1955) 286.
A half-page vignette introduces a scattering of names of very early women healers.

157. Lenden, E. ["On Women in Nursing and Medicine"]. Deutsche Rundschau, 7 (1879) 126-248. (Ger)
Following a brief review of the development of nursing as a separate profession, the author describes, with voluminous notes, the establishment of the still shaky foothold of women in medicine in various countries. Among the first women doctors were Elizabeth Blackwell, Miss Garrett and Sophia Jex-Blake in England, Miss Zakrzewska and Emily Blackwell in America, and Charlotte Heidenreich in Germany; their struggles for acceptance and freedom to practice are described at some length in the text and notes. Many, like the Russians, had to get their educations in foreign countries. The third part of the article details the status of medical education for women at the time it was written. The desire for medical education met generally with little enthusiasm on the part of the medical and academic establishments. Women were still considered by many to be suited only to nursing

and midwifery. Before the battle could be won, elementary and premedical education for girls would have to be made equal to that offered boys. This struggle is a part of the greater movement for the emancipation of women in general.

158. Lipinska, Melanie. [History of Women Physicians from Antiquity to Present]. Librairie G. Jacques & C., Paris, France, 1900, 586 pp. (Fre)
This world history of women in medicine is divided into six parts: primitive times, antiquity, middle ages, modern times, nineteenth century, and 1890-1900. The discussion of women in medicine is prefaced by a review of the primitive concepts of illness and medicine and the religious and social beliefs on which these concepts were based. The development of primitive medicine is traced from the appearance of the sorcerer through the witch doctor to the emergence of the doctor priest. It is stated that the involvement of women in medicine largely depended on the status of women in a given society--a view illustrated by the examination of women's status in primitive cultures, including the tribes of Africa, Australia, and North America. Throughout the work Dr. Lipinska emphasizes women's social status and its effects on the medical training available to women. Section 2, "Antiquity," covers Egypt, Greece, and Rome. Section 3, "The Middle Ages," charts the progress made by medical women in Salerno, Germany, France, England, and Poland from the 13th to the 15th centuries, and describes the medical involvement of religious orders as typified by St. Hildegarde of Germany. "Modern Times," section 4, covers the period from the 16th through the 18th centuries: this section is particularly interesting for its analyses of medical studies of French women and the effects of the French revolution on the status of women. Section 5, "The Nineteenth Century," describes the beginnings of the women's movement in Europe and the U.S., women's involvement in battlefield medicine, medical education for women in the U.S., and the founding of the Female Medical College at Philadelphia. The acceptance of women in medical colleges in Switzerland, France, England, and Russia is also traced. The volume culminates with a review of the progress of women doctors in the last ten years of the 19th century and a description of the activities of medical missionaries in the Orient. This book, written by a woman physician, includes a bibliography.

159. Lipinska, Melinie. [Women and the Progress of the Medical Sciences]. Masson & Cie., Paris, France, 1930, viii, 235 pp. photo., ports. (Fre)
This book, divided into five sections, traces the part played by women in medical care from primitive times to the early 20th century. "The Primitive Period" discusses prehistoric medicine; "Antiquity," the classical period; "Middle Ages," the Italian schools, the German developments, and the effects of the feudal system; "Modern Times to the 19th century"

traces the rise, decline, and early steps to reestablishment of the practice of medicine by women in European countries between about 1500 and 1800. The final section, "The 19th and 20th Centuries," describes the struggle for admission to medical schools and for the right to practice from 1800 through World War I and the years immediately following it. This book contains very little documentation. [A 285-page Polish edition was published in Warsaw, Poland in 1932.]

160. Loomis, Metta May. "The Contributions Which Women Have Made to Medical Literature." New York Medical Journal, 100 (12 September 1914) 522-524.
When women have been able to practice medicine and do research, they have distinguished themselves, and their observations and research have had lasting value. Women do not receive credit for the work they have contributed to medicine. The author concludes that "Women writers should claim all to which they are justly entitled, seeing to it that the credit for their contributions is not placed on the wrong side of the account owing to their failure to sign articles for publications with their given name."

161. Lovejoy, Esther Pohl. Women Doctors of the World. The Macmillan Company, New York, 1957, x, 413 pp. photos., ports.
This study of women in medicine begins with ancient Greece and ends with 1949. It briefly surveys women doctors in the Middle Ages and Renaissance and the struggle to admit women to medical education in the 18th and 19th centuries. Other chapters are devoted to Lydia Folger Fowler, the first American woman to receive an M.D. (from Rochester Eclectic Medical College, New York); the history of Woman's Medical College, Philadelphia; the Blackwell sisters and their founding of the New York Infirmary; medical women in Boston and Chicago, from Michigan to the Pacific Coast, and in Canada; the beginnings of medical education for women in Britain (a chapter is devoted to Sophia Jex-Blake); and women's activities in continental Europe, the Balkans and Near East, the Far East, Australia and New Zealand, Africa, and Latin America. There are chapters arranged historically, dealing with women doctors in World War I, World War II, and the postwar period, as well as an account of the American Women's Hospitals. The book, based on the writings of women doctors and worldwide medical school records, contains hundreds of names and many photographs of both American and foreign women physicians. There is a lengthy index.

162. Loyola, Sister M. "Women in Medicine." Catholic World, 157 (May 1943) 156-164.
Asserting that "from the very beginning Christianity took an affirmative attitude toward the study and practice of medicine by women," Sister Loyola presents examples of Christian women healers and physicians. Among those mentioned: Fabiola,

who, following her conversion to Christianity, practiced medicine in Rome and in the Holy Land; Macrina who, with her brother St. Basil, managed 347 church-connected hospitals in Constantinople; St. Bridget of Ireland (c. 525); Trotula, of 11th-century Salerno; and St. Hildegarde, "the most independent and learned" of all the medieval medical women. Following the Middle Ages, "secularization of the universities, the gradual decay of the true Christian spirit, and the neo-paganism of the Renaissance" resulted in the exclusion of women from medicine. The women who took up the struggle for medical education in the 18th and 19th centuries are profiled, and the Catholic Church's role in women's education is emphasized.

163. McKibbin-Harper, Mary. "Editorial Comment." Women in Medicine, 60 (April 1938) 10.
Praise and respect for Kate Campbell Hurd-Mead's monumental History of Women in Medicine is the emphasis of this editorial, encouraging every woman doctor to "get it into circulation. It has a bearing on our status. It is our professional family tree!"

164. MacMurchy, Helen. "Medicus et Medica [Part I]." American Medicine, 7 (6 February 1904) 231-234. (Special Articles.)
This history of medical education for women covers the founding of the Woman's Medical College of Pennsylvania and Hospital, the New York Infirmary for Women and Children and its Medical College for Women, the Northwestern University Woman's Medical College (Chicago) and the Chicago Hospital for Women, the Woman's Medical College of Baltimore, the New England Female Medical College and the New England Hospital for Women and Children, the Women's Medical College of Toronto, the London School of Medicine for Women; and the admittance of women to medical studies at Johns Hopkins University Medical Faculty, and Edinburgh University (Scotland).

165. Macy, Mary Sutton. "Medical Women, in History and in Present Day Practice: [Part I]." New York Medical Journal, 104:5 (29 July 1916) 193-198. (Original Communications.)
[This article also appears in the Woman's Medical Journal, 27:4 (April 1917) 79-86.]

166. Macy, Mary Sutton. "Medical Women, in History and in Present Day Practice: [Part II]." New York Medical Journal, 104:6 (5 August 1916) 257-259.
This article concludes with a partial list of women entitled to be called "well known in their specialties."

167. Marks, Geoffrey and Beatty, William K. Women in White. Charles Scribner's Sons, New York, New York, 1972,

239 pp. illus., ports.
This work reviews the role of women in medicine from ancient
healers to their status in the U.S. in the present decade. It
is divided into three sections. The first is a 20-page review
of early practice, including midwifery. The second section
focuses on women in modern medicine and uses brief biographies of outstanding physicians to illustrate the 19th-century
struggle for education and training, principally in the U.S.
Included here are Elizabeth Blackwell, Elizabeth Garrett Anderson, Mary Putnam Jacobi, Emily Dunning Barringer, and
Alice Hamilton. There is also a reference to the mysterious
Dr. James Barry, who served as inspector general of the
British army (1856-65) and was found to be a woman upon
"his" death. A third section discusses women in related
fields--such as Florence Nightingale and Dorothea Dix. The
epilogue gives brief notes on outstanding contemporary women physicians in the U.S. There is a selected bibliography
and name index.

168. "Medical Women in the Past." Clinical Excerpts, 14:7 (1940)
        3-12. illus.
      Spanning several continents and the past 2000 years, this
      article mentions the names of many prominent medical wo-
      men. It concentrates on the founding of women's medical col-
      leges in America and the opening of established medical
      schools to women.

169. "A Medico-Literary Causerie: The Evolution of the Medical
        Woman [Part I]." Practitioner, 52 (February 1896) 288-
        292.
      Noting that the "evolution of the medical woman is all but
      complete," this article glances back at the history of the
      movement. Mentioned are the "traces" of the medical woman
      of ancient Rome and Greece, Trotula and the School of Saler-
      no, women healers of the Middle Ages, and the modern pio-
      neers in America.

170. "A Medico-Literary Causerie: The Evolution of the Medical
        Woman [Part II]: Concluded." Practitioner, 52 (April
        1896) 407-412.
      Beginning with the pioneering work of Elizabeth Garrett-An-
      derson, this article goes on to review Sophia Jex-Blake's
      "siege" of the University of Edinburgh and the initiation of
      women's medical education in Switzerland, Russia, and France.
      The current status of women's medical studies and practice
      in several countries is discussed.

171. Minor, T. C. "The Doctresses of Medicine." Interstate
        Medical Journal, 8 (March 1901) 97-108. port.
      Between 1899 and 1900, the Paris school had 29 French wo-
      men and 100 women students from other countries enrolled.
      "Is this right? Is it a misfortune?" The author reviews the
      history of women in medicine, from Agnodice, the Athenian

woman who assumed a male disguise to practice medicine, through Henrietta Faber (who also impersonated a male in order to care for the wounded), the 19th-century widow of a French officer, to the beginning of the 20th century, when Russian and Anglo-Saxon female physicians "overrun Asia, many in the guise of missionaries." [This article is a translation from the French.]

172. Peo, Evalene E. "Women in the Profession: President's Annual Address." Woman's Medical Journal, 16:7 (July 1906) 109-110. (Presentation, State Society of Iowa Medical Women, Des Moines, Iowa, May 1906.)

173. Percival, Eleanor. "Women in Medicine." Canadian Medical Association Journal, 23 (September 1930) 436-438.

174. Potter, Marion Craig. "'Medical Women of Yesterday.'" Woman's Medical Journal, 26:6 (June 1916) 160-162. (Address, Annual Meeting, Medical Women's National Association, Detroit, Michigan, 13 June 1916.)
In this review of the first medical women in modern times, Dr. Potter highlights the names of those who pioneered the difficult way so that other women who wanted medical training could obtain it. Not all these women left written work behind: some preferred instead to put their energies into talking to women who might become doctors and into practicing medicine. Those named include: Alice Freeman Palmer, Elizabeth Blackwell, Elizabeth Garrett Anderson, Emily Blackwell, and Sarah Read Adamson Dolley. Each of these women made significant contributions to the progress of women in medicine.

175. Power, Eileen. "Some Women Practitioners of Medicine in the Middle Ages." Proceedings of the Royal Society of Medicine, 14 (21 December 1921) 20-23.
Eileen Power discusses primarily Trotula of Salerno and Jacoba Felicie, the extent of their "practice," and the opinions of their contemporaries toward women healers. In conclusion, Powers also mentions Joan du Lee, an English woman doctor mentioned in an unpublished petition to King Henry IV in the early 15th century.

176. Reddy, D. V. S. "Centenary of Eve's Entry into Medical Schools and Colleges." Journal of Indian Medical Association, 17:2 (November 1947) 42-44.
The careers of Elizabeth Blackwell, Elizabeth Garett [sic] Anderson, Clara Swain, and Mary Scharlieb are surveyed. The early medical education of women in India is contrasted with Indian women physicians' present status.

177. Reeve, Arthur B. "Famous Women Doctors and Their Pioneer Work." McCall's Magazine, (January 1912) 28-29, 60-61. ports.

While two generations ago there were scarcely ten women
physicians in the United States, today "there must be considerably more than ten thousand." This brief history of
women's victory in medicine focuses on the lives of Drs.
Elizabeth and Emily Blackwell, Elizabeth Garrett Anderson,
Sophia Jex-Blake, Mary Pierson Eddy (the only woman physician in Turkey), and Yamei Kin (a well-known practitioner
in China).

178.   Ruben, R. J. " Women in Medicine: Past, Present and Fu-
       ture. " Journal of the American Medical Women's Asso-
       ciation, 27:5 (May 1972) 251-259. tables. (Address,
       Barnard College, Columbia University, New York, 4 No-
       vember 1971.)
       Historical data and statistics (both available elsewhere) for
       present and future trends are reiterated.

179.   Sandelin, Ellen. ["On the Status of Female Doctors in Vari-
       ous Countries"]. Hygiea, 63 (1901) 297-325. (Swe)
       The author reviews briefly the history of women in medicine
       in Greece and Rome and in the various European countries to
       the middle of the 19th century. She then discusses at length
       the developments of the second half of the 19th century in
       each country, with comments and notes on outstanding or pio-
       neering women and the institutions they were related to. For
       the United States, this includes Elizabeth Blackwell and the
       Woman's Medical College, the "Philadelphia Hospital," the
       Women's Hospital of Philadelphia, the New York Infirmary
       for Women and Children and other institutions. In England
       the pioneers included Elizabeth Garrett-Anderson, who with
       Dr. Blackwell founded the London School of Medicine for Wo-
       men; in Scotland, Sophia Jex-Blake. By the end of the cen-
       tury, a number of medical schools in Great Britain were
       open to women. The first women in Indian medical schools
       entered Madras in 1875, but much of the medical care for
       women came from foreign doctors and hospitals established
       by compassionate foreigners. Russian women were among
       the first to study medicine, although they had to leave their
       own country to do so, usually going to Switzerland. They
       were not permitted into the established schools at home, but
       in 1872 special courses were opened for them in St. Peters-
       burg. The Swiss and French schools attracted more foreign
       than native women--mostly Russians, Americans, and English.
       Schools were open to women in Italy, Greece, Spain, Portu-
       gal, but few took advantage of them. Holland and Belgium
       were among the first to permit women practitioners; Austria
       among the last. The history of the acceptance of women in
       Scandinavia is considered at length.

180.   Schönfeld, Walther. [Women in Occidental Medicine from An-
       tiquity to the End of the 19th Century]. Enke, Stuttgart,
       1947, viii, 176 pp. illus., ports. (Ger)
       This historic overview of women in medicine deals not only

with the role of female physicians but also with the influence
of female saints and priestesses, trained dilettantes, and mid
wives on the development of occidental dilettante. The book
spans from antiquity to the 19th century. After a short description of the social and scientific background of every period or century, the author gives a series of biographies of
women. For the period after 1600, the biographies are
grouped by country; a short general description of the individual countries precedes each biography (which also includes
those of quacks). The book, which contains an extensive bibliography and a series of illustrations, is indexed.

181. Schwartz, Adolf W. "Likenesses of Women Physicians on
      Stamps." Journal of the American Medical Women's
      Association, 14:2 (February 1959) 142-144. facsim.
      Various women physicians who have appeared on different
      countries' postage stamps are named. A vignette is given
      for each. Hygeia, daughter of Aesculapius, is found on a
      New Zealand and Greek stamp. An Elizabeth Blackwell
      stamp to commemorate the centenary of her enrollment in
      medical school was not approved by the U.S. Post Office in
      1947. Suzanna Orelli, Ph.D. and holder of an honorary de-
      gree of doctor of medicine from the University of Zurich,
      Switzerland appears on a Swiss postage stamp. Two honor-
      ary doctors of medicine appear on postage stamps: Queen
      Elina of Italy and Marie Curie of Poland. Queen Elisabeth
      of the Belgians graduated from the University of Leipzig in
      1900 with a degree of doctor of medicine. Her likeness ap-
      pears on Belgium postage.

182. Scoutetten, Henri. ["The History of Women Physicians from
      Antiquity to the Present"]. La France Medicalé, 14:
      98/99 (1867) 331-336. (Fre)
      More than half of this paper is devoted to women healers of
      ancient times, from the midwives of the biblical Hebrews
      through the Egyptians, Indians and Chinese, the Romans,
      Arabs of the Middle Ages, and midwives of medieval France.
      Throughout the Middle Ages the common people of France de-
      pended on quacks, "healers," and poorly trained midwife-
      nurses. In more recent times some women have achieved
      the rank of physician, such as Mme. Boivin who, with her
      professor son-in-law, wrote a textbook on uterine diseases.
      In the book, published in 1837, the author title appears as
      follows: "Mme. Boivin, doctor of medicine, decorated with
      the gold medal of civil merit of Prussia." In recent times,
      America, England, and Switzerland have accepted women as
      physicians and even established women's medical colleges.
      The author thinks that women are suited by nature for sooth-
      ing pain and rescuing the unfortunate, but not for medicine or
      surgery except perhaps for women's diseases and minor sur-
      gery. If a woman has enough spirit to earn a doctorate, she
      would not be refused in France, but this article's author
      states that he would not accept her; let women fill the role
      assigned them by nature.

183.   Selmon, Bertha. "Medical Opportunity for Women Spreads
           Abroad." Medical Woman's Journal, 54:2 (February
           1947) 45-49, 56. (History of Women in Medicine.)
        Continuing this series on the history of women in medicine,
        Dr. Selmon quotes entirely from James R. Chadwick's 1879
        article entitled "Study and Practice of Medicine by Women"
        (International Review, October 1879). Chadwick covers the
        situation of medical women in various other countries.

184.   Steinberger, S. ["The History of Women Physicians"].
           Gynaekologia (Budapest), (1902) 36-41. (Hun)
        [Article not examined by editors.]

185.   Stenhouse, Evangeline E. "Women: Patients and Physicians."
           Journal of the American Medical Women's Association,
           7:9 (September 1952) 333-339. illus. (Inaugural Address,
           American Medical Women's Association, Chicago, Illinois,
           9 June 1952.)
        The author organizes her presentation around women in the
        "very early days" and women physicians of her day. Begin-
        ning with ancient and medieval times, the author works her
        way to the present discussing women as patients and healers,
        as depicted in art and records.

186.   Van Hoosen, Bertha. "Romance of the Medical Education of
           Women in England." Medical Woman's Journal, 32:8
           (August 1925) 224-225. (Editorial.)
        Women physicians in England and America should be aware
        of "how close the ties between [them] must always be."
        Elizabeth Blackwell was British and after working for the
        rights of women to practice medicine in the United States,
        she returned to England where she became the first woman
        physician registered to practice. In her honor, American
        medical women are endowing the Elizabeth Blackwell bed in
        the George Washington Ward of the Royal Free Hospital in
        London.

187.   Walker, Jane. "The Return of Women to Medicine." Con-
           temporary Review, 137 (January 1930) 46-50. (Address,
           London School of Medicine for Women, London, England,
           1 October 1929.)
        Reviewing the historical facts and the legends of medical wo-
        men of ancient and medieval times, Dr. Walker offers evi-
        dence to support one of her own speculations: that a woman
        doctor wrote the "Book of Ecclesiastes." Dr. Walker then fo-
        cuses upon three pioneers of the modern medical women's
        movement: Elizabeth Blackwell, Elizabeth Garrett Anderson,
        and Sophia Jex-Blake. Of the three women, Dr. Walker be-
        lieves Jex-Blake is "in some ways the most brilliant, with
        a large measure of genius ... you either disliked her in-
        tensely or you would be prepared to go with her to prison and
        to judgment." Finally, praise is given to male champions of
        women's right to enter the medical profession.

188.   Walsh, James J. "Women in the Medical World." New Yor
         Medical Journal, 96 (28 December 1912) 1324-1328. (A
         dress, Commencement, Woman's Medical College of
         Pennsylvania, Philadelphia, Pennsylvania, 29 May 1912.)
         Dr. Walsh points out that contrary to the increasingly popu-
         lar belief that this is the first time in history women have
         had an opportunity for the fullest education, there have been
         a series of epochs of flourishing feminine education in the
         history of humanity. Beginning with Plato, Dr. Walsh dis-
         cusses these epochs. General advice to the new graduates
         concludes the article.

189.   Whitten, Kathryn M. "Women and the Practice of Medicine.
         Medical Woman's Journal, 50:11 (November 1943) 273-
         276. (Address, Annual Convention, Women's Medical So-
         ciety of the State of New York, 1943.)
         There have been women healers since earliest times. Wheth
         er their work was obscured or brought into the light (as was
         done during times of stress), women have been working "in
         a very practical way" with the sick. Dr. Whitten reviews
         the history of women in medicine from the earliest time
         through the present, and concludes with a personal account
         of her own experiences when she first went to Fort Wayne,
         Indiana as a physician.

190.   "Who Was First Woman Physician?" Journal of the Ameri-
         can Medical Association, 230:12 (23-30 December 1974)
         1707. (International Comments.)
         The issuance of a U.S. postage stamp honoring Elizabeth
         Blackwell as the first woman physician in the Western Hemi-
         sphere created controversy within the West German press.
         Although it was not claimed that Dr. Blackwell was the world
         first woman physician, West Germans pointed out that Dr.
         Dorothea Christiane Erxleben (née Leporin) graduated in Ger-
         many in 1754.

191.   Wollstein, Martha. "The History of Women in Medicine."
         Woman's Medical Journal, 18:4 (April 1908) 65-69.
         Following her review of medical women's history, which be-
         gins in ancient times and encompasses events in many coun-
         tries, Dr. Wollstein notes that modern women doctors suffer
         most from a lack of hospital appointments.

192.   "Women Doctors: An Historic Retrospect." Contemporary
         Review, 108 (October 1915) 504-510.
         The European War and the increased activity of women phy-
         sicians make this an interesting moment to glance at the his-
         tory of women doctors. This article scans the accomplish-
         ments of women healers in ancient times to the present, de-
         voting much attention to Drs. Elizabeth Blackwell, Elizabeth
         Garrett-Anderson, and Sophia Jex-Blake. A discussion of
         the entrance into medicine of Indian girls mentions one Hindu
         doctor, Rukmabai, who faced imprisonment rather than ratify

the marriage made for her as a child.   Another physician, Dr. Krishnabai, presides over an Indian hospital and is an expert surgeon.   The war will undoubtedly have a beneficial effect on women in medicine, notes the author, who concludes that a woman physician comes very close to being a perfect human being.

193.   "Women in Medicine." World Medical Journal, 11:1 (January 1964) 43.   (Editorial.)
This article is a discussion of how to make the best use of the pool of medical womanpower. Surprise is expressed at the hostility toward pioneering 19th-century women physicians, and a lament is voiced that somewhere, particularly in the Christian world, something went wrong and women were relegated to more "menial" tasks in medical care.

194.   "Women Who Practiced Medicine in Ancient Times." North American Med. Chir. Review, 5 (1861) 372, 560.
[Article not examined by editors.]

SOUTH, CENTRAL, LATIN AMERICA AND MEXICO

195.   Beauperthuy de Benedetti, Rosario. [Women and Medicine: Work of Incorporation as Numbered Individual to Occupy Chair Number 22.   With a Critique of the Work by Carlos R. Travieso, Numbered Individual of the Venezuelan Society of the History of Medicine and of the National Academy of Medicine]. [Sociedad Venezolana de Historia de la Medicina?], Caracas, Venezuela, 1970, 29 pp. illus., facsims., port. (Spa)
This is an oration delivered by Dr. Beauperthuy on the occasion of her installation as the first woman to become a full member ["numbered individual"] of the Venezuelan Society of the History of Medicine (12 March 1970). A biographical sketch in Travieso's critique notes that she is a corresponding member of the French Society of the History of Medicine and in 1966 received the Burgky Prize of the French Academy of Medicine for her research and publication on her ancestor, Louis D. Beauperthuy, discoverer of the vector of yellow fever. Beauperthuy gives a brief sketch of women in medicine from the ancient Greeks to the 18th century, followed by a biography of Elizabeth Blackwell, first woman to receive an M.D. degree, and some comments on early students at Zurich and Paris. The first woman medical student at the Central University in Caracas was Virginia Pereira Alvarez, who eventually graduated from Woman's Medical College of Pennsylvania. The first woman to graduate in medicine was Lya Inberg, in 1936, although two women had received degrees in 1912 and 1929 on the basis of medical studies in Europe. In 1969, of 311 M.D.s graduating from the Central University, over 80 were women.

196. "Women Physicians in Brazil." Women in Medicine, 90 (October 1945) 16.
A very brief "history" of women physicians in Brazil is given.

USSR

197. Bazanov, V. A. and Pavluchkova, A. V. ["From 'Schools for Midwives' to 'Courses for Women Physicians' (On the Centennial of Education for Women Physicians)"]. Akusherstvo i Ginekologiia (Moskva), 48 (November 1972) 74-76. (Rus)
The first midwifery school in Russia was opened in 1757. It offered courses only in German, and no clinical subjects were included in the curriculum. During its first 20 years, 35 midwives finished their training in this school in Moscow, and 168 completed training in a similar school in Petersburg. By the end of the 18th century, clinics were attached to the schools for clinical practice, but even in the mid-19th century the level of education was still low. The first women, N. P. Suslova and M. A. Bokova, were admitted to medical studies at the university in 1862, but the revolutionary movement in Russia put an end to these studies. In 1872 a special department was opened at the Medico-Surgical Academy, on a four-year experimental basis; its graduates were given the right to practice medicine in the fields of gynecology, pediatrics, and venereal diseases. In 1876 the courses were transferred to the Nicolaev Military Hospital where they were called "Women's Medical Courses." The five-year curriculum included various subjects; 959 women completed this course. The courses were closed in 1882, and it was not until 15 years later, in 1897, that the Women's Medical Institute was established.

198. Belitskaia, E. La. ["Higher Medical Education of Women in Russia (1872-1972)"]. Askepii (Sofia), 3 (1974) 114-119. (English Abstract.) (Rus)
[Article not examined by editors.]

199. Belitskaia, E. La. ["Polyclinical Service in Prerevolutionary Petersburg and the Participation of Women Physicians. (On the Centenary of Higher Medical Education for Women in Russia)"]. Sovetskoe Zdravookhranenie, 31:10 (1972) 64-68.
[Article not examined by editors.]

200. Dionesov, S. M. ["Pages from the History of the Education of Women Physicians in Russia in the 19th Century"]. Sovetskoe Zdravookhranenie, 29 (1970) 63-68. (Rus)
In anticipation of the 100th anniversary of the founding of the first Courses for the Education of Women as Midwives, the author reviews the history of their origin, existence, and abolition. The courses were associated with the Imperial

Medical-Surgical Academy of Russia. In 1870 the chief of
the Academy and two other professors appealed to the Medical Council for the right of women to study medicine, pointing out the advantages to be gained. Permission was given
in 1872 by the Minister of Defense to open the courses for a
four-year probationary period, and this decision was confirmed in 1876. The Tsarist authorities were concerned
about the political views of the women. For this reason and
because of the financial problems faced by the courses, they
were transferred to the Nicolaev Military Hospital. In May
1881 the resignation of Defense Minister D. A. Milutin sealed
the fate of the courses, which were closed down by the new
minister on July 31, 1882. During the almost 15 years the
courses were in existence, 691 women graduated and became physicians.

201. Karnaukhova, E. I. ["On the Beginning of Medical Education
for Women in Russia"]. Sovetskoe Zdravookhranenie
(Moskva), 21 (1962) 48-52. (Rus)
[Article not examined by editors.]

202. Nekrasova, E. [From the Past of the Courses for Women:
Part I. The Lubyanskie Courses in Moscow; Part II.
The Physicians' Courses in Petersburg]. Moscow, USSR,
1886, 99 pp. (Rus)
Although (at the time this book was written) the courses for
women had been in existence for only about 20 years, the
memory of their origin was fading. Dedicated to the memory
of the author's sister, V. S. Nekrasova, one of the first Russian women in medicine, the book recalls the founding and
early years of the two schools. After much effort and struggle by Russian women desiring higher education, official permission was given by the minister of public education to open
the Lubyanskie Courses for Women. Part I describes the
founding, activities, curriculum, teachers, financial problems,
administration, and significance to the times, of the courses.
Many women received their education in the sciences which
enabled them later to get into higher educational establishments. Many of them became teachers, some in these same
courses; others entered the medical courses and became physicians. Part II describes the effort leading to the establishment of the medical courses for women in Petersburg and the
life of the first students there. The first appeal for the right
of women to study medicine was dated 1864. After many
years of discussions and struggle, the doors of the Medical-
Surgical Academy of Petersburg were opened to women on
November 1, 1872; there they could take courses in histology,
anatomy, botany, physics, and chemistry. Initially called
Courses for Scientific Midwives, they later became the Women's Medical Courses. The author reviews admission requirements, curriculum, teaching, conditions of life, and the
number of graduates from 1877 to 1880 and the hardships they
endured. Sixty women graduated from the courses during the

first year. Many of the students became practicing physicians. At the time of the writing of this book, 24 women, pioneers of medical education in Russia, were engaged in practical work as "Zemzki Vrach."

203. Okunkova-Goldinger, Z. and Ladova, Rosalia M., trans.
"The History of Medical Education of Women in Russia."
Woman's Medical Journal, 12:3 (March 1902) 51-54.
This is the first of two articles on the development of education for women physicians in Russia. Women's medical education began when the government's medical department formalized instruction for midwives in 1757, including the admission of midwives to university clinics. In 1872 an anonymous gift was given to the military department for a woman's medical college in connection with the Military Medical Academy. In the same year Alexander II decreed the establishment of a separate four-year course for learned midwives in connection with the Imperial Medico Chirurgical Academy. In 1876 a fifth year was added to the course, equalizing the training of women with that of men. However, the program was then transferred from the Academy to the Nikolaevsky Hospital and became a separate school. Funds for the operation of the school were not appropriated, and attempts were made to get the city government of St. Petersburg to operate it. In 1895 the rules and regulations for the Medical Institute for Women received confirmation and sanction of the emperor. In 1897 the Institute opened in St. Petersburg. Of 264 applicants, 188 were accepted; 75 of these were college graduates and assistant physicians.

204. Okunkova-Goldinger, Z. and Ladova, Rosalia M., trans.
"The History of Medical Education of Women in Russia:
The Work and Status of Medical Women of Russia."
Woman's Medical Journal, 12:4 (April 1902) 79-82.
This, the second of a two-part article, documents the certification and work of women physicians in Russia in the 19th century. In 1878 Alexander II authorized the issuance of temporary certificates to women physicians who took state examinations until such time as a suitable form for a diploma could be agreed upon. These certificates were in effect for 20 years until Nicholas II confirmed a Senate resolution authorizing women physicians to receive the same degree and privileges as men physicians. During the Turko-Russian War, 42 women entered military medical service. In 1897 they were commanded to the Red Cross Society. Aside from military service, women physicians carried on active practices in the provinces. Data from 1893 show there were 313 women physicians in the 409 states or counties with self-government. In Turkestan there were six hospitals with women physicians at the head of each. Data from 1882-83 show 11 women physicians as school inspectors of primary schools. It was also reported that women physicians in the cities gave service gratis to hospitals, infirmaries,

and other charitable institutions.   For example, from 1878
to 1890 women physicians in St. Petersburg received no remuneration for their services from the city government.

205.   Rozova, K. A.   ["The First Medical School for Women in
          Russia"].   Feldsher Akush, 37 (July 1972) 35-38.   (Rus)
       The first "practical" midwives' schools were opened in Rus-
       sia in the 18th century.   In 1861 the first two women medical
       students, M. P. Suslova and M. A. Bokova, were admitted
       to the Petersburg Medical Surgical Academy.   In the year
       1872 there were 44 Russian women studying abroad; that year
       saw the founding of the first women's medical higher school
       in Russia.   Its primary aim was to prepare "scientific" mid-
       wives.   The course lasted four years and the students paid
       50 rubles a year.   In 1876 the courses were transferred to
       the Nicolaev Military Hospital, given the name of Women's
       Medical Courses, and extended to five years.   The last class
       graduated in 1887.   The Women's Medical Institute was
       opened in Petersburg at the end of the 19th century, and after
       1905 Women's Medical Schools were opened in Odessa, Kiev,
       Moscow, and Kharkov.   At present there are 668,000 physi-
       cians in the Soviet Union, 70 per cent of them women.

206.   Shibokov, Anatotii Aleksovich.   [The First Medical Women
          in Russia].   Medical Publishing Company, Leningrad,
          USSR, 1961, 119 pp.   illus., ports.   (Rus)
       According to the annotation on the title page, this pamphlet
       was written to appeal to a wide variety of readers; it de-
       scribes the patriotism and self-sacrifice of prerevolutionary
       Russian nurses and the first women physicians, the struggle
       for women's medical education, and the contributions of med-
       ical women in the Crimean and Russo-Turkish Wars.   Most
       of the text is devoted to the training and activities of nurses
       and feldschers (field paramedics who handle minor medical
       problems); the last chapter, on "Women's Medical Education
       in Russia at the End of the 19th Century," contains a section
       on the early development of medical schools.   The Women's
       Medical Courses at Petersburg, started in 1872, attached to
       the Nikolaev Military Hospital in 1876, and closed in 1882,
       graduated classes ranging from five in 1876 to 88 in 1887.
       In 1892 there were 568 women doctors in Russia, about half
       of them in government service or institutional practice.

207.   Stochik, A. M. and Ponetaeva, N. E.   ["History of Higher
          Medical Education of Women in Russia"].   Zdravookhra-
          nenie Rossiiskoi Federatsii, 16 (September 1972) 37-41.
          (Rus)
       Medical education for women in Russia was first considered
       in 1861.   After very many discussions and a private donation
       of 50,000 rubles, four-year courses were finally opened in
       July 1872 at the Medico-Surgical Academy to train "scientific
       midwives."   The courses received no state financial support.
       Many outstanding medical doctors taught there.   In 1876 the

courses were transferred to the Nikolaev Military Hospital and the curriculum was increased to five years. In 1883 the women graduated from these courses and were given the title of physician. During the first ten years, 959 women were admitted to the courses; 434 were still studying in 1883, and 281 had completed the five-year course. The courses were closed in 1882 because of financial problems, but in 1897 the Women's Medical Institute was founded. Although many famous scientists taught there, the graduates did not enjoy the rights of graduates of other medical faculties. It was not until 1904 that they could work in all hospital departments or become professors. The first year, 188 women were enrolled, and the number increased to 1256 in 1913-14. In 1906 a medical faculty was opened at the Higher Women's Courses in Moscow; 1060 women graduated from this faculty before the 1917 revolution. There were also medical faculties at the universities at Derpt, Warsaw, Kazan, and Charkov. In 1918 all these special establishments for women were closed because they now enjoyed equal rights with men.

208. Tikotin, M. A. "Students at the First Petersburg Women's Medical Institute in the First Russian Revolution." Sovetskoe Zdravookhranenie, 4 (1975) 69-71. [Article not examined by editors.]

209. Zikeev, P. D. ["On the History of the Struggle for Higher Medical Education for Women in Russia"]. Klinicheskaia Meditsina (Moskva), 47 (October 1969) 151-154. (Rus) Two letters to Nadezhda Vasilyevna Stasova, founder, director, and chief coordinator of the Higher Education Courses for Women in Petersburg, are presented, one from I. M. Sechenov, the second from Sechenov's wife, M. A. Sechenova-Bokovaya, dated September 15, 1889 and October 18, 1889 respectively. Both letters show great sympathy and concern for one of the forms of social movement in the second half of the 19th century--the struggle of Russian women for their right to higher professional education-- as well as warmth and appreciation of Stasova's work. The author also presents a short history of the foundation and work of the school, its financial and social problems, and its battle with the Russian government for existence. N. Stasova was finally removed from her position by the tsarist authorities. She tried to find comfort in working for Sunday (vocational) schools, but found it difficult to reconcile herself to her situation. N. Stasova was a woman of great energy and modesty and was truly devoted to her work, full of love and faith in the irresistible strength of truth. She died on September 27, 1895.

UNITED STATES

210. Barringer, Emily Dunning. "Fifty Years Ago." Journal of the American Medical Women's Association, 6:8 (August

1951) 315-316.
A reminiscence of life in the United States at the turn of the century initiates this article, which continues on to a brief remembrance of Dr. Emily Blackwell, and concludes with an elucidation of the work and spirit of Mary Putnam Jacobi.

211.   Barringer, Emily Dunning. "Nineteen Forty-One and the Woman Doctor." Women in Medicine, 73 (July 1941) 8-13.
With elaborate analogy to an artist painting a picture, the author sketches in broad strokes the last several decades of history of women physicians in the United States, as well as the situation as it existed in 1941 for women physicians.

212.   Blake, John B. "Women and Medicine in Ante-Bellum America. (The Fielding H. Garrison Lecture)." Bulletin of the History of Medicine, 39:2 (March-April 1965) 99-123. (37th Annual Meeting, American Association for the History of Medicine, Bethesda and Washington, April 30, 1964.)
A well-documented discussion of Elizabeth Blackwell, women's rights, and the struggles of women in medicine, with a substantial section on the emergence of various 19th-century medical schools and their respective attitudes toward women in medicine constitutes this article.

213.   Bloch, Harry. "Women's Role in Medicine in Early Colonial Times." New York State Journal of Medicine, 75:5 (April 1975) 770-772. (History of Medicine.)
Following a brief and general review of the position and lack of education for women in early colonial times, this article describes women's contributions as healers, nurses, apothecaries, herbalists, and midwives.

214.   Daniel, Annie S. "Shall Women Study Medicine." Medical Record, 94 (16 November 1918) 850-853. (Presentation, Woman's Medical Association of New York City, October 16, 1918.)
Women studying medicine in the 19th century, their struggles and successes, are cited in this article. Dr. Daniel speaks also of the difficulties women physicians had in securing admission to medical societies.

215.   "Difference of Opinion." Medical Woman's Journal, 34:9 (September 1927) 272.
Quotes are extracted from an article by Rollin Lynde Hartt, later reprinted in its entirety. ["The Woman Physician: Has She Arrived after Her Long and Adventurous Struggle?" Medical Woman's Journal, 34:10 (October 1927) 302-307.]

216.   Donegan, Jane Bauer. Midwifery in America, 1760-1860: A Study in Medicine and Morality. Syracuse University, Syracuse, New York, 1972, vii, 304 pp. (Ph.D. thesis.)
The years 1760 to 1860 witnessed a revolution in obstetrics:

the introduction of forceps (which only men were trained to use) and the replacement of untrained female midwives by trained male obstetricians just as women were becoming too "modest" to appreciate their attentions. This dissertation shows how the problem of female modesty led to formal training of women midwives in the 1850s, many of whom then outraged men by becoming qualified physicians. Harriot Hunt, Martha Sawin, Lydia Folger Fowler, and other women physicians are discussed, as is the opening of American medical colleges to women.

217. Drouillard, Louisa C. "Women in the Medical Profession." Transactions of the Medical Society of Tennessee: 62nd Session, (1895) 234-245.
In this, the first paper delivered by a woman physician before the Medical Society of Tennessee, the history of medical women in the United States is divided into seven periods: (1) female midwifery in the colonial period, (2) complete exclusion of females from the profession during the Revolution, (3) a period of general reaction, (4) formation of medical colleges for women, (5) struggle for entrance into the reputable colleges, (6) founding of hospitals where women could receive clinical training, and (7) struggle for official recognition in the profession. A discussion of the paper by members of the medical society follows.

218. Furman, Bess. "Portraits Honor Medical Women." Journal of the American Medical Women's Association, 12:12 (December 1957) 443-444. ports.
This article is a reprint from the October 27, 1957, issue of the New York Times. The exhibit of medical women at the Medical Museum of the Armed Forces Institute of Pathology "goes back to a facsimile of the most ancient known pictorial record of a woman doctor," c. 3000 B.C. The prized item of the exhibit is a portrait of Dr. Mary Edwards Walker, by J. B. Hudson, depicting (according to the historian in charge of the exhibit) Dr. Walker's role as a Civil War spy.

219. Guion, Connie M. "Contribution of Medical Women to Society." Journal of the American Medical Women's Association, 15:8 (August 1960) 764-770. (Address, Women's Medical Association of New York City [Branch Fourteen], November 4, 1959.)
The study of medicine has been a natural pursuit for women through the ages--and periodically their aspirations have turned to struggles as "men have conspired to prevent them from doing so." After a cursory look at women in medicine before Blackwell, the author turns her attention to Elizabeth Blackwell's efforts to obtain a medical education and to found the New York Infirmary for Women and Children. Florence Sabin's professional life and contributions are also followed, from her internship in medicine at Johns Hopkins through her professorship there, her eventual work at the Rockefeller

Institute for Medical Research, and her ultimate return to and work in Denver, Colorado. The author gives credit for her detailed account of the life of Florence Sabin to Eleanor Bluemel's The Life of Florence Sabin.

220.   Hartt, Rollin Lynde. "The Woman Physician: Has She Arrived After Her Long and Adventurous Struggle?" Medical Woman's Journal, 34:10 (October 1927) 302-307.
"While it may be true that the number of medical women in the entire country is not equal to the number of medical men in the city of New York, the time will come when this condition will be changed." Evidence to support the author's belief that women physicians have indeed "arrived" includes historical facts, little-known anecdotes, and opinions of present-day educators. [The article also appears in Century Magazine, July 1927.]

221.   Henderson-Smathers, Irma. "Medical Women of North Carolina." Medical Woman's Journal, 56:10 (October 1949) 43-44. (History of Women in Medicine.)
This article introduces a series of articles about women physicians of North Carolina. Its "faith that one man is as good as another" aided the state in assuming "the lead in recognizing its women doctors." North Carolina Medical College, which existed from 1886 to 1913, admitted women to classes in 1902 and graduated its first woman in 1912. The North Carolina Medical Society granted a woman membership in 1872, becoming one of the first four state societies to do so. Dr. Henderson-Smathers opens her series with the biography of a male, Dr. John Dickson. It was in his home in Asheville, North Carolina that Elizabeth Blackwell began to "read medicine," preparing herself for entering medical school.

222.   "An Historical Masterpiece." Medical Woman's Journal, 46:5 (May 1939) 148. (Editorial.)
Praise is given to Dr. Annie Daniel for her series of articles on the history of the New York Infirmary, the first of which appears in this month's Journal. ["'A Cautious Experiment.' The History of the New York Infirmary for Women and Children and the Women's Medical College of the New York Infirmary; Also Its Pioneer Founders: 1853-1899."] Dr. Daniel's research often led, as she put it, "into an attic, a cellar, and to more than one graveyard." This journal's editors call the resulting articles "an intimate, authentic history" that hopefully will inspire young women physicians with appreciation for the work of pioneer medical women.

223.   Holloway, Lisabeth M. "O Pioneers!" Philadelphia Medicine, 71:10 (October 1975) 407-411.
The author, curator of the historical collections of the library at the College of Physicians of Philadelphia, discusses the history of women's medical colleges and coeducational medical

schools in the United States as well as medical education
abroad. In 1870 the U.S. census showed that 525 of 62,383
physicians and surgeons were female. The 1890 census reveals that of 103,482 white physicians and surgeons, 4,424
were female (572 of those were born abroad); colored physicians (Chinese, Japanese, and Indians) numbered 1,190 males
and 133 females; and Negro physicians numbered 794 male
and 115 female. The author points out the interesting fact
that by 1890 Howard Medical School had graduated only 19
women, and Meharry did not admit women at all. "Where
did these 298 non-white women doctors come from?"

224. Hurd-Mead, Kate Campbell. Medical Women of America: A
Short History of the Pioneer Medical Women of America
and of a Few of Their Colleagues in England. Froben
Press, New York, New York, 1933, 95 pp. photo.,
ports.

This history of early women physicians in the U.S. and England also includes brief histories of the gradual opening of
medical colleges to women, of women's hospitals, and the
admission of medical women to hospital positions and medical
societies. It surveys women physicians in research and
teaching, as specialists, missionaries, and writers, and in
the American Women's Hospitals. A survey of the Medical
Woman's National Association in 1931 showed that of 162 women physicians, only three had retired because of marriage.
Most were in public health, obstetrics and gynecology, or
pediatrics. An appendix gives the autobiography of Elizabeth
Cushier, gynecologist and friend of the Blackwells. Many
portraits and an index are included.

225. Irwin, Inez Haynes. "Medicine." In: Angels and Amazons:
A Hundred Years of American Women. Doubleday, Doran
& Company, Inc., Garden City, New York, 1933, 133-
162.

This recounting of women's post-Civil War struggles for medical education includes examples of persecution by male students. The founding of the Chicago Women's Medical College
and the opening of other schools to women are described.
One section tells of the opening of medical societies to women and their admission to specialties and institutional practice. A concluding section on the history of nursing in America mentions several women physicians.

226. Irwin, Inez Haynes. "They Become Doctors." In: Angels
and Amazons: A Hundred Years of American Women.
Doubleday, Doran & Company, Inc., Garden City, New
York, 1933, 42-50.

This chapter reviews details of the lives of American women
physicians between 1840 and 1860. Mentioned are Ann Preston and Hannah Longshore, graduates of the Woman's Medical
College of Pennsylvania's first class of 1852, and Sarah
Adamson and Mrs. Gleason, the earliest women graduates of

the Eclectic School, Rochester. Details of struggles for medical education are recounted for Emily and Elizabeth Blackwell, Harriet Hunt, Mary Putnam Jacobi, and Marie Zakrzewska.

227. Jacobi, Mary Putnam. "Woman in Medicine." In: Woman's Work in America. Edited by Annie Nathan Meyer. Henry Holt and Company, New York, New York, 1891, 139-205.

The history of women's struggle to enter the full practice of the medical profession is summarized by Dr. Jacobi, herself one of the pioneers of this movement. She divides the history of medical women into seven periods: (1) the colonial period of exclusively female midwifery, (2) the revolutionary period of emerging interest in medical art and education, from which women were excluded, (3) a period of reaction led by Samuel Gregory, (4) the emergence of special medical schools for women, (5) the appearance on the scene of women demanding to be educated as full physicians--Harriot Hunt, Emily and Elizabeth Blackwell, Marie Zakrzewska, Ann Preston, and Emmeline Cleveland, (6) the founding of hospitals where women could receive clinical training, and (7) the struggle for official recognition in the profession. The first colleges and hospitals where women could receive training are discussed. Contemporary statistics regarding women in medicine are cited. Many early women physicians from various parts of the country are treated in the light of their individual contributions.

228. Jacobson, Beverly and Jacobson, Wendy. "Only Eight Percent: A Look at Women in Medicine." Civil Rights Digest, 7:4 (Summer 1975) 20-27. illus.

There are many deterrents to women becoming physicians in the United States. One indication of that is the fact that women comprise only 8 per cent of the profession. Even as more women enter medicine, few achieve top hierarchical positions. Women were respected healers in the American colonies, but the medical schools founded after the first in 1765 were run "by university-trained, upper class white males, educated at the great medical centers of Germany, France, and Britain," and women were excluded. Later, few women could afford the expense and time it took the Blackwell sisters to become doctors and found hospitals. After Flexner's influential report on medical schools, many schools--which had admitted women--closed. The institutions with the best facilities and endowments tended to be exclusively male. Training for midwives was obstructed. Women have to be careful when entering medicine that they do get positions in the hierarchy and that their favorite specialties do not get designated as "female."

229. Kaufman, Martin. "John Stainback Wilson and Female Medical Education." Journal of the History of Medicine,

28:4 (October 1973) 395-399.   (Notes and Events.)
One of the few male physicians who advocated medical education of women, John Stainback Wilson wrote several arguments in support of his beliefs.   This footnoted article reviews and analyzes Wilson's arguments and places them in
historical context.

230.   Keefer, Dorothy Campbell.   "Women in the BUSM: a Brief
              History."   Boston University Medical Center Centerscope,
              (July/August 1971) 4.   port.   (Women in Medicine.)
       Created in 1848, the Boston Female Medical College was the
       first American medical school for women.   In 1851 the insti-
       tution was renamed New England Female Medical College.
       Boston University School of Medicine (BUSM), which absorbed
       the New England Female Medical College, graduated its
       first class in 1874 (two of the five graduates were women).
       In this brief history, the educational struggles of Elizabeth
       Blackwell are recalled.   It is noted that after Blackwell's
       graduation in 1849 a century passed before "all medical
       schools admitted women on an equal basis with men."

231.   Keegan, B.   "Women in Medicine."   Illinois Medical Journal,
              147:4 (April 1975) 382-383.
       [Article not examined by editors.]

232.   Love, Minnie C.   "History of the Women Practitioners of
              Colorado."   Colorado Medical Journal, 8:4 (1902) 147-
              150.
       [Article not examined by editors.]

233.   McKibbin-Harper, Mary.   "Indian Medicine Women."   Medical
              Woman's Journal, 35:10 (October 1928) 286-287.
       Dr. McKibbin-Harper tells of a few facts she learned about
       Indian medicine women from Derrick and Eunice Lehmer, In-
       dian lore researchers.

234.   McNutt, Sarah J.   "Response to the Toast 'Pioneers of Yes-
              terday in Medicine.': At the Banquet of the Women's
              State Medical Society, May 5, 1919."   Woman's Medical
              Journal, 29[19]: 9 (September 1919) 191-192.
       Dr. McNutt reviews the advances of six pioneer women phy-
       sicians.   "In 1872," adds Dr. McNutt, "a new star arose
       and burst upon the world in a great brilliance--Dr. Mary
       Putnam Jacobi."   The many "firsts" of Dr. Jacobi are enu-
       merated.

235.   Marshall, Clara.   "Fifty Years in Medicine."   Virginia Med-
              ical Semi-Monthly, (27 January 1899) 1-18.   (Reprint.)
              (Presentation, National American Woman's Suffrage Asso-
              ciation, 16 February 1898.)
       Dr. Marshall surveys the advances made by medical women
       since Elizabeth Blackwell's graduation a half century ago.
       She touches upon the admission of women to medical schools

and the founding of women's schools, as well as the admission of women to medical societies--particularly the American Medical Association. A summary of the American woman physician's present status examines the following: the contribution of women to medical literature; women's success in competitive examinations for hospital posts, medical school admissions, and before state examining boards; the results of women's work in hospitals and private practice; and women's professional recognition.

236. Mason-Hohl, Elizabeth. "Early California and Its Medical Women." Women in Medicine, 78 (October 1942) 14-16.
A sketchy history of California's medical heritage is traced up to the practice of Dr. Elizer Pfeifer Stone in Nevada City in 1957. From this point forward a catalogue is given of women physicians' names and the "firsts" many of them accomplished: Dr. Charlotte Blake Brown was instrumental in founding the Pacific Dispensary for Women and Children in San Francisco; Dr. Willella Howe Waffle was the first woman to practice in Los Angeles County; Dr. Rose Talbot Bullard, in 1903-1904, served as president of the Los Angeles County Medical Association; and Dr. C. Annette Buckel, having served the army in the 1860s, worked with the Blackwells as well as with Dr. Marie Zakrzewska in Boston and went ultimately to California where, upon her death, she left a legacy to be used for child psychology.

237. Mason-Hohl, Elizabeth. "History of Women in Medicine." Medical Woman's Journal, 52:10 (October 1945) 33-34.
This article outlines the format to be employed for future "History of Women in Medicine" articles appearing in the Journal.

238. "Medical Education of Women in Cincinnati." Journal of the American Medical Women's Association, 9:12 (December 1954) 401-403. illus.
Medical instruction for women in Cincinnati, Ohio became available in 1883 when the Cincinnati College of Medicine first admitted women students. In 1886 women were separated from the men when a separate department was created and named the Woman's Medical College of Cincinnati. In 1890 this department became a separate institution by obtaining a charter of its own. The Laura Memorial College was founded in 1885 by Alexander McDonald as a memorial to his daughter, Laura McDonald Stolls, who died in childbirth. Laura Memorial College absorbed the Woman's Medical College of Ohio. Alexander McDonald hoped that this College would help to train women physicians who would acquire "knowledge and skill to keep other women from early, and possibly preventable, death."

239. Morantz, Regina. "The Lady and Her Physician." In: Clio's Consciousness Raised: New Perspectives on the History

of Women. Edited by Lois W. Banner and Mary Hartman. Harper & Row Publishers, Inc., New York, New
York, 1974, 38-53.
In this paper, the author criticizes the supposition--most
commonly held by feminist historians--that 19th-century Amer
ican male physicians were hostile to female patients and that
they expressed their animosity by employing painful and ineffective medical practices. To explore how some Victorian
women viewed their roles, Morantz further discusses the
ideas of early women physicians. Quotes by Elizabeth Blackwell, Ann Preston, Marie Zakrzewska, Harriot Hunt, and
Mary Putnam-Jacobi show that they "were not out to vindicate
their oppressed sisters as much as to refine and purify Victorian society." The early women physicians' attitudes mir-
rored those of their male counterparts, Morantz points out.
"These professional women were not modern-day feminists,
charging the barricades of male privilege, but were very much
Victorian women, prisoners of their own time and culture."

240. More, V. "Dr. Elizabeth Bass Assembles Notable Collection." Mississippi Doctor, 21 (August 1943) 83-84.
This article discusses the Elizabeth Bass collection of material on women in medicine. [Article not examined by editors.]

241. Mosher, Eliza M. "The History of American Medical Women." Medical Woman's Journal, 29:10 (October 1922)
253-259. ports.
Dr. Mosher's own biographical sketch precedes her article on
Elizabeth Blackwell. This article is the first in a series of
histories of medical women which will be presented by the
Journal. The biography of Dr. Mosher begins with her commencement of medical studies in 1869 at the New England
Hospital for Women and Children, and follows the vicissitudes
of her career to 1922. Following this sketch, Dr. Mosher's
historical article covers the activity of Drs. Elizabeth and
Emily Blackwell, and Dr. Marie Zakrzewska.

242. Packard, Francis R. "Women in Medicine." In: History of
Medicine in the United States: Volume II. Paul B. Hoe-
ber Inc., New York, New York, 1932, 1222-1227.
This brief review of women's role in American medical his-
tory is found in the appendix of Packard's comprehensive text-
book. A biographical sketch of Drs. Elizabeth Stone [sic]
Blackwell and Emily Blackwell includes discussion of the
founding of the New York Infirmary for Women and Children.
Also described is the history of the founding of the Woman's
Medical College of Pennsylvania and the important role of
Dr. Clara Marshall. The New York Medical College and
Hospital for Women is shown to have been incorporated chiefly
through the efforts of Clemence Sophia Lozier.

243. Pioneer-Pacesetter-Innovator: The Story of The Medical College of Pennsylvania. The Newcomen Society of North

America, New York, New York, 1971, 27 pp. photos. , port.

This historical survey of the first medical college for women in the United States details the growth of the school from its modest beginnings in two rented rooms in 1850, to a modern $19-million facility. Many of the heroes of its success story are women, and the booklet reviews the progress of the school during the tenure of various deans: Ann Preston, Rachel Bodley, Clara Marshall, Martha Tracy, Marion Fay, and Glen Leymaster.

244. Pope, Emily F. ; Call, Emma L. ; and Pope, C. Augusta.
      The Practice of Medicine by Women in the United States.
      Boston, Massachusetts, 1881, 12 pp. (Presentation,
      American Social Science Association, Saratoga, 7 September 1881.)
      [Item not examined by editors.]

245. "Post Office Honors First Woman Doctor on 125th Anniversary of her Hobart M. D. Degree. " Association of Episcopal Colleges News, 12:2 (April 1974) 3. facsim.
      One hundred and twenty-five years to the day after Elizabeth Blackwell received her medical degree from Geneva College (on 23 January 1849), "inside the same four walls of the Presbyterian Church in Geneva where Elizabeth received her diploma in 1849, the United States Post Office, the City of Geneva, and Hobart [formerly Geneva] and William Smith Colleges joined in paying her tribute on the occasion of the issue of a special United States 18¢ postage stamp in her honor. " At this same celebration, Dr. Frances Keller Harding was presented with the Elizabeth Blackwell Award.

246. Reeve, J. C. "The Entrance of Women into Medicine. "
      Western Reserve Medical Journal, 3 (1894-1895) 345-362.
      [Article not examined by editors.]

247. [Reid, Ada Chree]. "Women Physicians and Nurses. " Journal of the American Medical Women's Association, 4:6
      (June 1949) 253. (Editorial.)
      The association between women physicians and nurses is traced from Elizabeth Blackwell's relationship with Florence Nightingale, through the Civil War, to Dr. Marie Zakrzewska's founding of the New England Hospital for Women and Children in Boston.

248. Selmon, Bertha L. "The Boston Story: [Part I]. " Medical Woman's Journal, 53:2 (February 1946) 47-49. (History of Women in Medicine.)
      This history of women in medicine in Boston opens with a discussion of women midwives and nurses. Social climate, e.g. , Victorian prudery, which made it difficult for women to formally enter medical courses, is touched upon. Following a mention of the founding of the New England Female Medical College is a description of Harriot Kezia Hunt's youth.

249.   Selmon, Bertha L.   "The Boston Story (Continued). "   Med-
       ical Woman's Journal, 53:3 (March 1946) 40-42.   (His-
       tory of Women in Medicine.)
       This history of Boston medical women reproduces corres-
       pondence between Harriot K. Hunt and O. W. Holmes, dean
       of the medical faculty of Harvard University.   Asking for
       permission to attend medical lectures at Harvard, Hunt
       stresses the need for qualified women physicians to attend
       those of her sex.   She describes her intense desire for for-
       mal medical knowledge and writes, "Your refusal in the city
       of my birth, education, and life, seemed unjust to me.... "
       Although the faculty agreed to permit Hunt, and male Negroes
       to attend lectures in the fall of 1850, the [white] male stu-
       dents revolted against it.   Their letter to the faculty deplores
       the thought of Hunt appearing in the medical lecture room
       "where her presence is calculated to destroy our respect for
       the modesty and delicacy of her sex. "   Hunt withdrew her
       application.   In 1853 the Medical College of Philadelphia con-
       ferred upon her an honorary medical degree.   Following the
       biography of Harriot Hunt is a profile of Marie Zakrzewska
       and a mention of the women who staffed the newly organized
       New England Hospital for Women and Children.

250.   Selmon, Bertha [L].   "Early Development of Medical Oppor-
       tunity for Women in the United States. "   Medical Wo-
       man's Journal, 54:1 (January 1947) 25-28, 60.   (History
       of Women in Medicine.)
       A continuation of this series from earlier volumes of the
       Journal, this article reviews the women's medical colleges
       which were dealt with in previous installments.   A discus-
       sion of coeducational institutions which admitted women, fol-
       lows.   Lucinda Susannah (Capen) Hall, an 1852 graduate of
       the Worcester [Massachusetts] Medical Institution, is pro-
       filed, using excerpts from an article by Frederick C. Waite.
       This is followed by Chadwick's view of 19th-century medi-
       cine and women's place therein.

251.   Selmon, Bertha L.   "Early History of Women in Medicine. "
       Medical Woman's Journal, 52:3 (March 1945) 38-42.
       (History of Women in Medicine.)
       Dr. Selmon covers briefly the professional career of Emily
       Blackwell and Marie Zakrzewska and presents excerpts from
       Rachel Baker's accounts of the New York Infirmary for Wo-
       men and Children.

252.   Selmon, Bertha L.   "History of Women in Medicine. "   Med-
       ical Woman's Journal, 52:1 (January 1945) 39-40, 52.
       This first in a series of articles on the history of medical
       women begins by discussing "The Sunrise of Women in Medi-
       cine" (1840-1870), when women, as well as medicine itself,
       were beginning to " 'crack the shell of tradition. ' "   Dr. Sel-
       mon quotes from Kate Hurd-Mead's Medical Women of Amer-
       ica and discusses midwifery as the antecedent to women as
       physicians.

253. Shryock, Richard Harrison. "Women in American Medicine."
Journal of the American Medical Women's Association,
5:9 (September 1950) 371-379. (Lecture, College of Physicians, Philadelphia, April 14, 1950.)
This lecture, delivered upon the occasion of the centenary of
the Woman's Medical College of Pennsylvania, analyzes trends
and issues surrounding women in American medicine in the
preceding 100 years. Dr. Shryock discusses factors which
originally favored women in medicine, those factors which opposed them, major trends, and the outcome of these trends.

254. Sloop, Mary Martin. "An Outline of Work among Mountain
Whites of North Carolina." Bulletin of the Woman's
Medical College of Pennsylvania, 65:5 (March 1915) 38-
39.

255. Waite, Frederick C. "Early Medical Service of Women."
Journal of the American Medical Women's Association,
3:5 (May 1948) 199-203. ports.
This article gives a brief description of the medical education
of women in the U.S., particularly in the Western Reserve
(that area of land that is now northeastern Ohio).

256. Waite, Frederick C. "The Medical Education of Women in
Cleveland (1850-1930)." Western Reserve University
Bulletin, No. 16 (15 September 1930) 1-29. tables.
A history is given of the women who attended and graduated
from the medical colleges of Cleveland, Ohio which include
among others: Cleveland Medical College [later Case Western Reserve University] and the homeopathic schools of Cleveland. For all their pioneering efforts in accepting women,
two per cent women graduated from Cleveland medical schools
from 1843 to 1930 while women graduates from homeopathic
schools reached 12.5 per cent.

257. Waite, Lucy. "Women in the Medical Profession." Medical
Herald, 16 (December 1897) 449-452.
[Article not examined by editors.]

258. Welsh, Lilian. "The Significance of Medicine as a Profession for Women." Bulletin of the Woman's Medical College of Pennsylvania, 74:1 (January 1924) 3-9. (Address,
Seventy-fourth Annual Session, Woman's Medical College
of Pennsylvania, 26 September 1923.)
The history of the Woman's Medical College of Pennsylvania
is followed by a discussion of the motivation of women to
study medicine, a motivation manifested in the desire "to advance the well-being of women and children." The history of
medical education for women in the United States is set in
the social and political context of the time. The article concludes with a discussion of the medical opportunities available for women.

259.   Wilder, Dora Lee.   "Woman in the Field of Medicine."   Jour
         nal of the Tennessee State Medical Association, 2 (1909-
         1910) 323-325.
         A woman physician today "stands on an equal plane with her
         brother physician," and this happy circumstance is due to the
         efforts of pioneer women in medicine--women like Elizabeth
         Blackwell, Elizabeth Garrett, and Hannah Longshore.   Be-
         cause of prejudice, it was necessary to form women's med-
         ical colleges, such as those in Pennsylvania and New York,
         e.g., when a 19th-century University of Michigan professor
         was asked whether women were to be admitted to the medical
         school he answered, "No, thank God; they can only enter
         there in the pickling vat."   Now women physicians are found
         everywhere, and there are more than 10,000 practicing in the
         United States.   The article is a brief summary of the history
         of women in medicine.

BIOGRAPHIES

Specific physicians of the 19th and 20th centuries
are the subjects of this section. Comprehensive
life histories are included, as well as articles which
list educational and career data, and material which
consists of biographical segments about travel and
other experiences. (Material focusing only on one
aspect of a physician's life, i.e., missionary activity or war work, can be found in the classification
which relates to that activity.) Fictionalized accounts of the lives of historical figures are also included in this section.

260. Adamson, Rhoda H. B. "Elsie M. Chubb: M.D. Lond.,
B.A. South Africa, D.P.H. 28 September, 1958." Journal of the Medical Women's Federation, 41:1 (January
1959) 52-53. (Obituary.)
Dr. Chubb studied at the London School of Medicine for Women and, in 1920, obtained a post in Cape Province, South
Africa organizing the school inspection service of "about
56,000 scholars."

261. Back, Marjorie. "Elizabeth Dill Russell, B.Sc., M.R.C.S.,
L.R.C.P." Medical Women's Federation News-Letter,
(March 1928) 71. (Obituary.)

262. Emanuel, Vera and Martin, Peter. "Mis' Lady Doctor."
Saturday Evening Post, (15 June 1946) 12 passim, photos.
port.
As a wife and mother living in a Johannesburg suburb, "with
servants cheap and plentiful, time hung heavy on my hands,"
writes Vera Emanuel, recalling her motivation to obtain a
medical degree. She set up office in Newclare, a section of
Johannesburg, and became "Mis' Lady Doctor" to "the dis-
eased, superstition-ridden blacks, half-whites and Orientals
of what must be one of the ugliest and most primitive slums
in the world." Dr. Emanuel details many of her interesting
adventures and medical cases. Although she personally encountered only one instance of white resentment of her racial-
ly-mixed practice, Dr. Emanuel writes that the question of
adequate medical care for South Africa's black population
"can't be answered by nervous coughs and by changing the
subject."

263. Klenerman, Pauline. "Impressions of a Recent Trip to the
United States of America." Medical Woman's Journal,
56:12 (December 1949) 32-35.
Dr. Klenerman, a pediatrician in Durban, South Africa, reminisces about the medical schools and hospitals she visited in
the United States.

264. van Heerden, Petronella. [The 16th Hill]. Tafelberg, Cape
Town, South Africa, 1965. port. (Afr)
"Petronella van Heerden was born on a farm in the Boer Republic of the Orange Free State. After the Anglo-Boer War,
Emily Hobhouse, who worked among the women in the concentration camps, gave Petronella a copy of John Stuart Mill's
book, The Subjugation of Women, which interested her and
led her to seek a university education. The Consul for the
Netherlands in the Free State informed her about a bursary

for Boer students to study in Holland. With this bursary and
an allowance given to her by her father, she set off for Holland to study medicine. The book tells of her adventures and
struggles in Holland, and of her return to South Africa, where
she practiced medicine in the Orange Free State for many
years. " [English summary provided to the editors by Dr.
Isabel Robertson, Medical Women's International Association
vice president for Africa.]

ASIA

265. Dall, Caroline Healey. The Life of Dr. Anandabai [sic] Joshee,
        a Kinswoman of the Pundita Ramabai. Roberts Brothers,
        Boston, Massachusetts, 1888, 187 pp. port.
      Born in Poona, India in 1865, Anandibai Joshee married at
      the age of nine. "The first unconverted high-caste Hindu wo-
      man to leave her country," she graduated from the Woman's
      Medical College of Pennsylvania in 1886 and became the first
      Hindu woman to receive an M.D. in any country. That same
      year, she was appointed physician-in-charge of the female
      wards of the Albert Edward Hospital, Kolhapur, India. Af-
      flicted with tuberculosis, Dr. Joshee died in 1887, at the age
      of 22. Letters written by Dr. Joshee form a major portion
      of this biography.

266. "Dr. Afable of Manila Admitted to A.C.S. " Medical Woman's
        Journal, 54:5 (May 1947) 46. (News Notes.)
      A biography is given of Dr. Trinidad Afable, a Philippine
      Islands physician who was, in 1947, admitted to the American
      College of Surgeons.

267. "Dr. Anandibai Joshee. " Medical Missionary Record, 1:12
        (April 1887) 291.
      This brief article quotes from a Poona, India newspaper,
      which announces the return home of Anandibai Joshee, fol-
      lowing her graduation from the Woman's Medical College in
      Philadelphia.

268. "Dr. Honoria Acosta-Sison: A Philippines Medical Pioneer. "
        World Medical Journal, 11:1 (January 1964) 36.
      The first native woman physician in the Philippines (1910),
      Honoria Acosta-Sison has also made several contributions in
      her specialty, obstetrics and gynecology.

269. "Dr. Rukhmabai: A Pioneer Medical Woman of India. "
        World Medical Journal, 11:1 (January 1964) 35-36. port.
        (International Figures ... in 20th Century Medicine.)
      Following a review of the first indigenous Indian women who
      received formal medical degrees and returned to India to
      practice, Dr. Rukhmabai's medical service to women and
      children which began in Bombay in 1895, is described.

270.   Fahimi, Miriam. "Homa Shaibany, M.B.B.S., First Woman
          Surgeon of Iran." Journal of the American Medical Wo-
          men's Association, 7:7 (July 1952) 272-273. port. (Al-
          bum of Women in Medicine.)
       The first and, at the time of this article, the only Persian
       woman surgeon, Dr. Shaibany was also the first woman phy-
       sician to go to England for medical study (which she did on
       a government scholarship). She was brilliant in anatomy,
       morphology, embryology, and neurology and took a degree in
       human anatomy and morphology. After World War II, she re-
       turned to her homeland to meet with "great opposition" from
       the male gynecologists and surgeons. Ultimately she was
       asked by Princess Shamse to equip, organize, and administer
       a hospital for the Red Cross. This hospital was set up in
       Teheran.

271.   "First Chinese Woman Physician in Hong Kong." Journal of
          the American Medical Association, 78:8 (1922) 591.
          (Medical News--Foreign.)
       This very brief news item identifies Dr. Hoashoo, a graduate
       of Edinburgh University, as the first Chinese woman to set up
       practice in Hong Kong.

272.   "First Indian Woman Physician." Missionary Review of the
          World, 55 (July 1932) 447.
       [Article not examined by editors.]

273.   Fischer, Golda. "Medical Women in Israel: Some Interest-
          ing Personalities." Journal of the American Medical Wo-
          men's Association, 7:5 (May 1952) 181-183. ports.
       Part II in a series of three articles presents brief biograph-
       ical sketches of some of the first women physicians in what
       is now the State of Israel. The outstanding accomplishments
       of each are mentioned. [Part I in this series deals with his-
       torical perspectives, and Part III with professional activity.]

274.   Flemming, Roberta M. "Pierra Hoon Vejjabul, M.D.: First
          Woman Doctor of Thailand." Journal of the American
          Medical Women's Association, 6:7 (July 1951) 279. port.
          (Medical Women Around the World.)
       Defying tradition and convention, overcoming family disapprov-
       al and poverty, Dr. Pierra Hoon Vejjabul graduated from the
       Faculty of Medicine of the University of Paris in 1932, re-
       turning to Thailand in 1937 to become her country's first wo-
       man doctor. Associated with Thailand's Ministry of Public
       Health, "Dr. Pierra" found herself in the unique position dur-
       ing the war of owning two houses of prostitution in her ef-
       forts to control venereal disease and "educate and elevate"
       the prostitutes. She founded her own maternity and child wel-
       fare hospital, has adopted 35 children (all girls but one), and
       began publishing the first magazine for women and children in
       Thailand. The name "Vejjabul" means great woman doctor
       and was bestowed upon her by the premier of Thailand.

275. J. B. G. "Daphne Chun Wai Chan, O. B. E. , Hon. D. Soc. Sc. ,
        M. B. , B. S. , (Hong Kong), F. R. C. S. (Edinburgh),
        F. R. C. O. G. , J. P. " University of Hong Kong Gazette,
        19:6 (1 August 1972) 78-81.
      Dr. Chun's retirement as professor of obstetrics and gyne-
      cology at the University of Hong Kong prompted this biogra-
      phy.

276. King, Gordon. "An Episode in the History of the University
        of Hong Kong: The First Daphne W. C. Chun Lecture. "
        University of Hong Kong Supplement to the Gazette, 20:
        6 (1 August 1973) 1-9. table.
      The experiences of Hong Kong medical students during the
      war include mention of the women who obtained M. D. s between
      1942 and 1950. Professor King, who himself escaped from
      war-torn Hong Kong by a route planned by Dr. Daphne Chun,
      credits the safety of the Hong Kong medical students to her
      efforts.

277. Kobayashi, Aya. [A Woman Doctor among the Outcasts].
        Iwanami Publishers, Tokyo, Japan, 1962, iv, 206 pp.
        figs. , illus. , tables. (Jap)
      Aya Kobayashi begins the book with her childhood remem-
      brances, especially during grammar school when she learned
      about the special group of people in Japan called "eta, " who
      were ostracized and treated as outcasts. The "eta" people
      suffered discrimination in every area of society. In July
      1950, Dr. Kobayashi passed her national medical examinations
      and the following March went to work as a physician at Yo-
      shida Clinic which treated the "eta" people. Writing about
      her experiences with the "eta, " she hopes others will be more
      understanding of the plight of these people.

278. "Ma Chung Ho Kei, M. B. , B. S. (Hong Kong), F. R. C. O. G. "
        University of Hong Kong Gazette, 19:6 (1 August 1972)
        78.
      This biography of Dr. Ma was prompted by her appointment
      as professor of obstetrics and gynecology at the University
      of Hong Kong.

279. Memant (Mlle). ["Dr. Anandibai Joshee"]. Revue Encyclo-
        pédique, (1896) 488-489. port. (Fre)
      Yamuna Joshee was born in Poona in March 1865, daughter
      of a rich Brahmin landed proprietor. She was very preco-
      cious, and at the age of five demanded a tutor to study San-
      skrit. In March 1874 she married Gopal Vinyak, a widower
      20 years older than she, and took the given name of Anandi-
      bai. After the death of a newborn son in 1878, she deter-
      mined to devote herself to the alleviation of suffering among
      Indian women, who were never treated by male doctors ex-
      cept in extreme cases. Her husband approved, but she met
      great opposition from others to her desire to attend medical
      school. She finally entered the Woman's Medical College of

Pennsylvania in 1883, and although plagued by ill health, received her doctor of medicine degree at a large reception in
her honor in 1886. She was the first high-caste Hindu woman to receive this degree anywhere in the world. Her heal
was not improved by a stay in Colorado and became worse o
the long voyage home. She returned to her family home,
where she died in February 1887. Her ashes were buried in
America.

280.   Nagatoya, Yoji. "Dr. Keiko Okami: Japan's First Female
        Medical Student Who Studied Abroad." Journal of the
        American Medical Women's Association, 15:12 (December
        1960) 1175-1177. photo.
        Keiko Okami studied medicine at the Woman's Medical Colleg
        of Pennsylvania because, until the end of World War II, "it
        was practically impossible for women in Japan to receive a
        medical education" in their own country. Dr. Okami's "life
        story" is presented in abbreviated form, followed by a dis-
        cussion of medical women in Japan.

281.   Porter, Sarah K. "A Japanese Woman Physician in Court."
        Medical Missionary Record, 9:10 (October 1894) 218.
        When Dr. Hishakawa began treatment of a typhoid fever pa-
        tient, she promptly reported the case to the health bureau,
        but her report received no recognition. Later, for failure
        to report the patient, she was taken to court. Her lawyer
        informed the court that because Dr. Hishakawa was a Chris-
        tian, she "cannot be induced to tell a falsehood." She was
        acquitted.

282.   "Professor Daphne Chun Wai-Chan." University of Hong
        Kong Gazette, 19:4 (9 March 1972) 53-54.
        Dr. Chun's many "firsts" as a physician, as a woman, and
        as a Chinese are included in this tribute to her.

283.   "Professor Daphne Wai-Chan Chun, M.B., B.S. (H.K.),
        F.R.C.S. Ed., F.R.C.O.G." University of Hong Kong
        Gazette, 4:5 (25 June 1957) 37.
        Dr. Chun is the first woman professor to be appointed since
        the University of Hong Kong's foundation in 1911.

284.   "Rosie Young Tse-Tse, M.D. (Hong Kong), F.R.C.P., J.P."
        University of Hong Kong Gazette, 21:6 (1 September 1974)
        102-103.

285.   Wilson, Dorothy Clarke. Take My Hands: The Remarkable
        Story of Dr. Mary Verghese. McGraw-Hill Book Com-
        pany, Inc., New York, New York, 1963, 216 pp.
        Mary Verghese graduated from the Christian Medical College
        at Vellore, India, where--influenced by the ideals of its
        founder, Dr. Ida Scudder--she became a surgeon. Shortly
        after graduation, an accident made Dr. Verghese a paraplegic.
        This biography focuses on how she overcame her physical

handicap, learning to perform delicate operations while seated
in her wheelchair, and how she became a rehabilitation specialist. Emphasized is the role played by her Christian faith
in reconstructing her life. "Without the accident," Dr. Verghese is quoted as saying, "I might have been only an ordinary doctor."

286.   Yoshioka, Yayoi. [The Story of Medical Education for Wo-
          men in Japan]. [n. p.], 1926. photos., port. (Jap)
Among other information, photos of the funeral and memorial
services for Dr. Yayoi Yoshioka constitute a substantial portion of this book. Dignitaries, faculty, and staff of the hospital came to pay tribute and respect to Dr. Yoshioka. From
the services at the hospital to the Aoyama Cemetery, where
she was buried, family, relatives and friends sang her school
song, burned incense in her memory, and spoke of her life
and service in medicine. Dr. Yoshioka's biography is attached. She was the recipient of a number of awards and
honors from the Emperor of Japan. Some of the certificates
are photographed. Pictured also is the scroll from which her
eulogy was read at the funeral.

AUSTRALIA & NEW ZEALAND

287.   "Annie Jean MacNamara." Medical Journal of Australia, 2:
          10 (5 September 1970) 472-476. (Obituary.)
This obituary consists of accounts of and tributes to the life
of Dr. MacNamara from several persons who knew her.

288.   Baker-McLaglan, Eleanor Southey. Stethoscope and Saddle-
          bags. [New Zealand ?], 1962.
[Book not examined by editors.]

289.   Barrie, Susan. "Mary Puckey, M.D." Medical Woman's
          Journal, 56:8 (August 1949) 38-39, 42. port.
Dr. Puckey is chief executive officer and medical superintendent of the Rachel Forster Hospital in Sydney, Australia.
The hospital, founded by Drs. Lucy Gullett and Harriet Biffin, caters to women and children and is staffed by women
physicians.

290.   Cohen, Lysbeth. Dr. Margaret Harper: Her Achievements
          and Place in the History of Australia. Wentworth Books,
          Sydney, New South Wales, 1971. 47 pp. port.
Intimate biographical detail relates Dr. Harper's family background and her professional experiences. Early years of
practice found Dr. Harper continually beset by the debarment
of, or at best "dim view" of, women as hospital residents
and interns. In 1922 Dr. Harper and four other medical women founded the Rachel Forster Hospital in Sydney--staffed
by women for the treatment of women and children. Dr.
Harper's hospital assignments over the years and her burgeon-

ing interest in the health of the newborn and the education of mothers regarding child care are traced from her 1907 appointment as resident to the Royal Hospital for Women in Paddington, through her tenure at the Royal Alexandra Hospital for Children at Camperdown. Her lifelong concern for "Mothercraft" evolved over these years and she consulted, lectured, and wrote prolifically on the subject. In 1930 Dr. Harper was the first person to describe the difference between coeliac disease and cystic fibrosis of the pancreas.

291. De Garis, Mary C. Clinical Notes and Deductions of a Peripatetic: Being Fads and Fancies of a General Practitioner. Ballière, Tindall and Cox, London, England, 1926, xvi, 176 pp. chart.
In her introduction, Dr. De Garis states that her book resulted from "a clinical stocktaking of [her] twenty years of a wandering practice in Victoria, Queensland, New South Wales, England, and Macedonia." From a general practitioner's point of view and from "the woman's angle," Dr. De Garis presents her "pet obsessions" and experiences with obstetric subjects and various diseases. Case reports illustrate the material. "Practical Notes and Sundry Reflections" offer suggestions to the young physician in rural practice. A final chapter describes her experience with the Scottish Women's Hospitals in Macedonia. An index is included.

292. "Dr. Harriet Clisby." Medical Woman's Journal, 37:11 (November 1930) 320.
At the time this article was written, Harriet Clisby, a native of Australia who had acquired her medical training in England and who had practiced in America, had just turned 100 years old. Before she heard that it was possible for women to become doctors, she and a friend had founded Australia's first magazine, The Interpretator, and later edited another, The Southern Phonographic Magazine. Giving up her regular practice in the 1880s, Dr. Clisby went to Geneva where she founded a woman's organization, the "Union des Femmes."

293. "Eleanor Southey Baker-McLaglan." New Zealand Medical Journal, 70 (October 1969) 272. (Obituary.)
Dr. McLaglan (1879-1969), who became in 1903 the sixth woman in New Zealand to qualify in medicine, wrote a book about her career, titled Stethoscope and Saddlebags (1962).

294. "Flying Angels of Australia." Journal of the American Medical Women's Association, 10:8 (August 1955) 286.
A half-page article on Drs. Freda Gibson and Merna Mueller's flying emergency medical service in South Australia. Each year the two doctors average more than 100 trips treating 1,250 patients and spending up to 300 hours actual flying time. At the time this article was written, these two women were the only women doctors in Australia (and perhaps the world) to operate a flying doctor service together.

295. Gordon, Doris. Backblocks Baby-Doctor; an Autobiography.
      Faber & Faber Limited, London, England, 1955, 254 pp.
      port.
      One of the first two women students to earn their degrees at
      Otago University Medical School, Doris Gordon received train-
      ing as a house surgeon and practiced as a public health offi-
      cer and as an obstetrician. Dr. Gordon and her husband
      eventually bought a private practice in Stratford, New Zealand,
      where the Drs. Gordon introduced pure chloroform inhalation
      to help relieve the pain of childbirth. This auboiograph-
      ical account gives the flavor of both life and medical practice
      in New Zealand.

296. Gordon, Doris. Doctor Down Under. Faber and Faber, Lon-
      don, England, 1958, 190 pp.
      This autobiography covers the practice of Doris Gordon in
      New Zealand from World War I until her retirement in the
      1950s. Her experiences document the progress of medical
      practice in that country during that period. Although Dr.
      Gordon was a surgeon, obstetrics dominate the case histories
      given in this book. While she apparently worked among the
      Maoris, this experience is covered in an earlier book, Back-
      blocks Baby-Doctor. Dr. Gordon, with her physician husband,
      established the Marire Hospital in Stratford, New Zealand.
      There are no illustrations, indexes, or references in this
      personal narrative.

297. Hercus, Sir Charles and Bell, Sir Gordon. "Women of the
      Otago Medical School." In: The Otago Medical School
      Under the First Three Deans. E. & S. Livingstone Ltd.,
      Edinburgh, Scotland, 159-165. ports.
      Brief biographies of women who attended Otago Medical School
      in Dunedin, New Zealand are included in this article. There
      are portraits of Emily Siedeberg, the first woman student
      there and later an obstetrician; Margaret Cruickshank, a high-
      ly respected country practitioner of medicine; and Muriel
      Bell, lecturer in the department of physiology.

298. Horan, Margaret B. "A Goodly Heritage: An Appreciation
      of the Life and Work of the Late Dr. Helen Mayo."
      Medical Journal of Australia, 1:8 (20 February 1971)
      419-424. photo., ports. (Original Articles.) (The
      Fifth Helen Mayo Lecture of the Mothers and Babies'
      Health Association of South Australia, Adelaide, Austra-
      lia, 2 October 1970.)
      One of the founders of the Mothers and Babies' Health Asso-
      ciation, Helen Mayo was active throughout her professional
      life in maternal and child welfare. She helped establish the
      School for Mothers to help women complement their maternal
      instinct with concern for the total physical, mental, and
      moral welfare of their children.

299. The Lilian Helen Alexander Memorial in the University of

Melbourne. Ford Press, Carlton, Australia, [n.d.],
11 pp.

Events leading up to the admission of women medical student
at the University of Melbourne, and activities of several Aus
tralian women physicians are incorporated into this biography
of Dr. Alexander. The University's memorial to her is a
bas-relief in marble.

300. Little, Marjory. "Some Pioneer Medical Women of the Uni-
versity of Sydney." Medical Journal of Australia, 2:11
(13 September 1958) 341-350. facsim., photo., ports.
(Post-Graduate Oration, Post-Graduate Committee in
Medicine, University of Sydney, Sydney, Australia, 14
May 1958.)

The medical school of the University of Sydney "never made
any difference" between men and women students. Upon grad
uation, however, medical women faced severe difficulty in ob
taining practical experience in hospitals. The story of medical women in Australia began in 1865, when an American
physician--Wilhelmina Ferguson--applied for medical board
registration in Victoria (her qualifications were rejected). In
1885, Dagmar Berne entered the University of Sydney's medical school. Not until 1895, however, did the first women--
Isa F. Coghlan and Grace T. Robinson--graduate in medicine
(Dr. Berne completed her studies in England). This article
goes on to give biographies of several notable Australian women physicians, and also presents histories of hospitals and
other organizations they founded.

301. Manson, Cecil and Manson, Celia. Doctor Agnes Bennett.
Michael Joseph Ltd., London, England, 1960, xv, 189 pp.
photos., port.

This biography of Dr. Bennett was compiled from her own
reminiscences, diaries, letters, and news clippings. The
book begins with background information on Dr. Bennett's
family and her decision to study medicine at the Medical College for Women in Edinburgh, Scotland, where she experienced the feelings of frustration and "exasperation over the
handicaps which the women students suffered at that time."
Her professional activities in Wellington, New Zealand and at
St. Helen's Hospital are recounted. Dr. Bennett served in
World War I, after which she returned to Wellington, where
she took up the cause of antenatal care. At the age of 66
she joined a nurse-friend and began a "flying doctor" service
to provide care to people in the northern territories of Australia. When World War II broke, Dr. Bennett, now 68,
helped form the Women's War Service Auxiliary and then
served aboard the ship Port Alma as surgeon. An epilogue
by Dr. Agnes Bennett concludes the work. The book is indexed.

302. "Margaret Harkness McLorinan." Medical Journal of Australia, (19 November 1932) 642-643. port. (Obituary.)

303.   "Marjory Little." Medical Journal of Australia, 2 (31 Au-
        gust 1974) 338-339. port. (Obituary.)
        Details of Dr. Little's life and career are given by Dr. Ethel
        Durie. Dr. Little served with the British Expeditionary
        Forces in France during World War I. Returning to her
        homeland of Australia after the war, Dr. Little set up a pri-
        vate pathology practice in Sydney and worked with Professor
        Welch at the University of Sydney. In 1958 she delivered the
        Annual Postgraduate Oration in the Great Hall of the Univer-
        sity of Sydney, and was the only woman ever invited to de-
        liver the Oration.

304.   Preston, Frances I. Lady Doctor: Vintage Model. A. H.
        & A. W. Reed, Wellington, New Zealand, 1974, 159 pp.
        photos.
        Frances Preston, M.B., Ch.B., was one of New Zealand's
        earliest women doctors, having graduated from the Otago Med-
        ical School, Dunedin, in 1922. Her autobiography was written
        "to cast ... light on the circumstances and difficulties of
        medical practice for a woman in the 1920s." Her medical
        service included locum, hospital, and sanatorium work in
        Dunedin (with Dr. Muriel Bell), New Plymouth, Rotorua, and
        the Hokianga. She fought not only disease, but prejudice
        against women in medicine, and her memoirs abound with
        anecdotes about the practice of rural, sometimes primitive,
        medicine. A threatened miscarriage once brought Dr. Pres-
        ton to a remote area, four hours journey from Rawene,
        Hokianga. A heavy rain made the return trip impossible un-
        til the next day so Dr. Preston found herself holed up in a
        tiny room off the kitchen. In the morning her host presented
        her with uncooked eggs and bacon saying only, "Breakfast."
        It seems that "being the only able-bodied woman about, I
        was expected to do the cooking." Eventually, Dr. Preston
        left medicine and "plunged with enthusiasm into learning to
        be ... an efficient farm-wife: a career no less demanding
        and exhausting than the one I had abandoned." Thus began
        her long-lived involvement with the Women's Division of Fed-
        erated Farmers Movement, a rural community service dedi-
        cated to improving "the lot of women living lonely lives on
        remote farms." The last chapter contains brief biographical
        notes about more than two dozen of the earliest medical wo-
        men in New Zealand, including both speculation and statistics
        on impediments to continuing practice for women physicians.
        Appendix I lists these women chronologically by year of grad-
        uation from medical school, and Appendix II offers names of
        drugs used in the Pleasant Valley Sanatorium in 1925. An
        index is included. The book is illustrated with personal pho-
        tographs.

305.   Skirving, R. Scot. "Dagmar Berne: The First Woman Stu-
        dent in the Medical School of the University of Sydney."
        Medical Journal of Australia, (14 October 1944) 407-409.
        photos., port.

Georgina Dagmar Berne (1866-1900) studied medicine in Sydney but completed her courses in London (the author of this article does not know at which school). In 1895, she "put up her plate" in Sydney. A tuberculous condition cut short her promising medical career.

306.   Stewart, Marian. "New Zealand's First Woman Doctor: Emily H. Siedeberg McKinnon, M. D. " Journal of the American Medical Women's Association, 4:10 (October 1949) 440. port.
Emily Hancock Siedeberg McKinnon received her degree in 1896. She was a founding member of the Dunedin branch of the Society for the Protection of Women and Children in 1899. From 1905 to 1938, she was medical superintendent of St. Helen's Maternity Hospital, Dunedin, a training school for midwives and the first hospital in New Zealand to institute an antenatal clinic. Dr. McKinnon was made a Commander of the British Empire in 1949.

CANADA

307.   Abbott, Maude E. S. "Autobiographical Sketch (1928). " McGill Medical Journal, 28 (1959) 127-152.
[Article not examined by editors.]

308.   "Augusta Atowe Gullen, M. D. " In: 100 Years of Medicine: 1849-1949. Modern Press Limited, Saskatoon, Saskatchewan, 1949, 25.
Augusta Stowe Gullen was the first woman to study and graduate in medicine in Canada, having received her degree from Victoria University in 1883. Brief notes on her life as doctor and suffragist are offered.

309.   Beattie, Lillian M. "Maude Abbott: Canadian Pathologist. " University of Western Ontario Medical Journal, 24:3 (May 1954) 89-98.
This anecdotal history of Maude Abbott's life begins with her early years and medical education. Dr. Abbott's work with congenital heart disease is also discussed.

310.   Beregoff-Gillow, Pauline. A Doctor Dares to Tell: The Inside Story of Medicine. Comet Press Books, New York, New York, 1959, xv, 207 pp.
Aware that the writing of her book might be construed a "severely unethical act, " Dr. Beregoff-Gillow presents an exposé of the "closed hospital" system and its "self-seeking practices. " ("A 'closed hospital' is one which makes its facilities available only to members of the medical staff of that hospital, and they alone may admit and treat the patients while they are in that institution. ") The author discusses her situation as a woman physician and gives a detailed view of the closed hospital, its practices, and the personal experi-

ences she has had with this system of health care. In conclusion, Dr. Beregoff-Gillow offers her recommendations on
what can be done to correct the system.

311.   Bett, W. R. "Cardiac Pioneers. Maude Abbott (1869-1940)."
        Chest and Heart Bulletin, 22 (1959) 37.
        [Article not examined by editors.]

312.   Buck, Ruth Matheson. The Doctor Rode Side-Saddle. Mc-
        Clelland and Stewart Limited, Toronto, Canada, 1974,
        175 pp. photos., ports.
        Elizabeth Matheson's story as a frontier doctor in the terri-
        tory of Saskatchewan, Canada, from 1898 to 1918 is told
        by her daughter (one of nine children). Dr. Matheson at-
        tended the Women's Medical College, in affiliation with
        Queen's University, but abandoned her medical studies tem-
        porarily when she married. Indeed, much of the book is
        about her husband, John Matheson. "Of all the activity that
        filled Elizabeth's days, it was the work that she shared with
        her husband [missionary to the Cree Indians] that meant most
        to her." Together they worked to build up St. Barnabas
        Anglican Mission at Onion Lake, where Elizabeth taught the
        Indian children. One incident illustrates the isolation and
        primitive conditions which are part of the picture of pioneer
        life on the prairies which the book portrays: when Elizabeth
        was pregnant with her second child, she developed a severe
        mastitis. It became necessary to make an arduous three-day
        trip to Battleford to see a doctor. Upon arriving, she found
        that both the town's doctors were at a banquet at the Queen's
        Hotel, where there wasn't a man sober. The doctor who
        finally came in haggard the next morning was the police sur-
        geon. He muttered, "Badly swollen," pulled out a scalpel,
        and stabbed the "throbbingly painful breast. Blood and pus
        spurted the length of the small room. Elizabeth fainted."
        Eventually, John Matheson "resolved to send her away to re-
        sume her studies," because a doctor was needed at his mis-
        sion. She studied at Ontario Medical College and practiced
        for five years without being registered, having several chil-
        dren during that time. Finally, she graduated from Manitoba
        Medical College and secured her registration. "She was cer-
        tain that her registration came because of John Matheson's
        signature on the cheque." She established her practice and,
        traveling frequently to see patients, "the doctor and her beautiful
        pacing mare became known throughout the country." Although
        a postscript tells us that Elizabeth lived to be 92 in 1958, the
        narrative essentially ends with John Matheson's death.
        Many personal photographs illustrate the text. A bibliography
        is included.

313.   Buck, Ruth Matheson. "The Mathesons of Saskatchewan Dio-
        cese." Saskatchewan History, 4 (1960) 41-62. photos.,
        ports., table.
        Four Mathesons distinguished themselves in missionary en-

deavors in the Anglican diocese of Saskatchewan beginning in
1877. Elizabeth Beckett, who had interrupted her medical
studies to marry John Matheson, agreed to resume her studie
because it became evident that a doctor was needed at her
husband's mission. In 1898 she graduated from the Women's
Medical College in Toronto and began her practice at Onion
Lake. After John's death she was appointed assistant medical inspector in the Winnipeg public schools.

314.   "Charlotte Whitehead Ross, M.D." In: 100 Years of Medi-
            cine: 1849-1949. Modern Press Limited, Saskatoon,
            Saskatchewan, 1949, 32. photo.
        Dr. Ross was the first woman physician to practice in Mon-
        treal (after graduating from the Woman's Medical College in
        Philadelphia in 1875), but the bulk of her career was spent
        in Whitemouth, Manitoba, where she treated many accident
        cases in the lumber camps. Other biographical details are
        presented in this brief article.

315.   Chase, Lillian A. "Dr. B. Chone Oliver." Medical Woman'
            Journal, 54:9 (September 1947) 51. (News Notes.)
        This obituary gives a brief recounting of Dr. Oliver's pro-
        fessional activities. Dr. Oliver, a 1900 graduate of the Uni-
        versity of Toronto, was active in medical missions work in
        India.

316.   "Correspondence." Medical Woman's Journal, 32:9 (Septem-
            ber 1925) 260-xi.
        [A woman physician] describes being stationed in Bonnie Bay,
        Newfoundland during the time when nurses and physicians used
        snowshoes to see their cases, lived in wood-heated log cabins
        and were in need of more trained medical assistance. One
        of the difficulties of her job that she identifies is the fact that
        all the government nurses are English. "I wish we could
        convince the Governor that Newfoundland nurses would be bet-
        ter. But the Governor is always English."

317.   Currie, Muriel G. "Some Canadian Women in Medicine."
            Nova Scotia Medical Bulletin, 34:7 (July 1955) 268-271.
        Brief sketches of the careers of 14 Canadian women physi-
        cians, all born in the late 1800s, are provided. Dr. Mar-
        garet Ellen Douglas practiced in Winnipeg, served overseas
        during the war, and took a leading part in women's organiza-
        tions. Dr. Maria T. Anguin was the first woman to prac-
        tice in Halifax. Dr. Annie Isabel Hamilton also practiced in
        Halifax, then went to China. Dr. Blaycock was the first wo-
        man to obtain a degree in surgery in Quebec. Dr. Mary
        Mackay was one of the first women graduates in medicine
        from the University of Toronto. Dr. Jane Heartz Bell even-
        tually took over Dr. Anguin's practice. Dr. Maude Elizabeth
        Seymour Abbott distinguished herself in cardiology. Dr.
        Clara May Olding practiced in Saint John, Chester, and Hali-
        fax. Dr. May Lelia Randall practiced pediatrics in Sydney.

Dr. Helen MacMurchy was the first woman physician admitted to the staff of the Toronto General Hospital (in 1901). Dr. Victoria Sara Ernst practiced in Bridgewater for 30 years. Dr. Florence Maude O'Connell and Dr. Minna May Austen both spent one term in China. Dr. Jemima MacKenzie practiced and directed an orphanage in India.

318. Currie, Muriel G. "Some Canadian Women in Medicine: Part II." Nova Scotia Medical Bulletin, 34:8 (August 1955) 298-299.
Second in a series of sketches of Canadian women physicians, this article includes, among others, Mary Mackenzie, Ada Wallace (first woman coroner in Manitoba), Elinor F. Black (first Canadian woman appointed professor of obstetrics and gynecology at the University of Manitoba), and Thelma S. Miner (first woman medical health officer in Saskatchewan).

319. Daley, Dorothy E. "Memorial to Marion Hilliard (1902-1958)." Journal of the American Medical Women's Association, 14:1 (January 1959) 62. port.
Having authored A Woman Doctor Looks at Love and Life, which was a compilation of a series of articles she had written for a Canadian magazine on women's problems, Marion Hilliard was associated with the Women's College Hospital in Toronto, and was, for the last ten years of her life, chief of the obstetrics and gynecology department.

320. "Dr. Abbott Joins the Editorial Staff." Medical Woman's Journal, 44:4 (April 1937) 107. (Editorial.)
A thumbnail sketch is given of Dr. Maude E. S. Abbott of Montreal, Canada.

321. "Dr. Abbott's Place in Medicine." Medical Woman's Journal, 48:7 (July 1941) 200-202, 217.
The author discusses Maude Abbott's professional interests and her personality.

322. "Dr. Helen MacMurchy: Former Chief of the Child Welfare Division of Canada." Medical Woman's Journal, 41:6 (June 1934) 165-166. port.
Helen MacMurchy, who received her M.D. from the University of Toronto in 1901, served from 1920 to 1934 as chief of the Division of Child Welfare in Canada's Department of National Health. A resumé is given of her education, appointments, and published books and pamphlets.

323. "Dr. M. Ellen Douglas." Medical Woman's Journal, 45:9 (September 1938) 281.
Presented is an abbreviated biography of Margaret Ellen Douglas (whose portrait appears on the front cover of this issue of the Journal). Dr. Douglas is a 1905 graduate of the Ontario Medical College for Women.

324. "Dr. Maude Abbott. " Medical Woman's Journal, 47:10 (Octo-
         ber 1940) 310. (Editorial.)
      The death of Maude Abbott on September 2, 1940 prompted
      the Montreal Daily Star to voice esteem for her personal at-
      tributes and professional triumphs. The tribute is reprinted
      here in its entirety.

325. Douglass, M. Ellen. "A Pioneer Woman Doctor of Western
         Canada. " Manitoba Medical Revue, 27 (1947) 255-256.
      [Article not examined by editors.]

326. Dubin, Nathan I. "Maude Abbott: Pioneer Woman Doctor.
         Founder of MCP's First Full-time Departments of Path-
         ology and Bacteriology. " Alumnae News [Medical College
         of Pennsylvania], 26:1 (February 1975) 12-13.   port.
      A review of Maude Elizabeth Seymour Abbott's career empha-
      sizes her activities at the Woman's Medical College of Penn-
      sylvania.   The author, who was a student of Dr. Abbott's at
      McGill University, tells of his personal admiration for her.
      "I little thought I would follow in her footsteps at W. M. C. , "
      writes Dr. Dubin, now the College's professor of pathology.

327. "Elizabeth Smith Shortt, M. D. " In: 100 Years of Medicine:
         1849-1949.   Modern Press Limited, Saskatoon, Saskatch-
         ewan, 1949, 17.
      Brief biographical notes are given on the life of Elizabeth
      Shortt, one of Canada's earliest pioneer women doctors.   She
      graduated from Queen's University in 1884 and outlined at
      length "the indignities and difficulties to which women stu-
      dents of those days were subjected. " Dr. Shortt was active
      in public health and woman suffrage.

328. "Emily Howard Stowe ... Pioneer. " In: 100 Years of Medi-
         cine: 1849-1949.   Modern Press Limited, Saskatoon,
         Saskatchewan, 1949, 14.   photo.
      Emily Howard Stowe was the first Canadian woman to practice
      medicine (having graduated in 1868 from the Women's New
      York Medical School) and was a pioneer leader in the suffrage
      movement.   Dr. Stowe decided to study medicine after the
      birth of her three children.   She was, however, refused ad-
      mittance to Toronto University because of her sex.   After
      being told that the doors of the University were not open to
      her, she responded: "Then I will make it the business of
      my life to see that they will be open, that women may have
      the same opportunities as men. "

329. Gilmore, Hugh R. "Dr. Maude Abbott's Scrapbook: Histor-
         ical Notes of the International Association of Medical
         Museums. " Laboratory Investigation, 6:1 (1957) 89-94.
         port.
      In 1907, Dr. Abbott helped to found the International Associa-
      tion of Medical Museums; she served as first secretary and
      treasurer, holding the office until her death in 1940, and also

edited the Association's Bulletin from 1907 to 1938. In 1955, the organization's name changed to International Academy of Pathology. Most of the information contained in this article concerns the Association and its journal (now, Laboratory Investigation).

330. Gray, Jessie. "In Memoriam: Jessie McGeachy, M. D." Journal of the American Medical Women's Association, 21:5 (May 1966) 417.
President of the Federation of Canadian Medical Women in 1959, Jessie McGeachy was the Canadian representative on the editorial board of the Journal of the American Medical Women's Association when she died in 1966.

331. Guest, Edna. "Maude Abbott, 1869-1940: Her Contribution to Cardiology." Journal of the American Medical Women's Association, 5:2 (February 1950) 74. (Album of Women in Medicine.)

332. H. L. S. "Appreciation: Roberta Bond Nichols." Nova Scotia Medical Bulletin, 45:12 (December 1966) 333.
Roberta Bond received her M. D. degree in 1925 from Dalhousie University. She practiced in Newfoundland and Halifax, Nova Scotia.

333. Hacker, Carlotta. "Jennie Trout: An Indomitable Lady Doctor Whose History Was Lost for a Half-Century." Canadian Medical Association Journal, 110:7 (6 April 1974) 841, 843, 857. illus.
Carlotta Hacker [who wrote The Indomitable Lady Doctors, Clarke Irwin & Co., Toronto, Canada, 1974] describes her often-frustrated efforts to track down biographical background on Jennie Gowanlock Trout. A contemporary of Emily Stowe, Canada's first woman physician (practicing in Toronto in 1867), Dr. Trout apparently practiced in Toronto in the 1870s and was "very likely" Canada's second woman physician. Despite the "curiously silent" records, Hacker managed to glean several facts about Jennie Trout's life. An 1875 graduate of Woman's Medical College in Philadelphia, Dr. Trout was licensed with Ontario's College of Physicians and Surgeons that same year, becoming the first woman listed on that register. Although no Canadian medical school admitted women, the Toronto School of Medicine admitted Emily Stowe and Jennie Trout to one session so they could fulfill the country's medical registration requirements. The two women were friends who together championed women's rights. Jennie Trout's association with Dr. Stowe, however, contributed to her historical obscurity. In 1883, as if in rivalry, the two established separate medical schools for women. The rivalry persisted, and the famous Stowe family avoided mentioning Dr. Trout in their family papers. Another reason for Dr. Trout's obscurity was her move--15 years before her death --to Los Angeles, California.

334.   Harvey, Ruth A. Johnstone. "Isabel I. Thomas Day, M.D.,
           R.R.C." Journal of the American Medical Women's
           Association, 10:7 (July 1955) 256. port.
        This article offers a descriptive sketch of the life of Dr. Day
        "a very much beloved physician and surgeon in her adopted
        home, Vancouver, British Columbia."

335.   Harvey, Ruth A. Johnstone. "Marjorie Bennett, M.D.,
           F.A.C.A." Journal of the American Medical Women's
           Association, 10:7 (July 1955) 255. port. (Album of Wo-
           men in Medicine.)
        Marjorie Bennett was president of the Federation of Medical
        Women of Canada in 1954-1955.

336.   "Helen MacMurchy, M.D." Medical Woman's Journal, 47:3
           (March 1940) 92.
        A Canadian physician and social reformer, Dr. MacMurchy
        wrote for several medical journals and lectured in Canada,
        the U.S., and England. (Her portrait is on the front cover
        of this issue of the Journal.)

337.   "Helen Reynolds Ryan, M.D." In: 100 Years of Medicine:
           1849-1949. Modern Press Limited, Saskatoon, Saskatch-
           ewan, 1949, 37. port.
        Helen Reynolds Ryan was the first woman to become a mem-
        ber of the Canadian Medical Association (1880s). While still
        a child, she determined to become a doctor so that she and
        her brother could practice together, and indeed they did car-
        ry on a joint practice for a time in Mount Forest. Eventual-
        ly, she married and opened a practice in Sudbury.

338.   Hind, E. Cora. "Dr. Amelia Yeomans." Manitoba Messen-
           ger, (June 1913) 9.
        [Article not examined by editors.]

339.   "Honor Conferred Upon a Canadian Medical Woman." Med-
           ical Woman's Journal, 37:9 (September 1930) 261-262.
        Augusta Stowe-Gullen was the first Canadian female to study
        medicine in Canada and to take a medical degree from a
        Canadian university. During her lifetime she was always
        committed to equal suffrage educationally, medically, legal-
        ly, and politically.

340.   Jones, R.O. "Eliza P. Brison, 1881-1974." American
           Journal of Psychiatry, 131:6 (June 1974) 720. (In Me-
           moriam.)
        Dr. Brison worked as a psychiatrist in Nova Scotia.

341.   "Lillian A. Chase, M.D." Medical Woman's Journal, 51:4
           (April 1944) 35.
        Lillian Chase (whose portrait appears on the front cover of
        this issue of the Journal) graduated in medicine from the Uni-
        versity of Toronto. In 1942 she was appointed captain in the
        Royal Canadian Army Medical Corps.

342.   MacDermot, H. E.   Maude Abbott: A Memoir.   The Mac-
            millan Company of Canada Limited, Toronto, Canada,
            1941, xi, 264 pp.   photos., ports.
        Maude Abbott was "a striking figure in Canadian social and
        medical history."   After failing to gain admission to the med-
        ical school of McGill University in Montreal, her undergrad-
        uate alma mater, she took her medical training at Bishop's
        College, whose students received their hospital training from
        the McGill teaching staff at the Montreal General Hospital.
        Her goal was to join the medical faculty at McGill, which
        she eventually did.   In 1898 she was appointed assistant cur-
        ator of the medical museum at McGill--the beginning of what
        later became an important project in her life: her develop-
        ment of the Osler Catalogue of the Circulatory System.   Her
        museum involvement led to her organizing of the International
        Association of Medical Museums, and she was long the ed-
        itor of its Bulletin.   In 1923 she accepted the chair of path-
        ology at the Woman's Medical College of Pennsylvania, but
        only for two years, after which she returned to McGill.   The
        museum had always been at the core of her work at McGill,
        and she was put in charge of the Medical Historical Museum,
        an outgrowth of her former work there.   Her area of special
        interest was congenital heart disease, and her Atlas of Con-
        genital Cardiac Disease illustrates "the extensive consultant
        correspondence which grew up between her and clinicians all
        over the North American continent and to some extent in
        England and on the Continent."   In addition to her contribu-
        tions to the field of cardiology, Dr. Abbott is remembered
        for being a vital stimulus to others working in her field.   In-
        cluded are an index and three appendixes, one of which is a
        bibliography of her publications.

343.   McGeachy, Jessie A.   "Elinor Black, M. D."   Journal of
            the American Medical Women's Association, 7:10 (Octo-
            ber 1952) 394.   port.   (Album of Women in Medicine.)
        Elinor Black was the first Canadian woman physician to be
        appointed as a chairperson of a department of obstetrics and
        gynecology with the full rank of professor.   Two women doc-
        tors were important medical models and mentors in helping
        her to decide to become a doctor: Lillias Cringan-McIntyre
        and Geraldine Oakley.   When Dr. Black received her M. D.
        degree in 1930, she considered that she might have to earn
        her living as a stenographer because that profession would
        have offered her a more comfortable living.

344.   MacKay, Jean Sinclair.   "Elizabeth Beatty, M. D."   Mission-
            ary Monthly, (May 1940) 207-208.
        [Article not examined by editors.]

345.   MacKenzie, K. A.   "Doctor Annie Maxwell Fulton, 1848-1889:
            The First Nova Scotian Lady to Receive a Medical De-
            gree."   Nova Scotia Medical Bulletin, 27:4 (April 1948)
            109.   port.

Although a Canadian native, Dr. Maxwell-Fulton obtained her M.D. at the Woman's Medical College of Pennsylvania and practiced medicine in Michigan.

346.   MacL. , E.   "An Appreciation: Dr. Florence J. Murray. "
        Nova Scotia Medical Bulletin, (June 1975) 101.   port.

347.   MacMurchy, Helen.   "Dr. Abbott's Place in Medicine. "
        Bulletin of the Academy of Medicine, Toronto, 14 (1941)
        259-264.
        [Article not examined by editors.]

348.   "Maude E. Abbott, M.D. , LL.D. " In: 100 Years of Medi-
        cine: 1849-1949.   Modern Press Limited, Saskatoon,
        Saskatchewan, 1949, 28.   port.
        Maude Abbott, long associated with McGill University, is
        best known for her research on cardiac disease and for her
        development of a system of classification for medical muse-
        ums.   Biographical information is presented in this brief
        article.

349.   "Maude Elizabeth Seymour Abbott. " Medical Woman's Jour-
        nal, 43:8 (August 1936) 216.
        Listed are the professional credentials of Dr. Abbott (whose
        portrait appears on the front cover of this issue of the Jour-
        nal).

350.   "Maude Elizabeth Seymour Abbott: B.A. (McGill), M.D.
        (Bishop's), L.R.C.P. &S. (Edin), M.D. (McGill, Hon.),
        F.R.C.P. (Canada), LL.D. (McGill, Hon.). " Medical
        Woman's Journal, 47:10 (October 1940) 312-314.
        This biography concentrates on Dr. Abbott's technical writing.
        A bibliography of her published works concludes the article.

351.   Murray, Florence J.   At the Foot of Dragon Hill.   E. P.
        Dutton & Company, Inc. , New York, New York, 1975,
        xiii, 240 pp.
        Born in 1894 in Nova Scotia, Florence Jessie Murray went to
        the Far East in 1921 as a Presbyterian medical missionary.
        During the Japanese occupation of Korea, Dr. Murray was
        placed under house arrest, and in 1942 was deported--ex-
        changed by the Japanese for prisoners of war.   In 1947 she
        returned to her work in Korea and there spent the next 22
        years.   In this book, Dr. Murray tells of her first two dec-
        ades in Manchuria and Korea.   In the preface, she provides
        information on her family background and her medical and
        graduate medical education, and the motivation behind her
        life's work.

352.   Nichols, R. Bond.   "Early Women Doctors of Nova Scotia. "
        Nova Scotia Medical Bulletin, 29 (January 1950) 14-21.
        Prior to 1910, Nova Scotia produced over 30 women medical
        graduates.   By 1949, Dalhousie University alone had granted

medical degrees to 55 women. A biographical sketch of Dr.
Jane L. Heartz Bell is given.   Dr. Bell, who received her
M. D. degree in 1893, was, at the time of this article, "the
only one of the seven Nova Scotia women graduates of ...
Women's Medical College of New York living in Nova Scotia. "
A biographical sketch is also given of Dr. Annie Hamilton,
who practiced medicine in Halifax.   Other women mentioned
are Mary Mackay, one of the first women graduates in medicine of Trinity College, University of Toronto; Dr. Jemina
Mackenzie, a graduate from Dalhousie; Dr. Alice Symonds;
Katharine Mackay; and Victoria Sara Ernst.   Anecdotes are
given of the lives of many of the women mentioned.   About
Victoria Sara Ernst we are told: "She led her final year,
but because she was a woman, she was not allowed to intern.
Demanding her rights, she was told, 'Very well but you will
have to sleep with the other interns. ' On her graduation day,
as she went up to get her degree, her classmates rose in a
body and sang, 'God Save Our Gracious Queen!' "

353.   "Nora Livingston and Maude Abbott. " Calgary Associate
          Clinic Historical Bulletin, 22 (1958) 228-235.
          [Article not examined by editors.]

353a.   "Proceedings at the Academy of Medicine of Toronto on the
          Occasion of the Presentation of a Portrait of Dr. Helen
          MacMurchy, C. B. E. , by the Federation of the Medical
          Women of Canada, January 9, 1940. " Medical Woman's
          Journal, 47:3 (March 1940) 70-74.
          A presentation address by Dr. Maude Abbott pays tribute to
          Helen MacMurchy's character as well as her many accom-
          plishments in the field of maternal and child health care.
          Also published are the texts of addresses by Dr. Edna M.
          Guest, president of the Federation; Dr. D. E. Robertson,
          president of the Academy of Medicine; and Dr. MacMurchy.

354.   Robinson, Marion O.   Give My Heart: The Dr. Marion Hil-
          liard Story.   Doubleday & Company, Inc. , Garden City,
          New York, 1964, 348 pp.   photos. , ports.
          Once, on the verge of quitting medical school, Marion Hil-
          liard went into a delivery room and witnessed a birth for the
          first time: "She knew instantly that, for her, this was what
          life was all about. " Dr. Hilliard went on to realize her goal
          to be known as " 'not just a good woman doctor, but a good
          doctor. '" Eventually she became chief of the obstetrics and
          gynecology department at Women's College Hospital in Toron-
          to.   She also led a career as an author.   When asked, after
          her book A Woman Doctor Looks at Love and Life was pub-
          lished (1957), how she as a single woman knew so much
          about marriage and sex, Dr. Hilliard replied, "It gives me
          an objective point of view. A married woman knows only
          one man. " This biography, detailing Dr. Hilliard's life
          from childhood to her death, contains many photographs, and
          has an index.

355.   Stewart, W. Brenton. "Women in Medicine." In: <u>Medicine</u>
        <u>in New Brunswick: A History of the Practice of Medi-</u>
        <u>cine in the Province of New Brunswick, and of the Men</u>
        <u>and Women Who Contributed to this History, Encompass-</u>
        <u>ing the Period of Time from Prior to the Arrival of the</u>
        <u>White Man in America to the Early Part of the Twenti-</u>
        <u>eth Century.</u> The New Brunswick Medical Society, New
        Brunswick, Canada, 1974, 86-91.
        A sketchy history of Canadian medical women, this chapter
        profiles Elizabeth C. Secord, the first qualified woman phy-
        sician practicing in New Brunswick. She received her M. D.
        in 1881 from Keokuk College (Michigan). Several other wo-
        men who practiced medicine in New Brunswick in the 19th
        and 20th centuries are mentioned. The author concludes that
        in view of these women's contributions, the "Medical Society
        of New Brunswick should welcome more attractive lady phy-
        sicians every year."

356.   "They Were First: Six Women Medical Pioneers." <u>Canadian</u>
        <u>Medical Association Journal</u>, 110:7 (6 April 1974) 840.
        (Medical History.)
        The six pioneers discussed in this article (their portraits ap-
        pear on the front cover of this issue of the Journal) are Dr.
        James Miranda Stuart Barry, the first woman to practice
        medicine in Canada; Dr. Emily Howard Stowe, the first
        Canadian woman to practice in Canada, and her daughter Au-
        gusta Stowe-Gullen, the first woman to hold a faculty position
        in Canadian medicine; Dr. Ethlyn Trapp, the first woman
        president of a provincial medical association and of the Na-
        tional Cancer Institute of Canada; Dr. Bette Stephenson; and
        Dr. Jennie Trout.

357.   White, Agnes H. T. "Jane Heartz Bell, M.D." <u>Journal of</u>
        <u>the American Medical Women's Association</u>, 6:2 (Febru-
        ary 1951) 62. port. (Album of Women in Medicine.)
        Jane Heartz Bell started a general practice in Halifax in 1898
        with a special interest in diseases of women and children.
        Besides being a doctor, she was also active in civic affairs.

358.   White, Paul D. "Maude E. Abbott, 1869-1940." <u>American</u>
        <u>Heart Journal</u>, 23:4 (April 1942) 567-575.
        This article was written to present some of the "most per-
        tinent quotations" made by various people about Maude Abbott,
        as well as to offer a useful bibliography of Dr. Abbott's pub-
        lications on cardiovascular disease.

CHINA

359.   "An Appeal for Medical Help in China." <u>Medical Woman's</u>
        <u>Journal</u>, 30:3 (March 1923) 92-93.
        Dr. Ida Kahn of Nanchang writes of the appalling conditions
        arising out of the civil war and pleads for American women
        physicians to come to her aid in China.

360. "Dr. Jamei Kin, China's Foremost Woman Physician. " Wo-
       man's Medical Journal, 27:3 (March 1917) 61.
       Jamei Kin, daughter of Christian Chinese parents who lived
       near Shanghai, came to the United States with American mis-
       sionaries and received her medical education at the Women's
       Medical College of the New York Infirmary for Women and
       Children. At the time this article was written, Dr. Kin was
       a government official in China where she headed the Pei-Yang
       Woman's Medical School and Hospital, and was visiting physi-
       cian to the Widows' Home, the Girls' Refuge, and the Infant
       Asylum. [This article also appears in the Bulletin Medical
       Women's Club of Chicago, 5:11 (July 1917) 4.]

361. "Dr. Y. May King [sic]. " Medical Missionary Record, 2:4
       (August 1887) 80-82. port.

362. "Fair Chinese Doctors from the University of Michigan. "
       Double Cross and Medical Missionary Record, 11:7 (July
       1896) 152.
       Meiyie Shie [also known as Mary Stone] and Ida Kahn are the
       first Chinese girls to graduate from the University of Michi-
       gan.

363. Han, Suyin. Birdless Summer: China. Autobiography. His-
       tory. G. P. Putnam's Sons, New York, New York, 1968,
       347 pp. map, photos. , port.
       This third autobiographical volume by Han Suyin (Rosalie
       Chou) covers the years from 1938 to 1948. She describes
       the spirit and politics of China during this tumultuous period
       and her strong personal feelings about the course of events--
       the Japanese invasion, Chiang Kai-shek's activities, and the
       rise of communism. Against this background, her own life
       unfolds: an unhappy marriage, work as a midwife in Chengtu,
       a career as a writer, adoption of a daughter, life as a diplo-
       mat's wife and medical student in London, and her year as
       house surgeon at the Royal Free Hospital. The book closes
       with her decision to leave London and return to Hong Kong and
       possibly to China.

364. Han, Suyin. The Crippled Tree: China. Biography, History.
       Autobiography. G. P. Putnam's Sons, New York, New
       York, 1965, 461 pp. map, photos. , ports.
       In her search for a deeper understanding of her own Chinese
       heritage, Dr. Han Suyin wrote this sweeping history of China
       covering the years from 1885 to 1928. Although she eventual-
       ly graduated in medicine from the University of London, this
       first volume of her autobiography covers only her early years
       as a Eurasian child in Peking.

365. Han, Suyin. A Mortal Flower: China. Autobiography, His-
       tory. G. P. Putnam's Sons, New York, New York, 1966,
       413 pp. map, photos. , ports.
       " 'I am going to be a doctor, Mama. ' Mama counted the

stitches in her knitting.... 'Papa, I am going to be a doctor.' 'A doctor? It's very difficult to be a doctor if you are a woman.' 'She is making up stories as usual,' said Mama." But the story came true. In this second volume of her autobiography, Han Suyin tells of her early education in Peking, her experiences as a Eurasian at Yen Ching University, her years studying medicine in Belgium (1935-1938), and her decision to return to China in spite of the mounting Japanese peril. The author tells the story of her life against the backdrop of a crucial period of Chinese history and offers invaluable insights into events occurring around her--the rise of Chiang Kai-shek, his split with Mao Tse-tung, and the Japanese invasions of first Manchuria, then China itself.

366. "Hu King Eng, Graduate of an American College." Woman's
      Medical Journal, 6:11 (November 1897) 334-346.
      Dr. Hu King Eng, the only female Chinese to graduate from
      an American medical college (Woman's Medical College of
      Pennsylvania, 1890), was born in 1866 to a military mandarin
      father. Her grandfather's was the second Chinese family to
      convert to Christianity. Dr. Hu was recently appointed first
      physician to the private household of Li Hung Chang, China's
      grand viceroy.

367. Katscher, Leopold. ["The First Chinese Female Physician"].
      Schweizerische Medizinische Wochenschrift, 13:1 (2 Janu-
      ary 1932) 16. (Ger)
      This article commemorates the 70th birthday of the first
      Chinese woman physician, Dr. Dschamei Kin. She studied
      medicine in New York and worked among the Chinese immi-
      grants before returning to her fatherland in 1905. In China
      she introduced modern medical knowledge and techniques. Be
      cause of resistance to new ideas, she had to adapt to a more
      traditional framework. She started by training nurses and
      midwives in order to create extensive health services. She
      publicly fought opium trade and was a pioneer for women's
      education at all levels.

368. Lewis, Robert E. "Chinese Women Physicians." Outlook,
      (4 March 1911) 517-518. (Letters to the Outlook.)
      The letter-writer, General Secretary of the YMCA, corrects
      an Outlook editorial stating that Dr. Yamei Kin is the only
      Chinese woman physician who graduated from an American
      medical college. Among the Chinese women he mentions are
      Dr. Hu-King-Eng (an alumna of Woman's Medical College in
      Philadelphia), Drs. Ida Kahn and Mary Stone (both graduates
      of the University of Michigan, 1896), and Drs. Li, Wong,
      and Tsao.

369. Lin, Chiao-chih. "The Party Keeps Me Young." In: New
      Women in New China. Foreign Languages Press, Peking,
      People's Republic of China, 1972, 21-30. photo.
      Lin Chiao-chih (a.k.a. Dr. Khati Lim) heads the gynecology

and obstetrics department of Peking's Capital Hospital (formerly the Peking Union Medical College Hospital), and serves on the standing committees of both the National People's Congress and the Chinese Medical Association. Writing this autobiographical account at age 70, Dr. Lin recalls how she remained "cool and aloof ... [ignoring] the ridicule I got as a woman breaking into the medical profession," while studying in England and the United States, and at Peking's Union Medical College, which was run by U.S. imperialists who gained scientific knowledge by performing experiments with drugs and bacteria on Chinese patients. Women's emancipation and the gradual eradication of class distinctions following China's liberation in 1949 inspired Dr. Lin to reexamine her role and attitudes as a physician. She realized that her prerevolution goal to "be a good person ... a doctor with a conscience" was a meaningless ideal: "In a society where classes exist, an ideal which takes no class view is only a dream"; and without a class view, "even if one possesses most superior medical skill one cannot make real use of it." Becoming a revolutionary medical worker meant reaching an understanding of the proletarian workers' needs and hopes, learning to "cure their physical ills while they treat my sick thinking." To Dr. Lin, the work of a people's doctor means sharing medical knowledge with the masses and uniting the people to struggle together in the socialist revolution.

370. McLean, Mary H. Dr. Li Yuin Tsao: Called and Chosen and Faithful. Published by the author, St. Louis, Missouri, 1925, 96 pp. photos., ports.
A graduate of Woman's Medical College of Pennsylvania (1911), Li Yuin Tsao interned at the Mary Thompson Hospital for Women and Children in Chicago. In 1912, she took charge of the Friends' Hospital in Nanking, China. Dr. Tsao lectured extensively to Nanking citizens in matters of public health, and instructed women medical students in Ginling College for Women. Her experiences in medical school and the hospitals in which she worked are described. The book's prevailing theme centers on Dr. Tsao's Christian faith, from how Satan attempted to thwart her medical studies, to how her faith aided her career. Included are several posthumous tributes to her, written by Drs. Clara Marshall and Bertha Van Hoosen, among others.

371. "Mary Stone, M.D." Medical Woman's Journal, 50:7 (July 1943) 182.
Dr. Mary Stone (whose portrait appears on the front cover of this issue of the Journal) was born in Kiu Kiang, Central China, in 1873, the daughter of "Mother" Stone who was the first Chinese woman in Central China to become a Christian. Dr. Mary Stone graduated in 1896 from the Medical Department of the University of Michigan. This biography retells incidents in the life of Dr. Stone, who returned to China to live and work.

372.   "Meigii Shie and Ida Kahn." Double Cross and Medical Mis-
            sionary Record, 11:11 (November 1896) 237.
        A detailed account is presented of Meigii Shie [Mary Stone]
        and Ida Kahn's graduation ceremonies from the University of
        Michigan and of their plans for the immediate future.

373.   Sawyers, Martha. "Pity Them Not." Collier's, (17 Novem-
            ber 1945) 81. illus.
        The author recalls her impression of Dr. Anna M. Y. Chow,
        a Chinese woman physician in Kunming.

374.   Sheets, Emily T. "Doctor Mary Stone: 'The Lady Doctor.'"
            Woman's Medical Journal, 29 [19]:2 (February 1919) 24-
            26.
        Born in 1873 in a Chinese Methodist parsonage in Kuikiang,
        Dr. Stone graduated in medicine from the University of Mich-
        igan. This biography concentrates on her work in China as
        a reform movement leader, a missionary, and a surgeon in
        the Elizabeth Skelton Danforth Memorial Hospital in Kuikiang.

375.   [Wong, Helena]. "Helena Wong, M.D." Medical Woman's
            Journal, 48:11 (November 1941) 357.
        Dr. Helena Wong (whose portrait appears on the front cover
        of this issue of the Journal) was born in Wuchow, Kwangsi,
        China and received her medical training at Hackett Medical
        College (later Canton Christian University) in Canton.

EUROPE, EASTERN

376.   Bazanov, V. A. and Vladimirova, G. A. ["The 'Russian
            Colony' in Zurich"]. Sovetskoe Zdravookhranenie, 28
            (1969) 71-76. (Rus)
        The authors describe the University of Zurich in the mid-
        19th century, especially the life of the Russian colony. N. P.
        Suslova was the first Russian woman medical graduate; the
        second was M. A. Bokova, who graduated in 1871. In 1872
        there were 44 Russian women medical students in Zurich.
        Many of them later became physicians. Among them were
        N. O. Ziber-Shumova, later a prominent biochemist in Peters-
        burg; E. O. Shumova-Simanovskaya, a physiologist who worked
        with Pavlov; and P. V. Putyata-Kershbaumer, the first wo-
        man physician in Austria. All these students were deeply in-
        volved in the revolutionary movement; they were forced to
        leave Zurich in 1873 by a special order of the Czar. In
        1872 the Russian government opened the Women's Medical
        Courses in Petersburg.

377.   Bucar, F. ["The First Croatian Woman Physician"]. Lijec-
            nicki Vjesnik, 66:2 (1944) 27+. (Cro)
        [Article not examined by editors.]

378.   Czajecka, Boguslawa and Jasicka, Janina. ["The First Wo-

man to be Graduated from the Jagiellonian University--
Helena Donhaiser-Sikorska (1873-1945)"]. Przeglad Lekarski, 27 (29 October 1971) 671-675. photo. (Pol)
Helena Donhaiser-Sikorska, the first female medical student at
the University of Krakow, was born the daughter of a Krakow
architect on April 25, 1873. After numerous difficulties she
gained admission to the Medical Faculty at Krakow in 1899
and became a medical doctor in 1906. She married Professor Sikorska in 1902. From 1906 to 1911 she worked as
assistant to Professor Bujwida in a variety of fields, including
bacteriology. From 1914 to 1921 she served in the army and
in 1927 was appointed an expert on the Krakow Medical Committee. She received several state decorations for her long
career and many contributions to the health of the Polish
people. She died on June 5, 1945.

379.   Dettelbacher, Werner. ["Dr. Marie Siebold--One of the First
        Women Doctors in Serbia, in Turkey, and in Egypt"].
        Munchener Medizinische Wochenschrift, 115:45 (November
        1973) 2051-2053. port. (Ger)
"Marie Siebold, born in St. Petersburg, studied in Zurich
and Bern from 1870-1874 and qualified in 1874. She first
obtained recognition as a surgeon in a military hospital in
Serbia during the Russo-Turkish War of 1877/78 and then
practiced in Belgrade from 1878-1888. Exiled for safety reasons, she was active in Constantinople for 17 years, until a
harem intrigue led to her expulsion. After unsuccessful practice in Belgrade, she was active in Egyptian hospitals from
1907. On the outbreak of war in 1914, she returned to Serbia and was imprisoned by the Bulgarians with a military
hospital in Albania." [journal summary.]

380.   Dionesov, S. M. ["Russian Zurich Students (From the His-
        tory of Medical Education of Russian Women)"]. Sovet-
        skoe Zdravookhranenie, 30 (1971) 68-72. (Rus)
In the late 1850s and early 1860s the striving of women for
higher education and in particular for medical education became very noteworthy in Russia. Since such education was
forbidden, and only a few exceptions were allowed--such as
Anna Kleiman (Odessa), Rosalinda Simonovich (Petersburg)
and Kashevarova--women had to go abroad to continue their
medical education. They preferred Zurich because of the
emigrant group already there. In 1865 Knyazhnina and N. P.
Suslova, and in 1868 M. A. Bokova and A. Serebrennaya,
went to Zurich and became physicians. In the winter of 1871-
72 there were 17 Russian women students in Zurich, in the
summer there were 43, and the number steadily increased.
They also became very much interested in political and social
problems and learned about the class struggle and the working
class movement, for Zurich had become one of the centers of
the Russian revolutionary movement. Many of them became
very active. The Russian government grew concerned about
their political activities and influenced the Swiss authorities

to force the Russian women to leave by January 1874. Some
transferred to other universities; a few stayed in Zurich.
One, A. Lukanina, graduated in 1875 and received her physician's diploma in Philadelphia the next year. These women proved that they could study science and medicine as
successfully as men.

381.   [Dobrski, Konrad]. ["Miss Dr. Anna Tomaszewicz and the
       Warsaw Medical Society"]. Zdrowie, 1:15 (1878) 194.
       (Pol)
       [Article not examined by editors.]

382.   ["Dr. Anna Tomaszewicz-Dobrska"]. Przeglad Poranny, 13:
       131 (1918) 4. (Obituary.)
       [Article not examined by editors.]

383.   ["Dr. Anna Tomaszewicz-Dobrska: Obituary"]. Kurier War-
       szawski, 98:164 (1918) 7.
       [Article not examined by editors.]

384.   Dominik, M. ["Dr. Halina Jankowska"]. Przeglad Lekarski,
       23 (1967) 229-236.
       [Article not examined by editors.]

384a. ["Emeritus Dr. Elena Dérerová, M.D."] Československá
       pediatrie, 25:1 (January 1970) 34. (Slo)
       A remarkable woman and physician, Elena Dérerová worked
       in Bratislava as a pediatrician for many years. She was in-
       terested in a variety of medical problems: along with chil-
       dren's diseases, she also took an interest in prevention and
       treatment of diseases in old age. In August 1957, she was
       given the title of Honorary Physician. Elena Dérerová, a
       wonderful representative of her socialist country, retires on
       pension and her colleagues wish her well.

385.   Filar, Zbigniew. Anna Tomaszewicz Dobrska: A Leaf from
       Polish Medical History. Polish Society of the History of
       Medicine, Warsaw, Poland, 1959, 263 pp. facsim., pho-
       tos., ports. (Pol)
       Anna Tomaszewicz was the second Polish woman to become
       a physician, the first to practice in Poland. Born in 1854,
       she determined in her early teens to study medicine, in spite
       of the objections of her family. She studied in Zurich in
       1871-77 and after brief postgraduate studies in Vienna, Ber-
       lin, and Petrograd, she returned to Warsaw. She met and
       overcame opposition from the local medical society and the
       establishment in Petrograd [Poland was part of Russia at the
       time] and in 1882 was made chief of Lying-in Hospital Num-
       ber 2 in Warsaw, a position she held until the institution was
       closed in 1911. She also carried on a large private practice
       and was deeply involved in charitable and social work activ-
       ities. She was a founding member of the Society of Polish
       Culture and an active advocate of women's rights. She died

in 1918, exhausted by her active and difficult life, and especially her work during the war. Appendixes give: an ancestry record; autobiographical note; letters to her son, her sister, and her friend Eliza Orzeszkowa.

386. ["The First Hungarian Woman Doctor"]. A Het, 2 (1895)
      781. (Hun)
      [Article not examined by editors.]

387. ["The First Hungarian Woman Gynecologist"]. Ui Idok, 1
      (1897) 506. (Hun)
      [Article not examined by editors.]

388. Gavrilovic[j], Vera S. ["The First Two Serbian Women Doctors of Medicine"]. Acta Historica Medicinae Pharmaciae Veterinae, (1967) 65-72. photos., ports. (Ser)
      "In Serbia, the old fashioned patriarchal notions, as far as the education of women was concerned, were a governing factor for a very long time. Dositej Obradovic was the first to point to the necessity of education for Serbian women. He believed that no nation can strive to become a cultural nation if 'their women remain in the darkness of commonness and barbarity.' Therefore, he demanded that special attention be extended to the education of women. In this paper, the author deals with the first two women physicians in liberated Serbia, who completed their medical studies in Zurich, Switzerland. Because of government regulations, woman doctors at that time could not hold jobs in Serbian state service, but could only work on their own. Dr. Draga Milosevic-Ljocic (1855-1926) was born in Sabac, in West of Serbia. She finished the High School for Girls in Belgrade and went on to study medicine in Zurich, where she obtained her degree of 'doctor of medicine, surgery and midwifery (obstetrics), and eye diseases.' In June 1876, when Serbia became engaged in war with Turkey, she took part as a student of medicine in the battle of Sumatovac, serving as a lieutenant of the medical corps of the Serbian army. After the end of the wars that Serbia waged for its independence (1876-1878), Dr. Ljocic was very active. She devoted much effort to the organization of the Society of Women Doctors. She set up a Mothers' Association in Belgrade, where she was both the physician and the first chairman. Dr. Marija Vucetic-Prita (1866-1954) was born in a well known family at Pancevo, near Belgrade, where she went to school. She obtained her secondary education in Zurich, Switzerland, where she completed also her medical studies since, at that time, being a girl, she could not either go to a high school or study medicine in Serbia itself. In 1893 she began to work as a doctor in a hospital at Sabac. She wrote a number of articles for the Srpski archiv za celokupno lekarstvo (the Serbian Archives for Medicine), as well as for medical annuals (Pancevo, Zagreb, Novi Sad). During the First World War she worked as a doctor in a reserve hospital in

Kragujevac, then in Pristina in 1915, and finally in Prokuplje
where the hospital was dissolved. After retreating with the
Serbian army through Albania, Dr. Prita reached Italy, where
from she went to Switzerland, where she worked as a doctor
in Lausanne. In the summer of 1918, Dr. Prita went to
Toulon, France, where she worked as a doctor of the Toulon
Detachment of Disabled Soldiers. She returned to her native
land in 1919. She accomplished an immense job in public
health services. She helped very much to build the Dr. Elsie
Inglis Memorial Hospital in Belgrade. In the International
Society of Women Doctors she worked as the representative
of the Belgrade Society of Women Doctors. She was also a
founder of the Women's Party. She died in active duty as a
very old woman. " [Article English summary.]

388a. Gavrilovicj, Vera S. ["Nadezda Stanojevicj, M.D., First
 Woman-Pediatrician in Our Country"]. Srpski Arhiv za
 Celokupno Lekarstvo, 103:4 (April 1974) 335-340. facsim., port. (Ser)
Dr. Nadezda Stanojevicj was born August 3, 1887, in Pirota.
After finishing high school in Belgrade in 1905, she went to
Petersburg, Russia to study medicine. She graduated in
1911 and returned to Belgrade where she worked in a clinic
as an intern. During the war, in 1914-1915, she worked in
the reserve in Uzhitsa, Valjevo, Chachka, and again in Bel-
grade. In 1919 she went abroad to specialize in pediatrics,
studying in Rome and Paris and in other cities along the way.
In Paris she worked in the clinic of the Hôpital des Enfants
Malades. She returned to Belgrade with her diploma in 1920
and worked there as a pediatrician with Dr. A. Stampary.
She retired in 1953. Dr. Stanojevicj has been awarded many
Yugoslavian orders and medals in honor of her work.

389. Gavrilovicj, V[era S.] ["Oldest Serbian Woman Physician--
 Katitsa Jakshicj-Radulaski"]. Srpski Arhiv za Celokupno
 Lekarstvo, 102:10-11 (October-November 1974) 843-845.
 port. (Ser)
Katitsa Jakshicj-Radulaski was born in Glini on November 1,
1884. After completing school in Zagreb, she went to Zurich,
where she studied medicine. In 1908 she became a physician
in Zagreb and later moved to Sarajevo. In 1912-1913, during
the Balkan Wars, she joined the army, where she was mainly
engaged in sanitation; she was awarded the Order of St. Sava
for her work. In 1914-1918 she worked in a Zagreb clinic.
She later went to Paris for advanced studies, and then practiced in various pediatric institutions in her home country.
She retired in October 1948. Her 90th anniversary is being
observed this year [1974].

390. Harris, Harry. "The Little Czech Woman in Black. " Medical Woman's Journal, 54:8 (August 1947) 58-59.
Dr. Vlasta Kalalova-DiLotti tells in her own words of the
"cruelties of World War II" during which time her husband,

son, and daughter were killed in Czechoslovakia by the Nazis retreating from Russia.

391.   Jasinska, W. ["Some Remembrances of Dr. Wandzie Star-
        kowskie"]. Przeglad Lekarski, 22 (1966) 237-238. (Pol)
        [Article not examined by editors.]

392.   Jaworski, Jozef. ["Dr. Anna Tomaszewicz-Dobrska"]. Ga-
        zeta Lekarska, 53:27 (1918) 215-216. (Obituary.) (Pol)
        [Article not examined by editors.]

393.   Jaworski, Józef. ["Dr. Anna Tomaszewicz-Dobrska"].
        Zdrowie, 34:10 (1918) 272-273. (Obituary.) (Pol)
        [Article not examined by editors.]

394.   ["Jubilee of a Doctor"]. Liječničkog Vjesnicka, 47:5 (May
        1925) 125-126. (Slo)
        February 28, 1925, was the 70th birthday of Dr. Draga Ljocic-
        Milosevic. She studied medicine in Zurich and received the
        doctoral degree in 1879, but the Ministry of Internal Affairs
        in her native land refused to recognize the degree. With a
        colleague, Dr. Vladana Gjorgjevic, and others, she formed
        a society to advocate the admission of women to the medical
        qualification tests given to male medical graduates. The
        state, however, at the urging of the medical establishment,
        decreed that foreign medical degrees would not be recognized.
        It was only after a long difficult struggle that the law was
        changed and Ljocic-Milosevic was able to devote her life to
        the practice of obstetrics and to the Women's Medical Society.
        She is to be congratulated on a long life spent in service to
        women in her native Belgrade.

395.   Katona, Ibolya. ["The First Hungarian Woman Doctor"]. Az
        Orszagos Orvostorteneti Konyvtar Kozlemenyei, 2 (1956)
        80-98. (Hun)
        [Article not examined by editors.]

396.   Klodzinaki, S. ["Dr. Dorota Lorska"]. Przeglad Lekarski,
        23 (1967) 236-241. (Pol)
        [Article not examined by editors.]

397.   Koscialkowska, W[ila]. ["Eliza Orzeszkowa: Biographical
        Sketch"]. Klosy, 32:812 (1881) 35. (Pol)
        This biographical sketch is apparently continued in issue num-
        ber 813 (p. 54-55) and issue number 814 (pp. 67-68). [Ar-
        ticle not examined by editors.]

398.   Lathrop, Julia. "A Married Woman of Genius." The Woman
        Citizen, (7 October 1922) 16. port. (What the Ameri-
        can Woman Thinks.)
        Dr. Radmila Miliovitch Lazarevitch, daughter of the first wo-
        man physician in Serbia, studied medicine in Zurich. This
        article recalls, from facts given by Dr. Lazarevitch, the
        story of Dr. Miliovitch, her mother.

399.   Lazar, Szini C.   ["Dr. Elena Puscariu: 1875-1965"].   Rev.
       Med. (Turgu Mures) , 12 (1966) 224-225.
       This article also appears in Orv. Szl. , 12 (1966) 214-215.
       [Article not examined by editors.]

400.   Madarasz, Erzsebet.   ["The First Hungarian Woman Doctor;
       a Memory of Vilma Hugonnai"].   Magyar Noi Szemle, 3
       (1937) 2-7.   (Hun)
       [Article not examined by editors.]

401.   Marko, Miklos.   ["The First Hungarian Woman Gynecologist"].
       Vasarnapi Ujsag, 44 (1897) 22.   (Hun)
       [Article not examined by editors.]

402.   "News Notes."   Medical Woman's Journal, 55:1 (January
       1948) 50.   port.
       A biography is given of Dr. Antoinette Popovici, a specialist
       in internal medicine in Bucharest, Rumania.

403.   "Notes from the Woman's Medical College of Pennsylvania."
       Medical Woman's Journal, 54:3 (March 1947) 56.
       Mention of Dr. DiLotti's talk at the College headlines these
       news items, most of which deal with recent graduates' appoint-
       ments.   Dr. Vlasta Klalova DiLotti is a surgeon and under-
       ground leader from Czechoslovakia.

404.   Podgorska, Klawe Zofia.   ["Women Physicians from War-
       saw"].   Archiwum Historii Medycyny, 28:3 (1965) 243-
       250.   (Pol)
       Before World War I Poland was part of Russia, so women who
       wished to study medicine generally did so in Russia or, like
       many Russian women, in Switzerland.   The author discusses
       the careers of ten Polish women who began to practice medi-
       cine during that period.   Anna Tomaszewicz-Dobrska was born
       in 1854 in Mlawie and studied in Warsaw, Petersburg, and
       Zurich.   She practiced obstetrics and pediatrics in Warsaw
       for many years.   Teresa Ciszkiewicz studied medicine in War-
       saw and Berne and received her diploma as a doctor of medi-
       cal sciences in 1879.   She practiced gynecology in Warsaw
       and died in 1920.   Elzbieta Downarowicz, a neurologist, was
       the first woman accepted into the Warsaw Medical Society (in
       1896) .   Stanislawa Poplawska studied medicine in Warsaw
       and Zurich.   In 1907 she became the first woman staff phy-
       sician in Warsaw; she specialized in physiology and hygiene.
       Michalina Paschalis studied in Warsaw and Petersburg and
       practiced in Warsaw, Krakow, and Lodz.   In 1913 she be-
       came a staff physician at the Karola-Marii Hospital.   Justyna
       Budzinska-Tylicka was born in 1867, received her medical
       diploma in Paris in 1898, practiced pediatrics in Krakow and
       Warsaw.   She died in 1936.   Maria Ratynska studied in Swit-
       zerland, practiced pediatrics in Warsaw, and died in 1920.
       Marta Ehrlich was the first woman professor of medicine in
       Warsaw.   She studied in Berne, specialized in pediatrics, and

was appointed to the full professorship in 1938. Wanda Szcza-winska was born in 1866, studied in Geneva, and received a doctorate in natural sciences in 1891. She completed her medical education in Paris in 1902, then worked at the Sorbonne and at the Pasteur Institute. She then became a pediatrician and practiced in Warsaw from 1911 until her death in 1955. Natalia Zilberlast-Zandowa, a well-known neurologist and researcher, was a strong advocate of women's rights. The author notes that in 1938 there were 664 women practicing medicine in Warsaw.

405. Poglubko, K. A. ["Contribution to the Biography of A. Go-lovina--the First Bessarbian-Bulgarian Female Doctor"]. Askelpii, 1 (1970) 124-130. (Rus)
[Article not examined by editors.]

406. "Princess and Physician." Woman's Medical Journal, 5:4 (April 1896) 99.
Mlle. Beglarion, an Armenian princess with an M. D. degree, plans to build a hospital on her father's estate.

407. Przerwa, Tetmajer A. ["Helena Wolf ('Anka') and Janina Zachariasz, Doctors in the 'Zycie' Youth Organization"]. Przeglad Lekarski, 22 (1966) 234-236. (Pol)
[Article not examined by editors.]

408. Reti, Ende and Vilmon, Gyulane. ["Gleanings from the Medical Council Records"]. Orvostorteneti Kozlemenyek. Communications de Historia Artis Medicinae, [n. d.], 81-96. (Hun)
In studying the records of 1878-79, the authors came across notes on the first woman physician in Hungary, Vilma Hugonnai. While living in Switzerland with her husband, she became interested in medicine and started studying at the university there. She obtained her M. D. diploma in 1879 and returned to Hungary hoping to practice. This article recounts some of the struggles she went through before she was given a baccalaureate degree in 1881. The government finally recognized her medical degree in 1896 and allowed her to practice.

409. Sebesta, Vilma. "The Year Spent in the United States on the Mary Putnam Jacobi Fellowship of the Women's Medical Association of New York, 1937-38 (Second Part of Report)." Medical Woman's Journal, 46:1 (January 1939) 25-27.
Dr. Sebesta, of Budapest, reports on her year's work and studies in the United States, which was made possible by the Mary Putnam Jacobi Fund. She draws comparisons between the U. S. and Hungary, giving special attention to the differences in medical philosophies and practice.

410. Svejcar, J. ["In Memory of Grazyna Volna, CSc. "]. Ceskos-

lovenska Pediatrie, 29:12 (December 1974) 651. (Cze)
The distinguished pediatrician, Dr. Volna, died on June 13, 1974. She was born in 1919 in Poland, moved to Prague during the war, and obtained her degree at the Charles University in 1947. Until 1960 she was at the pediatric division of the Polyclinic and from 1965 at the Institute of Pharmaceutical Sciences in the University Department of Pediatrics. Her doctoral thesis in 1962 presented new observations and concepts on eczematous diseases in infants. Later she developed new immunological techniques and specialized in allergy; her advice and observations were much sought by colleagues. She published 40 papers in the field. Her sensitivity and highly cultured manner were much admired by patients, and her intelligence, skill, and dedicated energy made her work admired by fellow pediatricians. She was able to communicate in Czech, Polish, and Slovak. Her gracious skill and delicacy in human relations with patients are an irreplaceable loss.

411.   Szenajch, Wladyslaw. [Dr. Maria Ratynska. "Marynka"].
       Warsaw, Poland, 1932. (Pol)
       [Book not examined by editors.]

412.   Vida, Tivadar. ["Vilma Hugonnay"]. Orvosi Hetilap, 116:
       42 (19 October 1975) 2492-2494. port. (Hun)
       Vilma Hugonnay, the first Hungarian woman doctor, was born in 1847, the daughter of Count Kalman Hugonnay. In 1865 she married Gyorgy Szillassy and had a child who died at the age of six years, an event which stimulated her interest in pediatrics. While living in Zurich in 1872, she began to study medicine seriously, taking lectures from prominent doctors of the time. Because foreigners could not become physicians in Zurich at that time, she first matriculated in Latin and mathematics. After graduation, she became a nursing assistant to a professor at the medical school. She passed the oral examination for the diploma of Doctor of Medicine three years later, in February 1879. During this period she published two papers, one on tracheotomy in diphtheria and the other on the diagnosis and treatment of burns. When she returned to Budapest in 1879, she could not be recognized as a physician but was given a certificate as a midwife. She received a baccalaureate in 1881 and became an assistant at the Budapest Clinics to Professor Vince Wartha, whom she later married. When the Ministry of Culture finally recognized her Zurich degree in 1897, she began an extensive medical practice, treating 174 patients during the first six months. She died of heart failure in 1922. Her name is associated with major research progress in Hungarian medicine, as well as with improvement in the social and professional status of women.

413.   "Women Physicians in Germany." Woman's Medical Journal,
       5:11 (November 1896) 302.

Drs. Krayevska and Keck, two female physicians, have been
employed to attend to the Mohammedan population of Bosnia
and Herzegovina.

414.   "Yugoslav Woman Physician Stays on the Go in Her Roles of
         Clinician, Housewife, Mother." Medical Tribune, (4 Sep-
         tember 1974) 16-17. illus. (G. P. Around the World
         series.)
[Article not examined by editors.]

EUROPE, WESTERN

415.   Aggebo, Anker, ed. [Danish Physician Memoirs, Fourth Col-
         lection: Denmark's First Woman Physician, Nielsine Niel-
         sen's Reminiscences]. Nyt Nordisk Forlag, Arnold Busck,
         Copenhagen, Denmark, 1941, 162 pp. port. (Dan)
This is the fourth book in the series, the first devoted to a
single person. It has a brief foreword followed by an "Outline of the History of Women Doctors," which mentions many
notable women healers and physicians and contains a summary
of Nielsine Nielsen's career. The memoirs, previously unpublished, cover Nielsen's childhood, youth, and young womanhood, and her study-travels in the three years after her graduation. Her early interest in the women's movement probably encouraged her to petition the Ministry of Education for
admission to medical studies in 1874. When the medical
schools were opened to women by royal decree in 1875, following a vote of approval by the faculty, she was one of the
first to enroll. She received her doctoral degree in 1885
and, after her foreign study years, set up practice in Copenhagen in 1889. After the initial shock, the community accepted her for her abilities. She continued to be active in
the women's rights movement, but medicine was her life.
She practiced primarily in the fields of gynecology and venereology, and was appointed city venereologist in 1906.

416.   Aigner, Reinhold. ["Dr. Oktavia Aigner-Rollett, the First
         Woman Doctor in Graz: Biography of an Early Austrian
         Woman Physician"]. Historisches Jahrbuch der Stadt
         Graz, 2 (1969) 141-157. facsims., ports. (Ger)
The author, the youngest son of Dr. Rollett, included much
material from family archives. Oktavia Rollett was born in
Graz in 1877, daughter of a professor of physiology and histology at the University of Graz and later rector of the university. After graduation from the girl's lyceum in Graz,
she continued to study and take courses in languages until
she was admitted as a regular auditor in philosophy. She
switched to medicine in 1901 and completed the course in 1905
with distinction. She set up private practice in Graz in 1907,
and remained the only woman practicing there until 1915.
She also served as a school doctor and was the first woman
member of several medical organizations. In 1908 she mar-

ried Dr. Walter Aigner, for many years associated with the
Anatomical Institute at Graz; they had three sons. She remained in private practice for nearly 20 years, through the
1914 war. Beginning in 1925 she shifted to health insurance
work, again as one of the first women in the field. In 1935
she received the title of Medizinalrat, in recognition of her
service to her fellow citizens. She began to give up her
practice in 1949, at the age of 73, exhausted by the war year
and the growing burden of paperwork, and retired completely
at the beginning of 1953. In 1955, on the 50th anniversary
of her doctorate, she received a Golden Diploma from the
University--the first woman so honored. She died in May of
1959, one day before her 82nd birthday.

417.   "American Association of University Women Fellowships."
        Medical Woman's Journal, 55:2 (February 1948) 53-54.
        port.
        Five European women physicians received grants from the
        American Association of University Women to study in the
        U.S.: Drs. Anna M. Jorgensen, Sigrid Holm and Helene
        Ytting of Denmark; Dr. Helene Goudsmit of Belgium; and Dr.
        Ada Middelhoven of Holland. Biographies of these women
        focus on their war-time activities.

418.   Andreae, Horst. ["Maria Montessori, Physician and Edu-
        cator: On Her 100th Birthday"]. Agnes Karll Schwester,
        24 (October 1970) 412, 414. (Ger)
        Maria Montessori was born on 31 August 1870. As a child
        she was considered a mathematical prodigy. She was the
        first woman to study natural science and medicine in Rome
        and the first woman physician in the psychiatric clinic in
        Rome; she also studied philology and pedagogy. Her experi-
        ence in children's clinics, homes, and schools convinced her
        than even retarded children could learn more and better when
        teaching methods were adapted to the developmental rhythms
        of the individual child and that learning begins with the hands,
        not the brain. Her first school started in 1906 and her meth-
        ods soon spread throughout the world. She fled Italy's fascist
        dictatorship, traveling to India with her adopted son in 1933
        and returning to Europe after the end of the war. She died
        in Holland in 1952.

419.   Andreen, Andrea. [Karolina Widerström: Sweden's First
        Woman Doctor]. P. A. Norstedt and Sons, Stockholm,
        Sweden, 1956, 95 pp. illus., photos., ports. (Swe)
        Karolina Olivia Widerström, the first woman licenciate in
        medicine in Sweden, was born in Hälsingborg in December
        1856, daughter of a veterinary physician-medical gymnastics
        teacher. She entered medical studies at the Karolinska In-
        stitutet in 1881 and passed her candidate's examination in
        1884. The next year she and four friends took an extended
        walking tour of Norway, the first of many foreign travels.
        She passed her medical licenciate examination in 1888

and set up practice the next year. In addition to her private
practice, she was active in elementary education, sex education, and sexual hygiene teaching for children and adult women,
dress reform, and women's rights. She served on school
boards, was a town council member in Stockholm, and was
active in medical and women's organizations. She received
many honors, including an honorary doctorate in medicine
from the Karolinska in 1933. She died in March 1949, at
the age of 92. A name index and list of Dr. Widerström's
publications are included.

420.   Andreen, Andrea. "Women Doctors in Sweden." Journal of
          the American Medical Women's Association, 2:2 (Febru-
          ary 1947) 44. port.
        Karolina Widerström, Sweden's first woman doctor, received
        her degree in 1888. As a gynecologist in 1897, she started
        to help educate Swedish women on sex hygiene, and her lec-
        tures were later published as a book, Hygiene for Women,
        which was still used as a textbook at the time this article was
        written. She fought for the abolition of the law that regulated
        prostitution as an officially recognized profession. She ini-
        tiated the first open air classes for tuberculous children. A
        strong advocate of equal rights, she helped win the fight for
        women to get the vote, women's right to hold government
        positions, and their right to obtain equal pay. At the time
        this article was written there were 3,600 doctors in Sweden
        and 250 of them were women.

421.   Bartley, Eileen. "Eileen Mary Hickey: B.Sc., M.D.,
          D.P.H., F.R.C.P.I. 3 February 1960." Journal of the
          Medical Women's Federation, 42:2 (April 1960) 96-97.
          (Obituary.)
        Dr. Hickey received her M.D. degree in 1923 from Queen's
        University of Belfast. Details of her professional life are
        given herein.

422.   Canals, Dolores. "Manuela Solis, M.D.: The First Woman
          Doctor of Spain." Journal of the American Medical Wo-
          men's Association, 6:2 (February 1951) 61. port. (Al-
          bum of Women in Medicine.)
        The first Spanish woman to hold an official medical degree,
        Manuela Solis, born in Valencia in 1862, did postgraduate
        work under the great professors of her time in Paris: Pinard,
        Tarner, Varnier. When she went to Madrid with her husband,
        she experienced a good deal of prejudice which she overcame,
        and in 1906 she was elected a member of the Spanish Society
        of Gynecologists.

423.   Dangotte, C. ["The First Belgian Female Doctor: Isala van
          Diest (1842-1916)"]. Annales de la Société Belge d'His-
          torie Des Hopitaux, 5 (1967) 77-85. (Fre)
        Anne Catherine Albertine Isala Van Diest was born in Louvain,
        Belgium, the daughter of a doctor. She and her five sisters

and one brother all received the same education, an unusual circumstance for the times. After the death of the brother, Isala decided she wanted to be a doctor. She attended college in Berne, Switzerland, then returned to Louvain where she demanded admission to the medical school. When the rector offered her the opportunity to take only the physiology and midwifery courses, she returned to Berne and enrolled with 22 other women in the Faculty of Medicine there. The author notes that women were having better success in some other countries, citing Elizabeth Blackwell and Elizabeth Garrett who were both admitted to practice in England after studying in America. Van Diest received her diploma as doctor of medicine in 1877 with a thesis on a South American plant reputed to have medicinal properties. In 1880 the Free University at Brussels finally accepted women students, and in 1882-83 Van Diest registered for courses in surgery and obstetrics. She appeared on the list of practitioners for the Brussels district in 1884, continuing until 1903. She devoted much of her activity to social works, such as a society for public morality, the Belgian League for Women's Rights, and a home for "the repentant." Although she studied in a foreign country, she is considered the first Belgian woman doctor. The first woman graduate in medicine at Brussels was Clemence Everaert (in 1893), and the first at Ghent was Bertha DeVriese (in 1900).

424.   de Azevedo, Nair. "Domitila de Carvalho, M.D.: Physician-Poet of Portugal." Journal of the American Medical Women's Association, 6:7 (July 1951) 280. port. (Medical Women Around the World.)

Dr. Domitila de Carvalho's advanced studies were sponsored by Queen Amelia de Braganca, Queen of Portugal. Dr. de Carvalho graduated almost simultaneously in medicine, philosophy, and mathematics. During her career she introduced two bills which became law: one governing the admission of children to the cinema and the other providing for the teaching of hygiene and child care in all lyceums for women. She is a writer, a teacher, and a poet whose name had been chosen to be engraved on the Penedo da Saudade, "a place full of the traditions of Portugal's literary life."

425.   "Dr. Aletta Jacobs." Medical Woman's Journal, 45:6 (June 1938) 175.

Dr. Jacobs, the first woman to practice medicine in Holland, is profiled in this short article. (Her portrait appears on the front cover of this issue of the Journal.)

426.   "Dr. Alma Sundquist." Medical Woman's Journal, 46:2 (February 1939) 59.

A very brief biography profiles Dr. Sundquist, a noted Stockholm physician. (Her portrait is featured on the front cover of this issue of the Journal.)

427. "Dr. Dora Brucke-Teleky." Medical Woman's Journal, 44:10
        (October 1937) 291.
      Dr. Brucke-Teleky (whose portrait appears on the front cover
      of this issue of the Journal) was the first medical woman to
      be appointed assistant in the surgical clinic of Professor Ei-
      selberg in Vienna. She was also the first to be elected as a
      member of the scientific society, Gesellschaft der Aerzte, in
      Vienna. In addition, Dr. Brucke-Teleky founded the Vienna
      Medical Women's Association.

428. "Dr. G. Montreuil-Straus." Medical Woman's Journal, 45:
        10 (October 1938) 310.
      Germaine Montreuil-Straus founded the Committee for the
      Education of Women, a branch of the "French Society of San-
      itary and Moral Prophylactics." Shortly before this biogra-
      phy was written, Dr. Montreuil-Straus joined the Journal
      staff. (Her photograph appears on the front cover of this is-
      sue of the Journal.)

429. "Eugenia Delanoe, M.D." Medical Woman's Journal, 52:11
        (November 1945) 32, 54.
      Dr. Delanoe graduated in medicine from the University of
      Paris in 1910. In 1930 she became health officer for the
      French Protectorate hospital in Casablanca, Morocco, where
      she introduced smallpox vaccination.

430. ["A Female Physician in Vienna"]. Allg. Wiener Med. Ztg.,
        40 (1895) 488-489. (Ger)
      [Article not examined by editors.]

431. "The First Woman Police Physician in Vienna." Medical
        Woman's Journal, 36:6 (June 1929) 156.
      Dr. Helene Jokl was appointed first woman police physician
      in Vienna. Other firsts for women physicians in Viennese
      government posts are listed.

432. "Gladys M. Sandes, M.B., B.S., F.R.C.S." British Med-
        ical Journal, 1:5586 (27 January 1968) 255. port.
      (Obituary Notices.)

433. "Greek Doctor Receives Soroptimist Clubs Fellowship Award."
        Medical Woman's Journal, 56:9 (September 1949) 45.
      Among her other accomplishments in the field of psychiatry
      and neuropsychiatry, Dr. Dora Papara tested for the first
      time on humans, the effects of high-dosage hypertonic solu-
      tions injected in the veins. She performed this research
      while chief of the Women's and Children's Section of the
      Athens "Public Lunatic Asylum." Dr. Papara will study at
      the University of Pennsylvania Medical School.

434. Harlem, O. K. ["We Interview: Ida Nakling, General Prac-
        titioner, Strand"]. Tidsskrift for den Norske Laegefor-
        ening (Oslo), 84 (15 June 1964) 930-932. (Nor)
      [Article not examined by editors.]

435. Hayes, A. J., ed. <u>At Work: Letters of Marie Elizabeth</u>
      <u>Hayes, M. B. Missionary Doctor, Delhi, 1905-8.</u>
      Marshall Brothers Ltd., London, England, xii, 263 pp.
      maps, photos., port.
      Born in Ireland, Marie Elizabeth Hayes took her degree in
      the school of medicine connected with the Royal University.
      In addition to her residencies, she studied at the School of
      Tropical Medicine in London in preparation for work in India.
      At the time of her death in 1908 at the age of 33, Dr. Hayes
      had full charge of a mission hospital in Rewari, India. A
      ward in the St. Stephen's Hospital, Delhi, was named in her
      memory. This collection of Marie Hayes's letters, edited
      by her mother, also contains correspondence by Dr. Hayes's
      coworkers and a biographical foreword by G. R. Wynne,
      archdeacon of Aghadoe.

436. Heise, Agnete. "Alma Sundquist." <u>Kvinden og Samfundet,</u>
      56:2 (31 January 1940) 18. port. (Dan)
      Not only the women in the Swedish women's movement but
      women the world over will mourn the death of Alma Sund-
      quist. Born in 1872, she took her medical examinations in
      skin and venereal diseases. She served for a time as mu-
      nicipal venereologist and was a member of the commission
      on sex education. Despite her busy professional life, she
      found time to take a serious interest in the health and welfare
      of working women and to be active in the feminist movement.
      She was one of three physician representatives on the com-
      mittee of the first woman suffrage conference. In 1930 she
      was a member of a League of Nations commission, studying
      working conditions of women and children in the East. She
      was an active member of the Medical Women's International
      Association and its international president in 1934-1935. She
      also worked enthusiastically for full equality of women phy-
      sicians in Scandinavia.

437. "Honor Accorded a French Woman." <u>Medical Woman's Jour-</u>
      <u>nal,</u> 39:9 (September 1932) 230.
      M. Condat became, in 1923, the first woman in France to
      occupy the post of associate professor of medicine at the
      Faculté de Médecine de Toulouse. She was then appointed
      to the chair of therapeutics at that institution.

438. Hübsch, M. ["Dr. Pischinger"]. Österreichische Ärztezei-
      tung, 26:2 (25 January 1971) 155. (Ger)
      A brief obituary is presented of Dr. Olga Pischinger, who at
      the time of her death at 93 was one of the oldest physicians
      in Vienna.

439. Humpal-Zeman, Josephine. "Under the Kaiser." <u>Woman's</u>
      <u>Medical Journal,</u> 1:8 (August 1893) 164-165.
      The appointments of Drs. Anna Bayerova and Bohmuila Kec-
      tova as provincial physicians of Bosnia have advanced the
      hopes of women in medicine throughout the Austrian empire.

440. Hurd-Mead, Kate Campbell. "Doctoresse Legey of Maternité Indigène." Bulletin of the Medical Women's National Association, 24 (April 1929) 10.
At the time of this article, Dr. Legey was the pioneer woman physician in the French territories of Algeria and Morocco. Her accomplishments are cited.

441. Hurd-Mead, Kate Campbell. "Scandinavian Medical Women-- Then and Now: [Part 1]." Women in Medicine, 47 (January 1935) 16-19.
In the ancient graves of Scandinavian women are buried surgical instruments such as are not found in the graves of the men. In the Scandinavian literature are also found references to women serving as "surgeons, midwives, nurses, and makers of medicine." In Finland, it was 1870 before the first woman physician, a Russian named Mme. Chabanow [sic], was admitted to the medical school at Helsingfors. Today, ten per cent of the physicians in Finland are women. Denmark is treated more extensively in this article. In the 15th century, the University of Copenhagen was founded, and in 1875, the University opened its registry to women. Dr. Eli Moller [sic] was the first woman surgeon and obstetrician in Copenhagen. Dr. Marie Jorgensen-Krogh has done important work in metabolism. Dr. Estrid Hanses-Hein did work to "free her country from the curse of prostitution." Other important women physicians are mentioned. In Sweden, 1888 marked the date that Carolina Olivia Wiederstrom, the first woman doctor in this country, received her medical degree. She had a very successful practice in obstetrics and gynecology, and had a great interest in hygiene for women. Swedish physician Alma Sundquist, president of the International Association of Women, is a specialist in venereal diseases and sex hygiene.

442. Hurd-Mead, Kate C[ampbell]. "Scandinavian Medical Women --Then and Now (Continued)." Women in Medicine, 48 (April 1935) 15-16.
Norway is the final Scandinavian country discussed in this two-part report. In 1876, the first Norwegian university was open to women: today almost 10 per cent of each medical class are women. Helga Spangborg-Holth was the first woman to graduate from the medical school. Dr. Holth's areas of interest and special accomplishments are reviewed as well as those of other pioneer Norwegian medical women.

443. Irish Medical Association Journal, 34 (1954) 84. (Obituary Notice.)
An obituary notice is given for Dr. Dorothy Stopford Price. [Article not examined by editors.]

444. Irish Medical Association Journal, 37 (1955) 321. (Obituary Notice.)
An obituary notice is given for Dr. Kathleen Lynn. [Article not examined by editors.]

445.   Jacobs, Aletta H.   "Holland's Pioneer Woman Doctor."   Med-
        ical Woman's Journal, 35:9 (September 1928) 257-259.
        port.
        The first woman to study medicine in Holland, Aletta H.
        Jacobs obtained her degree in 1879 from the University of
        Groningen.   Dr. Jacobs was also "the first woman to inter-
        est herself in the conditions under which girls and women
        worked; the first to tackle the never-to-be-mentioned subject
        of prostitution; the first physician to establish a clinic for
        poor women, and the first to raise the issue of birth control.
        In addition, she led the women of Holland in the suffrage
        movement, and in the latter years of her life has worked
        equally hard for peace."

446.   Jadassohn, Werner.   ["Biography and Obituary: Aida Steiner-
        Wourlisch, M.D."].   Schweizerische Medizinische Wochen-
        schrift, 13:1 (2 January 1932) 16.   (Ger)
        This obituary for the 20th-century Swiss dermatologist, Aida
        Steiner-Wourlisch, recalls her training and especially her pro-
        fessional successes.   Dr. Wourlisch worked in particular in
        a campaign against venereal disease, an endeavor that called
        for numerous public speeches and other activities.   Her un-
        timely death at the age of 35 ended a very promising career.
        The article lists her scientific publications.

447.   Jelliffe, S. E.   "Madame Dejerine-Klumpke: 1859-1927."
        Bulletin of the New York Academy of Medicine [2nd se-
        ries], 4 (1928) 655-659.
        [Article not examined by editors.]

448.   Kalopothakes, Mary.   "Pioneer Medical Women in Greece."
        Bulletin of the Medical Women's National Association,
        42 (October 1933) 19-20.
        The work of the first woman to enter the Greek Medical
        School in the late 1800s is described.   Dr. Anthe Vassilaidon
        was appointed in 1902 as physician to the Woman's Prison,
        where she began a study of the prison psychology of women.
        Dr. Anna Katsigra devoted her career to school hygiene.
        She refused a lectureship in obstetrics in the University of
        Athens as she felt "the time not ripe for this step."   Dr.
        Vessalide Papgeorgion, another Greek pioneer medical wo-
        man, devoted herself to philanthropic organizations.   Dr.
        Angelique Panayotation was the first Greek woman graduated
        from the Medical School of the University of Athens.

449.   Landry, L. Thuillier.   "Dr. Dejerine Klumpke."   Medical
        Women's International Journal, 1:5 (November 1927) 47-
        48.   (Necrology.)   (Fre)
        The professional affiliations, honors, and writings of the emi-
        nent French neurologist Dr. Dejerine Klumpke are mentioned
        in this obituary.

450.   Lide, Frances.   "Belgian Doctor Receives Grant to Study

Here: Holds Fellowship at G. W. Hospital." <u>Medical</u>
<u>Woman's Journal,</u> 56:1 (January 1949) 63. port. (Notes
from the George Washington University.)
Dr. Eli Ann Hoebeke received a grant from the American
Association of University Women and is now a fellow in anesthesia at the George Washington University Hospital. Her experiences as a medical student in Belgium during the war are
described.

451. McKibben-Harper, Mary, ed. "Autobiography of Mary Ka-
      lopothakes, M. D. " <u>Bulletin of the Medical Women's Na-</u>
      <u>tional Association,</u> 42 (October 1933) 17-19.
Because the University of Athens would not allow women to
receive higher education in the early 1880s, Mary Kalopothakes went to Paris for her medical education. While she
was interested in anatomy, she specialized in children's diseases because that was the health care need in Greece. Dr.
Kalopothakes also founded the profession of nursing in Greece.
Active in public health work, she devoted special attention to
the prevention of tuberculosis. She also wrote a textbook for
school hygiene courses and edited a monthly journal, <u>Hygeia.</u>

452. <u>Madame Dejerine: 1859-1927.</u> Masson et Cie Editeurs,
      [Paris, France], 1929, 106 pp. photos. , ports. (Fre)
The publishers have collected in one volume a number of eulogies and obituaries of Augusta Dejerine-Klumpke, an outstanding neurologist, by her colleagues and former students.
They include a biography by Dr. André-Thomas (reprinted
from <u>Encephale</u>) , a eulogy given at a meeting of the French
Neurological Society by its president Gustave Roussy, three
eulogies given at her funeral, and 11 obituaries reprinted
from European and American journals, or presented at meetings of learned societies. Augusta Klumpke was born in San
Francisco, received her bachelor's degree at Lausanne, and
her medical training at Paris. She was the first woman extern and later the first woman intern in the hospitals of Paris.
She worked closely with her husband in research and writing
until his death in 1917, and continued her work alone and
with her daughter. She was a founding member and one-time
president of the French Neurological Society. With the help
of her daughter she established the Dejerine Foundation, with
a laboratory, library and museum which contain much of the
work of the husband and wife team. Neurologists the world
over mourn the loss of a personality rich in character and
in scientific achievement.

453. "A Memorial to Dr. Aletta Jacobs. " <u>Medical Woman's Jour-</u>
      <u>nal,</u> 38:9 (September 1931) 235.
A memorial dedicated to Aletta Jacobs, Holland's first woman physician and a leader of the suffrage movement, was
uncovered at the Westerveld, Holland, crematorium. Made
by a famous Dutch woman sculptor, the memorial shows the
figures of a woman and a man--Dr. Jacob's husband C. V.
Gerritsen--kneeling on the globe and holding a lighted torch.

454.   Michel, Auguste Marie. A Mutilated Life Story: Strange
            Fragments of an Autobiography. Sketches of Experiences
            as a Nurse and Doctor in an African Hospital, and in the
            American West. Published by Auguste Marie Michel,
            Chicago, Illinois, 1911, iii, 171 pp.
        Auguste Marie Michel, M.D., begins her autobiography by
        telling her experiences in Africa as a missionary nurse in
        the 1890s. Another chapter reprints a letter to President
        McKinley, in which she volunteered as a physician in the
        Spanish-American War. In this letter she describes herself
        as "perfectly fearless ... with the strength and build of a
        Venus," and "completely immune from all diseases." The
        largest part of the book consists of an account of a suit
        brought by Michel against an express company, which she ac-
        cused of stealing her autobiography. A third section is de-
        voted to short pieces espousing universal suffrage, praising
        the workers, and decrying the evils of capitalism. Several
        of her poems also appear. A short foreword gives details
        of her upbringing in France, her education at the National
        Medical University of Chicago, and her marriage. There is
        neither index nor bibliography.

455.   Montreuil-Straus, G. "Two Medical Women in Morocco."
            Medical Woman's Journal, 45:10 (October 1938) 287-294.
            photo.
        At its last annual banquet, the Association Française des
        Femmes Médecins heard the "story of the interesting and
        lively experiences of Mademoiselle Broido." Large extracts
        from her account of her medical career in Morocco form the
        major portion of this article. Another French physician who
        served in Morocco was Française Entz Legey, who died in
        1935. Dr. Legey's adventures and professional activities are
        also detailed.

456.   Nilsson, Ada. [Glimpses from My Life as a Doctor]. Natur
            Och Kultur, Stockholm, Sweden, 1963, 173 pp. photos.,
            ports. (Swe)
        In this anecdotal autobiography of one of Sweden's early wo-
        men doctors, Dr. Nilsson talks of her childhood, her early
        education and determination to be a doctor, her friends, her
        medical education and training, her practice, and some of
        her travels. She was active in women's rights and in the
        radical movements of the early 20th century and was a friend
        of some of the women radicals of the period, as well as of
        other celebrated women. An example is Alexandra Kollontay,
        the first accredited woman diplomatic representative from one
        country to another, minister from the Soviet Union to Norway
        in 1923 to 1925 and to Sweden from 1930 to 1945. Nilsson
        continued to practice until she was past 80, when she was
        forced by progressive blindness to retire. The book has no
        index.

457.   Pirami, Edmea. "An 18th Century Woman Physician."

World Medical Journal, 12 (1965) 154-155. port.
Maria Dalle [sic] Donne (1778-1842) "was the first woman in
the world to graduate in medicine and get a doctorate, which
she obtained in the University of Bologna."

458. Price, Mary C. "Rachel Ethel Bamford, J.P.: B.A., M.B.,
    B. Ch., B.A.O. Belfast. 25 September 1958." Journal
    of the Medical Women's Federation, 41:2 (April 1959)
    106. (Obituary.)
Dr. Bamford studied medicine at Queen's University, Belfast,
Ireland and received her M.B., B.Ch. in 1922.

459. "Queen Amelie of Portugal." Woman's Medical Journal, 16:
    3 (March 1906) 47. port.
A caption under Queen Amelie's portrait notes that she--a
doctor of medicine--will serve as honorary president of the
[1906] international medical congress.

460. Regnault, Paule and Stephenson, Kathryn L. "Dr. Suzanne
    Noël: The First Woman to Do Esthetic Surgery." Plas-
    tic and Reconstructive Surgery, 48:2 (August 1971) 133-
    138. illus., port.
Born in 1878, Suzanne Blanche Marguerite Gros Pertet Noël
received an M.D. from the Faculty of Medicine of Paris and
passed the "Internat des Hôpitaux de Paris" examinations in
1913. Following her second husband's death, she became an
ardent feminist, fighting for the franchise and women's
rights. She founded the first European chapter of the Soroptimist Association. In 1928 she received the "Légion d'hon-
neur" for her war contributions. The authors of her biography recall Dr. Noël's personality and describe her surgical
techniques. Dr. Noël, who herself had many face-lifts,
stressed the importance of physical appearance on the personality and "the value of fighting against the ugliness of age
to give one moral strength and confidence." This philosophy
is discussed in her first book, La Chirurgie Esthétique, Son
Rôle Social, published in 1926.

460a. Roussy, Gustave. [Eulogy of Madame Dejerine-Klumpke:
    1859-1927]. Printed by Imprimerie Lahure, Paris,
    France, 1928, 21 pp. port. (Fre)
"Remarks presented at the meeting of the Society of Neurology of Paris on 1 December 1927 by Professor Gustave Roussy, President of the Society." Mme. Dejerine, born Augusta
Klumpke in San Francisco and educated in Europe, is eulo-
gized as one of the great figures of modern neurology, one
of the founding members and most active workers of the
Neurological Society and its president during the war, and a
woman "of great learning and infinite goodness." She received her bachelor's degree at Lausanne and her medical
degree at Paris. She was the first woman extern (1882) and
intern (1886) at the Paris hospitals. She and her husband
worked so closely together that it is often impossible to iden-

tify their individual contributions to their many research projects and publications. With her daughter she established in
1920 a foundation--with laboratory, library, and museum of
neurology--in the Faculty of Medicine. She later established
a fund with the Society of Neurology for the encouragement of
original research in the field of neurology. This eulogy contains no index or bibliography.

461.   Ruys, A. Charlotte. "Pioneer Medical Women in the Nether-
        lands." Journal of the American Medical Women's Asso-
        ciation, 7:3 (March 1952) 99-101. ports.
        Dr. Aletta Henrietta Jacobs was the first woman physician in
        the Netherlands (c. 1878). She was militantly active in work-
        ing with the poor, with women's rights, and women's suffrage
        (which began in 1919 in the Netherlands). Other pioneer wo-
        men in the Netherlands are also discussed briefly.

462.   Satran, Richard. "Augusta Dejerine-Klumpke: First Woman
        Intern in Paris Hospitals." Annals of Internal Medicine,
        80:2 (February 1974) 260-264. port. (History of Medi-
        cine.)
        Born in 1859 in San Francisco, Augusta Dejerine-Klumpke
        lived most of her life in France and died in Paris in 1929.
        While a medical student at the Faculty of Medicine in Paris,
        she became the first to describe and elucidate mechanisms of
        lower brachial plexus palsy ("Klumpke palsy"). This biogra-
        phy also describes her struggles to secure an externship, and
        ultimately the first woman's internship, in the hospitals of
        Paris.

463.   Schnabel, Ilse. "Medical Practice Around the World: Pio-
        neer Medical Women of Switzerland." Journal of the
        American Medical Women's Association, 8:7 (July 1953)
        246-247. ports.
        Two Swiss women doctors, Drs. Anna Heer and Marie Hein-
        Vögtlin, and a nurse, Oberin Ida Schneider, founded the
        Schweizerische Pflegerinnenschule und Krankenhaus (Swiss
        school for nurses and hospital) in Zurich. Brief biographies
        of the lives of the doctors are given.

464.   Selvini, Mara. "Maria Montessori, M. D." Journal of the
        American Medical Women's Association, 7:2 (February
        1952) 64. (Medical Women Around the World.)
        Dr. Montessori took her medical degree at the University of
        Rome and began work in the education of abnormal children.
        Her methods were employed with normal children with the
        same "brilliant" results. Since 1931, International Con-
        gresses of Montessori Studies have been held annually.

465.   Selvini, Mara Palazzoli. "Myra Carcupino Ferrari, M. D."
        Journal of the American Medical Women's Association,
        12:2 (February 1957) 60. port. (Album of Women in
        Medicine.)

Founder (c. 1921) and president of the Italian Association of
Women Doctors, Myra Carcupino Ferrari held professional
positions in several welfare organizations.

466. Selvini, Mara Palazzoli. "Piera Locatelli, M. D." Journal
of the American Medical Women's Association, 8:7 (July
1953) 250. port. (Medical Women Around the World.)
Dr. Locatelli received her medical degree in 1924 from the
University of Pavia. Her work has been done in the field
of neurology, and in 1926 she received the Lallemand Prize
from the Academy of Science in Paris for her studies "in the
influence of the nervous system on the regeneration of organs
and tissues in animals of different species."

467. Sheppard, Amy and Ramsay, Mabel. "Florence Ada Stoney,
O. B. E. , M. D. , B. S. Lond. , D. M. R. E. Camb." Medical
Women's Federation News-Letter, (January 1933) 64-66.
(Obituary.)

468. Siebel, Johanna. [The Life of Dr. Marie Heim-Vögtlin, the
First Swiss Woman Physician: 1845-1916]. Rascher &
Cie. , Zurich, Switzerland, 1919, 275 pp. photos. , ports.
(Ger)
Marie Heim-Vögtlin was the first woman medical student of
Swiss birth, the first woman in Switzerland to receive a doctor's degree, and the first European woman to go through the
same education and examinations as male students to achieve
the doctorate. She was born on 7 October 1845, the daughter
of a pastor in the village of Boezen. After considerable struggle with ill health, with her family, and with public opinion,
she entered the medical courses at Zurich in 1868 and was
licensed in January 1873. The next year she defended her
dissertation and received her doctor of medicine degree. She
was married in 1875 to Albert Heim, a professor of geology.
Her favorite and first child, a son, was born in 1882, and a
daughter in 1886. Dr. Heim-Vögtlin maintained a busy practice throughout these years, as her interests in child care
became stronger. She was instrumental in the founding of a
woman's hospital and nursing school in 1899, and devoted
much of her time to the infant department. Through this she
became interested in the problems of adoption, as well as of
the family and home. She was active in the temperance movement for many years. She died in 1916, after a long illness.

469. Sorrel-Dejerine, Y. "Madame Dejerine Klumpke." Presse
Med. , 62:2 (1959) 1997-1999.
[Article not examined by editors.]

470. Steppanen, Anni. "Finland." Medical Woman's Journal, 55:
9 (September 1948) 26-29.
Dr. Steppanen, of Helsinki, tells of her experiences in Finland during the war. While admitting that "physicians rarely
understand high politics," she offers her opinion of the events
in her country during the past decade.

471. Svartz, Nanna. [Step by Step: An Autobiography]. Albert
      Bonniers, Stockholm, Sweden, 1968, 257 pp. photos.,
      ports. (Swe)
      This informal autobiography contains many anecdotes about
      Svartz's family, her travels, friends, and work. She was
      born in 1890 and started her medical studies in 1911 in a
      class of 16 men and two women. She defended her doctoral
      thesis, on anaerobic infections, in 1927. Her interests in-
      cluded infectious diseases and antibacterial agents, rheuma-
      tology, and especially bacteriology and immunology. She
      traveled to most of Europe--as well as Russia, the U.S. and
      Canada--to international congresses, and on visits to clinics
      and laboratories. Included in the book are her memories of
      the famous scientists she met and worked with, and some of
      the interesting patients she treated. The book contains no
      subject index, but does include a name index.

472. Vilar, Lola. Woman and Physician. Valencia, Spain, 1972,
      95 pp.
      Lola Vilar, a Spanish physician, headed the Spanish Associa-
      tion of Women Doctors. This booklet is a collection of her
      writings--poems, meditations, and essays on professional,
      social, and personal issues as perceived by her. Dr. Vilar
      collected them for presentation to her colleagues in the Span-
      ish Association of Women Doctors. Included in the book are
      poems and essays about women physicians (one essay is dedi-
      cated to Esther Pohl Lovejoy, another profiles Dr. Fe del
      Mundo, and others salute women medical missionaries). This
      English translation, encouraged by members of the Medical
      Women's International Association, contains frequent errors
      in spelling and grammar.

473. Widerström, Karolina. "Anna Stecksén." Dagny (1904) 375-
      377. (Obituary.) (Swe)

474. Widerström, Karolina. ["Memories of Dr. Anna Stecksén"].
      Svenska Lakaresallskapets Forhandlingar, 18:10 (1904)
      275-277. (Swe)
      A eulogy for Dr. Stecksén was presented by Dr. Widerström
      at the October 18 meeting of the [Swedish Medical?] Society.
      Anna Stecksén, born in 1870 in Stockholm, passed the med-
      ical candidate examination in 1893 and was licensed in 1897.
      After three years of additional study in Stockholm and abroad
      she presented her thesis on "Curtis' Blastomycete" and was
      granted a doctoral degree in 1900. She was deeply interested
      in the pathogenesis of cancer and did considerable research
      on the possibility of an infectious cause. Unfortunately, dur-
      ing her laboratory work she picked up an infection which first
      took the form of an acute otitis, then later, after she had re-
      turned to work, reappeared as endocarditis. During her ill-
      ness she was able to continue her research at times with her
      normal energy, but the illness cut short her promising career
      in October 1904.

475.   ["A Woman Doctor in Vienna"]. <u>Allgemeine Wiener Medizin-</u>
          <u>ische Zeitung</u>, 40 (1895) 488-489. (Ger)
       A news item from the Institute for Officers' Daughters in
       Hernels (Austria) announces that as of the beginning of the
       current school year a woman physician has been performing
       medical services for the students there. Georgine von Roth,
       daughter of a deceased field-marshall-lieutenant, studied med-
       icine and passed her qualifying examinations in Bern, Swit-
       zerland. The editorial writer comments that von Roth was
       originally appointed to teach natural sciences and to act as
       assistant director, and the duties of staff physician have been
       added; her foreign diploma has not yet been accepted for prac-
       tice in Vienna. Her appointment will add pressure for the
       solution of the question of legal recognition of women doctors.

476.   "The Work of Dr. Maria Montessori." <u>Woman's Medical</u>
          <u>Journal</u>, 21:9 (September 1911) 205.
       Maria Montessori was the first woman to receive a medical
       degree from the University of Rome. Her work in pedagog-
       ical psychology is the subject of this article.

GERMANY

477.   Biermer, Leopold. "Käthe Heinemann." <u>Nachrichtenbl. Dt.</u>
          <u>ges. Gesch. Med. Naturwiss. Technik.</u>, 22:2 (1972) 41-
          <u>42.</u> (Ger)
       Born in 1889 in Frankenberg, Käthe Heinemann studied in
       mathematics, physics, chemistry, mineralogy, botanics, and
       zoology and obtained a doctorate in pedagogy in 1922. She
       then worked in Breslau and Kassel but was dismissed in 1933
       for opposition to the national socialist regime. Although she
       studied medicine in Göttingen and passed the exams, the di-
       ploma and licensure were denied her. She therefore worked
       as a private assistant in pathology in Freiburg. In 1945 she
       became chief of internal medicine in the Kassel City Hospital
       and in 1948 she became director of the Institute of Pathology.
       She published several articles on medical history. After her
       retirement in 1954 she lived in Kassel, where she died on
       May 6, 1972.

478.   Boedeker, Elisabeth and Mayer-Plath, Maria. [<u>Fifty Years</u>
          <u>of Women's Appointments to Academic Positions in Ger-</u>
          <u>many: A Documentation of the Period 1920-1970</u>]. Ver-
          <u>lag Otto Schwartz & Co.</u>, Göttingen, Germany, 1974, xii,
          387 pp. (Ger)
       This is a listing, divided into prewar Germany-Federal Re-
       public and East Germany (DDR), of women who, after obtain-
       ing their doctorates, have taken higher examinations and be-
       come "dozents"--assistant professors in universities. Listings
       are by subject field, e.g., archeology, mathematics, medicine,
       philosophy. For each woman, data given include date and
       place of birth; address (if still in Germany) or date of emi-

gration or death (if not) ; date, place, and title of doctoral
dissertation; date, place, and title of inaugural dissertation;
teaching and other positions held; field(s) of specialization;
monographs and other publications; memberships and honors.
The chapters on medicine contain 91 names for Germany-
Federal Republic and 49 names for the DDR. Also included
are an overall statistical summary, a list of women dozents
who emigrated for political or racial reasons between 1932
and 1945, a combined name index to the total listing, a bibliography, and lists of East and West German universities and
technical universities. This book was sponsored by the German Association of University Women, the Federal Ministry
of the Interior (Women Section) , the Federal Ministry of Education and Science, and the German Science Writers' Association, Inc. A foreword is by Professor Werner Poels,
president of the College Association (Hochschulverband) . Dr.
Elisabeth Schwarzhaupt, chairman of the German Association
of University Women, wrote the introduction.

479. Dettelbacher, Werner. ["Josepha von Siebold and Her Daughter Charlotte--the First Women Obstetricians in Germany"
Münchener Medizinische Wochenschrift, 114:16 (April
1972) 788-791. facsims., port. (Ger)
Josepha Henning, born in Geismar (Eichsfeld) in 1771, was
trained in Goettingen and Duderstadt to manage her uncle's
large agricultural estates. At 22, Josepha married the physician Damian Siebold, with whom she worked as a midwife
and assistant, as the medical profession strictly excluded women from medical practice other than midwifery and kitchen-
help. (The only German woman to obtain her medical degree
in the 18th century, Dorothea Christiane Leporin, could only
do so with special permission by Frederic II of Prussia.)
When Damian Siebold became incapable of continuing his medical practice for mental reasons, Josepha began to study obstetrics in Wuerzburg, under her brother-in-law, Elias von
Siebold. In 1807, she obtained permission to practice obstetrics and pox vaccination from the Archducal Medical College
in Darmstadt and began an extensive country practice. In
1815, she was given the honorary doctorate in obstetrics by
the University of Giessen, the first woman in the history of
German universities to be granted this title. She carried on
a large and charitable practice until her death in 1849. Her
daughter, Charlotte Heidenreich-von Siebold, obtained her medical degree from Giessen University after successfully defend-
ing her thesis on ectopic pregnancy. She worked in Darmstadt and Giessen; like her mother, she was involved in charitable practice. In the spirit of her work, the women of
Darmstadt created the Heidenreich-von Siebold Foundation for
indigent expectant mothers which was continued until 1948.

480. Heusler-Edenhvizen, Hermine. "A Pioneer Woman Doctor in
Germany: Dr. Franziska Tiburtius." Medical Women's
International Journal, 1:5 (November 1927) 8-10.

Germany's first woman physician, Franziska Tiburtius, died
in May, 1927 at the age of 84. Dr. Tiburtius and her friend
and colleague Dr. Emilie Lehmus founded a polyclinic for
poor women in Berlin, and later, a nursing home for women.
Quotes excerpted from Dr. Tiburtius's autobiography are included in this obituary.

481.   Kashade, R.   ["Charlotte Heidenreich-von Siebold, Germany's
          First Woman Obstetrician"].   Janus, 42 (1938) 185-188.
          (Ger)
       Born in 1788 as the daughter of Josepha von Siebold, the first
       woman to obtain an honorary doctorate in obstetrics, Charlotte
       studied medicine in Goettingen and later in Giessen and re-
       ceived her medical degree in Darmstadt in 1814.   To obtain
       the degree of doctor of medicine she applied to Giessen Uni-
       versity, and was granted the right to defend her thesis in
       obstetrics on March 26, 1817.   The decision was preceded
       by some dispute as to whether a woman should be admitted
       at all, and if the traditional form of a public defense of the
       doctorate thesis should be used for women.   By insisting on
       the traditional procedure, Charlotte von Siebold created an
       important precedent for women medical doctors.   She became
       a very famous obstetrician and worked with many noblewomen.
       She also treated the poor, and after her death in 1859, the
       Charlotte Heidenreich-von Siebold Foundation was formed in
       commemoration of her services to the indigent.

482.   Köhnecke, Ingeborg.   ["No Dormitory for the Emancipated.
          Seventy-five Years of Female Medical Studies.   A Pio-
          neer: Dr. Franziska Tiburtius"].   Deutsches Arzteblatt,
          49 (6 December 1973) 3402-3406.   photo.   (Ger)
       This article is a brief biography of Dr. Franziska Tiburtius,
       written in commemoration of the 75th year after women were
       admitted to university studies in Germany.   The author de-
       scribes the hardships endured by Franziska Tiburtius and her
       colleague Emilie Lehmus because of their pioneer role as fe-
       male physicians.   The influence Tiburtius had on the future
       development of women's acceptance to professional life is
       stressed.

483.   Krüger, Gisela.   [The Importance of Charlotte Heiland, Called
          von Siebold, for Obstetrics in Her Time].   University of
          Berlin, Berlin, Germany, 1969.   (M. D. thesis.)   (Ger)
       After a short introduction to women's education, this thesis
       concentrates on the life and work of the 19th-century female
       physician Charlotte Heiland.   The book then extensively dis-
       cusses the merits of Heiland's medical thesis on ectopic
       pregnancies and quotes contemporary views of her work.
       There is a bibliography.

484.   Lange, Helene.   ["Our First Female Physicians"].   In:
          [Times of Struggle: Essays and Speeches of Four Dec-
          ades], 2 vol., Berlin, Germany, 1928.   (Ger)

As a co-founder of special high school courses for women, the author describes the success of two of her students who obtained medical degrees: Else von der Leyen and Irma Klausner. They were the first German women to obtain a medical degree from a German university after having undergone the same preparatory and medical training as their male colleagues. Although they both had a recognized high school diploma, the two women encountered considerable resistance when they wanted to register in medical school. But with the support of the women's movement, they successfully concluded their studies. In the view of the author, every woman at the university is a success of the women's movement. [This article first appeared in Die Frau, August, 1900.]

485.   La Roe, Else K.   Woman Surgeon: The Autobiography of Else
            K. La Roe, M.D.   Dial Press, New York, New York,
            1957, 373 pp.
In this autobiographical account, Dr. La Roe begins by relating incidents from her life in Germany which set her on the track of medicine. She continues to tell of wartime experiences, when she found herself playing hostess to Joseph Goebbels and Hermann Goering. Throughout the book, Dr. La Roe tells her story by means of the people she knew and the events which gave them their context--from her childhood in Heidenheim, Germany through the days of her Manhattan, New York medical practice. Dr. La Roe fills the pages of her book with case histories reflecting her life as a plastic surgeon. She covers such topics as her experiences with cancer patients, homosexuality, intersex, war victims, and women patients, per se.

486.   Lauer, Hans H.   ["Two Courageous Women for their Period:
            Josepha von Siebold and Her Daughter Charlotte Heiden-
            reich-von Siebold"].   Medizinscher Monatsspiegel, 2 (1966)
            29-31.   facsim., ports.   (Ger)
In this account of the lives of Josepha von Siebold and her daughter Charlotte Heidenreich von Siebold, the author emphasizes their professional work and their publications. He gives some insight into the training and the private life of Josepha von Siebold and shows the difficulties she encountered in obtaining payment for her work in pox vaccination. The author describes the studies of Charlotte Heidenreich in Goettingen and Giessen and her very successful obstetrical practice.

487.   Moenckeberg, A.   ["A German 'Hakima' in Yemen: A Diary"].
            Medizinische Klinik (Munchen), 58 (22 March 1963) 483-
            488.   (Ger)
[Article not examined by editors.]

488.   Platzer, Elisabeth.   ["Life Portrait: For the 80th Birthday
            of Dr. Ilse Szagunn"].   Müchener Medizinische Wochen-
            schrift, 109:37 (15 September 1967) 1914-1915.   port.
            (Ger)

Dr. Ilse Szagunn (née Tesch) was born on 16 September 1887 and even as a child had determined to become a doctor. Because women were not allowed to matriculate in medicine in Prussia, she started her medical studies in Heidelberg in 1908. Even after women were permitted in the school at Berlin, they had to take private courses--in anatomy, for example, because Professor Waldeyer refused to accept them in his classes. Ilse Tesch passed the state medical examination in 1913 and shortly thereafter married Walter Szagunn, a lawyer. Dr. Szagunn's primary professional interests have always been in the socio-medical problems, such as mother and child care, school medicine, and social welfare; she was a pioneer as a vocational school physician. Her activities as author, editor, and speaker have been concerned mostly with the health and welfare of the young, of women and especially of mothers. She was a member of the Prussian state board of health from 1921 to 1933. In 1945 she opened a medical practice in Berlin, in which she is still active. She was a founder of the German Society of University Women and is an honorary member of the German Society of Women Physicians and the Berlin Medical Society.

489. Schaefer, Romanus Johannes. ["Dr. Charlotte Heidenreich von Siebold, nee Heiland. In Commemoration of Her 150th Birthday: September 12, 1938"]. Munchener Medizinische Wochenschrift, 85:36 (9 September 1938) 1393-1397. port. (Ger)

Regina Josefa (Henning), widow of Georg Heiland, married the physician Johann Theodor Damian von Siebold in 1795. She studied obstetrics with her father-in-law and brother-in-law and in 1807 was authorized to practice obstetrics; in 1813 she was certified for the practice of obstetrics, vaccination, and as a teaching associate to her husband. In 1815 she was awarded the diploma of Doctor of Obstetric Arts honoris causae by the University of Giessen. Her daughter from her first marriage, Charlotte Heiland, who was adopted by von Siebold, began her instruction in anatomy, physiology, and midwifery. Charlotte was awarded a doctoral degree in obstetrics at Giessen in 1817, with a thesis on extrauterine pregnancy based on a case which she had helped treat. She built up a large practice in Darmstadt, assisted at the birth of the future Duke Ernst of Saxe-Coburg-Gotha in 1818 and of the future Queen Victoria in London in 1819, and consulted on the care of various pregnant princesses. She married a military surgeon, Dr. Andreas August Heidenreich, in 1829 and continued her practice and interest in maternity care until her death on July 8, 1859, at the age of 71.

490. Schmidt-Schütt, Margarete. [Doctor in Haiti]. Herbig, Berlin, Germany, 1942, 303 pp. photos. (Ger)

As an autobiography covering the three years of Dr. Schmidt-Schütt's life in Haiti (1923-1926), the book concentrates on the delivery of medical care in Haiti. The author worked as a primary care physician in Haiti and gives interesting accounts of her personal contacts with the population. She is acutely aware of the cultural differences between her and her patients and describes the numerous communication problems. In a chapter on medical experiences, she describes some of the common tropical diseases in Haiti and discusses several treatments and medications. She is equally interested in the influence of tropical climates on Europeans who work there and discusses her own experiences and studies on the subject. Photographs show hospital facilities and some landscape views.

491. Schönfeld, Walther. ["Franziska Tiburtius (1843-1927)"]. Pommersche Lebensbilder, 2 (1936) 296-301. port. (Ger)

Franziska Tiburtius and Emilie Lehmus, the first German women doctors certified in Zurich, settled in Berlin in 1876 without official permission--a truly revolutionary step for the time. Tiburtius was born in 1843 on the island of Ruegel. After finishing school, she taught in private families for several years, part of her plan to become a teacher and open a school in her home town. Later, while teaching in England, she became interested in medicine; an older brother was a doctor and his wife had been the first woman dentist in Berlin. She enrolled in the medical school in Zurich in 1871, and after graduation she and Lehmus set up practice in Berlin, although the city had denied both certification. In spite of ridicule, they stayed in the city and in 1878 founded the first polyclinic for women. Tiburtius continued in practice until 1907, when she retired but remained in Berlin. She died in 1927 in the women doctors' clinic to which she had devoted so much of her work.

492. Tiburtius, Franziska. [Memories of an Octogenarian]. C. A. Schwelschke and Sohn, Berlin, Germany, 1925, 223 pp. port. (Ger)

In this autobiography by the 19th-century German woman physician, Franziska Tiburtius, the author briefly describes her childhood in Northern Germany and her years in England where she worked as a governess. Writing about her years as a medical student in Zurich, where she was among the first women to be admitted to medical studies, she illustrates the tensions and the help and friendship of many professors and fellow students with anecdotes and letters. She then extensively narrates her work in Berlin where she founded a free women's clinic with her fellow student, [Emilie] Lehmus, and ran an extensive private practice. Throughout the book, the author analyzes the various problems and the gratifications of her contemporaries who, as women physicians, were pioneers in an almost exclusively male field.

GREAT BRITAIN

493. Acres, E. Louis. <u>Helen Hanson. A Memoir.</u> H. R. Allen-
      son, Ltd., London, England, 1928, 118 pp.
      Dr. Sybil Pratt writes about this book: "Mrs. Marston Acres,
      in her Memoir of Dr. Helen Hanson, gives us a vivid and sym-
      pathetic account of one to whom was indeed granted her heart's
      desire. No one who knew Helen Hanson could imagine her
      serving with anything less than her fullest capacity all the
      numerous and varied loyalties which claimed her allegiance.
      It was no easy task which confronted Mrs. Acres, when she
      set out, as she says herself, 'to visualize the Daughter, the
      Friend, the Christian, the Traveller, the Medical Woman in
      the hospital and the school, the Doctor on war service and
      the Suffragist.' ... As with so many women who enter the
      medical profession, the training was but a means to an end,
      and, as Mrs. Acres says, Helen Hanson's 'burning desire for
      service made her spread her energies over many departments in
      life instead of concentrating them on intensive work in one field.'
      'The Woman's Question,' we are told, 'was never far from her
      mind,' and yet it never became an obsession. The unlimited op-
      portunities for surgical experience to be gained in India filled
      her with enthusiasm...." [Book not examined by editors.]

494. Adamson, R. H. B. "Florence Stacey-Cleminson, M. B.,
      B. S. Lond." <u>Medical Women's Federation Quarterly Re-
      view,</u> (July 1935) 59-60. (Obituary.)

495. Aitken, Janet and Kennedy, Agnes. "Eve Attkins. M. B.
      B. E." <u>Journal of the Medical Women's Federation,</u> 45:
      4 (October 1963) 235-236. (Obituary.)

496. Anderson, Louisa Garrett. <u>Elizabeth Garrett Anderson:
      1836-1917.</u> Faber and Faber Limited, London, England,
      1939, 338 pp. photo., ports.
      This biography of Elizabeth Garrett Anderson, by her daugh-
      ter Louisa, mixes Dr. Garrett Anderson's personal and pro-
      fessional life from youth through retirement with the history
      of women in Great Britain during her lifetime. Dr. Garrett
      Anderson began her medical training at the Middlesex Hospital
      in London; but refused admission to formal education at Mid-
      dlesex, Oxford, Cambridge, and London, she studied private-
      ly, and finally was listed on the medical register as an
      L. S. A., having passed the apothecaries examination. She
      opened the St. Mary's Dispensary for Women in 1866. This
      later became the New Hospital for Women and Children, and
      finally was named the Elizabeth Garrett Anderson Hospital.
      In 1870, she obtained her M. D. from the University of Paris.
      Dr. Garrett Anderson was active in supporting admission of
      women to the University of Edinburgh. In 1883 she became
      Dean of the London School of Medicine for Women and held
      that office for 20 years. She then became president of the
      school, serving until her death in 1917. This biography in-
      cludes appendices of selected names and numbers of women

on the medical register in the late nineteenth century, and
enrollment figures for the London School of Medicine from
1887 to 1917. There are also biographical notes on persons
mentioned in the book, as well as an index and bibliography.

497.   Anderson, Olive M. "Elizabeth Garrett Anderson and Her
            Contemporaries." Journal of the Medical Women's Fed-
            eration, 40:3 (July 1958) 167-179. (Address, Ulster
            Medical Society, 21 November 1957.)
        Biographical sketches are presented of Elizabeth Garrett An-
        derson, Elizabeth Blackwell, and Sophia Jex-Blake. [This
        article also appears in the Ulster Medical Journal, 27 (1957)
        97-107.]

498.   Andrews, Mabel L. V. "Reminiscences of My Return to Med
            ical Work." Journal of the Medical Women's Federation,
            43:3 (July 1961) 126-127.
        This account by Dr. Andrews recalls her experience in re-
        turning to work after her marriage and the birth of two chil-
        dren forced her to leave medical practice. Dr. Andrews
        tells of her doubts and fears after having been away from
        hospital ward work for 18 years. "Looking back I realize
        how helpful it would have been to all concerned if some fa-
        cilities could have been available in the way of a refresher
        course to help to bring me up to date before returning to
        medicine."

499.   "Anna Broman, M. R. C. S., L. R. C. P." Journal of the Med-
            ical Women's Federation, 44:3 (July 1962) 129-130.
            (Obituary.)

500.   Baker, A. H. "Elizabeth Bolton: C. E. B., M. D." Journal
            of the Medical Women's Federation, 43:3 (April 1961)
            138-139. port. (Obituary.)
        Dr. Bolton was dean of the Medical School of the Royal Free
        Hospital from 1931 to 1945. She was educated at the London
        School of Medicine for Women and qualified in 1904 from the
        Royal Free Hospital.

501.   Balfour, Frances. Dr. Elsie Inglis. Hodder and Stoughton,
            London, England, [n.d.], 253 pp. ports.
        This biography of Elsie Inglis (1864-1917) tells of her up-
        bringing in India, Edinburgh, and Paris, and her medical
        education at the Edinburgh School of Medicine for Women
        (where women were not admitted to clinical work in the hos-
        pital except in two special women's wards). In Glasgow,
        wanting to study surgery, she fought for and won the right
        to attend classes with men. After her qualification in 1892
        she was house-surgeon in the New Hospital for Women in
        London; many of her letters dealing with conditions there
        are printed. Other letters support suffrage, advocate women
        as sanitary inspectors, etc. Later she practiced in Edin-
        burgh, where she obtained an M. D. (in 1899) when the Uni-

versity of Edinburgh finally admitted women to its examinations for degrees. She founded the Elsie Inglis Hospital, the
only maternity center run by women in Scotland. During
World War I she founded and led the Scottish Women's Hospitals in Serbia and Yugoslavia, and in Russia in 1917. There
is no index or bibliography.

502.   Balfour, M. I. "Elizabeth Bielby, M.D." Medical Women's
         Federation News-Letter, (November 1929) 56-58. (Obitu-
         ary.)

503.   Barclay, E. R. "Lilian Enid Watney, M.B., B.S. (Lond.)."
         Medical Women's Federation News-Letter, (January 1934)
         75-76. (Obituary.)
         Dr. Watney worked as a physician in China.

504.   Barrett, Florence E. and Berry, F. May Dickinson. "Dame
         Mary Scharlieb, D.B.E., J.P., M.D., M.S." Medical
         Women's Federation News-Letter, (November 1930) 71-
         76. (Obituary.)

505.   Bartley, Eileen. "Winifred Eileen Hadden: M.D., D.P.H.
         6 May 1960." Journal of the Medical Women's Federa-
         tion, 42A:3 (July 1960) 148-149. (Obituary.)
         Facts of both Dr. Hadden's personal and professional life are
         mixed in this brief obituary notice.

506.   Benson, Annette M. "Margaret Lamont, M.B., B.S. (Lond.),
         D.P.H. (Camb.)" Medical Women's Federation News-
         Letter, (January 1932) 65-66. (Obituary.)

507.   Bernard, Marcelle. "Catherine Chisholm, C.B.E., M.D.
         (Manchester), Hon. F.R.C.P." Journal of the Ameri-
         can Medical Women's Association, 8:6 (June 1953) 209.
         port. (Album of Women in Medicine.)
         Founder of the Duchess of York Hospital for Babies, Man-
         chester, England, Catherine Chisholm was the first woman
         to enter and, in 1904, to graduate from the Manchester Uni-
         versity School of Medicine, as well as the first woman gen-
         eral practitioner in that city. For postgraduate work she
         went to the United States and wrote a thesis on menstruation
         in adolescent girls. She was a founder of the British Med-
         ical Women's Federation and from 1928 to 1929 was president
         of this group. She worked hard to extend suffrage to women,
         and to promote the right of married women to work.

508.   Berry, (Lady). "Anaesthetic Reminiscences." Medical Wo-
         men's Federation News-Letter, (March 1928) 17-24.
         Relating her experiences as an anesthetist during the late
         1800s to the present, Dr. Berry gives her opinion of vari-
         ous anesthetics and procedures. She urges her female coun-
         terparts to become more active within the societies of anes-
         thetists, and make their work known in medical journals.

509.   Blackledge, Joan and Dixon, Dorothy. "Mona Macnaughton, M.A., M.D. 22nd May, 1964." Journal of the Medical Women's Federation, 46:3 (July 1964) 194-195. (Obituary.)

510.   Blair, Mary A. "Dr. Cecily Phelps, M.R.C.S., L.R.C.P." Medical Women's Federation Quarterly Review, (July 1936) 62-64. (Obituary.)

511.   Bolton, Elizabeth. "Helen Nora Payne: M.D., B.S. Lond., D.P.H. 24 August, 1958." Journal of the Medical Women's Federation, 41:1 (January 1959) 50-51. (Obituary.) This account of Dr. Helen Nora Payne's student and professional life is given by her former classmate and good friend.

512.   Bolton, Elizabeth; Orr, Ellen B.; Chisholm, Catherine; Martindale, Louisa; Carling, Esther; Thomson, St. Clair and Mead, Kate C. H. "Jane Harriett Walker, C.H., LL.D. J.P., M.D.: A Founder and First President of the Medical Women's Federation." Medical Women's Federation Quarterly Review, (January 1939) 17-25. (Obituary.) Each of the authors offers a brief tribute to Jane Harriett Walker, who introduced open air treatment of tuberculosis to England and directed the East Anglian Sanatorium at Nayland, near Colchester.

513.   Bothma, J. H. ["The First Women to Become Doctors Had to Be Nurses"]. South African Nursing Journal, 39 (March 1972) 10-12. (Afr) It is a little-known fact that the first two women to receive degrees of Doctor of Medicine--Elizabeth Garrett and Elizabeth Blackwell--both had to serve for a while as nurses before they could become recognized as physicians. Garrett, inspired by Blackwell's example, determined to become a doctor, but no medical school or hospital would accept her and no examining board would admit her. She proposed to the director of the Middlesex Hospital that she become a nurse there for a year, as a way of attending dissections and operations without being noticed. She also served as a nurse in the London Hospital during the five years of private instruction and demonstrations by which she studied medicine. She was finally admitted to the examination of the Society of Apothecaries and licensed by them to practice. Eventually she obtained an M.D. from the Sorbonne. Blackwell was accepted at Geneva Medical College, but the only hospital position she could get after graduation was in a "poorhouse" in Philadelphia that took in various "incorrigible characters." Later she served as a nurse at La Maternité in Paris. In London she met Florence Nightingale who offered her a position as head nurse in her hospital.

514.   Burgess, Alan. Daylight Must Come: The Story of a Cou-

rageous Woman Doctor in the Congo. Delacorte Press,
New York, New York, 1974, 297 pp. maps, photos.
This story begins with the capture and torture of Dr. Helen
Roseveare, British Protestant missionary and physician in
Zaire (Congo) during the Simba uprisings of 1964. Dr.
Roseveare and some of her colleagues were saved by mer-
cenaries and taken to England. She returned to continue her
work, which included the establishment of a medical school
for the Congolese at Nyankunde and the initiation of regional
medical care through the use of an airplane to fly physicians
from Nyankunde to surrounding community health centers.
Dr. Roseveare came to Zaire in 1953 at the age of 28. She
was born in England and received her medical degree at Cambridge. She worked under the auspices of the Worldwide
Evangelization Crusade. Photographs of Dr. Roseveare with
patients, colleagues, and students have been included. A map
of Zaire locates Nyankunde and other communities discussed
in the book.

515.   Burton, Katherine. According to the Pattern: The Story of
         Dr. Agnes McLaren and the Society of Catholic Medical
         Missionaries. Longmans, Green and Co., Inc., New
         York, New York, 1946, 252 pp.
Until 1936 canon law of the Roman Catholic Church forbade
women in religious orders to become doctors. This book
tells the story of the founding of the Society of Catholic Medical Missionaries through the biographies of Agnes McLaren,
who spearheaded the effort to support Catholic missionary activities with women physicians, and Anna Dengel, who fulfilled
Dr. McLaren's work. Dr. McLaren, a friend of Sophia Jex-
Blake, was born in Scotland in 1837. Long associated with
suffragist activities, she decided upon a medical career and
received her degree from the University of Montpellier in
1878. She then practiced in Cannes. In 1898 she converted
to Catholicism and began her efforts to provide women physicians for Catholic missions. She was helpful in achieving
the appointment of Elizabeth Bielby, also a Catholic convert,
to a mission in Rawalpindi, India. Anna Dengel, born in
Austria in 1892, received her M.D. degree from the University of Cork in 1919 and joined the mission in Rawalpindi,
India. She came to the United States for fund raising and in
1925 recruited Joanna Lyons to the service; Dr. Lyons was
the first American Catholic woman medical missionary in
India. Drs. Dengel and Lyons founded the Society of Catholic
Medical Missionaries in 1925. In 1941 the Society received
the approval of the Pope as a religious congregation with public vows. This history includes a bibliography and index.

516.   Campbell, Janet M. "Ethel Maud Stacy, L.S.A., M.B., B.S.
         Lond." Medical Women's Federation Quarterly Review,
         (January 1939) 83-84. (Obituary.)

517.   Campbell, Janet and Herzfeld, Gertrude. "Marguerite H.

Kettle, M. R. C. S., L. R. C. P." Medical Women's Federation Quarterly Review, (July 1939) 84-86. (Obituary.)

518. Campbell-Mackie, Mary. "Fifty Years as a Woman Doctor." South African Medical Journal, 13:44 (28 March 1970) 371-374.

When the centenary of the admission of women in medicine was celebrated in November 1965, pioneer women doctors were remembered as having confronted not only the prejudice of male doctors but also the prejudice of their own families. When Mary Campbell-Mackie entered Glasgow University in 1910, there were eight women students and about 300 men. As a resident, she had to eat by herself because the 18 male residents refused to eat with her. As the first woman doctor in Baghdad, she was able to enter the homes and care for the Arab Moslem women. Medical care can transcend the differences created by language, religion, and thought.

519. Campbell-Mackie, M. "Looking Back ... Fifty Years of Medicine as a Woman Doctor." South African Nursing Journal, 34:4 (April 1967) 12-14.

Dr. Campbell-Mackie discusses the utilization of medical women-power, the "many frustrations" of a woman who enters medicine, her first appointment, and her work in Baghdad.

520. "Caroline Gordon Lennox McHardy." Medical Women's Federation News-Letter, (July 1929) 80-81. (Obituary.)

Dr. McHardy graduated in 1922 from the London Hospital School.

521. Carter, R. Adelaide. "Harriet Rosa Delo Ford, M. B., D. O.: 12 March, 1960." Journal of the Medical Women's Federation, 42A:3 (July 1960) 150. (Obituary.)

522. Casson, Elizabeth and Wilson, Isabel G. H. "Margaret Scoresby-Jackson, M. D. Durh." Medical Women's Federation Quarterly Review, (January 1940) 65-66. (Obituary.)

523. "Cecilia F. Williamson, L. R. C. P. & S. I., F. R. C. S. I. 27th June, 1964." Journal of the Medical Women's Federation, 46:4 (October 1964) 260. (Obituary.)

524. Chadburn, Maud M. "Eleanor Davies-Colley, M. D., F. R. C. S." Medical Women's Federation Quarterly Review, (January 1935) 65-66. (Obituary.)

525. Chesser, Elizabeth Sloan. "Annabel Burdoch Gale, M. D." Medical Women's Federation News-Letter, (March 1931) 51-52. (Obituary.)

Dr. Annabel Burdoch Gale (formerly Clark) probably became the first woman appointed house physician to a mixed hospital when she joined the Macclesfield Infirmary in 1902. Because her appointment was followed by the resignation of the entire hospital staff, she carried on her hospital work with a male house surgeon until her resignation six months later.

526.   Chisholm, Catherine. "Kate King May-Atkinson, M.B. Ch.B."
          Medical Women's Federation News-Letter, (January 1934)
          73-74. (Obituary.)

527.   Christie, A. F. Mary. "Doreen Robinson, M.D., Ch.B.
          Edin." Medical Women's Federation Quarterly Review,
          (April 1935) 53-54. (Obituary.)

528.   Clark, Ida Clyde. "First Woman Doctor." Literary Digest,
          124 (Digest 1) :23 (7 August 1937) 23-24.
       The article on Dr. James Barry was reprinted from Coronet.
       Dr. Barry was Army Inspector General of Hospitals for Great
       Britain. At death, Dr. Barry was discovered to be a woman.
       Previously, no one had realized the truth of Dr. Barry's sex.
       When she entered college she was described as "'a frail look-
       ing young man'" who would not box and insisted upon being
       accompanied through rough neighborhoods.

529.   Coghill, Violet A. P. "Grace Giffen Dundas, F.R.C.S.,
          D.P.H., L.R.C.P., L.R.C.S. (Edin.)." Medical Wo-
          men's Federation News-Letter, (January 1934) 74. (Obit-
          uary.)

530.   Cormier, Hyacinthe M. [Miss Agnes McLaren of the Third-
          Order of St. Dominic, Doctor of Medicine]. Librairie
          Poussielgue, Paris, France, 1915. (Fre)
       [Book not examined by editors.]

531.   "Correspondence." Medical Women's Federation News-Letter,
          (July 1931) 79-80.
       This letter to the editor is in response to an obituary notice
       of Dr. Annabella Gale (formerly Dr. Daisy Clark) which
       stated that in 1902 she was appointed house physician to the
       Macclesfield Infirmary--the first woman to be given such a
       position in a mixed hospital. The letter writer informs the
       News-Letter that in 1890 Dr. Alice McLaren was appointed
       house physician to Leith General Hospital.

532.   "Daisy Annabelle Macgregor, M.D. Glasgow." Medical Wo-
          men's Federation News-Letter, (March 1928) 70. (Obitu-
          ary.)

533.   Dally, Ann. Cicely: The Story of a Doctor. Victor Gol-
          lancz Ltd., London, England, 1968, 238 pp.
       This biography of Cicely Williams, the first person to de-
       scribe the deadly disease kwashiorkor, tells of her early life
       in Oxford, England and her medical training there (which she
       was able to obtain thanks only to the absence of men students
       during World War I). The book recounts her experiences in

the Gold Coast (Ghana) , where she became interested in
tropical diseases in children, a specialty to which she devoted her life. She was transferred from Ghana to Singapore, where she found terrible malnutrition in babies. She
fought against company propaganda promoting the feeding of
babies with sweetened condensed milk at birth. The book describes her experiences as a prisoner of the Japanese during
World War II. After the war she joined the World Health
Organization as maternal and child health advisor, where she
emphasized educating mothers in childcare on an individual
level to prevent malnutrition and disease. Now in her seven-
ties, she has become an expert in family planning.

534.   "Dame Louisa Aldrich-Blake, D.B.E., M.S., M.D." Med-
            ical Woman's Journal, 33:3 (March 1926) 81.
        A posthumous tribute to Dame Louisa Aldrich-Blake, the first
        woman to obtain a Master of Surgery degree, highlights ma-
        jor achievements of her career.

535.   "Dame Mary Scharlieb, D.B.E., J.P., M.D., M.S. Lond."
            Medical Women's Federation News-Letter, (July 1926) 19.
        The announcement "of the bestowal of His Majesty the King
        of the honour of a Dame of the British Empire upon Dr. Mary
        Scharlieb" includes the text of a congratulatory letter by
        Christine Murrell, the Federation president.

536.   Dawson, Kathleen A. "Ethel Pryce, M.D., Ch.B." Medical
            Women's Federation Quarterly Review, (April 1937) 57.
            (Obituary.)

537.   "Dinner Given to Dr. Jane Walker, A Distinguished English
            Woman Physician, By the Women's Medical Society of
            New York City." Medical Woman's Journal, 30:12 (De-
            cember 1923) 375.
        In her speech before the Society, Dr. Walker expressed "great
        disgust regarding our American sleeping cars" and "deplored
        the fact that medical women are not organized in America as
        they are in England...."

538.   Dobbie, Mina L. "Gertrude Grogan, B.A., M.B., Ch.B.,
            B.A.O., R.U.I." Medical Women's Federation News-
            Letter, (November 1930) 80-82. (Obituary.)

539.   "Dr. Christine Murrell." Medical and Professional Woman's
            Journal, 41:2 (February 1934) 60.
        Christine Murrell was the first woman elected to the British
        Medical Association's Medical Council. Upon her death in
        1933, one published tribute to Dr. Murrell read, "... man's
        strength to comfort man's distresses was surely hers." A
        list of her professional activities is given.

540.   "Dr. Elizabeth Garrett Anderson--An English Pioneer." Wo-
            men in Medicine, 54 (October 1936) 22.

Elizabeth Garrett Anderson was the first woman doctor in England. While there was some "not unnatural family opposition, she found an ally in her father" in her desire to study medicine. Since she was not allowed to practice in any established hospitals at the time because she was a woman, she opened in 1866 a small dispensary, the beginning of the New Hospital for Women, which after her death was called Elizabeth Garrett Anderson Hospital. She was the first woman in England to gain the civic distinction of becoming mayor when she held that position in her home town of Aldeburgh in 1908.

541.   "Dr. Elizabeth Hurdon." Medical Woman's Journal, 43:9
          (September 1936) 248.
        Dr. Hurdon's biography is complemented by her portrait, which appears on the cover of this issue of the Journal.

542.   "Dr. Elizabeth Hurdon." Medical Woman's Journal, 48:3
          (March 1941) 92. (Editorial.)
        This brief memorial to Dr. Hurdon is presented upon the occasion of her death. (Dr. Hurdon's portrait appears on the front cover of this issue of the Journal.)

543.   "Dr. Elsie Inglis." Medical Woman's Journal, 44:6 (June
          1937) 171.
        Dr. Inglis (whose portrait appears on the front cover of this issue of the Journal) obtained her degree in 1892 at Edinburgh. She founded the Scottish Women's Hospital during World War I. This brief article gives an overview of Dr. Inglis's life during the war years.

544.   "Dr. Elsie Inglis: Founder of the Scottish Women's Hospitals, Died December 26, 1917." Women's Medical
          Journal, 28:1 (January 1918) 21.

545.   "Dr. Elsie Maud Inglis (1864-1917): Pioneer Scottish Woman Doctor and Founder of the Scottish Women's Hospitals, 1914. H. P. Tait, M.D., F.R.C.P., D.P.H." Journal of the Medical Women's Federation, 46:3 (July 1964) 170-174.

546.   "Dr. Fanny Jane Butler." Medical Missionary Record, 5:3
          (March 1890) 57-62.
        This article presents a biography of Dr. Butler, the first "fully equipped lady Medical Missionary" from England to India. (A portrait of Dr. Butler appears on page 46 of this issue of the Record.)

547.   "Dr. Hamilton Converts the Ameer." Woman's Medical Journal, 6:10 (October 1897) 319.
        Dr. L. Hamilton of Scotland serves as physician to the Ameer of Afghanistan's royal family. She has won the Ameer's approval to vaccinate the Afghan population.

548. "Dr. Louisa Martindale." Medical Woman's Journal, 42:11
        (November 1935) 309.
        Dr. Martindale (whose picture appears on the front cover of
        this issue of the Journal) studied at the London School of
        Medicine for Women, taking her M.B. and B.S. degrees in
        1890. She received her M.D. in Berlin.

549. "Dr. Mary B. Scharlieb." Medical Woman's Journal, 44:3
        (March 1937) 76.
        Dr. Mary Scharlieb (whose portrait appears on the front cov←
        of this issue of the Journal) graduated from the Royal Free
        Hospital in London and did extensive work in India. In 1916
        she helped form a woman's medical service for India. In
        1920 she was appointed one of the first woman magistrates
        in England.

550. "Dr. Mary Gordon: Supervisor of All Women's Prisons in
        England." Medical Woman's Journal, 27:1 (January 192(
        21. port. (Special Article.)

551. "Dr. Mary Scharlieb: President of the London School of
        Medicine." Medical Woman's Journal, 33:11 (November
        1926) 329-330. port.
        In 1866, Mary Bird Scharlieb left England for India, where
        her husband had chosen to practice law. Anxious to be of
        help to Indian women who unnecessarily suffered in childbirth
        she entered the Medical School in Madras, as one of four wc
        men students. Believing in the "'undesirability and folly of
        educating women to be doctors,'" the school's superintendent
        told the women that he could not prevent them from walking
        through the wards, since the government had sent them to th←
        college, but that he would not teach them. His attitude
        changed when the women proved themselves capable of han-
        dling the work. After three years' work in Madras, Dr.
        Scharlieb returned to England and obtained a degree from the
        Royal Free Hospital. Her many professional activities in
        England and in India are recounted. In her autobiography,
        Reminiscences, Dr. Scharlieb writes that her life "separated
        itself into three divisions: professional, home and social
        life and the growth and development of the medical woman's
        movement."

552. "Dr. Mary Walker." Lancet, 2:7896 (28 December 1974) 158
        Mary Walker discovered physostigmine in the 1930s and this,
        along with her observations of the properties of curare, "led
        her to make the most important British contribution to thera-
        peutic medicine up to that time." Nevertheless, she re-
        ceived little recognition for her work.

553. "'Dr. Scharlieb's Reminiscences.'" Medical Woman's Jour-
        nal, 31:9 (September 1924) 264-265.
        After going to India as the wife of an English barrister,
        Mary Scharlieb wanted to become a doctor to alleviate the

suffering she saw among the women of India who were forbidden the services of men physicians. Dr. Scharlieb was
one of the pioneer women surgeons not only in India but in
England as well. "She is inclined to the opinion that women
should confine themselves to midwifery and the diseases of
women and children, pointing out that there is ample scope
for women physicians and surgeons in this particular field."

554. "Dr. Violet Kelynack." Medical Woman's Journal, 47:11 (No-
        vember 1940) 341-342.
      Drs. Mabel Ramsay, Catherine Chisholm, and Elizabeth Bol-
      ton pay personal tributes to Violet Kelynack, who for 20 years
      served as medical secretary of the British Medical Women's
      Federation. In 1903 she won the degree of M. D., Ch. B.
      Edin., but married and never practiced medicine. Dr. Ram-
      say, writing of Dr. Kelynack's devotion to the rights of women
      to medical education, also describes the struggles of women
      students at Edinburgh University. (Dr. Kelynack's portrait
      appears on the front cover of this issue of the Journal.)

555. Doherty, Winifred J. "Jane E. Wood, M. B., B. S. Lond.,
        M. R. C. S., L. R. C. P." Medical Women's Federation
        News-Letter, (January 1932) 67. (Obituary.)

556. Dollar, Jean M. "D. Winifred Hall: M. B., Ch. B. Liverp.,
        F. R. C. S. Eng., F. R. C. S. Edin. 17 February, 1958."
        Journal of the Medical Women's Federation, 40:3 (July
        1958) 213-214. (Obituary.)
      This article enumerates the various facets of Dr. Hall's
      "definite personality": her ability to make brief but incisive
      observations at medical meetings, her insight into her pa-
      tients' troubles, her exact and careful surgical technique, and
      her invaluable advice to colleagues.

557. Dunnett, Agnes. "Madeline Phyllis Parker, L. M. S. S. A."
        Medical Women's Federation News-Letter, (March 1928)
        72. (Obituary.)

558. E. C. "Elizabeth Sykes, M. B., Ch. B. Sheffield." Medical
        Women's Federation Quarterly Review, (January 1943) 72-
        73. (Obituary.)

559. "Edith Neild, M. B." Medical Women's Federation News-Let-
        ter, (November 1927) 63. (Obituary.)
      Dr. Neild, who qualified in Edinburgh in 1898, was the first
      woman to be appointed house physician at the London Homeo-
      pathic Hospital.

560. "Elizabeth Garret [sic] Anderson, M. D." Medical Woman's
        Journal, 48:12 (December 1941) 384-385.
      This article presents a brief account of Elizabeth Garrett's
      early life and her decision to enter the field of medicine. In
      her thirties, Dr. Garrett married J. G. S. Anderson. They

had three children, the eldest of whom, Louisa, also entered the medical profession. The second half of this accou is devoted to the adult life of Dr. Louisa Garrett Anderson, who was active in the woman suffrage movement (initially in the non-militant faction and later with Mrs. Pankhurst, the militant leader). She and a friend, Dr. Flora Murray, formed the Women's Hospital Corps at the outbreak of war in 1914. After the war, Dr. Louisa Garrett Anderson and Dr. Flora Murray retired from practice and settled together at Penn in Buckinghamshire. (Dr. Louisa Garrett Anderson' portrait appears on the front cover of this issue of the Journal.)

561. "Elizabeth Hurdon, M. D." Medical Woman's Journal, 48:3 (March 1941) 93.
Dr. Hurdon (whose portrait appears on the front cover of this issue of the Journal) was one of the founders of the Marie Curie Hospital (London). She received her medical training at the University of Toronto and Johns Hopkins University. She taught at the latter institution for several year before offering her services to the war department. After the war, she returned to London, England.

562. "Elizabeth Jane Moffett. B. Sc., M. D. 22 September, 1960. Journal of the Medical Women's Federation, 43:1 (January 1961) 34-35. port. (Obituary.)

563. "Elsie Cooper: M. B., Ch. B. 17 April, 1958." Journal of the Medical Women's Federation, 40:3 (July 1958) 212. (Obituary.)

564. "Emily M. Spencer Mecredy: M. D., B. S. Lond. 4 December, 1958." Journal of the Medical Women's Federation, 41:2 (April 1959) 105-106. (Obituary.)
Dr. Mecredy received her medical training at the London School of Medicine for Women, obtaining her M. D. degree in 1910. This obituary notice recalls Emily Mecredy's personality as well as her professional activities.

565. Evans, Barbara. "Lucy Wills, M. D., B. S. 26th April, 1964." Journal of the Medical Women's Federation, 46:4 (October 1964) 261. (Obituary.)

566. Fancourt, Mary St. J. They Dared to be Doctors: Elizabeth Blackwell; Elizabeth Garrett Anderson. Longmans Green and Co. Ltd., London, England, 1965, xii, 148 pp. illus photos., ports.
This joint biography of Elizabeth Blackwell and Elizabeth Garrett Anderson turns on their meeting in London in 1859 when Blackwell inspired a determined Garrett to study medicine. It tells of the education of both women, the obstacles they overcame, and their professional careers. The book describe Blackwell as thinker and innovator and Garrett Anderson as

absorbed practitioner, and their common strengths, courage, and dedication despite their different personalities. The book includes several portraits and an index.

567. Farrer, Ellen M. "Hilda Crichton Bowser, B.Sc., M.B., B.S., M.R.C.S., L.R.C.P." Medical Women's Federation Quarterly Review, (July 1941) 63-64. (Obituary.)

568. Fay, Marion. "Memoir of Helen Ingleby: 1887-1973." Transactions and Studies of the College of Physicians of Philadelphia, 41 (April 1974) 314-315.
With Dr. Jacob Gershon Cohen, Helen Ingleby coauthored Comparative Anatomy, Pathology and Roentgenology of the Breast in 1960, after many years of research and teaching, including 20 years as chief of the department of pathology at the Woman's Medical College of Pennsylvania.

569. Fisk, Dorothy. "Sarah Gray, F.R.C.S.I., L.R.C.P. & S. Edin., L.R.F.P.S. Glas." Medical Women's Federation Quarterly Review, (April 1941) 58-59. (Obituary.)
Dr. Gray, in 1921-22, was elected the first woman president of the Nottingham and Notts Chirurgical Society.

570. Fitter, Clara. "Annie Christina Sutherland, M.D." Medical Women's Federation News-Letter, (July 1933) 53-54. (Obituary.)

571. G. M. K. "Constance Elaine Field, M.D., F.R.C.P., J.P." University of Hong Kong Gazette, 19:1 (January 1972) 9-10.
The founder of Hong Kong's Paediatric Society and the developer of a Department of Paediatrics within the [University of Hong Kong's] medical faculty, Dr. Field retired to England in 1971.

572. Gaffikin, Prudence E. "Edith Mary Guest, M.A. Oxon., M.D. Lond." Medical Women's Federation Quarterly Review, (April 1942) 59-60. (Obituary.)

573. "General Memoranda." Medical Women's Federation News-Letter, (November 1930) 88-89. port.
A portrait complements this biography of Dr. Harriet Clisby who, at the age of 100, is the world's oldest medical woman. Born in 1830, she obtained her M.D. in New York in 1865.

574. Gillett, Richenda. "Alice Brown, M.D. Brux., L.R.C.P. & S. Edin." Medical Women's Federation Quarterly Review, (April 1942) 58-59. (Obituary.)

575. Gillie, K. Annis. "Some Women Doctors I Met in the United States of America." Journal of the Medical Women's Federation, 43:4 (October 1961) 190-193.
K. Annis Gillie reminisces about her trip to the United

States where she visited hospitals and women doctors in New York, Boston, Philadelphia, Washington, D.C., Ann Arbor, Chicago, Minneapolis, St. Paul, and Houston.

576. Goodbody, Norah C. and Braid, Frances. "Mabel Donovan, M.D., Ch.B. Birm." Medical Women's Federation Quarterly Review, (January 1942) 55-56. (Obituary.)

577. Green, Pearl. "Monica Down, M.B., B.S." Medical Women's Federation News-Letter, (November 1927) 64. (Obituary.)
Dr. Down, who qualified in 1921 at the Royal Free Hospital, "was unselfish to an extraordinary degree, never putting herself first...."

578. Guthrie, Sylvia K. "Catherine Corbett: M.B., Ch.B., D.P.H. June 22, 1960." Journal of the Medical Women's Federation, 43:3 (April 1961) 141. (Obituary.)
Dr. Corbett was, with Catherine Chisholm, the first woman doctor to enter the Manchester Medical School.

579. H.M.P. and H.B.R. "Ethel Rowley, L.M.S.S.A." Medical Women's Federation Quarterly Review, (January 194? 56-57. (Obituary.)

580. Handley-Read, Eva. "Alice Marion Benham, M.D., B.S. Lond." Medical Women's Federation Quarterly Review, (July 1939) 86. (Obituary.)

581. Herzfeld, Gertrude. "Some Impressions of a Recent Visit to America." Medical Women's Federation News-Letter, (April 1933) 36-45.

582. Hogarth, Margaret and Fairfield, Letitia. "Jane H. Turnbull, D.B.E., M.D., B.S. Lond.: October 15, 1958." Journal of the Medical Women's Federation, 41:1 (January 1959) 46-48.
Dr. Turnbull was one of the pioneers in working for the reduction of maternal and infant mortality, and the organization for the welfare of mothers and children. She was a medical officer in the Ministry of Health in 1919 and in 1933 took over as senior medical officer upon Dame Janet Campbell's retirement. This article recalls her personal characteristics as well as her professional activities.

583. Hubert, Marjorie B. and Gillie, Annis. "Octavia Margaret Wilberforce. 19th December, 1963." Journal of the Medical Women's Federation, 46:1 (January 1964) 52-54. (Obituary.)

584. Hurd-Mead, Kate Campbell. "Elizabeth Garrett-Anderson: 1836-1917." Medical World, 58:7 (July 1940) 405-408. (Guest Editorial.)

585.   Hutton, I. Emslie. With a Woman's Unit in Serbia, Salonika
            and Sebastopol. Williams and Norgate Limited, London,
            England, 1928, 302 pp. photos., ports.
        A year after the war broke out, Isabel Emslie Hutton went to
        the Edinburgh war office and offered her services. But the
        "patronizing" RAMC officer could see no use for women doc-
        tors in a war. Dr. Hutton then approached the Scottish Wo-
        men's Hospitals, and in August 1915 joined a unit in France.
        It marked the beginning of several years of work with Scottish
        women's units that took her to such culturally diverse places
        as Serbia and Macedonia. Interwoven with descriptions of
        medical work are reports of the changing political scene (in-
        cluding Bolshevist activity in Russia and elsewhere) and of
        native customs. Many women physicians are mentioned.
        Photographs of coworkers, political figures, and hospitals il-
        lustrate Dr. Hutton's narrative, which contains the text of
        many letters written by the author. An index concludes the
        book.

586.   "Items of Interest." Woman's Medical Journal, 18:5 (May
            1908) 106-108.
        Among other items of interest is the announcement that Dr.
        Mary Louisa Gordon of London has been appointed as inspec-
        tor of prisons and assistant inspector of state and certified
        inebriate reformatories. It is the first time a woman has
        been given such a position.

587.   Ivens-Knowles, Frances and Joyce, Margaret. "Phoebe Mil-
            dred Bigland, M.D., D.P.H. Liverpool, M.R.C.P.
            Lond." Medical Women's Federation News-Letter, (No-
            vember 1930) 76-79. (Obituary.)

588.   "Jane Walker, C.H., M.D., LL.D." Lancet, (26 November
            1938) 1259-1261. port.
        Jane Harriett Walker gained fame for her work in the treat-
        ment of tuberculosis, and for her activities as a founder and
        active member of the Medical Women's Federation. Noted
        for her "vigorous, constructive Elizabethan courage" and for
        her unconventional appearance and mind, Dr. Walker was a
        magistrate for Suffolk county, a prolific writer, and a founder
        of Godstowe (a preparatory girls' school).

589.   Janisch, Ruth N. "Ada J. MacMillan, M.D." Medical Wo-
            men's Federation Quarterly Review, (April 1942) 60-61.
            (Obituary.)

590.   Janisch, Ruth N. "Hilda Byett, M.B., B.S., D.P.H." Med-
            ical Women's Federation Quarterly Review, (April 1942)
            61. (Obituary.)

591.   Jeffries, L. M. Blackett and Brown, Gwendolen. "Alice
            Sanderson Clow, M.D. (Lond.): July 29, 1959." Jour-
            nal of the Medical Women's Federation, [41]: 4 (October

1959) 218-219.
Dr. Clow received her M.D. from the London School of Medicine for Women in 1915. This obituary presents a brief
biography of her life.

592.   Jervis, J. Johnstone. "Gladys J. C. Russell, M.B., Ch.B
St. And., D.P.H. Manch." Medical Women's Federatio
Quarterly Review, (January 1943) 70-71. (Obituary.)

593.   Joyce, Margaret. "Ariel R. S. McElney, M.B., Ch.B."
Medical Women's Federation News-Letter, (January 1934
75. (Obituary.)

594.   "Julia Pringle: M.B., Ch.B. January, 1960." Journal of t
Medical Women's Federation, 42A:3 (July 1960) 147-148.
(Obituary.)
Dr. Pringle qualified in medicine in 1903. Shortly thereafte
she went to Baltimore and studied at Johns Hopkins under th
famous gynecologist, Professor Kelly.

595.   Kidd, Mary. "Helen Beatrice de Rastricke Hanson, M.D.,
B.S. Lond., D.P.H. Oxon." Medical Women's Federa-
tion News-Letter, (November 1926) 68-69. (Obituary.)
Kind words are offered by Mary Kidd on behalf of her friend
Helen Hanson, recently killed in an automobile accident. Dr
Hanson worked as a medical missionary in India and as a
school medical officer in London. She also served during th
war.

596.   Kirby, Percival R. "Dr. James Barry, Controversial South
African Medical Figure: A Recent Evaluation of His Life
and Sex." South African Medical Journal, 44:17 (25
April 1970) 506-516. illus., photo.
James Barry had a long career as a military doctor in the British colonies. Serving in Africa and the West Indies, he ended
his career as Inspector-General of Hospitals in Canada. He had
made a number of controversially strict administrative decisions about health care and sanitary conditions and the diet of
the sick wherever he supervised: he also presented significant
pharmaceutical official report on a plant that grew at the Cape
of Good Hope that successfully cured both syphilis and gonor-
rhoea. Included in this article are documents about his death
and sexual identification. The doctor who wrote James Barry's
death certificate, D. R. McKinnon, avoids mentioning a gender
pronoun. When the Registrar-General heard rumors that Dr.
Barry might have been a woman, he makes further inquiries of
Dr. McKinnon. In answer, the doctor writes that a woman who
performed the last offices for Dr. Barry said "that she had examined the body, and that it was a perfect female and farther
that there were marks of her having had a child when very
young...." The doctor himself adds, "But whether Dr. Barry
was male, female, or hermaphrodite I do not know, nor had I
any purpose in making the discovery...." The author concludes

from all the evidence that, "What is really important is that
he was reared, as far as we know, as a boy" and that he
was "definitely a male, though one who was unfortunately
feminine in external appearance."

597.   "Lady Barrett, C.H., C.B.E., M.D., M.S. Lond." Med-
             ical Women's Federation Quarterly Review, (October 1945)
             35-40. (Obituary.)
        Dr. Mary A. Blair, Professor Winifred C. Cullis, Miss
        Margaret M. Basden, Dr. Louisa Martindale, and "A Friend"
        join in paying tribute to Lady [Florence Willey] Barrett, dean
        of the London (Royal Free Hospital) School of Medicine for
        Women from 1926 to 1931.

598.   Ledgerwood, Hilary; Fairfield, Letitia and Cox, Alfred.
             "Christine Murrell: A Tribute." Medical Women's Fed-
             eration News-Letter, (January 1934) 68-71. (Obituary.)

599.   Leney, Lydia. "Isabel Hill, M.B., Ch.B. Edin." Medical
             Women's Federation News-Letter, (October 1933) 59-60.
             (Obituary.)

600.   Lewin, Octavia. "Elizabeth Knight, M.B., D.P.H." Med-
             ical Women's Federation News-Letter, (January 1934) 71-
             73. (Obituary.)
        Dr. Knight, who took the Bachelor of Medicine degree in
        1904 at the London University and did her medical work at
        the London School of Medicine for Women, actively partici-
        pated in the push for women's rights. Once, arrested and
        jailed for her political activity, she was ordered to scrub
        the cell's floor: when she finished, "there read across the
        floor, in letters strangely contrasting in colour with that of
        the areas she had neglected, the words 'Votes For Women.'"

601.   Lewis, Nancy R. "Kathleen Muir, M.D. 10 August 1962."
             Journal of the Medical Women's Federation, 44:4 (Octo-
             ber 1962) 169-170. (Obituary.)

602.   Lutzker, Edythe. "Edith Pechey-Phipson, M.D. Pioneer
             Woman of Victorian England and India." Warsaw-Cra-
             cow, (August 1965) 24-31.

603.   Lutzker, Edythe. Edith Pechey-Phipson, M.D.: The Story
             of England's Foremost Pioneering Woman Doctor. Ex-
             position Press, New York, New York, 1973, 259 pp.
             photos., ports.
        This is the first full length biography of Dr. Pechey, one of
        the five women who initiated the struggle for medical educa-
        tion for women in Great Britain. Edith Pechey, along with
        her better known colleague, Sophia Jex-Blake, and three oth-
        er women, was admitted to the University of Edinburgh in
        1869. In 1883, following a practice in Leeds, Dr. Pechey
        went to India under the auspices of the Medical Women for

India Fund. She worked at the Cama Hospital in Bombay, and then, in 1894, turned to private practice. She was an advocate of improved health and medical services for women, and of the banning of child marriages. In 1905 she left India with her husband and returned to England via Australia and Canada. She died in 1908 in England. One of the monuments to her work is the Pechey-Phipson Sanitarium for women and children near Nasik, India, which she and her husband founded and endowed. This work includes photographs, a bibliography, and an index.

604.   Lutzker, Edythe. "Edith Pechey-Phipson, M.D.: Untold Story." Medical History, 11 (1967) 40-45.

605.   Lutzker, Edythe. Some Missing Pages from the Histories of Nineteenth Century Medicine: [Paper presented at the 21st Congress of the History of Medicine, Siena, 22-28 September 1968]. Arti Grafiche E. Cossidente, Rome, Italy, 1970, 3 pp.
Edith Pechey-Phipson (1845-1908) is the subject of this biography.

606.   Lutzker, Edythe. "A Woman for All Seasons: Edith Pechey-Phipson, M.D." Journal of the Medical Women's Federation, 55:3 (October 1973) 136-139.

607.   MacDonald, J. Ramsay and Bone, Honor. "Ethel Bentham, M.P., J.P., M.D." Medical Women's Federation News-Letter, (March 1931) 48-51. (Obituary.)
Dr. Bentham was the first woman physician to become a member of Parliament. She obtained this honor when nearing 70 years of age, after three unsuccessful attempts. One of the founders of the Women's Labour League, Dr. Bentham was active in the woman suffrage movement. Mr. MacDonald, who wrote one of the tributes to Dr. Bentham, is the prime minister.

608.   McIlroy, Louise. "Mary Lauchline McNeill, M.B., Ch.B., Glasg." Medical Women's Federation News-Letter, (November 1928) 62-63. (Obituary.)
Dr. McNeill, who "had the mind of a poet and of a mystic," died in Africa where she served as a medical missionary.

609.   MacKenzie, Ridley. "'Doctor James Barry.'" Canadian Medical Association Journal, 21 (July 1929) 85-86. (Men and Books.)
Said to have qualified at Edinburgh at the age of 15, James Barry--a woman who masqueraded as a man throughout her medical career--ultimately became inspector-general of hospitals for the British army. This biography, which speculates that Dr. Barry was the granddaughter of a Scottish earl, concentrates on her life during the 1850s when she was stationed with the Montreal garrison. A strict vegetarian,

Dr. Barry was excessively vain and engaged in many quar-
rels. At social gatherings, she "invariably attached herself
to the best looking woman ... causing much annoyance to the
men present." She wore three-inch thick innersoles to add
to her height and wrapped towels around her body to disguise
her figure. When she was discovered upon death to be a woman, her previously arranged military funeral was counter-
manded.

610.   McLaren, Alice J. and Smith, E. D. Chalmers. "Elizabeth
       Helen Smith, M.D., Ch.B. Glas." Medical Women's
       Federation Quarterly Review, (April 1939) 74-75. (Obitu-
       ary.)

611.   McLaren, Barbara. Women of the War. George H. Doran
       Company, New York, New York, 1918, x, 160 pp. illus.,
       photos., ports.
       This is a collection of biographical sketches highlighting the
       work of outstanding British women in the war. Each biogra-
       phee is generally given a separate chapter and photograph.
       Of the 31 chapters, three include physicians. Louisa Garrett
       Anderson and Flora Murray were cited as the first women
       doctors to operate a military hospital (Endell Street, London).
       Elsie Inglis, founder of the Scottish Women's Hospitals, was
       included for this contribution and her special services in
       Serbia and Rumania. Florence Stoney was noted for her x-
       ray work in military hospitals.

612.   McLaren, Eva Shaw and Barton, Ethel M., ed. Elsie Inglis:
       The Woman with the Torch. Macmillan Company, New
       York, New York, 1920, xv, 80 pp. photos., ports.
       (Pioneers of Progress Series.)
       Dr. McLaren wrote this book upon the request of the Society
       for Promoting Christian Knowledge, the sponsors of the Pio-
       neers of Progress Series. A portion of the biography has
       been taken from the manuscript of a novel written by Dr.
       Inglis between 1906 and 1914, but never published. This
       novel, The Story of a Modern Woman, "very evidently ...
       expresses Elsie Inglis's views on life," and quotations are
       taken from it. This book begins with tributes to Dr. Inglis
       from various sources, followed by a description of the mileau
       in which she is seen as the central figure. A biographical
       account of Dr. Inglis's life covers her childhood, her med-
       ical career, her work with the Scottish Women's Hospitals,
       and her activities in Serbia and Russia. A brief bibliography
       of works related to the field of medicine, the spiritual as-
       pects of health, and men and women physicians is included.

613.   MacLaren, Gertrude D. "Annie T. Brunyate, M.D., B.S.
       (Dur.)." Medical Women's Federation Quarterly Review,
       (January 1938) 60-61. (Obituary.)

614.   MacMerchy [sic], Helen. "The Life of Sophia Jex-Blake,

M.D." Medical Woman's Journal, 27:7 (July 1920) 179-
185.

The "greatest English pioneer among medical women," Sophia
Jex-Blake found inspiration to study medicine when she met
Dr. Lucy Ellen Sewall at the New England Hospital for Women and Children. The two women became lifelong friends
and co-workers in medicine and in the women's cause. This
biography focuses upon Dr. Jex-Blake's struggle at Edinburgh
University. Her temperament and her physical appearance are
described as well. The information in this article comes
from Dr. Margaret Todd's book, The Life of Sophia Jex-
Blake.

615.   Macnicol, Mary. "Alexandra Mary Chalmers Watson, C.B.E.,
        M.D., C.M.: an Appreciation." Medical Women's Fed-
        eration Quarterly Review, (October 1936) 19-22. port.
Dr. "Mona" Chalmers Watson was the daughter of Mrs. Auckland Geddes, one of the original founders of the Medical College for Women, Edinburgh. Dr. Chalmers Watson was also
the niece of Dr. Elizabeth Garrett Anderson. An active supporter of the suffrage campaign, she was a member of the
Women's Social and Political Union.

616.   Malleson, Hope. A Woman Doctor: Mary Murdoch of Hull.
        Sidgwick and Jackson, Ltd., London, England, 1919, vii,
        231 pp. ports.
This biography of Mary Murdoch (1864-1915) of Hull, England,
based on her correspondence and recollections of friends and
relatives, gives a historical sketch of the London School of
Medicine, where she was posted briefly on graduation in 1892
from Edinburgh Medical College for Women. The rest of her
life, however, was spent in Hull, where she practiced privately and at first performed operations in private houses.
Later, in 1910, she became honorary assistant physician and
honorary senior physician at the Victoria Hospital for Children, after which many more women physicians were employed. She supported housing reform, creches, and schools
for mothers in prevention of illness. Many of her letters
dealing with her support of the suffrage movement and the
National Union of Women Workers are printed in the book.
There are numerous other quotations from her letters. Appendixes include eight lectures and addresses by her, and
reprints of her obituaries.

617.   Manton, Jo. Elizabeth Garrett Anderson. E. P. Dutton &
        Co., Inc., New York, New York, 1965, 382 pp. illus.,
        photos., ports.
This comprehensive biography of England's first woman physician is divided into two parts. The first half of the book,
"The Medical Student," describes Elizabeth Garrett Anderson's
family background, her decision to enter the medical profession, and her early struggles to obtain a medical education.
One chapter provides historical details on European women

healers.   Part Two, "The Physician," traces Dr. Garrett-Anderson's career from 1870 (when she obtained her M.D. from the Faculty of Medicine in Paris) to her death in 1917. The biography is based largely on previously unpublished materials from hospitals and medical schools where Dr. Garrett-Anderson worked, and on private letters and other documents of the Garrett and Anderson families.   Several appendixes containing letters, minutes, and records pertaining to Dr. Garrett-Anderson's medical studies, are included.   A list of sources is also given, as well as an index.

618.   "Marjory Winsome Warren, C.B.E., M.R.C.S., L.R.C.P. 5 September, 1960." Journal of the Medical Women's Federation, 42A:4 (October 1960) 197-199.   (Obituary.) Dr. Warren was one of the British pioneers in the field of geriatric medicine.   This article recalls her specific contributions to the profession.

619.   Martindale, Louisa.   "L. Martindale, M.D., B.S., J.P." Medical Woman's Journal, 31:6 (June 1924) 177-178. port. A gynecologist who used x-ray therapy, L. Martindale was one of the first two women to be appointed as Justice of the Peace to the Brighton Borough.   In 1921, Dr. Martindale was appointed president of the London Association of the Medical Women's Federation.

620.   Martindale, L[ouisa]. A Woman Surgeon.   Victor Gollancz Ltd., London, England, 1951, 253 pp.   port. This autobiography of L. Martindale tells of her medical education at the London School of Medicine and her world tour, during which she observed medical conditions in India, Ceylon, New Zealand, Australia, and the U.S.   In 1901 she became the partner of Dr. Mary Murdoch in Hull.   In 1906 she settled in Brighton and founded the New Sussex Hospital, because no other institution would accept women physicians. Each year she took her holidays abroad so she could do graduate work, which was impossible for women in England. She gives accounts of the Mayo Clinic, her consulting practice as an obstetrician/gynecologist in London, her trips to the conventions of the Medical Women's International Association of which she was president, and her research on uterine and cervical cancers.   She also includes an account of Dr. Mary Murdoch.   There is no index.

621.   Martindale, Louisa; Barrett, Florence E.; and McIlroy, A. Louise.   "Elizabeth Hurdon, C.B.E., M.D. Toronto." Medical Women's Federation Quarterly Review, (April 1941) 59-62.   (Obituary.) Dr. Hurdon is remembered by three friends who recall her outstanding work in cancer research.

622.   Martland, E. Marjorie.   "Marjorie Blandy, M.B., M.R.C.P."

Medical Women's Federation Quarterly Review, (January 1938) 59-60. (Obituary.)

623. Mears, Mary. "Isabella Mears, L. K. Q. C. P. I." Medical Women's Federation Quarterly Review, (January 1937) 60-61. (Obituary.)

624. Miller, Florence Fenwick. "Pioneer Medical Women [A Record and Remembrance]." Fortnightly Review, 122 (November 1924) 692-706.
Florence Fenwick Miller began medical studies at the University of Edinburgh (in 1869) shortly after the first five women entered medical courses there. Only 16 years old at the time, she remembers the bitter opposition to her and the other women students and, finally, the events which led to most of them giving up the struggle; her own parents removed her from school while most of the other women continued studies abroad. While detailing the Edinburgh events, the author describes the medical women involved: Sophia Jex-Blake, May Thorne, Edith Pechey. Women physicians who pioneered elsewhere also enter into the author's recollections, among them Elizabeth Blackwell, who in old age had a "deprecating ... manner [and] nearly exaggerated gentleness: as if accustomed to apologise for existing just as she was, wise and learned." Dr. Lucy Sewall's appearance struck the author as "quite alarming; she wore those terrible spectacles that show the entire eyeball magnified, and as she fixed this piercing gaze upon me I felt an insect under a microscope...."

625. Miracle, Marian. "A Woman Army Surgeon." Medical Pickwick, 1 (1915) 302.
James Barry, the physician who masqueraded as a man throughout her career, is the topic of this article. [Article not examined by editors.]

626. Mole, Joyce B. "Else Spiegel, M. D.: 6 April, 1960." Journal of the Medical Women's Federation, 42A:3 (July 1960) 149. (Obituary.)
In 1938, Else Spiegel qualified as a doctor in Berlin. A very abbreviated biographical sketch is presented.

627. Morton, Barbara G. "Selina Fitzherbert Fox, M. B. E.: M. D. Durham. 27 December, 1958." Journal of the Medical Women's Federation, 41:2 (April 1959) 106-107. (Obituary.)
Dr. Selina Fox was the founder of the Bermondsey Medical Mission in 1904, as well as one of the early women doctor pioneers in medico-social work in London. She also served, during the 1914-1918 war, as the first woman governor of Girls at Aylesbury.

628. "Mrs. Elgood." Medical Woman's Journal, 30:10 (October

1923) 309-310. port.
Sheldon Amos Elgood, who obtained her M.D. at London University in 1900, became the first woman physician to be appointed in the service of the Egyptian government. In Egypt, she opened the first outpatient department for women and children in a government hospital and was instrumental in founding the first free children's dispensaries in Egypt. For these and her many other activities, "Mrs. Elgood" was awarded the Decoration of the Nile, the Order of the British Empire, and several other honors.

629. "New Professor of Pathology at Woman's Medical College."
        Medical Woman's Journal, 32:10 (October 1925) 282.
Helen Ingleby was a member of the Royal College of Surgeons and the first British woman physician to be appointed Licensure to the Royal College of Physicians. At the time this article was written, she had just been appointed professor of pathology at the Woman's Medical College of Pennsylvania.

630. "Norah Hamilton, M.B.B.S., F.F.A.R.C.S. 19 November,
        1961." Journal of the Medical Women's Federation, 44:
        2 (April 1962) 82. (Obituary.)
Dr. Hamilton qualified in 1921 at Durham after which she joined her father in general practice.

631. "Obituary." Medical Women's Federation News-Letter, (July
        1926) 62-65.
Presented are brief tributes to the work and characters of Drs. Helen Louise Billett, Catherine Fraser, Mary Ethel Sim Scharlieb, and Kate Marion Vaughan.

632. "Obituary." Medical Women's Federation News-Letter, (July
        1927) 60-61.
Briefly reported are the deaths of Dr. Gladys M. R. Webster (a medical missionary to India); Caroline Matthews (an army surgeon who had been imprisoned during the last war); and Franziska Tibertius (Germany's first woman doctor).

633. "Obituary." Medical Women's Federation News-Letter, (July
        1928) 75-77.
Posthumous tributes are paid to Dr. Elizabeth Park Young Paterson, Isabel Elizabeth Imison, and Jane Henderson Ruthven.

634. "Obituary." Medical Women's Federation News-Letter, (July
        1930) 83-84.
Brief biographies are presented of Drs. Susan Campbell, a medical missionary to India for over 30 years, and May Pigott, a specialist in ultra-violet therapy and venereology, who died at the age of 33.

635. "Obituary." Medical Women's Federation News-Letter,
        (March 1929) 63-64.

Dr. Alice Vickery is profiled herein. "She was a born feminist and a strong supporter of the equal moral standard, political equality, equal divorce and equal guardianship of children, married women's right to property and other kindred topics."

636.   "Oldest Woman Doctor: Mentally Active at One Hundred
          Years." Medical Woman's Journal, 38:1 (January 1931)
          18.   port.
        British physician and journalist Harriet Clisby obtained her
        M.D. in New York in 1865.

637.   O'Neill, Frederick William Scott. Dr. Isabel Mitchell of
          Manchuria. 3d edition, London, England, 1918.
        [Book not examined by editors.]

638.   Orchard, Ethel. "Two Years Medical Practice in the White
          Tropics." Medical Women's Federation News-Letter,
          (January 1934) 38.
        A British physician, Dr. Orchard, received an appointment
        to treat the Aborigines in Barclay, North Queensland, Australia.

639.   Pam, Millicent. "Joyce E. Roffey: M.B., B.S. Lond.,
          M.R.C.S., L.R.C.P. 14 March, 1958." Journal of the
          Medical Women's Federation, 40:3 (July 1958) 214.
          (Obituary.)
        Dr. Roffey "was one of the first twelve students to go from
        the London School of Medicine for Women to St. Mary's Hospital, Paddinton, for her clinical years." In 1948 she helped
        form the Gillingham Welfare Association for the Care of the
        Aged Sick.

640.   Pantin, Amy. "Flora Levy. B.Sc. M.R.C.S., L.R.C.P.
          17th December 1962." Journal of the Medical Women's
          Federation, 45:2 (April 1963) 113-114.   (Obituary.)

641.   Parsons, Florence M. "Addie Wilkes: B.A. (Birmingham),
          M.R.C.S., L.R.C.P. 12 February, 1958." Journal of
          the Medical Women's Federation, 40:3 (July 1958) 215.
          (Obituary.)
        Dr. Wilkes qualified in 1928 at University College, London,
        and Charing Cross Hospital.

642.   Payne, Sylvia M. "Dr. Dorothea Nasmyth: M.A., M.D."
          Journal of the Medical Women's Federation, 42:2 (April
          1960) 98.   (Obituary.)
        Dr. Nasmyth, the first woman to read physiology in Oxford,
        was also the first woman general practitioner in Oxford.

643.   Pickard, Ellen and Stewart, Marguerite. "Margaret Thackrah, B.A., M.D., B.S., M.R.C.P." Medical Women's
          Federation Quarterly Review, (April 1937) 56-57.   (Obituary.)

644.   Pocock, Dorothy. "Muriel Marrat, M.R.C.S., L.R.C.P."
        Medical Women's Federation News-Letter, (November
        1926) 70. (Obituary.)
        Brief notes on Dr. Marrat's career are given in this obituary.
        At the time of her death, she had intended to start a prac-
        tice in Woking, where she had served as deputy assistant
        medical officer.

645.   "The President-Elect: Dr. V. Mary Crosse, O.B.E., M.D.
        (Lond.) D.P.H., M.M.S.A., D. Obst. R.C.O.G." Jour-
        nal of the Medical Women's Federation, 45:3 (July 1963)
        171-172.
        Dr. Crosse obtained her M.D. degree in 1930 from the Lon-
        don School of Medicine for Women. A history of her profes-
        sional career is given herein.

646.   "The President Elect: Dorothy McNair, M.D. London, F.F.A.,
        R.C.S." Journal of the Medical Women's Federation,
        44:3 (July 1962) 122-123.
        Elected president of the Medical Women's Federation (1963-
        64), Dr. McNair is profiled in this article.

647.   "The President-Elect: Georgiana M. Bonser, M.D. Manch.,
        F.R.C.P. Lond." Journal of the Medical Women's
        Federation, 40:3 (July 1958) 202-204.
        Dr. Bonser entered medical school at the age of 16 and in
        1920 qualified M.B., Ch.B. Her work in cancer research
        is known and appreciated worldwide.

648.   "The President-Elect: Sylvia Kema Guthrie, M.D. Manch.,
        M.R.C.P. Lond." Journal of the Medical Women's Fed-
        eration, [41]:3 (July 1959) 159.
        A native of Manchester, England, Sylvia Kema Guthrie re-
        turned there to work with children's health problems shortly
        after receiving her M.D. degree in 1926. This article an-
        nounces that she is president-elect of the Medical Women's
        Federation.

649.   "Professor Margaret Fairlie. LL.D., M.B., Ch.B., F.R.-
        C.S.ED., F.R.C.O.C. 12th July 1963." Journal of the
        Medical Women's Federation, 45:4 (October 1963) 237.
        (Obituary.)
        Dr. Fairlie, professor of midwifery at the University of St.
        Andrews from 1940 to 1956, is profiled in this obituary no-
        tice.

650.   Racster, Olga and Grove, Jessica. The Journal of Dr.
        James Barry. John Lane, the Bodley Head, London,
        England, [1932], 183 pp.
        The authors state that their main intention in publishing this
        fictionalized journal of James Barry was "to analyse and lay
        bare the mind of a woman who could keep up such a lifelong
        deception." They also confess concern about the danger "in

turning scanty fact into fiction." An appendix distinguishes
what facts they did uncover.

651. Radford, Muriel. "Amy Hodgson, M.D., D.P.H. (Liverpool)
      M.R.C.P. (London)." Medical Women's Federation News
      Letter, (March 1931) 52-54. (Obituary.)

652. Rae, Isobel. The Strange Story of Dr. James Barry: Army
      Surgeon, Inspector-General of Hospitals, Discovered on
      Death to be a Woman. Longmans, Green and Co., Lon-
      don, England, 1958, 124 pp. illus., ports.
      This book is presented as a factual biography of the life of
      Dr. James Barry. Certain questions are central to the life
      of Barry: "Was Barry, as rumour said, in fact a woman?
      ... could [she] have concealed her sex successfully for more
      than forty years? ... [if so] was she then, also, the first
      woman M.D. in Britain?" Isobel Rae focuses on Barry's
      professional competence her dedication, and her humanitari-
      anism, rather than on the "old romantic figure." This chron
      ological narrative is supported with excerpts of letters and
      papers from various sources, including the "Barry Papers"
      of the War Office. A bibliography for each chapter is given.
      The work is also indexed.

653. "Recognition Accorded English Medical Women." Medical
      Woman's Journal, 41:9 (September 1934) 249-250.
      In 1934 Helen M. M. Mackay was elected a fellow of the
      Royal College of Physicians of London--the first time in its
      400-year existence that a woman has been so honored. Lucy
      Wills of London was awarded the William Julius Mickle Fel-
      lowship for 1934. The award is given by the University of
      London to a University graduate who has done most to ad-
      vance medicine and science. Brief biographies of both phy-
      sicians are given.

654. Rew, Mabel. "Lady Hutton, C.B.E.: M.D. Edin. 11 Janu-
      ary, 1960." Journal of the Medical Women's Federation,
      42:2 (April 1960) 95. (Obituary.)
      Lady Hutton received her M.D. degree in 1912 in Edinburgh.
      She was a prolific writer and wrote several medical books
      as well as an account of her experiences with the Scottish
      Women's Hospitals during World War I: With a Women's
      Unit in Salonika, Serbia, and Sebastopol.

655. Riddell, (Lord). Dame Louisa Aldrich-Blake. Hodder and
      Stoughton Ltd., London, England, [n.d.], 91 pp. photos.,
      ports.
      Born in 1865, Louisa Aldrich-Blake entered the London
      School of Medicine for Women in 1887 and received her M.D.
      degree from London University in 1894. Her career was as
      a surgeon: 1895-1902 as assistant surgeon at the Elizabeth
      Garrett Anderson Hospital; 1895-1906 as anesthetist to the
      Royal Free Hospital (first woman to hold the post); and 1896-

1898 as surgical registrar at the Royal Free Hospital (first woman in that position). From 1902 to 1925 she rose from full surgeon to senior surgeon and consulting surgeon at the Elizabeth Garrett Anderson Hospital. Dame Louisa was dean of the London School of Medicine for Women from 1914 until her death in 1925.

656. Rolant-Thomas, Catherine M. "Dorothy Lancaster: M.B., B.S. May 7, 1961." Journal of the Medical Women's Federation, 43:3 (April 1961) 139-141. (Obituary.)
Dr. Lancaster, a dermatologist, founded a new department at the Caernarvon and Anglesey Infirmary in North Wales, and became the first woman consultant appointed to the honorary medical staff of that hospital.

657. Romieu, Claude. ["Agnes McLaren, First Woman Physician at the University of Montpellier"]. Monspeliensis Hippocrates, 31 (1966) 21-28. facsims., ports. (Fre)
Agnes McLaren started her medical studies in Edinburgh in 1873, at the age of 38 years. When the school was closed to women two years later, she went to Montpellier to complete her studies. She defended her thesis, "Flexions of the Uterus," and received her doctor of medicine degree in August 1878. The only place in the United Kingdom that would recognize her degree was Ireland, where she was licensed by the Royal College of Physicians in 1878. She did not remain in Britain, however, but returned to France, where she practiced primarily in gynecology and pediatrics. She converted to Catholicism at Lyons in 1898 and the next year joined the Third Order Dominicans. For the rest of her life her great ideal was the founding of an association of women physicians who would devote themselves to the care of women and children in the poor countries. In 1909, in her 72nd year, she traveled to India for the opening of a hospital in Rawalpindi, and in the next few years made five trips to Rome on behalf of a proposed new order of medical missionaries. She died in 1913, while preparing for yet another trip. The Medical Mission Sisters, founded after the war, now has more than 300 medical sisters and more than 60 hospitals throughout the world, especially in India.

658. "Rosa Bale, L.R.C.P.&S. Edin., L.R.F.P.S. Glas." Medical Women's Federation Quarterly Review, (January 1942) 54-55. (Obituary.)

659. Rose, Joan K. "Christina McCulloch Blaikie, M.B., Ch.B. Edin." Medical Women's Federation Quarterly Review, (October 1945) 40-41. (Obituary.)

660. Rose, Joan K. and Pringle, Julia. "Katherine Jane Stark Clark: M.D., Ch.B. Edin., D.P.H.: 6 October, 1958." Journal of the Medical Women's Federation, 41:1 (January 1959) 48-49. (Obituary.)

This brief biography of Dr. Clark is followed by a letter
from Dr. Pringle which discusses Dr. Clark's medical schoo
days.

661.   Russell, M. P.   "James Barry--1792(?)-1865: Inspector-
        General of Army Hospitals." Edinburgh Medical Journal,
        50:9 (1943) 558-567.
        Eighty-two years before Sophia Jex-Blake's fight won for wo-
        men admission to medicine at Edinburgh University, James
        Barry, disguised as a male, obtained her M.D. (in 1812)
        from that institution. She entered the Army Medical Service
        the following year, and after 46 years' service, achieved the
        rank of inspector-general of army hospitals. Drawing on ma
        terial from other sources, this biography follows the events
        in the career of Dr. Barry, offers physical and personality
        descriptions, and speculates about Dr. Barry's origin and
        her motivations for carrying out her remarkable sex imper-
        sonation for 73 years.

662.   Rutherford, N. J. C. "James (Miranda?) Barry." Journal
        of the Royal Army Medical Corps, 96-97 (May 1951)
        278-281.
        [Article not examined by editors.]

663.   St. John, Christopher. Christine Murrell, M.D.: Her Life
        and Her Work. Williams & Norgate Ltd., London, Eng-
        land, 1935, 133 pp. port.
        The most significant honor in the life of Christine Murrell
        was her election in 1933 to the General Medical Council of
        Great Britain as its first woman member. Dr. Murrell re-
        ceived the M.D. degree in 1905 from the University of Lon-
        don. She had a general practice in London's West End with
        Dr. Honor Bone. She was a member of the St. Marylebone
        Health Society, served in the Woman's Emergency Corps
        during World War I, was elected to the Council of the British
        Medical Association in 1924, and was president of the Med-
        ical Women's Federation in 1925. Dr. Murrell wrote "Wo-
        manhood and Health," published in 1923. This biography in-
        cludes a photograph of the subject. There are no references,
        bibliography, or index.

664.   Scharlieb, Mary. "Lillias Hamilton, M.D. Brux., L.R.C.P.,
        L.R.C.S. Edin." Medical Women's Federation News-
        Letter, (March 1925) 44-45. (Obituary.)
        Dr. Hamilton worked as a physician in Afghanistan. She also
        organized the Studley Horticultural College for women in agri-
        culture and domestic management, and served during the war
        in Serbia.

665.   Scharlieb, M[ary]. "The Pioneer of Women Practitioners,
        Elizabeth Garrett Anderson." Hospital (London), 63
        (1917) 270-272.
        [Article not examined by editors.]

666. Scharlieb, Mary. <u>Reminiscences.</u> Williams and Norgate,
London, England, 1924, xi, 239 pp. port.
Mary Scharlieb uses her diaries as a basis for recalling her
life as a young woman in India and her decision to become a
midwife-physician when she discovered all upper-class Indian
women, both Hindu and Moslem, were barred by their religion from being treated by male doctors. She tells of her
struggles to acquire this education in Madras in the 1870s,
recounts the extreme difficulty experienced by women wishing
to study medicine in England, and tells of her own struggle
to pass the required examinations and to obtain practical experience in Vienna, since no London hospital would accept
women. During a further five years in India, she founded
the Royal Victoria Hospital for Caste and Gosha women and
lectured at Madras Medical College. Upon her return to
England, her old friend Elizabeth Garrett-Anderson assisted
her in beginning a private practice when teaching posts were
closed to her because of prejudice, and finally obtained for
her the post of chief surgeon at New Hospital when Garrett-
Anderson retired. She mentions many women physicians encountered in her work and gives an extensive discussion of
Elizabeth Garrett-Anderson and of Florence Nightingale, who
especially encouraged her Indian projects. She mentions her
work on prenatal care and venereal diseases, and devotes a
chapter to the history of the London School of Medicine for
Women, where she states the student body has increased
since its founding from 14 to more than 500. She concludes
by giving qualifications for various specialties, such as public
health, medical missions, general practitioner, and consultant
and specialist.

667. Schw., W. ["The Male General Inspector of the British
Army Hospital Was--a Woman"]. <u>Kurz und Gut</u>, 6:5
(1972) 24. port. (Ger)
This article outlines the main events in the life of Dr. James
Barry, a woman who, disguised as a man, became Inspector-
General of Hospitals in the British army and an "officer and
gentleman" admired for "his" medical knowledge and conscientious work. The author very briefly describes Dr. Barry's behavior, especially underlining her "manliness" and the
difficulties she had because of her soprano voice. Dr. Barry,
born as Miranda Barry (an orphan), went to medical school
as a man and later joined the army. Her real sex was
known to one physician and probably to the highest army command. It was discovered during her autopsy (but not publi-
cized by the army) that she was a woman.

668. Smith, Mary Sloan. "Florence M. Robinson, M.B., Ch.B.
Glas." <u>Medical Women's Federation News-Letter</u>, (July
1931) 80. (Obituary.)

669. Soltau, B. Eleanor. "Edith Louisa Young, M.D." <u>Medical
Women's Federation News-Letter</u>, (March 1930) 62-63.

(Obituary.)

Dr. Young qualified in 1901 at the London School of Medicine. She spent 24 years in India as a medical missionary and built the Rohmatpur Hospital in Palwal.

670.   Stewart, Clara. "Kathleen Wilson, M.B., Ch.B." Medical Women's Federation Quarterly Review, (April 1942) 57-58. (Obituary.)

671.   Stewart, Clara. "Maude Elizabeth Seymour Abbott, B.A., M.D., F.R.C.P. Canada, L.R.C.P.E." Medical Women's Federation Quarterly Review, (January 1941) 63-64. (Obituary.)

672.   Stuart, Madeleine. "Winifred Drummond Cargill, M.B., Ch.B., D.T.M. & H." Medical Women's Federation News-Letter, (November 1930) 79-80. (Obituary.)

673.   Sutherland, Joan K. "Isabella Ferrier Pringle, M.D., F.R.C.P.E., D.P.H. 7th May 1963." Journal of the Medical Women's Federation, 45:4 (October 1963) 238. (Obituary.)

674.   Swanson, A. Maud. "Mary J. Pirret, M.D. Glas., D.P.H. Camb." Medical Women's Federation Quarterly Review, (January 1943) 71-72. (Obituary.)

675.   Sylk, Ellen. "Agnes Keen, L.R.C.P., L.R.C.S. Edinburgh, L.R.F.P.S. Glas." Medical Women's Federation News-Letter, (April 1933) 63. (Obituary.)

676.   Taylor, L. Dorothea. "Marie Moralt, M.B., B.S." Medical Women's Federation News-Letter, (January 1932) 66-67. (Obituary.)

677.   Thorburn-Johnstone, Mabel. "Refugee Work in Salonica." Medical Women's Federation News-Letter, (March 1928) 40-42.

Dr. Thorburn-Johnstone tells of her experiences as a physician with the Society of Friends in Greece.

678.   Thorne, May and Jex-Blake, Sophia. "Pioneer British Medical Women." Medical Woman's Journal, 33:6 (June 1926) 176-177.

After going to China in 1856, "Mrs. Isabel Thorne ... was led to the study of medicine solely by the fact that in her early married life she sorely felt the need of medical knowledge, as she was unable to get skilled medical knowledge for her children, and attributed the death of her first baby to the lack of such knowledge." In 1869, she gained admission as a medical student to the University of Edinburgh. In 1870, however, the University reversed its decision to open medical training to women. "Mrs. Thorne" is the first name on the student enrollment list of the London School of Medicine for Women, which was founded by Sophia Jex-Blake in 1874. Mary Edith Pechey was, in 1869, one of the first five women to matriculate in Edinburgh's medical training program, but because no British university would give medical degrees to women, she obtained her M.D. at the University of Bern. Dr. Pechey practiced in India from 1883 to 1905.

679. Todd, Margaret. The Life of Sophia Jex-Blake. Macmillan and Co., Ltd., London, England, 1918, xviii, 574 pp. ports.
This biography is divided into three parts: Sophia Jex-Blake's childhood and youth, her attempts to get a medical education and degree, and her subsequent practice. Dr. Jex-Blake is best known for leadership in the struggle for admission and examination of women medical students at the University of Edinburgh. In 1874 she founded the London School of Medicine for Women, in 1886 she opened the Edinburgh Hospital for Women and Children, and in 1888 she opened a medical school for women in Edinburgh. She was the first woman physician in Scotland. Both the text and appendixes are replete with letters, essays, and journal excerpts by the biographee. There is an index to this work.

680. "Veronica Catherine Jessica McPherson, M.B., CH.B. (GLAS.)." South African Medical Journal, 13:12 (1975) 2206. port.
This obituary notice for Dr. McPherson recounts her service in South Africa, as well as her origins and medical studies in Scotland.

681. "Violet Redman King, M.B., Ch.B. Leeds." Medical Women's Federation Quarterly Review, (July 1941) 64-65. (Obituary.)

682. Wade, Phyllis. "Marjorie Pearl Christine Greene (Mrs. P. P. Cole). M.B., B.S., D.M.R.E. 22nd May, 1964." Journal of the Medical Women's Federation, 46:4 (October 1964) 259. (Obituary.)

683. Walker, Jane. "Dame Mary Scharlieb, D.B.E., J.P., M.D., M.S." Medical Women's Federation News-Letter, (November 1930) 101-104. (Obituary.)
Dr. Walker, who describes herself as Mary Scharlieb's oldest living friend among women physicians, mingles personal reminiscences with the facts of Dr. Scharlieb's educational and professional accomplishments. "[Dr. Scharlieb] never had an operating knife in her hand till she was turned 40 years of age, and yet very shortly she became one of the six great abdominal surgeons of the world."

684. Walker, Jane H. "Dame Millicent Garrett Fawcett, G.B.E., J.P., LL.D." Medical Women's Federation News-Letter, (November 1929) 58-59. (Obituary.)

685.   Walker, Jane. "Dr. Jane Waterston." <u>Medical Women's</u>
        <u>Federation News-Letter</u>, (January 1933) 66-68. (Obitu-
        ary.)

686.   Watson, Anne Mercer; Stephen, James A.; Thompson, Constanc
        M.; Hutton, Isabel Emslie; and Innes, Elizabeth. "Apprecia
        tions of the Late Laura Stewart Sandeman, M.D." <u>Med-</u>
        <u>ical Women's Federation News-Letter</u>, (July 1929) 19-26.
        Dr. Sandeman, who obtained her M.D. in 1900, served with
        the Scottish Women's Hospitals during the war. She prac-
        ticed medicine in Aberdeen, Scotland, where she also ran
        twice as Parliamentary Unionist candidate; she was never
        elected to Parliament, because the people of Aberdeen "were
        threatened with the loss of their doctor...."

687.   Wauchope, Gladys Mary. <u>The Story of a Woman Physician.</u>
        John Wright & Sons Ltd., Bristol, England, 1963, vii,
        138 pp.
        Gladys Mary Wauchope was the first woman medical student
        at the London Hospital Medical College, having attended from
        1918 to 1921. Her autobiography begins with her ancestry,
        childhood, and leisurely Edwardian girlhood. Largely as a
        result of World War I, "which shattered the Edwardian world,
        she turned her thoughts to a career in medicine. As a stu-
        dent during the war, she often went "out on the district."
        After graduation, Dr. Wauchope practiced at the London for
        a time and then, in 1922, took a post as assistant to a coun-
        try doctor; then on to Queen Charlotte's Hospital, then back
        to the London. "By 1924 it was time for me to launch into
        practice." One chapter is devoted to medical personalities,
        including Dr. Florence Edmonds and Dr. Helen Boyle. World
        War II changed the character of her work--"less general prac
        tice, more hospital consulting work, and a continuous series
        of lectures to St. John Ambulance Brigades." Dr. Wauchope
        developed a special interest in diabetes and hypoglycemia and
        became a specialist in this field, contributing articles to en-
        cyclopedias and professional journals. In 1946 she became
        the eighth woman to be elected a fellow of the Royal College
        of Physicians in London. In 1948 the National Health Ser-
        vice began and she became a part-time consultant for them,
        giving up her general practice. At retirement age in 1954,
        she began teaching premedical courses in addition to her pri-
        vate consulting practice. The last chapter reflects on the
        overwhelming advances made in medical knowledge just during
        her own medical career. A bibliography and an index of
        names is included.

688.   Wilberforce, Octavia M. "Mary Addams Leslie-Smith. M.B.
        February 3, 1961." <u>Journal of the Medical Women's</u>
        <u>Federation</u>, 43:2 (April 1961) 75-77. (Obituary.)

689.   Williams, Ethel M. N. "Mabel R. Campbell, M.A., M.B.,
        Ch. B." <u>Medical Women's Federation Quarterly Review,</u>
        (January 1940) 64-65. (Obituary.)

690.   Williams, Ethel M. N.   "Mary Gordon, L.R.C.P.E., L.M."
        Medical Women's Federation Quarterly Review, (July
        1941) 63.   (Obituary.)

691.   "World's Oldest Woman Physician."   Medical Woman's Jour-
        nal, 36:9 (September 1929) 256.
        A brief biography is presented of Dr. Harriet Clisby of Lon-
        don, England, adjudged at the time of this article to be the
        oldest living woman physician at the age of nearly 100.   She
        received her M.D. degree in 1865 from the New York Med-
        ical School.

INTERNATIONAL

692.   Bass, Elizabeth.   "Dedications in Books by Medical Women."
        Journal of the American Medical Women's Association, 5:
        8 (August 1950) 328-329.
        Dedications often "give insight into the life of the author."
        Examples include Mary E. Walker's dedication to "The Prac-
        tical Dress Reformers, The Truest Friends of Humanity...";
        and Elizabeth Blackwell's dedication of an early work to "...
        That Ever-Living Manifestation of Divine Goodness, Our Lord,
        who is crucified afresh in every outcast woman."

693.   Bass, Elizabeth.   "These Were the First."   Journal of the
        American Medical Women's Association, 7:11 (November
        1952) 432.   (Album of Women in Medicine.)
        May Farinholt Jones was the first woman physician at the
        Mississippi State College for Women, the first woman doctor
        to take the Mississippi State Board medical examination, and
        the first woman physician admitted to the Mississippi State
        Medical Society.   In 1919 Anna Dengel was sent to India,
        where she became director of St. Catherine's Hospital for
        Women and Children.   The first of the Catholic sisterhood to
        practice medicine in conjunction with her religious duties,
        she founded the Society of Catholic Medical Missionaries.
        Receiving her medical degree in 1866, Susan La Flesche Pi-
        cotte, an Omaha, was the first Indian woman to study medi-
        cine in the United States.   Kying Yuo Me [sic] was the first
        native Chinese woman to receive a degree (in 1885) in the
        United States.   Specializing in obstetrics and gynecology,
        Helen MacMurchy, in 1901, became the first woman physician
        admitted to the staff of Toronto General Hospital.   An obste-
        trician, Sarah Windsor was the first woman to serve in the
        maternity department of Boston's Massachusetts Homeopathy
        Hospital and the first woman physician elected president of
        the Boston Homeopathic Medical Society.

694.   Bass, Elizabeth.   "These Were the First."   Journal of the
        American Medical Women's Association, 10:8 (August
        1955) 284.
        Dr. Consuelo Vadillo was the first woman in Yucatan to re-

ceive a medical degree. Dr. Bethenia Owens-Adair was one
of the first to decry constricting corsets, to urge swimming
and skating, and to advise against side saddles. She helped
obtain passage of a law in Oregon requiring medical examinations for all of those seeking marriage licenses. Dr. Edna
Lyle Thomas was the only woman physician in Australia who
visited her outlying patients by airplane. She instituted a
diphtheria immunization campaign. Dr. Mary Louise Jennings
was the first woman physician to practice in Geneva, New
York. Dr. Nettie L. Gerish organized the first Play Ground
Association in 1945.

695.   "Century of Service." Medical Woman's Journal, 56:2 (Feb-
          ruary 1949) 54-55. (News Notes.)
        The centennial of Elizabeth Blackwell's graduation from Gen-
        eva Medical School was celebrated by Hobart (formerly
        Geneva) and William Smith Colleges by presenting citations
        to 12 distinguished women doctors from the U.S., Canada,
        England, and France.

696.   "Honors for Medical Women." Bulletin Medical Women's
          Club of Chicago, 16:6 (February 1927) 7.
        Dr. Mabel E. Elliott is the only American woman doctor al-
        lowed to practice (and recently licensed) in Japan. Dr.
        Brian Garfield is the first woman surgeon in France.

697.   Hume, Ruth Fox. Great Women of Medicine. Random House,
          New York, New York, 1964, 268 pp. illus., photos.,
          ports.
        This collection of biographies of outstanding medical women
        includes Elizabeth Blackwell, Elizabeth Garrett Anderson,
        Sophia Jex-Blake, Mary Putnam Jacobi, as well as Florence
        Nightingale and Marie Curie. A final chapter on 20th-century
        women mentions Louise Pearce, Helen Taussig, Florence
        Sabin, Maude Slye, Anna Williams, Gerty Cori, Alice Hamil-
        ton, Estella Warner, Martha Eliot, Leona Baumgartner, Ci-
        cely Williams, and Frances Kelsey. A bibliography of
        sources and additional readings and an index have been in-
        cluded, as have many portraits and photographs of these wo-
        men physicians.

698.   "In Memoriam." Medical Woman's Journal, 40:2 (February
          1933) 55.
        Obituary notices on Dr. Jane Waterston and Dr. Marcena S.
        Ricker give a brief look at the professional activities of these
        women. Dr. Waterston practices in Cape Colony, Africa.
        Dr. Ricker was the physician of Susan B. Anthony.

699.   Knapp, Sally. Women Doctors Today. Thomas Y. Crowell
          Company, New York, New York, 1947, 184 pp. illus.
        This collective biography of women in medicine includes quo-
        tations from, and brief accounts of, the lives of 12 women
        physicians: Katherine Li, in 1947 a cancer surgeon at Wo-

men's Christian Medical College in her native Peking; Vesta
Rogers, a general practitioner who is quoted on the difficulty
of getting a medical education as a woman; Edith Summerskill,
British gynecologist and M.P.; Lena Edwards, a black obstetrician, who speaks of her problems in overcoming racial
and sexual barriers to a medical career; Ida Scudder, medical missionary who founded a medical college for women in
India (this chapter includes a recipe from an India witch doctor); Lauretta Bender, a psychiatrist who writes of her experiences with psychotic children; Emily Van Loon, a Philadelphia ear, nose and throat specialist; Katharine Elsom, a
nutritionist who specializes in vitamin treatment; Sophie Rabinoff, a public health physician in New York City; Hanna Hirszfeld, a Polish pediatrician who served in Serbia during World
War I and carried on an underground clinic in the Warsaw
ghetto during World War II; Barbara Stimson, O.B.E., an
American orthopedic surgeon who served in Britain's Royal
Army Medical Corps in World War II; and Rita Finkler, a
Russian-born endocrinologist.   The book contains no index or
bibliography.   Each chapter is headed by a portrait sketch of
its subject.

700.   "Medical Women of Today."   Medical Woman's Journal, 40:
          1 (January 1933) 18-19.
       Biographical sketches are presented of the professional lives
       of the following women: Dr. Mary E. Bates, a surgeon from
       Denver, Colorado; Dr. Dora Brucke-Teleky, an Austrian sur-
       geon; Dr. Alice Bryant, one of the leading otolaryngologists
       in the East; Dr. Frances Eastman Rose, a West Coast sur-
       geon; and Dr. Olga Stastny.

701.   "Medical Women of Today."   Medical Woman's Journal, 40:
          2 (February 1933) 45-46.
       Biographical sketches are presented of the professional lives
       of the following women: Dr. Martha Tracy, Dean of the Wo-
       man's Medical College of Pennsylvania; Dr. Ellen C. Potter,
       the first woman to occupy a position in a governor's cabinet;
       Dr. Paulina Luisi, the first woman graduate of the University
       of Montevideo and the first woman to obtain a medical degree
       in Uruguay; Dr. Mary T. Greene of Castile, New York; Dr.
       Mabel E. Gardner, an outstanding Ohio surgeon; and Dr. Har-
       riet Doane, the only woman physician in Pulaski, New York.

702.   Roth, Nathan.   "The Personalities of Two Pioneer Medical
          Women: Elizabeth Blackwell and Elizabeth Garrett An-
          derson."   Bulletin of the New York Academy of Medicine,
          47:1 (January 1971) 67-79.

SOUTH, CENTRAL, LATIN AMERICA
AND MEXICO

703.   "About the Author."   Medical Woman's Journal, 59:1 (Janu-

ary 1952) 15-16.   port.
This article gives biographical information on Dr. Maria
Luisa Aguirra, one of the authors of "Drepanocytic Anemia"
(an article appearing in this issue of the <u>Journal</u>).

704.   Beregoff-Gillow, Pauline. [<u>My Life in Colombia. Cartagena:</u>
<u>1922-1925, Research Student; 1932-1933, Teacher by In-</u>
<u>vitation.   My Calvary in Bogota, 1965-1973</u>].   Colombia,
1974?, 104 pp.   illus.   (Spa)
As the author's introduction says, this is not an autobiography
but the testimony of a profound love for the Colombian people.
It is also a testimony of her deep dislike for inefficiency and
corruption, as they appeared in her struggles to establish
and maintain the Arthur S. Gillow Foundation for Scientific
Research and Preventive Medicine in memory of her husband.
The book is written in the form of letters to her dead husband, the first part being anecdotal memories of her life in
Cartagena, her early career as a microbiologist, and her
education in Colombia, where she was the first woman to
earn an M.D. degree, and again in the United States.   After
her marriage she and her husband spent many years in research and practice in Canada.   On his death in 1964, she
returned to Colombia with the intent of establishing a research
institute, and much of the book is devoted to her struggles
with the Colombian authorities and the medical-scientific establishment over this project.   At the time of writing, the
Institute, which she had supported almost single-handedly,
was apparently in danger of closing for lack of money and
adequately trained help, and of being taken over by the Central Military Hospital.   There is no table of contents, index,
or bibliography for this work.

705.   Beregoff-Gillow, Pauline. [<u>The Only Love</u>].   Printed in Bo-
gota, Colombia, [n.d.], 137 pp.   (Spa)
This book is written as letters to the author's deceased husband, Dr. Arthur Gillow, on each anniversary of his death
and on numerous occasions between anniversaries, during the
years from 1965 to 1972.   The letters or essays discuss the
author's efforts to establish a "preventorium" or institute of
preventive medicine, the difficulties encountered in building it,
and the great problems in running it.   The latter include interference by governmental authorities, poorly trained staff,
and even thieving professional staff members.   In addition to
the discussions of the institute, but closely related, are discussions of the author's philosophy of medicine, which was
primarily that prevention of disease is the main objective,
rather than treatment after disease has occurred.   This work
contains no table of contents, index, or bibliography.

706.   Bernard, Marcelle. "Ines L. C. deAllende, M.D." <u>Journal</u>
<u>of the American Medical Women's Association</u>, 9:1 (Janu-
ary 1954) 30.   port.
Ines L. C. deAllende received her degree in 1934 in Argen-

tina. She worked as a member of the Institute of Physiology and then began researching and writing a number of articles in the field of endocrinology. Aparato Sexual Gemenina del Bufo Arenarum Hensel she wrote by herself, and with Dr. Orias she coauthored La Etiologia Vaginal Humana en Condiciones Normales y Patologicas, which was translated by George W. Coener for publication in the United States.

707.   Brodie, Jessie Laird. "Margarita Delgado de Solis Quiroga, M.D." Journal of the American Medical Women's Association, 7:10 (October 1952) 396. port. (Album of Women in Medicine.)

When the Pan American Medical Women's Alliance was founded in 1947, a Mexican, Margarita Delgado de Solis Quiroga, was active in this group and eventually became president. She was the first woman to hold a chair in abnormal psychology, pedagogic psychotechnic and physiology on the Faculty of Medicine. Other posts of importance in her career include professor in chief of physiological and biological research of the Medical Faculty, head of the biology department of the Institute of Hygiene, and chief of scientific research in the Department of Health.

708.   Brodie, Jessie Laird. "Maria Luz Donoso de Carrasco, M.D." Journal of the American Medical Women's Association, 13:8 (August 1958) 347. port. (Album of Women in Medicine.)

A Bolivian, Maria Luz Donoso de Carrasco is president-elect of the Pan American Medical Women's Alliance. She was the first woman to receive an M.D. degree from the Universidad Mayor de San Andres of La Paz (1941). In 1956, with the help of the Bolivian Red Cross, she organized a day-care center for children of working mothers.

709.   Brodie, Jessie Laird. "Tegualda Ponce, M.D." Journal of the American Medical Women's Association, 9:1 (January 1954) 29. port. (Album of Women in Medicine.)

A president of the Pan American Medical Women's Alliance, and a native of Chile, Tegualda Ponce's professional specialty was primarily obstetrics and gynecology.

710.   "Dr. Pauline Luisi--Member of Disarmament Conference." Medical Woman's Journal, 39:3 (March 1932) 67-68.

A native of Uruguay, Pauline Luisi was the first South American woman representative to the League of Nations and was Uruguay's representative to the 1932 disarmament conference at Geneva. Her other distinctions include being the first woman doctor in Uruguay and serving as head of the clinic at the Medical Faculty of Montevideo. She advocated the revising of history textbooks so that the concept of settling differences between countries by arbitration rather than war, would be presented. She also served on the League of Nations' International Committee of Experts on white slave traffic as well as on the consultative commission for the protection of children and young people.

711.   "Dra. Elvira Rey Chilia: Physician-Surgeon; President of
            Cuban Medical Women's Association." Medical Woman's
            Journal, 54:2 (February 1947) 24, 44. port.
        Dr. Chilia received her M.D. degree in Havana, Cuba in
        1940. This article profiles Dr. Chilia's education and pro-
        fessional affiliations.

712.   "Dra. Margarita Delgado de Solís." Medical Woman's Jour-
            nal, 57:3 (March 1950) 27-28. port.
        Margarita Delgado, a president of the Pan American Medical
        Women's Alliance, was the first woman to hold a chair in the
        "Introduction to Psychology of Abnormals," Psychotechnic
        Pedagogie and Physiology of the Faculty of Medicine. She
        worked for a number of years with juvenile delinquents at the
        Woman's Reformatory of Mexico City.

713.   "Dra. Ruth Wresinski Tichauer: Vice President for Bolivia,
            P.A.M.W.A." Medical Woman's Journal, 57:9 (Septem-
            ber 1950) 24-25. photo.
        Ruth W. Tichauer went to Bolivia originally intending to be a
        professor of social medicine but worked in a number of gov-
        ernment programs instead, including helping to set up the
        Department of Nutrition. She became a Bolivian citizen and
        set up a general practice as well as becoming a vice presi-
        dent of the Pan American Medical Woman's Alliance.

714.   "Dra. Tegualda Ponce Vargas." Medical Woman's Journal,
            53:11 (November 1946) 39. port.

715.   "The First Mexican Woman Medical Student." Double Cross
            and Medical Missionary Record, 11:2 (February 1896) 29.
        Petra Borilla Toral (whose portrait appears elsewhere in this
        issue) is the first Mexican woman to study to be a medical
        missionary in the U.S., or probably in any land.

716.   Georgi, Audrey Adele. "Mexican Woman Physician." Med-
            ical Woman's Journal, 54:2 (February 1947) 51-53, 62.
        This article presents a biography of Dr. Consuelo Vadillo
        Gutiérrez, the first woman to graduate from Merida Medical
        College in Mexico. The author attributes Dr. Vadillo's re-
        fusal to conform and active fighting of prejudice to the fact
        that she was able to do postgraduate work at several medical
        colleges in the U.S. (i.e., Johns Hopkins University, Wo-
        man's Medical College of Pennsylvania, and New York's Co-
        lumbia University).

717.   Lara, Maria Julia de. [Laura Martinez de Carvajal y del
            Camino: First Female Medical Graduate in Cuba. On
            the 75th Anniversary of her Graduation (15 July 1889)].
        Havanna, Cuba, 1964, 125 pp. (Publications in the His-

tory of Public Health, Number 28.) (Spa)

Laura Martinez de Carvajal was the first Cuban woman to
graduate in medicine from the University of Havana and the
first woman doctor to practice in Cuba, specializing in ophthalmology. If social progress is the result of individual progress, women in Cuba owe much to her determination and devotion, which set an example for others to follow. Laura
Martinez was born in Havana on August 27, 1869. She
learned to read by the age of four, received a bachelor's degree at 13, became a licenciate in physiomathematical sciences at 18 and in medicine at 19. Five days after her graduation she married Enrique Lopez Veitia, an oculist, and
they worked together in the Clinic of Medical Specialists in
Havana and on a textbook of clinical ophthalmology for over
twenty years, until Enrique's death in 1910. She bore seven
children and was interested in music, poetry, and needlework,
as well as keeping up her practice. Some years after her
husband's death, she moved to a home in the country where
she became interested in gardening and fruit growing, and
where she and her daughter Maria set up a school for poor
workers' children, which they maintained for about twenty
years. She died in January 1941. There is a marble bust
of Laura Martinez in the Carlos Finlay Historical Museum of
the Academy of Sciences in Havana, and her home, "El Re-
tiro," is part of a tourist circuit. The author's concluding
review of the history of women in medicine in Cuba, includes
mention of an Enriqueta Faber who practiced for many years
as a man. The appendix lists women who graduated in medicine from the University of Havana to 1964.

718.   Lobo, F. B. ["Rita Lobato: The First Woman Medical
            Graduate in Brasil"]. Revista Hist., 42 (1971) 483-485.
            (Por)
        [Article not examined by editors.]

719.   "News Notes." Medical Woman's Journal, 55:8 (August 1948)
            53.
        Among information given on several women in this column is
        a biography of Esperanza Oteo de Hoogh, a graduate of the
        National Medicina School of Mexico, and currently director
        of Mexico's Department of Education Social Work Office.

720.   "Prof. Ag. Dra. Maria Luisa Saldun de Rodriquez [sic]."
            Medical Woman's Journal, 54:8 (August 1947) 37-38, 67.
            port.
        Dr. Saldun de Rodriguez is the first woman in Uruguay to
        obtain the title of "Professor Agregado" at the Medical School.
        Her various professional activities, memberships, and honors
        are cited in this article.

721.   Silva, Alberto. [The First Woman Doctor of Brazil]. Irmãos
            Pongetti, Rio de Janeiro, Brazil, 1954, 243 pp. facsim.,
            photos., ports. (Por)

The author, a historian at the University of Bahia, started
the research that led to this book after a radio program in
Rio de Janeiro mistakenly identified the first Brazilian woman
doctor as Ermelinda Lopes de Vasconcelos. Ermelinda graduated from the University of Rio de Janeiro in 1888, while
Rita Lobato Velho Lopes received her doctor of medicine degree from the University of Bahia in 1887. The book describes Lopes' early life and student days in some detail,
with extensive quotations from university archives and contemporary news sources to prove that she was the first woman in Brazil to achieve a doctorate. Lopes, Vasconcelos,
and Antonieta Cesar Dias started medical school together;
Dias also received her degree from Rio de Janeiro. The
first women doctors in some of the other South American
countries were Eloisia (Eloiza) Dias Inzunzo (Chile, 1866),
Cecilia Guierson (Argentina, 1889) and Paulina Luisi (Uruguay,
1908). The book includes a list of all of the 131 women who
received diplomas in medicine from the University at Bahia
from 1887 to 1951; 20 of these in the years through 1931 submitted theses and received doctoral degrees but all after that
date received only diplomas in medicine.

USSR

722.   Barkman, E. and Vasilievskaya, O.   ["Anniversary of a Dis-
          tinguished Physician (1889-1969) Lyudmila Sergeevna
          Bogolepova"].   Sovetskoe Zdravookhranenie, 28:9 (1969)
          82-83.   port.   (Rus)
        Lyudmila Sergeevna Bogolepova graduated from the Moscow
        Higher Women's Courses in 1913.   In 1921 she was appointed
        a member of the board of health of the city and participated
        in the organization of new medical services, such as mother
        and child care, school health, and sanitoria.   She was es-
        pecially interested in occupational diseases and their preven-
        tion.   From 1925 to 1932 she was director of the Scientific
        Research Institute for Occupational Diseases.   In 1933 she
        began to teach at the First Moscow Medical Sechenov Institute,
        then for seven years taught at the Central Institute for the
        Advanced Training of Physicians.   In 1948 she was given the
        title of professor.   From 1946 to 1962 Bogolepova was as-
        sistant to the director of the Central Scientific Research In-
        stitute of Sanitary Education.   Bogolepova delivered many pub-
        lic lectures on her particular interests: the prophylaxis of
        occupational disease and the education of the people in better
        care of their own health.   She also wrote more than 100 pub-
        lications, the most important being "Sanitary Education and
        Self-Activity of the Population" (1957); "Scientific Works in
        the Field of Sanitary Education and Hygienic Education of the
        People" (1967); and "Methods of Scientific Works on Hygienic
        Education of the People" (1965).   She guided many scientists
        in writing and defending their dissertations.   For many years
        she was a member of the executive committee of the Interna-

tional Union of Sanitary Education and is now an honorary member of this organization. She has received the Order of Lenin and many medals of the USSR.

723. Bisiarina, V. P. ["Contribution of Women Physicians to the Study of Marginal Pathology"]. Klinicheskaia Meditsina (Moskva), 53:8 (August 1975) 15-18. (Rus)
Diseases which are regarded as marginal for some parts of Siberia are described, and the contributions of women pediatricians working in the area to their management are pointed out. Women physicians studied the clinical manifestations, variations, and course of brucellosis, opisthorchosis, endemic goiter, and tularemia in children. They introduced into practice new and effective methods of treatment and prophylaxis of these diseases. These methods resulted in a sharp reduction of morbidity in children; many severe forms of the diseases disappeared, and the course of some has changed favorably. Nine women physicians are mentioned; most of them were associated with the Omsk Medical Institute.

724. Dionesov, S. M. [V. A. Kashevarova-Rudneva, Russia's First Female Physician]. Wissenschaft, Moscow, USSR, 1965, 103 pp. facsims., ports. (Rus)
The author recalls the life of Varvara Alexandrovna Kashevarova-Rudneva, born Nafanova in 1844, an outstanding Russian woman of the 19th century and a pioneer of women's medical education. The book is based mostly on her autobiographical notes. The first chapter is about the early history of women's education in Russia, the second discusses her childhood and youth. She entered the Institute for Midwives in Petersburg in 1861, graduated in 1862, and was appointed midwife of the Bashkirskoye Kazach'e Voisko. She continued her medical education at the Medical-Surgical Academy in Petersburg during the years 1863-1868. V. Kashevarova (her first husband's name) received her physician's diploma in December 1868 and was awarded a gold medal for excellence in her studies. In 1870 she married M. M. Rudneva, a teacher. She defended her thesis at the Medical-Surgical Academy on May 25, 1876 and became the first woman doctor of medicine educated in Russia. Together with her husband, she participated in the First International Medical Congress in the summer of 1876 in Philadelphia. She left Petersburg in 1881 and died in Staraya, Russia in 1889. The book contains an index of dates and highlights of Dr. Kashevarova-Rudneva's life, and a list of her published works, as well as 101 references and footnotes.

725. "First World Health Assembly: Maria Dmirievna Kovrigina, M.D." Journal of the American Medical Women's Association, 3:10 (October 1948) 425. port.
This is a very brief biographical note on Dr. Kovrigina, deputy to the minister of health in the USSR and delegate to the first World Health Assembly in Geneva.

726.   Gevorkov, A. A. and Farkhadi, R. R. ["First Women Phy-
        sicians in the Samarkand Regions"]. Sovetskoe Zdra-
        vookhranenie (Moskva), 20:11 (1961) 61-63. (Ger)
        [Article not examined by editors.]

727.   Hurd-Mead, Kate Campbell. "Dr. Anna N. Shabanoff, Pio-
        neer Woman Physician of Russia." Bulletin of the Med-
        ical Women's National Association, 28 (April 1930) 11-
        12.
        Anna N. Shabanoff obtained her medical degree in Finland at
        the University of Helsingfors where she was the first woman
        medical student. In 1872, the Military Medical Academy of
        St. Petersburg opened its doors to women and Anna returned
        to her homeland to finish her studies (in 1878) but did not
        have the right to practice. Dr. Shabanoff and other women
        physicians founded the Women's Medical Institution for the ed-
        ucation of women physicians. She also helped organize hos-
        pitals in Russia as well as the first day nursery for the chil-
        dren of working women in St. Petersburg. Dr. Shabanoff
        was the founder and permanent president of the Russian Wo-
        men's Society, as well as founder and first president of the
        Women's League for Peace. In addition to these activities,
        Dr. Shabanoff produced many and varied scientific works.
        She provided the first scientific work in medicine by a woman
        physician, The Metabolism in Children.

728.   Korchilava, D. S. H. ["Varvara Nikolaevna Kipiani: the
        First Georgian Woman Physiologist"]. Sovetskoe Zdra-
        vookhranenie, 31 (1972) 86-87. (Rus)
        The name of V. N. Kipiani, the first woman physiologist in
        Georgia, was well-known in Europe at the beginning of the
        20th century. She was born in 1879 in Kutaisi and studied in
        Tiblisi. After graduation she taught for four years. She
        then left for Brussels to join her father, a professor of law
        and sociology at the university there. After passing her en-
        trance examinations and enrolling in the medical department
        of the university in 1901, she met the woman teacher and
        professor of psychophysiology, Ioteiko, who greatly influenced
        her career. During her student years she worked in Ioteiko's
        laboratory and for the Revue Psychologique, published by
        Ioteiko. From 1905 to 1913 Kipiani produced 22 important
        publications and worked in a variety of fields, which included
        studying the role of sugar in muscle work, the psychology of
        the deaf, dumb, and blind, and other problems in psychology
        and pedagogics. She participated in many international con-
        gresses and was the recipient of honorary awards, medals,
        and diplomas. Beginning in 1911 Kipiani was chairwoman of
        the Georgian section of the Belgian Museum of International
        Exhibits. She also taught Georgian and Russian and provided
        financial help to Russian students.

729.   Magilnitskii, S. G. ["First Women-Ophthalmologists in South-
        ern Russia in the 19th Century"]. Oftalmologicheskii

Zhurnal, 29:1 (1974) 73-76. (Rus)
Four women ophthalmologists are discussed. Olga Arkad'evna
Mashkovtseva (1851-1933) was a graduate of the Higher Medical Courses for Women in Petersburg in 1878 and started
her practice in Cherepovets. In 1887 she moved to Simfero-
pol, where she worked for 46 years, combining practice with
scientific work, mostly on glaucoma and trachoma, and lecturing. She was elected to participate in the work of the
Ninth All-Union Congress of Ophthalmology in Moscow on 1
November 1926. Evgenia Elizarovna Dikanskaya graduated
from the Petersburg Medical Courses for Women in 1883 and
became the first woman ophthalmologist in Herson. She specialized at the Eye Hospital of Magavli and at the Raukhfus
Hospital, but chose to return to Herson instead of pursuing a
teaching career. She headed two expeditions to remote depths
of the Zakaspiiskaya and Orenburgskaya provinces to fight eye
diseases. In 1903 she opened an eight-bed eye hospital. She
saw 150,000 patients and performed 1500 major operations
during her 40 years in Herson. She was a highly educated
woman, loved music and sculpture, and published many scientific reports. She was an active board member of the physicians' society in Herson and of the Odessa ophthalmologic
circle and participated in the Congress of Ophthalmologists
in Moscow in 1913. The first woman ophthalmologist in
Kishinev, Julia Alexandrovna Kvyatkovskaya, started her practice in 1894. During one of Dikanskaya's expeditions, she
performed 225 operations. She later (May 1899) opened an
eye hospital, where 200 patients were seen daily. During
one four-year period she saw 12,500 outpatients and 899 in-
patients. Her major publication, "Laceration of the Sclera
with Subconjunctival Dislocation of the Crystalline Lens in the
Only Eye," based on her own experience, was published in
1909. The first woman ophthalmologist in Samarkand was
Shmits. She operated an eye clinic, where she saw 21,783
outpatients and performed 574 operations, mostly for trachoma.
She had to function as surgeon, nurse, pharmacist, and jani-
tor of the hospital. In 1900 she published a detailed report
on her work in Samarkand from November 1898 to November
1899.

730. Nesterenko, A. I. ["The First Heroes of Medical Work--
        Women Physicians"]. Klinicheskaia Meditsina (Moskva),
        53:8 (August 1975) 151-153. (Rus)
    During 1928-29 five women physicians were awarded the hon-
    orary title of "Hero of Labor." They are A. N. Shabanova,
    A. A. Krasuskaya and A. A. Eltsina from Leningrad, M. S.
    Prokofeva from Tombov, and M. T. Zalivako from Pskov.
    Their merits and their outstanding services to the fields of
    medicine they worked in are briefly described.

731. ["Olga Yaroslavovna Rezhabek (On Her 70th Birthday)"].
        Arkhiv Patologii, 30:2 (1968) 94-95. port. (Rus)
    Dr. Rezhabek was born 23 June 1897 into the family of a

medical doctor. In 1915 she started to work as a nurse in
Rostov-on-Don. In 1921 she graduated from the medical
faculty of Donskoi University and worked at the same faculty
in the department of pathological anatomy until 1932. In 1933
she was invited to teach in Ashkhabad in the Turkmen SSR.
There she took an active part in organizing the medical institute. Since 1951 she has been the head of the Department of
Pathological Anatomy of this institute. She has published
more than 50 works in this field. She defended her first dissertation in 1937 and the second in 1945. She became the
first woman doctor of medical science and Professor of the
Republic. Professor Rezhabek is now retired, an Honorary
Worker, but remains active in scientific, Party, and social
life. She has been awarded many Orders of the Soviet Union.

732.   Popova, A. P. ["A. P. Popova, M. D."]. Sovetskoe Zdra-
         vookhranenie, 24 (1965) 61-62. (Rus)
       [Article not examined by editors.]

733.   ["Professor Eugeniia Nikolaevna Tretjakova"]. Pediatriia,
         49 (March 1970) 85-86. port. (Rus)
       The students and colleagues of E. Tretjakova congratulate
       her on the occasion of her 70th birthday and the 46th anni-
       versary of her scientific teaching and medical activities.
       Having graduated from the medical department of the Tomsk
       University in 1924, she became a pediatrician and combined
       her practical work with teaching medicine. In 1937 she de-
       fended her candidate's thesis, and in 1955 her doctoral thesis.
       She is an author of 70 works on pediatrics. Her main fields
       of interest are rheumatism, tubercular meningitis, and non-
       specific diseases of the respiratory tract in children. Tret-
       jakova has been an active participant of many congresses,
       conferences, and symposia in the USSR and abroad. She has
       combined her scientific and pedagogical work with public and
       social activities. She has been awarded the title of Honoured
       Physician and the Order of the Red Banner.

734.   Sechenov, I. M. ["Correspondence of I. M. Sechenov and
         M. A. Bokova-Sechenova"]. Nauchnoe Nasledstvo, 3
         (1956) 233-264. (Rus)
       A series of 45 letters written by Sechenov over a period of
       28 years are collected. They were written from Paris
       (three letters dated October 1862 to February 1863), Graz
       (22 letters from October 1867 to March 1868), Petersburg
       (14 letters; March 1886 to April 1887), and Moscow (Septem-
       ber 1889-February 1890). The letters describe Sechenov's
       life and scientific work during this period, describe his atti-
       tude toward women's education, and give advice and help to
       his wife in her own scientific work.

735.   Skachilov, V. A. ["A. I. Veretennikova's Stay in Bashkiria
         (On the 100th Anniversary of the Beginning of Medical
         Education for Women in Russia)"]. Sovetskoe Zdravoo-

khranenie, 32:4 (1973) 70-75. (Rus)
[Article not examined by editors.]

736. Strashun, I. D. ["The First Steps of Russian Women Physicians"]. Sovetskoe Zdravookhranenie, 7 (1960) 73-78.
(Rus)
Now that Soviet women physicians enjoy equal rights with men,
the author recalls the first women doctors in Russia and the
hardships they had to overcome. Suslova and Kashevarova
were the first ones board qualified to practice in all fields
of medicine. Bokova was allowed to practice only obstetrics,
gynecology, and pediatrics. All of the 19 women graduates
of the Courses for Women Physicians in Petersburg in the
years 1872-1882 participated in the Russo-Turkish War and
showed great courage; V. S. Nekrasova lost her life in the
war. At home, however, they met many obstacles in the
way of practice, and hostility from officials, although the
people needed their help badly. All went through humiliation
and suspicion for their desire to practice medicine. These
women included V. P. Matveeva, Mashkovtseva, and Yanov-
skaya in the Novgorod Province; N. Semyanovskaya and An-
geleva in Tambov Province; Kochurova in the Nizhegorod
Province; S. Bolot, S. Gasse, and A. Arkhangelskaya in
Moscow Province. There were exceptions: in Tver (Kalinin)
Province V. Bednyakova, the daughter of a state councillor,
and in Kharkov Province S. Sharkhovaya, from a noble family, were allowed to practice with relatively little complica-
tion.

737. "A Woman in the Russian Council." Bulletin Medical Wo-
men's Club of Chicago, 5:11 (July 1917) 3.
Dr. Schischkina Yavein, head of the Defenders of Women's
Rights (the Russian suffrage organization) was, at the be-
ginning of the war, chief of a hospital unit supported by
Russian women.

738. Zabludovskaia, Elena Davydovna. [V. A. Kashevarova-Rud-
neva]. Meditsina, Moscow, USSR, 1965. (Rus)
[Book not examined by editors.]

739. Zikeev, P. D. ["The Diploma of N. P. Suslova (on the
100th Anniversary of Her Doctoral Thesis)"]. Klinicheskaia Meditsina (Moskva), 46 (November 1968) 147-
149. (Rus)
In December 1867 the medical world of Russia learned the
exciting news from Zurich of the successful defense of the
doctoral thesis by the young Russian woman physician Nadezhda Prokofievna Suslova, who had recently graduated from the
Medical Department of the University of Zurich. The thesis
was titled "Contribution to the Knowledge of the Lymphatic
Heart." The author describes the obstacles facing the Russian women of that time in their struggle for acceptance in
the study of medicine and medical sciences. The battle was

at least partly won in 1897 when the tsarist government
opened the Women's Medical Institute. The image of N. P.
Suslova inspired other Russian women to cope with the hardships they endured in their studies.

UNITED STATES

740. "AMWA Presents...." Journal of the American Medical Wo-
        men's Association, 14:10 (October 1959) 923. port.
      An otolaryngologist, Suzanne Howe was appointed the first wo
      man physician to become a civilian consultant to the First
      Army.

741. "AMWA Presents...." Journal of the American Medical Wo-
        men's Association, 15:6 (June 1960) 607. port.
      A surgeon, Jane Cooke Wright's major professional area of
      concern has been researching a chemotherapeutic agent that
      will be able to cure human cancer. Her father, also a doc-
      tor, had initiated this research at the Harlem Hospital where,
      since his death, she has continued as director. Since her
      husband has formed the first life insurance company in Ghana,
      West Africa, Dr. Wright visited there and wrote a survey of
      the medical situation for the U.S. State Department. She was
      a recipient of the Spence Chapin award in 1958 for her ex-
      cellent results in treating the Wilms tumor in children.

742. "AMWA Presents...." Journal of the American Medical Wo-
        men's Association, 15:8 (August 1960) 792. port.
      Dr. Eileen B. McAvoy, a 1952 graduate of Baylor University
      College of Medicine, was the first woman to intern with the
      U.S. Army Medical Corps (at the U.S. Army Hospital in
      Waltham, Massachusetts).

743. "AMWA Presents ... Dr. Margaret J. Giannini." Journal of
        the American Medical Women's Association, 15:10 (Octo-
        ber 1960) 995. port.
      A pediatrician, Margaret J. Giannini was a pioneer in working
      with retarded children. Amita, Inc., an organization that
      recognizes contributions of American women of Italian origin,
      presented her with their Woman of the Year award c. 1960.

744. "AMWA Presents ... Eva F. Dodge, M.D.: First Woman
        Professor Emerita at University of Arkansas Medical
        School." Journal of the American Medical Women's As-
        sociation, 19:10 (October 1964) 870-872. port.
      A member of the obstetrics and gynecology faculty at the Uni-
      versity of Arkansas Medical School, Eva F. Dodge was the
      first woman to be honored as a professor emerita there. The
      fifth woman to receive a medical degree from the University
      of Maryland Medical School, her father's alma mater, she
      became the first woman to be given a rotating internship and
      a residency in obstetrics at the University Hospital in Balti-

more. She was also the first woman to have a medical practice in Winston-Salem, North Carolina, where she organized and directed a maternity clinic at the City Hospital and later expanded a County Maternity Clinic at the Baptist Hospital with the Public Health Service for rural users. She helped to establish Planned Parenthood services in maternity clinics in other areas of the South as well. From 1962 to 1964 she was elected president of the Pan American Medical Women's Alliance. Early in her career she was offered a professorship at Woman's Christian Medical School in Shanghai, China.

745. "A. Parks McCombs, M.D." Medical Woman's Journal, 52: 8 (August 1945) 43.
Dr. McCombs (whose portrait appears on the front cover of this issue of the Journal) received her medical degree in 1929 from Cornell University Medical College.

746. "Additional Honors for Dr. Van Hoosen." Medical Woman's Journal, 34:10 (October 1927) 309.
When the Medical Woman's Journal editors asked Dr. Van Hoosen to furnish a list of her degrees, to their surprise, an LL.D. had been added to her honors--and the degree had been conferred over a year ago [1926]. "No better proof of the innate modesty of our junior editor could be advanced."

747. "Adelaide Ward Peckham, M.D." Medical Woman's Journal, 48:10 (October 1941) 323.
Dr. Adelaide Ward Peckham (whose portrait appears on the front cover of this issue of the Journal) began her study of medicine in 1882. Her career is followed in the course of this article, from her alma mater, the Women's Medical College of the New York Infirmary for Women and Children, through her studies at the University of Pennsylvania and Johns Hopkins University, to her faculty appointment at the Woman's Medical College of Pennsylvania.

748. "Adele Schwartz, M.D." Medical Woman's Journal, 53:8 (August 1946) 59, 49.

749. Alexander, Ida M. "A Woman Doctor in France." Journal-Lancet, 39 (15 April 1919) 201-203.
A country doctor from the United States, Ida M. Alexander, was assigned to a tuberculosis clinic in Paris where she saw from 25 to 35 women, children, and babies each day. Because of crowded conditions in the sanatoria and a general lack of information about tuberculosis on the part of the public, Dr. Alexander considered this disease "the giant destroyer of France."

750. Alexander, Leslie L. "Susan Smith McKinney, M.D., 1847-1918. First Afro-American Woman Physician in New York State." Journal of the National Medical Association, 67:2 (March 1975) 173-175. photo., table. (Medical History.)

Susan Smith McKinney was the first Negro woman physician
in Brooklyn and New York State, and the third in the U. S.
She was graduated in 1870 from the New York Medical Col-
lege for Women as valedictorian of her class. She prac-
ticed in Brooklyn for 24 years and during that period was a
member of the staff of the New York Medical College and
Hospital for Women and was an organizer and staff member
of the Brooklyn Woman's Homeopathic Hospital and Dispensary
She took postgraduate work at the Long Island Medical College
Hospital in Brooklyn and was a member of the Kings County
Medical Society and the New York State Homeopathic Medical
Society. Dr. McKinney was also official physician to the
Brooklyn Home for Aged Colored People. In 1895 she left
New York to accompany her second husband, an army chap-
lain, to Montana and Nebraska, where she was also licensed
to practice. In 1898 she became resident physician and facul-
ty member at Wilberforce University, Ohio, where she remained until her death. A junior high school in Brooklyn
was named in her honor.

751. "Alice Stone Woolley, M. D." Medical Woman's Journal, 51:
      7 (July 1944) 34.
      Recently inaugurated president of the American Medical Wo-
      men's Association, Alice Stone Woolley (whose portrait ap-
      pears on the front cover of this issue of the Journal) re-
      ceived her M. D. from the University of Maryland College
      of Physicians and Surgeons.

752. "Alice Stone Woolley, M. D." Medical Woman's Journal, 53:
      12 (December 1946) 42. port.
      This biography focuses on Dr. Woolley's professional and
      social affiliations.

753. Allee, Ann Silver, comp. A Contribution to the Reshaping
      of Values: A Story of Vision and Courage, in Tribute
      to Eleanor Bertine, 1887-1968. The Orchard, Bridge-
      water, Connecticut, March 1, 1968, 9 pp.
      A reminiscence of the International Conference of Women
      Physicians held on 15-25 October 1920 includes "Synopsis of
      contents" of the proceedings of this conference. Dr. Eleanor
      Bertine's contributions to this conference, her paper on
      "Health and Morality in the Light of the New Psychology,"
      is discussed, as well as her participation in the discussion
      period following the papers on "Adaptation of the Individual
      to Life."

754. "Alma Dea Morani, M. D., F. A. C. S." Medical Woman's
      Journal, 53:7 (July 1946) 53. port. (News Notes.)
      Dr. Morani received a $1500 fellowship for further study
      and work in her specialty, plastic surgery.

755. "Alma Dea Morani, S. B., M. D., F. A. C. S." Medical Wo-
      man's Journal, 52:2 (February 1945) 50.

Dr. Morani (whose portrait appears on the front cover of
this issue of the Journal) received her M.D. degree in 1931
from the Woman's Medical College of Pennsylvania in Philadelphia. She is an eminent plastic surgeon and is the only
woman member of the Society of Plastic and Reconstructive
Surgery.

756.   Alpha Kappa Alpha Sorority, Inc. Heritage Series #4: Wo-
        men in Medicine. Alpha Kappa Alpha Sorority, Inc.,
        Chicago, Illinois, 1971, 32 pp.   ports.
The women physicians whose biographies appear in this pamphlet "are a representative group" of the approximately 200
black female physicians living and practicing in the United
States. The successors of Dr. Susan McKinney Steward,
the first black woman awarded a doctorate of medicine from
New York Medical College (1879), are Dr. M. Mitchell Bateman, a 1946 graduate of the Woman's Medical College of
Pennsylvania; Dr. Dorothy L. Brown, one of three black women who are fellows of the American College of Surgeons,
as well as the first black woman legislator in the state of
Tennessee; Dr. Elizabeth B. Davis, who graduated in 1949
from the College of Physicians and Surgeons, Columbia University, New York City; Dr. Helen O. Dickens, a 1952 recipient of the Distinguished Daughter of Pennsylvania Award;
Dr. Lillian Dove, who attended Meharry Medical College from
1913 to 1917; Dr. Effie O. Ellis, who has held several federal government positions and state appointments; Dr. M.
Joycelyn Elder, assistant professor of pediatrics at the University of Arkansas School of Medicine; Dorothy Boulding
Ferebee, who received her M.D. degree from Tufts University School of Medicine, and who came from a family of
seven lawyers; Dr. Angella D. Ferguson, a faculty member
at Howard University; Dr. Audrey Forbes, honored many
times for her outstanding contributions to the field of medicine; Dr. Margaret E. Grigsby, a prolific writer on medical
topics and professor of medicine at Howard University; Dr.
Jean L. Harris; Dr. Alicia E. Hastings; Dr. Xa Cadenne Hill;
Dr. Edith Irby Jones, the first black student admitted to the
University of Arkansas School of Medicine; Dr. Margaret
Morgan Lawrence; Dr. F. Pearl McBroom; Dr. Helen Payne;
Dr. Mildred E. Phillips; Dr. Jeanne Spurlock, the first black
person and first woman to receive the Strecker Award presented annually by the Institute of the Pennsylvania Hospital for
outstanding contributions in psychiatric care and treatment; Dr.
Mary A. T. Tillman; Dr. Maggie Walker; Dr. Ethel Sutton Weiseger; Dr. Jane C. Wright; Dr. Lois A. Young, the first black
woman admitted to the University of Maryland College of Medicine (M.D. 1960); and Dr. N. Louise Young. Education,
professional appointments, honors, awards, professional and
civic affiliations, and hobbies are given for each woman in
this pamphlet.

757.   Alsop, Gulielma Fell. Deer Creek: The Story of a Golden

Childhood. The Vanguard Press, Inc., New York, New York, 1947, 310 pp.

This is a memoir of the childhood of Gulielma Fell Alsop (a 1908 graduate of the Woman's Medical College of Pennsylvania). Its title is taken from the location of her grandmother's summer home in Pennsylvania, where the author spent much of her childhood. There is little in the book related to the author's future medical education or career, save an indication that she wanted to be a missionary in China. Her father replied that she had better study medicine. There are no dates, references, or photographs in the book.

758. Alsop, Gulielma Fell. "Rachel Bodley, 1831-1888: Chemist-Scientist; Third Woman Dean of the Woman's Medical College." Journal of the American Medical Women's Association, 4:12 (December 1949) 534-536. port. (Album of Women in Medicine.)

Rachel Bodley, a chemist and scientist, became the first woman professor of chemistry on the faculty of the Philadelphia Female Medical College in 1865. "At that time, in the eyes of the world, the entire venture of women in the field of medicine was a frail and insignificant thing, hardly worth the opposition it had aroused in the Philadelphia County Medical Society, hardly worth considering as a life career." In 1874 Rachel L. Bodley was appointed third woman head of the Female Medical College. She invited the first foreign student at that school to live with her, a young Brahman, Mrs. Annandibai Joshee. "Rachel Bodley came to the college when the importance of science in the medical curriculum was beginning to be felt. She, as well as Ann Preston, should be counted among its founders, as the firm foundation of science was needed for the stabilization of the curriculum."

759. "Always at the Front." Medical Sentinel, 13:7 (July 1905) 140.

According to this brief article, Dr. Mae H. Cardwell was the first woman physician on the staff of a Portland, Oregon hospital, the first president of the Portland Medical Club, the first woman treasurer of the State Medical Society, and the first woman physician to hold public office (as a member of the Portland City Health Board)--to mention just a few of her professional distinctions.

760. Anderson, M. Camilla. "New AMWA President, 1959-1960; Jessie Laird Brodie, M.D." Journal of the American Medical Women's Association, 14:7 (July 1959) 604. port.

761. Andriole, Vincent T. "Florence Rena Sabin--Teacher, Scientist, Citizen." Journal of History of Medicine and Allied Sciences, 14:3 (July 1959) 320-347.

This biography of Florence Rena Sabin was awarded the Ida and Henry Schuman Medical Historical Essay Prize for 1958.

Beginning with Sabin's birth in a Colorado mining camp, the essay discusses her early decision to study medicine, her research and teaching career at Johns Hopkins, her work in hematology and immunology at the Rockefeller Institute, and her energetic career in public health in her native Colorado during the last decade of her life.

762. "Angeline Frances Simecek, M.D." Medical Woman's Journal, 48:7 (July 1941) 216.
Dr. Simecek (whose portrait appears on the front cover of this issue of the Journal) graduated from the University of Nebraska College of Medicine in 1933. Upon receipt of the Mary Putnam Jacobi fellowship in 1936, Dr. Simecek chose to study at the University of Charles in Prague, Czechoslovakia. Her professional affiliations are included in this brief biography.

763. "Anita Gelber, M.D." Medical Woman's Journal, 51:11 (November 1944) 33.
Dr. Gelber (whose portrait appears on the front cover of this issue of the Journal) worked as a nurse for several years before studying medicine. The 1927 graduate of Rush Medical College specialized in dermatology.

764. "Anita Newcomb McGee, M.D." Woman's Medical Journal, 5:1 (January 1896) 27. (Biographical Series.)

765. "Ann Preston, M.D." Woman's Medical Journal, 10:9 (September 1900) 381-383. (Biographical.)
This biographical sketch of the life of Ann Preston tells of her sheltered Quaker girlhood, her graduation from medical school at the age of 39, and her work as educator and administrator at the Woman's Medical College of Pennsylvania.

766. "Anna E. Blount, M.D." Medical Woman's Journal, 32:6 (June 1925) 173. port.
Anna E. Blount became the president of the Medical Women's National Association. Frances Eastman Rose from Spokane, Washington was president-elect, which gave the west coast representation.

767. "Annie Sturges Daniel." Medical Woman's Journal, 51:9 (September 1944) 36. (Editorial.)
In this article, the Journal editors eulogize Dr. Daniel, whose history of the New York Infirmary for Women and Children was serialized by this publication. [The history is entitled "A Cautious Experiment...."]

768. "Another First." Medical Woman's Journal, 50:10 (October 1943) 256-257. port. (Section on War Service.)
Dr. Frances Phillips received the first navy commission for a woman physician in Southern California. Dr. Phillips's professional activities are briefly mentioned.

769. "Another First for DAR: The Dr. Anita Newcomb McGee
         Award." Daughters of the American Revolution Maga-
         zine, 101:3 (March 1967) 247-248. ports.
      The Dr. Anita Newcomb McGee Award was given by the Na-
      tional Society, Daughters of the American Revolution (DAR)
      to Captain Linda A. Bowman, U.S. Army nurse. The award
      is named in honor of Dr. McGee, who organized the Army
      Nurse Corps during the Spanish-American War. A brief
      biography of Dr. McGee is presented.

770. "The Appointment of Dr. Mary E. Wooley." Medical Wo-
         man's Journal, 39:2 (February 1932) 40.
      President of Mt. Holyoke College, Mary E. Wooley was ap-
      pointed by President Hoover to the Geneva Disarmament Con-
      ference. In response to a question about the power of wo-
      men to bring about world peace, she said, "'... I believe
      that part of their strength and their effectiveness as peace
      advocates lies in the very fact that they have not had the ex-
      perience in directing affairs that men have had. Their imag-
      ination is not cramped by the traditions of the case--that war
      has always been and therefore must always be. Their atti-
      tude is that it must stop. Here, as many times before, wo-
      men rush in successfully where masculine angels fear to
      tread.'"

771. "Armina Sears Hill: Medical Woman of the Month." Journal
         of the American Medical Women's Association, 5:6 (June
         1950) 246. port.
      "She helped with the pioneer work among poor families,
      teaching the preparation of milk formulas, cleanliness, and
      baby care in the clinics at the University of Chicago Settle-
      ment House and at the Women and Children's Hospital, then
      known as the Mary Thompson Hospital.... In 1912, Dr. Hill
      organized a clinic for adolescent girls at the Mary Thomp-
      son Hospital...."

772. Arnold, Jeannie Oliver. "Fifty-Two Years a Doctor." Med-
         ical Woman's Journal, 51:7 (July 1944) 27-28.
      A brief autobiography by Dr. Arnold, who received her M.D.
      degree in 1891, includes anecdotes of her practice in Provi-
      dence, Rhode Island.

773. Arthurs, Ann Catherine. "In Memoriam: Jean Crump, M.D.
         (1892-1963)." Journal of the American Medical Women's
         Association, 18:9 (September 1963) 739. port.
      Dr. Crump was a graduate of the Woman's Medical College
      of Pennsylvania where she served as professor of pediatrics.
      A pioneer in pediatric allergy, she served as president of
      both the Philadelphia and Pennsylvania Allergy Societies.

774. "Awards for Distinguished Teaching: Drs. O'Grady and Zap-
         pala Honored." School of Medicine Commentary: Uni-
         versity of California, Davis, 1:4 (November 1972) 1.
         ports.

One of five recipients of "Citations for Distinguished Teaching" on the UCD campus, Dr. Lois F. O'Grady is associate professor in the department of internal medicine.

775.   Bainbridge, Lucy Seaman. "One of the Pioneer Women in
         Medicine." Medical Woman's Journal, 28:3 (March 1921)
         75-78.   port.
       Cleora Augusta Seaman received her doctor of medicine degree from the Western Homeopathic College (Cleveland) in 1860, at the age of 46.   In 1869 she established the Seaman Free Dispensary.   Dr. Seaman died that same year.   This biography contains anecdotes of her personal and professional life.

776.   Baker, Josephine. "Annie Sturges Daniel, M.D.: 1858-
         1944." Medical Woman's Journal, 51:9 (September 1944)
         34-35.
       Sixty years of Dr. Daniel's life were filled with her responsibility as director of the outpatient department of the New York Infirmary for Women and Children.   In that post she championed prison reform and the elimination of tenement houses and sweatshops.   Following Josephine Baker's personal tribute to Dr. Daniel is a reprint of the obituary which appeared in the New York Times, and a poem entitled "Tenement Angel," dedicated to Dr. Daniel's memory.

777.   Baker, Rachel. "Elizabeth Blackwell: The First Woman
         Doctor." Journal of the American Medical Women's
         Association, 2:3 (March 1947) 136-138.   photo., port.
       A brief, episodic sketch of Blackwell's life; from her early home environment, through her professional life, to her death in 1910.

778.   Baker, Rachel. The First Woman Doctor: The Story of
         Elizabeth Blackwell, M.D.   Julian Messner Inc., New
         York, New York, 246 pp.   illus.
       This biography of Elizabeth Blackwell was written for adolescent readers.   More than one half of the text is devoted to her early family life, teaching career, and her decision to become a physician.   The remainder of the book concentrates on her internship at La Maternité in Paris, and the founding and operation of the New York Infirmary.   The book contains an index, but no bibliography.   Assistance from the New York Infirmary and the New York Academy of Medicine Rare Book Room were acknowledged by the author.

779.   Baker, S. Josephine. Fighting for Life. The Macmillan
         Company, New York, New York, 1939, 264 pp.   photos.,
         ports.
       In this autobiography, dedicated to Dr. Annie Sturges Daniel, S. Josephine Baker tells of her early determination to become a physician, her education at New York Infirmary Medical College and the women physicians who influenced her, and her

first experience in public health with the New York City Department of Health in Hell's Kitchen. She tells of her conviction that well-baby care for the prevention of disease was
more important than care after illness hit. In 1908 she
proved this point by visiting mothers on the lower east side,
which decreased the death rate by 1,200. She set up free
milk clinics, licensed midwives, and taught the use of silver
nitrate to prevent blindness in newborns. She recounts her
experiences treating the poor families of New York, and
throughout discusses the effect of her sex on her career.
The book includes a summary of her experiences in the College Equal Suffrage League, for which she went to the White
House and lobbied President Wilson. An index concludes the
work.

780.   Ball, Elizabeth B. "A Mother's Vision." Medical Woman's
        Journal, 53:1 (January 1946) 39-43, 58. port.
        Crediting her decision to study medicine to her mother's in-
        fluence, Dr. Ball (a 1907 graduate of the University of Illi-
        nois Medical School) recalls her own childhood and her many
        professional activities as a pediatrician in Quincy, Illinois.

781.   Bancroft, Jessie Hubbell. "Eliza M. Mosher, M.D." Med-
        ical Woman's Journal, 32:5 (May 1925) 122-129. ports.
        For Eliza M. Mosher to become a doctor after her mother
        had first said to her, "I would just as soon think of paying
        to have thee shut up in a lunatic asylum as to have thee stud
        medicine," is a reflection of her determination throughout her
        whole professional career. Dr. Mosher was among the first
        five women to be admitted to the University of Michigan Med-
        ical School. Giving up private practice, she became the first
        resident physician at the new State Reformatory Prison for
        Women at Sherborn, Massachusetts and later superintendent of
        that institution. Returning to private practice, Dr. Mosher
        combined that practice with being resident physician at Vas-
        sar College. She later became dean of women at the Uni-
        versity of Michigan, where she developed a physical education
        program for women. She was one of the founders of the
        American Posture League for which she designed an enterop-
        tosis belt and a kindergarten chair. She helped to organize
        the Medical Women's National Association, and she wrote a
        book on personal hygiene entitled, Health and Happiness, a
        Message to Girls. Her "record is that of a pioneer, facing
        for the first time new situations, new needs, finding her own
        solution for the problems, with the courage of her own con-
        victions, a constructive power that was not only original,
        but so entirely in accordance with all that the latter years
        have developed for such needs, that one marvels at the
        breadth and insight and efficiency of it all."

782.   "Banquet in Honor of Dr. Rosalie Slaughter Morton: Winter
        Park, Fla., June 13, 1934--Cleveland, Ohio." Medical
        Woman's Journal, 41:8 (August 1934) 224-225. port.

783.   "Banquet Tendered to Eliza M. Mosher, M.D., on Her Com-
            pletion of Fifty Years in the Practice of Medicine."
            Medical Woman's Journal, 32:5 (May 1925) 132-144.
        At this banquet, friends and colleagues reminisce about Dr.
        Mosher's contributions to medicine and society over her long
        influential career, as well as their friendship with her.

784.   Barker-Ellsworth, Alice. "In Memoriam: Dr. Margaret
            Vaupel-Clark." Medical Woman's Journal, 39:3 (March
            1932) 71.
        In 1900, Margaret Vaupel-Clark created a method to measure
        the mental and physical well-being of children that was used
        at the Iowa State Fair. As a result of the effectiveness of
        this program, a women's and children's building was erected
        on the state fair grounds. Through her work and influence,
        a chair of eugenics for the scientific preparation of parent-
        hood was established at the University of Iowa.

785.   Barringer, Emily Dunning. Bowery to Bellevue: The Story
            of New York's First Woman Ambulance Surgeon. W. W.
            Norton & Company Inc., New York, New York, 1950,
            262 pp. photo.
        Emily Dunning Barringer's autobiography concentrates on the
        brief period of her life from 1902 to 1905 (when she retired
        as chief of staff of the Gouverneur Hospital in New York
        City). She joined the Gouverneur as an ambulance surgeon
        in 1902, following a well publicized and arduous battle to se-
        cure a position there. Born in 1876, she did her undergrad-
        uate work at Cornell University and received her M.D. de-
        gree from Cornell following study at the Medical College of
        the New York Infirmary. She was guided in her education
        and medical training by Mary Putnam Jacobi. In her later
        career, Dr. Barringer served with the American Women's
        Hospitals and worked on behalf of the American Medical Wo-
        man's Association to secure commissions for women physi-
        cians in the army and navy. The final chapter ends on a ro-
        mantic note, with the newly-married Drs. Barringer sailing
        off to Europe and a "limitless horizon." [This book was the
        basis for an MGM motion picture, The Girl in White.]

786.   Barsness, Nellie N. "Highlights in Careers of Women Phy-
            sicians in Pioneer Minnesota." Journal of the American
            Medical Women's Association, 13:1 (January 1958) 19-22.
        The article briefly discusses many firsts for women physi-
        cians in Minnesota.

787.   Barsness, Nellie N. "History of Medicine: Highlights in
            Careers of Women Physicians in Pioneer Minnesota."
            Journal of the American Medical Women's Association,
            2:11 (November 1947) 524-525.
        This article deals primarily with the life and work of Dr.
        Martha G. Ripley, who practiced in the late 19th century in
        Minneapolis. She was active in the suffrage movement and

in changing the Age of Consent Law from ten to 18 years.
Dr. Mary Jane Snoddy Whetstone is also mentioned. She was
the second woman to practice medicine in Minneapolis, the
first woman to be elected a vice-president of the State Medical Association, the first woman to be appointed to the staffs
of two city hospitals and, along with Dr. Mary Hood, headed
the first staff of the Northwestern Hospital for Women and
Children.

788.   Bartholow, Roberts. New York Medical Journal, 5:2 (May
       1867) 167-170. (Letters to the Editor.)
       The author, a late assistant-surgeon (captain) of the United
       States Army, reminisces about his encounters with Mary
       Walker. When he first met her in Washington at Lincoln Gen
       eral Hospital, she functioned in "some pretended inspectorial
       capacity" which he perceived as functioning in fact as "spy
       and informer." At Chattanooga he also encountered Dr. Walk
       er when she appeared for employment as medical officer be-
       fore the medical director of the army of the Cumberland.
       Dr. Bartholow was a member of the medical board that ex-
       amined her qualifications. He remembers that "she betrayed
       such utter ignorance of any subject in the whole range of
       medical science, that we found it a difficult matter to conduct
       an examination. The Board unanimously reported that she
       had no more medical knowledge than any ordinary housewife,
       that she was, of course, entirely unfit for the position of
       medical officer, and that she might be made useful as a
       nurse in one of the hospitals." He interprets her riding
       about outposts alone one day as a fully intended maneuver on
       her part to be captured and forwarded to Richmond. Depart-
       ment headquarters thought that she could spy with more facil-
       ity as a medical officer and as a woman.

789.   Bass, Elizabeth. "Alma Matilda Lautzenheiser Rowe, M.D."
       Journal of the American Medical Women's Association,
       7:6 (June 1952) 223. port. (Album of Women.)
       An advocate of foundation garments that conformed to the
       natural lines of the body instead of the tight corsets that
       contracted at the waist and pushed the abdominal organs
       downward, Alma Matilda Lautzenheiser Rowe started study-
       ing medicine in 1889 at the Woman's Medical College, North-
       western University. She also believed that babies should not
       be confined by the then fashionable lengthy baby clothes.

790.   Bass, Elizabeth. "Another Past President: Louise Tayler-
       Jones. President 1928-1929." Women in Medicine, 90
       (October 1945) 21-22. port.
       Dr. Tayler-Jones, a 1903 graduate of Johns Hopkins School
       of Medicine, is remembered by the author as "the gentle wo-
       man, quiet yet forceful and farsighted, a good companion, a
       convincing campaigner" who, "because of her love for little
       children and pity for them ... selected the practice of pedi-
       atrics."

791.   Bass, Elizabeth. "Belle Anderson Gemmell, M.D." Journal
        of the American Medical Women's Association, 7:2 (Feb-
        ruary 1952) 66. port. (Album of Women in Medicine.)
        Belle Anderson Gemmell, born in 1863, kept records of her
        experience as a student, and the early history of the med-
        ical profession in Utah, where her father was a pioneer phy-
        sician. Her medical training proved especially valuable in
        1901 when she went with her husband to live in the mining
        districts of Zacatacas in Mexico and helped the villagers.

792.   Bass, Elizabeth. "Clara Israeli, M.D." Journal of the
        American Medical Women's Association, 11:3 (March
        1956) 108. port. (Album of Women in Medicine.)
        Some facts of the life of Dr. Clara Israeli, a bacteriologist
        and pathologist, are given.

793.   Bass, Elizabeth. "Elizabeth Comstock, M.D." Journal of
        the American Medical Women's Association, 11:2 (Febru-
        ary 1956) 77. port. (Album of Women in Medicine.)
        Dr. Comstock's father, "a staunch believer in opportunities
        for women," encouraged his daughter (born in 1875) to study
        medicine. She was the first woman physician to be presi-
        dent of the Tri-County Medical Society of Buffalo, Trem-
        pealeau and Jackson counties [New York State].

794.   Bass, Elizabeth. "Esther Pohl Lovejoy, M.D." Journal of
        the American Medical Women's Association, 6:9 (Septem-
        ber 1951) 354-355. port. (Album of Women in Medi-
        cine.)
        An "impressionistic sketch" of Dr. Lovejoy is presented.
        She was the first woman to head a health department of a
        large United States city (Portland, Oregon).

795.   Bass, Elizabeth. "Florence Rena Sabin, M.D." Journal of
        the American Medical Women's Association, 5:11 (Novem-
        ber 1950) 466-467. port. (Album of Women in Medi-
        cine.)
        One of the most highly respected researchers in anatomic re-
        search and experimental work in tuberculosis, Florence Rena
        Sabin also authored a widely used medical text, Atlas of the
        Medulla and Mid-Brain (1901). The first woman to be ap-
        pointed to the faculty of Johns Hopkins, she achieved the rank
        of professor of histology. She was the first woman president
        of the American Association of Anatomists. After Dr. Sabin
        retired, she returned to her home state of Colorado where
        she advocated preventive health care. In 1949 Dr. Sabin,
        then commissioner of health and charities, Denver, Colorado,
        was elected a vice-president of the American Public Health
        Association.

796.   Bass, Elizabeth. "It Runs in the Family: Three Sisters Who
        Were Physicians." Journal of the American Medical Wo-
        men's Association, 9:2 (February 1954) 45-47. illus.

The author cites families in which multiple members, especially sisters, were physicians. A few salient facts for each life are given.

797. Bass, Elizabeth. "Kate Campbell Hurd Mead, M.D." Journal of the American Medical Women's Association, 11:4 (April 1956) 155. port. (Past Presidents of AMWA.)
This article is a short biography of Dr. Hurd-Mead, a medical historian and the author of A Short History of the Pioneer Medical Women of America and A History of Women in Medicine.

798. Bass, Elizabeth. "L. Rosa Hirschmann Gantt, M.D." Journal of the American Medical Women's Association, 11:3 (March 1956) 109. port. (Past Presidents of AMWA.)
Rosa Hirschmann Gantt was the first woman physician to practice in Spartanburg, South Carolina. Her professional commitments included improving health and welfare conditions in rural areas by instituting traveling health trucks, medical inspection of schools, social hygiene programs, playgrounds, tuberculosis prevention measures, and many community movements. She helped extend the work of the American Women's Hospitals to the mountain regions of North and South Carolina and Kentucky. One of the first women members of the Southern Medical Association, she also served as president of the American Medical Women's Association in 1932. By appointment, she served under three presidents of the U.S. and under five governors of South Carolina.

799. Bass, Elizabeth. "Leisure Hours." Women in Medicine, 66 (October 1939) 9-12.
Elizabeth Blackwell, author of Pioneer Work and Counsel to Parents on the Sex Education of Children, adopted an orphan child, Katherine Barrie, because "medical solitude is really awful at times." Her colleague and friend, Marie Zakrzewska, describes many pleasant walks the two women took together. Dr. Elizabeth Cushier and Dr. Emily Blackwell lived together for 18 years and shared a summer home in Maine as well as travels. A pioneer medical woman in Scotland, beginning her career in 1865, Sophia Jex-Blake, "gave [her] greatest affection and sympathy" to the working women and girls in the clinics she established. She retired from medicine to start a dairy farm. Marie E. Zakrzewska came to America from Germany because the only degree she could earn there was midwifery. Her autobiography, A Woman's Quest, describes the hardships she endured. She retired to a country home which became a social center for her German and American friends. Mary Putnam Jacobi enjoyed her vacation by getting up at daybreak to write and read for the rest of the day.

800. Bass, Elizabeth. "Mary McKibbin Harper." Women in Medicine, 62 (October 1938) 8-10. port.

Receiving her degree in 1899, Mary McKibbin Harper specialized in obstetrics and gynecology. She was especially
active on behalf of crippled and blind children and founded a
"Tiny Tim Bed" in the Women and Children's Hospital in
Chicago and the Dickens Society which was both a literary
and philanthropic organization. Co-editor of the Medical Reviews, she edited three special numbers devoted entirely to
women's work. For twelve years from October, 1926, she
edited the Bulletin of the Medical Women's National Association.

801. Bass, Elizabeth. "Mary Ryerson Butin, M.D." Journal of
the American Medical Women's Association, 7:6 (June
1952) 222-223. port. (Album of Women in Medicine.)
Encouraged by her mother to study medicine, Mary Ryerson
[Butin] graduated from the Woman's Medical College of Chicago in 1881. She became the first woman member of the
Nebraska State Medical Society. In 1902 Dr. Butin was appointed city and county health officer in Madera, California--
the first instance of a woman receiving such an appointment
in the United States.

802. Bass, Elizabeth. "More Than One Hundred Years Ago."
Journal of the American Medical Women's Association,
7:10 (October 1952) 380-383. (Address upon receipt of
Alumnae Achievement Award, Woman's Medical College
of Pennsylvania, Philadelphia, June 11, 1952.)
After a brief introduction which mentions the author's Women
in Medicine collection at the Rudolph Matas Library of the
Tulane School of Medicine, Dr. Bass gives "cameo sketches"
of several women who practiced medicine in the United States
during the first half of the 19th century, and the circumstances under which they practiced.

803. Bass, Elizabeth. "Pioneer Women Doctors in the South."
Journal of the American Medical Women's Association,
2:12 (December 1947) 556-560.
This article consists of a collection of brief biographical
sketches taken from other sources.

804. Bass, Elizabeth. "Virginia Meriwether Davies, M.D." Journal of the American Medical Women's Association, 4:11
(November 1949) 504. port.
Facts of Dr. Davies' career are presented, as they were
gleaned from press clippings and personal accounts given by
Dorothy Dix, Dr. Davies' cousin. Dr. Davies' mother, although a Southerner, was an abolitionist and friend of Lucy
Stone. Her teachers at the Medical College of New York Infirmary were the founders, Emily and Elizabeth Blackwell.
Dr. Davies carried on a thriving medical practice until three
weeks before her death at the age of 87.

805. Bates, Mary Elizabeth. "Letters to the Editor." Medical

Woman's Journal, 53:5 (May 1946) 38, [41].
Mary Bates points out that the obituary of Dr. Josephine A.
Jackson, which appeared in the Journal's April 1946 issue
(p. 53) erroneously stated that Dr. Jackson was the first woman intern at Chicago's Cook County Hospital. Dr. Bates,
however, was Cook County's first woman intern, beginning
her service in 1881 at the age of 20. She describes her internship and mentions the women interns who followed her
lead.

806.   Battino, Barbara. "Esther Clark: Accomplishment Is Her
          Trademark." Stanford M.D., 11:4 (Fall 1972) 20-21.
          port.
       Esther Bridgman Clark, a 1925 Stanford Medical School grad-
       uate, in 1927 became the first pediatrician to service the San
       Mateo-San Jose, California area. Pioneering in the concept
       of group practice, she joined an internist and two surgeons
       in Palo Alto, California and formed the nucleus for what de-
       veloped into the Palo Alto Medical Clinic, which now supports
       140 physicians. Early in her 45-year career, she campaigned
       for immunization against smallpox, diphtheria, whooping cough
       and tetanus. The city's infant death rate dropped significantly
       by 1937, and newspapers credited Dr. Clark with making Palo
       Alto "the safest place in the world for a baby to be born."
       In 1953 she established the Children's Health Council (CHC)
       in Palo Alto for the treatment of retarded and physically and
       emotionally handicapped children. She also urged the Ameri-
       can Academy of Pediatrics to initiate a Child Accident Pre-
       vention Committee, on which she served for four years. At
       the age of 72, Dr. Clark--who always believed in the im-
       portance of developing interests and activities to complement
       one's professional life--left practice to begin "a vigorous re-
       tirement that includes African safaris and wildlife photogra-
       phy."

807.   Baumann, Frieda. "Memoir of Ruth Hartley Weaver."
          Transactions and Studies of the College of Physicians of
          Philadelphia, 41 (April 1974) 316-317.
       Ruth Hartley Weaver was graduated from the Woman's Medi-
       cal College of Pennsylvania in 1917 as the youngest in her
       class. This memoir reviews her career in public health and
       her professional activities and accomplishments in Philadel-
       phia until her retirement in 1960.

808.   Baumann, Frieda. "Memorial to Ellen Culver Potter, M.D.
          (1871-1958)." Journal of the American Medical Women's
          Association, 13:7 (July 1958) 296-297.
       Dr. Potter was the first resident physician at the Hospital of
       the Woman's Medical College in 1904. Her long list of ap-
       pointments and accomplishments is reviewed.

809.   Baumann, Frieda. "Memorial to Louise Pearce, M.D. (1885-
          1959)." Journal of the American Medical Women's Asso-
          ciation, 15:8 (August 1960) 793. port.

810. "Beatrix A. Bickel, M.D." Medical Woman's Journal, 52:
       12 (December 1945) 37.
       Dr. Bickel (whose portrait appears on the front cover of this
       issue of the Journal) graduated from the Cleveland Medical
       College (Ohio) in 1896. She practiced in Hamburg, Germany
       at the turn of the century. As a result of the war, Dr.
       Bickel had difficulty regaining her American citizenship and
       returning to the United States. By 1923 she was employed
       by the U.S. Public Health Service and also served as chief
       librarian of the Army Medical Library until her retirement
       in 1942.

811. Beatty, Geneva. "Dorothy Hewitt, M.D." Journal of the
       American Medical Women's Association, 10:12 (Decem-
       ber 1955) 438. port. (Album of Women in Medicine.)
       Dorothy Hewitt was one of the founders of the Long Beach
       branch of the American Medical Women's Association. She
       practiced obstetrics for a while in the Frontier Nursing Ser-
       vice. Later Dr. Hewitt was a founding member of the Amer-
       ican Academy of Obstetrics and Gynecology.

812. Beatty, J. "So That Mothers May Live: American Woman,
       Dr. Ida Scudder, Who Tackled the Problem of Furnish-
       ing Women Doctors for Indian Women." Reader's Digest,
       43 (November 1943) 101-104.
       [Article not examined by editors.]

813. "Belle Anderson Gemmell, M.D.: Our Fifty Years in Prac-
       tice Club." Medical Woman's Journal, 49:8 (August
       1942) 254.
       Belle Anderson Gemmell, one of three sisters to acquire a
       medical degree, practiced for fifty years. She was an early
       associate editor of the Medical Woman's Journal and also
       authored a history of the Medical Profession in Utah-1857
       to 1880 based on her father's notes and experiences as a doc-
       tor. (Dr. Gemmell's portrait appears on the front cover of
       this issue of the Journal.)

814. Benetar, Judith. Admissions: Notes from a Woman Psy-
       chiatrist. Charterhouse, New York, New York, 1974,
       219 pp.
       The protagonist describes the book she is planning to write:
       "... it's partly documentary, partly autobiography, partly
       just, well, 'musing,' I guess." And she claims the book's
       message will be that "psychiatrists are human, too," and
       "we're all in this thing of life together." Judith Benetar is
       the pseudonym of a woman psychiatrist in New York City.
       She has written a memoir of her personal and professional
       life, her patients and colleagues, her failing marriage, and
       her lover. The reader learns not only about Dr. Benetar's
       patients, but also about her feelings regarding those patients;
       not only about the clinical aspects of her life as a psychia-
       trist, but also about how her profession affects her personal

life. Thus, when she loses a patient to suicide, the doctor
herself must be treated. And when an emergency case is
brought in, she reprimands the patient with a very human,
"Stop it, will you! You're scaring the shit out of us!"

815.   Bennett, Jane E. "Dr. Ruth." Missouri Alumnus, 62:3
        (March-April 1974) 20-23. photos., ports.
        A 1906 graduate of the University of Missouri School of Medi-
        cine, Ruth Seevers at 90 is probably the oldest practicing wo-
        man physician in Missouri. Dr. Seevers has no intention of
        retiring after 67 years of general practice.

816.   Bennett, Ruth Blount. "Anna Ellsworth Blount, M.D." Jour-
        nal of the American Medical Women's Association, 12:3
        (March 1957) 86. port. (Past Presidents of AMWA.)
        Anna Ellsworth Blount was president of the American Medical
        Women's Association from 1925 to 1926, then known as the
        Medical Women's National Association. Some of her fields
        of interest during her career include woman suffrage, eugen-
        ics, social hygiene, and sex education. In 1895 she was af-
        filiated with Hull House.

817.   Bernard, Marcelle [T]. "Elaine Pandia Ralli, M.D." Jour-
        nal of the American Medical Women's Association, 7:4
        (April 1952) 152. port. (Album of Women in Medicine.)
        Receiving her degree in 1925, she has spent a large portion
        of her professional life researching metabolism functions in
        such areas as nutritional disturbances and diabetes. She was
        placed in charge of reorganizing New York City hospitals' out-
        patient services to improve clinic services and to decrease
        the need for hospitalization of ambulatory patients.

818.   Bernard, Marcelle [T]. "Eleanor Anderson Campbell, M.D.
        Co-Founder of the Judson Health Center, New York."
        Journal of the American Medical Women's Association,
        6:10 (October 1951) 401-402. port. (Album of Women
        in Medicine.)
        When Eleanor Anderson was a young girl, she visited some
        tenements and never forgot the "cold-water flats, dirty chil-
        dren, and over-worked mothers.... Even though she later
        married, had a daughter, and enjoyed an interesting social
        life, she still felt a strong desire to serve the unfortunate."
        To do "free medical social service work where the need was
        greatest," Eleanor Anderson Campbell helped to found a clinic
        in Judson Memorial Church, which later moved and became
        Judson Health Center.

819.   Bernard, Marcelle [T]. "Elizabeth Bass, M.D." Journal of
        the American Medical Women's Association, 8:9 (Septem-
        ber 1953) 310. port. (Album of Women in Medicine.)
        Finishing her medical degree in 1904, Elizabeth Bass was the
        first woman appointed to the teaching staff of Tulane Univer-
        sity School of Medicine in 1911, four years before women

were admitted as students there. She was a professor of
clinical laboratory diagnosis and associate professor of clinical medicine. Among her "firsts as a woman" include the
following: secretary of the Orleans Parish Medical Society
from 1920 to 1922, an officer of the Southern Medical Association as chairman of the section of pathology in 1939.
From 1921 to 1922 she was president of the American Medical Women's Association. Dr. Bass founded and maintained
a collection, "Women in Medicine," at the Matas Medical
Library of Tulane University.

820.   Bernard, Marcelle [T]. "Ella A. Mead, M.D." Journal of
       the American Medical Women's Association, 11:6 (June
       1956) 220. port. (Album of Women in Medicine.)
Receiving her medical degree in 1903, and having made a
study in which she found 75 per cent of the children in a
school system handicapped in 1912, Dr. Mead foresaw the
need for child guidance clinics. She was instrumental in
establishing a nursing service in Weld County, Colorado. As
a result of the 1947 Sabin Law, the county health department
was organized, and Dr. Mead was appointed assistant health
department medical officer in 1948 in charge of vital statistics.

821.   Bernard, Marcelle [T]. "Estella Ford Warner, M.D." Jour-
       nal of the American Medical Women's Association, 6:7
       (July 1951) 284. port. (Album of Women in Medicine.)
Receiving her medical degree in 1918, Estella Ford Warner,
at the beginning of her career, worked primarily in public
health services concerned with children's medical care and
treatment. In 1932 she became the first woman physician to
receive a commission in any of the uniformed services when
she became an officer in the United States Public Health Service. As a staff member of the Public Health Service, she
worked among the Native Americans in New Mexico, Colorado,
and Arizona as well as California. In 1951 Dr. Warner went
to Beirut, Lebanon to assume the duties of regional public
health representative in the Near East under the Point 4 program. She established a school of public health at the American University in Beirut.

822.   Bernard, Marcelle [T]. "Helen Margaret Wallace, M.D."
       Journal of the American Medical Women's Association,
       7:12 (December 1952) 464. port. (Album of Women in
       Medicine.)
Helen M. Wallace, who received her medical degree in 1937,
was appointed director of the Bureau for Handicapped Children by the New York City Department of Health.

823.   Bernard, Marcelle T. "Jeanne Cecile Bateman, M.D."
       Journal of the American Medical Women's Association,
       6:4 (April 1951) 148. port. (Album of Women in Medi-
       cine.)

Dr. Jeanne Cecile Bateman, appointed clinical instructor in
medicine at George Washington University in 1948, was also
appointed chief investigator in the George Washington University grant-supported study of the use of intra-arterial injections of nitrogen mustard to control cancer.

824.   Bernard, Marcelle T.   "Lillie Rosa Minoka Hill, M.D."
        Journal of the American Medical Women's Association,
        11:7 (July 1956) 261.   port.   (Album of Women in Medi-
        cine.)
Lillie Rosa Minoka, a graduate of the 1899 class of the Woman's Medical College of Pennsylvania, was a Mohawk Native
American who was raised by Quakers in Philadelphia.   She
married Charles Hill, an Oneida Native American and went to
live on the Oneida Reservation in Wisconsin after having practiced for five years.   Her husband did not allow her to have
a regular practice, but he did want her to care for neighbors
and relatives which she did do.   In 1934 she applied for a
license to practice medicine in Wisconsin.   In the Oneida
language she is known as "You-da-gent" which means, "she
who carries aid."

825.   Bernard, Marcelle [T].   "Lunette I. Powers, M.D."   Journal
        of the American Medical Women's Association, 6:5 (May
        1951) 194.   port.   (Album of Women in Medicine.)
Since Lunette I. Powers received her degree in 1900, she has
delivered 5,000 babies in Muskegon, Michigan and served as
general practitioner there.

826.   Bernard, Marcelle T.   "Mabel M. Akin, M.D."   Journal of
        the American Medical Women's Association, 11:4 (May
        1956) 190.   port.   (Past Presidents of AMWA.)
This article presents a catalogue of Mabel Akin's achievements, memberships, and honors.

827.   Bernard, Marcelle [T].   "Mary Louise Tinley, M.D."   Jour-
        nal of the American Medical Women's Association, 8:12
        (December 1953) 417.   port.   (Album of Women in Medi-
        cine.)
Mary Louise Tinley was born of parents who had migrated
to Council Bluffs, Iowa from Ireland.   After receiving her
medical degree in 1894, she returned to Council Bluffs to be
a general practitioner.

828.   Bernard, Marcelle [T].   "Mary Martin Sloop, M.D."   Journal
        of the American Medical Women's Association, 7:5 (May
        1952) 184.   port.   (Album of Women in Medicine.)
Mary Martin Sloop started a school in Crossnore, North
Carolina in 1911 for educating and giving health care to the
people of the mountains.   By 1952 this educational institution
had expanded from a "humble shack" to "20 buildings on 260
acres of land."

829. Bernard, Marcelle [T]. "Nelle S. Noble, M.D." Journal
      of the American Medical Women's Association, 7:11 (No-
      vember 1952) 430. port. (Album of Women in Medi-
      cine.)
      Nelle S. Noble, the first woman to intern at Methodist Hos-
      pital in Des Moines, Iowa, practiced general medicine and
      obstetrics for 44 years, retiring in September, 1949, having
      treated four generations of families in that city.

830. Bernard, Marcelle T. "Nellie O. Barsness, M.D." Jour-
      nal of the American Medical Women's Association, 8:4
      (April 1953) 151. port. (Album of Women in Medicine.)
      Dr. Barsness was one of the first women physicians in Min-
      nesota. She served during World War I in the French army.

831. Bernard, Marcelle T. "Olga Frances Stastny, M.D." Jour-
      nal of the American Medical Women's Association, 8:11
      (November 1953) 380. port. (Past Presidents of AMWA.)
      Receiving her medical degree in 1913, Olga Frances Stastny
      practiced a great variety of medicine: rehabilitation, anes-
      thesiology, preventive medicine, clinical medicine, obstetrics
      and gynecology. For some of her career she worked abroad
      in Czechoslovakia, France, and Greece. From 1930 to 1931
      she served as president of the American Medical Women's
      Association.

832. Bernard, Marcelle [T]. "Rebecca Parrish, M.D. Founder
      of the Mary Johnston Hospital, Manila, Philippine Islands."
      Journal of the American Medical Women's Association,
      6:8 (August 1951) 317-318. photo., port. (Hospitals
      Founded by Women Physicians.)
      Receiving her medical degree in 1901, Rebecca Parrish went
      into foreign missionary work in Manila in 1906 and became
      the first woman physician to practice in the Philippines. At
      the end of that year, she established the Bethany Dispensary,
      an outpatient clinic. In 1908 she was able to found the Mary
      Johnston Hospital which later had wards for children, mater-
      nity, medical and surgical health care and service, as well
      as a ward for crippled children, and a nursing school. In
      the Battle of Manila (1945), the Mary Johnston Hospital was
      destroyed. It was rebuilt in 1950.

833. Bernard, Marcelle [T]. "Ruth A. Parmelee, M.D." Jour-
      nal of the American Medical Women's Association, 9:2
      (February 1954) 53. port. (Album of Women in Medi-
      cine.)
      In 1912 Ruth A. Parmelee received her medical degree and,
      after finishing her training, began her medical career in the
      Near East under the American Board of Foreign Missions in
      1914. She was the first woman physician to settle in Turkey's
      Euphrates River Valley [in modern times]. In 1923 she was
      affiliated with the American Women's Hospitals in Thessalon-
      ika, Greece, and from 1925 to 1941 she was a hospital direc-

tor at Athens, until she was forced to evacuate and returned to the United States. She worked with the Athens Municipal Hospital to help lay the foundation for the first school of nursing under government auspices. It opened in 1938. She prepared an English-Greek lexicon of medical, psychological, and special terms and an "Outline of Hygiene" in Greek. She worked in Greek and Yugoslav refugee camps in Egypt, Syria, and Palestine from 1943 to 1948, when she joined the staff of Pierce College, Elleniko, Greece.

834.   Bernard, Marcelle [T]. "Sophie Rabinoff, M.D., M.S.P.H." Journal of the American Medical Women's Association, 7:8 (August 1952) 311. port. (Album of Women in Medicine.)
Receiving her degree in 1913, Sophie Rabinoff did a residency in pediatrics at the New York Home for Hebrew Infants and then went to Palestine with the Hadassah Medical Group, where she organized a children's hospital and clinic for Arab and Jewish children. When she returned to the United States, she soon became interested in public health. In 1939 Dr. Rabinoff was appointed health officer in charge of the East Harlem Health District and started a constructive "whispering" campaign to spread the word about diphtheria immunization wherever mothers and babies congregated--parks, sidewalks, etc. In 1952 Dr. Rabinoff was appointed professor of public health and industrial medicine at the New York Medical College.

835.   "Bertha [L]. Selmon, M.D." Medical Woman's Journal, 52:1 (January 1945) 54.
Dr. Selmon (whose portrait appears on the front cover of this issue of the Journal) spent 21 years (1903 to 1924) as a medical missionary in China. Dr. Selmon's professional activities and affiliations are noted.

836.   "Bertha L. Selmon, M.D." Medical Woman's Journal, 56:2 (February 1949) 43, 49. port.
Bertha Eugenia Loveland Selmon, a 1902 graduate of American Medical Missionary College, died in January 1949. This brief article tells of Dr. Selmon's work in China and Michigan, and her research and writing of histories of women in medicine.

837.   "Bertha Shafer, M.D., Harriet Cory, M.D." Medical Woman's Journal, 53:8 (August 1946) 26-28. ports.
Biographies are presented of Bertha Meserve Shafer and Harriet S. Cory upon the occasion of their election to honorary life membership in the American Social Hygiene Association.

838.   Best, Katharine and Hillyer, Katharine. "Colorado's Little Doctor." Coronet, 25 (March 1949) 99-103. illus.
This article discusses Dr. Florence Rena Sabin's work in public health in Colorado.

839.   "....Beyond the Call...."   Chironian, 30:1 (Summer 1968)
          21-22.   port.
       Under a program sponsored by the American Medical Asso-
       ciation, Dolores Fiedler served as an obstetrician and gyne-
       cologist to civilians in war-torn Vietnam.   The 1953 graduate
       of New York Medical College discusses the problems of being
       a physician in Vietnam "with only 1,500 native doctors to
       help."

840.   "Biographical Note."   Journal of the American Medical Wo-
          men's Association, 1:9 (December 1946) 297.
       Alice Stone Woolley practiced general medicine and was presi-
       dent of the American Medical Women's Association from 1944
       to 1945.

841.   Bittner, Christina.   ["Doctor Elizabeth Blackwell"].   Tribune
          Medicale, (December 1953).   (Fre)

842.   [Blackwell, Alice Stone].   "An Early Woman Physician."   The
          Woman's Journal, 37 (6 October 1906) 1, 158a-159b.
          port.
       This biography of Dr. Emily Blackwell discusses her ances-
       try, her medical education, and her cofounding of both the
       New York Infirmary for Women and Children and the Medical
       College of the Infirmary.

843.   Blackwell, Anna.   "Elizabeth Blackwell."   English Woman's
          Journal, (14 February 1858).   (Letter to the Editor.)
       [Article not examined by editors.]

844.   Blackwell, Elizabeth.   Pioneer Work in Opening the Medical
          Profession to Women.   Longmans, Green, and Co., Lon-
          don, England, 1895, ix, 265 pp.
       This autobiography covers Blackwell's life from her birth in
       1821, to 1876.   It is topically organized as follows: early
       family life, earning money for study, study in America, study
       in Europe, practical work in America, and visits to England
       in 1858 and 1869.   The work draws heavily on her correspon-
       dence and journals, many entries and letters being entirely
       reproduced.   Outstanding among the friends and associates
       mentioned are Lady Noel Byron, Florence Nightingale, Cor-
       nelia Hussey, Marie Zakrzewska, Elizabeth Garrett, and
       Sophia Jex-Blake--as well as her sister, Dr. Emily Black-
       well.   Appended is a letter from Dr. Stephen Smith, a class-
       mate of Blackwell's at Geneva, on medical coeducation of the
       sexes (dated 1892).   Also appended: a poem "in honour of
       the fair M.D.," the first annual report of the New York Dis-
       pensary for Poor Women and Children (1855), and a list of
       addresses and publications which indicate England's "'search
       after righteousness.'"   [An Everyman's Library edition
       (1914?) includes a supplementary chapter by Robert Cochrane
       which covers Blackwell's final years and her death in 1910,
       and also provides information on the status of women's med-

ical education in 1914.   An introduction by M. G. Fawcett
places Blackwell in historical perspective and is followed by
a comprehensive list of her publications and speeches.]

845.   Blain, M.   "Florence Nightingale and Elizabeth Blackwell."
            South African Nursing Journal, 34:2 (February 1967) 7-9.
        The author feels that although both Blackwell and Nightingale
        should be equally well-known as trailblazers for the women
        of the world, many have never heard of Elizabeth Blackwell.
        Dr. Blackwell's struggle for a medical education is reviewed
        and certain events compared with events in Florence Nightin-
        gale's life.

846.   Blake, John B.   "Mary Gove Nichols, Prophetess of Health."
            American Philosophical Society, Proceedings, 106 (1962)
            220-223.
        [Article not examined by editors.]

847.   Bland, Bessie Farinholt.   "May Farinholt Jones, M.D."
            Medical Woman's Journal, 52:6 (June 1945) 56-57.
        After the death of her husband, May Jones studied medicine
        and graduated in 1897 from the Medical College of Baltimore
        (Maryland).   She was the first woman physician at the Mis-
        sissippi State College for Women, the first woman ever ad-
        mitted to the Mississippi State Medical Association, and the
        first woman to take the state board medical examination in
        Mississippi.

848.   Block, Jean Libman.   "The Doctor Was an 'Adventuress.'"
            Today's Health, 48:8 (August 1970) 20-21, 63.   illus.
        Dr. Esther Pohl Lovejoy (1869-1967) is the subject of this
        biography.

849.   Block, J[ean] L[ibman].   "Father-Daughter Surgical Team."
            Good Housekeeping, 151 (September 1960) 32, passim.
            illus.
        [Article not examined by editors.]

850.   Bluemel, Elinor.   Florence Sabin: Colorado Woman of the
            Century.   University of Colorado Press, Boulder, Colo-
            rado, 1959, 238 pp.   photos., ports.
        This biography of Florence Rena Sabin, based on her person-
        al papers, recounts her struggles for a medical education at
        Johns Hopkins University, her long career as professor of
        anatomy and histology at Johns Hopkins, the years from 1925
        through 1938 when she set up and headed the Department of
        Cellular Studies at the Rockefeller Institute for Medical Re-
        search, and her retirement years when she fought for and
        saw passed the "Sabin Health Bills," giving Colorado one of
        the best public health programs in the U.S.   In Denver, her
        public health work resulted in a 50 per cent drop in the tu-
        berculosis rate and a 90 per cent drop in syphilis cases.
        Among other topics discussed are her work for women's suf-

frage in Baltimore during the early twenties and her research work on anatomy, lymphatics, tuberculosis, and cellular processes. An extensive bibliography and index conclude the work. Several portraits appear throughout.

851. Bodly [sic], Rachael. "Emeline H. Cleveland." Woman's Medical Journal, 10:10 (October 1900) 425-426. (Biographical.)
This biography of Dr. Cleveland, who died in 1878, was extracted from a memorial address by Dr. Bodley.

852. Booth, Alice. "Dr. Florence Rena Sabin: The First Woman in America to Reach a Commanding Position in the Field of Medical Research." Good Housekeeping, 92 (June 1931) 50-51, 198, 200, 202. port. (America's Twelve Greatest Women.)
This portrait of Dr. Sabin, the first woman to be elected to the National Academy of Sciences and to be made a full member of the Rockefeller Institute for Medical Research, is a recounting of the events which led Dr. Sabin to her prominent position in medicine. The article quotes Dr. Sabin's opinions on various aspects of medicine and life.

853. Bourdeau-Sisco, Patience S. "Amanda T. Norris Ninety-Four Years Young." Medical Woman's Journal, 50:7 (July 1943) 188. port.
The oldest woman doctor in Maryland, 94-year-old Amanda T. Norris, graduated from the Woman's Medical College of Pennsylvania in 1880.

854. Brackett, Elizabeth R. "Mildred G. Gregory, M.D." Journal of the American Medical Women's Association, 8:3 (March 1953) 111. port. (Album of Women in Medicine.)
Mildred G. Gregory is probably the only woman physician in New Jersey who was director of a hospital. After she was certified by the American Board of Pediatrics in 1942, she chose to practice solely pediatrics and became involved with hospital administration.

855. Branson, Helen Kitchen. "The Doctor from Meharry." Medical Woman's Journal, 52:5 (May 1945) 36-37, 60.
Dr. Edna L. Griffin serves the Mexican and Negro population of Pasadena, California. This article describes the blatant discrimination practiced against the Negro in California, and Dr. Griffin's "uphill fight" for a medical education and practice. The hospitals in Pasadena will either refuse to admit Negro patients or insist upon their being kept in private rooms if they are admitted.

856. Branson, Helen Kitchen. "The Woman Who Can't Be Downed." Medical Woman's Journal, 57:5 (May 1950) 34-35.
Determined that poor people who did not even have a nickel for transportation to get to the public health clinic in down-

town Los Angeles should have easy access to adequate health
care, Ruth Temple entered the Los Angeles Health Department in 1924. By 1934 she set up a demonstration clinic in
the needed district and at last, in 1941, the city established
a municipal polyclinic to supplement her private work. The
Southeast District Health Association, a nonprofit educational
facility, cooperated with the municipal polyclinic operated by
the city. At the time this article was written there was an
educational program, then called the Community Health Association, carried on jointly by city officials and the Southeast
District.

857.   "British and American Medical Officer." Medical Woman's
          Journal, 51:3 (March 1944) 32. (Section on War Ser-
          vice.)
       A profile of Achsa M. Bean, who graduated in 1936 from the
       University of Rochester School of Medicine, focuses upon her
       activities in the British and American Medical Corps.

858.   Brodie, Jessie Laird. "Career Satisfactions of a Physician."
          American Soroptimist, 33:8 (May 1960) 6-7. photos.,
          port.
       Dr. Brodie discusses her desire to become a physician, her
       concept of what women in medicine should be, and her
       thoughts on combining marriage and medicine.

859.   Brodie, Jessie Laird. "Dorothy Boulding Ferebee, M.D."
          Journal of the American Medical Women's Association,
          15:11 (November 1960) 1095. (Album of Women in Medi-
          cine.)
       When Dorothy Boulding Ferebee graduated from Tufts Univer-
       sity in 1924, she could not find a place to serve her intern-
       ship until she won first place in a competitive examination
       after graduation. An early president of the National Council
       of Negro Women, she was also medical director of a health
       clinic on plantations in Mississippi, as well as a founder and
       organizer of the South East Settlement House in Washington,
       D.C. Dr. Ferebee is the only woman physician holding the
       position of chief of a large coeducational university's (How-
       ard's) health service.

860.   Brodie, Jessie Laird. "Sarah D. Rosekrans, M.D." Jour-
          nal of the American Medical Women's Association, 13:8
          (August 1958) 346. port. (Album of Women in Medicine.)
       A president of the Pan American Medical Women's Alliance,
       Sarah Didriksen Rosekrans also was president, or chief of
       staff, of Neilsville's (Wisconsin) Memorial Hospital. She
       shared her practice with her husband.

861.   Brody, Irwin A. "The Decision to Study Medicine." New
          England Journal of Medicine, 252:4 (27 January 1955)
          130-134.
       A portion of this article examines the motivations of specific

women who entered the medical profession. Among the pioneer women physicians, one finds examples of "the crusading spirit and the conscious sense of dedication to a righteous cause." The generation following the Blackwells and Zakrzewska, however, entered the profession "in a more natural manner," as opposition to women's ambitions lessened. Several women--including Drs. Elizabeth Cushier, Rosalie Slaughter Morton, and S. Josephine Baker--are quoted.

862.   Brooks, Benjy F. "Goldie Suttle Ham, M.D." Journal of
        the American Medical Women's Association, 16:1 (January 1961) 67. port. (Album of Women in Medicine.)
Goldie Suttle Ham was the first woman in a residency in Houston.

863.   Brown, Adelaide. "The History of the Development of Women in Medicine in California." Medical Woman's Journal, 33:1 (January 1926) 17-20.
Reprinted from the May 1915 issue of California and Western Medicine, this article describes the struggles and accomplishments of several pioneer women physicians in California.

864.   Brown, Elizabeth B. "Esther M. Greisheimer, Ph.D.,
        M.D." Journal of the American Medical Women's Association, 10:5 (May 1955) 180. port. (Album of Women in Medicine.)
Author of Physiology and Anatomy, a widely used textbook in colleges and schools of nursing, Esther Greisheimer has been the woman professor in Temple University's Medical School to work with, advise, and entertain women students. She herself studied voluntary nerve impulses with Max Cremer, glycogen formation with Lovatt-Evans, and cardiac output under different types of anesthesia by means of the Cuvette oximeter.

865.   Brown, Harrison J. "Boat and Buggy Doctor." Medical Woman's Journal, 56:7 (July 1949) 21-22. port.
This article about Agnes Barlow Harrison relates her experiences as a student at the University of Michigan Medical School, from which she graduated in the 1880s, and as a physician in the Puget Sound area of Washington.

866.   Brown, Sara W. "Colored Women Physicians." Southern Workman, 52:12 (December 1923) 580-593.
Dr. Rebecca Cole was the first non-white graduate from the Woman's Medical College of Pennsylvania (M.D., 1867). She served as superintendent for several years in the Government Home in Washington for children and old women.

867.   Brunner, Lois. "Art in Surgery." Philadelphia Magazine, (December 1950) 36-37, 51. photo.
Dr. Alma Dea Morani, whose hobby is sculpture, studied plastic surgery because to her it was "the perfect fusion of

'art and medicine.'" She is on the staff of five Philadelphia hospitals, chiefly Woman's Medical College Hospital, and she is interested in educating the public on the basic purpose of plastic surgery: cosmetic considerations are secondary to "the reconstruction and the rehabilitation of the damaged part of the human anatomy."

868.   Brussel, James A. "Pants, Politics, Postage, and Physic." Psychiatric Quarterly Supplement, 35 (Part 1, 1961) 332-345.
Reviewing the extraordinary personal history of Mary Edwards, the author, a psychiatrist, diagnoses her as paranoid, "representing a compromise with reality unwelcomingly thrust upon a militant and determined ego that revolted against its sex, rebelling--not in a mere turn to homosexuality--but in an open, and as complete as possible, switch to the opposite sex. At best, Mary Walker was a poorly adjusted and chronically unhappy wretch of a woman." He credits her with several practical and beneficial contributions to the everyday life of America: the return receipt for registered mail, and the inscribing of a return address on an envelope.

869.   Bryant, Ruby F. "D.A.R. Founder of the Army Nurse Corps." Daughters of the American Revolution Magazine, 86:4 (April 1952) 435-436, 454. port.
A biography is given of Dr. Anita Newcomb McGee, founder of the Army Nurse Corps.

870.   Bryant, W. S. Felicia Autenried Robbins, M.D., 1869-1950. Privately printed, New York, New York, 1951, 12 pp. [Item not examined by editors.]

871.   Bryson, Louise Fiske. "Elizabeth Bradley Bystrom, M.D., 1852-1906." Woman's Medical Journal, 16:6 (June 1906) 93-94.

872.   Burt, O. W. Physician to the World: Esther Pohl Lovejoy. Messner, New York, New York, [c 1973], 189 pp. [Book not examined by editors.]

873.   Bushnell, Katharine C. Dr. Katharine C. Bushnell. Rose and Sons, Salisbury Hartford, 1930.
This brief autobiographical sketch was written by Dr. Bushnell in Shanghai. [Item not examined by editors.]

874.   Butler, A. S. G. Portrait of Josephine Butler. Faber, London, England, 1954.
[Book not examined by editors.]

875.   Butler, Miriam. "Ann Catherine Arthurs, M.D." Journal of the American Medical Women's Association, 15:3 (March 1960) 291. port. (Album of Women in Medicine.)

Dr. Arthurs began her medical career in 1921 when she entered Johns Hopkins University as a student. She transferred after one year to the Woman's Medical College of
Pennsylvania from which she graduated in 1925, and where
she held the rank of associate professor in the Department
of Otolaryngology for 25 years.

876. "Cajun Country's George and Ethel Smith." The Mayo Alum-
     nus, 11:3 (July 1975) 32-36. photos.
     Dr. Ethel Smith, a Mayo-trained surgeon, practices medicine
     with her husband George in Lafayette, Louisiana. Biograph-
     ical information and a description of life and practice in
     Lafayette constitute this article.

877. Calderone, Mary S. "Physician and Public Health Educator."
     Annals of the New York Academy of Sciences, 208 (15
     March 1973) 47-51.
     This autobiographical account of Mary Calderone's career as
     a doctor includes reminiscences from a professor who re-
     membered her at medical school: "She never used the fact
     that she was a woman, but never forgot it." With a degree
     in public health, she became medical director of the Planned
     Parenthood Federation of America, when male doctors refused
     to take the job because they perceived it as a position without
     a future. When she left Planned Parenthood to form the Sex
     Information and Education Council of the U.S. (SIECUS), she
     was replaced with "two male physicians, each of whom earned
     more than I was earning after eleven years of service....
     At SIECUS I have always received adequate compensation."
     She feels that "there are as many points of difference between
     men and men and women and women as there are between
     men and women. For either sex to use these differences
     against the other sex is self-defeating for both sexes."
     [This article is part of a series on "Successful Women in
     the Sciences: An Analysis of Determinants."]

878. Calverley, Eleanor T. My Arabian Days and Nights. Thom-
     as Y. Crowell Company, New York, New York, 1958,
     viii, 182 pp.
     Eleanor Calverley was Kuwait's first woman physician. She
     went there in 1912 with her missionary husband, opened a
     dispensary, and practiced 18 years. She was a graduate of
     the Woman's Medical College of Pennsylvania. Her dispen-
     sary and services to Arab women were the forerunners of the
     Olcott Memorial Hospital, which in 1955 was headed by Mary
     Bruins Allison, also a graduate of the Woman's Medical Col-
     lege of Pennsylvania. This autobiography was written follow-
     ing a 1955 re-visit to Kuwait by Dr. Calverley in which the
     contrasts between the pre- and post-oil-rich society of Ku-
     wait are drawn. A glossary of Arabic terms is included.

879. Campion, N. R. "Amazing Doctor Guion." Look, 25 (12
     September 1961) 98-100. illus.
     [Article not examined by editors.]

880. Campion, Nardi Reeder and Stanton, Rosamond Wilfley.
      Look to This Day! The Lively Education of a Great Wo-
      man Doctor: Connie Guion, M.D. Little, Brown and
      Company, Boston, Massachusetts, 1965, 308 pp. photos.,
      ports.
      This biography of the first woman professor of clinical medi-
      cine in the U.S. (Cornell Medical College) concentrates on
      Connie Guion's youth and premedical career in teaching at
      Sweet Briar and Wellesley. Born in 1882 in North Carolina,
      Connie Guion received her M.D. degree from Cornell Med-
      ical College in 1917. She interned at Bellevue, practiced for
      one year at the Waverley Sanitarium in Columbia, South Caro-
      lina, and returned to Bellevue in 1919. This book ends at
      that time, but the foreword tells the reader that Dr. Guion
      achieved recognition in her later career as the first woman
      member of the medical board of the New York Hospital.
      The Connie Guion Building of the New York Hospital, Cornell
      Medical Center, was the first hospital building in the U.S.
      named for a living woman physician. An index and many pho-
      tographs of Dr. Guion have been included.

881. "Cancer Center Added to Guadalupe's Service." Medical Wo-
      man's Journal, 56:7 (July 1949) 55.
      Headed by its first woman chief of medical staff, Dr. An-
      toinette Le Marquis, San Diego's Guadalupe Clinic opened a
      cancer clinic for women. "Little, slim and dark-eyed, this
      busy little physician," Dr. Le Marquis, is profiled.

882. "Candidates for Office 1976: To Be Elected at the 1975
      AMWA Annual Meeting." Journal of the American Med-
      ical Women's Association, 30:9 (September 1975) 385,
      388-390. ports.
      Biographies, complemented by portraits, are presented of
      nine women physicians who have been nominated for various
      offices of the American Medical Women's Association.

883. "Captain Loizeaux First Woman Physician Commissioned in
      European Area." Medical Woman's Journal, 51:3 (March
      1944) 32. (Section on War Service.)

884. "Carrie M. Hayward." Woman's Medical Journal, 16:6
      (June 1906) 92-93. port. (Obituary.)
      Dr. Hayward was an 1897 graduate of the Woman's Medical
      School of Chicago. Dr. Hayward's personal qualities are
      discussed and sympathy is extended to Dr. Louise Acres, Dr.
      Hayward's close friend and household companion during the
      last ten years.

885. Cary, Helen A. "Jessie Laird Brodie, M.D." Journal of
      the American Medical Women's Association, 7:10 (Octo-
      ber 1952) 395. port. (Album of Women in Medicine.)
      Chosen president-elect of the Pan American Medican Women's
      Alliance for 1953, Jessie Laird Brodie began her pediatrics

practice in an office in her home so that she might have
close supervision of her three children. In 1928 her prize
senior surgical thesis, which incorporated original research
material on congenital pyloric stenosis, was published in the
Journal of the American Medical Association.

886.   Cass, Victoria. "New AMWA President--1960-1961: Claire
        F. Ryder, M.D., M.P.H." Journal of the American
        Medical Women's Association, 15:7 (July 1960) 688.   port.
        Working with the Massachusetts Department of Health in 1947,
        Claire F. Ryder pioneered two programs: a pilot study of
        the distribution and utilization of hospital beds under the first
        Hospital Survey and Construction Act and the establishment
        and administration of the first State Multiphasic Screening
        Clinic, whose name changed to the Health Protection Clinic.
        She has specialized in developing home care and restorative
        services to handicapped older people in the United States
        Public Health Service.

887.   "Centennial of a Trailblazer." Journal of the American Med-
        ical Women's Association, 4:3 (March 1949) 125-128.
        ports.
        Marking the 100th anniversary of the graduation of Elizabeth
        Blackwell from the medical department of what is now Hobart
        College, the College honored twelve distinguished women phy-
        sicians "In recognition of the contributions made by the wo-
        men doctors of our own country and the rest of the world to
        the science, practice, and teaching of medicine...." A por-
        trait along with a brief vignette is provided for each of the
        twelve recipients. Five Elizabeth Blackwell Citations were
        also awarded by the New York Infirmary for Women and Chil-
        dren. A brief sketch of each of the five women to receive
        this citation is included.

888.   Chambers, Peggy. A Doctor Alone. A Biography of Eliza-
        beth Blackwell: The First Woman Doctor. 1821-1910.
        The Bodley Head, London, England, 1959, vii, 191 pp.
        illus., photos., ports.
        In this biography of Elizabeth Blackwell, the author devotes
        a major portion of the book to Blackwell's friends and col-
        leagues: her sister Emily, Marie Zakrzewska, Elizabeth
        Garrett-Anderson, Mary Putnam Jacobi. The book contains
        no index.

889.   Chapman, Rose Woodallen. Dr. Mary Wood-Allen: A Life
        Sketch. Ruby I. Gilbert, Chicago, Illinois, 1908, 96 pp.
        ports.
        This is a biographical memoir of Dr. Mary Wood-Allen,
        written by her daughter. Dr. Wood-Allen was born in Ohio,
        studied medicine in Vienna, and received her M.D. degree
        from the University of Michigan in 1875. She edited a jour-
        nal called American Motherhood and was active in the Wo-
        man's Christian Temperance Union as a lecturer. Photo-

graphs of Dr. Wood-Allen are included.   There are no references, citations, bibliography, or index.

890.   Charlton, Ethel.   "Margaret Ewart Colby, M.D. President
        Iowa Medical Women's Social Society."   Woman's Medical Journal, 11:7 (July 1901) 267-268.
        This biographical sketch of Dr. Colby focuses upon the factors related to her medical career.

891.   "Childhood and School Days.   Marie Zakrzewska, M.D."
        Woman's Medical Journal, 10:12 (December 1900) 509-511.   (Biographical.)

892.   "Chinese Woman Physician Hopes to Establish Hospital in
        Canton."   Medical Woman's Journal, 32:8 (August 1925) 228.
        Rose Goong Wong was the first American-Chinese woman to pass the New York State Medical Board and the first American-Chinese woman doctor to practice in San Francisco.
        "Born in San Francisco, she had to fight the prejudice of the East which her parents held for the modern and scientific ways of the West."

893.   "Cincinnati Girl Is Medical Sister."   Medical Woman's Journal, 55:4 (April 1948) 50.   (News Notes.)
        Sister M. Marcella Du Brul, a graduate of the University of Cincinnati Medical College and a member of the Medical Mission Sisters, is helping to open the first mission of that society in Africa--the Holy Family Dispensary, Berekum, Ashanti district, Gold Coast.

894.   "Clare N. Reese, M.D."   Medical Woman's Journal, 52:5
        (May 1945) 40.
        Dr. Reese (whose portrait appears on the front cover of this issue of the Journal) reported for duty at the U.S. Navy Hospital at San Diego, California.   A brief resumé of Dr. Reese' professional activities is given.

895.   Cleaves, Margaret A.   The Autobiography of a Neurasthene.
        Richard G. Badger, The Gorham Press, Boston, Massachusetts, 1910, 246 pp.
        In this book Dr. Cleaves chronicles what she has never been able to discuss with family or professional associates--the mental and physical anguish of her neurasthenic condition.
        Despite living an active life, she was plagued by sleeplessness, ennui, lack of appetite, a chronic fatigue of mind and body--only partially explained by a persistent anemia and injury to an auditory nerve.   Learning to conserve a limited supply of energy was the basic challenge.   The telling of this story was a form of therapy for the author, but another purpose was to help remove "the sting and opprobrium which the essential neurasthene bears...."

896.   "Cleveland Cancer Medal Awarded: Dr. Elise Strang L'Es-
          perance Receives the 1942 Clement Cleveland Award;
          Niece of Chauncey Depew, with Her Sister, Was Founder
          of Clinic for Disease." Medical Woman's Journal, 49:
          10 (October 1942) 305.

897.   Cloyes, S. A. The Healer: The Story of Dr. Samantha S.
          Nivison and Dryden Springs, 1820-1915. DeWitt Histor-
          ical Society of Tomkins County, Inc., Ithaca, New York,
          1969, 64 pp.
       [Book not examined by editors.]

898.   Cobb, W. Montague. "Anna Bartsch-Dunne, 1876- ." Jour-
          nal of the National Medical Association, 60:2 (March
          1968) 161-162. (Medical History.)
       Dr. Anna Bartsch-Dunne (whose portrait appears on the front
       cover of this issue of the Journal) graduated in 1902 from
       Howard University and in 1903 became a faculty member here.
       A list of the Anna Bartsch-Dunne Scholarship recipients is
       given. [Howard University Medical School women students
       are eligible.]

899.   Cobb, W. Montague. "E. Mae McCarroll, A.B., M.D.,
          M.S.P.H., 1898- . First Lady of the NMA." Journal
          of the National Medical Association, 65:6 (November
          1973) 544-545. facsim. (Medical History.)
       Dr. McCarroll (whose portrait appears on the front cover of
       this issue of the Journal) graduated in 1925 from Woman's
       Medical College of Pennsylvania. In 1946 she became the
       first Afro-American physician appointed to the staff of the
       Newark (New Jersey) City Hospital. She later became deputy
       health officer for that city.

900.   "Colonel Margaret D. Craighill: Colonel Margaret D. Craig-
          hill Returning As Dean of W.M.C." Medical Woman's
          Journal, 53:5 (May 1946) 33-34. port.
       This biography of Dr. Craighill, the first woman to be com-
       missioned as an officer in the U.S. Army, concentrates on
       her military service.

901.   "Colorado Crusader." Time, (28 October 1946) 78. port.
       This brief article discusses Dr. Florence Rena Sabin's im-
       pact on the public health department of Colorado.

902.   Colver, Alice Ross and Birdsall, Helen Brant. Dream within
          Her Hand. Macrae Smith Company, Philadelphia, Pennsyl-
          vania, 1940, 309 pp. ports.
       In this biography of Cornelia Brant, author Alice Colver
       wanted to prove it was possible to successfully combine a
       career with marriage and motherhood. The book describes
       Cornelia Chase's childhood in a Quaker family in Newark,
       New Jersey, and how her early dream of becoming a doctor
       was subordinated to an early marriage. Her dream revived

again after three children; she persuaded her husband to let
her attend the New York Medical College and Hospital for
Women, where she graduated in 1903. She spent the rest of
her life as a general practitioner specializing in physical
therapy, while carrying on her family life. The book contains a brief bibliography of secondary sources.

903. Comandini, Adele. Doctor Kate: Angel on Snowshoes. The
      Story of Kate Pelham Newcomb, M.D. Rinehart & Com-
      pany, Inc., New York, New York, 1956, 339 pp. photos.
      This is an autobiography of Kate Newcomb, a specialist in
      obstetrics and gynecology, born in 1886, who gave up medicine
      for ten years after poor treatment had killed her first child.
      She resumed practice in Rice Creek, northern Wisconsin,
      when she realized how few doctors there were in the area.
      She tells of her medical education in Buffalo and gives ex-
      periences of her life in the "backwoods," where the nearest
      hospital was a 55-mile drive away. No index or bibliography
      appear in the work.

904. "Commissioner of Public Welfare of the State of Pennsylvania:
      First Woman to Occupy a Position in a State Cabinet."
      Medical Woman's Journal, 30:9 (September 1923) 274.
      port.
      A biography is presented of Ellen C. Potter, who graduated
      in 1903 from the Woman's Medical College of Pennsylvania.

905. Comstock, Elizabeth. "Margaret Caldwell, M.D." Journal
      of the American Medical Women's Association, 9:7 (July
      1954) 235. port. (Album of Women in Medicine.)
      Receiving her degree in 1876 from the Woman's Hospital
      Medical College at Northwestern University, Margaret Cald-
      well opened up a general practice in 1878 in Waukesha, Wisc.,
      which had become famous for its mineral springs. She was
      the first woman to become president of the Waukesha County
      Medical Society.

906. Comstock, Elizabeth. "Maude Glasgow, M.D." Journal of
      the American Medical Women's Association, 8:1 (January
      1953) 26. port.
      Receiving her medical degree in 1901 from Cornell, Maude
      Glasgow became active in institutional health programs by
      serving as medical inspector in the New York Department of
      Health and establishing a medical service for the New York
      Telephone Company. She has authored leaflets for the De-
      partment of Health as well as written books which include
      Life and Law, The Scotch-Irish, The Subjection of Woman,
      and the Problems of Sex. In the Problems of Sex she pro-
      poses that women were the first doctors and that in the earli-
      est civilizations women were rulers, and when they were,
      there were no wars.

907. "Connie M. Guion, M.D." Journal of the American Medical
      Women's Association, 6:6 (June 1951) 244. port. (Al-

bum of Women in Medicine.)
One of the first recipients of the Elizabeth Blackwell Award
(1949) for her work in internal medicine, Dr. Guion was a
teacher of clinical medicine. She was appointed chief of the
Medical Clinic (1929) and was made professor of clinical
medicine (1946) at Cornell University Medical College.

908. "Consciousness-raising Is Not Analysis." Jefferson Medical
        College: Alumni Bulletin, 24:1 (Fall 1974) 19-20. port.
      A biography of Merle Edelstein, a psychiatrist in private
      practice, includes her views on therapy--especially therapy
      for women. Warning against the harmful effects of the fem-
      inist movement's consciousness-raising groups, Dr. Edel-
      stein adds that "being chauvinized is only a symptom of the
      woman's real problem."

909. "Contract Surgeon." Medical Woman's Journal, 49:11 (No-
        vember 1942) 345.
      In 1918 Dr. Gertrude F. McCann was hired by the United
      States government as a contract surgeon. She had received
      her training as a fellow in pathology and bacteriology at the
      Rockefeller Institute. Dr. McCann describes her work as a
      contract surgeon.

910. "Contract Surgeon: Dolores Mercedes Pinero, M.D., San-
        turce, Puerto Rico." Medical Woman's Journal, 49:10
        (October 1942) 310, 324.
      Practicing in Puerto Rico when World War I broke out,
      Dolores Mercedes Piñero wanted to contribute her medical
      training to the war effort; thus she became a contract sur-
      geon.

911. "Contract Surgeon Loy McAfee." Medical Woman's Journal,
        49:9 (September 1942) 276, 294.
      A medical editor, Loy McAfee became a contract surgeon in
      1918. When her contract was annulled in 1921, Dr. McAfee
      returned to editing. In 1930 she worked for the government
      in the historical section of the Army War College and later
      served with the Army Medical Library. In 1926 Dr. McAfee
      acquired a law degree. Much of the information presented
      in this article was taken from the April, 1941 issue of The
      Military Surgeon.

912. "Cordelia Agnes Greene, M.D." Woman's Medical Journal,
        15:4 (April 1905) 80-81. (Obituary.)

913. Corea, Gena. "Dorothy Reed Mendenhall; 'Childbirth Is Not
        a Disease.'" Ms., 11:10 (April 1974) 98-100, 102-104.
        photos., port. (Lost Women.)
      Dorothy Mendenhall, in 1926, traveled to Denmark to study
      child-delivery practices. In the U.S. at this time, childbirth
      was the second leading cause of death in women between the
      ages of 15 and 44--the rate in Denmark was much lower. Dr.

Mendenhall discovered that in Denmark midwives delivered
most babies. Her report and consequent work in this area
revolutionized childbirth practices in the U.S. A considerable portion of this article is devoted to Dr. Mendenhall's
education at Johns Hopkins University School of Medicine.

914.   Cote, Marie M. "Obstetrics in Burma." Woman's Medical
            Journal, [8]:10 (October 1899) 347-349. (Obstetrical De-
            partment.)
        Dr. Cote relates a few of her experiences as a physician
        ministering to Burmese women.

915.   Coutard, Vera L. "Hepsy's Need Gave Crossnore a School."
            Independent Woman, 28:6 (June 1949) 162-164. photos.
        Dr. Mary Martin Sloop, a graduate of the Woman's Medical
        College of Pennsylvania, settled with her doctor husband in
        the remote village of Crossnore in North Carolina in 1911
        and proceeded to found a school for children in the area.

916.   Cox, Pearl Bliss. "Pioneer Women in Medicine: Michigan
            XV." Medical Woman's Journal, 56:4 (April 1949) 46-
            51. facsim., ports. (History of Women in Medicine.)
        This article [one in a series of articles about Michigan wo-
        men physicians], presents brief biographies of several women
        physicians who graduated with the 1896 class of the Univer-
        sity of Michigan's medical department. Women who gradu-
        ated from other medical schools but practiced in Michigan
        are also profiled.

917.   Cox, Pearl Bliss. "Pioneer Women in Medicine: Michigan
            XVI." Medical Woman's Journal, 56:5 (May 1949) 48-51,
            64. (History of Women in Medicine.)
        This article [one in a series of articles about Michigan wo-
        men physicians] concentrates on the lives of several women
        who obtained M.D.s in 1898 and 1899.

918.   Cox, Pearl Bliss. "Pioneer Women in Medicine: Michigan
            XVII." Medical Woman's Journal, 56:6 (June 1949) 26-
            29, 56. (History of Women in Medicine.)
        Several women who obtained medical degrees in 1899 and
        1900 are profiled in this installment [one in a series of ar-
        ticles about Michigan women physicians].

919.   Cox, Pearl Bliss. "Pioneer Women in Medicine: Michigan
            XVIII." Medical Woman's Journal, 56:7 (July 1949) 38-
            41. (History of Women in Medicine.)
        Several women who received M.D.s in 1900 are the subject
        of this installment [one in a series of articles about Michigan
        women physicians].

920.   Cox, Pearl Bliss. "Pioneer Women in Medicine: Michigan
            XIX." Medical Woman's Journal, 56:9 (September 1949)
            41-45. (History of Women in Medicine.)

This article [the final installment in a series about Michigan women physicians] opens with a review of the series. The remainder of the article is devoted to the lives of women who obtained M.D.s in 1900 and practiced for some time at the Battle Creek Sanitarium.

921.   Crawford, Mary M. "Medical Women in the News: Elise S.
        L'Esperance, M.D." Journal of the American Medical
        Women's Association, 3:7 (July 1948) 310-311. port.
President of the American Medical Women's Association from 1948-1949, Elise L'Esperance was graduated from the Women's Medical College of the New York Infirmary for Women and Children in 1899, where she continued to be supportive after she began her professional career. She was the first woman to attain the rank of assistant professor in the Department of Pathology of Cornell University Medical College. Her specialty was the origin, treatment, and prevention of malignant tumors. With her sister, Kate Depew Strang, she founded in 1932 the Strang Cancer Clinic at the New York Infirmary, which helped patients and helped young physicians get special training. In 1937 she planned and established the first cancer prevention clinic at the Infirmary. After she received numerous awards for her work in cancer, Cornell appointed her assistant professor in the Department of Preventive Medicine.

922.   Crocker, Geraldine H. "Ethel Hill Sharp, M.D. (1876-
        1952)." Journal of the American Medical Women's Association, 19:12 (December 1964) 1068.
Ethel Hill Sharp's mother was county superintendent of the Women's Christian Temperance Union (WCTU) and wanted her daughter to pursue her commitment to temperance. Dr. Sharp was active in WCTU during her professional life.

923.   Curcio, Mary R. "Dr. Baumann Retires." Journal of the
        American Medical Women's Association, 18:1 (January
        1963) 40-41. port.
A biographical sketch is presented of Dr. Frieda Baumann upon the occasion of her retirement as editor of the Journal of the American Medical Women's Association. Dr. Baumann was the first woman to be appointed chief of a medical service at Philadelphia General Hospital.

924.   Curtis, Annie N. "In Memoriam: H. Frances Sercombe,
        M.D., Formerly of Milwaukee, Wis.; The Women's Medical College of Chicago, Class of '81." Medical Woman's
        Journal, 32:3 (March 1925) 89.
"She did not break new ground nor reach marked heights in her work, yet something in her quality calls forth both those words. If we do not look for too much, we find more."

925.   Cushier, Elizabeth M. "In Memory of Dr. Emily Blackwell."
        Woman's Medical Journal, 21:4 (April 1911) 87-89. (Pre-

sentation, Fifth Annual Meeting, Women's Medical Society of New York State, 10 March 1911.)

926.   Cushier, Elizabeth M. and Thelberg, Elizabeth B., ed.
        "Autobiography of Dr. Elizabeth Cushier." Medical Re-
        view of Reviews, 39:3 (March 1933) 121-131.
        Writing this autobiography at the age of 93 (one year before
        her death), Elizabeth M. Cushier recalls her childhood en-
        vironment and its influence upon her decision to study medi-
        cine. She describes her experiences as a student, and later
        a staff physician and surgeon, at the New York Infirmary for
        Women and Children. Dr. Cushier fondly remembers her
        friendship with Emily Blackwell, their travels and vacations,
        and the homes they shared from 1882 until Dr. Blackwell's
        death in 1910. Following the autobiography is a personal
        tribute to Dr. Cushier by Elizabeth Thelberg.

927.   D. K. "The Late Medical Degree to a Female." Boston
        Medical and Surgical Journal, 40 (1849) 58-59.
        The author expresses his opinion that Elizabeth Blackwell has
        been induced to depart from her "appropriate sphere" by en-
        tering the medical field. [Article not examined by editors.]

928.   Dale, James G. Katherine Neel Dale: Medical Missionary.
        Wm. B. Eerdmans Publishing Co., Grand Rapids, Mich-
        igan, 1943, 216 pp. photos., ports.
        Katherine Neel Dale graduated from the Woman's Medical
        College of Pennsylvania in 1897. She went to Ciudad del
        Maiz, San Luis Potosi, Mexico as a medical missionary of
        the Associate Reformed Presbyterian Church in 1898. She
        worked in San Luis Potosi, primarily at Rio Verde where a
        hospital was built, for the next 14 years. Following a fur-
        lough in the U.S., Dr. Dale returned to Tampico, Mexico in
        1919 and practiced for 11 years. In 1930 she went to Tama-
        zunchale, where she continued her practice until her death
        in 1941. This biography, written by her minister-husband in
        the year following her death, emphasizes Dr. Dale's mission-
        ary calling and dedication. There are several photographs
        of patients, of the region, and of Dr. Dale.

929.   Dall, Caroline H. and Zakrzewska, Marie E. A Practical
        Illustration of "Woman's Right to Labor;" or, A Letter
        from Marie E. Zakrzewska, M.D., Late of Berlin,
        Prussia. Walker, Wise, and Company, Boston, Massa-
        chusetts, 1860, 167 pp.
        Caroline [Healy] Dall describes the events leading up to and
        following publication of her treatise, Woman's Right to Labor.
        She tells of her life's objective to inspire women with "de-
        sire for thorough training to some special end," and of her
        frustration at being unable to find an example of a woman
        who led "a life flowing out of circumstances not dissimilar
        to [ordinary women], but marked by a steady will, an un-
        swerving purpose." (Florence Nightingale's father had a

title; Dorothea Dix had money and time; George Sand "wasn't
respectable"). Then, in 1856, Dall met Marie Zakrzewska:
"A woman born to inspire faith." Dall and Mary L. Booth
persuaded Zakrzewska to publish an autobiographical manuscript written originally in 1859 as a letter to Booth. In the
letter, Zakrzewska writes of her childhood in Berlin, her
medical education, and her work in America. In the comments following Zakrzewska's letter, Dall reminds readers
that "the possibilities of a Zakrzewska lie hidden in every
oppressed girl."

930.   Danforth, I. A. "Marie Josepha Mergler." Woman's Med-
            ical Journal, 11:8 (August 1901) 291-293. (Original Arti-
            cles.) (Memorial Services, Union Park Congregational
            Church, Chicago, Illinois, 26 May 1901.)
        Dr. Danforth, a faculty member of the Women's Medical Col-
        lege [Chicago] when Marie Josepha Mergler was a student,
        recalls Mergler's "remarkable self-poise and iron-will" as
        well as the "queenly--yet womanly--grace" she displayed as
        a medical student before hostile audiences. He then pictures
        Dr. Mergler "in her splendid maturity" as a surgeon and an
        expert in female diseases. In seeking her consultation, Dr.
        Danforth faced ridicule from his medical brethren, but he
        "coveted her steady hand, her quick and unerring judgment,
        her self-poise and absolutely unruffled demeanor...."

931.   Daniel, Annie Sturgis [sic]. "An Appreciation. Dr. Mercy
            N. Baker." Woman's Medical Journal, 29[19]: (January
            1919) 13. (Editorial.)

932.   Daniel, Annie Sturgis [sic]. "'A Cautious Experiment.' The
            History of the New York Infirmary for Women and Chil-
            dren and the Women's Medical College of the New York
            Infirmary; Also Its Pioneer Founders: 1853-1899."
            Medical Woman's Journal, 46:5 (May 1939) 125-131.
        This, the first in a series of articles by the same title, is
        primarily a record of Elizabeth Blackwell's struggle to enter
        medicine and her early years in the medical profession. Por-
        tions of letters, and newspaper excerpts which announce the
        incorporation of the Female Medical College of Pennsylvania,
        speculate as to Dr. Blackwell's possible role in that institu-
        tion. A biography is also given of lawyer and philanthropist
        Charles Butler, who served as the first president of the New
        York Infirmary for Women and Children (1853-1864).

933.   Daniel, Annie Sturges. "'A Cautious Experiment.' The His-
            tory of the New York Infirmary for Women and Children
            and the Women's Medical College of the New York In-
            firmary; Also Its Pioneer Founders: 1853-1899." Med-
            ical Woman's Journal, 48:7 (July 1941) 197-199, 216.
        This article [part of a series on the New York Infirmary]
        presents excerpts from Infirmary reports (1871-1881). These
        excerpts cover different aspects of the life of Dr. Mary Put-

nam Jacobi--her ancestry, education, teaching, and medical
practice, among other topics.

934.   Daniel, Annie Sturges. "Dr. Marie Louise Chard." Medical
          Woman's Journal, 45:4 (April 1938) 114.
        This biography of Marie Chard includes the text of a letter
        by Emily Blackwell. The picture of Dr. Chard on the front
        cover of this issue of the Journal was taken at the time of
        her graduation in 1895 from the Women's Medical College of
        the New York Infirmary.

935.   Daniel, Anne S[turges]. "Dr. Mary Putnam Jacobi: A Med-
          ical Pioneer." Medical Woman's Journal, 27:6 (June
          1920) 159-161. (Presentation, Annual Meeting, Woman's
          Medical Association of New York State, March 22, 1920.)
        Quotes from Dr. Jacobi's commencement address at Women's
        Medical College of the New York Infirmary in May 1883, il-
        lustrate Jacobi's high ideal of the medical profession and her
        concern about women's advancement within it. This review
        of Jacobi's professional accomplishments focuses upon her
        contributions to medical literature.

936.   "Daughters of Science: Dr. Rose Wistein, Cedar Rapids,
          Iowa." Medical Woman's Journal, 36:7 (July 1929) 182-
          184. port.
        This biography of Dr. Rose Wistein covers her life from her
        birth and early years in Czechoslovakia, through her move
        as a young girl to the United States and her subsequent study
        of medicine, to her professional life as a physician. Anec-
        dotes of her life are included.

937.   "Daughters of Science: Kate A. Mason Hogle, M.D." Med-
          ical Woman's Journal, 37:9 (September 1930) 256-257.
          port.

938.   Davidson, Gisela K. "Reflections of a Woman Physician
          After 34 Years of Practice in the State of Maine." Jour-
          nal of the Maine Medical Association, 63:6 (June 1972)
          103-104, 112.
        An Austrian refugee who had graduated from the Medical
        School of the University of Vienna, Dr. Davidson began her
        residency in 1938 at a State of Maine institution for the treat-
        ment of tuberculosis. In this reminiscence, Dr. Davidson
        discusses the comparative time away from practice spent by
        women physicians (who leave to have children) and male phy-
        sicians (who leave to enter military service). She also dis-
        cusses the low percentage of women in medicine, the con-
        tributions women in medicine can make, and her opinions
        about a proposed new medical school in Maine for which the
        state has not consulted women physicians.

939.   Davis, Loda Mae. "Her Job Is World Health." Medical Wo-
          man's Journal, 56:6 (June 1949) 41-43. port.

The former associate chief of the (U.S.) Children's Bureau, Martha M. Eliot, has been appointed assistant director general of the United Nations World Health Organization (WHO). Dr. Eliot was the only woman to sign the constitution of WHO. She was the first woman president of the American Public Health Association and has received acclaim for her many accomplishments in the field of maternal and child health. In addition to her professional activities, Dr. Eliot's personal life and physical appearance are detailed. A poetry lover, her first cousin is T. S. Eliot. Dr. Eliot and her close friend, Dr. Ethel C. Dunham (an internationally known pediatrician), plan to share a house in Geneva, Switzerland.

940. Davis, Paul J. "Mary Putnam Jacobi." Journal of the American Medical Women's Association, 21:6 (June 1966) 506-508.
Reprinted from the article "Doctors Afield" in the New England Journal of Medicine, 273 (November 4, 1965) 1036-1038, the emphasis in this article is on Mary Putnam Jacobi's prolific writings.

941. "Dean Marion Fay, Ph.D." Medical Woman's Journal, 59:7 (July 1952) 21-22, 24. photo. (Women in Medicine.)
This biography of Dr. Fay, dean of Woman's Medical College of Pennsylvania, is based on an interview with her in her office at the College.

942. "Death of a Pioneer Woman Physician." Medical Woman's Journal, 29:6 (June 1922) 117.
Frances Armstrong Rutherford (1839-1922) graduated from the Woman's Medical College of Pennsylvania in 1865.

943. "Death of Dr. Clemence S. Lozier." Medical Missionary Record, 3:5 (September 1888) 129.

944. "Delivering Babies Hasn't Lost Its Thrill." Jefferson Medical College: Alumni Bulletin, 24:1 (Fall 1974) 21-22. port.
Profiled is Dr. Gwen Kaplow (M.D., 1966).

945. Dempsey, Lillian E. "After Fifty Years." Medical Woman's Journal, 53:12 (December 1946) 45-49. port.
Dr. Dempsey, who graduated in 1896 from the University of Oregon Medical School, recalls incidents from her childhood and from her medical practice in Vallejo, California.

946. Dickerman, Marion. "Harriet M. Doane: 1872-1940." Medical Woman's Journal, 47:5 (May 1940) 155.
A personalized tribute to Dr. Doane, a general practitioner, is made on the occasion of her death in March 1940.

947. "Dinner to Dr. Esther Rosencrantz." Medical Woman's Journal, 51:2 (February 1944) 39. (News Notes.)

Dr. Rosencrantz was honored upon the occasion of her retirement after 30 years of service at the University of California Medical School. The 1904 graduate of Johns Hopkins was a noted collector of, and speaker on, the works of Sir William Osler.

948. Dissosway, Carolyn F.-R. "Mary Putnam Jacobi, M.D. (1842-1906)." New York State Journal of Medicine, 74: 10 (September 1974) 1854-1855. (History of Medicine.)

949. "Distaff and the Caduceus." Journal of the American Medical Women's Association, 16:7 (July 1961) 534-535.
A review of "the accomplishments of the first pioneering women in the field of medicine in Texas." Very brief sketches of a general nature. The information on many of the women was taken from George Plunkett Red's book, The Medicine Man in Texas.

950. "A Distinguished Graduate: Mary G. Fulton, M.D., Medical Missionary to China." Bulletin of the Woman's Medical College of Pennsylvania, 67 (December 1916) 21-23. photo.

951. "Distinguished Representatives of Michigan's Woman MDs." Michigan Medicine, 74:2 (January 1975) 20-23. ports.
This is a collection of brief biographical sketches of 25 women physicians practicing in Michigan in 1974. Data included for each biographee are medical specialty, teaching affiliation (if any), medical school attended, years in practice, marital status, size of family (if any), profession of spouse (if married), outstanding accomplishments, awards, honors, and recognitions. Twenty-three of the biographies are accompanied by photographs. Among the subjects are Gertrude B. Gregory, first woman physician hired by Ford Motor Company, and Marjorie Peebles-Meyers, "Outstanding Physician of the Year" (1968) of the Michigan State Medical Society.

952. "Dr. Abbott Leaves Post at Women's [sic] Medical College for McGill University." Medical Woman's Journal, 32: 8 (August 1925) 226.
After serving a professorship and holding the chair of pathology and bacteriology for two years on the faculty of the Woman's Medical College of Pennsylvania, Maude E. Abbott returned to McGill University where she was a lecturer in pathology.

953. "Dr. Adelaide Brown." Woman's City Club Magazine, (September 1940) 22-23. (Obituary.)
The daughter of Dr. Charlotte Brown (founder of the San Francisco Children's Hospital), Adelaide Brown distinguished herself in public health work in San Francisco.

954. "Dr. Agnes Eighelberger [sic]: President Elect of the State

Society Iowa Medical Women." Woman's Medical Journal, 18:7 (July 1908) 150.   port.
Dr. Eichelberger graduated from the Woman's Medical College, Chicago, in 1888.

955.   "Dr. Alice Barker-Ellsworth." Women in Medicine, 58 (October 1937) 23-24.   port.
Dr. Barker-Ellsworth was one of the pioneer workers for sex education in public schools.

956.   "Dr. Alice Butler." Medical Woman's Journal, 36:10 (October 1929) 279.
This obituary notice for Dr. Alice Butler gives a listing of Dr. Butler's affiliations within a biographical framework.

957.   "Dr. Alice Hamilton." Medical Woman's Journal, 43:10 (October 1936) 280.
Dr. Hamilton was a medical consultant for the United States Department of Labor at the time this sketch was written.
(Her picture appears on the front cover of this issue of the Journal.)

958.   "Dr. Alice S. Woolley." Journal of the American Medical Women's Association, 1:9 (December 1946) 296.
(Reprinted from the Poughkeepsie New Yorker of Monday, November 18, 1946.)   Three women physicians from Poughkeepsie have been presidents of the American Medical Women's Association: Grace N. Kimball, Elizabeth B. Thelberg, and Alice Stone Woolley.

959.   "Dr. Alma Morani Elected 2nd President of AWHS." Viewpoint: The Woman's Medical College of Pennsylvania, 22:3 (Summer 1967) 1, 6.   port.

960.   "Dr. Alma Vedin." Medical Women's Journal, 32:2 (February 1925) 56-57.   port.
Alma Vedin spent a large proportion of her medical career as anesthetist on the faculty of the New York Infirmary for Women and Children and the New York Hospital.

961.   ["A Doctor! An English Woman, Maria Walker"]. El Siglo Medico, (1866) 783.   (Spa)
This brief note on Dr. Mary Walker covers her New York practice, her receipt of the Medal of Honor, and her wearing of male attire.

962.   "Dr. Angenette Parry." Medical Woman's Journal, 46:6 (June 1939) 185.
Graduating from the Women's Medical College of the New York Infirmary in 1891 at the age of 34, Dr. Parry served over 20 years as an obstetrician at the New York Infirmary. For four years, she headed the obstetrical department of the American Women's Hospital at Kolskinia, Greece.   A listing

of her numerous memberships in professional and social organizations is given, and Dr. Parry's portrait appears on the
front cover of this issue of the Journal.

963.   "Dr. Ann Preston." Medical Woman's Journal, 43:12 (De-
          cember 1936) 333.
       A brief biography is given of Dr. Preston (whose portrait
       appears on this month's Journal cover).

964.   "Dr. Anna Forest Rowe: Established First Hospital for Wo-
          men and Children in Brooklyn." Medical Woman's Jour-
          nal, 28:3 (March 1921) 80.
       Dr. Rowe founded the Lucretia Mott Dispensary and Infirmary.
       The hospital was dissolved in 1892 by a special legislative
       act, because "Dr. Rowe wore herself out by service, and ...
       it was necessary to remove her from it almost by force."

965.   "Dr. Anna H. Voorhis." Medical Woman's Journal, 54:11
          (November 1947) 49.
       This brief article recounts an incident in the life of Dr.
       Voorhis. In 1932 Dr. Voorhis sailed on the ship American
       Merchant. During the voyage, the ship's doctor died sudden-
       ly. Dr. Voorhis, being the only other physician on board,
       was asked to pronounce the doctor dead. Dr. Voorhis was
       then appointed ship's doctor for the duration of the voyage:
       had there been no doctor aboard, the ship would not have been
       permitted to dock but would have had to remain in quarantine
       for three weeks.

966.   "Dr. Anna Hubert." Medical Woman's Journal, 46:4 (April
          1939) 120.
       Dr. Hubert (whose portrait appears on the front cover of this
       issue of the Journal) graduated in 1911 from Johns Hopkins
       Medical School. In 1914, she made the first medical survey
       of women prisoners on Welfare Island, New York City.

967.   "Dr. Anna Shaw." Bulletin Medical Women's Club of Chi-
          cago, 7:11 (July 1919) 2-3.
       This obituary notice highlights the life of Dr. Anna Howard
       Shaw, honorary president of the National American Woman
       Suffrage Association.

968.   "Dr. Anna W. Williams." Medical Woman's Journal, 43:6
          (June 1936) 160.
       A distinguished bacteriologist, Dr. Anna W. Williams was
       an 1891 graduate of the Women's Medical College of the New
       York Infirmary. (Her portrait appears on this issue's cover.)

969.   "Dr. Anne Walter Fearn." Medical Woman's Journal, 46:9
          (September 1939) 287.
       An 1893 graduate of Woman's Medical College in Pennsylvania.
       Anne Walter Fearn devoted 40 years to work in China. She
       died in 1939--two weeks before her autobiography, My Days

of Strength, was published. Dr. Fearn's portrait appears on
the front cover of this issue of the Journal.

970.   "Dr. Annie R. Ranes." Bulletin of the Medical Women's
       Club of Chicago, 19:9 (June 1931) 22-23. port.

971.   "Dr. Barbara Fish." New York University Medical Quarterly,
       26:3 (Winter 1971) 6. port. (New Professors.)
       Dr. Fish has been promoted to professor of child psychiatry
       at the University.

972.   "Dr. Barrett." Bulletin Medical Women's Club of Chicago,
       13:8 (April 1925) 5.
       This obituary of Dr. Kate Walker Barrett gives her profes-
       sional and social affiliations. "At the last Democratic Na-
       tional Convention it was Dr. Barrett who made one of the
       best nominating speeches naming Carter Glass for the presi-
       dency."

973.   "Dr. Caroline M. Purnell: Former Commissioner to Ameri-
       can Women's Hospitals in France." Medical Woman's
       Journal, 30:3 (March 1923) 78-79. port.

974.   "Dr. Caroline Sanford Finley." Medical Woman's Journal,
       44:5 (May 1937) 139.
       Dr. Finley (whose portrait appears on the cover of this issue
       of the Journal) graduated in 1901 from Cornell Medical School.
       During the war, Dr. Finley offered her services and those of
       a small group of medical women to the United States--in any
       capacity the government wished to use them. This offer was
       refused. The French government, meanwhile, accepted the
       group which formed the nucleus of the Women's Over-Seas
       Hospitals. Dr. Finley's post-war work is also discussed.

975.   "Dr. Carrie Johnson Acquitted." Woman's Medical Journal,
       6:4 (April 1897) 99.
       Dr. L. Carrie Johnson of Pueblo, Colorado was found not
       guilty of a murder charge. Dr. Johnson had been accused
       of performing "a criminal operation" upon a woman which
       caused the woman's death.

976.   "Dr. Catharine MacFarlane." Club Woman's Journal, 7:5
       (February 1941) 6. port.
       A recounting of Dr. MacFarlane's professional activities con-
       stitutes this article, written on the occasion of Dr. MacFar-
       lane's receipt of the Gimbel Philadelphia Award.

977.   "Dr. Catherine N. Hinterbuchner Appointed Chairman of the
       Department of Rehabilitation Medicine." Chironian, 86:
       4 (Summer-Fall 1971) 35. port.
       Catherine Nicolaides Hinterbuchner became the first woman
       physician in the U.S. to chair a department of rehabilitation
       medicine when she was appointed to that post by New York

Medical College.   She is a 1951 graduate of the University of
Athens.

978.   "Dr. Charlotte Blake Brown."   Medical Woman's Journal, 44:
          4 (April 1937) 108.
          Dr. Brown (whose portrait appears on the front cover of this
          issue of the Journal) graduated in 1874 from the Woman's
          Medical College of Pennsylvania.   Dr. Brown, with a group
          of friends, founded what was to develop into the Children's
          Hospital of San Francisco, which provided the first training
          school for nurses on the Pacific Coast.

979.   "Dr. Cleora Seaman."   Medical Woman's Journal, 44:8 (Au-
          gust 1937) 231.
          Dr. Seaman (whose portrait appears on the front cover of
          this issue of the Journal) instigated the founding of a med-
          ical college for women in Cleveland, Ohio.   In 1870, the
          Cleveland Hospital College incorporated the woman's college.

980.   "Dr. Connie M. Guion."   Medical Woman's Journal, 43:1
          (January 1936) 21.
          In addition to this brief biography of Dr. Guion, her portrait
          is on the front cover of this issue of the Journal.

981.   "Dr. DeVore Served in Hawaii."   Medical Woman's Journal,
          49:10 (October 1942) 322.   (News Notes.)
          Louise DeVore, in Honolulu by chance when Pearl Harbor
          was bombed, volunteered her services to the U.S. military.
          At first serving as an anesthetist, she eventually replaced a
          ranking hospital staff officer.   While she assumed the respon-
          sibility of the post and served in full capacity, she did not
          receive the rank and pay commensurate with this function.
          Her commanding officer tried unsuccessfully to obtain a com-
          mission for her.

982.   "Dr. Edith Loeber Ballard."   Medical Woman's Journal, 56:
          3 (March 1949) 60.   (In Memory.)
          A graduate in medicine from Cornell, Edith Loeber Ballard
          was one of the first women surgeons in the South to perform
          major operations.

983.   "Dr. Eleanor B. Kilham."   Medical Woman's Journal, 44:9
          (September 1937) 257.
          Dr. Kilham (whose portrait appears on the front cover of
          this issue of the Journal) received her M.D. degree in 1882
          from the New York Infirmary for Women and Children.   Dur-
          ing World War I, Dr. Kilham worked with the American Com
          mittee for French Wounded in Paris, at Noyon.

984.   "Dr. Elisabeth Larsson Gracefully Retires from the Race with
          Old Doctor Stork after 35 Years."   Alumni Journal
          [Loma Linda University], 42:2 (March 1971) 25-26.   pho-
          to., port.

Dr. Larsson was born in the village of Gronviken, Brache, in central Sweden. She received her M.D. degree from Loma Linda University (California) and became an instructor in obstetrics and gynecology at that university in 1935. Among her numerous honors is that of having been elected to the Swedish Medical Society.

985.   "Dr. Elise S. L'Esperance." Medical Woman's Journal, 43:
        4 (April 1936) 104.
        Given are the professional associations and accomplishments of noted pathologist Elise L'Esperance (who is honored with her portrait on the cover of this month's Journal).

986.   "Dr. Eliza H. Root." Medical Woman's Journal, 42:12 (De-
        cember 1935) 341.
        Dr. Eliza H. Root (whose portrait appears on the front cover of this issue of the Journal) graduated in 1882 from North-western University Woman's Medical College of Chicago. Dr. Root was one of the first editors of the Journal.

987.   "Dr. Eliza M. Mosher." Medical Woman's Journal, 42:4
        (April 1935) 108.
        This memorial highlights events in the professional life of Dr. Mosher, the first woman student to enter the University of Michigan Medical School, receiving her degree in 1875.

988.   "Dr. Eliza M. Mosher: Memorial." Bulletin of the Medical
        Women's National Association, 23 (January 1929) 6-13.
        port.
        The first dean of women at the University of Michigan, Eliza M. Mosher was previously resident physician in the Massa-chusetts Prison for Women as well as a college lecturer and college resident physician. Dr. Mosher also helped to es-tablish the American Women's Hospitals. As a prison phy-sician, she equipped and organized a new hospital with mater-nity and nursery departments. "In a period when many of the so-called 'women's rights reformers' injured their cause by a dress and manner aggressively harsh, unlovely and mas-culine, Dr. Mosher retained a sweet dignity in both that made a strong impress and did much to overcome prejudice against higher education and larger activity for women." This article consists of tributes from a variety of people who knew Dr. Mosher.

989.   "Dr. Elizabeth Blackwell, Early Life, to Graduation in 1849."
        Woman's Medical Journal, 10 (1900) 261-264. (Biograph-
        ical.)

990.   "Dr. Elizabeth Blackwell, from Graduation to 1853." Wo-
        man's Medical Journal, 10:7 (July 1900) 296-298. (Bio-
        graphical: Sketches of the Life and Work of the Pioneer Women in Medicine.)
        After graduation, Elizabeth Blackwell continued to attend lec-

tures in Philadelphia and to pursue additional clinical training in Europe. While working at La Maternité in Paris, she
suffered an eye infection and as a result, became blind in
one eye. After her sister Emily Blackwell was graduated
from medical school in Cleveland, Ohio, Elizabeth joined her
in New York. There she began, in 1852, a course of lectures on the physical education of girls which was published
in book form as The Laws of Life in Reference to the Physical Education of Girls. In 1853 she established a dispensary
in a poor quarter near Tompkin's Square. "The first seven
years were full of difficulties. There was no medical companionship, the profession stood aloof and society was dis-
trustful of the innovation. Insolent letters occasionally came
to her by post to her helpless discomfiture."

991.   "Dr. Elizabeth Blackwell, Professional Career." Woman's
          Medical Journal, 10:8 (August 1900) 340-343. (Biograph-
          ical.)

992.   "Dr. Elizabeth Crosby to Join Anatomy." University of Ala-
          bama Medical Center Bulletin, 8 (April 1964) 8, 5.
          port.
        This article, written on the occasion of Dr. Crosby's appoint-
        ment as professor emeritus in the anatomy department at the
        University of Alabama, gives Dr. Crosby's professional back-
        ground, her memberships, honors, and awards, as well as
        a number of her medical publications.

993.   "Dr. Elizabeth Mason-Hohl." Medical Woman's Journal, 47:
          8 (August 1940) 256.
        Dr. Mason-Hohl (who is pictured on the front cover of this
        issue of the Journal) belongs to numerous civic and medical
        organizations and enjoys a large medical practice in Holly-
        wood, California. The 1915 graduate of the University of
        Nebraska's medical school also translated Trotula of Salerno.

994.   "Dr. Ella M. S. Marble, Washington, D.C." Woman's Med-
          ical Journal, 5:3 (March 1896) 69. (Biographical Se-
          ries.)
        In addition to Dr. Marble's medical practice and her literary
        and philanthropic work, she established the first gymnasium
        for women and children in Washington, D.C.

995.   "Dr. Ellen A. Wallace." Medical Woman's Journal, 53:4
          (April 1946) 53.
        Ellen Alfleda Wallace was the first physician to work for tu-
        berculosis prevention in New Hampshire.

996.   "Dr. Ellen Culver Potter." Bulletin of the Medical Women's
          National Association, 25 (July 1929) 5. port.
        After her experience in settlement work, Ellen Culver Potter
        became a physician. She taught gynecology and medicine for
        a while and then worked in public health, specializing in child

health, child welfare, and female prison health care. She
was a president of the Medical Women's National Association.

997.   "Dr. Emily A. Hill, Pioneer Physician of Bowling Green,
         Ohio." Woman's Medical Journal, 12:8 (August 1902)
         191.

998.   "Dr. Emily Dunning Barringer." Medical Woman's Journal,
         44:11 (November 1937) 323.
         Dr. Barringer (whose portrait appears on the front cover of
         this issue of the Journal) received her M.D. degree in 1901
         from Cornell Medical School. In this brief sketch, Dr. Bar-
         ringer's professional activities, honors, and awards are
         covered.

999.   "Dr. Esther Lovejoy, New Chairman of the American Women's
         Hospitals." Woman's Medical Journal, 29[19]:8 (August
         1919) 163. port.

1000. "Dr. Florence Brown Sherbon." Medical Woman's Journal,
         45:5 (May 1938) 142.
         In addition to this concise biography of Dr. Sherbon, her
         portrait is given on the front cover of this issue of the Jour-
         nal.

1001. "Dr. Florence Sabin." Medical Economics, 25:12 (September
         1948) 49-51.
         [Article not examined by editors.]

1002. "Dr. Frances Eastman Rose." Medical Woman's Journal,
         32:8 (August 1925) 226. port.
         At the time this article was written, Francis Eastman Rose
         was president-elect of the Medical Woman's National Associa-
         tion [which later became the American Medical Women's
         Association].

1003. "Dr. Geertruida J. Thorbecke." New York University Med-
         ical Quarterly, 26:3 (Winter 1971) 6-7. port. (New Pro-
         fessors.)
         Just promoted to professor of pathology, Dr. Thorbecke is a
         1950 graduate of the University of Groningen, The Netherlands.

1004. "Dr. Grace Kimball and Her Work for Armenia." Double
         Cross and Medical Missionary Record, 11:10 (October
         1896) 203-206.
         Dr. Kimball, who first went to Armenia in 1882, tells of
         her work experience in that country.

1005. "Dr. Harriet M. Doane." Medical Woman's Journal, 47:5
         (May 1940) 156.
         Dr. Doane (whose portrait appears on the front cover of this
         issue of the Journal) graduated from the Syracuse University
         School of Medicine in 1896.

1006.   "Dr. Helen Baldwin." Medical Woman's Journal, 47:12
            (December 1940) 372-373.
        After graduating from the New York Infirmary Medical
        School in 1892, Helen Baldwin (whose portrait appears on
        the front cover of this issue of the Journal) took postgradu-
        ate work at Johns Hopkins University and became one of
        the first women to work with Drs. Osler, Welsh, Kelly,
        and Halsted. Her career as instructor, researcher, and
        practitioner is detailed.

1007.   "Dr. Helen Morton, Boston, Mass." Woman's Medical Jour
            nal, 28:11 (November 1918) 238-239. port.
        "One of the first ambulances sent to France by the Ameri-
        can Women's Hospitals was given in memory of Dr. Helen
        Morton, of Boston...." A brief biographical sketch of Dr.
        Morton is given.

1008.   "Dr. Helen Taussig: Pediatrician With a Heart." Medical
            World News, (22 October 1965) 94-97, 100, 104-106.
            photos.
        This biographical summary of Dr. Taussig's career tells of
        her great contribution to the field of cardiology, the "blue
        baby operation," her part in averting a thalidomide disaster
        in this country, and her election as first woman president
        of the American Heart Association.

1009.   "Dr. Hetty K. Painter, Niece of John Brown (with her daugh
            ter)." Nebraska History Magazine, 23:1 (January-March
            1942) 72. photo.
        This photograph is accompanied by a brief description of Dr.
        Painter, who was a Union spy during the American Civil
        War; she also served as a nurse and as a doctor.

1010.   "Dr. Ida S. Scudder." Medical Woman's Journal, 45:7
            (July 1938) 212.
        Following her graduation from Cornell University Medical
        School (1899), Dr. Scudder began her life work in India.
        In addition to this brief biography, a portrait of Dr. Scud-
        der appears on the front cover of this issue of the Journal.

1011.   "Dr. Isabel Cobb: Her Times and Ours." Journal of the
            Oklahoma Medical Association, 53 (1960) 129-130. port.
        [Article not examined by editors.]

1012.   "Dr. Jane Wright Associate Dean." Journal of the National
            Medical Association, 59:5 (September 1967) 383. port.
            (Briefs.)

1013.   "Dr. Jane Wright on National Advisory Cancer Council."
            Journal of the National Medical Association, 59:1 (Janu-
            ary 1967) 58. port. (Briefs.)

1014.   "Dr. Jane Wright Wins Smith College Medal." Intercom,

2:6 (1968) 6.   port.
Jane C. Wright is a cancer researcher, a medical advisor
to Ghana, Kenya, and Tanganyika, and a recently appointed
associated dean of New York Medical College.

1015.   "Dr. Jane C. Wright Returns to NYMC As Associate Dean."
        Intercom, 1:4 (1967) 1, 8.   port.
        The first black woman to be appointed an associate dean at
        a medical school [New York Medical College], Dr. Wright
        has made notable contributions in cancer research and chemo-
        therapy.   Dr. Wright's private life as "Mrs. David D.
        Jones" keeps her "very feminine despite her demanding pro-
        fession."   As the New York Post described her in an April
        22 [1967] article: "She has elfin good looks, a schoolgirl's
        giggle, and an insatiable appetite for work."

1016.   "Dr. Josephine A. Jackson."   Medical Woman's Journal,
        45:1 (January 1938) 19.
        A graduate of Northwestern University Woman's Medical
        School (1896), Dr. Jackson confines her work in La Jolla,
        California to conferences only, using the spare time for
        writing.   (Her portrait appears on the front cover of this
        issue of the Journal.)

1017.   "Dr. Josephine B. Neal."   Medical Woman's Journal, 43:2
        (February 1936) 46.
        Dr. Neal (whose picture appears on the front cover of this
        issue of the Journal) graduated in 1910 from Cornell Uni-
        versity Medical College.

1018.   "Dr. Kazmierczak Honored."   Buffalo Physician, (Winter
        1973) 49.   port.
        Mary J. Kazmierczak, the first Polish woman to graduate
        from a New York State medical school, gets credit for start-
        ing the first successful mass immunization program (Buf-
        falo's 1920 diphtheria epidemic) and for helping to establish
        St. Rita's Home for Children (1930).

1019.   "Dr. Leona Baumgartner."   Medical Woman's Journal, 47:9
        (September 1940) 279.
        A Yale University graduate (Ph.D., 1932; M.D., 1934), Dr.
        Baumgartner (whose portrait appears on the front cover of
        this issue of the Journal) has obtained diversified profes-
        sional experience as an instructor and an administrator.   In
        1940 she became director of the maternal and child health
        activities in the New York City Health Department.   This
        listing of her affiliations includes bibliographical information
        on 29 of her published works.

1020.   "Dr. Leslie S. Kent, Eugene, Named President-Elect of
        O.S.M.S.:   First Woman Ever to Be Chosen Head of
        a State Medical Society."   Medical Woman's Journal,
        54:12 (December 1947) 37.

Dr. Kent was chosen president-elect of the Oregon State
Medical Society--her term to begin September 1948. A
one-paragraph biographical sketch is given.

1021. "Dr. Lillian K. P. Farrar." Medical Woman's Journal,
           43:7 (July 1936) 190.
        Dr. Farrar (whose picture appears on the front cover of
        this issue of the Journal) graduated from Cornell University
        Medical College in 1896. Her many "firsts" as a surgeon,
        medical instructor, and administrator are listed.

1022. "Dr. Louise B. Deal." Medical Woman's Journal, 38:7
           (July 1931) 185-186.
        An 1894 graduate of Cooper Medical College (now Stanford
        Medical School), Louise B. Deal was founder and first
        president of the Women Physicians Club of San Francisco,
        the Society for the Advancement of Women in Medicine
        and Surgery, vice-president of the San Francisco County
        Medical Society, chairman of the Child Hygiene Committee
        of the Federation of Women's Clubs, and Past Worthy
        Matron of the Order of Eastern Star.

1023. "Dr. Louise Pearce." Medical Woman's Journal, 43:3
           (March 1936) 72.
        Dr. Pearce is acclaimed for her research in venereal dis-
        eases. (Her picture appears on the front cover of this is-
        sue of the Journal.)

1024. "Dr. Lucy Porter Sutton." Medical Woman's Journal, 46:7
           (July 1939) 217, 221.
        Personal and professional interests of Dr. Sutton, a 1919
        graduate of Cornell Medical School, are given along with a
        list of scientific books and articles that she authored. (Dr.
        Sutton's portrait appears on the cover of this issue of the
        Journal.)

1025. "Dr. Lucy Sewell." Medical Woman's Journal, 44:2 (Febru-
           ary 1937) 49.
        Dr. Sewell (whose portrait appears on the front cover of
        this issue of the Journal) was inspired to study medicine
        through the influence of Marie Zakrzewska. After schooling
        in Boston, Dr. Sewell studied under physicians in London
        and Paris, returning to work at the newly established New
        England Hospital for Women and Children in Boston.

1026. "Dr. Lulu Hunt Peters." Medical Woman's Journal, 37:11
           (November 1930) 321.
        Lulu Hunt Peters was the author of Diet and Health with a
        Key to the Calories, Diet for Children, and a syndicated
        newspaper column on diet and health.

1027. "Dr. Mabel Elliott to Open Big Station to Fight Disease in
           Near East." Bulletin Medical Women's Club of Chi-

cago, 11:6 (February 1923) 6.
Dr. Elliott announced that she would "install, finance, and
direct the largest medical quarantine station in the world on
the island of Macronisi" (30 miles south of Athens, Greece).

1028.　"Dr. Margaret D. Craighill." Medical Woman's Journal,
　　　　48:1 (January 1941) 24.
　　　Dr. Craighill (whose portrait appears on the front cover of
　　　this issue of the Journal) received her M.D. degree in
　　　1924 from Johns Hopkins University. Dr. Craighill's edu-
　　　cation, professional appointments, and affiliations are given.

1029.　"Dr. Margaret F. Butler." Medical Woman's Journal, 39:1
　　　　(January 1932) 16. port.
　　　Margaret F. Butler served in her specialty, otolaryngology,
　　　on the faculty of the Woman's Medical College of Pennsyl-
　　　vania from 1896 until her death on October 16, 1931.

1030.　"Dr. Margaret H. Polk: Missionary to China for Thirty
　　　　Years." Medical Woman's Journal, 36:4 (April 1929)
　　　　102. port.
　　　Graduating from the Woman's Medical College of Pennsyl-
　　　vania in 1892, Dr. Polk sailed for China after four years
　　　of medical practice in the United States. In Soochow at the
　　　Woman's Medical School, Dr. Polk undertook the training
　　　of women physicians. In 1911, Dr. Polk, who had always
　　　been interested in the woman suffrage movement, withdrew
　　　from the church "because laity rights were not granted to
　　　women." As an independent missionary, she, in 1913, be-
　　　gan private practice in Shanghai.

1031.　"Dr. Margaret Witter Barnard." Medical Woman's Journal,
　　　　45:3 (March 1938) 79.
　　　Complementing her portrait on the cover of this month's is-
　　　sue of the Journal is this biography of Dr. Barnard, which
　　　lists her many professional affiliations. At the time, Dr.
　　　Barnard was director, District Health Administration, De-
　　　partment of Health, New York City.

1032.　"Dr. Marion Craig Potter." Medical Woman's Journal, 45:
　　　　8 (August 1938) 247.
　　　Listed are the professional interests and affiliations of this
　　　1884 graduate of the University of Michigan Medical School.
　　　Dr. Potter's portrait appears on the front cover of this is-
　　　sue of the Journal.

1033.　"Dr. Marjorie Peebles Myers [sic]." Journal of the Nation-
　　　　al Medical Association, 61:1 (January 1969) 98. port.
　　　　(Professional News-Personal.)
　　　Dr. Meyers is profiled briefly in this article. Her educa-
　　　tional background, honors and awards, and professional af-
　　　filiations are listed. In 1968, Dr. Meyers received the Ne-
　　　gro Life History Award and was also chosen Outstanding

Physician of the Year by the Michigan State Medical Society.
She was also the first woman of her race to graduate from
Wayne State University Medical School.

1034.   "Dr. Marshall Appointed V. A. Chief of Staff." MCG Today,
          4:2 (Fall 1974) 30. port.
          With her appointment as chief of staff at the Lenwood Divi-
          sion of the VA Hospital in Augusta, Georgia, Louie Frances
          Woodward-Marshall became the only woman holding this
          position in the Veteran's Administration's 171 hospitals. A
          profile of the 1948 graduate of the University of Georgia
          School of Medicine (now the Medical College of Georgia)
          concludes with the observation that "no title holds more
          meaning for Lou than 'Grandma.' "

1035.   "Dr. Mary A. Smith." Medical Woman's Journal, 42:9
          (September 1935) 252.
          Dr. Mary Smith (whose picture appears on the front cover
          of this issue of the Journal) graduated in 1881 from the Med-
          ical College of the New York Infirmary. She was one of
          the few women at that time to be admitted to membership
          in the American College of Surgeons.

1036.   "Dr. Mary E. Bates." Woman's Medical Journal, 9:1 (Jan-
          uary 1899) 11-12.
          The Journal welcomes Dr. Bates as a member of the editor-
          ial staff. A brief biography of her mentions the fact that
          she was the first woman to intern at Cook County Hospital
          in Chicago.

1037.   "Dr. Mary E. Dennis." Medical Woman's Journal, 45:12
          (December 1938) 376.
          Dr. Dennis (whose portrait appears on the front cover of
          this issue of the Journal) graduated from the University of
          California's medical school in 1897. She remained in gen-
          eral practice in Los Angeles for 36 years, with the excep-
          tion of three years spent on Catalina Island, "where her
          patients included wealthy yachtsmen, royalty, and mere
          fishermen." A founder of the Medical Women's Society of
          Los Angeles County, Dr. Dennis wrote many articles ad-
          vocating sterilization of the unfit, and stricter marriage
          laws.

1038.   "Dr. Mary Greene Completes 50 Years Service at Sanitari-
          um." Medical Woman's Journal, 55:2 (February 1948)
          51. (News Notes.)
          Mary T. Greene came to the sanitarium [in Castile, New
          York] in 1897 to assist her aunt, Dr. Cordelia A. Greene,
          "for a few weeks" and has been there since.

1039.   "Dr. Mary H. McLean." Medical Woman's Journal, 37:7
          (July 1930) 208-209. port.
          Determined to become a practicing physician, Mary H. Mc-

Lean went to St. Louis to open an office after she obtained
her medical degree and had to visit 46 rooming houses or
boarding houses before she could find one that allowed her
to hang her shingle.   During the St. Louis World's Fair in
1904, she was one of the sponsors of the Emmaus Home for
Girls, which had been organized "to care for young women
who had been lured to the city under false pretenses."

1040.   "Dr. Mary Ketring." Double Cross and Medical Missionary
           Record, 14 (October 1899) 167.   port.
         Dr. Ketring is a medical missionary in China.

1041.   "Dr. Mary M. Crawford." Medical Woman's Journal, 45:
           2 (February 1938) 49-50.
         A graduate of Cornell Medical College (1907), Mary Craw-
         ford is medical director at the Federal Reserve Bank of
         New York.   (Her portrait appears on the front cover of this
         issue of the Journal.)

1042.   "Dr. Mary M. Davenport." Medical Missionary Record, 2:
           10 (February 1888) 248-251.   port.

1043.   "Dr. Mary O'Malley, President-Elect M.W.N.A." Medical
           Woman's Journal, 39:5 (May 1932) 127.
         The United States government appointed Mary O'Malley the
         first woman Chief of Women's Services.   She served in this
         position at St. Elizabeth's Hospital in Washington, D.C.
         She became president elect of the Medical Women's National
         Association.

1044.   "Dr. Mary R. H. Lewis." Medical Woman's Journal, 45:
           11 (November 1938) 343.
         A 1911 graduate of Woman's Medical College of Pennsyl-
         vania, Dr. Lewis later served as medical director and
         superintendent of that institution's hospital.   (Her picture
         appears on the front cover of this issue of the Journal.)

1045.   "Dr. Mary Sorenson." Wisconsin Medical Journal, 57:10
           (1958) 28.   port.
         [Article not examined by editors.]

1046.   "Dr. Mary T. Greene Sanitarium: 100 Year Celebration."
           Medical Woman's Journal, 56:6 (June 1949) 21-25.
           photos., ports.
         This history of the Sanitarium in Castile, New York in-
         cludes a biography of Dr. Cordelia A. Greene, who took
         over "The Water Cure" (as the institution was formerly
         called) from her father in 1864.   Her niece, Dr. Mary T.
         Greene, assumed the Sanitarium duties in 1897.

1047.   "Dr. Mary Walker." Bulletin Medical Women's Club of
           Chicago, 7:7 (March 1919) 2-3.
         This obituary notice highlights some of the events and honors
         in Dr. Walker's "picturesque career."

1048.   "Dr. Mary Walker's Eccentric Dress Drew Attention from
         Her Real Achievements." The Literary Digest, (15
         March 1919) 94.
         While Mary Walker was most famous during her lifetime
         for wearing the more comfortable and healthful clothing of
         men rather than the dress of women, she made other con-
         tributions that tend to be overlooked: for heroic medical
         services during the Civil War she received the Medal of
         Honor; she was a pioneer for woman suffrage; she sold her
         hair to help a woman who was "financially embarrassed";
         and she created the inside neckband on men's shirts which
         "protects the flesh from being rubbed by the collar-button."
         Dr. Walker took a great deal of physical abuse because she
         dressed as a man, and the suffragettes ostracized her.
         "She was too queer, and the suffs, so long the target of
         ridicule, had in self-defense to avoid being chummy with
         the woman who actually did the thing they were constantly
         caricatured as doing."

1049.   "Dr. Nora Johnson Ross, 1926 South Lawndale Avenue, Died
         Friday, December 1, 1916." Bulletin Medical Women's
         Club of Chicago, 5:4 (December 1916) 5. (Obituary.)

1050.   "Dr. Olga Stastny: President-Elect." Bulletin of the Med-
         ical Women's National Association, 25 (July 1929) 6.
         port.
         This article presents a brief biography of Dr. Stastny, a
         1913 graduate of medicine at the University of Nebraska,
         and president-elect of the Medical Women's National Asso-
         ciation.

1051.   "Dr. Peck Honored by British." Medical Woman's Journal,
         50:9 (September 1943) 245-246. port. (News Notes.)
         This article is offered upon the occasion of Dr. Eleanor
         Kellogg Peck becoming the first woman physician to present
         a paper before the annual meeting of the British Pediatric
         Association. The subject of Dr. Peck's paper, as well as
         the names of those in attendance at the Association meeting,
         is given. Dr. Peck graduated from the College of Physi-
         cians and Surgeons, Columbia University.

1052.   "Dr. Rebecca Lee, First Negro Woman Medical Graduate."
         Bulletin, Medico-Chirurgical Society of the District of
         Columbia, Inc., 41:1 (January 1949).
         Recent research indicates that Rebecca Lee was the first
         Negro woman to receive a medical degree (New England
         Female Medical College, Boston, 1864). Two other early
         Negro women medical graduates were Rebecca Cole (Wo-
         man's Medical College, Philadelphia, 1867) and Susan Maria
         Smith McKenney Steward (New York Medical College and
         Hospital for Women, 1870).

1053.   "Dr. Roselyn Payne Epps." Journal of the National Med-

ical Association, 66:3 (May 1974) 271. port. (Professional News.)
Dr. Epps (M.D., Howard, 1955) was one of six recipients of the Federal Women's Award for 1974.

1054.   "Dr. Rosina Wistein." Bulletin of the Linn County Medical Society, (8 April 1937) 13. port.

1055.   "Dr. S. Josephine Baker." Medical Woman's Journal, 30: 6 (June 1923) 190-191. (Editorial.)
This editorial laments Dr. S. Josephine Baker's retirement as director of child hygiene, New York City Department of Health.

1056.   "Dr. S. Josephine Baker: President Medical Woman's National Association." Medical Woman's Journal, 42:7 (July 1935) 199.
This biographical sketch of Dr. Baker focuses mainly on her professional activities.

1057.   "Doctor Sarah Adamson Dolley." Woman's Medical Journal, 18:4 (April 1908) 86-87.
Among Dr. Dolley's many accomplishments are these: the second American woman to obtain a full medical diploma (after being refused admittance by 13 colleges); the first U.S. woman intern with full hospital service; organizer and first president of the first U.S. society of women physicians (the Blackwell Medical Society of Rochester, New York).

1058.   "Dr. Sarah Adamson Dolley." Woman's Medical Journal, 20:1 (January 1910) 17-18. (Editorial.)
Dr. Dolley, who graduated in medicine in 1851, died on December 27, 1909.

1059.   "Dr. Sarah Adamson Dolly [sic]." Medical Woman's Journal, 43:11 (November 1936) 304.
Sarah Adamson became the second woman to graduate in medicine in America (Eclectic School of Medicine in Rochester, New York, 1851). A biography is presented (and her portrait appears on this month's Journal cover).

1060.   "Dr. Stella Chess." New York University Medical Quarterly, 26:3 (Winter 1971) 6. port. (New Professors.)
Dr. Chess has made many contributions to the field of child psychiatry.

1061.   "Doctor Strikes." Medical Woman's Journal, 51:10 (October 1945) 52. (News Notes.)
Dr. Elizabeth Heyes resigned as company physician for the Shawmut Mining Company in Illinois because of "'intolerable'" sanitary conditions. "'I want to live under decent conditions or get out'" said Dr. Heyes. Meanwhile, 350 miners walked out because they would not work without a company doctor.

1062.   "Dr. Sue Gould Resigns Post with County." Medical Wo-
              man's Journal, 54:10 (October 1947) 57.   port.   (News
              Notes.)
         This article, reprinted from the Hudson Register, Hudson,
         New York, praises Dr. Gould for her work as commission-
         er of the Columbia County Health Department.

1063.   "Dr. Violette Bergere." Medical Woman's Journal, 33:10
              (October 1926) 300-301.   port.
         Dr. Bergere, who also holds a Doctor of Philosophy degree,
         received her Doctor of Medicine degree from the University
         of Montpellier, France, in 1917. In 1919, she became
         associate director of the Polish White Cross, and in 1920
         served as a surgeon on the Russian front at Minsk. Dr.
         Bergere founded the Emergency Hospital in Warsaw. She
         is now writing a book dealing with political conditions in
         Poland.

1064.   "Dr. Virginia Apgar." The Stethoscope [Columbia-Presby-
              terian Medical Center], 29 (September 1974) 6.   port.
              (Obituary.)

1065.   "Dr. Wilhelmina Afton Ragland." Medical Woman's Journal,
              46:8 (August 1939) 254.
         A very brief biography is given of Dr. Ragland, a 1909
         graduate of the Woman's Medical College of Pennsylvania.
         (Dr. Ragland's portrait appears on the front cover of this
         issue of the Journal.)

1066.   "Doctor Yarros Honored." Medical Woman's Journal, 49:6
              (June 1942) 194. (News Notes.)
         Rachelle S. Yarros, a pioneer in the field of social hygiene,
         helped to establish one of the earliest teaching clinics in
         Chicago, the American Social Hygiene Association, and the
         first pre-marital and marital consultation service under the
         Social Hygiene League. She wrote a book, Modern Woman
         and Sex, and was also active in advocating birth control as
         a necessary part of medical advice and care. Dr. Yarros
         was granted honorary life membership in the American So-
         cial Hygiene Association.

1067.   "Doctress in Medicine." Boston Medical and Surgical Jour-
              nal, 40 (1849) 25-26.
         An account of the graduation of Elizabeth Blackwell consti-
         tutes this article. [Article not examined by editors.]

1068.   Dole, Mary Phylinda. A Doctor in Homespun: Autobiogra-
              phy of Mary Phylinda Dole, B.S., M.D. Published by
              the author, 1941, 165 pp. illus., photos., ports.
         This book, states its introduction, "... is a part of the life
         story, told with directness and simplicity, of a New England
         country girl to whom many things happened." Some of those
         happenings in Mary Phylinda Dole's life included graduating

from Mount Holyoke College (to which she maintained a life-long loyalty), obtaining an M.D. from Woman's Medical College of Baltimore, and interning at the New England Hospital for Women and Children. Writing this autobiography at the age of 78, Dr. Dole recalls her studies at these institutions, and profiles the distinguished medical women who influenced her career. An illness forced Dr. Dole to stop practicing medicine in 1927. It was then she took up weaving, a craft which brought her many financial and personal rewards. Interwoven among anecdotes and facts are references to the advantages of remaining unmarried and of having the support and friendship of other women. The illustrated book includes an introduction by another Mount Holyoke graduate.

1069.   Donahue, Julia. "Fifty Years in Medicine (1892-1942)."
        Medical Woman's Journal, 52:3 (March 1945) 43-44.
        ports.
        This autobiographical account by Dr. Julia Donahue discusses her activities as a medical missionary in China. Returning to the United States, Dr. Donahue continued her missionary work at home before accepting a position at Massillon State Hospital in 1921. She worked as a physician there for nearly 20 years.

1070.   "Dorothy Boulding Ferebee, M.D., 1898- ." Journal of the
        National Medical Association, 62:2 (March 1970) 177.
        (Medical History.)
        The 46-year medical career of Dr. Ferebee (whose portrait appears on this month's cover of the Journal) included many responsible posts in civic and professional organizations.

1071.   "Dorothy S. Jaeger, M.D." Medical Woman's Journal, 53:
        1 (January 1946) 36.
        Dr. Jaeger (whose portrait appears on the cover of this month's Journal) teaches pediatrics at George Washington University and practices her specialty in Washington, D.C.

1072.   "Dorothy Wells Atkinson, M.D.: Medical Woman of the
        Month." Journal of the American Medical Women's
        Association, 4:8 (August 1949) 354-355. port. (Medical Women in the News.)
        Dr. Atkinson, president of the American Medical Women's Association, served as delegate to the Sixth International Congress of Medical Women at Amsterdam in 1947. A San Francisco physician, she taught at the University of California Medical School and was affiliated with the San Francisco Hospital for Women and Children.

1073.   Dorpat, Klarese. "New AMWA President-1965." Journal
        of the American Medical Women's Association, 20:1
        (January 1965) 49. port.
        A specialist in psychosomatic medicine, Bernice Sachs was

the president of the American Medical Women's Association
in 1965. Her special commitment to women in medicine includes a "belief that women have qualities such as compassion, empathy, tolerance, and stamina which uniquely qualify them to practice medicine. In doing so, they need not
deny their femininity, but rather make good use of it."

1074.   Doyle, Helen MacKnight. A Child Went Forth: The Auto-
            biography of Dr. Helen MacKnight Doyle with a Fore-
            word by Mary Austin. Gothan House, Inc., New York,
            New York, 1934, 364 pp.
        A major portion of this autobiography, which begins in 1878
        when "Nellie" MacKnight was a child, concentrates on her
        youth and family relationships. Helen MacKnight Doyle,
        who graduated from Toland Hall in San Francisco at age
        20, reminisces about her medical practice in the desert re-
        gions of California.

1075.   Drew, Nellie L. "Career of Dr. A. A. Starbuck." Med-
            ical Woman's Journal, 54:9 (September 1947) 45-46.
        Dr. Starbuck obtained her M. D. degree in 1906 from Boston
        University. She was the first doctor to discover the pres-
        ence of acetone in urine without sugar, although the paper
        discussing her findings was denied publication by the Massa-
        chusetts Medical Journal as it was "contrary to their teach-
        ings." An English medical journal ultimately published the
        paper. Dr. Starbuck runs a resort in the Berkshires in the
        summertime and has a general practice in New England.

1076.   Drooz, Irma Gross. Doctor of Medicine. Dodd, Mead &
            Company, [n. p.], 1949, 308 pp.
        In her autobiography, Irma Gross Drooz, a neuropsychia-
        trist, gives a detailed account of her education at the New
        York University College of Medicine from 1938 to 1942 and
        her internship in surgery at Beth Israel Hospital, where she
        was only tolerated in the operating room because she did
        all the preoperative workups. She gives many details of
        her residencies in neurosurgery and neurology at Mount Sinai
        Hospital. The book ends with her residency at the New York
        State Psychiatric Institute and her first job in Fayetteville,
        North Carolina. She concludes with her hopes for future
        work in preventive psychiatry and the treatment of mental
        illness. No bibliography or index appear in the book.

1077.   Dunnahoo, Terry. Emily Dunning: a Portrait. Reilly &
            Lee Books, Chicago, Illinois, 1970, 142 pp.
        Written for young people, this fictionalized biography of
        Emily Dunning concentrates on her mother's influence in her
        decision to enter medicine and upon the struggle to obtain
        that medical education. She entered Cornell University Med-
        ical School in 1899, where, according to the author, she
        welcomed male opinions on medicine, an influence she had
        missed while studying in an all-woman school (the Medical

College of the New York Infirmary for Women and Children).
An adventurous account is given of Dr. Dunning's work as
ambulance surgeon of New York's Gouverneur Hospital. The
book's "Epilogue" tells of her marriage to Ben Barringer,
her later professional activities, and her death in 1961.

1078.   Dutton, William S. "A Mighty Little Woman But She's All
         Grit!" American Magazine, (March 1928) 16 passim.
         photos. , port.
         Dr. Harriet G. McGraw attended Lincoln Medical College in
         Lincoln, Nebraska. She and her second husband moved to
         Tyron, Nebraska where she is the only physician for miles.
         This article describes Dr. McGraw's life, from her difficult
         childhood, personal tragedies, and professional ambitions,
         to practice in Tyron.

1079.   Dyer, Helen M. "In Memory: Mary Jane Walters." Med-
         ical Woman's Journal, 54:9 (September 1947) 50-51.
         (News Notes.)
         A list of professional appointments is included in this obitu-
         ary of Dr. Walters, reprinted from the Goucher Alumna
         Quarterly.

1080.   East, Marion Reed. "Women Physicians of Oregon." Jour-
         nal of the American Medical Women's Association, 19:3
         (March 1964) 228-231.
         This article highlights Oregon women physicians: sources
         are mentioned from which information was taken, primarily
         Olof Larsell's book The Doctor in Oregon.

1081.   "Eccentric Esthetes: The Remarkable Dr. Claribel Cone,
         M.D." Medical Newsmagazine, 4:2 (1960) 94-99. illus.,
         port.
         [Article not examined by editors.]

1082.   Eddy, Mary Pierson. "A Busy Woman." Woman's Medical
         Journal, 6:1 (January 1897) 12.
         Dr. Eddy, the only woman permitted by the Turkish empire
         to practice medicine in that country, describes her work.

1083.   Edward, Mary Lee. "Anna Hubert, M.D." Journal of the
         American Medical Women's Association, 12:1 (January
         1957) 30. port. (Album of Women in Medicine.)
         In her youth, Anna Hubert was fond of mountain climbing.
         Hubert Glacier, in the Olympic National Forest, is named
         after her. In 1913 she became resident at the New York
         Infirmary for Women and Children and remained affiliated
         with that institution as a surgeon and specialist in gynecol-
         ogy until her death in 1956. It is attributed to Dr. Hubert
         that she was one of the leaders who held the Infirmary to-
         gether and kept it from closing that she built up a depart-
         ment of surgery and gynecology at a time when a woman
         trying to practice surgery received no encouragement, that

she was a pioneer among the women surgeons of the world.
She was also surgeon of the Kate Depew Strang Clinic from
the date of its opening in 1933. She was the first person
to make a medical survey of the needs of women prisoners
at Welfare Island in New York City (in 1914).

1084.   Edwards, Linden F. "Dr. Mary Edwards Walker (1832-
              1919); Charlatan or Martyr? Part I." Ohio State Med-
              ical Journal, (September 1958) 1160-1162. (The His-
              torian's Notebook.) (Presentation, meeting of the Amer-
              ican Association for the History of Medicine, Williams-
              burg, Virginia, 8 May 1957.)
A strong advocate of women's rights, Mary Edwards Walker
was the first woman to practice medicine in Columbus, Ohio,
the first woman to serve on an army surgical staff in time
of war (when she served with the northern forces during the
Civil War), and the first woman to receive the Congressional
Medal of Honor.

1085.   Edwards, Linden F. "Dr. Mary Edwards Walker (1832-
              1919); Charlatan or Martyr? Part II." Ohio State Med-
              ical Journal, 54 (1958) 1296, 1298.
Although Mary Walker was a registered practitioner of medicine, her main claim to fame is as an eccentric who dressed
in male attire and gave popular lectures on dress reform,
woman suffrage, capital punishment, smoking and drinking,
and the prevention of infanticide. For a short time, she
operated a tuberculosis sanitarium and a school for the prevention of the disease, and during her career as a practitioner in Rome, New York, she founded a woman's colony
called "Adamless Eden." Her fortunes declined and eventually she had to resort to appearances at dime museums for
her livelihood.

1086.   Edwards, Muriel. "Emma K. Willits, M. D." Journal of
              the American Medical Women's Association, 5:1 (Janu-
              ary 1950) 42-43. port. (Album of Women in Medicine.)
When Emma Willits enrolled in medical school, "women medical students ... were no longer herded behind screens in
the classroom, but they were still referred to as 'hen medics' and occasionally hooted at by their male confreres." In
response to a male surgeon's remark early in her career--
"What do you expect to do with hands like that?"--she responded, "I will use skill instead of brute force." Indeed,
her distinguished career as surgeon at San Francisco's
Children's Hospital from 1897 as a resident, with a few
years off for private practice, until her retirement in 1941
attests to that skill.

1087.   Egan, Lenora Horton. "Dr. Lillias Horton Underwood of
              Korea." Medical Woman's Journal, 32:7 (July 1925)
              200-201.
When Lillias Horton sailed for Korea in 1887, after having

obtained her medical degree under the auspices of the Presbyterian Church, she became the first woman doctor to practice in that country. The king had initially invited a woman
doctor to care for the queen and the court babies. Dr.
Underwood, however, also perceived her responsibilities as
including the establishment of public health care. She
helped to found a dispensary "where every sort of ailment
was attended to, from pulling teeth to operations for cata-
ract."

1088.   "1880 U-M Grad. Bethenia Owens: Physician, Feminist,
            and Social Reformer." The University of Michigan Med-
            ical Center Alumni News, 1:4 (Fall 1975) 3.   port.
         Dr. Owens received her medical education from the Eclectic
         Medical College of Philadelphia. Arriving in Portland, Ore-
         gon, she was ridiculed, and her consequent attempts to enter
         Jefferson Medical College (Philadelphia) were frustrated.
         She then entered the University of Michigan Medical School,
         and in 1880 at the age of 40, she received her M.D. de-
         gree and returned to Portland. This brief biography fol-
         lows her life through her marriage at the age of 14, her
         subsequent divorce and reclaiming of her maiden name (a
         courageous step in 1859), her medical education and practice,
         and concludes with her death at the age of 88.

1089.   "Eleanor R. Izquierdo, M.D." Journal of the American
            Medical Women's Association, 11:10 (October 1956)
            379.   port.   (Album of Women in Medicine.)
         A recipient of the first Kate Hurd Mead Alumnae Award of
         the Woman's Medical College of Pennsylvania, Eleanor R.
         Izquierdo has been active in teaching and research in the
         fields of pathology and neuropathology.

1090.   "Eleanor Scott, M.D." Medical Woman's Journal, 48:5
            (May 1941) 156.
         Dr. Eleanor Scott (whose portrait appears on the front cover
         of this issue of the Journal) received her M.D. from Cornell
         University in 1935. This biography gives Dr. Scott's educa-
         tion, professional activities, and hobbies.

1091.   Elia, Joseph J. "Alice Hamilton--1869-1970." New England
            Journal of Medicine, 283:18 (29 October 1970) 993-994.
            (Editorial.)
         This "historical essay" praises and provides examples of
         Dr. Hamilton's "solitary yet formidable explorations into
         the occupational hazards of a newly industrialized America
         and her commitment to the social reform movements of her
         time...."

1092.   "The Elizabeth Blackwell Centennial." Medical Woman's
            Journal, 56:3 (March 1949) 17-26.   facsim., photo.,
            ports.
         A special convocation held in January [1949] by Hobart and

William Smith Colleges cited 12 women doctors of the U.S.,
Canada, England, and France on the 100th anniversary of
Elizabeth Blackwell's graduation. Biographies and portraits
of the award recipients are presented, and a description of
the ceremony is given.

1093.   "Elizabeth Blackwell Centennial: 1847-1947." Medical Wo-
              man's Journal, 54:11 (November 1947) 34-35. illus.,
              port.

1094.   "Elizabeth Blackwell, M.D." Medical Woman's Journal,
              33:1 (January 1926) 21-22. port.
          "The new hope for the world that I see dawning with the
          advent of womanhood into the realm of independent thought
          and equal justice makes me very happy," wrote Elizabeth
          Blackwell in a New Year's greeting to her sister-in-law and
          friend, Lucy Stone. Dated 1887, the letter was given to the
          Medical Woman's Journal editors by Lucy Stone's daughter,
          Alice Stone Blackwell. Following a reprint of the letter is
          an account of the life of Dr. Antoinette Brown Blackwell,
          sister-in-law of Drs. Elizabeth and Emily Blackwell, fellow
          worker with Susan B. Anthony and Lucy Stone, and an or-
          dained minister.

1095.   "Elizabeth Blackwell, M.D." Medical Woman's Journal, 47:
              4 (April 1940) 126.
          This abbreviated mention of Dr. Blackwell's accomplishments
          is complemented by a portrait of her (which appears on the
          front cover of this issue of the Journal).

1096.   "Elizabeth Burr Thelberg, M.D." Medical Woman's Journal,
              42:6 (June 1935) 169. port.
          This obituary notice lists Dr. Thelberg's professional ac-
          tivities and affiliations. Dr. Thelberg was resident physician
          at Vassar College since 1887. In 1884, she received her
          medical degree from the Women's Medical College of the
          New York Infirmary for Women and Children.

1097.   "Elizabeth Hamilton-Muncie, M.D." Medical Woman's Jour-
              nal, 54:5 (May 1947) 44-45.
          This biography of Dr. Hamilton-Muncie discusses her deter-
          mination to enter medicine--a goal of which she firmly in-
          formed her husband before their marriage. When her sec-
          ond child was three years old, she entered the New York
          Medical College and Hospital for Women. As a surgeon, she
          performed the first Pratt hysterectomy (a vaginal hysterec-
          tomy technique). She is the author of the book Four Epochs
          of Life, a sex education book. A list of her most notable
          lectures concludes this article.

1098.   "Elizabeth Kittredge, M.D." Medical Woman's Journal, 50:
              10 (October 1943) 367.
          Dr. Kittredge (whose portrait appears on the front cover of

the Journal) received her M.D. degree from Johns Hopkins University (Baltimore, Maryland) in 1922. A brief biography of Dr. Kittredge is given in this article.

1099.   "Elizabeth McSherry, M.D." Good Housekeeping, 161 (September 1965) 54-55+. illus.
[Article not examined by editors.]

1100.   "Elizabeth Mason-Hohl, M.D." Medical Woman's Journal, 49:3 (March 1942) 89-90.
Newly appointed editor of the Journal, Elizabeth Mason-Hohl (whose portrait appears on the front cover of this issue of the Journal) graduated in 1915 from the University of Nebraska. Her numerous professional activities are mentioned.

1101.   "Elizabeth Newcomer, M.D." Medical Woman's Journal, 52:6 (June 1945) 51.
Dr. Newcomer (whose portrait appears on the front cover of this issue of the Journal) specialized in the radiologic treatment of cancer. She is the only woman physician in radiology in Denver, Colorado.

1102.   "Ellen C. Potter, M.D.: Medical Woman of the Month." Journal of the American Medical Women's Association, 4:2 (February 1949) 85. port. (News of Women in Medicine.)
Dr. Potter, recipient of the W. S. Terry, Jr. Memorial Merit Award of the American Public Welfare Association, did extensive work in social welfare and was active in prison work, geriatrics, and many other areas of public concern.

1103.   "Ellen Culver Potter, M.D." Medical Woman's Journal, 49:12 (December 1942) 386-387.
The professional resumé of Ellen Culver Potter (whose portrait appears on the front cover of this issue of the Journal) is reproduced in this article. Some of the highlights of her career include: being the first woman to hold a position as cabinet officer in a state cabinet (as secretary of welfare, Department of Welfare of Pennsylvania); writing numerous articles on public welfare and public health administration; being medical director and director of classification of various New Jersey penal and correctional institutions and institutions for the feebleminded; and, in 1929-1930, being president of the American Medical Women's Association.

1104.   "Ellen E. Mitchell, M.D." Medical Missionary Record, 5:10 (October 1890) 203-205.
Born in 1829, Dr. Mitchell worked as a nurse during the Civil War, obtained her M.D. from the Women's Medical College in New York in 1871, and is now a medical missionary in Maulmain, Burma.

1105.   Elliot, H. B. "Woman as Physician." In Eminent Women

of the Age, Being Narratives of the Lives and Deeds
of the Most Prominent Women of the Present Generation. By James Parton, et al. S. M. Betts, Hartford, Connecticut, 1869, 513-550.
Short biographies are given of Clemence S. Lozier, Elizabeth Blackwell, Harriot K. Hunt, Hannah E. Longshore, and
Ann Preston.

1106.   Elliott, Mabel Evelyn. Beginning Again at Ararat. Fleming
        H. Revell Company, New York, New York, 1924, 341
        pp. photos., port.
        Dr. Elliott served in a prominent position as director of
        the Near East division of the American Women's Hospitals
        during the world war. This book is a record of her work
        in the Near East and her thoughts on medical care, human
        suffering, imperialism, and war. The book is full of de-
        scriptions of refugees--the treatment of women and children
        by Turkish men, and the hardships and physical abuse borne
        out of custom by these women. Dr. Elliott's personality is
        gradually unfolded through the pages of this work. The book
        contains an "appreciation" by Grace N. Kimball, president
        of the Medical Women's National Association. There is no
        index.

1107.   "Elvira DeLiee, M.D." Medical Woman's Journal, 48:4
        (April 1941) 118.
        Dr. DeLiee (whose portrait appears on the front cover of
        this issue of the Journal) is the holder of the Mary Putnam
        Jacobi Fellowship for 1938-39 and is a fellow in medicine
        at the New York University College of Medicine. This
        brief article gives Dr. DeLiee's professional interests.

1108.   "Emily Dunning Barringer, M.D." Medical Woman's Jour-
        nal, 49:7 (July 1942) 219-220.
        As president of the American Medical Women's Association
        from 1941 to 1942, Emily Dunning Barringer has been es-
        pecially active in trying to obtain equal rank and equal pay
        for women physicians in the Medical Reserve Corps of the
        United States Army and Navy. When she became New York
        City's first woman ambulance surgeon in 1902, she opened
        up the opportunity for women to hold internships in New
        York City hospitals. (A portrait of Dr. Barringer appears
        on the cover of this issue of the Journal.)

1109.   "Emily Dunning Barringer: President AMWA." Women in
        Medicine, 73 (July 1941) 7. port.
        A gynecologist, Emily Dunning Barringer was the first wo-
        man physician to be a delegate from the New York State
        Medical Society to the House of Delegates of the American
        Medical Association. In 1941 she became president of the
        American Medical Women's Association. Her work on gonor-
        rhea was featured at a scientific exhibit of the American
        Medical Association.

1110.   "Emma Dawson Parsons." Medical Woman's Journal, 51:
         11 (November 1944) 26-27. port.
         Born in 1859, Emma Dawson (later Parsons) was a frail
         child, and "her chief incentive in studying medicine was to
         acquire the knowledge that would enable her to make use of
         her limited store of strength to the best advantage." A
         graduate of Woman's Medical College at Chicago, Dr. Par-
         sons worked extensively in electrotherapy and practiced med-
         icine in Waterloo, Iowa for 40 years. In addition to her
         many professional activities, Dr. Parsons was a "spirited
         public citizen" and a shrewd business woman who maintained
         financial and administrative interest in several corporations.

1111.   "Emma Selkin-Aronson, M.D." Journal of the American
         Medical Women's Association, 9:4 (April 1954) 124.
         port. (Album of Women in Medicine.)
         Emma Selkin-Aronson was on the attending staff of the New
         York Infirmary for Women and Children and was active in
         its reopening in 1924 after it had been used as a reconstruc-
         tion hospital for soldiers. She also worked at the Bronx
         Hospital.

1112.   "Estella Ford Warner, M.D." Medical Woman's Journal,
         52:10 (October 1945) 50-51. port.
         Dr. Warner graduated from the University of Oregon School
         of Medicine in 1918. Shortly thereafter she went to Europe
         and served as a medical officer in the YWCA.

1113.   "Ester I. McEachen, M.D." Medical Woman's Journal, 51:
         8 (August 1944) 38-39.
         Dr. McEachen (whose portrait appears on the front cover of
         this issue of the Journal) graduated from the University of
         Nebraska College of Medicine in 1927. She practices pedi-
         atrics while participating in a variety of social and profes-
         sional organizations in Nebraska.

1114.   "Esther Loring Richards, M.D." Medical Woman's Journal,
         48:8 (August 1941) 253.
         Dr. Richards (whose portrait appears on the front cover of
         this issue of the Journal) received her M.D. degree in 1915
         from Johns Hopkins University. A brief resumé is herein
         given of her education and professional activities.

1115.   "Esther Pohl Lovejoy, M.D." Journal of the American Med-
         ical Women's Association, 10:4 (April 1955) 132-133.
         port. (Past Presidents of AMWA.)
         Dr. Lovejoy, a graduate of the University of Oregon Medical
         School, went with her brother and husband in 1897 to Alaska
         during the gold rush. Both her husband and brother lost
         their lives there. She later established a scholarship fund
         for medical students (one third of whom should be women)
         at the University of Oregon Medical School. Dr. Lovejoy
         was a member of the Portland Board of Health where she

made local headlines by leading a campaign against rats,
the carriers of bubonic plague. She served during World
War I in France with the American Red Cross and was
decorated by five nations for her work.

1116.   "Esther Pohl Lovejoy, M.D." Medical Woman's Journal,
            51:6 (June 1944) 33-34. port.
         Upon the 50th anniversary of Esther Clayson Pohl Lovejoy's
         graduation from the University of Oregon Medical School (in
         1894), the Journal summarizes Dr. Lovejoy's professional
         activities and honors. "She is a dynamic speaker, a fear-
         less and just leader; a writer who makes even poverty, war,
         and desolation romantic; a friend and advisor incomparable
         ...."

1117.   "Eugen Kahn Awardee Selected, Joins Faculty." BCM: In-
            side Baylor Medicine, 6:9 (October 1975) 3.   port.
         Historical background on the Eugen Kahn Award, presented
         by Baylor College of Medicine's psychiatry department for
         scholarship and service as a psychiatry resident, is given,
         along with biographical information on Dr. Virginia David-
         son, who in 1975 became the second woman to receive the
         award since its 1964 inception. Reflecting upon her psy-
         chiatry residency, Dr. Davidson says, "I was allowed to
         struggle and not be done in by it...." Her major interests
         concern drug addictions and the psychiatric problems of
         women.

1118.   "Evelyn Witthoff, M.D." Medical Woman's Journal, 52:7
            (July 1945) 44.
         This article presents a very brief biography of Dr. Witthoff,
         a graduate of the Medical School at the University of Illinois
         (Chicago). In 1941, Dr. Witthoff sailed for India where
         she served as a medical missionary.

1119.   "Exhibit on Medical Women in Oregon." Journal of the
            American Medical Women's Association, 15:4 (April
            1960) 400-401. photos.
         One of the more popular window displays prepared by the
         Committee on Oregon Medical History of the Oregon State
         Medical Association in honor of Oregon's centennial year
         included photographs and memorabilia of Drs. Esther P.
         Lovejoy, Leslie Swigart Kent, Mary Anna Cooke Thompson,
         Bethenia Owens-Adair, and Jessie Laird Brodie. Each of
         these women's major contribution is given a sentence in
         this brief article.

1120.   "F. Muriel Ramsey, M.D." Medical Woman's Journal, 52:
            3 (March 1945) 50.
         Dr. Ramsey (whose portrait appears on the front cover of
         this issue of the Journal) wrote a novel entitled Evergreen,
         a characterization of a woman physician. Her professional
         activities and affiliations are given in this article.

1121.   Fabricant, Noah D., ed. <u>Why We Became Doctors</u>. Grune
             & Stratton, New York, New York, 1954, x, 182 pp.
         This collection of 50 autobiographical sketches, two to three
         pages each, describes each subject's reasons for entering
         medicine. Seven of the subjects are women, and all the in-
         formation was drawn from their published autobiographies
         (listed in the bibliography). Rosalie Slaughter Morton, daugh-
         ter of a Virginia gentleman, chose medicine as an opportun-
         ity to lead a useful life; family opposition strengthened rath-
         er than diminished that ambition. Elizabeth Blackwell first
         considered a medical career upon the suggestion of a ter-
         minally ill woman friend. She overcame her distaste for
         biology and physiology, and resisted the constraints of mar-
         riage; her determination to become a physician became a
         moral crusade for her. Emily Dunning Barringer cited the
         birth of her brother when she was eight years old as the
         childhood incident which instilled in her a desire to help
         the sick and suffering. The difficult birth had brought skilled
         obstetricians into the Dunning home and commanded the as-
         sistance of the youngster to fetch medical supplies. Anne
         Walter Fearn was attracted to medicine by an unknown wo-
         man physician's conversation which she overheard on a train
         trip to San Francisco. A family friend arranged for her to
         meet several women doctors in San Francisco who served as
         models and inspired her to select medicine as an alternative
         to the life of a social butterfly. Josephine Baker, who head-
         ed the New York City Health Department for more than 25
         years, cited her interest in medicine as possibly stemming
         from treatment for an orthopedic injury in childhood. Fam-
         ily opposition stiffened her will to pursue a medical educa-
         tion and career. Alice Hamilton and her sister were forced
         to consider self-supporting careers due to dwindling family
         finances. She selected medicine because it offered freedom
         from work in any given institution such as a school and
         would not require working under superiors. Alfreda Withing-
         ton had lost her family and a brother to consumption before
         a second brother became stricken. She accompanied him on
         his treatment in the Adirondack Mountains; his death instilled
         in her the need to follow a medical career.

1122.   Fairbanks, Virgil F. "Doctor Ashby of Virginia: An Ad-
             miring Profile." <u>The Mayo Alumnus</u>, 11:2 (April 1975)
             28-33. facsims., port.
         The oldest living graduate of the Mayo Graduate School of
         Medicine, Dr. Winifred Mayer Ashby celebrated her 95th
         birthday in October of 1974. A biographical sketch of Dr.
         Ashby is presented.

1123.   "Fanny C. Hutchins, M.D." <u>Medical Woman's Journal</u>, 51:
             7 (July 1944) 38. (In Memory.)
         This obituary notice mentions the professional and social
         activities of Dr. Fanny Collins Hutchins, a Cleveland, Ohio
         practitioner.

1124.   Fearn, Anne Walter. My Days of Strength: An American
             Woman Doctor's Forty Years in China. Harper &
             Brothers, New York, New York, 1939, vii, 297 pp.
             photos. , ports.
         In her autobiography, Anne Walter Fearn gives details of
         her early life in Louisiana and education at Woman's Med-
         ical College of Pennsylvania, from which she graduated in
         1893. After graduation she went to a mission hospital in
         Soochow, China; she tells of her experiences in a country
         where surgery was almost unknown, where male doctors
         never took obstetrical cases, and where cholera patients
         chewed copper coins as a cure. In 1895 she found the
         Soochow Hospital Medical College. Later in Shanghai she
         founded her own hospital, the Fearn Sanatorium. She tells
         of her experiences during the fall of the Manchu Dynasty in
         1911 and gives many examples of Chinese customs and med-
         ical practices.

1125.   "Fifty Year Club: Sara Craig Buckley, M.D." Medical Wo-
             man's Journal, 49:10 (October 1942) 317-318.
         This article reviews the developments in medicine during
         Sara Craig Buckley's lifetime. Before she began practicing
         in Chicago, she married Edmund Buckley and together they
         went to Europe to study and visit hospitals. In 1886 they
         went to Kyoto, Japan, where Dr. Buckley was an assistant
         in a hospital for seven years. Her two sisters, Anna Craig
         and Marion Craig-Potter, became physicians as well.

1126.   "Fifty Years in Practice Club." Medical Woman's Journal,
             49:7 (July 1942) 220-221.
         This article recognizes the fifty-year medical career of
         Jane Robbins. In reminiscing about her medical student
         days, Dr. Robbins mentions that she was one of the pioneers
         in helping to establish the first social club for school girls.

1127.   Figueredo, Anita V. "Antoinette Le Marquis, M.D." Jour-
             nal of the American Medical Women's Association, 14:
             6 (June 1959) 530-531. port. (Album of Women in
             Medicine.)
         "Dr. Le Marquis exemplifies those characteristics that
         make for greater acceptance and recognition of women phy-
         sicians by male colleagues." She is "a dainty, very fem-
         inine, soft-spoken woman." Her chief interest lies in the
         area of diseases of women and children.

1128.   "First Woman Army Doctor in Africa." Medical Woman's
             Journal, 51:3 (March 1944) 33. (Section on War Ser-
             vice.)
         Dr. Margaret M. Janeway's educational background and mili-
         tary service record are noted.

1129.   "First Woman Commissioned Officer in the Medical Corps,
             U.S. Army." Medical Woman's Journal, 50:6 (June

1943) 140-141. port.
This article presents biographical data on Dr. Margaret D.
Craighill upon her commission as the first woman officer
in the U.S. Army Medical Corps (rank of major). She
comes to this commission from her deanship at the Woman's
Medical College of Pennsylvania.

1130. "The First Woman Coroner Elected in United States. Dr.
Grace M. Norris, of Utica, N.Y., Has the Distinction
of Being the First Woman Physician Elected to the
Office of Coroner." Woman's Medical Journal, 29[19]:
12 (December 1919) 256.

1131. "The First Woman Physician Among Her People." Medical
Missionary Record, 4:6 (October 1889) 126.
Susan LaFlesche, a graduate of Woman's Medical College in
Philadelphia and an Omaha Indian, returns to her people
armed with scientific medicine and Christianity.

1132. "First Woman Surgeon in U.S. Public Health Service." Medical Woman's Journal, 39:9 (September 1932) 229.
Estelle Ford Warner was the first woman to be appointed a
surgeon "on the same basis as other surgeons in the United
States Public Health Service...."

1133. "Firsts." Medical Woman's Journal, 52:1 (January 1945)
56-57. (News Notes.)
Among the "firsts" of various women physicians whose names
are given in this article are Dr. Sue H. Thompson, the first
woman county health commissioner in New York State, and
Dr. Allen Daisy Emery, the first woman medical graduate
in Texas.

1134. Fleming, Alice. Doctors in Petticoats. J. B. Lippincott
Company, Philadelphia, Pennsylvania, 1964, 159 pp.
This collection of biographical sketches outlines the accomplishments of ten distinguished women physicians of the 19th
and 20th centuries. Marie Zakrzewska emigrated to this
country from Germany in 1853, determined to become a doctor. With the help of Elizabeth Blackwell she attained her
goal, founded a hospital in Boston, and became a pioneer
in the cause of assisting women bent on careers in medicine.
Mary Putnam Jacobi worked with Zakrzewska at the New
England Hospital for Women and Children and ultimately devoted her life to teaching and research. Emily Dunning
Barringer, encouraged by Jacobi, graduated from Cornell
Medical College and became, in 1902, the first woman to
intern at Gouverneur Hospital in New York City. Clara
Swain pioneered in medical mission work in India around the
turn of the century and built a hospital at Bareilly. Alice
Hamilton became a pathologist, worked with Jane Addams at
Hull House, and made significant contributions to the study
of occupational diseases. Another pathologist, Louise Pearce,

became a fellow at the Rockefeller Institute in 1913 and
helped to develop a new drug, tryparsamide, for the treatment of African sleeping sickness. Sara Jordon distinguished herself in the field of gastroenterology at the Lahey
Clinic in Boston, beginning in 1923, and became known as
the patron saint of ulcer victims. Karen Horney, who died
in 1952, is best known for her work in psychoanalysis, developing new concepts of neuroses and rejecting Freud's
pessimistic view of human nature. Leona Baumgartner was,
in the 1950s, New York's first woman commissioner of
health and as such had to worry about the health and welfare of approximately eight million people. Connie Meyers
Guion, as one of the most respected faculty members of
Cornell Medical College until her retirement in 1952, was
the first woman in America to have a hospital building
named after her--a five-story building which houses most
of New York Hospital's 86 different clinics.

1135.   Fletcher, Grace Nies. The Fabulous Flemings of Kathman-
         du: The Story of Two Doctors in Nepal. E. P. Dutton
         & Co., Inc., New York, New York, 1964, 219 pp.
         map, photos.
This joint biography of Dr. Bethel Fleming and her husband
describes her efforts as a medical missionary in India and
Nepal, where she set up a medical clinic in Kathmandu.   In
1956 she founded Shanta Bhawan, the first comprehensive
hospital in Nepal.   The book gives many details of social
and medical conditions in India and Nepal and recounts Dr.
Fleming's recruitment of Dr. Elizabeth Miller to serve in
Shanta Bhawan.   The book is based upon the author's interviews with Drs. Fleming and Miller in Nepal.   There is no
index or bibliography.

1136.   "Florence R. Sabin Honored for Statecraft, Education, Sci-
         ence." Rockefeller Institute Quarterly, 3:1 (1954) 3.
         photo.
The statue of Florence Sabin (by Joy Buba of New York)
was placed in Statuary Hall in Washington, D.C.

1137.   "Florence R. Sabin, M.D." British Medical Journal, 2:
         4843 (31 October 1953) 997-998. (Obituary.)
This brief obituary notice for Dr. Florence R. Sabin mentions her professional "firsts" and quotes Simon Flexner,
who referred to her as "'the greatest living woman scientist
and one of the foremost scientists of all time.'"

1138.   "Florence Rena Sabin, M.D., New York City." Medical
         Woman's Journal, 37:1 (January 1930) 1-2. port.
         (Special Article.)
In response to Florence Sabin's receiving the annual Pictorial Review Achievement Award in 1928, this biographical
sketch was written.   Florence Sabin was the first scientist
to make a complete study of the development of the lym-

phatic system; to discover the development and processes of the blood-cell; and to discover the functions
of the monocyte. As a woman she earned a great many
firsts in medicine: the first woman to be admitted to and
graduated from Johns Hopkins Medical University; the first
to be admitted as an intern and also as teaching faculty
there; the first woman to be admitted to European research
laboratories; and the first woman to be made a member of
the U.S. National Academy of Science. Dr. Sabin was also
the first woman to become a member of the Rockefeller Institute for Medical Research.

1139.   Floyd, Olive. Doctora in Mexico: The Life of Dr. Kather-
         ine Neel Dale. G. P. Putnam's Sons, New York, New
         York, 1944, 270 pp.
         After Dr. Katherine Neel Dale graduated from the Woman's
         Medical College of Pennsylvania in 1897, and completed her
         internship, she accepted her first appointment as medical
         missionary in the little Mexican city of Ciudad del Maiz.
         This biography of her life tells how she and her minister
         husband served the Mexican people for over forty years--
         part of that time in Rio Verde, where she built up an ex-
         tended practice and eventually organized a hospital. After
         a temporary exile during the revolution, the Dales were back
         in Mexico in 1919, spending ten years in Tampico, where in
         one year the Doctora treated 18,500 patients. Eventually
         new government decrees hampered their work there. After
         a period of planning and vacationing in their native South
         Carolina, the Dales went on to found the Mexican Indian
         Mission, including a school for Indian girls and a school for
         Indian boys, at Tamazunchale. Into this project she poured
         her energy until her death in 1941 at age 68. The schools
         continued to thrive.

1140.   "For Black Women: Medicine Is Opportunity, Challenge."
         BCM: Inside Baylor Medicine, 11:8 (August 1971) 2.
         "I know I have two blows against me--being a woman, and
         being black.... I am proud of what I am and will not wor-
         ry about what problems I have to face because if I do I will
         defeat my cause," says Thelissa Harris. She and Judith
         Craven, the first two black women to enroll in Baylor's
         medical school, briefly discuss their reasons for choosing
         medicine as a career, and the problems of successfully
         combining the roles of wife, mother, and physician. After
         completing medical training, both women plan to serve the
         black community.

1141.   Foulks, Sara E. "Sara Foulks, M.D." Medical Woman's
         Journal, 51:5 (May 1944) 36-37, 41.
         Sara E. Foulks (whose portrait appears on the front cover of
         this issue of the Journal) relates events and accomplishments
         of her life as well as her philosophy of life. A graduate of
         the Woman's Medical College of Pennsylvania, Dr. Foulks

was serving in the New York State Department of Health
when she wrote this brief autobiography.

1142.   Fox, Christie. "Dr. McCoy Gets High Navy Rank." Med-
            ical Woman's Journal, 51:3 (March 1944) 33. (Section
            on War Service.)
         A graduate of the University of Pennsylvania Medical School,
         Bernice McCoy received the rank of lieutenant commander
         in the Naval Reserve Medical Corps.

1143.   "Frances C. Van Gasken." Medical Woman's Journal, 46:
            12 (December 1939) 377.
         Dr. Van Gasken graduated from the Woman's Medical Col-
         lege of Pennsylvania in 1890 and later became an instructor
         at that college, specializing in internal medicine. Her por-
         trait appears on the front cover of this issue of the Journal.

1144.   Frye, Maude J. "In Memoriam: Response to Toast." Wo-
            man's Medical Journal, 18:4 (April 1908) 89.
         Dr. Mary Wood-Allen, Electa B. Whipple, and M. Eliza-
         beth Schugens are eulogized in this article.

1145.   Gage, Simon Henry and Gage, Asa Franklin. Mary Gage-
            Day, M.D. A Memorial Tribute: Compiled by Her
            Brothers. The Sun Company, Mohawk, New York, 1935,
            34 pp. port.
         Dr. Gage-Day (born in Worcester, New York in 1857) was
         granted her M.D. degree from the University of Michigan
         in 1888. Her biography is followed by a list of the many
         organizations to which she belonged, as well as a bibliogra-
         phy of her publications. Excerpts from a letter to her fam-
         ily recall an incident near Dodge City, Kansas, where she
         and her husband were working. A reproduction of the fun-
         eral rites, including tributes to Dr. Gage-Day, concludes
         this memorial.

1146.   Gambrell, W. Elizabeth. "Amey Chappell, M.D.: Thirty-
            fifty President of the American Medical Women's Asso-
            ciation." Journal of the American Medical Women's
            Association, 6:9 (September 1951) 356. port.
         Dr. Chappell began practice in 1932 in Atlanta, Georgia,
         facing the dual handicaps of a general financial depression
         and local prejudice. A list of her memberships and achieve-
         ments is included.

1147.   Gardner, Emily. "Projects Sponsored by Medical Women
            [Part I]." Medical Woman's Journal, 40:4 (April 1933)
            96.
         Dr. Gardner tells how she utilized her $1,000 Mary Put-
         nam Jacobi Fellowship of which she was the 1931-32 recip-
         ient. Dr. Gardner tells of her studies and work in London.

1148.   Gardner, Emily. "Projects Sponsored by Medical Women

[Part II]." <u>Medical Woman's Journal</u>, 40:5 (May 1933) 118-119.
Dr. Gardner describes her work in London and her studies in Vienna, which were made possible through the Mary Putnam Jacobi Fund.

1149.   Gardner, Mabel E.   "Bertha Van Hoosen, M. D.:   First President of the American Medical Women's Association." <u>Journal of the American Medical Women's Association,</u> 5:10 (October 1950) 413-414.   photo., port.
The many and various "firsts" of Dr. Van Hoosen are mentioned.   A descriptive biography follows.

1150.   Gardner, Mabel E.   "Helena T. Ratterman, M. D." <u>Journal of the American Medical Women's Association</u>, 9:12 (December 1954) 412.   port.
Dr. Ratterman, a native of Cincinnati, Ohio, instituted and developed prenatal clinics throughout the city.   She was interested in perpetuating opportunities for other women to achieve and served as president of the American Medical Women's Association in 1942-1943.   She also established the Cincinnati Medical Women's Club.

1151.   Gardner, Penney.   "APFME Summer Fellowship."   <u>Buffalo Physician,</u> (Summer 1968) 28-29.   photos.
Dr. Gardner recalls one summer during medical school training which she spent on a General Practice APFME Fellowship.

1152.   Gates, Irene.   <u>Any Hope, Doctor?</u>   Blandford Press, London, England, 1954, 192 pp.
Early chapters of this autobiography describe Irene Gates's training at Woman's Medical College of Pennsylvania from 1923 to 1927, including clinic work in South Philadelphia and her internship at Philadelphia General Hospital, where the women interns were in charge of the nurses' infirmary in addition to their regular work.   She tells of struggles with her conscience during her early practice with a society dermatologist in New York City, which led her to found a settlement clinic on New York's East Side and to work in the Medical Relief Bureau for the "new poor."   The remainder of the book describes her private practice after 1931 in New York, where she was associated with a large clinic [unnamed] in the medical department.   Dr. E. T. C. Milligan of Harley Street, London, wrote a foreword recommending Dr. Gates's philosophy of affectionate concern and help for patients in establishing a sound home life.

1153.   Gay, Claudine Moss.   "Presentation of the Elizabeth Blackwell Annual Award, 1973."   <u>Journal of the American Medical Women's Association</u>, 29:1 (January 1974) 48. photo.
This award was presented to Dr. Alice D. Chenoweth.

1154. Geib, M. Eugenia. "Camille Mermod, M.D." <u>Journal of</u>
      <u>the American Medical Women's Association,</u> 9:9 (Sep-
      tember 1954) 298. port. (Album of Women in Medi-
      cine.)
      A brief, descriptive account of Dr. Mermod's life, which
      highlights her medical experiences in various parts of the
      country.

1155. German, William J. "Louise Eisenhardt: 1891-1967."
      <u>Transactions of the American Neurological Association,</u>
      92 (1967) 311-313. (Obituary.)
      Dr. Eisenhardt's career in neurosurgery and neuropathology
      as a researcher, teacher, and writer was heavily influenced
      by and entwined with the career of Harvey Cushing. Before
      graduating with honors in 1925 from Tufts Medical School,
      Louise Eisenhardt played an active role in completing Dr.
      Cushing's book, <u>Tumor of the Nervous Acusticus.</u> Later,
      as neuropathologist to Dr. Cushing, she coauthored other
      works. In Boston, Dr. Eisenhardt supervised the assembly
      of the Brain Tumor Registry and pursued "a never-ending
      follow-up study of Dr. Cushing's patients." For many
      years she served as an editor for the <u>Journal of Neuro-</u>
      <u>surgery.</u>

1156. "Gertrude Seabolt, M.D." <u>Medical Woman's Journal,</u> 50:
      4 (April 1943) 101.
      Dr. Gertrude Seabolt (whose portrait appears on the front
      cover of this issue of the <u>Journal)</u> devoted many years of
      her practice to the problems of student health. This arti-
      cle gives a brief biography, as well as a listing of Dr.
      Seabolt's professional affiliations.

1157. Gibson, Julia R. <u>A Cry from India's Night.</u> Publishing
      House of the Pentecostal Church of the Nazarene, Kan-
      sas City, Missouri, 1914, 216 pp. photos., port.
      The purpose of this book is to bring the readers "into liv-
      ing contact with the people [of India]" through Dr. Gibson's
      own personal experiences. [Dr. Gibson was a 1915 graduate
      of the Woman's Medical College of Pennsylvania.] Chapters
      in the book discuss Hindu customs, the caste system, the
      condition of women, and other aspects of life in India. The
      book contains no index.

1158. Gillie, Annis. "Elizabeth Blackwell and the 'Medical Reg-
      ister' From 1858." <u>British Medical Journal,</u> 2 (22
      November 1958) 1253-1257. photo., ports. (Presiden-
      tial Address, Metropolitan Counties Branch, British
      Medical Association, 1958.)
      This article discusses Elizabeth Blackwell's family, her
      "urge towards medicine," her graduation from Geneva Col-
      lege in 1849, her welcome in London in 1850, and her
      work in America. Dr. Blackwell achieved the distinction
      of having her name appear on the first Medical Register

(published in 1858). A portion of the article tells of conditions for medical women in Great Britain and the "courageous group" of women physicians in London, headed by Sophia Jex-Blake. Concluding this article is a look at the issue of registration of women physicians in England in the 19th century.

1159.   Glasgow, Maude. "Maude Glasgow: Donor of the Janet M. Glasgow Scholarship Fund." Women in Medicine, 74 (October 1941) 10-12. ports.
An autobiographical account by Dr. Glasgow who, coming to New York from Northern Ireland, entered nurses training. After nursing for a short time, she decided to pursue a medical career. This article, a personal account of certain aspects of that career, ends with a listing of the author's medical articles which have been published "from time to time."

1160.   Glasgow, Maude. "Maude Glasgow, M.D. (An Autobiography)." Medical Woman's Journal, 51:3 (March 1944) 34-36.
Dr. Glasgow (whose portrait appears on the front cover of this month's Journal) describes the events leading up to her graduation from medical school in 1901, her subsequent professional appointments, and her personal health problems. Recalling her activities as a suffragette, she concludes this autobiography with the warning that "enfranchisement was but a step toward equality...." A bibliography of Dr. Glasgow's published works is included in the article.

1161.   Goldowsky, Seebert J. "Rhode Island's First Woman Physician." Rhode Island Medical Journal, 54 (November 1971) 546-549. port.
Biographical information is given on Dr. Martha Mowry, who practiced in Providence, Rhode Island for over 40 years. A note on Julia A. Beverly, probably the second woman physician to practice in Rhode Island, concludes the article.

1162.   Goodcell, Roscoe. "Marie Antoinette Bennette, M.D." Medical Woman's Journal, 54:10 (October 1947) 48-50.
This article presents an anecdotal biography of Dr. Bennette, a San Bernardino, California physician. The author is Dr. Bennette's nephew.

1163.   Goodwin, Occa Elaine. "Pearl Smith, M.D." Journal of the American Medical Women's Association, 9:5 (May 1954) 171. port. (Album of Women in Medicine.)
Dr. Smith was, at the time of this article, attending pathologist at the San Francisco Children's Hospital.

1164.   Gordon, Elizabeth Putnam. The Story of the Life and Work of Cordelia A. Greene M.D. The Castilian, Castile, New York, 1925, 208 pp. photos., ports.

The opening chapters of this memoir of Cordelia Greene
(1831-1905) describe her early life as a Quaker in upstate
New York, the beginnings of her career as a schoolteacher,
her conversion to Methodism, and her training at Woman's
Medical College of Pennsylvania in the 1850s. Dr. Greene
founded Castile Sanatarium, Castile, New York for the treatment of women patients. Assisting her were Drs. Clara
Swain, Caroline Stevens, Mary I. Slade, Jessica W. Findlay, and her niece Dr. Mary T. Greene. Later chapters
include accounts of her by her children and patients; excerpts from her letters; quotations and homilies expressing
her religious outlook; testimonials from friends including
Frances Willard, the Reverend Anna Ward Shaw, and Dr.
Marie Zakrzewska; and excerpts from her diaries during
trips through the Panama Canal and to Hawaii. Concluding
chapters deal with the founding of the Cordelia Greene Library, the life of Dr. Mary T. Greene, testimonials to
Mary Greene, and an account of social activities at the sanatarium and at the founder's day celebration in 1925. Several portraits appear throughout the book. There is no index.

1165.   Gosswiller, Richard. "A Girl Becomes a Doctor." Today's
          Health, 47:6 (June 1969) 29-33. photos.
          This article gives a view of one "girl" who is becoming a
          doctor. Dale King Phelps is the article's central subject,
          and the author tells us that "no one would mistake attractive
          Dale King Phelps for one of the guys [as] her eyes are
          large, her smile winning, her figure indisputable." Ms.
          Phelps's reasons for entering medical school are given
          along with her experience of applying for admission.

1166.   "Grace E. Rochford, M.D." Journal of the American Med-
          ical Women's Association, 5:12 (December 1950) 500.
          port. (Album of Women in Medicine.)
          A surgeon, Grace E. Rochford received her degree in 1906.
          In 1919 she was appointed to the surgical staff of the New
          England Hospital for Women and Children; in 1944 surgeon-
          in-chief; and in 1950 consulting surgeon.

1167.   "Grace N. Kimball, M.D." Medical Woman's Journal, 49:
          12 (December 1942) 391-392.
          In 1882 Grace N. Kimball went to Van (a city of Armenia
          in Turkey), sponsored by the American Board of Foreign
          Missions. Because she found that the greatest demands
          made upon her came from the sick, she realized she needed
          training in medicine and so returned to the United States
          where she was graduated from the Women's Medical Col-
          lege of the New York Infirmary. Returning to Van, Dr.
          Kimball initiated and developed the Industrial Relief organ-
          ization which distributed food and clothing throughout the en-
          tire province of Van. When Dr. Kimball returned to the
          U.S., she settled in Poughkeepsie, New York, where she

was active in providing hospital care for tubercular persons. She also helped found Bowne Memorial Hospital.

1168.   Grad, Marjorie A. "Cincinnati Women Physicians." The Woman Physician, 25:11 (November 1970) 735-736.
Names and experiences of a selection of Cincinnati women physicians are presented.

1169.   "Great Names in Chicago Medicine: Frances Dickinson." Chicago Medicine, 64 (10 March 1962) 24.
[Article not examined by editors.]

1170.   Gridley, Marion. Medical Woman's Journal, 56:2 (February 1949) 55. (News Notes.)
A brief biography is given of Lucille Johnson-Marsh, who is "three quarter Indian" and practices pediatrics in Miami, Florida.

1171.   Griscom, Mary W. "Pioneer Medical Women: A Few Interesting Biographical Sketches." Medical Woman's Journal, 38:7 (July 1931) 183-185. port.
Upon learning that she had cancer, Emeline Cleveland persuaded Anna E. Broomall to specialize in obstetrics and succeed her as professor of obstetrics at Woman's Medical College (Philadelphia). An 1871 graduate of Woman's Medical, Dr. Broomall studied midwifery in Germany "at a time when among the usual requirements for entrance were that the applicant should herself have had a baby." At Woman's Hospital in Philadelphia, she pioneered in abdominal surgery; hospital managers "stipulated that one of the men consultants should always be present" during her operations, but that requirement was later abandoned. Throughout her distinguished career as physician, teacher, and administrator, Dr. Broomall "never refused a case because it might not mean money; never failed to see possible advancement of other women; used every influence to open all possible avenues of new work for the [women medical] graduates."

1172.   Griscom, Mary W. "Surgery in the Wilderness." Atlantic Monthly, 137 (May 1926) 668-670.
Dr. Griscom tells anecdotes of her work in Chinese villages: the threat of tigers and robbers, the lack of adequate medical supplies, the patients' fear of "Western" medicine, and the problem of not knowing the Chinese language.

1173.   "Gullattee Trustee of Wesleyan University." Journal of the National Medical Association, 62:1 (January 1970) 77-78. port. (Briefs.)
A biography of Dr. Alyce McLendon Chenault Gullattee is given on this occasion of her election to the board of trustees of Wesleyan University (Middletown, Connecticut)--the first black woman to be so appointed.

1174.   Haffner, V. B.   "A Half-century in the Life of a Woman
            Physician." Nebraska Medical Journal, 60:6 (June 1975)
            197-199.
        This autobiographical article begins with Dr. Haffner's fam-
        ily and educational background. In 1925 Dr. Haffner re-
        ceived her M. D. degree from Boston University School of
        Medicine. She served her internship in Allentown, Pennsyl-
        vania, where she eventually set up a general practice. "I
        immediately confronted discrimination and prejudice due to
        my sex." Dr. Haffner encountered hostility from her col-
        leagues and from the townspeople in this community, and
        her practice was slow in starting. "Gradually, however,
        the Pennsylvania Dutch husbands gave their wives permission
        to see me professionally as they didn't like the idea of a
        man doctor examining their women." Dr. Haffner proceeds
        to discuss some of her patients and the fees she charged
        them.

1175.   Hall, Alice K.   "Beulah Cushman, M. D." Journal of the
            American Medical Women's Association, 7:3 (March
            1952) 109. port. (Album of Women in Medicine.)
        Dr. Cushman, an ophthalmologist, has practiced in Mil-
        waukee, Tacoma, Washington, and Chicago. She was grad-
        uated from the University of Illinois College of Medicine in
        1916.

1176.   Hamilton, A.   "Mollie Turpin Became an M. D. to Help the
            Poor; Project Concern." Good Housekeeping, 174
            (April 1972) 66+. illus.
        [Article not examined by editors.]

1177.   Hamilton, Alice.   Exploring the Dangerous Trades: The
            Autobiography of Alice Hamilton, M. D.   Little, Brown
            and Company, Boston, Massachusetts, 1943, 433 pp.
            illus.
        The autobiography of Alice Hamilton, the pioneer of indus-
        trial medicine in the U. S., concentrates on the years from
        1910 to 1942. Following graduation from the University of
        Michigan Medical School, study and research in Munich and
        at the Johns Hopkins University, Dr. Hamilton became a
        resident of Hull House in Chicago (in 1889). There she was
        introduced to the labor movement and to the problem of in-
        dustrial diseases. In 1910 the governor of Illinois appointed
        her to the Occupational Disease Commission; this Commis-
        sion was to survey the extent of industrial illness in the
        state. In 1912 she undertook a federal study of lead poison-
        ing. She remained in government service to study the muni-
        tions industry during the first world war. In 1918 Dr. Ham-
        ilton joined the Harvard faculty as an assistant professor of
        industrial medicine. In 1924 Dr. Hamilton accepted an invi-
        tation from the Soviet Union to review the state of industrial
        medicine there, and in the same year she was appointed to
        the Health Commission of the League of Nations. The story

of her research and medical work is interwoven with that of
her role as observer and participant in the social, political,
and international events that marked the first 40 years of
the 20th century.   This autobiography includes an index,
helpful in identifying significant persons and events in her
field.

1178.   Hanaford, Phebe A.   Daughters of America; or, Women of
            the Century.   True and Company, Augusta, Maine, 1882,
            730 pp.   illus., ports.
         Included in this book is a 24-page chapter which discusses
         many women physicians of 19th-century America.

1179.   "Hannah E. Longshore, M.D."   Woman's Medical Journal,
            11:12 (December 1901) 427-428.   (Biographical.)

1180.   Hano, Helene.   "Red and Black Star: Under the Quaker
            Emblem Medical Women Find New Areas of Service."
            Medical Woman's Journal, 56:7 (July 1949) 31-35.
         Three women physicians associated with the Society of
         Friends are profiled: Shirley Gage, who had charge of the
         Quaker hospital in Chungmou (Honan Province), China;
         Margaret Dann, who acted as medical officer for several
         refugee camps in postwar Europe; and Virginia Alexander,
         one of the five black woman doctors in Philadelphia.

1181.   Hansen, O. S.   "The Girl Who Didn't Go to China."   Jour-
            nal-Lancet (Minneapolis), 83 (February 1963) 69-70.
         H. Hartig is the subject of this article.   [Article not ex-
         amined by editors.]

1182.   Harper, Anita Wilson.   "Twenty-Five Years at St. Eliza-
            beth's."   Medical Woman's Journal, 37:10 (October
            1930) 288.
         Mary O'Malley's 25 years as director of the Women's Ser-
         vice in St. Elizabeth's Hospital was marked by a celebra-
         tion held on 2 September 1930.   Under her leadership,
         nearly 100 women physicians received psychiatric training.
         Dr. O'Malley's extensive bibliography includes studies of
         psychoses caused by such exogenous toxemias as carbon
         monoxide poisoning, and bromism.   In her remarks before
         the gathering, Dr. O'Malley said that the women doctors
         who had left St. Elizabeth's had all received the same pay
         that men had received for the same work.

1183.   "Harriet Carswell McIntosh."   Medical Woman's Journal,
            46:11 (November 1939) 348.
         A listing of Dr. McIntosh's training, appointments, member-
         ships, and published articles is given.   (A portrait of this
         1918 graduate of Woman's Medical College of Pennsylvania
         appears on the front cover of this issue of the Journal.)

1184.   "Harriet E. Garrison, M.D., Dixon, Ill."   Woman's Med-

ical Journal, 5:4 (April 1896) 105-106. (Women Physicians and Surgeons.)

1185.   "Harriet Kizia [sic] Hunt." Woman's Medical Journal, 10:
        5 (May 1900) 202-205. (Biographical.)

1186.   Hawkins, Lucy Rodgers. "North Shore Personalities."
        Wilmette Life, (13 October 1938) 28-29. port.
        Mary G. Schroeder bore seven children. "The seventh ir-
        ritated my husband ... I could not cope with his attitude
        and the small ones," she says, recalling the events that led
        to her nervous breakdown, her stay in two sanitariums, and
        her husband's decision "to rear the children himself and dis-
        pense with the companionship of his wife." Mrs. Schroeder
        went on to "turn her heartbreak into professional channels."
        She obtained a medical degree from Rush Medical College
        and studied under Carl G. Jung in Switzerland. A psychia-
        trist, Dr. Schroeder ran her own sanitarium and is now a
        consultant at Elgin Hospital and a faculty member of Rush.

1187.   Hay-Cooper, L. Life of Josephine Butler. Macmillan
        Company, New York, New York, 1922.
        [Book not examined by editors.]

1188.   Hays, Elinor Rice. Those Extraordinary Blackwells: The
        Story of a Journey to a Better World. Harcourt, Brace
        & World, Inc., New York, New York, 1967, 349 pp.
        photos., ports.
        Excerpts from the Blackwell family papers, including let-
        ters and daily journals, supply much of the detail for this
        account of Hannah and Samuel Blackwell and their 13 chil-
        dren--nine of whom lived to maturity. The professional and
        personal lives of Drs. Emily and Elizabeth Blackwell are
        recounted. They, along with their sisters-in-law Lucy Stone
        (an out-spoken feminist) and Antoinette Brown (the first or-
        dained woman minister), are profiled as rebellious "new wo-
        men." The gains these women made and the price they paid
        for being innovators provide the focus of this group biogra-
        phy. An extensive bibliography lists manuscripts and special
        collections as well as periodicals and books. A thorough in-
        dex concludes the work.

1189.   Hazzard, Florence Woolsey. "Bertha Selmon, M.D. (1877-
        1949)." Medical Woman's Journal, 56:8 (August 1949)
        47-52.
        The author reminisces about working with Bertha Selmon on
        the Medical Woman's Journal. The major portion of the
        article, however, gives anecdotes of Dr. Selmon's marital
        life, her work as a missionary in China, and her book,
        They Do Meet.

1190.   Hazzard, Florence Woolsey. "Eliza Mosher--Dean of Wo-
        men." Michigan Alumnus Quarterly Review, 52:24 (27

July 1946) 358-367. illus.
Dr. Eliza Mosher graduated from the Department of Medicine at the University of Michigan. In 1896 she became dean of women at the University. This article covers Dr. Mosher's accomplishments (and trials) in that position and her eventual decision to resign in favor of returning to the practice of medicine. In preparation for this return, Dr. Mosher took medical courses at the University.

1191.   Hazzard, Florence Woolsey. "Pioneer Women in Medicine: Spread to the States Prior to 1900." The Medical Woman's Journal, 55:2 (February 1948) 38-43, 68. (History of Women in Medicine.)
A biography is given of Dr. Eliza Mosher, from her childhood through her death in 1928.

1192.   Heggie, Barbara. "Ice Woman." New Yorker, (6 September 1941) 23-26, 29-30. port. (Profiles.)
Dr. Mary Engle Pennington is an authority on matters connected with the refrigeration of perishable food stuffs. She developed techniques used in the storage and distribution of many foods and helped implement the Pure Food and Drug Act by serving as first chief of the Food Research Laboratory established in 1907 by the U.S. Department of Agriculture. Dr. Pennington's present work as well as her professional background are discussed herein.

1193.   "Helena of Dakota: Helena Knauf Wink, M.D.; Jamestown, N.D." Medical Woman's Journal, 37:4 (April 1930) 99-101. illus.
Helena Knauf Wink was a pioneer general practitioner in Jamestown, North Dakota during the days when there were surface wells, poorly built houses, poor ventilation, and no sanitation. Worry over loss of crops, and hardships of every description, resulted in sickness and added to the already heavy burden of the pioneer.

1194.   Hemenway, Ruth. "Dr. Mary E. Carleton." Medical Woman's Journal, 34:2 (February 1927) 41-42.
Mary Eline Carleton graduated from Syracuse University Medical School in 1886 and went to China the following year. There, she built two hospitals: Woolston Memorial Hospital in Foochaw City, and the Nathan Sites Memorial Good Shepherd Hospital in Mintsing. Dr. Carleton encountered many difficulties, including a shortage of medical supplies and the unfamiliarity of the Chinese people with Western medicine and their suspicion of it.

1195.   Henderson-Smathers, Irma. "Catherine C. Carr, M.D." Journal of the American Medical Women's Association, 11:2 (February 1956) 76. port. (Album of Women in Medicine.)
Dr. Carr received her medical degree in 1919 from Johns

Hopkins University. This article lists her many memberships and club affiliations, some of which follow: she
served as secretary of the board of directors, Asheville
Colored Hospital; as secretary of the board of directors of
Asheville Traveler's Aid; and as treasurer of the class of
1914, Bryn Mawr College. Dr. Catherine C. Carr was
also section president of the Asheville Biltmore Needle Work
Guild.

1196.   Henderson-Smathers, Irma. "Medical Women of Illinois."
            Medical Woman's Journal, 59:3 (March 1952) 34-36.
            (History of Women in Medicine.)
         Brief biographies are given for three Illinois women physi-
         cians: Dr. Alice Bunker Stockham, Dr. Sarah Hackett
         Stevenson, and Dr. Sarah Ann Chadwick Clapp.

1197.   Henderson-Smathers, Irma. "Medical Women of Illinois."
            Medical Woman's Journal, 59:4 (April 1952) 39-40.
         Two Illinois women physicians are profiled in this article:
         Dr. Harriet C. Beringer Alexander and Dr. Julia Cole Black-
         man.

1198.   Henderson-Smathers, Irma. "Medical Women of Illinois."
            Medical Woman's Journal, 59:5 (May 1952) 41-42. (His-
            tory of Women in Medicine.)
         Brief biographical sketches are given of Drs. Mary Harris
         Thompson, Lucinda Carr, and Leila Gertrude Bedell.

1199.   Henderson-Smathers, Irma. "Medical Women of North
            Carolina." Medical Woman's Journal, 56:11 (November
            1949) 38-42. photo., ports. (History of Women in
            Medicine.)
         Biographies of four women are presented in this article [the
         second in a series of articles about women physicians of
         North Carolina]. Susan Dimock, who received her medical
         degree in 1863 from the University of Zurich, received an
         honorary membership in the North Carolina State Medical
         Society in 1872. She was head of the New England Hospital
         when, in 1875 at the age of 28, she drowned in a shipwreck.
         Annie Lowrie Alexander, an 1884 graduate of Woman's Med-
         ical College of Pennsylvania, became in 1887 the first wo-
         man to practice medicine in North Carolina. Elma Allen
         Travis graduated from the University of Michigan Medical
         School in 1883 and received her North Carolina medical
         license in 1888. Lucia Redding Thompson's North Carolin-
         ian birthplace was her only association with that state. An
         1891 graduate of Woman's Medical College, Dr. Thompson
         led an unusual life for a woman of her time. A divorcee,
         she put her three children in the care of her sister in order
         to study medicine. While specializing in obstetrics in
         Paris, she got into heavy debt but made a dramatic financial
         recovery while gambling at Monte Carlo. Dr. Thompson re-
         turned to the states and established a practice in Philadel-

phia. She also investigated the bubonic plague in the Far
East, under the auspices of the U.S. government.

1200.   Henderson-Smathers, Irma. "Medical Women of North
            Carolina." Medical Woman's Journal, 56:12 (Decem-
            ber 1949) 36-38. port. (History of Women in Medi-
            cine.)
          In this installment [one in a series of articles on women
          physicians of North Carolina], biographies given include that
          of Anna M. Gove, who was head physician at Woman's Col-
          lege of the University of North Carolina from 1893 until
          1937. Lucy Hughes-Brown, an 1894 graduate of Woman's
          Medical College of Pennsylvania, practiced medicine in both
          North Carolina and South Carolina; at her death in 1911, she
          was said to be the "only colored woman physician in South
          Carolina." Clara Ernull Jones, after becoming mother to
          seven children, studied medicine at the age of 43. An 1894
          graduate of Woman's Medical College of Pennsylvania, Dr.
          Jones served as head of the women's wards at the State
          Hospital for the Negro Insane (Goldsboro) for 26 years.
          Olivia M. Nelson practiced medicine in Asheville, North
          Carolina, but left the city and the practice of medicine and
          "went on the stage as a chorus girl and became one of the
          original Floradora Sextette."

1201.   Henderson-Smathers, Irma. "Medical Women of North Caro-
            lina." Medical Woman's Journal, 57:1 (January 1950)
            43. (History of Women in Medicine.)
          Dr. Lula C. Fleming "(colored)," was appointed a mission-
          ary to Africa by the American Baptist Missionary Union in
          1887, going to Palabala station of the Congo Mission. Ida
          M. Wilson, once superintendent of St. Peter's Hospital in
          Charlotte, North Carolina, was in government service in
          Fayetteville, North Carolina during the influenza epidemic
          of 1918, but probably did most of her practice in Ohio.

1202.   Henderson-Smathers, Irma. "Medical Women of North Caro-
            lina." Medical Woman's Journal, 57:2 (February 1950)
            38-40. port. (History of Women in Medicine.)
          Joy Harris Glascock graduated from Women's Medical Col-
          lege in Baltimore in 1896. After passing her board examina-
          tions with the second highest rating in her class and receiv-
          ing her North Carolina medical license in 1900, Sallie Bor-
          den, another North Carolina woman physician, took care of
          emergency cases at the small emergency hospital in Golds-
          boro. She abandoned the practice of medicine to marry Dr.
          Paul Churchill Hutton. A specialist in ophthalmology,
          Louise Merrimon Perry conducted an eye clinic for Ashe-
          ville's health department from 1942-1946 on a voluntary basis.
          Other community services included work at the Flower Mis-
          sion and the Lindley Home for Fallen Women.

1203.   Henderson-Smathers, Irma. "Medical Women of North Caro-

lina." <u>Medical Woman's Journal,</u> 57:3 (March 1950)
    37-38. (History of Women in Medicine.)
A relative of Tom Dixon, author of <u>The Clansman,</u> Delia
Dixon Carroll was a leader in the movement for the establishment of a home for delinquent women in North Carolina. She is quoted as having said, "If there has ever been
any prejudice to a woman physician in Raleigh or North
Carolina, I have never discovered it." Drs. Lucy C. Jones
and Edith B. Blackwell are also profiled in this article.

1204.   Henderson-Smathers, Irma. "Medical Women of North
            Carolina." <u>Medical Woman's Journal,</u> 57:4 (April 1950)
            37-39. ports. (History of Women in Medicine.)
Having attended many medical lectures with her husband,
Catharine Phoebe Hayden received her own medical degree
after he died in his senior year. May S. Miles's practice
was of a general character, restricted to women and children especially in the fields of school and college health,
athletics, and preventive medicine. Under the sponsorship
of the United Presbyterian Church, Alice Johnson went to
Port Said, Egypt, to do medical work. "Dr. Johnson was
small and slight in stature and when she lived in Asheville,
wore very masculine looking clothes, but after her studies
in psychology in Boston, her style of dress changed considerably to the feminine mode. Never, however, did her
mind or strong personality change."

1205.   Henderson-Smathers, Irma. "Medical Women of North
            Carolina." <u>Medical Woman's Journal,</u> 57:5 (May 1950)
            42-44. port. (History of Women in Medicine.)
Mary Lapham, having assumed her father's given business
and bank after he died, was a successful businesswoman before she became a doctor. In medicine, she was a pioneer
in the therapeutic use of artificial pneumothorax in pulmon-
ary tuberculosis. She did important and interesting work
with specimens of lung tissue and was disappointed that she
had not been able to interest anyone else in carrying forward this line of research. Mary Martin Sloop founded,
with her husband in Crossnore, an extensive educational
facility for mountaineer boys and girls.

1206.   Henderson-Smathers, Irma. "Medical Women of North
            Carolina." <u>Medical Woman's Journal,</u> 57:6 (June 1950)
            35-36. (History of Women in Medicine.)
Eulalie M. Abbott received her North Carolina medical li-
cense in 1904. Lois Boyd Gaw served as a college physi-
cian and anesthetist during her professional medical career.
"Since retiring, she lives at her home, 'Pine Shadows,'
Sanford, North Carolina, as Mrs. Harry Gaw." Helen W.
Bissell received her North Carolina State license in 1908.
After Irene Thornton Nesbitt married in 1914, she moved to
Texas, and after having some babies of her own, specialized
in pediatrics. Before she married, Bess Violet Puett Jones

had a large general practice, particularly among women and
children in her home town of Dallas, North Carolina. After
she married in 1918, she retired from active practice.
"Her husband writes the author that after marriage her medical skill was incidentally used frequently in her service as
pastor's wife in rural North Carolina communities especially during the influenza epidemic and was of great value to
him and to the people of his pastorates."

1207.   Henderson-Smathers, Irma. "Medical Women of North
            Carolina." Medical Woman's Journal, 57:7 (July 1950)
            37. (History of Women in Medicine.)
The North Presbyterian Mission sent Nettie Donaldson to
China, where she first helped to open a new station at Su-
tsierr-Ku and where she met and married the Reverend
Mark B. Grier.

1208.   Henderson-Smathers, Irma. "Medical Women of North
            Carolina." Medical Woman's Journal, 57:8 (August
            1950) 41-42. (History of Women in Medicine.)
Several physicians who practiced medicine in North Carolina
are mentioned.

1209.   Henderson-Smathers, Irma. "Medical Women of North
            Carolina." Medical Woman's Journal, 57:9 (September
            1950) 36. (History of Women in Medicine.)
Netta May Waite, Charlotte Rozelle, and Portia McKnight,
who was the first woman to graduate from the North Carolina Medical College, are among the physicians mentioned
in this article.

1210.   Henderson-Smathers, Irma. "Medical Women of North
            Carolina." Medical Woman's Journal, 57:10 (October
            1950) 30-31. (History of Women in Medicine.)
From 1916 to 1921 Margaret Whiteside served the Presbyterian Mission Board at the Nancy Tribord Hospital at
Montgomery, Punjab, India. After Marianna Parker married, her husband, also a doctor, "often consulted Mrs.
Nicholson in his cases for she was a very outstanding physician."

1211.   Henderson-Smathers, Irma. "Medical Women of North
            Carolina." Medical Woman's Journal, 57:11 (November
            1950) 32, 34. port. (History of Women in Medicine.)
In 1914 Martha Hayward became the first woman to receive
a North Carolina medical license by reciprocity (from Illinois). Margaret Castex Sturgis could not serve in the service during World War I when her husband, also a doctor,
went to serve because the war department rules against
foreign service of any kind for wives of men employed in
this way. Dr. Sturgis became surgical resident in the New
York Hospital, and served on the faculty of the Woman's
Medical College of Pennsylvania. Juanita Lea, who ran a

general practice in Tyron, North Carolina, owned and operated a commercial vineyard.

1212.   Henderson-Smathers, Irma. "Medical Women of North
            Carolina." Medical Woman's Journal, 57:12 (Decem-
            ber 1950) 35-38. port. (History of Women in Medi-
            cine.)
        In 1917, Louise M. Ingersoll, sponsored by the Southern
        Methodist Women's Board of Missions, went to Soochow,
        China. "Playing hospital with my dolls was my childhood
        pre-occupation. I had, by surreptitious means, acquired
        an old-fashioned medical book from which I instructed the
        favorite doll, always in my imagination--a woman physician,
        very charming and attractive, probably a wish fulfillment
        in hopeful anticipation of my own personality.... While I
        was two years old I attended a party and heard a mission-
        ary, just returned from China, tell many interesting things
        of life there. At once, I fell in love with China and finally
        decided that some day I would go there to do something
        splendid for the women and children." After many adven-
        tures and some bouts of ill health, Dr. Ingersoll returned
        to the United States to practice in Asheville until she re-
        tired in 1942.

1213.   Henderson-Smathers, Irma. "Medical Women of North
            Carolina." Medical Woman's Journal, 58:1 (January-
            February 1951) 31-33. ports. (History of Women in
            Medicine.)
        Margery J. Lord served Asheville in several medical ways:
        as physician for the school system, Dr. Lord "made a
        systematic study of remediable medical defects in school
        children causing them to do poor work" and educated the
        parents to rectify their children's defects. Dr. Lord be-
        came public health officer for Asheville in 1941. When
        Connie M. Guion was graduated from Cornell Medical School
        in 1917, she received the Polk prize for being first in her
        class in general eficiency. She is now chief of the General
        Medical Clinic of the outpatient department of New York
        Hospital.

1214.   Henderson-Smathers, Irma. "Medical Women of North
            Carolina." Medical Woman's Journal, 58:2 (March-
            April 1951) 33-35. ports. (History of Women in Med-
            icine.)
        In May 1943 Margaret D. Craighill became the first woman
        commissioned in the Army Medical Corps, receiving the com-
        mission of major, and in August 1945, the promotion to lt.
        colonel. Dr. Craighill's military service included being a
        consultant (1944-46) to the surgeon general for health and
        welfare of women in Washington, and her overseas service
        included visiting all the theaters of war (flying completely
        around the world) inspecting conditions of women in the
        army. She is now chief of service of the Menninger Psy-

chiatric Clinic, in charge of the medical care of women
veterans at the Winter Hospital. Rosa Hirschmann L.
Gantt, an ophthalmologist, was the first woman physician
to practice in Spartanburg, South Carolina. She did pioneer
public health work in South Carolina in antituberculosis, the
medical inspection of schools, and social hygiene.

1215.   Henderson-Smathers, Irma. "Medical Women of North
         Carolina." Medical Woman's Journal, 58:3 (May-June
         1951) 31-32. (History of Women in Medicine.)
         Cora Zetta Corpening was the first woman to take a pre-
         medical course at Mars Mill College, the only woman stu-
         dent in her class at Tulane Medical School and at the Uni-
         versity of North Carolina, the first woman to intern at St.
         Vincent's Hospital in Norfolk, Virginia, and the first wo-
         man to matriculate in the medical school of the University
         of North Carolina. Annie T. Smith, a general practitioner,
         is also profiled in this article.

1216.   Henderson-Smathers, Irma. "Medical Women of North
         Carolina." Medical Woman's Journal, 58:4 (July-Au-
         gust 1951) 27-28. port. (History of Women in Medi-
         cine.)
         Orra Miller Henderson received her medical degree from
         the University of Michigan in 1925 and interned at Los
         Angeles General Hospital. Katherine Baylis MacInnis was
         the first person in South Carolina to be certified by the
         board in allergy and was the first woman to be appointed
         to the board of regents of the American College of Allergy
         (March 1948). Caroline L. Hilborn published and lectured
         on temperance and evangelistic issues. In her last 25
         years, Dr. Hilborn engaged in general practice.

1217.   Henderson-Smathers, Irma. "Medical Women of North
         Carolina." Medical Woman's Journal, 58:5 (September-
         October 1951) 31-32. port. (History of Women in
         Medicine.)
         Blanch Nettleton Epler originated the City Laboratory in
         Kalamazoo, Michigan, and as city bacteriologist established
         milk standards. From 1929 to 1933 Dr. Epler contracted
         with the U.S. Coast Guard through the U.S. Public Health
         Service to practice general medicine for 50 miles off the
         Hatteras Banks Islands of North Carolina. Catherine Cross-
         Gray practiced general medicine in Delaware.

1218.   Henderson-Smathers, Irma. "Medical Women of North
         Carolina." Medical Woman's Journal, 58:6 (November-
         December 1951) 31-32, 34. (History of Women in Med-
         icine.)
         Several woman physicians of North Carolina are profiled in
         this article, including Lula Marjorie Disosway, who was the
         first woman intern at the James Walker Memorial Hospital,
         Wilmington, North Carolina.

1219.   Henderson-Smathers, Irma. "Medical Women of North
               Carolina." Medical Woman's Journal, 59:1 (January
               1952) 38-39. (History of Women in Medicine.)
         Brief biographies are presented of three North Carolina wo-
         men physicians.

1220.   Henderson-Smathers, Irma. "Medical Women of North
               Carolina." Medical Woman's Journal, 59:2 (February
               1952) 27-28. (History of Women in Medicine.)
         Biographies are given of Drs. Maude Stoovall Pressley,
         Elizabeth Hunter Ellis, Mary Cabell Warfield, and Eliza-
         beth R. Vann.

1221.   Hendricks, Anne M. "Memorial to Anna R. Darrow, M.D."
               Journal of the American Medical Women's Association,
               15:1 (January 1960) 75-76. port.
         At the age of twenty, Anna R. Darrow married Charles
         Darrow and "settled down to be a dutiful wife and mother."
         Later they both decided to study medicine together. They
         enrolled in Kirksville School of Osteopathy from which they
         graduated two years later, "she highest in the class and
         her husband second highest." They both entered medical
         school then and graduated in 1909. They then moved to
         Florida and practiced in the area around Lake Okeechobee.
         Dr. Anna R. Darrow immortalized her experience in this
         region in an art painting which won second prize in the 1947
         Mead Johnson contest at the AMA convention.

1222.   "Here Is Your Life: A Tribute to Elisabeth Larsson.
               Friends, Colleagues, Patients Pay Honor to Noted Wo-
               man Doctor." Alumni Journal [Loma Linda University],
               42:3 (May 1971) 8-11. photos.
         This article describes the program held in honor of Dr.
         Larsson upon the occasion of her "semi-retirement." Dr.
         Larsson has been practicing for 35 years at the White
         Memorial Medical Center in Los Angeles, California. Dr.
         Larsson's accomplishments are cited, as are the names of
         those who participated in the program.

1223.   "Hertha Tarrasch, M.D." Medical Woman's Journal, 53:2
               (February 1946) 33.
         Born in Berlin, Germany in 1900, Hertha Tarrasch had an
         operatic career on the European stage before studying medi-
         cine. Now a noted lecturer, researcher, and practicing
         psychiatrist in Philadelphia, Dr. Tarrasch is a 1941 grad-
         uate of the Woman's Medical College of Pennsylvania.

1224.   "High Honor Conferred upon Dr. Josephine Walter in Elec-
               tion as Trustee of New York Infirmary for Women and
               Children." Woman's Medical Journal, 24:7 (July 1914)
               145.

1225.   Hill, Emma Linton. "Early Medical History." Medical

Woman's Journal, 51:7 (July 1944) 25-26, 30.
Dr. Hill, a 1902 graduate of the University of Illinois Medical College, describes her family life and her medical
practice in Oswego, Kansas. (This autobiography is published posthumously; Dr. Hill died in an automobile accident in 1943.)

1226.   Hobson, Sarah M. and Rockhill, Margaret H.   "The Glory
             of Service."   Medical Woman's Journal, 31:7 (July
             1924) 210-211.   port.
Julia Holmes Smith "left her medical course in Boston University unfinished when she came to Chicago with her husband in 1874."   Dr. Smith has been an active contributor
to medical programs and contributed a section in gynecology
to Arndt's System of Medicine.   She was the first woman
appointed to fill an unexpired term as trustee of the University of Illinois in the 1880s.   Eliza M. Mosher was appointed resident physician of the Massachusetts Reformatory
Prison by the governor of that state, who stated that she
was the only woman he was willing to appoint and considered
that if a man were to be put in the position, it would set
the cause of women in the state of Massachusetts back 20
years.

1227.   Hollingshead, Frances.   "Ohio Women in Medicine--a Bio-
             graphical Note."   Ohio Medical Journal, 41 (1945) 829-
             831.
[Article not examined by editors.]

1228.   "Honor Conferred upon an American Medical Woman."   Wo-
             man's Medical Journal, 22:9 (September 1912) 209.
Dr. Harriet C. B. Alexander of Chicago was unanimously
elected an associate foreign member of the French Society
of Medico-Psychiatry.   The Society's report, which describes Dr. Alexander's professional activities and published
papers, calls her "an equal and original talent."

1229.   "An Honor Worthily Bestowed."   Woman's Medical Journal,
             26:3 (March 1916) 69-70.
The mayor of Chicago appointed Bertha Van Hoosen to the
staff of the Municipal Tuberculosis Sanatorium.   Such appointments of women to the staffs of city, county, and state
hospitals are rare.   A copy of the letter of appointment is
reproduced.

1230.   "Honorary Quotarian Wins Lasker Award for 'Inspiring Ap-
             plication of Preventive Medicine to Cancer Control.'"
             The Quotarian, 29:6 (December 1951) 6.   port.
One of the three 1951 Lasker awards presented by the American Public Health Association went to Catharine Macfarlane,
known as "Kitty Mac" among her friends at Woman's Medical College of Pennsylvania.

1231.   "Honored for Health Work." Medical Woman's Journal, 38:
        7 (July 1931) 179.
        Olga Stastny was named Noguchi medalist of 1931 by the
        Nebraska State Medical Association.

1232.   "Honors for Dr. Daisy Robinson, of New York." Woman's
             Medical Journal, 28:7 (July 1918) 168. port.
        This article is written upon the occasion of Dr. Daisy M.
        Orleman Robinson's receipt of the Medal of Honor (gold
        medal for epidemics) from the minister of war of France.
        A brief biographical sketch of Dr. Robinson follows this
        announcement.

1233.   "Honors to a Distinguished Woman." Medical Woman's
             Journal, 39:2 (February 1932) 42-43. port.
        One of comparatively few women surgeons holding member-
        ship in the American College of Surgeons, Bertha Van Hoo-
        sen is the only medical woman holding a full professorship
        in an obstetrical department of a coeducational university.

1234.   Hoover, Nancy. "Dr. Anna Easton Lake: First Lady Phy-
             sician Appointed to the White House." Journal of the
             American Medical Women's Association, 17:11 (Novem-
             ber 1962) 906-907.
        The story of Dr. Anna Easton Lake, born in 1849, has been
        passed down by her family in the oral tradition. Dr. Lake's
        in-laws greatly disapproved of her profession and referred to
        her as "'that Damned Yankee that married Albert.'" She
        and her husband lived on fashionable Charles Street in Balti-
        more where, ignoring social protocol, she turned the ground
        floor of their home into a free dispensary where she treated
        handicapped children. Her husband eventually quit the fam-
        ily firm and devoted his time to making orthopedic appli-
        ances for his wife's use in her work. Through Dr. Mary
        Walker, Anna Easton Lake received the presidential appoint-
        ment to attend President Grover Cleveland's daughter, a
        victim of cerebral palsy.

1235.   Hoskins, Mrs. Robert. Clara A. Swain, M.D. First Med-
             ical Missionary to the Women of the Orient. Woman's
             Foreign Missionary Society, Methodist Episcopal Church,
             Boston, Massachusetts, 1912, 31 pp. photos., ports.
        Clara Swain, first woman medical missionary in India, was
        graduated from the Woman's Medical College of Pennsylvania
        in 1869 at the age of 35. She had previously taught school
        and worked in the Castile Sanitarium in New York. She
        accepted a call to the mission of Methodist Episcopal Church
        in Bareilly, India, in 1870. There she trained Indian wo-
        men in medicine and opened the first women's hospital in
        India (1874). In 1885 Dr. Swain went to Khetri, India, to
        attend to the wife of the Rajah. She remained in service
        there until 1895, with the exception of a furlough to the U.S.
        in 1888-89. Dr. Swain left India in 1896 but returned for

an 18-month visit in 1906 to celebrate the 50-year jubilee
of the Methodist Mission.   She returned to rest in the Castile Sanitarium and died in Castile in 1910.

1236.   "The Housewife as Surgeon."   Jefferson Medical College:
          Alumni Bulletin, 24:1 (Fall 1974) 18.   port.
          The only female surgical resident at Jefferson, Virginia
          B. Clemmer cares for her daughter (although her husband
          helps), does all the housework, and makes a full dinner
          every night.   Other details of Dr. Clemmer's life are given
          in article.

1237.   Houston-Patterson, Anne.   " 'Fifty Three Years a Doctor.' "
          Medical Woman's Journal, 51:8 (August 1944) 31-32.
          Three months after her graduation from the Women's Med-
          ical College of Baltimore in 1891, Anne Houston-Patterson
          sailed for China because she had always wanted to be a
          missionary.   She recalls some of her most interesting cases.

1238.   Hunt, Harriot K.   Glances and Glimpses; or Fifty Years
          Social, Including Twenty Years Professional Life.
          John P. Jewett and Company, Boston, Massachusetts,
          1856, xii, 418 pp.
          Harriot Kezia Hunt presents her life, "not so peculiar in
          any one thing, as quietly and connectedly linking many
          things."   She states that she exhibits none of her "interior
          self....   Even now I stand in conscious hiddenness."   Hunt
          details her family's background preceding her own birth in
          1805 and tells of her childhood and her experiences as a
          teacher.   The illness of her sister consequently turned both
          their minds to the study of anatomy and physiology (Hunt's
          sister later married and abandoned medical study).   The
          record of Hunt's medical career involves details of her ap-
          plication for admittance to medical lectures at Harvard
          (1850).   Debarred from obtaining a "regular" degree, Hunt
          nonetheless carried on a medical practice.   In 1853 the Fe-
          male Medical College in Philadelphia conferred an honorary
          degree on Hunt, who reflects, "Courtesy and respect had
          led many of my patients for many years to address me as
          Dr., but the recognition of that College was very pleasant
          after eighteen years practice.   It led me to ask these ques-
          tions: How many males are practising on an honorary de-
          gree?   Did they wait as many years for it?"   Also included
          in this book is the chronicle of Hunt's social concerns: her
          persistent public protest of taxation (against women) without
          representation and her abhorrence of racial inequalities.
          Foremost in her concerns were women's rights to education,
          careers, and remuneration for all women's work including
          domestic labor.   She illustrates women's lamentable social
          position through stories about her patients.   Noting that the
          American Revolution gave freedom to the white man only,
          Hunt demands another revolution--purer, more universal.
          She recalls her thrill at attending a statewide women's rights

convention in Worcester, Massachusetts (1850). She also describes the prominent women of the age, many of them her acquaintances: Antoinette Brown, Lucy Stone, Lucretia Mott, and Marie Zakrzewska.

1239. Hunter, Gertrude T. "Pediatrician." Annals of the New York Academy of Sciences, 208 (15 March 1973) 37-40. A thoughtful reflection by Dr. Gertrude T. Hunter on the determinants which influenced her success in pediatrics as a woman and as a black. [This article is part of a series on "Successful Women in the Sciences: An Analysis of Determinants."]

1240. Hurd, Annah. "Record of Early Minnesota Medical Women." Journal of the American Medical Women's Association, 13:1 (January 1958) 23. The author lists "firsts" of women physicians in Minnesota medicine.

1241. Hutton, Isabel Emslie. Memories of a Doctor in War and Peace. James H. Heineman, Inc., New York, New York, [192?]. [Book not examined by editors.]

1242. "Hyla S. Watters, M.D." Medical Woman's Journal, 52:3 (March 1945) 27-29. photo., port. Dr. Watters served with the Methodist Mission Board in Wuhu, China. Her experiences in China are recounted in this article.

1243. "In Memoriam." Bulletin Medical Women's Club of Chicago, 2:10 (3 June 1914) 3. Dr. Julia Dyer Merrill began her medical career at Western Reserve University (Cleveland, Ohio) and received her M.D. degree in 1895 from Northwestern University Women's Medical School in Chicago (Illinois). Her appointments and affiliations are listed.

1244. "In Memoriam." Medical Woman's Journal, 39:4 (April 1932) 103. port. Dr. Isabel M. Meader graduated from Woman's Medical College of Chicago in 1887. She lived and practiced in Watertown, New York and, in 1900, started the first pathology laboratory in that city.

1245. "In Memoriam: Ada Chree Reid, M.D. 1895-1974: Editor-in-Chief, JAMWA (1947 to 1952)." Journal of the American Medical Women's Association, 29:7 (July 1974) 334. port. A few of Dr. Reid's professional affiliations are briefly mentioned.

1246. "In Memoriam: Annie Sturgis Daniel." Women in Medicine,

86 (October 1944) 22.

Dr. Daniel, graduated in 1879 from the medical school of the New York Infirmary for Women and Children, subsequently practiced in that Infirmary, ministering primarily to the poor.

1247.   In Memoriam: Clemence Sophia Lozier, M.D., [n.p., 1888?], 71 pp. port.

This memoir of the life of Dr. Clemence S. Lozier, founder of the New York Medical College and Hospital for Women, is offered by her daughter, Dr. A. W. Lozier. It consists of a series of eulogies delivered on behalf of Clemence Lozier. First is an address by the compiler upon presentation of a bust of her mother to the New York City Suffrage League. Then follows extracts from an address at the New York Medical College and Hospital for Women by Dean Phoebe J. Wait, M.D. Of particular interest is a tribute by Elizabeth Cady Stanton. Also included are: extracts from a eulogy by Hamilton Willcox, an obituary read by Dr. Harriette C. Keatinge before the New York County Homeopathic Association, resolutions by the board of trustees, faculty, and alumnae association of the New York Medical College and Hospital for Women and by the New York City Woman Suffrage League, and obituaries from the New York Evening Post and the New York Press.

1248.   "In Memoriam: Dr. Anna E. Broomall." Bulletin of the Medical Women's National Association, 32 (April 1931) 16-17.

Dr. Broomall, an 1871 graduate of the Woman's Medical College of Pennsylvania, in 1878 became head of the Department of Obstetrics at the College. In 1882 she established the Woman's Medical College Maternity Hospital in Philadelphia.

1249.   "In Memoriam: Dr. Clara Marshall." Bulletin of the Medical Women's National Association, 32 (April 1931) 16.

Dr. Marshall was the first woman to enter and graduate from the Philadelphia College of Pharmacy and Science. She took a medical degree at the Woman's Medical College of Pennsylvania (1875) where she ultimately became dean.

1250.   "In Memoriam: Dr. Hattie Elizabeth Alexander." The Stethoscope, 23 (July 1968) 3. port.

Dr. Alexander was responsible for the development of rabbit antiserum for the first effective treatment of bacterial meningitis. She was (in 1964) president of the American Pediatric Society. This article lists her many professional affiliations.

1251.   "In Memoriam--Ella B. Everitt, M.D." Bulletin of the Woman's Medical College of Pennsylvania, 72:4 (March 1922) 5-15. port.

Tributes to Dr. Everitt are given by the board of corporators, the hospital staff, the board of management, and the students of the Woman's Medical College of Pennsylvania, as well as by her colleagues, friends, and the dean of the College, Clara Marshall. A poem about Dr. Everitt by Julia H. Johnston, of the Business Women's Christian League, concludes the tribute.

1252. "In Memoriam: Helen Baldwin, M.D." Journal of the American Medical Women's Association, 1:2 (May 1946) 61. port.
Past-president of the medical board of the New York Infirmary for Women and Children, Dr. Baldwin was one of the first women physicians to study under Drs. Osler, Welch, Halsted, and Kelly at Johns Hopkins University Medical School. From 1896 to 1912 she worked in pathological chemistry in the laboratories of Dr. Christian Herter, a pioneer in biochemistry.

1253. In Memoriam: Mary Harris Thompson. Chicago Hospital for Women and Children, Board of Managers, Chicago, Illinois, 1896, 59 pp. photos.
Mary Harris Thompson founded the Chicago Hospital for Women and Children in 1865 and was instrumental in establishing the Woman's Medical College in Chicago, which opened in 1870. This booklet is a memorial testimony to her work and includes a brief biography, testimonies of various individuals and civic and professional groups in her behalf, and a history of the hospital. Dr. Thompson began her medical studies at the New England Female Medical College, worked at the New York Infirmary for Women and Children, and finally graduated from the New England Female Medical College. She began her practice in Chicago in 1863. Following her death in 1895, the hospital board voted to rename the institution the Mary Thompson Hospital of Chicago. This sketch also notes that Dr. Thompson invented a surgical needle used by many physicians.

1254. In Memoriam: Mrs. Charlotte Denman Lozier, M.D., Died January 3, 1870. Press of Wynkoop & Hallenbeck, New York, New York, [1870?], 33 pp. port.
Charlotte Denman Lozier began her studies at the New York Medical College for Women in 1864 and received her degree from that institution in 1869, having attended part-time in the intervening years. She was assistant professor of anatomy and physiology at that school until her death in 1870. Dr. Lozier was also first vice-president of the National Workingwomen's Association. This booklet is a collection of memorial tributes to her and reprints of newspaper obituaries.

1255. "In Memory." Medical Woman's Journal, 51:3 (March 1944) 39.

Martha Cleveland Dibble was a cofounder of the Women's and Children's Hospital in Kansas City, Missouri. This brief obituary notice supplies other facts about Dr. Dibble's life.

1256. "In Memory." Medical Woman's Journal, 51:12 (December 1944) 38. port.
The subject of this obituary notice is Dr. Fredericka C. Zeller, "an unusual character" who graduated from Northwestern University (Chicago, Illinois), traveled extensively, and practiced medicine in Peoria, Illinois.

1257. "In Memory." Medical Woman's Journal, 52:5 (May 1945) 53, 60. port.
Dr. Elsie Fox received her medical degree in 1911 from Cornell University. Her special interest lay in x-ray techniques, theory, and practice.

1258. "In Memory." Medical Woman's Journal, 52:7 (July 1945) 55.
Dr. Elizabeth Campbell graduated in 1895 from the Medical College of the University of Cincinnati (Ohio). She organized the Cincinnati Visiting Nurse Association and the Cincinnati Committee on Maternal Health. Dr. Campbell was also the first woman physician elected to the staff of a hospital in Cincinnati (Christ Hospital).

1259. "In Memory." Medical Woman's Journal, 53:3 (March 1946) 49. port.
Sarah Ellen Palmer graduated in 1880 from the Woman's Medical College of Pennsylvania. Among the first to perform caesarean sections, Dr. Palmer was a distinguished surgeon and lecturer.

1260. "In Memory." Medical Woman's Journal, 54:5 (May 1947) 46, 48.
Dr. Ida Shively Nelson, the first woman to receive a Bachelor of Science degree at Battle Creek College, graduated from the Medical College of Northwestern University [Michigan].

1261. "In Memory." Medical Woman's Journal, 55:6 (June 1948) 43.
Beatrice Pearce-Dickinson, who graduated from Northwestern Women's Medical College in 1887, practiced in Ketchikan, Alaska from 1908 until her death in 1948.

1262. "In Memory." Medical Woman's Journal, 56:6 (June 1949) 55.
This memorial to Dr. Elizabeth M. Van Cortland Hocker mentions her educational background and professional and social affiliations.

1263.   In Memory of Dr. Elizabeth Blackwell and Dr. Emily Black-
            well: January Twenty-Fifth MDCCCCXI, Academy of
            Medicine, New York. The Knickerbocker Press, New
            York, New York, [1911?], 90 pp.
        Dr. Stephen Smith opens the series of memorial addresses
        by recalling the admittance and course of study of Elizabeth
        Blackwell at Geneva Medical College. Dr. Smith was pres-
        ent in the class at Geneva when the dean received the letter
        from an eminent Philadelphia physician requesting the Col-
        lege permit Elizabeth Blackwell to be admitted and to be
        permitted to graduate. The faculty was unanimously op-
        posed to the admission of a woman but did not want the re-
        sponsibility of opposing the eminent Philadelphia physician,
        so they asked the class to decide (only one dissenting vote
        from the class would keep her out). In an uproarious man-
        ner and as a lark, the class voted a unanimous "Aye."
        When Blackwell became a class member, the entire class
        ceased its usual disruptive antics and in her presence con-
        ducted themselves with unusual decorum. Alice Stone Black-
        well, niece of Emily and Elizabeth, recalls the personalities
        of her aunts, both of whom were shy and reserved with a
        great deal of courage and kindness. Mrs. Henry Villard,
        a member of the board of trustees of the New York In-
        firmary for Women and Children, talks about the work of
        Emily Blackwell with the Infirmary. Dr. William H. Welch,
        former dean of Johns Hopkins University Medical School,
        devotes his attention to women in medicine and Dr. Black-
        well's desire to enter the field and to provide an opportun-
        ity for other women to do likewise. Dr. Abraham Jacobi,
        the "father of pediatrics" in America, discusses Dr. Eliza-
        beth Blackwell's scientific and medical interests. Dr.
        Gertrude B. Kelly memorializes Dr. Emily Blackwell as
        a great teacher.

1264.   In Memory of Mary Putnam Jacobi. [New York] Academy
            of Medicine, New York, New York, [1907?], vii, 85 pp.
        This memorial booklet, compiled by the Women's Medical
        Association of New York City, contains the texts of speeches,
        poems, and excerpts of Dr. Jacobi's writing delivered at a
        memorial service in her honor on 4 January 1907. Eulogies
        were delivered by William Osler, Elizabeth M. Cushier,
        Felix Adler, Florence Kelley, Charles L. Dana, and Rich-
        ard Watson Gilder. Dr. Emily Blackwell's tribute was read
        by Emily Dunning Barringer. The Women's Medical Asso-
        ciation of New York City announced the establishment of the
        Mary Putnam Jacobi Fellowship to aid women in postgradu-
        ate hospital work, an area in which Dr. Jacobi had felt wo-
        men suffered the most discrimination.

1265.   "In Memory: One of the First." Medical Woman's Journal,
            49:12 (December 1942) 391.
        This two-part article on Grace Niebuhr Kimball [reprinted
        from the Poughkeepsie New Yorker of 19 and 23 November

1942] gives a brief description of Dr. Kimball's motivation
to enter medicine and her accomplishments in the profession (she was the first woman appointed to the Poughkeepsie
Board of Health, worked in the antituberculosis campaign,
and served on the board of trustees and as president of the
Samuel and Nettie Bowne Memorial Hospitals).

1266. "In Memory: Dr. Fanny Hurd Brown; Passed on January
24, 1945." Medical Woman's Journal, 52:4 (April 1945)
55.
After Dr. Hurd Brown's graduation from the Medical Department of the University of Michigan in 1891, she went to
Korea to practice under the backing of the Detroit Presbyterian Missionary Society.

1267. Ingersoll, Louise M. and Burns, Margaret V. "Margery
J. Lord, M.D." Medical Woman's Journal, 51:9 (September 1944) 38.
Margery Juline Lord (whose portrait appears on the front
cover of this monthls Journal) holds the position of health
officer in Asheville, North Carolina.

1268. "Isabel M. Scharnagel, M.D." Medical Woman's Journal,
48:2 (February 1941) 54.
Dr. Scharnagel (whose portrait appears on the front cover
of this issue of the Journal) received her M.D. degree from
Rush Medical College (Chicago) in 1931. She was the first
resident in pathology at the New York Infirmary for Women
and Children. In 1932 she was awarded the Mary Putnam
Jacobi Fellowship and studied radiation therapy at Radium-
hemmet in Stockholm, Sweden. Upon her return to the U.S.
in 1933, she became the first resident at the Kate Depew
Strang Cancer Clinic. A list of her professional affiliations
and her publications is given.

1269. "It's Been Rewarding: But a Daughter Would Have Been
Nice." MCG Today, 5:1 (Fall 1975) 6. port.
Dr. Lois Taylor Ellison is profiled in this brief article.
A graduate of the Medical College of Georgia, she is the
mother of five children, and has recently been appointed
provost at the Medical College of Georgia.

1270. Jacobi, Mary Putnam. Mary Putnam Jacobi, M.D.: A
Pathfinder in Medicine. With Selections from Her Writings and a Complete Bibliography. Edited by the Women's Medical Association of New York City. G. P.
Putnam's Sons, New York, New York, 1925, xxxii, 521
pp. port.
The life of Mary Putnam Jacobi is described through the
vehicles of a biographical chapter, her Paris letters to the
Medical Record (1867-1870), selections from her writings,
and a complete bibliography. "The Women's Medical Association of New York City, desires to perpetuate the memory

of the work done by one of its founders ... a zealous worker for this advancement of the medical education of women."
Her life as physician, teacher, and author is outlined.   An
index is provided.

1271. Jacobi, Mary Putnam. "The Obituary of the Author."   Med-
          ical Record, 10 (1875) 357-358.
       The article preceding this obituary was entrusted to Dr.
       Jacobi just before Susan Dimock's death in a shipwreck. Dr.
       Jacobi writes of Dr. Dimock's modesty, simplicity, "soft-
       ness and elegance of appearance," and her "Puritan auster-
       ity of character."

1272. "Jane C. Wright '45: Appointed Associate Dean."   Chiron-
          ian, 29:2 (Summer 1967) 25-27.   port.
       As the newly-appointed associate dean of the New York Med-
       ical College, Jane Wright became the first Negro woman to
       hold such a position.   A 1945 graduate of that college, Dr.
       Wright is a cancer researcher and was a medical advisor
       with the African Research Foundation.   Excerpts from her
       report, A Visit to Kenya and Tanganyika in 1961, are in-
       cluded in this biography.

1273. "Jean C. Mendenhall: Contract Surgeon World War I."
          Medical Woman's Journal, 50:6 (June 1943) 161.
       A brief resumé of Dr. Mendenhall's professional education
       and career is herein given.

1274. "Jefferson's First Alumna."   Jefferson Medical College:
          Alumni Bulletin, 24:1 (Fall 1974) 14.   photo.
       Nancy Szwec Czarnecki was among the first class of women
       to graduate from Jefferson (class of 1965).   She and her
       husband share a general practice in Philadelphia.

1275. Jeffery, Mary Pauline.   Dr. Ida: India.   The Life Story
          of Ida S. Scudder, M.D., B.Sc., F.A.C.S., K.I.H.
          President, Medical College for Women, Vellore, India.
          Fleming H. Revell Company, New York, New York,
          1938, 212 pp.   photos., ports.
       [This book, the first of three about Dr. Scudder by Dr.
       Jeffery, was followed by Ida S. Scudder of Vellore: An
       Appreciation of Forty Years of Service in India, Mysore
       City, India, 1939; and Ida S. Scudder of Vellore: The Life
       Story of Ida Sophia Scudder, 1951, both books by Wesley
       Press and Publishing House.   The illustrations, prefaces,
       and minor additions to the text in the 1939 and 1951 editions
       update this original biography.   A full annotation to Jeffery's
       biography of Dr. Scudder appears in this bibliography under
       the citation of the 1951 edition.]

1276. Jeffery, Mary Pauline.   Ida S. Scudder of Vellore: An Ap-
          preciation of Forty Years of Service in India.   Wesley
          Press and Publishing House, Mysore City, South India,

[1939], xiv, 138 pp. photos., ports.
[Jeffery's original biography of Dr. Scudder was published
in 1938 in New York City; also, a "jubilee edition" was
published in 1951. This edition differs from that version
only in the illustrations, preface, and minor additions to
the text. A full annotation to Dr. Jeffery's biography appears in this bibliography under the citation of the 1951 edition.]

1277.   Jeffery, Mary Pauline. Ida S. Scudder of Vellore: The Life
            Story of Ida Sophia Scudder. Wesley Press and Publish-
            ing House, Mysore City, India, Jubilee Edition, 1951,
            xiv, 226 pp. photos., ports.
        This "jubilee edition" of Jeffery's first biography of Ida
        Scudder updates the earlier book and commemorates the
        50th anniversary of Dr. Scudder's work in Vellore, India
        [the 1938 and 1939 editions are cited elsewhere in this bib-
        liography]. Ida Scudder, born into a medical missionary
        family that had served in India for two generations, went to
        Vellore following graduation from Cornell Medical College
        in 1899. Her numerous contributions to public health and
        education included development of the Mary Taber Schell
        Memorial Hospital (begun in 1902) and the Christian Medical
        College (established in 1918). A nursing school, other hos-
        pitals and health services also grew out of her work. She
        has been compared with Albert Schweitzer in her talent,
        zeal, energy, and dedication. There are many photographs
        of Dr. Scudder, the hospital and college buildings in various
        stages of development, staff, graduates, patients, and
        friends. There is no index or bibliography.

1278.   Jeffery, M[ary] Pauline. "Letter to Editor." Medical Wo-
            man's Journal, 53:6 (June 1946) 52.
        Pauline Jeffery, a physician and a writer (Ida S. Scudder of
        Vellore), provides autobiographical information on her own
        educational background and current activities in India, as
        well as on Dr. Scudder's present involvements. Dr. Jef-
        fery apologizes that her own biography "is not very exciting
        as I have been fighting tuberculosis for the past fifteen
        years...."

1279.   "Jennie McCowen, A.M., M.D." Woman's Medical Journal,
            11:7 (July 1901) 265-267. (Biographical.)

1280.   Jennings, Dana C. "Lady Doctor: Alumna, Teacher, Phy-
            sician, Mother, Friend, Author ... Effie Faye Cashatt
            Lewis, M.D., U.S.D. '19, First Woman Graduate."
            Medicine ... News from the USD School of Medicine and
            Medical School Alumni Information, 3:3 (October 1975)
            6-7, 12. photos., ports.
        Dr. Lewis became, in 1919, the first woman to graduate
        from the University of South Dakota [USD] College of Medi-
        cine. During her medical school days as the lone woman

student, she used to think "'My girl voice is like a black
skin in a roomful of whites.'" As for the women's liberation movement, Dr. Lewis believes the more flamboyant
leaders of the movement are "... bludgeoning too many triv-
ialities. What harm is there in being whistled at, for example? Our being sex objects to men is one of the facts of
nature that will not change...." Dr. Lewis's marriage to
another physician with whom she had three children, is described in her book Doc's Wife (she also wrote four other
books). Following 20 years of professional inactivity, Dr.
Lewis practiced medicine in Iowa.

1281.   Jerger, B. "Someday She'll Be a Doctor: Suzanne Eggle-
            ston, U.C.L.A." Today's Health, 37 (November 1959)
            28-32. illus.
        [Article not examined by editors.]

1282.   "The Johnny Appleseed of AMWA: Dr. P. S. Bordeau-Sis-
            co." Journal of the American Medical Women's Asso-
            ciation, 16:3 (March 1961) 230.
        Dr. P. S. Bordeau-Sisco was active in helping to organize
        various women's medical groups: the Seventh-Day Adventist
        Sanatorium at Iowa Circle, District of Columbia; a Women's
        Medical Society in the District of Columbia; and Women's
        Medical Society of Maryland.

1283.   Johnson, Edith E. Leaves from a Doctor's Diary. Pacific
            Books, Palo Alto, California, 1954.
        [Book not examined by editors.]

1284.   Johnson, Evelyn. "New York Alumni ... She Kept 'em
            Laughing." Old Oregon, 38:1 (August-September 1957)
            15. photo.
        This article recalls Dr. Lovejoy's "spellbinding barrage of
        early medical school recollections" which she delivered at
        the special dinner staged by the Oregon Alumni Club of
        New York.

1285.   Johnston, Helen. "Mary Putnam Jacobi." Journal of the
            American Medical Women's Association, 1:4 (July 1946)
            118-122. (Inaugural Address, Annual Meeting, Ameri-
            can Medical Women's Association, San Francisco, June
            1946.)
        Incidents and accomplishments in the life of Mary Putnam
        Jacobi are presented.

1286.   Johnston, Malcolm Sanders. Elizabeth Blackwell and Her
            Alma Mater: The Story in the Documents. W. F.
            Humphrey Press Inc., Geneva, New York, 1947, 29 pp.
        This brief sketch prints excerpts of her "Autobiographical
        Sketches," journal, and correspondence to show Elizabeth
        Blackwell's progress from a pariah at the beginning of her
        years at Geneva College to, on commencement day, "feeling

more thoroughly at home in the midst of these true hearted
young men [her fellow graduates] than anywhere else in
town."

1287.   Johnstone, Rutherford T. "Climate for Exploration." Ar-
        chives of Environmental Health (Chicago), 3 (November
        1961) 559-561. port. (Editorials.)
        Dr. Johnstone recalls his association with Dr. Alice Hamil-
        ton, "the first lady of industrial hygiene and toxicology."
        A militant who believed in Richard Ely's program of so-
        cialism, Dr. Hamilton picketed with industrial strikers and
        avidly supported the accused anarchists Sacco and Vanzetti.
        A few medical contemporaries viewed her as being "pink,"
        recalls Dr. Johnstone, who himself was warned against
        associating with her. Dr. Hamilton's idealism and profes-
        sional activities are further described.

1288.   Jones, D. E. Sanapia: Comanche Medicine Woman. Holt,
        Rinehart and Winston, [c 1972], xvii, 107 pp. (Case
        studies in cultural anthropology.)
        [Book not examined by editors.]

1289.   Jones, Grace G. "Bertha Tapman Shamer, M.D." Jour-
        nal of the American Medical Women's Association, 11:8
        (August 1956) 295. port. (Album of Women in Medi-
        cine.)
        Dr. Shamer served as woman physician for the juvenile
        court from 1915 to 1925. She was one of the first doctors
        in Baltimore to administer salvarsan in the treatment of
        lues.

1290.   Journal of the American Medical Women's Association, 19:
        5 (May 1964) 404. (Album of Women in Medicine.)
        Marion Fay, a Ph.D. and professor of physiology, retired
        as president and dean of the Woman's Medical College of
        Pennsylvania in January 1964, after being affiliated with the
        College since 1935. She was the only woman to be presi-
        dent and dean at a medical school in the western hemi-
        sphere.

1291.   Judson, Eliza E. Address in Memory of Ann Preston,
        M.D. Delivered by Request of the Corporators and
        Faculty of the Women's [sic] Medical College of Penn-
        sylvania, March 11th, 1873. [Philadelphia, Pennsyl-
        vania? 1873], 29 pp.
        [Item not examined by editors.]

1292.   "Julia Woodzicka, M.D." Medical Woman's Journal, 49:
        10 (October 1942) 320-321.
        A portrait of Julia Woodzicka appears on the cover of this
        issue of the Journal. This article is primarily an auto-
        biographical reminiscence of Julia Woodzicka's experiences
        as a country doctor in the pioneering community of Royalton,
        Wisconsin.

1293.   "K. Frances Scott, M.D.: Medical Woman of the Month."
        Journal of the American Medical Women's Association,
        3:11 (November 1948) 481.   port.   (Medical Women in
        the News.)
        Elected president of the National Federation of Business and
        Professional Women's Clubs, Inc., K. Frances Scott (most
        of whose professional career has been spent in college health
        services) said in her inaugural address, "We must take up
        willingly and wholeheartedly the responsibilities that go
        with rights, put away the childish passing of resolutions and
        the sponsoring of causes without accepting the responsibil-
        ity for putting them into effect."

1294.   Kaltreider, Nancy B.   "The Hazards of Feminine Physician-
            hood."   Harvard Medical Alumni Bulletin, 50:1 (Septem-
            ber/October 1975) 10-13.   cartoons.
        Three Harvard medical graduates who rank motherhood
        equally with their careers tell how they have handled their
        dual roles.   They are Marian Woolston Catlin (M.D., 1955),
        Lesley Bunim Heafitz (1965), and Jean Emans (1970).

1295.   "Kate B. Karpeles."   Medical Woman's Journal, 46:3
            (March 1939) 91.
        Following her graduation from Johns Hopkins in 1914, Dr.
        Karpeles (whose portrait appears on the front cover of this
        issue of the Journal) became the first woman to intern at
        Garfield Memorial Hospital in Washington, D.C.

1296.   "Kate B. Karpeles, M.D."   Medical Woman's Journal, 48:
            9 (September 1941) 287.
        Dr. Karpeles (whose portrait appears on the front cover of
        this issue of the Journal) was encouraged by her father,
        himself a doctor, to study medicine.   After graduating from
        Goucher in 1909, she went on to receive her M.D. at Johns
        Hopkins University in 1914.   Dr. Karpeles's difficulties in
        obtaining an internship are recounted, as well as profes-
        sional appointments she ultimately held.

1297.   "Kate Campbell Mead, M.D.: President of the Medical Wo-
            men's National Association, Inc."   Medical Woman's
            Journal, 31:6 (June 1924) 178-179.   port.
        A gynecologist, Dr. Mead was active in milk station work.

1298.   "Katharine C. Bushnell, M.D."   Medical Woman's Journal,
            51:11 (November 1944) 29-30.   port.
        Following graduation from Woman's Hospital Medical College,
        Chicago [1879], Katharine C. Bushnell went to China as a
        medical missionary.   Frances E. Willard later asked Dr.
        Bushnell to work with the Purity Department of the Woman's
        Christian Temperance Union.   Her work in that position
        "gave her notoriety over the world for her investigation of
        white slavery and opium."   Dr. Bushnell's extensive writings
        are mentioned, and the text of a tribute to her written by
        Elizabeth Blackwell is included.

1299.   "Katherine C. Manion, M. D.: President-Elect Medical Wo-
        men's National Association, Inc." Medical Woman's
        Journal, 31:6 (June 1924) 179. port.
        Katherine C. Manion practiced medicine in Portland, Ore-
        gon, limiting her practice to diseases of women and chil-
        dren. "Dr. Manion is a woman's woman, was a prominent
        suffrage exponent and ... also bears the distinction of being
        one of the six women doctors of Portland, Ore., who of-
        fered their services to the Surgeon General for war ser-
        vices at the beginning of the World's War, and was refused
        on account of her sex."

1300.   "Kathryn M. Whitten, M. D." Medical Woman's Journal,
        50:11 (November 1943) 288.
        Dr. Whitten (whose portrait appears on the front cover of
        this issue of the Journal) received her medical education in
        15 different universities throughout the world. She prac-
        ticed surgery in Fort Wayne, Indiana and has written a book
        entitled The Horses of the Sun--an account of the life and
        work of a fictitious woman physician.

1301.   Katzeff, Miriam. "Letitia Douglas Adams, M. D." Journal
        of the American Medical Women's Association, 10:6
        (June 1955) 216. port. (Album of Women in Medicine.)
        Dr. Adams, a fellow of the American College of Surgeons
        and past chief of the surgical department at the New England
        Hospital for Women and Children in Boston, combines ob-
        stetrics and medical practice with her surgical skills.

1302.   Kelly, [Howard Atwood]. "Women in Medicine." Johns
        Hopkins Hospital Bulletin, 7:59-60 (February-March
        1896) 50-52. (Hospital Historical Club: Meeting of
        January 13, 1896.)
        Speaking to the society about Elizabeth Blackwell's book,
        Pioneer Work in Opening the Medical Profession to Women,
        Dr. Kelly highlights the facts and anecdotes he found par-
        ticularly interesting. He calls the autobiography "a striking
        chapter in the history of medicine," and adds that no other
        movement, in terms of "rapidity and force," can compare
        with the advancement of women in medicine.

1303.   Kerr, Laura. Doctor Elizabeth. Thomas Nelson & Sons,
        New York, New York, 1946, 208 pp.
        This is a fictional biography of Elizabeth Blackwell for
        young readers. It covers her childhood, education, career,
        writing, and public life. Emphasis is given to her rela-
        tionships with her sisters, her adopted daughter, and a few
        professional associates.

1304.   Kimball, Grace N. "Autobiographical Sketch." Medical
        Review of Reviews, 41:8 (August 1935) 393-398.
        Dr. Kimball traces her life from her work in the mission
        fields of Van, Turkey (where she traveled at the age of 26)

to her entry into medicine in 1888 and her subsequent return to Turkey. Her experiences as a physician in Van
constitute the major portion of this sketch. In 1896 Dr.
Kimball returned to the United States and took a position
as assistant resident physician at Vassar College. She resigned this position in 1898 and opened a general practice
in Poughkeepsie, New York.

1305.   King, John W. and King, Caroline R. "Early Women Phy-
             sicians in Vermont." Bulletin of the History of Medi-
             cine, 25:5 (September-October 1951) 429-441.
         A search of almanacs and directories in Vermont determined
         that 26 women who had graduated from medical colleges
         practiced in that state prior to 1900. Outstanding among
         them was the first Vermont woman physician, Emily A.
         Varney-Brownell, who graduated from the Woman's Medical
         College of Pennsylvania in 1855. She was also the first
         woman to be admitted to clinics at the Jefferson Medical
         College in Philadelphia. Emma Huddah Callendar, a gradu-
         ate of the New England Female Medical College (1869), was
         the first woman admitted to the Vermont Medical Society
         (1874) and was also the first woman to present a scientific
         paper to that society. Elizabeth Malleson, a Woman's Med-
         ical College graduate in 1887, was the second woman li-
         censed by the state medical society; she did not, however,
         become a member. Anna E. Barker, an 1891 Woman's
         Medical College graduate, was the second woman member
         of the medical society. A complete list of names, their
         schools, and places of practice is included in the text.
         Data cited for the article include census records from 1870
         to 1900, Walton's Vermont Register and Farmer's Almanac,
         and minutes of the state medical society meetings.

1306.   King-Salmon, Frances W. House of a Thousand Babies:
             Experiences of an American Woman Physician in China
             (1922-1940). Exposition Press, Jericho, New York,
             1968, 168 pp.
         When Frances King graduated from medical school in 1921,
         she learned of a new medical college being organized in
         Shanghai to train Chinese women physicians. She was in-
         trigued with the idea of going among "a really needful peo-
         ple as a teacher as well as a doctor." Having grown up
         on a farm in a pioneer community in South Dakota as one
         of ten children, Dr. King felt prepared to reach out for
         new, if foreign, adventures. "I went as my forebears had
         trekked into the Great Plains--as a pioneer." After a year
         of immersing herself in Chinese language and culture, Dr.
         King did her internship in obstetrics and taught physiology
         at Margaret Williamson Hospital in Shanghai--otherwise
         known as the House of a Thousand Babies, because of its
         reputation as a maternity hospital for abnormal deliveries.
         Having worked under Dr. Florence Kraker, who was on
         short-term appointment as acting head of the obstetrical de-

partment from Woman's Medical College in Philadelphia,
Dr. King, still in her first year of medical practice, "was
suddenly acting head of a department of obstetrics of over
one thousand deliveries a year, 35 per cent of them abnormal." She was determined to repudiate the mission
board's lament: "We've sent beautiful women and ugly women, older women and younger women, but we lose them
all [to marriage]" and one missionary's congratulatory comment to the board: "... you have sent more women to be
wives of our missionaries than any other board." Nevertheless, around 1930, she met and worked with and married
Robert J. Salmon, a chemist/pharmacologist at St. John's
Medical School, Shanghai. Together they watched political
conditions change in China, as Japan invaded. Dr. King-
Salmon and her two children set sail for San Francisco in
November 1940, expecting to return when conditions improved. The men stayed behind to try to prevent the university from collapsing. Eventually, Robert was interned
in a Japanese concentration camp, and Dr. King-Salmon,
never losing her love for China, lived for five years "like
so many American women during the war--working, bringing up children, alone, never knowing whether I was a
widow." Her husband returned, but neither was ever to
see China again.

1307.   Kinney, Dita H. "Dr. Anita Newcomb McGee and What She
         Has Done for the Nursing Profession." Trained Nurse
         and Hospital Review, (March 1901) 129-134. port.
        Born in 1864, Anita McGee married and bore two children
        before taking a medical degree in 1892 from Columbia Uni-
        versity, Washington, D.C. When the Spanish-American War
        broke in 1898, Dr. McGee evolved and directed a hospital
        corps of nurses under the National Society of the Daughters
        of the American Revolution. She was also appointed an
        assistant surgeon in the army (only one other woman, Mary
        Walker, had ever held that distinction). Excerpts of Dr.
        McGee's reports to the DAR are quoted in this article.
        This biography notes that she is an authority on American
        communistic societies and active in the American Associa-
        tion of Advanced Science.

1308.   Kittredge, Elizabeth. "A. Frances Foye, M.D." Journal
         of the American Medical Women's Association, 6:11
         (November 1951) 450. port. (Album of Women in Med-
         icine.)
        Dr. Foye was a general practitioner for the wives and chil-
        dren of foreign envoys and Washington social and political
        families. She successfully diagnosed and delivered triplets
        in 1950.

1309.   Kittredge, Elizabeth. "Amy J. Rule, M.D. (1870-1946)."
         Journal of the American Medical Women's Association,
         19:1 (January 1964) 54. port.

"Dr. Amy J. Rule was a tall, well-built woman with a warm
personality ... [who] felt very strongly about smoking and
drinking." She practiced medicine in Washington, D.C.

1310.   Kittredge, Elizabeth. "Eva F. Dodge M.D." Journal of
            the American Medical Women's Association, 15:11 (No-
            vember 1960) 1096. port. (Album of Women in Medi-
            cine.)
         Dr. Dodge was the first woman to serve an internship and
         residency in obstetrics and gynecology in the University
         Hospital of the University of Maryland (Baltimore) Medical
         School. She served as acting professor of obstetrics at the
         Woman's Christian Medical College in China. She was also
         the first woman physician to practice in Winston-Salem,
         North Carolina. Her fields of interest and many member-
         ships are listed.

1311.   Kittredge, Elizabeth. "May Davis Baker, M.D." Journal
            of the American Medical Women's Association, 6:11
            (November 1951) 451. port.
         Dr. Baker entered Columbian College (now George Washing-
         ton University) for her medical training in the late 1800s
         but transferred to Howard National University because of
         the pressure she felt at Columbian, a school where women
         "were not too welcome." After fifty years of practice, Dr.
         Baker retired only to be pressed into service again during
         World War II. After the war, at the age of 80, she took
         and passed the Pennsylvania State Boards.

1312.   Kleiner, Charlotte A. "Frances Bartlett-Tyson, M.D."
            Journal of the American Medical Women's Association,
            12:10 (October 1957) 356. port. (Album of Women in
            Medicine.)
         Dr. Bartlett-Tyson interned at Blockley Hospital (now Phila-
         delphia General) at the turn of the century, a great honor
         for that period. After her marriage, Dr. Bartlett-Tyson,
         upon her husband's request, retired from medicine; in 1918,
         however, a delegation of townspeople in Leonia, New Jersey
         (the Tysons' home since 1913) prevailed upon her to return
         to active practice.

1313.   Knapp, Sally. "Ida Scudder." Christian Observer, (26 Oc-
            tober 1949) 5-6. illus., port.
         The life of Dr. Ida Scudder, granddaughter of the first
         American missionary to India and herself a medical mis-
         sionary, is recalled: her birth in India, education in the
         U.S., and eventual return to India to minister to the sick.
         Various cases of illness and superstition handled by Dr.
         Scudder are retold.

1314.   Knauber, Connie. "Philadelphian of the Month: Dr. Cath-
            arine Macfarlane, Champion of Cancer Research."
            Philadelphia, 35:12 (December 1948) 28, 47. photos.

1315.   Knauf, John. "Daughters of Science: Helena of Dakota:
         Helena Knauf Wink, M.D., Jamestown, N.D." Medical
         Woman's Journal, 37:4 (April 1930) 99-101. illus.,
         photos.
         A biographical sketch of Dr. Helena Knauf Wink of North
         Dakota, this article presents an adventurous account of in-
         cidents in Dr. Wink's life. A photograph of Dr. Wink with
         her two physician sisters, Theresa K. Abt and Mary K.
         McCoy, is included.

1316.   Kneen, B. D. "She Walks with the People, Dr. Frances
         Eastman Rose." Independent Woman, 14 (April 1935)
         115+.
         [Article not examined by editors.]

1317.   Knight, Charlotte. "Prettiest Doctor in the Fleet." Col-
         lier's, (11 November 1950) 26-27+. photos.
         The first woman medical officer ever ordered to sea by the
         navy, Bernice Walters serves as anesthesiologist and sur-
         geon on board the USS Consolation, off the war-torn Korean
         coast. Lieutenant Commander Walters, nicknamed "Burma"
         due to her desire to live in some "weird place," flew
         with the Women's Auxiliary Service Pilots (WASPs) before
         signing with the navy.

1318.   Koelsch, F. ["Alice Hamilton, a Life for Occupational
         Medicine. A Comparison of the History of Occupational
         Medicine in the United States"]. Zentralblatt für Arbeit-
         smedizin und Arbeitsschutz, 9 (1959) 188-191. port.
         (Ger)
         [Article not examined by editors.]

1319.   "'Komapsumida' Is Korean for 'Thank You': An Interview
         with Roberta Rice." The Mayo Alumnus, (April 1968)
         1-3. illus., photo.
         Dr. Rice, a Mayo Clinic alumna, discusses her background,
         her decision to go to Korea as a medical missionary, and
         her philosophy of missions and medical practice.

1320.   Korman, Belle. "Carolyn Nicholas MacDonald, 1887-1942."
         Women in Medicine, 77 (July 1942) 29-30.
         This article is an account of a woman who suffered through
         many hardships to become a physician and then gave as
         fine personal attention to her patients as she gave medical
         attention.

1321.   Krasne, B. "Dr. Phyl. and Mother M.D.: Lady Phyllis
         Cilento." Independent Woman, 28 (February 1949) 45-
         46+.
         [Article not examined by editors.]

1322.   Kress, Lauretta Eby and Kress, Daniel Hartman. Under
         the Guiding Hand: Life Experiences of the Doctors

Kress. College Press, Washington, D.C., 1932, 240
pp. photos., ports.
This is a personal memoir of the life of Dr. Lauretta Eby
Kress as spent in practice with her husband. Dr. Kress
began medical studies at the Battle Creek (Michigan) Sanitarium in 1890 and received her M.D. degree from the
University of Michigan in 1894. Her obstetrics practice
was undertaken within the Seventh Day Adventist mission.
In 1899 Dr. Kress went to England, and was in Australia
from 1900 to 1907. She then returned to the U.S. for service in Washington, D.C., Loma Linda, California, and
Chicago, Illinois. Her longest service was in Takoma
Park, Maryland at the Washington Sanitarium. Her daughter, Ora Kress Mason, is a graduate of the George Washington University Medical School.

1323.   Kubie, Lawrence S. "Florence Rena Sabin, 1871-1953."
         Perspectives in Biology and Medicine, 4 (Spring 1961)
         306-315.

1324.   Kusta, Charlotte E. "Anna M. Young, M.D." Medical
         Woman's Journal, 53:2 (February 1946) 34.
         A specialist in pathology, Dr. Young (whose portrait appears
         on the front cover of this month's Journal) became the first
         woman ever elected to serve on the board of directors of
         the Cleveland Academy of Medicine.

1325.   Larsell, O. The Doctor in Oregon. Binfords & Mort,
         Portland, Oregon, 1947.
         [Book not examined by editors.]

1326.   Latham, Vida A. "Jane Downes Kelly Sabine, M.D.,
         F.A.C.S." Medical Woman's Journal, 57:9 (September
         1950) 40-41.

1327.   Lathrop, Virginia T. "Margery Lord, M.D." Journal of
         the American Medical Women's Association, 8:8 (August
         1953) 276. port. (Album of Women in Medicine.)
         A short biography of Dr. Margery Lord, the first woman
         to become a public health officer in North Carolina (1940),
         notes that she had been a community physician in Montreal
         and, during World War II, worked with the reorganization
         of venereal disease control clinics.

1328.   LeMarquis, Antoinette. "Viola J. Erlanger, M.D." Jour-
         nal of the American Medical Women's Association, 20:
         5 (May 1965) 482. port. (Album of Women in Medi-
         cine.)
         "A lady in the truest sense of the word, well-born, well-
         bred, and well-educated," Dr. Erlanger practiced in Cleve-
         land, Philadelphia, Chicago, and San Diego.

1329.   Lentz, J. "America's First Woman Physician: Elizabeth

Blackwell." Today's Health, 42 (January 1964) 36-37+.
[Article not examined by editors.]

1330.   "Leona Baumgartner, M.D." Modern Medicine, (9 Novem-
         ber 1964) 75-76. (Contemporaries.)
Dr. Baumgartner's philosophy as well as her professional
accomplishments are given herein. "The 62-year-old pediatrician plainly thrives at the cutting edge of social progress."

1331.   "Leona Baumgartner M.D., Ph.D." Medical Woman's
         Journal, 52:10 (October 1945) 44.
Dr. Baumgartner (whose portrait appears on the front cover
of this issue of the Journal) earned both her Ph.D. and her
M.D. at Yale University in 1932 and 1934 respectively.   A
very brief account of her medical activities is given.

1332.   "Leslie S. Kent, M.D.: Medical Woman of the Month."
         Journal of the American Medical Women's Association,
         4:1 (January 1949) 42-43. port. (Medical Women in
         the News.)
The first woman president of the Oregon State Medical Society and, according to the Journal, the first woman president of any state medical society, Leslie Kent carried on
a general practice.

1333.   L'Esperance, Elise S. "In Memoriam." Journal of the
         American Medical Women's Association, 1:9 (December
         1946) 295-296. port.
A brief tribute is given to the memory of Dr. Alice Stone
Woolley, "a distinguished woman, definitely feminine in
dress and thinking, which added greatly to the charm of
her brilliant mind."

1334.   "Letitia Westgate, M.D." Medical Woman's Journal, 52:
         4 (April 1945) 51-52. port.
A letter from Letitia Westgate to the Journal gives Dr.
Westgate's present status as well as introduces the news
clipping which follows. This clipping, reprinted from the
DeKalb [Illinois] Chronicle (May 1900), gives a biography
of Dr. Westgate, including a description of her work as
originator, administrator, and physician at the hospital she
designed in DeKalb, Illinois.

1335.   Lewis, Faye Cashatt. Doc's Wife. The Macmillan Com-
         pany, New York, New York, 1940, 198 pp.
Faye Cashatt Lewis had an M.D. of her own, from the
same school and year as "P.B." (an endearing term for
"Poor Bill," her husband). But Dr. Lewis decided that if
both she and her husband were addressed as "Doctor," the
residents of Ridgefield, Iowa would get confused. "After
all, the practice was to be his; anything I did of a professional nature was to be as his assistant...." Although the

townspeople never completely accepted Dr. Lewis as a fully
qualified physician, they believed "if schools trained women
physicians," that training would lean more to the nursing
than the healing art.   Eventually, Dr. Lewis came to be
looked upon as a "spare" doctor and was called upon when
"P.B." was unavailable.   In her book, Dr. Lewis describes
five years of her life as "Doc's wife" in rural Iowa.

1336.   Lewis, Harriet M.; Gerrish, Frederic H.; and Dyer,
Florence M. "Mary Alice Avery, M.D., of Portland."
Transactions of the Maine Medical Association, (1905)
418-421.   port.   (Necrology Report.)

1337.   "Lieutenant Commander Bernice McCoy, M.C., U.S.N."
Medical Woman's Journal, 51:12 (December 1944) 38.
The first woman medical officer to report for duty at the
United States Naval Hospital, San Diego, California, Dr.
McCoy received her medical degree from the University of
Pennsylvania Medical School in 1924.   (She is honored with
her portrait on the front cover of this issue of the Journal.)

1338.   Lightbody, Georgia Meaus. "Fighting the Devil." In: 100
Years of Medicine: 1849-1949. Modern Press Limited,
Saskatoon, Saskatchewan, 1949, 5-7. ports.
This brief biography of Elizabeth Blackwell relates her difficulties in getting admitted to medical school; she was finally accepted at Geneva Medical College where her presence
as the only woman transformed "this class from a band of
lawless desperadoes to gentlemen." She reassured her religious mother about her intentions in pursuing medicine by
writing that her only concern is "just to kill the devil,
whom I hate so heartily" and that what she was doing was
"living religion all the time."

1339.   Lindemann, Lillian C. "Emily Gardner, M.D., F.A.A.P.,
1899-1956." Journal of the American Medical Women's
Association, 12:11 (November 1957) 414. port. (Album of Women in Medicine.)
Dr. Gardner was the first woman to serve as president of
the Richmond Tuberculosis Association (1945-1947), and the
first woman to be chairman of the Richmond City Board of
Health.

1340.   Link, Eugene P. "Elizabeth Blackwell, Citizen and Humanitarian." Woman Physician, 26:9 (September 1971) 451-
458.
The author presents results of original research into the
nonmedical aspects of Blackwell's life: e.g., social orientation, religious influences, social medicine, and moral reform.

1341.   Link, Eugene P. "The Psychosomatic Outlook of Doctors
Abraham and Mary Putnam Jacobi." Journal of the

American Medical Women's Association, 7:12 (December 1952) 455-456. ports.

Mary Putnam Jacobi organized the first consumers' organization in America and was a leading proponent of woman suffrage. One way she applied her medical training for the rights of women was to examine the nature of psychosomatic complaints that women express in such works as "The Prophylaxis of Insanity" which "recognized the influence of social surroundings, the bearings of responsibilities and tensions, upon mental disease.... To overcome religious or political manias which she felt also contributed to mental disease, she recommended more practical, meaningful experiences for the patient, experiences in real activity with more basic satisfaction." In another essay, "The Question of Rest for Women During Menstruation," she not only pointed out the sociosomatic aspect of the cycle of menstruation, but she also attacked the contemporary idea that menstruation is a female weakness. "After careful study and research, she concluded that women do not need rest at this period and are not, thereby, inferior to men. She also noted that women who are interested in their work and who are not made useless by social patterns resembling a harem have less dysmenorrhea than others. Moreover, she indicated that celibacy increases menstrual pain and emphasized that this point has been overlooked. In our social arrangements, she added, celibacy implies, for the woman, social failure."

1342.   Lipinska, M. ["A Pioneer in America: Dr. Elizabeth Blackwell"]. Presse Medicale, 37:27 (3 April 1929) 443. (Fre)

Elizabeth Blackwell was born in Bristol, England in February 1821 and came with her family to America at the age of eleven years. She taught school and became interested in social problems such as slavery and woman suffrage. While teaching in Kentucky and in Charlestown [sic], South Carolina, she devoted her spare time to studying medicine and anatomy. She applied to every medical school in the country and was turned down or ignored by all except the college of medicine at Geneva, New York. The initial hostility of the Geneva townspeople gradually turned to benevolence in the face of her calm and dignified demeanor, and at her graduation in January 1849 an estimated 20,000 people came to see her receive her degree. After graduation she went to England, where she was accepted at St. Bartholomew's Hospital in all services except gynecology; to Paris, where she contracted a purulent ophthalmia that cost her the sight of one eye; and to Preissnitz's institute at Grafenberg in Silesia, where she became interested in physical therapy and gymnastics. She returned to New York and set up a clinic for women and children in 1853. Later she founded a small hospital which eventually became the New York Infirmary and Medical College for Women: she was

joined in this project by her sister Emily and by Mme.
Zakrzewska. Eventually Elizabeth Blackwell returned to
England to the chair of gynecology at the Women's Medical
College in London founded by Sophia Jex-Blake. She died
in May 1910 at her retirement home in Hastings.

1343.   "Lodi's Beloved Lady Physician Mamie Guthrie Pallesen Re-
        tires Following 45 Years of Practice." Alumni Journal
        [Loma Linda University], 42:2 (March 1971) 24, 26.
        port.
        This article gives a biographical account of Dr. Pallesen's
        life, from her early desire to be a missionary in India,
        through her medical education at Loma Linda University
        (California), to her professional activities.

1344.   Logie, Iona Robertson. "Dr. Sue of Columbia County."
        Medical Woman's Journal, 53:8 (August 1946) 24-25, 49.
        port.
        Canadian-born Sue Hurst Thompson Gould graduated in 1928
        from Rush Medical College. She was the first woman M.D.
        in the United States to direct a public health district (in
        Michigan). This biography discusses Dr. Gould's public
        health work in Columbia County, New York, and presents a
        chronological record of her professional career.

1345.   "Louise Wong, M.D." School of Medicine Commentary:
        University of California, Davis, 3:3 (August 1974) 8.
        photo. (Medical School Profiles.)
        Dr. Wong graduated at the head of her class at Davis and
        received the Janet M. Glasgow Scholastic Citation of the
        American Medical Women's Association.

1346.   Lovejoy, Esther P. "Kate Campbell Hurd-Mead (1867-
        1941)." Bulletin of the History of Medicine, 10:2
        (July 1941) 314-317. port.
        This biography focuses upon Dr. Mead's career as a writer
        and historian, and how "she honored herself by honoring
        women in her chosen profession and tracing their work from
        the remote past."

1347.   Lovejoy, Esther Pohl. "Mary Elizabeth Bates, M.D."
        Journal of the American Medical Women's Association,
        10:4 (April 1955) 134. port. (Album of Women in
        Medicine.)
        Completing her M.D. degree requirements in 1881 at the
        age of 20, Dr. Mary Elizabeth Bates went on to become
        the first woman intern at Cook County Hospital. In 1891
        she moved to Denver, where she promoted the passage of
        laws for the protection of women and children.

1348.   Lovejoy, Esther Pohl. "Mathilda K. Wallin, M.D." Jour-
        nal of the American Medical Women's Association, 7:1
        (January 1952) 30. port. (Album of Women in Medi-
        cine.)

Born in Sweden in 1858, Dr. Wallin came to the United
States in 1888 and received her M.D. degree in 1893 from
the Women's Medical College of the New York Infirmary
for Women and Children.

1349.   Lucas, Chris. "Barbara Craig: Class of 1976." School of
        Medicine Commentary: University of California, Davis,
        2:4 (April 1973) 12-13. photos. (Medical School Pro-
        files.)

1350.   Lucas, Chris. "Janwyn and Jack Funamura." School of
        Medicine Commentary: University of California, Davis,
        2:2 (February 1973) 4-5. photos. (Medical School Pro-
        files.)

1351.   "Lulu C. Fleming, M.D." Double Cross and Medical Mis-
        sionary Record, 14 (September 1899) 161-162.
        Dr. Fleming (1862-1899) labored as a medical missionary
        in the Congo.

1352.   Lynch, Frank W. "In Memory: Margaret Schulze." Med-
        ical Woman's Journal, 50:5 (May 1943) 132.
        Dr. Schulze's medical interests lay in gynecological pathol-
        ogy. In 1932 she presented a paper on granulosa-cell tu-
        mors of the ovary before the first meeting of the Pacific
        Coast Gynecologic Society: this study was "one of the first
        satisfactory papers on this subject in American literature."

1353.   Lynn, Ethel. The Adventures of a Woman Hobo. George
        H. Doran Company, New York, New York, 1917, 296 pp.
        A series of misfortunes in the life of Dr. Lynn and her
        husband led to a daring scheme. First, the San Francisco
        earthquake destroyed her growing practice and her husband's
        position. Then, after moving to Chicago they were struck
        by the panic of 1907. Finally, Dr. Lynn learned she had
        incipient tuberculosis. "To live in a hovel; to drag my
        weary body for miles in search of work; to cough my lungs
        out--this will be my life in Chicago.... Oh, my beautiful,
        my California!" So they packed a few belongings and headed
        west--on a tandem bicycle! Their adventures, complete
        with furtive railroad hops as they huddled in boxcars, are
        recounted in diary fashion. The pair reached California,
        but no hint is given regarding their subsequent fortunes.

1354.   Lyons, Dorothy J. "Paula Horn, M.D." Journal of the
        American Medical Women's Association, 13:6 (June
        1958) 257. port. (Album of Women in Medicine.)
        Paula Horn served as assistant medical director of the Los
        Angeles County General Hospital, 1934-1940. As an ob-
        stetrical consultant in contagious diseases, she started
        helping women with poliomyelitis give birth. As a result
        of having helped to deliver a baby in a respirator case by
        cesarean section in 1948 during a poliomyelitis epidemic,

she was asked to present a paper on "Pregnancy Compli-
cated by Poliomyelitis" to the International Congress of
Gynecology and Obstetrics, in Geneva, Switzerland.

1355.   "M. D., Mrs. and Mme. Trustee." Jefferson Medical Col-
            lege: Alumni Bulletin, 24:1 (Fall 1974) 15.   port.
         A member of Jefferson's board of trustees, Dr. Marie Oli-
         vieri Russell is a pediatric hematologist.

1356.   "Mabel Grier Lesher, M.D." Medical Woman's Journal,
            54:3 (March 1947) 53.   port.   (News Notes.)
         Dr. Lesher received her M. D. degree from Johns Hopkins
         Medical School.   Her professional activities and appoint-
         ments are herein presented.

1357.   "Mabel M. Akin, M.D." Medical Woman's Journal, 52:4
            (April 1945) 50.
         Dr. Akin (whose portrait appears on the front cover of this
         issue of the Journal) is profiled in part through an excerpt
         from Who's Who Among the Women of the Nation.

1358.   MacDonald, Carolyn N.   "A Medical Summer in Europe."
            Medical Review of Reviews, 41:12 (December 1935) 633-
            640.
         Dr. MacDonald relates incidents and observations from her
         travels and studies in Europe just prior to World War II.
         Dr. MacDonald especially discusses life and medical matters
         in Germany.

1359.   Macfarlane, Catharine.   "Elizabeth S. Waugh, M.D.: Thir-
            ty-fourth President of the American Medical Women's
            Association." Journal of the American Medical Women's
            Association, 5:10 (October 1950) 415.   port.
         Elizabeth S. Waugh was a specialist in obstetrics and gyne-
         cology.   A list of her professional affiliations is given.

1360.   Macfarlane, Catharine.   "Martha Tracy, M.D.: Dean Emer-
            itus, Woman's Medical College of Pennsylvania, 1876-
            1942." Medical Woman's Journal, 49:4 (April 1942)
            102-105.   port.
         A professor of hygiene, then professor of preventive medi-
         cine, and from 1917 to 1940, dean of the Woman's Medical
         College, Martha Tracy ended her career working for the
         Philadelphia Department of Health.   Under her direction,
         community health defense squads were being organized in
         each defense zone of the city after Pearl Harbor.   Her
         closest friend was Dr. Ellen C. Potter.

1361.   Macfarlane, Catharine.   "Memoir of Martha Tracy." Trans-
            actions and Studies of the College of Physicians of Phil-
            adelphia, 10:3 (December 1942) 179-181.
         This memoir is concluded with a list of scientific and other
         writings of Dr. Tracy.

1362.   Macfarlane, Catharine. "Memorial to Margaret Castex
         Sturgis (1885-1962)." Journal of the American Medical
         Women's Association, 18:4 (April 1963) 322-323. port.
         Margaret Castex Sturgis served on the faculty of the Wo-
         man's Medical College of Pennsylvania in the gynecology de-
         partment.   A tribute to her by Samuel B. Sturgis, her hus-
         band, includes, "To Margaret and to my mother, the two
         women in my life, I owe that in life which I have enjoyed
         or accomplished."

1363.   Macfarlane, Catharine and Ratterman, Helena T. "Mabel
         E. Gardner, M.D." Journal of the American Medical
         Women's Association, 9:12 (December 1954) 411. port.
         (Past Presidents of AMWA.)
         Dr. Gardner was recipient of the Elizabeth Blackwell Medal
         (an award for the outstanding woman physician of the year),
         principally for her services to the Association in establish-
         ing junior branches in medical schools.

1364.   McFerran, Ann. Elizabeth Blackwell: First Woman Doc-
         tor.   Grosset & Dunlap, New York, New York, 1966,
         175 pp. illus. (Pioneer Books.)
         Part of the "Pioneer Books" series, this book for young
         readers traces Elizabeth Blackwell's life from the time she
         was a young girl in England, to her death in 1910.   Empha-
         sized are the influences upon Dr. Blackwell's character:
         her father ("Elizabeth is, in every way her father's daugh-
         ter"), a hatred of slavery, and a belief in women's rights.
         Cartoon-like illustrations complement the text, which contains
         fictionalized dialogue.

1365.   McGraw, Harriet G. "'Lady Dr. DaFoe.'" Medical Wo-
         man's Journal, 51:9 (September 1944) 30-33, 37. port.
         The first Icelandic woman to graduate in medicine, Harriet
         G. McGraw received two M.D.s: from Bennett Medical
         College (1907) and from Loyola University (1908).   In this
         autobiography she recalls her two decades of general prac-
         tice in rural Nebraska and a high point in her life--being
         a guest of Mrs. Roosevelt at the White House.

1366.   McGrew, Elizabeth A.; Bennett, Granville A.; Hick, Ford K.;
         and Tucker, B. Fain. "Memorial Service for Carroll
         La Fleur Birch: August 9, 1969, The Methodist Tem-
         ple, Chicago, Illinois." Journal of the American Med-
         ical Women's Association, 24:10 (October 1969) 822-
         825.
         Active in the American Medical Women's Association, Car-
         roll La Fleur Birch was honored by having an award named
         after her.   The award is given to the woman medical stu-
         dent submitting the best scientific manuscript.   Dr. Birch
         had great interest in parasitology, hematology, and the
         genetic aspects of hemophilia.   In the College of Medicine
         at the University of Illinois, she worked in the hospital

wards, research, and teaching laboratories of pathology and
microbiology. She did studies dealing with malaria, leprosy,
sleeping sickness, and certain diseases caused by intestinal
parasites. While in India, she helped reorganize the control and administration of the Lady Hardinge Medical College
and Hospital for Women and Children in New Delhi.

1367.   McGuinness, Madge C. L.   "Mary Theresa Greene, M. D."
         Journal of the American Medical Women's Association,
         10:2 (February 1955) 66. port. (Album of Women in
         Medicine.)
         Dr. Greene, as one of the pioneer medical women of west-
         ern New York, founded Riverside Hospital, which later be-
         came Lafayette General Hospital in Buffalo. The only wo-
         man physician in Wyoming County, New York at the time,
         she served as president of the Wyoming County Medical
         Society.

1368.   McKibbin-Harper, Mary.   "Anna E. Broomall, M. D. (1847-
         1931)."   Medical Review of Reviews, 39:3 (March 1933)
         132-139.
         This article illustrates how closely connected the history
         of the Woman's Medical College of Pennsylvania is with the
         life of Anna E. Broomall: as student (graduating in 1871),
         as professor, obstetrician, and surgeon. In addition to de-
         tails of Dr. Broomall's education and 32-year career, in-
         formation about her personality and avocations is provided
         through reminiscences by Drs. Kate Mead and Mary Gris-
         com.

1369.   McKibbin-Harper, Mary.   The Doctor Takes a Holiday:
         An Autobiographical Fragment.   The Torch Press,
         Cedar Rapids, Iowa, 1941, 349 pp. photos. (A Book-
         fellow Book.)
         Dr. McKibbin-Harper--who for 12 years edited Women in
         Medicine, the publication of the American Medical Women's
         Association--dedicated this book to the Association. The
         book, one of several she has written about her travels,
         was "culled from a diary covering travel of nearly two
         years ... and yet other visits in the Near East" during the
         mid-1920s. The material was updated through correspon-
         dence to include data from the 1930s. Although observations
         of Palestine, Egypt, Malaya, Sarawak, and Japan are in-
         cluded, the text emphasizes India and China. The author's
         perspective is a combination of sociology, history, tourism,
         and professional views of medical practice and the role of
         medical women in each country. References to sociocul-
         tural conditions which prevent indigenous people from prac-
         ticing birth control typify her observations. There are a
         few photos of tourist sights and medical situations. Al-
         though there are frequent references to women physicians
         visited by the author, no name index is included.

1370.   McKibbin-Harper, Mary. "In Memoriam: Lulu Hunt Peters,
         M.D." Medical Review of Reviews, 41:8 (August 1935)
         428-431.
         A 1909 medical graduate of the Southern University of Cali-
         fornia, Lulu Hunt Peters was the first woman intern at the
         Los Angeles County Hospital. A specialist in dietetics, Dr.
         Hunt wrote a syndicated newspaper column on diet and
         health, as well as two well-known books, Diet and Health,
         a Key to the Calories, and Diet for Children. Dr. Peters
         died in 1930.

1371.   McKibbin-Harper, Mary. "Kate Campbell Hurd-Mead: 1876-
         1941." Women in Medicine, 72 (April 1941) 20. port.
         Kate Campbell Hurd-Mead's major contribution was her His-
         tory of Women in Medicine, which serves as a "professional
         family tree" for women doctors. Using the most approved
         methods of research, she documented "that women were
         learned physicians four thousand years ago." This obituary
         includes two brief articles by Kate Hurd-Mead: "Trotula's
         Gynecology and Obstetrics" and "History of Medicine."
         [Both these articles appear independently under Dr. Hurd-
         Mead's name in the HISTORY OF WOMEN IN MEDICINE sec-
         tion of this bibliography.]

1372.   McKibbin-Harper, Mary. "A Medical Woman Looks at
         China." Medical Review of Reviews, [35]:11 (November
         1929) 565-578.
         The author, who went to China in 1926, records her ob-
         servations of Chinese lifestyles, and reports on Chinese
         medical practices.

1373.   McKibbin-Harper, Mary. "A Medical Woman Looks at
         Mother India." Medical Review of Reviews, 35:9 (Sep-
         tember 1929) 457-476.
         The author mixes personal observations of Indian customs
         and living conditions with an informal report of hospitals
         and schools and the work of British and Indian women phy-
         sicians.

1374.   McNutt, Sarah J. "Medical Women, Yesterday and Today."
         Medical Record, 94:4 (27 July 1918) 135-139. (Original
         Articles.) (Presentation, Meeting, Women's New York
         State Medical Society, Albany, New York, 20 May
         1918.)
         Recalling her experiences as a student at the Women's
         Medical College of the New York Infirmary for Women and
         Children, and as an intern at the Infirmary, Dr. McNutt
         tells of her love and respect for Dr. Emily Blackwell. In
         1888, Dr. McNutt obtained a charter from the state legisla-
         ture to open Babies' Hospital in New York City. Medical
         care there was supervised by her and her sister, Dr. Julia
         G. McNutt. Concluding her speech, Dr. McNutt summarizes
         the present status of women physicians. She notes that

over 40 coeducational medical colleges in the United States
admit women on the same basis as men. And of the more
than 6,000 American women physicians, over 2,000 (over
30 per cent) have registered for war relief.

1375.   Macy, Mary Sutton. "Isabelle Thompson Smart, M.D."
         Medical Woman's Journal, 51:5 (May 1944) 28, 39.
         port.
         Dr. Smart worked as medical examiner of mentally defec-
         tive children for the New York City Board of Education.

1376.   "Madame President." New England Journal of Medicine,
         237:20 (13 November 1947) 749-750. (Editorial.)
         This article gives the family background and a brief biogra-
         phy of Dr. Martha May Eliot, an advocate of governmental
         support for health services for all people.

1377.   Maisel, Albert Q. "Dr. Sabin's Second Career." Survey
         Graphic, 36 (February 1947) 138-140. port.
         An eminent anatomist, Florence Rena Sabin divided her
         "first career" between teaching at Johns Hopkins University
         (1902-1925) and scientific study as a member of the Rocke-
         feller Institute for Medical Research (1925-1938). Retired
         in her home state of Colorado, the 73-year-old physician
         was asked to head a subcommittee on health. Called back
         into action by Colorado's high disease and death rates, Dr.
         Sabin fought for health reform through legislation: "Every-
         body but Florence Sabin calls them the Sabin bills." [This
         article appears in condensed form in Reader's Digest, (May
         1947) 9-12.]

1378.   "Major Margaret Janeway, M.C., A.U.S." Women in Med-
         icine, 87 (January 1945) 15-16. port.
         Margaret Janeway joined the U.S. army in 1942 as a con-
         tract surgeon (the army was not commissioning women med-
         ical officers) and was assigned to the WACs. Her respon-
         sibility was to inspect the medical facilities of all WAC
         installations in Africa and Italy. After the war, she was
         attached to the Women's Health and Welfare Unit, Office of
         the Surgeon General, Washington, D.C.

1379.   "Malnutrition in Africa." Buffalo Physician, (Fall 1975)
         26-28. photos.
         Dr. Charlotte Catz describes her African tour, during which
         she lectured on medical and nutritional topics. She cur-
         rently supervises research funding at the National Institute
         of Health and Human Development.

1380.   Mann, Helen and Velin, Connie. "International Women's
         Year--A Time for Appreciation." Vital Signs, (October
         1975). ports.
         At St. Joseph Mercy Hospital in Ann Arbor, Michigan [Vi-
         tal Signs is a publication of this hospital], 77 per cent of

the total hospital employees are women. Four of these women are interviewed during this International Women's Year.
Dr. Kathryn Richards, a surgeon, is one of those interviewed. This article gives biographical information on Dr.
Richards, a graduate of the University of Michigan Medical
School, as well as her opinions on topics of health care.
Dr. Richards feels that the fact that she is a woman is not
an obstacle in her dealings with fellow surgeons, because in
the "Ann Arbor setting" many women work in previously
male-dominated fields.

1381.   Manton, Ann P. D. "Esther E. Bartlett, M.D." Journal
        of the American Medical Women's Association, 10:6
        (June 1955) 217. port. (Album of Women.)
        As an anesthesiologist who studied under Ralph M. Waters,
        the father of anesthesiology, Dr. Bartlett's primary inter-
        ests lie in furthering the medical education of women phy-
        sicians at the New England Hospital in Boston.

1382.   Marble, Ella M. S. "The First Pan-American Medical
        Congress--Some of the Women Who Took Part." Wo-
        man's Medical Journal, 1:11 (October 1893) 199-201.
        During the Congress, held in September [1893], Dr. Eliza
        H. Root of Chicago read a paper on midwifery "and the de-
        sirability of a national law for the extermination of this
        class." Dr. Marble recalls her delight in noticing the "in-
        tense interest expressed on every masculine face" in the
        audience during Dr. Root's presentation. Dr. Sarah Hackett
        Stevenson, who "believes that the time has passed when it
        is necessary to have much if anything exclusively for wo-
        men," also read at this Congress a paper in which women
        physicians were "invited" to stand "shoulder to shoulder
        with their brothers." Other women who attended the con-
        ference are mentioned in this report.

1383.   "Marcelle Bernard, M.D. '44: The First Woman President."
        Chironian, 27:2 (February 1966) 15, 17. port.
        An alumna of New York Medical College's class of 1944,
        Marcelle Bernard became the first woman president of the
        1700-member Bronx County Medical Society. She has been
        a general practitioner in the Bronx for 15 years. "Dr.
        Bernard regards her success in a difficult profession, es-
        pecially against the prejudicial odds, not in an 'I told you
        so' Carrie Nation fashion, rather ... with the character-
        istic grace and femininity of the most attractive lady she
        is....'"

1384.   "Margaret C. Lewis M.D." Medical Woman's Journal, 49:
        5 (May 1942) 153.
        A graduate of Boston University Medical School, Dr. Lewis
        (whose portrait appears on the front cover of this issue of
        the Journal) serves as health and safety advisor on the Girl
        Scout national staff.

1385.   "Margaret Castex Sturgis, M.D." Medical Woman's Jour-
             nal, 50:2 (February 1943) 56.
          Dr. Sturgis (whose portrait appears on the front cover of
          this issue of the Journal) graduated in 1915 from the Wo-
          man's Medical College of Pennsylvania.   This article gives
          a brief professional biography of Dr. Sturgis.

1386.   "Margaret H. Rockhill." Medical Woman's Journal, 48:6
             (June 1941) 183.   (Editorial.)
          This editorial mourns the loss of Margaret H. Rockhill,
          who, although she never studied medicine herself, founded
          the first medical journal edited by and published for women.

1387.   "Margo Longo Still Does It Her Way." The Mayo Alumnus,
             11:3 (July 1975) 36-39.   port.
          Dr. Longo is a Mayo-trained surgeon who, with George and
          Ethel Smith, set up a surgical practice in Lafayette, Louisi-
          ana.   A brief biographical sketch of Dr. Longo is presented.

1388.   "Marguerite Patricia McCarthy, M.D." Medical Woman's
             Journal, 50:6 (June 1943) 155-156.
          Dr. McCarthy (whose portrait appears on the cover of this
          issue of the Journal) came from a family in which the fath-
          er believed in equality for women (her mother died when
          Dr. McCarthy was four years old).   Dr. McCarthy's sister
          studied law, and she herself graduated from the Woman's
          Medical College of Pennsylvania in 1929.   This article gives
          biographical data.

1389.   "Marie E. Zakrzewska, M.D.:   From Berlin to Life in New
             York." Woman's Medical Journal, 11:4 (April 1901)
             135-138.   (Biographical.)

1390.   "Marie E. Zakrzewska, M.D.:   Life in School of Midwifery.'
             Woman's Medical Journal, 11:2 (February 1901) 57-59.
             (Biographical.)

1391.   "Marie E. Zakrzewska, M.D.:   Life in the Hospital and Its
             Untimely Ending." Woman's Medical Journal, 11:3
             (March 1901) 91-94.   (Biographical.)
          The events leading up to Zakrzewska's departure for Amer-
          ica in 1853 are described.

1392.   "Marie E. Zakrzewska, M.D.:   Life Purposes Realized."
             Woman's Medical Journal, 11:6 (June 1901) 220-222.
             (Biographical.)
          "Throughout the history of the New England Hospital the
          life work of Dr. Zakrzewska is woven and interwoven like
          a thread of gold that lends brilliancy and value to the insti-
          tution."

1393.   "Marie E. Zakrzewska, M.D.:   Meets Dr. Blackwell and
             Enters Medical College." Woman's Medical Journal,
             11:5 (May 1901) 181-184.   (Biographical.)

1394.   "Marie E. Zakrzewska, M.D. The Interregnum." Woman's
         Medical Journal, 11:1 (January 1901) 10-12. (Biograph-
         ical.)

1395.   Marie Elizabeth Zakrzewska, 1829-1902. A Memoir. New
         England Hospital for Women and Children, Boston,
         Massachusetts, 1903, 30 pp. ports.
         This memorial was prepared by the directors of the New
         England Hospital for Women and Children. It traces the
         ancestry and life of Dr. Marie Elizabeth Zakrzewska, born
         in Berlin, Prussia in 1829. Dr. Zakrzewska's personality
         is revealed through anecdotes, and her eventual professional
         successes are outlined, beginning with her appointment in
         1852 as chief accoucheuse at the Berlin School of Midwifery.
         In 1853 Marie sailed for America, where she was to meet
         Elizabeth and Emily Blackwell with whom she cofounded the
         New York Infirmary for Women and Children. Moving to
         Boston, she also founded the New England Hospital for Wo-
         men and Children. Dr. Zakrzewska died on May 12, 1902,
         and this memoir concludes with a reprint of her funeral
         address which she herself had written.

1396.   "Marie Elizabeth Zakrzewska, M.D." Woman's Medical
         Journal, 12:6 (June 1902) 134-137. port. (Obituary.)
         By her own request, Dr. Zakrzewska's funeral service
         excluded religious ceremony. A farewell address to her
         friends, written by Dr. Zakrzewska several months before
         death, was read at the ceremony by Mrs. Emma Merrill
         Buller. The text of that address, along with a tribute to
         her memory by William Lloyd Garrison, is presented in
         this article.

1397.   "Marie J. Mergler, M.D." Woman's Medical Journal, 11:8
         (August 1901) 301-302. (Biographical.)
         Born in Bavaria, Marie Mergler graduated in 1879 from Wo-
         man's Medical College of Chicago. She held several faculty
         positions at her alma mater. In 1882, Dr. Mergler be-
         came one of the first two women to be appointed to the at-
         tending staff of Cook County Hospital. In 1889, she was ap-
         pointed dean of Northwestern University. A distinguished
         diagnostician and abdominal surgeon, Dr. Mergler made
         many contributions to medical literature. She died at the
         age of 50 in May, 1901.

1398.   Marshall, Clara. "Ann Preston, M.D.: A Biographical
         Sketch." Bulletin of the Woman's Medical College of
         Pennsylvania, 65:5 (March 1915) 6-9. port.

1399.   Marshall, R. R. "The First Lady President of a State
         Medical Society." Rocky Mountain Medical Journal, 59
         (November 1962) 35-36.
         [Article not examined by editors.]

1400.   "Martha Eliot, M.D." Journal of the American Medical
             Women's Association, 3:10 (October 1948) 424. port.
         Martha Eliot, associate chief of the Children's Bureau of
         the Federal Security Agency, was the first woman elected
         as president of the American Public Health Association.
         As a pediatrician during the depression and during World
         War II, she was concerned with the health, nutrition, and
         welfare of mothers and children, and under her direction
         from 1932 to 1947 the largest public medical care program
         for mothers and infants was initiated in the United States.
         These programs especially helped wives and children of the
         enlisted men in the lower pay brackets of the armed forces.

1401.   Martin, Elisabeth. "Amy Garrison Kimball, M.D." Jour-
             nal of the American Medical Women's Association, 9:3
             (March 1954) 92. port. (Album of Women in Medicine.)
         Although both of Amy Garrison Brown Kimball's parents
         were physicians, they would not support her desire to be-
         come a doctor, so she had to make her own arrangements.
         She was one of the first women medical students to attend
         the University of Michigan Medical College, one of the first
         women physicians to become a member of the American
         Medical Association, and one of the founders of the Home
         of the Friendless and the Children's Free Kindergarten.
         In 1900 she was the only woman physician from the United
         States to attend the Thirteenth Congress of International
         Medicine.

1402.   Martin, Elisabeth. "Annie Laurie Sawyer." Journal of
             the American Medical Women's Association, 3:2 (Febru-
             ary 1948) 80. (History of Medicine.)
         Annie Laurie Sawyer had a large solo practice in gynecology
         and obstetrics in Atlanta from 1901 to 1930.

1403.   Martindale, Louisa. "Dr. Kate Campbell Mead, of Had-
             dam, Connecticut, U.S.A." Medical Women's Federa-
             tion Quarterly Review, (April 1941) 62-63. (Obituary.)

1404.   Marting, Esther C. "American Medical Women's Associa-
             tion: In Memoriam." Journal of the American Med-
             ical Women's Association, 11:9 (September 1956) 319-
             320.
         Dr. Maude Glasgow, a pioneer in public health and pre-
         ventive medicine, and Dr. Elizabeth Bass, who worked
         throughout her life "to perpetuate the achievements of wo-
         men in medicine," are profiled.

1405.   "Mary Bacon, M.D." Medical Woman's Journal, 51:2
             (February 1944) 36.
         Dr. Bacon (whose portrait appears on the front cover of
         this issue of the Journal) "was the first and is now the only
         woman on the staff of Bridgeton Hospital," Bridgeton, New
         Jersey.

1406.   "Mary Dugan Ardery: President Elect State Society of Iowa
        Medical Women."   Woman's Medical Journal, 14:7
        (July 1904) 147.   port.

1407.   "Mary Ellen Hartman, M.D. Appointed Assistant Dean at
        Woman's Medical College of Pennsylvania."   Journal of
        the American Medical Women's Association, 21:8 (Au-
        gust 1966) 677.   port.
        In 1966 Mary Ellen Hartman was appointed assistant dean of
        the Woman's Medical College of Pennsylvania while she con-
        tinued to serve as assistant professor of anatomy, a post
        she has held since 1963.

1408.   "Mary Harris Thompson, M.D."   Woman's Medical Journal,
        11:9 (September 1901) 333-334.   (Biographical.)

1409.   "Mary J. Ross, M.D."   Journal of the American Medical
        Women's Association, 9:2 (February 1954) 52.   port.
        (Album of Women in Medicine.)
        Mary J. Ross received her medical degree in 1907.   She
        spent most of her medical career in Binghamton, New York
        where she delivered 3,200 babies or four per cent of the
        population of her community.   In 1919 she was instrumental
        in establishing the Well Baby Health Station, which served
        as a place where information about infant and postnatal care
        was disseminated to young mothers.   This program effec-
        tively decreased the infant mortality rate.   She did a great
        deal of unpublicized philanthropy, including devoting her time
        to this education program without pay until Binghamton took
        the program over in 1933.

1410.   "Mary Latimer James, M.D.:   Westchester, Pa."   Med-
        ical Woman's Journal, 52:10 (October 1945) 54-57.
        port.
        In this autobiography, Dr. James traces her life from her
        childhood in Gambier, Ohio through her college days at
        Bryn Mawr and Woman's Medical College of Pennsylvania.
        It was in Pennsylvania that Dr. James determined to be-
        come a medical missionary.   She served in Whiterocks,
        Utah on the Ute Indian Reservation, after which she went
        to China.   Dr. James discusses her work in China, es-
        pecially during the Nationalist revolution in 1911.

1411.   "Mary Luise Diez, M.D."   Medical Woman's Journal, 49:
        7 (July 1942) 223.   (News Notes.)
        Mary Luise Diez had been director of the Division of
        Child Hygiene, Massachusetts Department of Public Health,
        for thirteen years previous to her death on April 12, 1942.
        She was a recognized authority in the field of child hygiene
        and obstetrics.

1412.   "Mary M. Crawford, M.D.:   Medical Woman of the Month."
        Journal of the American Medical Women's Association,

4:5 (May 1949) 216.   port.   (News of Women in Medicine.)
A 1907 graduate of Cornell University's Medical College,
Dr. Mary Crawford "made history by being the first woman
to 'ride the ambulance' in Brooklyn for the Williamsburgh
Hospital." In 1918 she began work on the organization of
the medical division of the Federal Reserve Bank of New
York. A list of her accomplishments and affiliations is in-
cluded.

1413.   "Mary Priestly Rupert, M.D."   Medical Woman's Journal,
            47:1 (January 1940) 32.
        Mary Priestly Sheriff Rupert (whose portrait appears on the
        cover of this issue of the Journal) obtained her degree from
        the Woman's Medical College of Pennsylvania in 1904.   Con-
        tributions she made to her alma mater included organizing
        the Laboratory of Clinical Pathology and serving on the Col-
        lege's executive committee of the board.   Dr. Rupert died
        in 1939.

1414.   "The Mary Putnam Jacobi Fellowship."   Woman's Medical
            Journal, 21:4 (April 1911) 83.
        The first woman to benefit from the Fellowship is Dr. Alice
        Rohde, a 1910 graduate of the medical department of Johns
        Hopkins University.

1415.   "Mary Putnam Jacobi, M.D."   Woman's Medical Journal,
            16:9 (September 1906) 145-146.   (Editorial.)

1416.   "Mary Riggs Noble, M.D."   Medical Woman's Journal, 51:
            1 (January 1944) 32.
        Dr. Noble (whose portrait appears on the front cover of
        this month's Journal) graduated in 1901 from Woman's
        Medical College of Pennsylvania.

1417.   "Mary Theresa Greene, M.D."   Medical Woman's Journal,
            47:6 (June 1940) 184.
        Dr. Greene (whose portrait appears on the front cover of
        this issue of the Journal) received her M.D. at the Univer-
        sity of Michigan in 1890.   After the death of her aunt, Dr.
        Cordelia Greene in 1905, she became proprietor of the
        Greene Sanitarium in Castile, New York.

1418.   "Mary Townsend-Glassen, M.D."   Medical Woman's Jour-
            nal, 50:3 (March 1943) 78.
        Dr. Townsend-Glassen (whose portrait appears on the front
        cover of this issue of the Journal) practiced medicine in
        Phillipsburg, Kansas.   "It takes good health, altruism, en-
        thusiasm, and resiliency to practice medicine in Northwest-
        ern Kansas," says Dr. Townsend-Glassen.

1419.   "Mary Victoria Dryden, M.D."   Medical Woman's Journal,
            54:1 (January 1947) 53.   port.   (In Memory.)

Dr. Dryden studied medicine "in obedience to her mother's wishes," and received her M.D. degree from the University of Michigan in 1898. This brief obituary cites Dr. Dryden's professional activity.

1420. [Mason-Hohl, Elizabeth]. "Bertha L. Selmon, M.D.: 1877-1949." Medical Woman's Journal, 56:3 (March 1949) 35-36.
This obituary of Dr. Selmon mentions her stipulation in her will that another woman physician should take over her records, office, and medical practice in Battle Creek, Michigan.

1421. [Mason-Hohl, Elizabeth]. "Editorial." Medical Woman's Journal, 56:10 (October 1949) 27.
Caroline Louise Avery, who practiced medicine in San Jose, California from 1900 to 1948, died in August [1949]. She willed her eyes to the Stanford University Eye Bank.

1422. Mason-Hohl, Elizabeth. "Rosetta Sherwood Hall: Fifty Years in Practice." Medical Woman's Journal, 49:2 (February 1942) 52. (Editorial.)
An 1889 graduate of the Woman's Medical College of Pennsylvania, Dr. Hall is a "teacher, medical missionary, founder of four hospitals and a medical school, a wife and mother, a revered doctor who at the age of 77 practices actively in her home town."

1423. M[ason]-H[ohl], E[lizabeth]. "Twenty-Five Years Ago: May, 1925." Medical Woman's Journal, 57:5 (May 1950) 40-41. port.
Eliza M. Mosher was for 20 years senior editor of the Medical Woman's Journal. Her editorship initiated the exchange of information and was an impetus to the organization of the women in the medical profession. "Her leadership and example has now at long last given a 'press' and a resultant Pan American Medical Women's Alliance for the scientific, social, and fraternal cooperation of the women doctors of the Americas."

1424. [Mason-Hohl, Elizabeth]. "In Memory." Medical Woman's Journal, 53:4 (April 1946) 53.
Josephine A. Jackson (1865-1945), the first woman intern of Cook County Hospital, turned her Pasadena, California home into a laboratory where she "rehabilitated scores of psychoneurotics."

1425. Mason-Hohl, Elizabeth. "In Memory." Medical Woman's Journal, 54:6 (June 1947) 53.
Dr. Alice Barker-Ellsworth graduated in 1902 from the University of Michigan School of Medicine. She practiced in California. This article presents biographical data on Dr. Barker-Ellsworth.

1426.   "Mathilda Kristina Wallin, M.D." Medical Woman's Jour-
            nal, 49:11 (November 1942) 350.
        Born in Sweden, Mathilda Kristina Wallin came to the United
        States in 1888 and was graduated from the Women's Med-
        ical College of the New York Infirmary for Women and Chil-
        dren in 1893. In this article, which summarizes her pro-
        fessional career, some of her many contributions are high-
        lighted. After the Spanish War, she took charge of a pri-
        vate hospital on Long Island for convalescent soldiers.

1427.   "Maud Conyers Exley: 1876-1924." Bulletin of the Woman's
            Medical College of Pennsylvania, (January 1925). port.

1428.   "May Votaw, M.D." The University of Michigan Hospital
            Star, 23:3 (March 1975) 8. photo.

1429.   "A Medical Romance." Medical Woman's Journal, 55:12
            (December 1948) 61.
        Drs. Ronald and Mary Price have a joint medical practice
        in Armour, South Dakota. As both physicians are pilots,
        they fly seriously ill patients to the Mayo Clinic.

1430.   "Medical School Faculty Honors Dr. Lovejoy." Medical
            Woman's Journal, 51:6 (June 1944) 34.
        This review of Esther Pohl Lovejoy's career [published in-
        itially by a Portland, Oregon newspaper] was prompted by
        a formal tribute to her by the University of Oregon Med-
        ical School in March 1944.

1431.   "Medical School Was Worth the Wait." Jefferson Medical
            College: Alumni Bulletin, 24:1 (Fall 1974) 20-21. port.
        A senior medical student at Jefferson, Joan Simpson has a
        "three-fold minority status": she is a black, a woman, and
        older than the maximum age limit for admission.

1432.   "Medical Student and Interne: Mary Bennett Ritter, M.D.,
            1886." In: Recollections of Cooper Medical College:
            1883-1905. Stanford Medical School, Stanford, Cali-
            fornia, 1964, 1-8, port.
        Dr. Ritter's reminiscences of student days at Cooper Med-
        ical College (now Stanford University's medical department)
        include vivid descriptions of dissecting and surgery experi-
        ences. She spent one Fourth of July alone in the dissecting
        room, getting ahead on an assignment, windows open wide
        because of the odor. "Every few minutes a sheet would be
        blown off, revealing a grinning partially dissected head or
        a seemingly moving foot." During a gruesome cancer opera-
        tion "a student fainted. Soon another; and then a third.
        The three men were stretched out on the floor and no fur-
        ther attention was paid to them.... The two women students
        did not faint and thus disgrace the sex." Anecdotes are re-
        lated about four pioneer women physicians in California:
        Euthanesia S. Meade, Charlotte Brown, C. Annette Buckel,
        and Sarah I. Shuey.

1433.   "Medical Woman of the Month."   Journal of the American
         Medical Women's Association, 3:9 (September 1948)
         372.   port.   (Medical Women in the News.)
         A recipient of many awards for her research in biochem-
         istry, particularly her work on carbohydrate metabolism
         and enzyme reactions, Gerty T. Cori shared the Nobel
         Prize in Physiology and Medicine with her husband Carl,
         and with Bernardo Alberto Houssay of Buenos Aires, for
         their work in 1947 on the synthesis of glycogen.

1434.   Medical Woman's Journal, 56:2 (February 1949) 59.
         Else K. LaRoe, a 1923 graduate of medicine at the Uni-
         versity of Heidelberg and a former leader in the German
         women's movement, recalls an encounter with Hitler.
         Shortly before he came into power, Dr. LaRoe met him in
         her woman's magazine office.   "He told her women were
         good for two things only, to cook and to bear children, and
         she ordered him out of the office."   Dr. LaRoe now is a
         plastic surgeon in New York, and is married to an oil ex-
         ecutive.

1435.   "Medical Women in the News: Catharine Macfarlane, M.D."
         Journal of the American Medical Women's Association,
         3:6 (June 1948) 270.   port.
         Dr. Macfarlane was the first woman to be elected to the
         College of Physicians in Philadelphia and the first woman
         elected as president of the Obstetrical Society of Philadel-
         phia.   Cancer control research was inaugurated by her at
         the Woman's Medical College of Pennsylvania.

1436.   "Medical Women of Today."   Medical and Professional
         Woman's Journal, 40:7 (July 1933) 194-195.
         Biographical sketches are presented of the professional
         lives of the following women: Dr. Connie M. Guion, Dr.
         Catharine Macfarlane, Dr. Zella White Stewart, and Dr.
         Dolores Perez Marchand, the only medical woman, at the
         time of this article, in Ponce, Puerto Rico.

1437.   "Medical Women of Today."   Medical Woman's Journal,
         39:11 (November 1932) 288-289.
         Josephine Baker organized the first Child Health Bureau
         and in 1922 was the first woman to be associated with the
         League of Nations in a professional capacity [other than
         clerical and secretarial].   An expert in industrial medicine,
         Alice Hamilton wrote Industrial Poisons in the United States
         and in 1927 was appointed to the League of Nations' Health
         Committee by the United States.   In recognition of her work
         with sick and destitute refugees through the American Wo-
         men's Hospital established at Pireaus, Greece, the Greek
         government gave a decoration to Angenette Parry.   Active
         in public health work as well as being the only woman mem-
         ber of the French Society of Dermatology and Syphilology to
         which she was appointed in 1909, Daisy M. O. Robinson in-

troduced the Noguchi test of serum diagnosis in France in
1909. "... by her consecration to [her] work [Florence
Rena Sabin] has attained a position in the world of science
second to few men."

1438.   "Medical Women of Today." Medical Woman's Journal,
         39:12 (December 1932) 309-310.
         Bertha Van Hoosen was the only medical woman holding a
         full professorship in an obstetrical department of a coeduca-
         tional university at the time this article was written, as
         well as being one of the comparatively few women surgeons
         holding a membership in the American College of Surgeons.
         Dr. Van Hoosen was elected the first president of the Med-
         ical Women's National Association in 1915, became a mem-
         ber of the editorial staff of the Medical Woman's Journal,
         and was instrumental in the organizing of the International
         Medical Women's Association. Georgine Luden worked at
         the Mayo Clinic and Mayo Foundation in cancer research
         and in 1923 joined the staff of the Medical Woman's Journal.
         The first and only woman in the world to hold a position
         as head of a department of social hygiene, Rachelle Yarros
         was also the first woman physician to occupy a chair of ob-
         stetrics on a co-educational faculty. When she lived in
         Chicago during the early days of her career, "she preferred
         to work among the poor people of the city, and there was
         an abundance of such work in the territory in which Hull
         House was located, where Dr. Yarros lived and where the
         major portion of her work was done." As clinical director
         of the Women's Service of St. Elizabeth's Hospital, Wash-
         ington, D. C. Mary O'Malley made it possible for over 100
         women physicians to prepare to become psychiatrists. Au-
         thor of The Woman Doctor and Her Future, the British
         physician, Louise Martindale, was one of the first two wo-
         men to be appointed Justice of the Peace at the Brighton
         Borough, and served as president of the London Association
         of the Medical Women's Federation.

1439.   "Medical Women of Today." Medical Woman's Journal, 40:
         3 (March 1933) 68-69.
         Biographical sketches are presented of the professional lives
         of the following women: Dr. Rosalie S. Morton, the first
         woman physician to be appointed by the American Medical
         Association (AMA) as an officer in one of its sections, Dr.
         Maude E. Abbott, Dr. Elizabeth B. Thelberg, and Dr.
         Lillian H. South, the first woman physician to be elected
         an officer of the AMA.

1440.   "Medical Women of Today." Medical Woman's Journal,
         40:4 (April 1933) 92-93.
         Biographical sketches are presented on the professional
         lives of the following women: Dr. Florence Brown Sherbon,
         Dr. Marion Craig Potter, and Dr. Belle Anderson Gem-
         mell.

1441.   "Medical Women of Today." Medical Woman's Journal, 40:
        5 (May 1933) 116-117.
        Biographical sketches are presented of the professional ac-
        tivities of the following women: Dr. Vida A. Latham (M. D.,
        D. D. S.), Dr. Lena K. Sadler, Dr. Susanne Sanderson, and
        Dr. Barbara Hunt.

1442.   "Medical Women of the Year." Journal of the American
        Medical Women's Association, 12:12 (December 1957)
        445-449.   ports.
        Francis Bartlett-Tyson did general practice in West Phila-
        delphia and was appointed chief of the Gynecology Clinic of
        Woman's Hospital.   After marriage in 1909 to William Ty-
        son, she retired from practice on request of her husband.
        After doing volunteer work for the Red Cross for several
        years, and after World War I had drained most of the doc-
        tors from her community of Leonia, New Jersey, she was
        solicited by a delegation of townspeople to return to active
        practice.   She became the first school physician and town
        health officer in Leonia and successfully used toxoid treat-
        ments against diphtheria and as a result was effective in
        eliminating this disease from that community.   Madelaine
        Ray Brown, a victim of multiple sclerosis, lost the sight in
        her left eye and in 1954 was confined to a wheel chair:
        "This has not interfered with her work.   It is her ambition
        to continue with her teaching of Harvard students and with
        her work at the Massachusetts General Hospital." In 1954
        Dr. Brown received the Elizabeth Blackwell Award of the
        New York Infirmary for her work in neurology.   Clara G.
        Cook and Mary Margaret Frazer were both active in civic
        and medical organizations.   Mary J. Kaymierczak was active
        in child health clinics in Buffalo, New York, and with or-
        phanages, and in 1939 she helped to establish St. Rita's
        Home for Exceptional Children which gained recognition
        through the book, My Son's Story.

1443.   "Medical Women of the Year." Journal of the American
        Medical Women's Association, 13:1 (January 1958) 30.
        port.
        Dr. Kathleen Carmen Jones was, in 1955, chosen by Baylor
        University as one of the outstanding women graduates.   In
        1953 Dr. Jones was chosen by the Baptist Foreign Mission
        Board as the first mission doctor to Indonesia.

1444.   "Medical Women of the Year." Journal of the American
        Medical Women's Association, 13:12 (December 1958)
        512-521.   ports.
        Thelma Brumfield Dunn was one of six women physicians
        selected by the State Department to represent American
        medicine in Russia.   Dr. Dunn has devoted most of her life
        to the study of cancer.   "She is, without doubt, the world
        authority on the pathology of mice.   Investigators in this
        field from all over the world consult her.   Her morphologic

classification of mammary tumors and leukemia in mice is
used widely as standard reference." A biochemist, Eleanor
Mary Humphreys, explored the many problems presented by
diabetes before the days of insulin. Later in her career,
she taught pathology and from 1943-44 was president of the
Chicago Pathological Society. One of four women physicians
who received commissions during World War I as first
lieutenants, Lydia Bauer Hauck was also active during
World War II, sending food and clothing to women physicians
in Europe. An obstetrician, Helena T. Ratterman was
president of the American Medical Women's Association.
Janet Sterling Baldwin researched and created complete care
programs for children with cardiac disease. Lauretta Bender authored "Visual Motor Gestalt Test and Its Clinical
Use" and four volumes of "Bellevue Studies," from 1952 to
1956. She has contributed to scientific literature in the
fields of child psychiatry, clinical psychiatry, clinical neurology, neuropathology, pathology, psychology, Gestalt psychology, projective techniques in observation and treatment
of children, and education. Ruth E. Wagner owned and operated a 20-bed hospital for ten years. She has been concerned with community service and anticipated that over-
crowded housing would result in water shortages and problems of sanitation. She also helped to preserve vacant land
to be used for recreational purposes for future generations.
Employed by the Georgia Department of Public Health, Clara
B. Barrett became director of the Tuberculosis Control Division. Geneva Beatty has helped individuals in the under-
developed countries of the world through giving of her knowledge and skill to various hospitals supported by the College
of Medical Evangelists. As chief medical officer at the
Federal Reformatory for Women at Alderson, West Virginia,
in 1929 Edda Von Bose's responsibilities included heading
the Reformatory's Venereal Disease and Addiction Clinics
and treating as many as 2,000 at one time; she acquired
an extensive background in, and material on, drug addiction.
Ella Avery Mead started her career in public health in
Weld County, Colorado as city health officer.

1445.   "Medical Women of the Year." Journal of the American
          Medical Women's Association, 14:12 (December 1959)
          1098-1108. ports.
          Sara E. Branham was chief of the Section on Bacterial
          Toxins of the National Institutes of Health and a pioneer in
          the field of bacteriology. Camille Mermod was president
          of the American Medical Women's Association, 1954-1955;
          1956-1957. "So many of [Edith Rebecca Hatch's] private
          patients were treated at Millard Fillmore Hospital [Buffalo]
          that its lying-in room was fondly dubbed 'the Hatch-ery' by
          the staff." Margaret Noyes Kleinert was a pioneer in the
          field of otolaryngology and instrumental in the establishment
          of a special collection on women in medicine at the Women's
          Archives at Radcliffe College, Cambridge, Massachusetts.

Katharine Dodd worked in child welfare in Russia for nine
months under the auspices of the American Friends Service
Committee and American Women's Hospitals. Several other
women are profiled.

1446.   "Medical Women of the Year." Journal of the American
         Medical Women's Association, 17:3 (March 1962) 254-
         261. ports.
         Eleven women are presented as the Medical Women of the
         Year; a brief biographical sketch of each is given. Sketches
         include training, specialties, professional activities, honors,
         awards, and memberships.

1447.   "Medical Women of the Year ... 1955." Journal of the
         American Medical Women's Association, 10:11 (Novem-
         ber 1955) 394-403. ports.
         Among the women mentioned in this article are Josephine
         Renshaw, recognized for her "efforts ... to improve the re-
         lations between the public and the medical profession."
         Marie Ortmayer is recognized for "her research and ac-
         complishments in the field of gastroenterology." Mabel E.
         Gardner has been active in the American Medical Women's
         Association. Elaine Pandia Ralli has done significant re-
         search and teaching in the area of metabolic disturbances
         and nutritional diseases. Hilda H. Kroeger, a pediatrician
         and administrator, helped design an efficient labor and de-
         livery room suite in Pittsburgh's Elizabeth Steel Magee Hos-
         pital and has been active as well with the American Com-
         mittee on Maternal Welfare. Mary J. Ross started a free
         baby clinic in Binghamton, was city physician in that city,
         "the first woman to receive this appointment," and served
         for 20 years as "Examiner in Lunacy." Ruth M. Kraft was,
         among other "firsts," the first woman physician to serve as
         camp doctor for the New York Herald Tribune camp at
         Loomis, New York in the summer of 1938; the first woman
         physician to become chief of pediatrics at Grace Hospital,
         Detroit (1949); the first woman to be made an honorary
         registered pharmacist by the Board of Pharmacy of the
         State of Michigan, in 1951; and first resident sent from New
         Haven Hospital to the University of Pennsylvania Hospital.
         Elizabeth Mason-Hohl was nominated in 1954 (and renom-
         inated in 1955) for her "untiring efforts to further women
         in medicine." She was a cofounder and past president of
         the Pan American Medical Women's Alliance. One of the
         first women doctors in Minnesota, Nellie O. Barsness spe-
         cialized in radiology when x-ray machines were first intro-
         duced, and in otolaryngology. She was director for the
         Women's Christian Temperance Union for several years in
         Minnesota. Berta M. Meine was selected for her services
         to the Woman's Hospital in Philadelphia. Harriet E. Gil-
         lette was named for "her insight and farsighted approach to
         the needs of the cerebral palsied and the aged." Mary B.
         Olney is executive director and originator of a camp estab-

lished in 1938 for diabetic children.   Because of her work
as a "mountain doctor" and her work with school children
in the Asheville, North Carolina schools studying medical
defects that cause students to do poor work, and helping
parents correct the unsatisfactory conditions, she was honored as Medical Woman of the Year.   She was the first woman to be appointed a health officer in North Carolina.
Harriett Hardy has done extensive work in preventive medicine in the field of radioactive materials, lead poisoning,
silicosis, asbestosis, and has made the most extensive contributions of any worker in the study of beryllium poisoning.
May Owen has been active in various community and medical organizations in Texas.

1448.   "Medical Women of the Year ... 1956." Journal of the
          American Medical Women's Association, 11:12 (Decem-
          ber 1956) 434-441. ports.
Carolyn S. Pincock's principal professional interest has been
the Luetic Clinic for syphilitic children at the Children's
Hospital in Washington, D.C.   She was the first civilian doctor in Washington to use penicillin during the early days of
World War II.   Vida Annette Latham came to the United
States from England.   Receiving her D.D.S., and later her
M.D., she was the first woman to lecture on tropical medicine at the Woman's Medical College of Pennsylvania and
the first woman to serve as an elected delegate from the
Royal Societies in London for the convocation at the University of Chicago.   Among her many firsts is president of the
first World Columbian Dental Congress.   A woman doctor
who became chief emeritus of, and consultant to, the department of endocrinology at the Newark Beth Israel Hospital, Rita S. Finkler said upon being named Medical Woman
of the Year, "My daughter and my grandchildren are my
greatest and proudest achievements."   A radiologist, Esther
C. Marting specialized in tumor diagnosis and radiation
therapy.   Helen Johnston, a gerontologist, has been active
in the American Medical Women's Association (AMWA) as
president (1946-47) and as a representative to the International Association.   Viola G. Brekke was chief pathologist
and director of laboratories at Highland Park General Hospital in Detroit.   Ruth Hartley Weaver was instrumental in
getting tuberculosis surveys into the Philadelphia public
schools, wrote a series of articles in Philadelphia Medicine
interpreting the school health program to medical authorities,
and was working to introduce psychiatric programs into the
public schools.   Helen Knudsen helped administer a federal
aid program to 56 hospitals and public health centers in
Minnesota.   Alice Hamilton researched occupational disease
and worked at Hull House.   She received her award "not
only for excelling in the field of medicine but also for her
shining example to all of us of how to grow old gracefully."
Mary Mitchell Henry delivered about 5,700 babies and was
active in many civic organizations as well as several medical
societies.

1449.   Medical Women's International Association. Esther Pohl
         Lovejoy, M.D., Founder and First President, Medical
         Women's International Association. MWIA Golden Ju-
         bilee Souvenir. The Philippine Medical Women's Asso-
         ciation, Quezon City, Philippines, 1970, 15 pp.
         [Pamphlet not examined by editors.]

1450.   "Meet the Dean: Marion Fay." MD, 6:8 (August 1951)
         324-326. photos.
         Marion Fay, Ph.D., dean of the Woman's Medical College
         of Pennsylvania, is interviewed herein.

1451.   Melampus. "Dr. Mary Walker and Lady Physicians." The
         National Reformer, 9 (1867).
         [Article not examined by editors.]

1452.   Melville, Mildred McClellan. "Dr. Florence Rena Sabin:
         Woman with Two Careers." Today's Health, 31 (Feb-
         ruary 1953) 42-43, 64-65. port.

1453.   Memoir of Susan Dimock, Resident Physician of the New
         England Hospital for Women and Children. John Wilson
         & Son, Cambridge, Massachusetts, 1875, 103 pp.
         This book is a collection of memorial tributes to and a bio-
         graphical sketch of Susan Dimock, who died in 1875 at the
         age of 28 in a shipwreck while en route to Europe. Born
         in North Carolina, Dr. Dimock initiated her medical studies
         at the New England Hospital for Women and Children in 1866.
         She twice applied to Harvard and was twice refused admis-
         sion. She completed her studies at the University of Zurich
         in 1871. In 1872, Dr. Dimock returned to the New England
         Hospital for Women and Children to take charge of the insti-
         tution.

1454.   "Memorial Meeting, Dr. Elizabeth Blackwell and Dr. Emily
         Blackwell. Held in Academy of Medicine, New York,
         January 25, 1911. Special Report." Woman's Medical
         Journal, 21:2 (February 1911) 21-27. ports.

1455.   "Memorial Membership." Women in Medicine, 51 (January
         1936) 25. port.
         Dr. Mary Harris Thompson was "'the first woman surgeon
         who performed capital operations entirely on her own re-
         sponsibility.'" In 1865 she founded the Mary Thompson
         Hospital (Women and Children's) of Chicago. In 1869 she
         founded a Woman's Medical College and in 1874 a nurse's
         training school, "the first in the middle west." A brief
         account is given of the original hospital and its subsequent
         locations.

1456.   "Memorial Tablet for Dr. Emily Blackwell." Woman's
         Medical Journal, 25:11 (November 1915) 253. (Editor-
         ial.)

Victor David Brenner has designed a bronze medallion that has been placed in the New York Infirmary for Women and Children to honor Emily Blackwell.

1457.   "Memorial to Dr. Beulah Cushman (1890-1964)." Journal of
         the American Medical Women's Association, 19:11 (No-
         vember 1964) 979-980. port.
         Dr. Beulah Cushman, an "eminent ophthalmologist," re-
         ceived her M.D. degree in 1916 from the College of Medi-
         cine of the University of Illinois.

1458.   "Memorial to Doctor Dennis." Medical Woman's Journal,
         45:11 (November 1938) 344.
         A tribute to Mary E. Dennis (1870-1938) includes facts about
         her family background and her medical practice in Los An-
         geles and Catalina Island.

1459.   Menendian, Rose V. "Bertha Van Hoosen: A Surgical
         Daughter's Impressions." Journal of the American
         Medical Women's Association, 20:4 (April 1965) 349-
         350.
         This article consists of a personal view of Dr. Van Hoosen
         by one of the women who trained under her.

1460.   Menendian, Rose V.; Gardner, Mable E.; and Lovejoy,
         Esther Pohl. "Bertha Van Hoosen, M.D." Journal of
         the American Medical Women's Association, 12:1 (Janu-
         ary 1957) 22-24. port.
         This article is a tribute to Dr. Van Hoosen by three wo-
         men physicians who knew her in the capacity of friend,
         teacher, and in relation to her work with the MWIA, re-
         spectively.

1461.   Mermod, Camille. "Judith Ahlem, M.D.: Thirty-Seventh
         President of the American Medical Women's Association."
         Journal of the American Medical Women's Association,
         8:9 (September 1953) 311. port.
         Born on a Winnebago Indian reservation in Nebraska, Dr.
         Ahlem traveled extensively and practiced at the Livermore
         Sanitarium in Livermore, California.

1462.   Mermod, Camille. "Memorial to Emily Dunning Barringer
         (1877-1961)." Journal of the American Medical Women's
         Association, 16:12 (December 1961) 958. port.
         This article presents a brief sketch of the life of Dr. Emily
         Dunning Barringer, "a champion of women physicians' rights
         and the first woman to serve on the staff of a general mu-
         nicipal hospital in New York City."

1463.   Merritt, Emma L. "Address Delivered by Dr. Emma L.
         Merritt at a Banquet Given by Women Physicians, Oc-
         tober 11, 1924, in Honor of the Eighty-Third Birthday
         of Dr. Lucy Maria Field Wanzer." California and

Western Medicine, 23 (May 1925) 599-601. port.
The first woman to graduate from a California medical
school (Toland College, 1876), Dr. Wanzer also became
the first woman member of the San Francisco Medical Society. This article describes her childhood, the opposition
she encountered in medical school from faculty and students,
and her early practice among the poor ("gradually she got a
better class [of patients]").

1464.   Mesnard, Elise Marie. [Miss Elisabeth Blackwell and the
        Women Physicians.]. Bordeaux, France, 1889. (Fre)
        [Article not examined by editors.]

1465.   Miles, May S. "Joy Harris Glascock, M.D." Medical Wo-
        man's Journal, 53:6 (June 1946) 55. (In Memory.)

1466.   Miller, Deborah W. "Where There Is a Will, There Is a
        Way." Harvard Medical Alumni Bulletin, 50:1 (Septem-
        ber/October 1975) 18-22. photos., ports.
        To Drs. Marion Woolston Catlin, Lesley Bunim Heafitz, and
        Jean Emans, being a mother is as important as being a phy-
        sician. The three women--all alumnae of Harvard Medical
        School--tell how they achieved a workable combination of
        their dual roles.

1467.   Miller, Helen Markley. Woman Doctor of the West: Ber-
        thenia Owens-Adair. Messner, New York, New York,
        1960, 191 pp.
        [Book not examined by editors.]

1468.   Miller, Janet. Jungles Preferred. Houghton Mifflin Com-
        pany, Boston, Massachusetts, 1931, 321 pp. photos.
        Janet Miller kept a daily journal of an adventure that began
        with an expedition through the Belgian Congo to a mission
        located deep within central Africa, where she was stationed
        for three years. Dr. Miller (an American) adapted that
        journal into this book, which describes medical cases en-
        countered and the people to whom she ministered. Personal
        reflections and reactions, and descriptions of plant and ani-
        mal life comprise a major portion of the work.

1469.   Miller, Janet Goucher. "Charlotte Soutter Murdoch Young."
        Medical Woman's Journal, 54:8 (August 1947) 64-65.
        Dr. Young received her M.D. degree from the Woman's
        Medical College of Baltimore in 1902. This article, writ-
        ten upon the occasion of her death, gives biographical in-
        formation on Dr. Young.

1470.   Miller, Neal. "Lillian Heath, M.D. (Mrs. Lou J. Nelson)."
        Rocky Mountain Medical Journal, (December 1962) 48-
        49. photo.
        Receiving her medical degree in 1893, Lillian Heath re-
        turned to Rawlins, Wyoming Territory, where her parents

had settled as pioneers in 1877. Potential patients did not
readily accept Dr. Heath, as indicated by one lady who
said, "I expect to call her but I do not expect to pay her."

1471.   Minney, Doris. "Mary Elizabeth Bates, M.D." Medical
            Woman's Journal, 55:7 (July 1948) 30-31, 64.   port.
         This article is based on an interview with Dr. Bates at the
         age of 87. The first woman to intern at Chicago's Cook
         County Hospital, Dr. Bates recalls the pranks of male in-
         terns and discrimination she experienced there. In 1891
         she moved to Denver, where she practiced until two years
         ago. Now she works as a secretary at the Colorado Hu-
         mane Society. Dr. Bates's philosophies of life and medical
         practice are included.

1472.   "Miriam Butler, M.D." Medical Woman's Journal, 53:3
            (March 1946) 50.
         Dr. Butler (whose portrait appears on the front cover of
         this month's Journal) is an assistant professor at the Wo-
         man's Medical College of Pennsylvania.

1473.   Miskowiec, O. L. "Medicine to Match Our Mountains: A
            Story of the Life of Florence Rena Sabin." Rocky
            Mountain Medical Journal, 59 (April 1962) 40-45,
            passim.
         [Article not examined by editors.]

1474.   Morani, Alma D. "Elizabeth McLaughry, M.D., New Wil-
            mington, Pa." Medical Woman's Journal, 53:1 (Janu-
            ary 1946) 33-34.   port.
         An 1894 graduate of the Woman's Medical College of Penn-
         sylvania, Elizabeth McLaughry studied further with several
         famous physicians in the U.S. and Europe. She founded
         the Overlook Sanitarium in New Wilmington, Pennsylvania
         in 1910. In addition to giving her professional activities,
         this article mentions Dr. McLaughry's avocations and her
         healing philosophy as well, i.e., "the desirability of using
         'Religion' as a therapeutic measure."

1475.   Morani, Alma Dea. "A Eulogy to Esther P. Lovejoy."
            Journal of the American Medical Women's Association,
            22:10 (October 1967) 770-773.   port.
         A tribute to Esther P. Lovejoy, founder and director of the
         American Women's Hospitals Service for fifty years, and
         organizer and first president of Medical Women's Internation-
         al Association. Facts from Dr. Lovejoy's curriculum vitae
         are included.

1476.   Morani, Alma Dea. "New AMWA President--1958-1959:
            Katharine W. Wright, M.D." Journal of the American
            Medical Women's Association, 13:7 (July 1958) 287.
            port.
         Dr. Wright received her M.D. degree from George Wash-

ington School of Medicine, and was board certified in psychiatry in 1945.

1477.   "More than Fifty Years in Practice Club." Medical Wo-
            man's Journal, 49:3 (March 1942) 88-89. (Editorial.)
        Tribute is paid to Belle Constance Eskridge (1859-1941),
        the first woman surgeon in Houston, Texas.

1478.   "More than Fifty Years in Practice Club." Medical Wo-
            man's Journal, 49:4 (April 1942) 123, 128.
        Daisy Maude Orleman Robinson (1869-1942), who distinguished
        herself as a surgeon in France during World War I, was
        later associated with the United States Public Health Service.

1479.   "More than Fifty Years in Practice Club." Medical Wo-
            man's Journal, 49:5 (May 1942) 151-152.
        Praising Annie Sturges Daniel's 63-year medical career,
        this article focuses upon her writing of the history of the
        New York Infirmary for Women and Children.

1480.   "More than Fifty Years in Practice Club." Medical Wo-
            man's Journal, 49:6 (June 1942) 191.
        A biography of Sarah Adamson Dolly [sic] (1829-1909) fo-
        cuses on her founding, in 1886, of the New York State Wo-
        men's Medical Society. The 1851 graduate of the Central
        New York Medical School also influenced legislation concern-
        ing the appointment of women physicians to the staffs of
        state hospitals. Dr. Dolley's social and professional activ-
        ities are reviewed.

1481.   "More than Fifty Years in Practice: Frances Carothers
            Blanchard of Illinois." Medical Woman's Journal, 50:
            6 (June 1943) 156, 161.

1482.   Morris, James Polk. "Elizabeth Bass, M.D. (1876-1956):
            Tulane's Woman Pioneer in Medicine." Tulane Medi-
            icine: Faculty and Alumni, 5:1 (Spring 1973) 4-6.
            ports.
        Dr. Bass's many achievements and her relationship with
        Tulane University School of Medicine are recounted. Dr.
        Bass helped found what later became the Sara Mayo Hospital
        in New Orleans, Louisiana. She was very concerned with
        women's role in medicine and developed a collection in this
        area, which she donated to the Rudolph Matas Library at
        Tulane.

1483.   Morrison, Ann. "Elizabeth Blackwell: The Early Years."
            Journal of the American Medical Women's Association,
            21:2 (February 1966) 143-146.
        Fact and conjecture combine in this "narrative" of Eliza-
        beth Blackwell's early years.

1484.   Morton, Rosalie Slaughter. A Doctor's Holiday in Iran.

Funk & Wagnalls Company, New York, New York, 1940,
335 pp. illus., photos.
In her autobiography, A Woman Surgeon, Rosalie Slaughter
Morton stated her intention to travel to, and study social
conditions of, Iran. This book recounts the history of ancient Persia and describes how rapid social advances have
affected present-day Iran. Observations of work performed
in clinics and missions include mention of specific (mostly
foreign) women physicians. A major portion of the book
deals with the status of women in Iran. Hugh S. Cumming,
retired U.S. surgeon-general, wrote the foreword.

1485.   Morton, Rosalie Slaughter. A Woman Surgeon: The Life
         and Work of Rosalie Slaughter Morton. Frederick A.
         Stokes Company, New York, New York, 1937, 399 pp.
         port.
Rosalie Slaughter graduated from the Woman's Medical College of Pennsylvania in 1897. Her medical career, as a
surgeon and in public health and humanitarian activities, is
documented in this autobiography. During World War I, she
served in Salonica and Serbia and was initial chairman of
the War Service Committee of the American Medical Women's Association, which founded the American Women's
Hospitals. Following the war she organized a program for
Serbian students to come to the United States for higher
education. Her private practice was primarily in New York,
though she began in Washington D.C., and in later years
moved to Florida. This work, though filled with significant
names and events, does not contain an index. The narrative of her professional life is interwoven with personal experiences.

1486.   Mosher, Clelia Duel. "Again in the Running. A Series of
         Sketches from Observations Made by the Author During
         Her Service in France." Medical Woman's Journal,
         28:5 (May 1921) 128-130.

1487.   Mosher, Clelia Duel. "All in the Day's Work. A Series
         of Sketches from Observations Made by the Author Dur-
         ing Her Service in France." Medical Woman's Journal,
         28:4 (April 1921) 95-96.

1488.   Mosher, Eliza M. "Caroline M. Purnell, M.D. An Appre-
         ciation." Bulletin of the Woman's Medical College of
         Pennsylvania, 73:4 (April 1923) 3-4. port.
Dr. Purnell, whose death in 1923 prompted this biography,
was an 1887 graduate of Woman's Medical College of Pennsylvania and the "foremost woman surgeon of Philadelphia."

1489.   Mosher, Eliza M. "Dr. Elizabeth Blackwell [Part I]." Wo-
         man's Medical Journal, 20:7 (July 1910) 155-157.
The facts presented in this article, as well as in the other
articles of this four-part series on the life of Elizabeth

Blackwell, were largely excerpted from Blackwell's Pioneer
Work in Opening the Medical Profession to Women.

1490.   Mosher, Eliza M. "Dr. Elizabeth Blackwell [Part II]."
        Woman's Medical Journal, 20:8 (August 1910) 174-177.
        port.

1491.   Mosher, Eliza M. "Dr. Elizabeth Blackwell [Part III]."
        Woman's Medical Journal, 20:9 (September 1910) 188-
        190.

1492.   Mosher, Eliza M. "Dr. Elizabeth Blackwell [Part IV]."
        Woman's Medical Journal, 20:10 (October 1910) 208-
        210.
        Dr. Blackwell's failing health and her death in June 1910
        are the subjects of this article (the final in a four-part
        series). A list of Dr. Blackwell's writings is appended.

1493.   Mosher, Eliza M. "The History of American Medical Wo-
        men." Medical Woman's Journal, 29:10 (October
        1922) 253-259. ports.
        Brief biographies, complemented with portraits, are pro-
        vided on Drs. Eliza M. Mosher, Elizabeth and Emily Black-
        well, and Marie Zakrzewska.

1494.   Mosher, Eliza M. "The History of American Medical Wo-
        men." Medical Woman's Journal, 29:11 (November
        1922) 292-296. ports.
        This installment [one in a series of articles about American
        women physicians] sketches the lives of the following physi-
        cians: Sarah Adamson Dolly [sic], the second woman to
        graduate in medicine in the U.S.; Ann Preston, the first
        dean of a woman's medical college; Emeline Horton Cleve-
        land, the first woman to graduate in medicine in Ohio; and
        Mary Putnam Jacobi, the first woman admitted to member-
        ship in the New York Academy of Medicine.

1495.   Mosher, Eliza M. "The History of American Medical Wo-
        men." Medical Woman's Journal, 29:12 (December 1922)
        332-334. ports.
        This article presents biographical sketches of four pioneer
        medical women: Lucy E. Sewall, Susan Dimock, Charlotte
        Blake Brown, and Helen Morton.

1496.   Mosher, Eliza M. "The History of American Medical Wo-
        men." Medical Woman's Journal, 30:1 (January 1923)
        19-21. port.
        This installment [one in a series of articles about Ameri-
        can women physicians] gives biographical sketches of the
        following physicians: Mary H. Thompson, founder of the
        Mary Thompson Hospital in Chicago; Rachael Bodley, "the
        first woman scientist of her day"; Helen Webster, the first
        woman member of the Dutchess County Medical Society of

New York State; and Marie Mergler, the first woman to
successfully compete with men for the appointment of intern
in Cook County Hospital.

1497.   Mosher, Eliza M.   "The History of American Medical Wo-
               men."   Medical Woman's Journal, 30:2 (February 1923)
               57-59.   ports.
           This article [one in a series of articles about American wo-
           men physicians] presents biographies of three women: Dr.
           Cordelia Green [sic], who managed a sanatarium in Castile,
           New York; Dr. Sarah Hackett Stevenson, the first woman
           delegate to the AMA; and Dr. Clara A. Swain, the first
           medical missionary sent to the Orient by an American mis-
           sionary society.

1498.   Mosher, Eliza M.   "The History of American Medical Wo-
               men."   Medical Woman's Journal, 30:3 (March 1923)
               88-90.   ports.
           This article focuses on the lives of three early women phy-
           sicians: Cleora A. Seaman, first woman graduate of the
           Cleveland Homeopathic College; Amanda Sanford, first wo-
           man to receive a degree from the University of Michigan;
           and Juliet Hanchelt, founder of Chicago's first maternity
           ward.

1499.   Mosher, Eliza M.   "The History of American Medical Wo-
               men."   Medical Woman's Journal, 30:5 (May 1923) 150-
               151.   port.
           This article [one in a series of articles about American
           women physicians] offers biographies of Dr. Amelia Wilkes
           Lines (the first woman to practice medicine in Brooklyn,
           New York) and Dr. Frances Armstrong Rutherford (the first
           woman to open a medical office in Grand Rapids, Michigan).

1500.   Mosher, Eliza M.   "The History of American Medical Wo-
               men."   Medical Woman's Journal, 30:6 (June 1923)
               186-189.   ports.
           This installment [one in a series of articles about Ameri-
           can women physicians] gives biographical sketches of Agnes
           Eichelberger (founder of the Florence Crittenden Home in
           Sioux City, Iowa) and of Elizabeth Frances Kearney (a gen-
           eral practitioner).

1501.   Mosher, Eliza M.   "The History of American Medical Wo-
               men."   Medical Woman's Journal, 31:1 (January 1924)
               14-16.   ports.
           Receiving her medical degree in 1881, Mary Alma Smith
           shared her practice and living arrangements with her friend,
           Emma Culbertson, who received her medical degree from
           the University of Zurich.   They were both appointed at-
           tending surgeons at the New England Hospital.   Chloe Annette
           Buckel was active in forming and becoming the first presi-
           dent of the first milk commission in California which ex-

cluded tuberculous cows from the dairy. Dr. Buckel opened
a school of cookery in her own house, which resulted in
manual training becoming a part of the public school system
of Oakland. She inspired the founding of the "Mary R.
Smith Trust" to build cottage homes for brain damaged and
mongoloid children and was one of the directors of the institution from its beginning to the time of her death. "So
keen was her concern for defective children that at her
death she left a sum of money which should provide special
training for such children. This fund was used to aid in establishing fellowships at Leland Stanford University for the
study of feeble-minded children, the first of its kind created
in California." She bought a lot in the "Piedmont Hills" to
find peace and quiet and built a house, "to which, with her
beloved friend, Charlotte Playter, she retired some years
before her death."

1502.   Mosher, Eliza M. "The Passing of Dr. Radcliff." Medi-
         cal Woman's Journal, 31:5 (May 1924) 139-140. port.
         A remarkable woman and doctor, Sue Radcliff was treasurer
         for the American Women's Hospitals Committee of the Med-
         ical Women's National Association since 1917. She "car-
         ried the responsibility of accounting for its receipts and
         signed all checks for its disbursements, aggregating upwards
         of $2,000,000, without a single discrepancy being found in
         her account by any auditor."

1503.   Moss, Margaret Steel. "Ellen C. Potter, M.D., F.A.C.P."
         Public Administration Review, 1:4 (Summer 1941) 351-
         362.
         This article relates incidents in Ellen Potter's life which
         lead up to her medical studies and revealed her courage and
         determination. The article continues in an anecdotal style
         to describe her public health career, which began in 1920
         when she accepted the position of chief of the Pennsylvania
         State Child Health Division.

1504.   "Mrs. Maria Collins Douglass, M.D." Double Cross and
         Medical Missionary Record, 14 (September 1899) 161.
         Dr. Douglass (1833-1899) graduated from Woman's Medical
         College in Philadelphia in 1882 and then ministered to the
         "souls and bodies of Burmese women."

1505.   Mühl, Anita M. "Letters to the Editor." Medical Woman's
         Journal, 49:8 (August 1942) 260-263.
         Anita M. Mühl, a doctor from San Diego, California, went
         to Australia in 1938 as a visiting lecturer in psychiatry at
         the University of Melbourne. In this letter she describes
         her experiences as an American with a German name in
         security-conscious Australia during 1941. She observes that
         Australian medical women were serving in the army with
         full pay, were entitled to wear the same uniforms as men,
         and had equal responsibility with the men. She also dis-

cusses her return to San Diego and some of the changes
there since she left.

1506.   "Mühl, Anita M." <u>Medical Woman's Journal</u>, 50:9 (Septem-
          ber 1943) 243.
          Dr. Mühl (whose portrait appears on the front cover of this
          issue of the <u>Journal</u>) graduated in 1920 from Indiana Uni-
          versity.   She was the first woman ever to have made first
          place on the Indiana state board examinations.   In 1923 she
          obtained her Ph. D. from George Washington University.
          Dr. Mühl has published many articles and two books on the
          emotional factors in medicine.

1507.   "Named President of College." <u>Medical Woman's Journal</u>,
          53:11 (November 1946) 8.   port.
          Dr. Louise Pearce, a graduate of Johns Hopkins University
          Medical School, is profiled upon her appointment as presi-
          dent of the Woman's Medical College [of Pennsylvania].

1508.   "Nancy Vuckovich, M. D.:   Class of 1972." <u>School of Medi-
          cine Commentary: University of California, Davis</u>, 2:5
          (July 1973) 13.   photo.   (About Alumni.)

1509.   "Near East Heroine." <u>Medical Woman's Journal</u>, 31:11
          (November 1924) 323.   port.
          After serving as medical director of the Near East Relief,
          and chief of the American Women's Hospital, Mabel Elliott
          returned from medical service in Turkey, Syria, Greece,
          and the Aegean Islands to teach at the Woman's Medical
          College of Pennsylvania.   While she was active in the Near
          East, she wrote a book about the political, social, and ra-
          cial situation in the Near East, <u>Beginning Again at Ararat</u>.

1510.   Nemir, Rosa Lee.   "The Harry Bakwin Memorial Lectures
          (New York University School of Medicine)." <u>Journal of
          the American Medical Women's Association</u>, 30:2 (Feb-
          ruary 1975) 87-88.   port.
          A long-time pediatrics professor at New York University
          Medical School, Harry Bakwin vigorously supported medical
          education of women.   This biography stresses his interac-
          tions with women physicians and mentions his wife, Ruth
          Bakwin, M. D.

1511.   "Nettie L. Gerish, M. D." <u>Medical Woman's Journal</u>, 52:
          9 (September 1945) 47-48.
          Dr. Gerish (whose portrait appears on the front cover of
          this month's <u>Journal</u>) graduated from the Ohio Miami Med-
          ical School in 1915.   Her numerous contributions in her
          specialty, pediatrics, are discussed.

1512.   "New Chairman Announced: Nancy E. Warner, M. D.,
          Stresses Research and Training." <u>USC Medicine</u>, 23:1
          (Winter 1973) 5-6.   photo., port.

It did not take "'Women's Lib'" for Nancy Elizabeth Warner, "a trim good looking woman," to become chairman of
the Department of Pathology at the University of Southern
California School of Medicine.

1513.   "A New Director Elected." Medical Woman's Journal, 50:
            12 (December 1943) 304.
         A brief biography of Dr. Florence Rena Sabin is given upon
         the occasion of her election as a director of the American
         Society for the Control of Cancer.

1514.   New York Medical Journal, 4 (January 1867) 314-316.
            (Varia.)
         This article quotes from notices that appeared in British
         journals about Mary Walker, who lectured in London's St.
         James Hall on "The Experiences of a Female Physician in
         College, Private Practive, and in the Federal Army." The
         editorials unanimously agreed that Dr. Walker deserved the
         ridicule her audience gave her. One reviewer assured that
         "the interruptions and jocularities she experienced were not
         an insult to her sex, but to her capabilities as a public lec-
         turer." Another suggested "as an attractive subject for her
         public entertainments, 'Why Not? or, Clitoridectomy and
         its Uses.'"

1515.   "News from George Washington University: Doctor and
            Bride Finish at Top of George Washington University
            Graduating Class." Medical Woman's Journal, 55:7
            (July 1948) 52. port.
         The Drs. Soyster--"23-year-old Peter and his sparkling,
         black-haired bride, Eliza"--plan to serve out their intern-
         ships and residencies together, and later share a medical
         practice. "Mrs. Soyster," née Shumaker, received the
         John Ordonaux Prize for having the highest scholastic stand-
         ing in the class. She was the first woman in the George
         Washington University's Medical School to receive the award.

1516.   "News Notes." Medical Woman's Journal, 50:6 (June 1943)
            158. port.
         An obituary of Dr. Marion Craig Potter lists her profession-
         al affiliations as well as other biographical data.

1517.   "News Notes." Medical Woman's Journal, 51:4 (April 1944)
            40. port.
         The career of Sophie Rabinoff, a 1913 graduate of Woman's
         Medical College of Pennsylvania and a district health officer
         in New York City, is detailed.

1518.   "News Notes." Medical Woman's Journal, 51:10 (October
            1944) 35. photo.
         Dr. Mary B. Allison's preparations for her new post at
         Minter Hospital in Bulsar, India are described.

1519.   "News Notes." Medical Woman's Journal, 51:12 (December
            1944) 37. port.
        An alumna of the Woman's Medical College of Pennsylvania,
        Mary Latimer James worked with the American Church Mis-
        sion in China for more than 30 years. She was superinten-
        dent of the Church Mission Hospital in Wuchang when it was
        seized by the Japanese in 1937. Dr. James returned to the
        United States and worked at the Pennsylvania Epileptic Hos-
        pital and Colony Farm at West Chester, where she reports
        to have encountered "multitudinous problems" in administra-
        tion and "no opportunity to get any satisfying scientific work
        done."

1520.   "News Notes." Medical Woman's Journal, 52:5 (May 1945)
            52. port.
        Dr. Ada Walker is an eminent physician in the field of path-
        ology. She received her medical education from Temple
        University and graduated in 1913.

1521.   "News Notes." Medical Woman's Journal, 52:7 (July 1945)
            54. port.
        Dr. Anna Boggs Watson graduated in 1894 from the Woman's
        Medical College of Pennsylvania. She and a classmate,
        Caroline Lawrence, were appointed by the Woman's Board
        of the United Presbyterian Church as medical missionaries
        in Egypt.

1522.   "News Notes." Medical Woman's Journal, 54:12 (December
            1947) 49. port.
        On September 19, 1947, the Colorado State Medical Society
        gave recognition to Dr. Ella A. Mead for her untiring med-
        ical service. Dr. Mead is briefly profiled in this article.

1523.   "News Notes." Medical Woman's Journal, 55:9 (September
            1948) 46-47.
        In addition to news on the activities of several women's
        associations, biographies are given of Florence R. Sabin,
        the first woman graduate of Johns Hopkins Medical School
        (M.D., 1900), and of Gussie Annice Niles, a Salem, Ore-
        gon practitioner who died in July 1948.

1524.   "News Notes." Medical Woman's Journal, 55:11 (November
            1948) 60.
        Among other "News Notes" is a report of Dr. Dorothea
        Lemcke's activities as the first woman physician to direct
        medical matters for a major unit of the Bell Telephone
        System. Heading a staff which includes 13 other physicians,
        Dr. Lemcke oversees the medical well-being of over 10,000
        AT&T employees.

1525.   "News Notes." Medical Woman's Journal, 55:12 (December
            1948) 44-45.
        In addition to obituaries and news of appointments, biogra-

phies are given of three women physicians: L. Rosa Minoka Hill, who works on the Oneida Reservation in Wisconsin; Lunette I. Powers, who just completed 50 years of
medical practice in Michigan; and Emma Boone Tucker, a
retired medical missionary.

1526.   "News Notes." Medical Woman's Journal, 56:1 (January
            1949) 41. port.
        Irene Susanne Pierre Francis, a graduate of Meharry Med-
        ical College, is a Negro who faced much prejudice and in-
        tolerance. Now at least half Dr. Francis's patients in
        Kingsport, Tennessee are white. "Pain," she explains, "is
        a great equalizer."

1527.   "News Notes." Medical Woman's Journal, 56:4 (April 1949)
            54-55.
        Among several other "notes" concerning specific women phy-
        sicians is a profile of Dr. Mary M. Crawford, medical di-
        rector for the Federal Reserve Bank of New York.

1528.   "News Notes." Medical Woman's Journal, 56:9 (September
            1949) 48-49.
        Among the news items in this month's column is a brief
        biography of Leslie Swigart Kent, believed to be the first
        woman president of a state medical society (Oregon). Also
        mentioned is Dr. Harriette Keatinge (1837-1909), whose
        extraordinary number of female physician relatives prompted
        Ripley to cite her in his "Believe It or Not" column.

1529.   "News Notes." Medical Woman's Journal, 56:11 (November
            1949) 43.
        The "News" opens with a reprint of the New York Herald
        Tribune editorial tribute to Dr. Ellen C. Potter. She was
        honored upon her retirement as deputy commissioner for
        welfare of New Jersey.

1530.   "News of Medical Women: Courage and Devotion Beyond
            the Call of Duty." Journal of the American Medical
            Women's Association, 3:1 (January 1948) 36-37. photo.
        An expatiation is given upon the painting by Dr. Anna Dar-
        row of Ft. Lauderdale depicting "Courage and Devotion Be-
        yond the Call of Duty." This painting was entered in the
        ninth annual medical art exhibit held in conjunction with the
        American Medical Association meeting in June of 1947. Dr.
        Darrow won second prize for this painting whose subject, a
        woman physician in the Florida Everglades, was taken from
        Dr. Darrow's own experience.

1531.   [Nichols, Mary Sargent (Neal) Gove]. Mary Lyndon; or,
            Revelations of a Life: An Autobiography. Stringer and
            Townsend, New York, New York, 1855, 388 pp.
        This book represents an autobiographical account of the au-
        thor's career. [Wrote Poe in The Literati, "She is, I think,

a Mesmerist, a Swedenborgian, a Phrenologist, a homeo-
pathist, and a disciple of Preissnitz."]

1532.   "1962 Medical Women of the Year." Journal of the Ameri-
         can Medical Women's Association, 18:1 (January 1963)
         81-88. ports.
         This article lists the women chosen by various branches of
         the American Medical Women's Association as Medical Wo-
         men of the Year.   The biographical sketch for each woman
         lists her honors, awards, affiliations and other pertinent
         data.   Included are Elizabeth R. Brackett; Helen Octavia
         Dickens, the first Negro woman to be made a fellow of the
         American College of Surgeons; Gertrude Engbring, the first
         woman to receive the Stritch Award (Loyola) for outstanding
         contributions to medicine; Ruth Hartgraves; Florence A. Kel-
         ler, who received her M. D. from the American Medical
         Missionary College and became in 1903 the first woman phy-
         sician in New Zealand; Ella Oppenheimer; Ada Chree Reid;
         Adelaide Romaine, the first woman to hold office in the New
         York County Medical Society, having been elected treasurer
         in 1960; Mabel Richards Tarbell; Hulda Evelyn Thelander;
         and Priscilla White, the first woman to give the Banting
         Memorial Lecture of the American Diabetes Association (in
         1960), and also the first woman to be elected to the council
         of the Association.

1533.   Noall, Claire. Guardians of the Hearth: Utah's Pioneer
         Midwives and Women Doctors.   Horizon Publishers,
         Bountiful, Utah, 1974, x, 189 pp.
         Women midwives and physicians in Utah are discussed in
         detail, with abundant social and religious historical informa-
         tion as context.   Various medical cases are cited, as well
         as their treatment, outcome, and the costs of different med-
         ical services.   Much of the information is gleaned from per-
         sonal journal entries.

1534.   Nobel, Nelle S. "Lena Kellogg Sadler, M. D." Journal of
         the American Medical Women's Association, 11:6 (June
         1956) 219. port. (Past Presidents of AMWA.)
         Dr. Sadler, a past president of AMWA, was one of the
         founders of the Chicago Council of Medical Women.   For
         25 years she lectured throughout the county on health and
         hygiene and, with her husband, Dr. William S. Sadler,
         "was a pioneer in the popularization of preventive medicine."
         She wrote How to Feed the Baby, and coauthored several
         other books with her husband.

1535.   Noble, Iris. First Woman Ambulance Surgeon: Emily Bar-
         ringer.   Julian Messner, Inc. , New York, New York,
         1962, 192 pp.
         This biography of Emily Dunning Barringer, the first woman
         ambulance surgeon, is mainly devoted to her education at
         Medical College of the New York Infirmary, Cornell Medical

School, and Bellevue Hospital. She applied for and won a
position as intern at a general hospital, Gouverneur, which
had never before accepted a woman. Subsequently she became surgeon in the horse-drawn ambulance where she endured taunts of passersby and a conspiracy by four male
doctors to force her resignation. The book deals only briefly with her later years when she became a specialist in
gynecological surgery and venereal disease. An index is
included.

1536. "Notes from the Woman's Medical College of Pennsylvania."
      Medical Woman's Journal, 54:4 (April 1947) 67.
      Dr. Barbara B. Stimson spoke at the Founder's Day cere-
      monies at the College. Dr. Minerva S. Buerk's appoint-
      ment as a fellow in venereology at Johns Hopkins Hospital
      in Baltimore, Maryland is also announced.

1537. "Notes from the Woman's Medical College of Pennsylvania."
      Medical Woman's Journal, 54:7 (July 1947) 33.
      In this news article, the death of Dr. Linda Bartels Lange
      is announced. Also announced is the awarding of a second
      diploma to Dr. Honoria Acosta-Sison of the Philippine Is-
      lands.

1538. "Obituary: Sarah Elizabeth Finch, 1881-1921." Medical
      Woman's Journal, 28:11 (November 1921) 286.

1539. Oblensky, Florence E. "Anita Newcomb McGee, M.D. (4
      Nov. 1864--5 Oct. 1940)." Military Medicine, 133:5
      (May 1968) 397-400. port. (Obituary.)
      Dr. Newcomb, the first woman member of the Association
      of Military Surgeons, served as an assistant surgeon during
      the Spanish-American War, and founded the Army Nurse
      Corps. She was active throughout her life in the National
      Society Daughters of the American Revolution. Dr. McGee
      was buried with full military honors in Arlington National
      Cemetery. In 1966 the Daughters of the American Revolu-
      tion approved a commemorative award of the Dr. Anita
      Newcomb McGee medal to a nurse chosen by the U.S. sur-
      geon general as the "U.S. Army Nurse of the year."

1540. O'Connor, Katheryn and Forbes, Lorna. "Student News."
      Medical Woman's Journal, 52:2 (February 1945) 56, 58,
      60. photos., port.
      In this article Dr. Sarah I. Morris, a retiring faculty mem-
      ber at the Woman's Medical College, is profiled.

1541. O'Connor, Katheryn and Forbes, Lorna. "Student News."
      Medical Woman's Journal, 52:4 (April 1945) 57. photo.,
      port.
      Dr. Helen Angelucci, a 1927 graduate of the Woman's Med-
      ical College of Pennsylvania, is profiled herein.

1542.   O'Connor, Katheryn and Forbes, Lorna. "Student News."
             Medical Woman's Journal, 52:6 (June 1945) 58-59. pho-
             to., ports.
         Dr. Irene Maher, a 1944 graduate of the Woman's Medical
         College of Pennsylvania, is profiled on the occasion of her
         appointment to the faculty of her alma mater.

1543.   O'Connor, Katheryn and Forbes, Lorna. "Student News."
             Medical Woman's Journal, 52:7 (July 1945) 56, 60. pho-
             to., port.
         This brief biography of Dr. Bernice Durgin, a graduate of
         the Woman's Medical College of Pennsylvania, is presented
         upon the occasion of her appointment to the faculty of the
         College.

1544.   O'Connor, Katheryn and Forbes, Lorna. "Student News."
             Medical Woman's Journal, 52:8 (August 1945) 54. pho-
             to., port.
         A brief biography of Dr. F. Marian Williams, a 1932 grad-
         uate of Syracuse University Medical School, is herein given.

1545.   Offenbach, Bertha. "Four of Us: Sketches of the Four
             Women Ophthalmologists of the Massachusetts Eye and
             Ear Infirmary." Journal of the American Medical Wo-
             men's Association, 21:7 (July 1966) 595-598. photo.,
             ports.
         Sketches of professional activity interspersed amid personal
         reflections comprise this article.

1546.   "Old Doc Anna: As Told by Dr. Anna Darrow." Journal
             of the Florida Medical Association, 55:8 (August 1968)
             749-756. fascim., photos., port.
         A pioneer woman doctor in Florida, Dr. Darrow began prac-
         ticing in Okeechobee in 1912. This autobiographical account
         includes examples of not only the variety of problems for
         which she was consulted, but also the traveling and living
         conditions and difficulties with which she contended in order
         to practice.

1547.   "Olga Stasny [sic], M.D." Medical Woman's Journal, 31:
             5 (May 1924) 140-141. port.
         Olga Stastny was director of the quarantine station conducted
         by the American Women's Hospitals on Marcronissi Island,
         which was Greek territory in 1918. In a report to the
         United States government by a committee investigating the
         work of relief organizations in Greece, Dr. Stastny's work
         contribution is mentioned. "On the black rocky slopes of
         this quarantine island there are rows upon rows of shallow
         graves in which are buried the victims of typhus and other
         diseases, and throughout the length and breadth of Greece
         there are thousands of Pontus refugees who are alive and
         well today as a result of this self-sacrificing, heroic effort
         on the part of this organization.

1548. "Olga Stastny, M.D.: Omaha, Neb." Medical Woman's
       Journal, 37:6 (June 1930) 147-149. port.
       A native of Czecho-Slovakia, Olga Stastny received her med-
       ical training and acquired citizenship in the United States.
       During the world war, Dr. Stastny raised funds for Franco-
       Serbian relief work. After the war, she was the first med-
       ical woman to do Czecho-Slovakian relief work. Dr. Stast-
       ny is about to become president of the Medical Women's
       National Association.

1549. Oliphant, Beverly A. "Recipients of the Janet M. Glasgow
       Awards for Academic Distinction, 1969." Journal of
       the American Medican Women's Association, 24:10 (Oc-
       tober 1969) 829-832. ports.
       Dr. Oliphant's autobiography is presented as part of this
       article; she was a 1969 graduate of the George Washington
       University School of Medicine.

1550. Olson, Avis M.: Jones, Sarah Van Hoosen; Gardner, Mabel
       E.; Strong, R. M.; Raven, Clara; Jameson, Florence I.;
       and Watson, Jeanne M. "Bertha Van Hoosen, M.D.
       (1863-1952)." Journal of the American Medical Women's
       Association, 18:7 (July 1963) 533-543. ports.
       Tributes to Bertha Van Hoosen constitute this section of an
       entire issue of JAMWA dedicated to her on the occasion of
       the hundredth anniversary of her birth. Sarah Van Hoosen
       Jones gives a personal reminiscence of her Aunt "Gubble."
       She recounts the closeness of Bertha, and Alice, her sister.
       Mabel E. Gardner describes Dr. Van Hoosen's "medical
       personality." Dr. Strong speaks of her tenure as head of
       the department of obstetrics at Loyola University, while Dr.
       Clara Raven relates incidents about "Dr. Van" from her
       acquaintance with her as first a medical student and later
       a friend. Florence I. Jameson relates some of Dr. Van
       Hoosen's many comments while working with her on the book
       Petticoat Surgeon, e.g., "If the Procrustean bed is too
       short, lengthen it. I always did." Concluding this section,
       Jeanne M. Watson tells of plans to build a suburban unit of
       Crittenton General Hospital, whose main building will be
       named after Bertha Van Hoosen.

1551. "On Her Golden Graduation Day." Medical Woman's Jour-
       nal, 54:8 (August 1947) 56.
       Dr. Martha G. K. Schetky, celebrating the fiftieth anniver-
       sary of her graduation from medical school, gives her views
       on women in medicine.

1552. "One of America's Finest Women Physicians." Medical Wo-
       man's Journal, 29:11 (November 1922) 293. port.
       Sue Radcliff's active professional life is the subject of this
       brief article.

1553. "One of the World's Great Citizens: S. Josephine Baker,

M.D., D.P.H., Director Bureau of Child Hygiene, Department of Health, New York City." Medical Woman's
Journal, 29:8 (August 1922) 180-182.   port.
This biography of Dr. Baker covers her professional activities, appointments, honors, and the testimonial held in her
honor on 25 April 1922.

1554.   Osborn, Stellanova.   "Great Lakes Pioneer in Medicine."
        Medical Woman's Journal, 54:1 (January 1947) 29-36,
        60.   ports.
        Dr. Margaret Ann Fannon Osborn was drawn magnetically
        toward "thinking Hippocratic."   Born in Ohio and orphaned
        at the age of six years, Margaret Fannon attended the
        Young Ladies Seminary at Xenia, Ohio, after which she
        took private lessons from Professor Brown.   He recognized
        Margaret's ability, dissuaded her from becoming a nurse,
        and guided her toward medicine.   This article traces the
        life and activities of Dr. Osborn and her husband, their in-
        terests and adventures.

1555.   Ostler, Fred J.   "America's First Woman Doctor."   Coro-
        net, 25:4 (February 1949) 177-180.   illus.
        Elizabeth Blackwell is saluted on the one-hundredth anni-
        versary of her graduation from Geneva Medical College.

1556.   "Our Beloved Senior Editor."   Medical Woman's Journal,
        32:5 (May 1925) 148-149.
        When Eliza M. Mosher became senior editor of the Medical
        Woman's Journal, she used the Journal to help organize
        medical women who had been so busy getting a foothold into
        the profession that they had not previously considered or-
        ganizing.   As a result of this influence, the Medical Wo-
        men's National Association [which later became the Ameri-
        can Medical Women's Association] was formed.   This or-
        ganization made significant contributions during the world
        war by means of the War Service Committee (which after-
        wards became the American Women's Hospitals).

1557.   "Our Fifty Year Doctor."   Medical Woman's Journal, 49:
        11 (November 1942) 351.
        Graduating from the University of Michigan in 1892, Jeanne
        Cady Solis wrote technical articles and taught on the faculty
        of her alma mater until 1907.   During this time she owned
        and operated the Ann Arbor Private Hospital for the Men-
        tally Disturbed.

1558.   "Our Fifty Year Doctor."   Medical Woman's Journal, 49:
        12 (December 1942) 387-389.
        Ellen Wallace's retirement was gradual as the result of a
        lifelong problem with deafness.   When she entered medical
        school, she was already deaf in one ear and became pro-
        gressively deaf in the other ear in the ten years after she
        obtained her degree.   Working closely with her sister, Dr.

Julia Eastman Wallace Russell, Dr. Wallace helped to found the New Hampshire Memorial Hospital for Women and Children in 1895. Dr. Wallace, state superintendent of health and hygiene for the Women's Christian Temperance Union, was also active in tuberculosis prevention, and in milk inspection.

1559.   "Our Lady Asclepiads." Journal of the National Medical Association, 60:2 (March 1968) 136-137, 163. ports. (Editorials.)
Noting that a Negro man graduated from an American medical college two years before Elizabeth Blackwell received her M.D., this article observes that women, like Negroes, fought much prejudice in gaining access to the professions. The editorial goes on to mention the "firsts" of Negro medical women and presents brief biographies on several women.

1560.   "Our Special Correspondent: Dr. Mary McKibben Harper." Medical Woman's Journal, 32:8 (August 1925) 225-226. port.
Although "considered one of the most capable women physicians in the country," Mary McKibben Harper did not practice medicine after she married. Dr. McKibben Harper is now on her way to Europe, Asia, and the Near East to visit and to interview leading medical women of these countries in order to write articles for the Journal.

1561.   Owens-Adair, B. A. Dr. Owens-Adair: Some of Her Life Experiences. Mann & Beach, Printers, Portland, Oregon, [n.d.], 537 pp.
Bethenia Owens was born in 1840 and migrated to Oregon with her family in 1843. She married at the age of 14, bore a son and was divorced at the age of 18, whereupon she began her elementary school education. She was employed as a teacher, and then became a milliner prior to her decision to enter medicine. She received a degree from the Eclectic School of Medicine and returned to Oregon. In 1878 she went to Philadelphia to study at Jefferson, but was advised to go instead to the University of Michigan which was coeducational. In 1880 she received her M.D. degree from Michigan. In her later professional life she also did postgraduate work at the University of Chicago. She practiced in Portland, Astoria, and Seaside, Oregon and in North Yakima, Washington. This autobiography devotes 100 of its over 500 pages to her life story; the remainder is a collection of addresses, lectures, correspondence, biographical sketches of family and associates, and other material.

1562.   Owens-Adair, Bethenia Angelina. A Souvenir. Dr. Owens-Adair to Her Friends. Christmas 1922. Statesman Publishing Company, Salem, Oregon, 1922.
[Item not examined by editors.]

1563.   Paolone, Clementina J.   "Isabel M. Scharnagel, M.D."
              Journal of the American Medical Women's Association,
              9:8 (August 1954) 268.   port.   (Album of Women in
              Medicine.)
         Dr. Scharnagel received her M.D. degree from Rush Med-
         ical College in 1931.   She became the first resident in path-
         ology at the New York Infirmary for Women and Children
         and the first resident (1933) of the newly founded Kate De-
         pew Strang Cancer Clinic.

1564.   Parkhurst, Genevieve.   "Dr. Sabin, Scientist: Winner of
              Pictorial Review's Achievement Award."   Pictorial Re-
              view, (January 1930) 2, 70-71.   photo.
         Florence Rena Sabin's current career activities and personal
         interests form a major portion of this biography.   Her "chief
         hobby" at present is involvement in the movement to bring
         the best medical care to those who cannot afford it.   She
         and other women physicians in New York City formed the
         "Gotham Hospital Plan," which endows the patient instead
         of the hospital.

1565.   Parmelee, Ruth A.   "Reminiscences of Twenty Years in the
              Near East."   Women in Medicine, 51 (January 1936) 20-
              23.
         A missionary child born in Turkey, Ruth A. Parmelee went
         to the United States for her A.B. and M.D. degree, return-
         ing to Turkey to do medical missionary work.   Dr. Parme-
         lee was the first woman physician to practice in the valley
         of the Euphrates River.   "Never was a sign of disrespect
         shown me, even though some of my Turkish women patients
         turned out to be in houses or sections of ill-repute."   Dr.
         Parmelee was especially concerned about educating mid-
         wives, whom she was asked by the Turkish director of pub-
         lic health to instruct.   "Two things only, I hoped to accom-
         plish with these middle-aged ignorant women--to impress
         upon them in the absolute necessity for scrubbing their
         hands, and to understand when to call in the help of a doc-
         tor."   She also devoted much time and energy to the Armen-
         ian refugees.   After political tensions forced her to leave
         the country, she helped establish a maternity hospital with
         100 beds in Saloniki, Greece, which was later called Amer-
         ican Women's Hospital for Women and Children.   Dr. Par-
         melee also helped to establish nurses' training programs.
         The reminiscence ends referring to her recent return to
         Greece "... and the fact that we foreigners must remain
         in the background while our Greek friends push ahead in the
         great movement for improving hospital organization and
         nursing care in their land."

1566.   Parrish, Rebecca.   Orient Seas and Lands Afar.   Fleming
              H. Revell Company, New York, New York, 1936, 152
              pp.
         Dr. Parrish recounts her experiences as a world traveler

and writes vivid descriptions of such places as the Philippines, Japan, China, India, Arabia, Egypt, Palestine, Istanbul, Italy, France, and Norway.

1567.   Parsons, John L. "Alice Hamilton: Pioneer in Industrial
        Medicine." Medical Economics, 20 (September 1943)
        44-46, 141, 143. port.
        After hearing a speech by Jane Addams, Alice Hamilton
        decided to make medicine her career, and the slums her
        sphere of activity. She obtained a medical degree (studying
        in the U.S. and Germany) and joined Miss Addams at Hull
        House, Chicago. Settlement work put her in contact with
        workmen and the often appalling conditions in which they
        worked. In 1910 Governor Deneen appointed Dr. Hamilton
        to the Illinois Occupational Disease Commission; with a staff
        of 20 young doctors, students, and social workers, Dr.
        Hamilton began her lifelong battle against industrial poisons.
        She became a detective, crusader, and medico; when strikes
        were brought about by inhumane working conditions, she
        often joined the picketlines. Appointed assistant professor
        of industrial medicine at Harvard Medical School, Dr. Ham-
        ilton had to promise not to insist on her right to use the
        Harvard Club, not to march in the procession or sit on the
        platform at commencement, and not to demand her quota of
        football tickets. In that position, Dr. Hamilton divided her
        time between Harvard and the Department of Labor. In
        1924 she visited Russia at the Soviet Department of Health's
        request, to survey industrial hygiene. In 1937-38 she in-
        vestigated the U.S. viscose-rayon industry. Dr. Hamilton
        considered her sex a help in her professional activities be-
        cause "'it seemed natural for a woman to put the case of
        the producing workman ahead of the value of the thing he
        was producing; in a man that would have been sentimentality
        or radicalism.'" The author, who takes much of his in-
        formation from Dr. Hamilton's newly published book Explor-
        ing the Dangerous Trades, concludes this biography with the
        observation that "without her womanly indignation, compas-
        sion, and zeal, the story of the control of poisons in the
        dangerous trades might have been entirely different."

1568.   "Part Time Pediatric Residency Approved." Woman's Med-
        ical College: Today, 1:6 (March 1970) 6. port.
        The first physician accepted for the College's new part-
        time pediatric training program is Ingrid Laszlo, "an at-
        tractive, German-born physician" and the mother of two.
        This article notes that while the program was established
        to meet the needs of women, qualified men will also be con-
        sidered.

1569.   "The Passing of Emily Blackwell." Woman's Medical Jour-
        nal, 20:9 (September 1910) 186.

1570.   "Past President Ellen Culver Potter, M.D." Bulletin of

the Medical Women's National Association, 29 (July
1930) 5-6.   port.
This article is a "categorically arranged" biography of Dr.
Potter, past president of the Medical Women's National
Association.

1571.   Pelzel, Jane Barksdale.   "I Was an MD Dropout."   Medical Opinion & Review, 7:1 (January 1971) 64-68.   illus.
"If five years is the half-life of medical knowledge, mine
had undergone triple decay, and I felt like Osler's mother,"
writes Dr. Pelzel, recalling her return to medical practice
after many years of staying at home with her family.   Dr.
Pelzel describes her regret at having dropped her career,
her search for retraining, the ways in which medicine had
changed in her absence, and the impact of her new lifestyle
on her family.

1572.   "Pennsylvania's Distinguished Daughters."   The Pennsyl-
vania Clubwoman, 43:2 (December 1955-January 1956)
14-16.   photo., ports.
Two women connected with the Woman's Medical College of
Pennsylvania numbered among the ten 1955 Distinguished
Daughters of Pennsylvania, as awarded by the Pennsylvania
Federation of Women's Clubs: Dr. Marion Spencer Fay
(Ph.D., Yale), dean of the College, and Dr. Ellen J. Pat-
terson, class of 1898.

1573.   Perrin, Edwin N.   "Bars on Her Shoulders."   Medical
Economics, (August 1954) 154-155.   port.
The first woman to serve as a "regular army" doctor, Captain Fae Adams graduated from the Woman's Medical College, Philadelphia.

1574.   "Personal."   Woman's Medical Journal, 6:12 (December
1897) 367-368.
Among the news items appearing in this column: Miss L.
M. Johnson, M.D. just became the first woman to be admitted to the Maryland College of Pharmacy; and Dr. Bertha
V. Thompson [sic], with her new appointment in Oshkosh,
became the first woman city physician in Wisconsin.   Biographical information is also provided on Dr. Eva Harding,
who holds the Materia Medica chair at a Kansas City homeopathic college, and Dr. Frieda Lippert, of New York City.

1575.   Petteys, Anna C.   Doctor Portia: Her First Fifty Years
in Medicine as Told to Anna C. Petteys.   Golden Bell
Press, Denver, Colorado, 1964, 315 pp.   photos.,
ports.
Portia McKnight was the first woman graduate of the North
Carolina Medical College (1912).   She married a Russian
agronomist and moved to Russia, where she practiced as a
school physician in Moscow from 1914 to 1917.   In 1917
Dr. McKnight Lubchenco, her husband, and their three chil-

dren fled Russia via Siberia, Port Arthur, and Japan.
They returned to the McKnight family home in Blythewood,
South Carolina where she undertook a general medical practice.   Dr. Lubchenco finally settled with her family in Hax-
tun, Colorado, where she continued her practice and ultimately became chief of staff of the Logan County Hospital.
She was awarded a fifty-year service pin by the Colorado
Medical Society.   This biography devoted four of its seven
chapters to Dr. Lubchenco's life in Russia, with emphasis
on socio-political, economic, and family affairs.   Three of
the five Lubchenco children, including one daughter, became physicians.

1576.   Phelan, Mary Kay.   The Story of Dr. Florence Sabin:
        Probing the Unknown.   Thomas Y. Crowell Company,
        New York, New York, 1969, x, 176 pp.
        Dr. Florence Sabin grew up in the gold-mining country of
        Colorado in the late 19th century.   She studied music and
        at one time expected to become a pianist.   Her interests
        later turned to science.   She attended Smith College and
        Johns Hopkins Medical School.   Then began a varied and
        impressive career of teaching, research, and, much later,
        public health work.   She made discoveries concerning the
        origin and development of the lymphatic system ("there were
        those who resented the fact that a woman was responsible
        for making such discoveries").   She later investigated the
        growth of blood vessels and the origins of blood cells in
        the embryonic stage.   Her research commanded such respect
        that she was invited to organize a new department of cellu-
        lar studies at the Rockefeller Institute for Medical Research,
        and it was her work there which "helped lay the groundwork
        for discovering drugs by which tuberculosis can be controlled
        today."   At the age of 74, Dr. Sabin began a new phase of
        her career: in 1945 she returned to Colorado to tackle the
        appalling public health problem there.   "'We think of our
        state as a health resort, yet we're dying faster than people
        in most states,'" she said after her initial investigation.
        She tackled her new job with such energy that the governor,
        in response to a reporter's question about getting some dif-
        ficult bills through the legislature, said: "'Brother, when
        it comes to those bills, why, I'll have the little old lady on
        my side.   There isn't a man in the legislature who wants
        to tangle with her.   She's an atom bomb.   She's a dynamo."
        During her lifetime, Florence Sabin was the recipient of
        many honors, including 15 honorary degrees.   She died on
        October 3, 1953.   The book contains a bibliography and an
        index.

1577.   Phifer, Mary H.   "L. Rosa H. Gantt, M.D."   Bulletin of
        the Medical Women's National Association, 33 (July
        1931) 9-10.   port.
        Dr. Gantt was a graduate of the Medical College of Charles-
        ton, South Carolina.   She did work in public health and,

during the war, she and her husband opened their home to
soldiers at Camp Wadsworth in Spartanburg, South Carolina.

1578.   Phillips, Bessie. "First Woman Doctor in the Army."
             Medical Woman's Journal, 51:1 (January 1944) 25-26.
             (Section on War Service.)
         A reprint from the New York Times Magazine (11 July 1943)
         profiles Mary E. Walker as the first woman army surgeon,
         and as a woman's rights activist who wore male attire and
         wore her hair in the fashion of a man's.

1579.   Phillips, Dennis H. "Women in Nineteenth Century Wiscon-
             sin Medicine." Wisconsin Medical Journal, 71 (Novem-
             ber 1972) 13-18. (Medical History Feature.)
         Dr. Laura J. Ross was the first woman member elected to
         the Milwaukee Medical Society (1869). Dr. Ross was a po-
         litical activist, helping to organize the Woman's Exchange
         for "education, aid, and safety for women in industry," as
         well as the first woman's suffrage convention in Wisconsin
         (1869). Dr. Margaret Caldwell of Waukesha, Wisconsin
         avoided political issues and became known as the dean of
         women physicians in the state at the time of her death in
         1938. Dr. Bertha V. Thomson of Necedah "possessed an
         almost mystic attraction to medicine from early childhood"
         and received her formal medical training at Chicago. She
         became city physician in Oshkosh, Wisconsin--the first wo-
         man in the U.S. to hold such a position. Dr. Maybelle M.
         Park (M.D. 1894) was the first woman in the state to serve
         as a county health physician; she was appointed to this post
         in 1898 at the age of 27. A number of other women physi-
         cians practicing in 19th-century Wisconsin are discussed,
         as well as the setting for medical practice in general in
         the state.

1580.   Phillips, Josephine Dirion. "New AMWA President--1962:
             Edith Petrie Brown, M.D." Journal of the American
             Medical Women's Association, 17:1 (January 1962) 57.
             port.
         Dr. Brown graduated first in her medical class of 60 stu-
         dents when she received her M.D. degree from George
         Washington University School of Medicine in 1927. Edith
         Brown had a general practice although she took graduate
         courses in several specialty areas and won a coveted intern-
         ship at Grace Hospital in Detroit and a residency in pedia-
         trics at Children's Hospital in Washington, D.C. "Dr.
         Brown typifies the general practitioner who tries to be
         broadly prepared for the constant expansion of medicine."

1581.   "Phoebe A. Ferris, M.D., 1869-1945." Medical Woman's
             Journal, 53:4 (April 1946) 47-48. port.
         A 1902 graduate of the Medical School of Syracuse Univer-
         sity, Phoebe A. Ferris took charge of the Mrs. William
         Butler Memorial Hospital in Baroda, India from 1917 to

1929.   Descriptions of her medical missionary work in India
make up the major portion of this biography.

1582.   "Phyllis MacNeil, M.D."   Journal of the American Medical
Women's Association, 17:4 (April 1962) 347.   port.
(Album of Women in Medicine.)
After having worked as a nurse's aide in the polio wards
and in Helen Taussig's cardiac patient care program in
January and February of 1944, Phyllis MacNeil went on to
earn her M.D. in 1948 and became a surgeon.   In 1944 an
epidemic of poliomyelitis struck Baltimore, and she worked
with hundreds of children in the acute stages of the disease.

1583.   "Physician and Counselor."   Bulletin of the Woman's Medical College of Pennsylvania, 82:4 (March 1932) 12-13.
(We Quote.)
Reprinted from the February, 1932 issue of National Altrusan, this article profiles Dr. Sarah Morris, who belonged
to the Madison, Wisconsin Altrusan Club.   A 1910 graduate
of the Woman's Medical College of Pennsylvania, Dr. Morris is a professor of preventive medicine at the College.

1584.   Pickett, Elizabeth P.   "Mary E. MacGregor, M.D."   Journal of the American Medical Women's Association, 13:
7 (July 1958) 304.   port.   (Album of Women in Medicine.)
Dr. MacGregor received her M.D. degree in 1922 from
Cornell Medical College.   She was an "active humanitarian"
and one of the few women at the time to be trained in and
to practice urology.

1585.   Piercy, Harry D.   "Marie Zakrzewska, Class of 1856."
Case Western Reserve Medical Alumni Bulletin, 33:4
(Fourth Quarter 19[69]) 14-15.   port.
One of the first four women accepted in 1854 at the Cleveland Medical College of Western Reserve University [now
Case Western Reserve University], Marie Zakrzewska made
a number of significant contributions as a woman in medicine.   In 1857 she helped to establish with Drs. Elizabeth
and Emily Blackwell the New York Infirmary for Women
and Children in New York.   There she introduced record
keeping on patients; recorded, in addition to the traditional
name and address, were sex, age, occupation, diagnosis,
and treatment of each case.   The New England Female Medical College of Boston invited her to be the first professor
in obstetrics.   When its hospital closed, she helped to organize a hospital for women and children, later called the
New England Hospital.   Under Dr. Zakrzewska's direction,
the New England Hospital was the first in America with a
school for nurses.   She is also credited with starting the
first hospital social service.

1586.   Pincock, Carolyn S.   "AMWA President, 1968: Alice Drew

Chenoweth, M. D." Journal of the American Medical
      Women's Association, 23:1 (January 1968) 20-21. photo.
This article was written on the occasion of Dr. Chenoweth's
investiture with the office of president of the American Medical Women's Association (AMWA). A brief outline of her
interests, affiliations honors, and awards is given.

1587.   Pincock, Carolyn S. "Presentation of the Camille Mermod
             Award, 1974." Journal of the American Medical Wo-
             men's Association, 30:2 (February 1975) 81.
A brief biography of Ruby Sears is given as this award
is presented, posthumously, to her. Dr. Minerva S. Buerk,
her sister, accepted the award in Ms. Sears's memory.

1588.   "Pioneer Medical Women." Medical Woman's Journal, 33:
             5 (May 1926) 145.
An 1891 graduate of the Eclectic Medical College, Sarah M.
Siewers worked for the abolition of war and capital punishment and for the furtherance of women's suffrage and temperance. Her poetry advocated women's rights.

1589.   "Pioneer Medical Women." Medical Woman's Journal, 33:
             8 (August 1926) 238-239. port.
"One of those intrepid souls who, in the face of adverse
public opinion and the open enmity of men in the medical
profession, broke down the prejudice against women in
medicine" was Eliza H. Root. An 1882 graduate of Northwestern University Woman's Medical College of Chicago,
Dr. Root served as one of the first editors of the Medical
Woman's Journal. She was a professor of obstetrics and a
dean at her alma mater, and practiced in Chicago for 30
years. "She was particularly devoted to the study of bird
life, although shy about revealing this love or indeed of
showing her feelings at all."

1590.   "Pioneer Medical Women." Medical Woman's Journal, 34:
             2 (February 1927) 55.
An abbreviated biography is given of Dr. Pauline S. Nusbaumer, secretary of the Alameda County [California] Medical Association at the time of her death in 1927.

1591.   "Pioneer Medical Women." Medical Woman's Journal, 34:
             3 (March 1927) 87.
A pioneer in welfare work for women and children, Jean
Turner Zimmerman founded the first haven for stranded
women and children. As president of the National White
Cross League, she became nationally known in 1909 when
she launched a campaign against white slave traffic. At
the time of her death in 1927, Dr. Zimmerman was operating the Chicago Woman's Shelter.

1592.   "Pioneer Medical Women: Dr. Susan La Flesche Picotte."
             Medical Woman's Journal, 37:1 (January 1930) 19-20.

Receiving her medical training in the East, and among the
first graduates of the Woman's Medical College of Pennsylvania, Susan La Flesche returned to her tribe, the Omahas,
in Nebraska where she served her people as the government physician. "Contrary to the ideas that are so often
promulgated at the present time, her home, husband, and
two children did not interfere with her engaging in a large
practice and making constant efforts in behalf of her people."
As a representative of the Omahas, she went to Washington to petition for a law forbidding the sale of liquor on the
Omaha and Winnebago reservations. She was the only Native American ever commissioned as a medical missionary
by the Presbyterian Board of Missions. She founded a hospital in Walthill, Nebraska as she said, "I believe in prevention of disease and hygienic care more than I do in giving or prescribing medicine, and my constant aim is to
teach these two things, particularly to young mothers....
My greatest desire in having the hospital built was to save
the little children."

1593.   "A Pioneer Returns." Journal of the American Medical
         Women's Association, 19:3 (March 1964) 232. photo.
         A very brief article tells of Dr. Esther Pohl Lovejoy's re-
         visit to Portland at the age of 93. Dr. Lovejoy had been
         the head of the Portland Department of Health (1909-1912),
         and the second woman to graduate from the University of
         Oregon Medical School (1894).

1594.   Platt, Lois I. "New AMWA President--1957-1958." Jour-
         nal of the American Medical Women's Association, 12:
         7 (July 1957) 224. port.
         A descriptive biography is given of Dr. Elizabeth Sartor
         Kahler, a "native Washingtonian." She received her M.D.
         degree in 1940 from George Washington University Medical
         School. Dr. Kahler's various professional and non-pro-
         fessional affiliations are included.

1595.   Plechl, Pia Maria. [The Cross and the Staff of Aescula-
         pius: Dr. Anna Dengel and the Medical Missionary
         Sisters]. Verlag Herold, Vienna, Austria, 1967, 227
         pp. photos. (Ger)
         Published in honor of the 75th birthday of Dr. Anna Dengel,
         the founder of the Catholic Medical Mission Society, this
         book deals with the biography of Dr. Dengel and with the
         development of the Society. The first part contains the
         story of Dr. Dengel's early training in Austria and Ireland,
         her work in India, and later the preparations for the Society
         in the United States, culminating in its formation in Wash-
         ington D.C. in 1925 and its later transfer to Fox Chase,
         Philadelphia. In the second half of the book, the author
         describes her personal experiences in observing the work of
         the Medical Missionary Sisters in Africa and Asia where
         they maintain numerous hospitals staffed by members of the

Society. The book emphasizes the social and medical problems encountered by the Sisters in their missionary work.
It contains numerous photographs and a list of the most important dates in the history of the Society, as well as a
bibliography.

1596.   Polk-Peters, Ethel. "Autobiographical Sketch." Medical
         Review of Reviews, 41:8 (August 1935) 405-409.
         Following graduation from the Woman's Medical College of
         Pennsylvania, Ethel Polk-Peters joined her aunt, Dr. Mar-
         garet Polk, at the Mary Black Hospital and Women's Med-
         ical College in Soochow, China. Dr. Polk-Peters organized
         a unit of Chinese and American women doctors and medical
         students to work with refugees in Siberia. She describes
         her adventures in Russia and her work as teacher and phy-
         sician in China, and later in the U.S.

1597.   Porth, Edna. "Helen Wynyard Bellhouse, M.D., M.P.H."
         Journal of the American Medical Women's Association,
         10:10 (October 1955) 361. port. (Album of Women in
         Medicine.)
         A pediatrician, Helen Wynyard Bellhouse was appointed di-
         rector of the Maternal and Child Health Division of the
         Georgia Department of Public Health in 1952. Grady Me-
         morial Hospital and Emory University School of Medicine
         appointed her visiting instructor in pediatrics in 1955. She
         is also administratively responsible for the nutrition de-
         partment of the Georgia Department of Public Health.

1598.   Potter, Ellen C. "Ella B. Everitt, M.D." Journal of the
         American Medical Women's Association, 9:6 (June 1954)
         204. port. (Album of Women in Medicine.)
         Ella B. Everitt was born in 1866 and died in 1922. She be-
         came professor of gynecology in 1902 at the Woman's Med-
         ical College of Pennsylvania and later became chief of
         staff at the newly founded Woman's College Hospital. She
         was responsible for the establishment of scholarships by
         various denominations at the Woman's Medical College for
         financing the training of medical women missionaries. A
         chapel connected to a hospital in China was established in
         her name.

1599.   Powell, Janet Travell and Wensel, Louise Oftedal. "Doctor
         Wife and Mother." Wellesley Alumnae Magazine, (No-
         vember 1953) 13-15, 36. cartoon, photo., port.
         Two Wellesley alumnae recall their motivations for becom-
         ing physicians, describe their present career activities,
         and tell how they have raised children and managed a house-
         hold while practicing medicine. Janet Travell teaches
         pharmacology at Cornell Medical College and has carried
         on a medical practice since 1933; Louise Oftedal Wensel
         specializes in psychiatry.

1600.   Poynter, Lida. "Dr. Mary Walker, M.D. Pioneer Woman
         Physician." Medical Woman's Journal, 53:10 (October
         1946) 43-51. (History of Women in Medicine.)
         One of the pioneer medical women, Mary Walker, acquired
         her medical degree in 1855 from Syracuse Medical College
         (a short-lived eclectic school and one of the few that in-
         augurated medical coeducation for women). An independent
         thinker, Dr. Walker became one of the first suffragists and
         was a very consistent feminist all the rest of her life. An
         advocate of dress reform, she wore some style of reform
         dress until 1877 when she began to wear full masculine at-
         tire, although she never tried to pass as a man. One of
         her contributions was organizing a relief association to en-
         able women who visited Washington, D.C. to look for rela-
         tives or friends among the soldiers, to have a respectable
         place to spend the night, and to look after prospective moth-
         ers among the unmarried women who frequently became
         homeless. She also left her influence at the Confederate
         prison where she was incarcerated. As a result of her
         complaints, the prisoners occasionally ate wheat bread and
         cabbage rather than the usual corn bread. She was one of
         the first women in the country to study law, and while she
         never practiced formally, she used her legal knowledge
         (without pay for herself) to help the poor, and thus was
         able to help veterans of the war or their dependents to se-
         cure pensions.

1601.   "President, Dr. S. Josephine Baker." Women in Medicine,
         49 (July 1935) 17. port.
         A very brief account of Dr. Baker's professional activities
         since her graduation in 1898 from the Women's Medical
         College in New York is given. Active in public health, Dr.
         Baker was appointed assistant to the commissioner of the
         New York City Health Department. In 1908 she founded the
         model Bureau of Child Hygiene. She also organized the
         Little Mothers' League and the first Federation of Children's
         Agencies in New York City. An active worker in the suf-
         frage movement and an advocate of women's rights, she once
         refused a lectureship at New York University because wo-
         men were not admitted as students to the postgraduate
         classes. As a result, the policy changed.

1602.   "President-elect L. Rosa H. Gannt, M.D." Bulletin of the
         Medical Women's National Association, 29 (July 1930)
         7. port.
         Dr. Gannt graduated in 1901 from the South Carolina Med-
         ical College in Charleston, with the first class to graduate
         women.

1603.   "The President-Elect of the Medical Women's National As-
         sociation." Medical Woman's Journal, 37:7 (July 1930)
         205. port.
         A listing of Dr. Gantt's affiliations and memberships is

herein given.   Dr. Gantt graduated in 1901 from the Medical College of South Carolina.

1604.   "President-Elect of the State Society Iowa Medical Women."
          Woman's Medical Journal, 17:7 (July 1907) 318-319.
          port.
          Kate A. Mason-Hogle is the subject of this article.

1605.   "President Olga Stastny, M.D." Bulletin of the Medical
          Women's National Association, 29 (July 1930) 6.   port.
          A biographical sketch of Dr. Olga Stastny is presented,
          with particular emphasis on her work during [World War I].

1606.   Prior, Mary A.   "Queen City Women: A Series of Life
          Sketches."   Woman's Medical Journal, 5:7 (July 1896)
          175-176.
          A number of Cincinnati, Ohio ["Queen City"] women physi-
          cians are profiled in this article, including Julia Carpenter,
          Juliet M. Thorpe, Mary Osborn.

1607.   "Problems of Sex."   Medical Woman's Journal, 56:12 (De-
          cember 1949) 47-48.   (Book Reviews.)
          Although this article is a book review of Maude Glasgow's
          Problems of Sex, a major portion is a biography of Dr.
          Glasgow.

1608.   Pryor, Helen B.   "The Second Time Around."   Journal of
          the American Medical Women's Association, 27:1 (Jan-
          uary 1972) 34-36.
          Dr. Hulda Thelander, appointed to the curriculum committee
          of the University of California Medical School, enrolled in
          and completed the entire medical school course in order that
          she might be qualified to make suggestions.   She was also
          interested in learning about advances in medical knowledge.
          In this article Dr. Thelander's comments and reactions are
          expressed.

1609.   "Psychiatric Lecture Series Honors Dr. Hilde Bruch."
          BCM: Inside Baylor Medicine, 5:3 (April 1974) 1.
          port.
          Dr. Bruch is a professor of psychiatry at Baylor College of
          Medicine in Houston, Texas.   The four people who were
          brought in to speak at the Houston Psychiatric Society's
          meetings in honor of Dr. Bruch are listed.   Brief biograph-
          ical information is given on Dr. Bruch, one of the world's
          leading authorities on emotional problems relating to eating.

1610.   Puckett, Pearl.   "She's Mom to Two Thousand American
          Flyers."   Independent Woman, (January 1946) 23, 32.
          illus., photo.
          The office of Margaret Chung, the first woman to practice
          modern medicine in San Francisco's Chinatown, is a kind of
          headquarters for 2,000 "fair-haired" flyers.   It all began

when the Japanese attacked China and some American fly-
ers told Dr. Chung that they would offer their services to
China. Convinced that Japan would also attack the U.S.,
Dr. Chung's "American birth triumphed over her Chinese
ancestry," and she advised the flyers to fight for their own
country. The legend of "Mom Chung" grew. Now her of-
fice is filled with souvenirs sent to her by American flyers.
Among the mementos: "fabric from the plane in which
Quentin Roosevelt met his death; a charred fragment of the
Hindenburg ... a piece of the fuselage from the Will Rogers-
Wiley Post plane ... the rising sun insignia from the first
Jap plane shot down in the attack on Pearl Harbor ... and
a pair of goggles, minus a lens shot out by Bruno Musso-
lini...."

1611. Purdy, Ann. "The Woman Doctor: A Personal Memoir."
        Stanford M.D., 7:2 (Spring-Summer 1968) 16-18. port.
       In what she calls an "embarrassed profile," Ann Purdy re-
       calls her childhood community which allowed women no legal
       rights, where she witnessed much suffering from epidemic
       diseases and dreamed of becoming a doctor. Majoring in
       premedical sciences at McGill University, she was "hissed
       in nearly every class." A professor told her she could not
       be admitted to embryology classes because she would be in
       danger of bodily injury. When her application to McGill
       Medical School was refused, "scuttlebutt from Montreal Wo-
       men's Club had it that the medical faculty had threatened
       mass resignations if a woman was admitted. The sentiment
       was that having had one Maude Abbott they did not want an-
       other." She was "accepted but not welcomed" at Johns Hop-
       kins Medical School "into which women had been bought on
       a 10 per cent quota by a wealthy Baltimore woman for a
       half million dollars when the Medical School was hard up."
       There is a listing of contributions to medicine made by wo-
       men Dr. Purdy admires. She herself is best known for
       having conducted the pediatric cardiac clinic at Stanford Uni-
       versity Hospitals from 1931 to 1952. At the time this ar-
       ticle was written, she was emeritus clinic professor of
       pediatrics at Stanford.

1612. Putnam, Ruth, ed. Life and Letters of Mary Putnam Ja-
        cobi. G. P. Putnam's Sons, New York, New York,
        1925, xvii, 381 pp. facsims., ports.
       "As a child, Mary was always the leader ..." and a leader
       she remained--in opening the field of medicine to women as
       well as in her work as physician, educator, and suffragist.
       The whole of her remarkable career is here presented
       largely in her own words, through liberal use of corres-
       pondence. With faithful attention to chronology, the story
       of her pursuit of a medical education unfolds: her 1865
       graduation from New York's School of Pharmacy and from
       the Woman's Medical College of Pennsylvania the following
       year, her triumphant battle to win a degree from the Ecole

de Médecine in Paris, culminating with winning second
prize for her thesis and receiving "très satisfait" on final
exams.   Upon her return to America, she was elected to
the Medical Society of the County of New York and began
teaching at the Women's Medical College of New York.
Mary had a flair for writing and published a number of
stories in addition to her scientific papers. She disdained
the "literary physician" reputation, however, and preferred
to devote her major efforts to her science. Both her talent
and her intellectual precociousness are evident in a story
she wrote at age nine, a fragment of which could also serve
as her epitaph: "I went into the great world; many were
the rebuffs I met with, but I conquered them and my purpose was gained. I have devoted my life to aiding my fellow men...." A record of her publications follows the
text; there is no index. Photographs of family members are
included.

1613.   Quain, Fannie Dunn. "Pioneering in North Dakota." Wo-
             men in Medicine, 50 (October 1935) 15-17. (From Med
             ical Review-Woman's Number III.)
         Fannie Dunn Quain, the first native of North Dakota to take
         a medical degree, wrote this autobiographical reminiscence.
         She founded the State Tuberculosis Association, a branch of
         the National Tuberculosis Association, and the first baby
         clinic in North Dakota. After recalling an especially vivid
         and harrowing adventure, she concludes, "these experiences
         which I have been asked to relate were a few of many in
         the life of a pioneer and appear to me only incidents as
         compared with the real issues and values of life. These,
         to my mind, are my son and daughter and the part that I
         took in the organization of the Girls' Gymnasium Club and
         the 'Original Crowd' organizations...."

1614.   Rea, Marion Hague. "Fifty Years Ago--Dr. Marie For-
             mad." Medical Woman's Journal, 43:5 (May 1936) 132-
             133.
         Dr. Formad's completion of 50 years of service at the Wo-
         man's Hospital of Philadelphia prompted a banquet in her
         honor and this article, which tells how she came from Mos-
         cow in 1883, studied at the Woman's Medical College of
         Pennsylvania, and became a distinguished surgeon, gynecolo-
         gist, and pathologist. (Marie Formad's picture appears on
         the front cover of this issue of the Journal.)

1615.   Redman, Helen C. "Women in American Radiology." Jour-
             nal of the American Medical Women's Association, 27:
             9 (September 1972) 475-481.
         This article reviews early women in radiology. "The rela-
         tionship of the radiologist to the clinical is ... generally
         not one of competition.... This seems to allow acceptance
         of the woman physician by even some of the most vocal anti-
         feminist males. Some even admit that such a woman physi-

cian is a woman." An increasing number of women in
radiology is seen as the trend of the future.

1616.   Reed, Marjorie E. "Lovisa I. Blaire, M.D." Medical
              Woman's Journal, 52:4 (April 1945) 56.
         A biographical sketch of Dr. Blair, a graduate of the Wo-
         man's Medical College of Pennsylvania, constitutes this
         article. Dr. Blair was born and practiced medicine in
         Wilkes-Barre, Pennsylvania, and played a major role in
         the development of the diphtheria prevention program in
         that city.

1617.   Rees, Florence M. "Dr. Jennie Brookings Clark." Med-
              ical Woman's Journal, 53:12 (December 1946) 57. (In
              Memory.)

1618.   Reid, Ada Chree. "Elise Strang L'Esperance M.D."
              Journal of the American Medical Women's Association,
              14:5 (May 1959) 432-433. photo., port.
         Dr. L'Esperance received her M.D. degree in 1900 from
         the Women's Medical College of the New York Infirmary.
         In 1910 she began her association with Professor James
         Ewing as his assistant. She founded, in 1932, the Kate De-
         pew Strang Tumor Clinic at the New York Infirmary.

1619.   Reid, Ada Chree. "Esther Pohl Lovejoy, M.D." Journal
              of the American Medical Women's Association, 22:8
              (August 1967) 545-546. port.
         Author of numerous books--The House of the Good Neighbor
         (1920); Certain Samaritans (1927 and 1934); Women Physi-
         cians and Surgeons (1939); and Women Doctors of the World
         (1957)--Esther Pohl Lovejoy was an active force in organ-
         izing women physicians for service overseas. As a result
         of this work, Dr. Lovejoy was instrumental in founding and
         became director of the American Women's Hospitals.

1620.   "Rita Sapiro Finkler, M.D." Medical Woman's Journal,
              49:4 (April 1942) 121-122.
         Dr. Finkler (whose portrait appears on the front cover of
         this month's Journal) graduated from the Woman's Medical
         College of Pennsylvania in 1915. An endocrinologist, she
         wrote extensively in her specialty. A bibliography of her
         published works is included along with a recounting of her
         many professional and social activities.

1621.   Ritter, Mary Bennett. More Than Gold in California:
              1849-1933. The Professional Press, Berkeley, Cali-
              fornia, 1933, 468 pp.
         Mary Bennett Ritter was one of the second generation of
         women physicians in California. She attended Cooper Med-
         ical College in San Francisco, interned at Children's Hos-
         pital under Charlotte Blake Brown, and in 1887 assumed
         the practice of Sarah I. Shuey in Berkeley. Other women

associated with her early career were Euthanasia Sherman
Mead and C. Annette Buckel. While practicing in Berkeley,
Dr. Ritter became involved in the role and care of women
students at the University of California. Her concern and
activity were later rewarded when the first dormitory for
women on that campus was named in her honor. Her husband's work as director of the Scripps Institution caused
them to move to La Jolla in 1909. At this point, Dr. Ritter's autobiography becomes absorbed in their life and
travel together and with her activities in civic roles.

1622.   Robinson, Victor. "Elizabeth Blackwell." Medical Life,
            35:7 (July 1928) 310-333. ports. (Medical Woman's
            Number.)
         [This biographical essay originally appeared under the title
         "America's First Doctress," in the Woman's Number of
         Medical Review of Reviews, August 1916; it was republished
         in Delaware State Medical Journal, September 1916.]

1623.   Robinson, Victor. "Mary Putnam Jacobi." Medical Life,
            35:7 (July 1928) 334-353. port. (Medical Woman's
            Number.)
         "The sisters Blackwell may have been more heroic, and the
         charming Susan Dimock ... may have been more picturesque,
         but no woman physician of the period approached Dr. Mary
         Putnam Jacobi in intellectual breadth and scope." This bio-
         graphical essay concentrates on the hundreds of writings by
         Dr. Jacobi.

1624.   Rockhill, Margaret H. "Memorial: Dr. Eliza M. Mosher.
            Pioneer Woman Physician and Senior Editor." Medical
            Woman's Journal, 35:11 (November 1928) 305-312.
            ports.
         "A Personal Tribute" by Margaret Rockhill precedes a
         lengthy narrative of Eliza Mosher's professional activities
         and personal attributes, and the text of the sermon delivered
         at Dr. Mosher's funeral.

1625.   Rockstro, Enid. "Winifred Ladds, M.D. (London)." Med-
            ical Women's Federation News-Letter, (November 1930)
            82.

1626.   Rogers, Fred B. "Martha Tracy (1876-1942): Exceptional
            Woman of Public Health." Archives of Environmental
            Health, 9 (December 1964) 819-821. port. (Histor-
            ical Note.)
         Martha Tracy's career as scientist, educator, and admin-
         istrator is briefly summarized. In 1917 she received her
         doctorate in public health from the University of Pennsyl-
         vania and, in the same year, was appointed dean of the Wo-
         man's Medical College of Pennsylvania. After retiring from
         the deanship in 1940, she was named assistant director of
         health for Philadelphia.

1627. Root, E. H. "The Degree Medicinae Doctor for Women in
       Rush Medical College." Woman's Medical Journal,
       [13]:5 (May 1903) 91-92. port.
       In an April [1903] commencement, Josephine Agnes Jackson
       became the first woman to receive a medical degree from
       Rush Medical College. Dr. Jackson graduated from North-
       western University Woman's Medical School (now closed) in
       1896 and interned at Cook County Hospital.

1628. Root, Eliza H. "Dr. Margaret Taylor Shutt." Woman's
       Medical Journal, 13:4 (April 1903) 69-70.
       Dr. Shutt of Springfield, Illinois possessed the double train-
       ing of law and medicine.

1629. Root, Eliza H. "Dr. Marie J. Mergler as Woman and
       Physician." Woman's Medical Journal, 11:8 (August
       1901) 293-297. (Remarks, Memorial Services, Union
       Park Congregational Church, Chicago, Illinois, 26 May
       1901.)

1630. Root, Eliza H. "Frances Emily White, M.D." Woman's
       Medical Journal, 14:5 (May 1904) 97-99. port.

1631. Root, Eliza H. "Sarah Hackett Stevenson, M.D." Woman's
       Medical Journal, 14:4 (April 1904) 76-78. port.
       Dr. Stevenson's recent stroke comes as a staggering blow
       to medical women everywhere.

1632. Rose, Blanche E. "Early Utah Medical Practice." In:
       Utah Historical Quarterly. Volume 10. Edited by J.
       Cecil Alter. Utah State Historical Society, Salt Lake
       City, Utah, 1942, 14-33.
       Brigham Young felt strongly that there was a need for wo-
       men physicians, and his opinions influenced many Mormon
       women in their choice of a profession. Romania Bunnell
       Pratt Penrose graduated from Woman's Medical College in
       Pennsylvania in 1877 and became the first "native daughter"
       to practice in Utah, specializing in diseases of the eye.
       Ellen B. Ferguson was probably the first woman physician
       in Utah and the first woman deputy sheriff in the United
       States. Martha Hughes Paul Cannon, in addition to being
       one of Utah's early women physicians, was the first woman
       in the United States to be elected a state senator. Ellis
       R. Shipp practiced in Utah after 1878, was a prolific writer,
       and is remembered for the courses in nursing and obstetrics
       which she organized and conducted. [This information on
       Utah women physicians is found within the chapter cited, on
       pages 27-32.]

1633. Rose, Katherine S. Ms., (December 1972) 4. (Letters to
       Ms.)
       The granddaughter of Dr. Mabel S. Ulrich writes to the ed-
       itors regarding the article about her grandmother ("A Doc-

tor's Diary," Ms., July 1972). Katherine Rose reports that
her mother dropped out of medicine for a journalistic career.
"Her work ended in the Women's Page and then marriage.
All those sexist problems cleaned up, eh?" Her grandmother, Mabel S. Ulrich, moved into other fields than medicine,
opening a bookstore/gallery which was frequented by local
struggling authors (Fitzgerald among them).

1634.   "Rose Minoka-Hill, M.D." Medical Woman's Journal, 56:
              9 (September 1949) 39-40. facsim., photo.
         This biography of Lillie Rosa Minoka-Hill, a Mohawk Indian
         who worked among her people, was prompted by her accep-
         tance of a medal from the Woman's Medical College of
         Pennsylvania. Her alma mater honored her as a 50-year
         graduate.

1635.   "Rosemary Shoemaker, M.D." Medical Woman's Journal,
              49:2 (February 1942) 53.
         Dr. Shoemaker (whose portrait appears on the front cover
         of this month's Journal) received her M.D. in 1933 from
         the University of Pennsylvania School of Medicine. She is
         the only woman practicing urology in southern California.

1636.   Rosen, George and Caspari-Rosen, Beate, comps. 400
              Years of a Doctor's Life. Henry Schuman, Inc., New
              York, New York, 1947, xvii, 429 pp.
         The purpose of this anthology was to present an informal
         portrait of the physician "not only as the Great Healer or
         Great Scientist ... but also as a citizen of everyman's
         world." Excerpts from the writings of more than 80 per-
         sonalities who contributed to the literature of medical auto-
         biography include the works of four women physicians:
         Elizabeth Blackwell, S. Josephine Baker, Alice Hamilton,
         and Rosalie Slaughter Morton.

1637.   Ross, Ishbel. Child of Destiny: The Life Story of the
              First Woman Doctor. Harper & Brothers, New York,
              New York, 1949, 309 pp. port.
         This biography of Elizabeth Blackwell is based on family
         papers and reminiscences of Alice Stone Blackwell, as well
         as New York Infirmary records and papers at Radcliffe,
         Syracuse, and Oxford. The book gives details of Dr. Black-
         well's early life and tells of her decision to become a phy-
         sician, partly to "recover full mental freedom" after falling
         in love with a man she felt too narrow and rigid for her un-
         conventionality. It covers her education at Geneva, in Paris,
         and in London, and her struggle to establish herself in New
         York, culminating in the founding of the New York Infirmary
         with Marie Zakrzewska, where she urged women to wear
         looser clothing, engage in physical activity, and learn sani-
         tation in order to improve their health. Other chapters dis-
         cuss her activities for the Sanitary Aid Commission supply-
         ing nurses for the Union Army, her return to England where

she founded hospitals, worked for the medical education of
women, and espoused various moral reforms. The book
contains many quotations from her letters and diaries, an
index, and a bibliography.

1638.   Ross, Nancy Wilson. "Post-Mortem Pioneer." Reader's
        Digest, 47 (July 1945) 73-75.
        Adapted from Ross's Westward the Women, this article
        dramatizes events in the life of Dr. Bethenia Owens.

1639.   Roy, J. H. "Pinpoint Portrait of Doctor Dorothy Boulding
        Ferebee." Negro History Bulletin, 25 (April 1962) 160.
        [Article not examined by editors.]

1640.   Rudd, Helga M. "The Women's Medical College of Chicago:
        Records of Professors and Instructors and Alumnae.
        1871-1895." Medical Woman's Journal, 53:8 (August
        1946) 50-54. (History of Women in Medicine, Bertha
        Selmon, ed.)
        This installment [the last of three articles about the College,
        which was later called the Northwestern University Woman's
        Medical College] presents biographies of many of the school's
        distinguished graduates.

1641.   "Ruth V. Hemenway, M.D." Medical Woman's Journal, 52:
        2 (February 1945) 33. port.
        Dr. Hemenway graduated from Tufts Medical School in 1921.
        After hearing Dr. Mary Stone speak on medical missionary
        work in China, Dr. Hemenway determined to go to China
        also. In 1923 she went to Fukien Province in China and was
        Mintsing Hospital superintendent from 1924 to 1935. Dr.
        Hemenway kept a diary of her China experiences between
        1923 and 1941. Excerpts from this diary are presented in
        serial form in various issues of the Journal, from 1945
        through 1948.

1642.   Ruud, Helen. "Dr. Eliza Roxana Morse." Bulletin of the
        Medical Women's Club of Chicago, 18:12 (September
        1930) 3-4. port.

1643.   Ryder, Claire F. "Alice Hamilton, M.D." Journal of the
        American Medical Women's Association, 11:11 (November
        1956) 413, 416. port. (Album of Women in Medicine.)
        Alice Hamilton was a pioneer in industrial medicine and
        brought the facts of industrial disease before the entire
        country. Her autobiography, Exploring the Dangerous Trades,
        was published in 1943. She taught, studied and lived at Hull
        House. She coauthored Industrial Toxicology with Dr. Har-
        riet L. Hardy.

1644.   [Ryder, Claire F.] "Living Portraits." Journal of the
        American Medical Women's Association, 16:7 (July 1961)
        536-538. (Presentation, Midyear Meeting, Board of Di-

rectors, American Medical Women's Association, Hot
Springs, Arkansas, 15 November 1959.)
This biography of Louise Taylor-Jones is presented as a
vignette without the subject's name being mentioned: readers can find her name in another section of the journal.
After her father died and her family suffered financial hardship, Louise Taylor-Jones was fortunate in having a supportive mother who believed "that good food and a good education were essential" and who "had always been a stanch
supporter of independence for women." Several experiences
in her life document the prejudice against women during her
lifetime. For example, on two different occasions she taught
classes and yet the institutions, Columbian University and the
Army Medical Museum, assumed that she would teach without having her name printed in their school catalogs. Columbian University refused to pay her at all. In 1915 she
established a Red Cross hospital in Serbia. While pediatrics
was a fairly new field, she specialized in it.

1645.   "S. Josephine Baker, M.D." Medical Woman's Journal, 52:
        5 (May 1945) 38-39. port.
        This memorial to Dr. Baker gives biographical data on this
        1898 graduate of the Women's Medical College of the New
        York Infirmary.

1646.   Sabin, Francene. "From Skates to Scalpels." Diversion
        (December/January 1975) 34-37. photos., port.
        Dr. Tenley Albright, a former Olympic gold-medalist, prac-
        tices surgery in Boston, Massachusetts. This article deals
        with Dr. Albright's skating career, her Olympic success
        while a junior at Radcliffe College (Massachusetts), and her
        eventual acceptance in the medical program at Harvard Uni-
        versity (Massachusetts). She discusses also her feelings on
        being a woman physician and the way in which others respond
        to her as such.

1647.   Safford, Pearl. "An Interview." Medical Woman's Journal,
        51:10 (October 1944) 29-34.
        The subject of this biography is Dr. Lydia Allen De Vilbiss,
        whose many activities as a public health specialist included
        innovative work in the fields of birth control, venereal dis-
        ease, child hygiene, and maternal health. Dr. De Vilbiss
        also wrote and lectured about public health problems.

1648.   Sahli, Nancy Ann. Elizabeth Blackwell, M.D. (1821-1910):
        A Biography. University of Pennsylvania, Philadelphia,
        Pennsylvania, 1974, liii, 468 pp. (Ph.D. thesis.)
        The author states in her preface the significance of her re-
        search into the life of Elizabeth Blackwell as presenting "a
        biography derived from primary source material" and "a
        corrective for the erroneous impressions" conveyed by other
        works on Blackwell, i.e., their focus on her American med-
        ical career, and their almost total neglect of Blackwell's

last 40 years of life. Sahli qualifies her speculation on the causes of Elizabeth Blackwell's behavior and states that she has tried to present as complete and balanced a picture of Elizabeth Blackwell's life as possible. Sahli begins with Blackwell's childhood, education, and medical practice; devotes a chapter to Blackwell in England from 1869-1879; continues with Blackwell's interest in moral reform; and concludes with a chapter on Blackwell's "Private Life, Retirement, and Death." The work is thoroughly footnoted and contains a bibliography and an index.

1649.   "Salvation Army." Medical Woman's Journal, 55:1 (January 1948) 46. port.
Dr. Mary Richardson, along with her husband, operates a Salvation Army hospital in Yong Dong, Korea. The husband and wife physician team have established similar hospitals in India. During the war, Mary Richardson took charge of employment of the handicapped in Philadelphia. She is now a major in the Salvation Army.

1650.   Sanes, Samuel. "Elizabeth Blackwell: Her First Medical Publication." Bulletin of the History of Medicine, 16:1 (June 1944) 83-88. facsim.
Elizabeth Blackwell's inaugural thesis, submitted for her M.D. degree at Geneva Medical College, was published in the Buffalo Medical Journal and Monthly Review of February 1849. Titled "Ship Fever," it became the first article published by a woman physician in the United States. Dr. Blackwell's writing style, in contrast to the "ornate and prolix style" of the day, was "forthright, plain and clear, practically journalistic." The content of the thesis reveals Dr. Blackwell's character and points of view, including "a feminine sensitivity to human suffering," and "a righteous desire for social and economic justice."

1651.   Sargent, Eva R. "Mary Gaston, M.D." Journal of the American Medical Women's Association, 10:8 (August 1955) 284. port. (Album of Women in Medicine.)
Dr. Mary Gaston helped found the Somerset Hospital in Somerville, New Jersey.

1652.   "Says Age Is Asset to Chicago Woman Physician." Medical Woman's Journal, 54:6 (June 1947) 51-52. port. (News Notes.)
This article profiles Dr. Helga M. Ruud, one of three Chicago women over 80 featured in an article in the International Altrusan.

1653.   Schaefer, Jane. "Ann Purdy, M.D." Journal of the American Medical Women's Association, 11:1 (January 1956) 42, 44. port. (Album of Women in Medicine.)
Entering McGill University for her premedical training, Dr. Purdy's troubles were enhanced by the almost daily hissing

and booing of her male classmates, who resented her presence." She entered Johns Hopkins University Medical
School and "sold her blood at intervals" to pay part of her
way.

1654.   Schoch, Agnes Selin. "Dr. Elizabeth Reifsnyder: Pioneer
         Woman Medical Missionary to China." Pennsylvania
         History, 9 (April 1942) 151-153.
         Born in 1858 to a "jolly, well-to-do Pennsylvania Dutch fam-
         ily," Dr. Reifsnyder graduated from the Woman's Medical
         College of Pennsylvania in 1881. She opened the Margaret
         Williamson Hospital in Shanghai, China.

1655.   Schwendener, Hattie. "Daughters of Science: Dr. Hattie
         Schwendener, St. Joseph, Mich." Medical Woman's
         Journal, 36:9 (September 1929) 242-244. port.
         An autobiographical account is given by Dr. Hattie Schwen-
         dener, born in 1858 in Nunda, New York. Dr. Schwendener
         recalls her home environment and the predisposing factors
         which lead to her medical education and subsequent gradua-
         tion in 1879 from Wooster University. Hattie Schwendener's
         father took the news of her desire to be a doctor in his
         stride and provided Hattie a year's preceptorship in his of-
         fice. Her mother, on the other hand, "shed secret tears"
         for her daughter's decision for a career: "she had antici-
         pated a pretty, domestically inclined, home companion, and
         I never qualified," writes Dr. Schwendener. An account of
         her student days and her years in practice is also given.

1656.   "Section on War Service." Medical Woman's Journal, 50:7
         (July 1943) 179. port.
         Dr. Eleanor Hayden's career as an actress in Broadway
         summer stock preceded her medical career. In 1931, "when
         the depression struck," she decided to pursue the study of
         medicine rather than "fight for maintenance of salary and
         billing" in the theater. In 1939 she received her M.D. de-
         gree from New York University School of Medicine. At the
         time of this article, Dr. Hayden was a first lieutenant in
         the WAAC Medical Corps.

1657.   "Section on War Service." Medical Woman's Journal, 50:
         10 (October 1943) 256.   port.
         In order to follow her husband into military service, Dr.
         Effie M. Ecklund of Chicago joined the first WAC training
         center at Fort Des Moines as contract surgeon with the U.S.
         Army Medical Corps. Data on Dr. Ecklund's medical and
         graduate medical education are given.

1658.   "Section on War Service." Medical Woman's Journal, 51:
         2 (February 1944) 27.   port.
         A 1929 graduate of Woman's Medical College of Pennsylvania,
         Martha Elizabeth Howe is a captain in the army, serving her
         assignment at Fitzsimons Hospital, Denver, Colorado.

1659. "Section on War Service." Medical Woman's Journal, 51:
         4 (April 1944) 35. photo.
       "Carrying on in the footsteps of her late husband, a medical
       officer who lost his life on Guadalcanal," Dr. Laura E.
       Weber goes on active duty in the navy's medical corps.

1660. "Section on War Service." Medical Woman's Journal, 51:7
         (July 1944) 31. port.
       The commissioning of Mildred M. Healy, M.D. as a lieuten-
       ant in the navy's medical corps, prompted this biography of
       her.

1661. "Section on War Service." Medical Woman's Journal, 51:8
         (August 1944) 33. ports.
       Biographies are given of two physicians, both newly com-
       missioned in the navy's medical corps: Ellen W. Feder
       and Margaret Stebbins.

1662. Selmon, Bertha L. "An All-Medical Family (Six Physicians)."
         Medical Woman's Journal, 52:7 (July 1945) 37-39, 53.
         photos.
       Excerpts from "Notes from the Pine Mountain Settlement
       School" (Harlan County, Kentucky) and from Dr. Emma
       Boose Tucker's journal constitute major portions of this
       biographical article on Dr. Tucker. Emma Boose and her
       husband, Francis Tucker, returned to the United States after
       serving as medical missionaries in China. All of their four
       children also became physicians.

1663. Selmon, Bertha L. "Beginning of Public Acceptance--Ann
         Preston's Story." Medical Woman's Journal, 52:8 (Au-
         gust 1945) 37-39, 42. port. (History of Women in
         Medicine.)
       A brief discussion of the names of women appearing in the
       1869 edition of Eminent Women of the Age, is followed by
       the Ann Preston excerpt from that book. Dr. Bertha L.
       Selmon's poem, "The Ideal is the Real," concludes this
       article.

1664. Selmon, Bertha [L]. "Blackwell Footsteps in Michigan."
         Women in Medicine, 67 (January 1940) 21-27.
       This article sketches the careers of 50 women physicians
       in Michigan in the nineteenth century. The biographies were
       limited to those women born in the first half of the century.
       They are presented according to the country or region in
       which the physicians practiced. Outstanding among them is
       the material on Helen Walker M'Andrew who was active in
       opening the University of Michigan to women in 1869.

1665. Selmon, Bertha L. "Did You Read About 'Mom' in January,
         1946, 'Independent Woman?'" Medical Woman's Journal,
         53:4 (April 1946) 70.
       "'Mom' to the boys in aviation," Dr. Margaret Chung grad-

uated from the University of California and specialized in
plastic surgery.

1666.   Selmon, Bertha L. "Early History of Women in Medicine."
          Medical Woman's Journal, 53:1 (January 1946) 44-48.
          facsim., port. (History of Women in Medicine.)
The second woman to graduate from an American medical
college was Lydia Folger Fowler, who received her degree
in 1850. Sarah Adamson Dolley, who graduated in 1851
from the Eclectic School at Rochester [New York], became
the third American woman physician. Also in 1851, a few
months after Dr. Dolley's graduation, Rachel Brooks Gleason obtained her M.D. In addition to biographies of these
three women, other early women medical graduates are discussed, quoting extensively from Kate Hurd-Mead's Medical
Women of America.

1667.   Selmon, Bertha L. "Fifty Year Club: Hattie A. Schwen-
          dener, M.D." Medical Woman's Journal, 49:9 (Sep-
          tember 1942) 286-287.
Hattie A. Schwendener was an early pioneer medical woman
who practiced for 50 years. She was active in medical work
with children, especially orphans.

1668.   Selmon, Bertha L. "Hannah E. Longshore M.D." Medical
          Woman's Journal, 52:9 (September 1945) 39-41. (His-
          tory of Women in Medicine.)
This biography of Dr. Longshore, a graduate of the first
class of women physicians at the first woman's medical college in the U.S., quotes extensively from Eminent Women
of the Age. Attitudes towards women as physicians are
quoted, as well as excerpts revealing Dr. Longshore's success as teacher and physician. Dr. Longshore's family back
ground is also briefly covered.

1669.   Selmon, Bertha L. "History of Women in Medicine." Med-
          ical Woman's Journal, 52:5 (May 1945) 29-33.
Excerpts from The Life and Letters of Mary Putnam Jacobi,
Woman's Work in America, Medical Women of America,
and other documents comprise this discussion of the life and
times of Dr. Jacobi.

1670.   Selmon, Bertha [L]. "History of Women in Medicine: Mich-
          igan V." Medical Woman's Journal, 55:4 (April 1948)
          31-34, 62. (History of Women in Medicine.)
Biographies are given of several women who, between 1875
and 1880, obtained medical degrees from the University of
Michigan.

1671.   Selmon, Bertha [L]. "History of Women in Medicine: Mich-
          igan VI. The Battle Creek Sanitarium Provides Oppor-
          tunity." Medical Woman's Journal, 55:5 (May 1948) 41-
          44, 59. (History of Women in Medicine.)

Biographies are given of several women physicians who were
associated with the Battle Creek Sanitarium, which gained
renown for its use of physiotherapy in the treatment of ailments.

1672.   Selmon, Bertha L. "History of Women in Medicine: Mich-
           igan X." Medical Woman's Journal, 55:10 (October
           1948) 46-52. photos., ports. (History of Women in
           Medicine.)
        The life stories are told of several Michigan medical wo-
        men who practiced during the late 19th century.

1673.   Selmon, Bertha L. "In Memory." Medical Woman's Jour-
           nal, 51:5 (May 1944) 41. port.
        A 1904 graduate of the American Medical Missionary Col-
        lege, Linda Gage Roth was dean of women and medical di-
        rector of the Battle Creek [Michigan] College.

1674.   Selmon, Bertha [L]. "In Memory." Medical Woman's
           Journal, 54:1 (January 1947) 52-53. photo.
        Dr. Katharene Wave Allee Flanagan was the first woman
        graduate of the Baltimore University School of Medicine
        (1899). A very brief biography of Dr. Flanagan is included
        as well as reference to a more extensive biography.

1675.   Selmon, Bertha L. "In Memory." Medical Woman's Jour-
           nal, 54:2 (February 1947) 43. port. (News Notes.)
        Dr. Nina Copeland Wilkerson graduated in 1929 from the
        University of Kansas School of Medicine. She was, at the
        time of her death in 1946, the only woman physician prac-
        ticing in Sturgis, Michigan.

1676.   Selmon, Bertha L. "'A Memorial Service in Memory of
           Dr. Elizabeth Blackwell and Dr. Emily Blackwell':
           1911 (From a little book contributed by Martha K. Wal-
           lin, M.D.)." Medical Woman's Journal, 52:6 (June
           1945) 36-39, 59. ports. (History of Women in Medi-
           cine.)
        The memorial service was held at the New York Academy
        of Medicine and sponsored by the Women's Medical Associa-
        tion of New York City.

1677.   Selmon, Bertha [L]. "Pioneer Women in Medicine: Mich-
           igan VII. Battle Creek Sanitarium (Continued)." Med-
           ical Woman's Journal, 55:6 (June 1948) 50-53. (History
           of Women in Medicine.)
        Biographies are presented of several women physicians who
        were associated with the Battle Creek Sanitarium.

1678.   Selmon, Bertha [L]. "Pioneer Women in Medicine: Michi-
           gan VIII. Battle Creek Sanitarium (Continued)." Med-
           ical Woman's Journal, 55:8 (August 1948) 48-52, 59.
           port. (History of Women in Medicine.)

Biographies are given of several women physicians who
served on the Sanitarium's staff.

1679.   Selmon, Bertha L. "Pioneer Women in Medicine: Michi-
             gan IX." Medical Woman's Journal, 55:9 (September
             1948) 38-43. ports. (History of Women in Medicine.)
        Given are biographies of several women who practiced med-
        icine in Michigan during the late 19th century.

1680.   Selmon, Bertha L. "Pioneer Women in Medicine: Michi-
             gan XI." Medical Woman's Journal, 55:12 (December
             1948) 38-43, 58. ports. (History of Women in Medi-
             cine.)
        Biographies of several women physicians are given.

1681.   Selmon, Bertha L. "Pioneer Women in Medicine: Michi-
             gan XII." Medical Woman's Journal, 56:1 (January
             1949) 48-52. port. (History of Women in Medicine.)
        Early women graduates of the University of Michigan Med-
        ical Department, and several women who practiced medi-
        cine in Michigan, are the subjects of this article.

1682.   Selmon, Bertha L. "Pioneer Women in Medicine: Michi-
             gan XIII." Medical Woman's Journal, 56:2 (February
             1949) 44-49. port. (History of Women in Medicine.)
        Biographies of several Michigan women physicians are pre-
        sented.

1683.   Selmon, Bertha L. "Pioneer Women in Medicine: Michi-
             gan XIV." Medical Woman's Journal, 56:3 (March 1949)
             42-46. port. (History of Women in Medicine.)
        Biographies of several early Michigan women physicians are
        presented in this installment.

1684.   Selmon, Bertha [L]. "Pioneer Women in Medicine: Spread
             to the States Prior to 1900." Medical Woman's Jour-
             nal, 54:10 (October 1947) 51-54, 64. port. (History
             of Women in Medicine.)
        In this installment on the history of women in medicine,
        Dr. Selmon traces the "widening stream of medical women
        to each individual state." The life of Helen Walker Mc-
        Andrew, M.D. is profiled in some depth.

1685.   Selmon, Bertha [L]. "Pioneer Women in Medicine: Spread
             to the States Prior to 1900." Medical Woman's Jour-
             nal, 54:12 (December 1947) 39-43. ports. (History of
             Women in Medicine.)
        Drs. Amanda Sanford, Helen Upjohn, Helen Frances Warner,
        Sarah Gertrude Banks, Margaret Cochrane Cooper, and
        Mary E. Green are among the Michigan women physicians
        profiled in this article.

1686.   Selmon, Bertha [L]. "Pioneer Women in Medicine: Spread

to the States Prior to 1900. Eastern Graduates Enter
the State of Michigan Before the University Opens to
Women (1870)." Medical Woman's Journal, 54:11 (November 1947) 40-44, 68. facsim., photo., ports.
(History of Women in Medicine.)
Dr. Mary Grover Clark, Dr. Anna M. Longshore Potts,
Dr. Frances Armstrong Rutherford, Dr. Mary P. Havens,
and Dr. Lucinda Sexton Wilcox are among the women profiled in this article.

1687.   Selmon, Bertha L. "Woman's Medical College of Pennsyl-
         vania." Medical Woman's Journal, 52:10 (October 1945)
         41-43. (History of Women in Medicine.)
This article [a continuation of a series on the College]
quotes from books by and about women physicians, from
valedictory addresses, and from alumnae association notes,
to paint a continuing history of Emeline Horton Cleveland
and Rachel L. Bodley, early graduates and forces at the
Medical College of Pennsylvania.

1688.   Selmon, Bertha L. "Woman's Medical College of Pennsyl-
         vania." Medical Woman's Journal, 52:11 (November
         1945) 47-49. (History of Women in Medicine.)
This third article in a series of four articles on the College deals with the medical career of Anna Broomall, professor of obstetrics from 1878-1903.

1689.   Selmon, Bertha [L]. "The Women's Medical College of Chi-
         cago: Northwestern University Woman's Medical Col-
         lege. The Founders." Medical Woman's Journal, 53:
         7 (July 1946) 43-45. (History of Women in Medicine.)
This article [the second of three articles about the College]
profiles, among others, Mary Harris Thompson. Dr.
Thompson, one of the founders of the Women's Medical College of Chicago, was the first woman in Chicago to perform
major surgical operations.

1690.   Sensenig, E. Carl and Humphrey, Tryphena. "Elizabeth C.
         Crosby." Alabama Journal of Medical Sciences, 6
         (October 1969) 357-363. port.
This article was inspired by the presentation to Dr. Crosby
of the Karl Spencer Lashley Award of the American Philosophical Society. Dr. Crosby's background, professional
activity, memberships, and honors are detailed in this article. She has had many honorary degrees conferred upon
her, including an honorary M.D. degree from the University
of Groningen, the Netherlands.

1691.   Severinghaus, E. L. "Emma D. Kyhos, M.D." Journal
         of the American Medical Women's Association, 13:9
         (September 1958) 381. port. (Album of Women in Med-
         icine.)
Dr. Kyhos received her medical degree from the University

of Wisconsin in 1931.   In 1941 Dr. Kyhos assisted Dr.
Severinghaus in human nutrition studies.   Dr. Kyhos was
the joint author of four articles for which "patients in
Wisconsin General Hospital and volunteer subjects in the
Wisconsin State Prison were the human material."   After a
year of nutrition study and relief work in Naples, Italy, Dr.
Kyhos returned to the United States to become the first full-
time physician for employees at the Hoffmann-La Roche
plant in Nutley, New Jersey.

1692.   Shamer, Bertha Tapman.   "Claribel Cone, M.D."   Journal
          of the American Medical Women's Association, 7:11
          (November 1952) 431-432.   port.   (Album of Women in
          Medicine.)
          Claribel Cone graduated from the Woman's Medical College
          of Baltimore in 1890, the first college south of the Mason-
          Dixon Line where women could receive medical training.
          After receiving her degree, she entered Johns Hopkins Hos-
          pital to work in the laboratory of Dr. William H. Welch,
          professor of pathology.   With her sister as companion, she
          went to Europe to study in foreign laboratories.   In Paris
          she saw her old friend, Gertrude Stein, who encouraged her
          to purchase the work of such struggling artists as Matisse,
          Picasso, Van Gogh, and Cezanne.   Through the joint will of
          Dr. Cone and her sister, the Baltimore Museum of Art re-
          ceived this vast collection as well as a bequest of $400,000
          for a new wing to install the collection permanently.

1693.   [Shanahan, Kathleen].   "Living Portraits."   Journal of the
          American Medical Women's Association, 16:8 (August
          1961) 615-616.
          This biography is of Dr. Eleanor T. Calverly, Kuwait's
          first woman physician.   It is presented as a vignette with-
          out the subject's name being mentioned: The reader can find
          her name in another section of the journal.   Dr. Calverly
          received her medical degree from the Woman's Medical Col-
          lege in Philadelphia.   In 1912, on New Year's Day, Dr. Cal-
          verly opened her dispensary in Kuwait and became the first
          woman medical missionary to the Arabian people.   She min-
          istered to Arabian women and children and news of her suc-
          cess spread.   "When it became known that the doctor lady
          was expecting her first child, the women accepted her as
          another woman."

1694.   Shaw, Anna Howard and Jordan, Elizabeth.   The Story of a
          Pioneer.   Harper & Brothers Publishers, New York,
          New York, 1915, 338 pp.
          Anna Shaw was a pioneer in many respects--literally so as
          a teenager in the Michigan wilderness in the 1860s.   De-
          spite extreme poverty, she graduated from Boston Univer-
          sity Theological School in 1878 and served as a pastor in
          Cape Cod for eight years.   After overcoming the resistance
          of her parishioners to a young woman pastor, she divided

her time between studies at the Boston Medical School and the two churches she served. During this period she also began lecturing for woman suffrage, which became the vital influence in her life. She campaigned vigorously in nearly every state for the right of women to vote. Anna Shaw, a colleague and close friend of Susan B. Anthony, recalls their work together in "the Cause."

1695.   "She Never Wanted to Be a Nurse." Jefferson Medical College: Alumni Bulletin, 24:1 (Fall 1974) 16-17. port.
Martina Mockaitis Martin came to Jefferson in 1957 to study nursing, and left Jefferson in 1968 with her M.D.

1696.   "She Works in Philadelphia: Dr. Anne Pike, Physician and Teacher of Medicine, One of Nearly Half a Million Women Who Work in the Country's 3rd Largest City--Profiled in September." Charm Magazine, (September 1953). photos., port.
This biography incorporates a historical and current description of Dr. Pike's alma mater--Woman's Medical College of Pennsylvania.

1697.   Sherbon, Florence Brown. "Pioneer Medical Women: Hail and Farewell!" Medical Woman's Journal, 36:2 (February 1929) 47-49. ports.
This article gives biographical information on Dr. Dora Ann Sweezey McGreagor, who in 1864 received her M.D. degree from the Woman's Medical College of Pennsylvania. Several anecdotes in the life of Dr. McGreagor are included, as is a letter to Dr. McGreagor from Dr. M. J. Scarlett (one of Dr. McGreagor's professors in medical school).

1698.   Sheriff, Hilla. "Letters to the Editor." Medical Woman's Journal, 49:5 (May 1942) 158.
Hilla Sheriff, who graduated in 1926 from the Medical College of South Carolina, offers her autobiography in this letter. She was closely connected with the American Women's Hospitals' activities in South Carolina.

1699.   Shmigelsky, Irene. "Ruth Renter Darrow, M.D., 1895-1956." Journal of the American Medical Women's Association, 12:8 (August 1957) 271. port. (Album of Women in Medicine.)
Dr. Darrow graduated from Rush Medical School. She had a particular interest in and did notable research on erythroblastosis.

1700.   "Significant Autobiographies: IV--The Woman Physician." Everybody's Magazine, 9 (August 1903) 226-231.
In this autobiographical account, an anonymous woman physician discusses her motivations towards medicine, her early training, and her first practice. Anecdotes of medical cases, antagonism of brother physicians, attitudes of patients,

and advice to the would-be woman physician, fill out this article.

1701.   Simecek, Angeline. "Report of Work Under Mary Putnam
        Jacobi Fellowship, 1936-37." Medical Woman's Jour-
        nal, 46:5 (May 1939) 153-154.
        Funding from the Mary Putnam Jacobi Fellowship permitted
        Dr. Simecek to work and study at the General Hospital in
        Prague, Czechoslovakia, where she developed an interest in
        the field of female sterility.

1702.   Singer, Joy Daniels. My Mother, the Doctor. E. P. Dut-
        ton & Co., Inc., New York, New York, 1970, 224 pp.
        This book consists of a biography and memoir of Anna
        Kleegman Daniels by one of her daughters. The narrative
        concentrates on the subject's early family life as a Jew in
        Russia and her role in the family as daughter, sister, wife,
        and mother following immigration to the U.S. in the early
        20th century. There is little discussion of her professional
        education at Cornell, her subsequent medical practice, or
        her role as a woman physician. There are sketches of in-
        cidents with patients to illustrate her relationships with
        them and her position on issues such as abortion. A Yid-
        dish glossary is appended.

1703.   "Sisters Forty-Six Years in Practice: Frances J. Henry,
        M.D. and Anna Henry McClung, M.D." Medical Wo-
        man's Journal, 52:6 (June 1945) 41-42, 48. ports.
        Dr. Frances J. Henry and Anna Henry McClung are sisters
        who have been in medical practice for 46 years, Dr. Fran-
        ces J. Henry in Kansas City, Missouri and Dr. Anna Henry
        McClung in Pattonsburg, Missouri. This article gives bio-
        graphical information on their lives.

1704.   "A Sketch from a Western Country Medical Woman's Life.
        (As a Preparatory School for War Service.)" Woman's
        Medical Journal, 27:8 (August 1917) 178-180.
        A woman doctor who has practiced in mining camps, lumber
        camps, and dredgers in California's El Dorado and Sacra-
        mento counties, describes the kinds of medical cases she
        encountered, the difficulties of travel, and other hardships
        she experienced over her 24-year career.

1705.   Sloop, Mary T. Martin and Blythe, Legette. Miracle in
        the Hills. McGraw-Hill Book Company, Inc., New York,
        New York, 1953, x, 232 pp. photos.
        Mary T. Martin Sloop was born and raised in North Caro-
        lina. She graduated from the Woman's Medical College of
        Pennsylvania in 1906 and interned the following year at the
        New England Hospital for Women and Children. In 1908
        she married, and she and her physician-husband practiced
        together in the hill country of North Carolina. They es-
        tablished a school at Crossnore to increase the educational

opportunities for youth in the region and counter the trend
of early marriages then prevalent. One of Dr. Sloop's
children, Emma Sloop Fink, also became a doctor. In
1951 Mary Martin Sloop was named American Mother of the
Year. This autobiography emphasizes the human interest
aspects of Appalachian life.

1706. Smith, Alice M. "Dr. Alice M. Smith's Annual Letter."
       Bulletin Medical Women's Club of Chicago, 14:5 (Janu-
       ary 1926) 6-7.
       Dr. Smith's letter comes from Tacoma, Washington, where
       she is involved in many public offices and is the woman
       member of the State Institutional Board of Health. Dr.
       Smith devotes much of her letter to a description of her lit-
       erary endeavors and reports that a play she has written,
       The Strength of the Weak, is in the hands of a New York
       agent.

1707. Smith, Joseph T. "Alice Ettinger, M.D." Journal of the
       American Medical Women's Association, 8:10 (October
       1953) 344. port. (Album of Women in Medicine.)
       Dr. Ettinger received her M.D. degree from the Univer-
       sity of Berlin. She was sent to Boston by Dr. H. H. Berg
       of Berlin in response to a request by Dr. Joseph H. Pratt
       to send a well-trained pupil to Boston to work with the
       Joseph H. Pratt Diagnostic Hospital. Dr. Ettinger, through
       her work with the rural hospitals in Maine, developed
       throughout that state "a keen interest in the practice of
       radiology."

1708. Smith, Katharine. "Della G. Drips, M.D." Journal of the
       American Medical Women's Association, 10:1 (January
       1955) 29. port. (Album of Women in Medicine.)
       Dr. Drips received her M.D. degree from the University of
       Minnesota, after which she went to the Mayo Foundation.
       In 1949, she retired. Throughout her career her special
       interest was gynecologic endocrinology, a field in which she
       did pioneer investigations. A list of her professional mem-
       berships is included.

1709. Smith, Stephen. "The Medical Co-education of the Sexes."
       Philanthropist, (August 1892) 3, 6.
       Dr. Smith retells the story of Elizabeth Blackwell's accep-
       tance and admission to Geneva Medical College (New York)
       from the point of view of a student in the class which voted
       for her admission. Dr. Blackwell was the first woman ad-
       mitted to a medical school in the United States.

1710. Snelgrove, Erle E. "The First Woman Doctor." Hygeia,
       (August 1949) 534-535, 567. ports.
       Portraits and biographical data are given on the 12 physi-
       cians who received Elizabeth Blackwell Centennial Citations
       at the Hobart and William Smith Colleges. The awards

were given following a radio salute to medical women by
Mrs. Franklin D. Roosevelt.

1711.   Snell, Elsie K. "Dr. Marie Zakrzewska, Memorial Mem-
         ber." Women in Medicine, 58 (October 1937) 25.
         Presented is a short biography of Dr. Zakrzewska who went
         to the United States from Poland in 1853. There she lived
         with her sister in "unbelievable poverty." She had hoped to
         find greater success in the U.S. than she had in Berlin with
         her midwifery degree. She found to her surprise that in
         America "women physicians were not recognized and held
         places inferior to a nurse." Eventually she met Elizabeth
         Blackwell who encouraged her to obtain a medical degree,
         which she did from the Cleveland Medical College. She
         went on to become the leading woman physician in Boston.

1712.   Snyder, Charles McCool. Dr. Mary Walker: The Little
         Lady in Pants. Vantage Press, New York, New York,
         1964, 166 pp. photos., ports.
         Born in 1832, Mary Edwards Walker obtained a medical de-
         gree in 1855 from the Syracuse Medical College. She mar-
         ried Albert Miller in a ceremony at which she appeared in
         trousers, refused to assume her husband's name, and ex-
         cluded from the ritual the wife's vow to obey her husband.
         The marriage did not last long. Dr. Walker went on to be-
         come a dress reform crusader, an assistant surgeon during
         the Civil War and winner of the Congressional Medal of
         Honor, a lecturer and author, and suffragette. She died at
         the age of 86. This biography, which contains references
         and an index, includes photographs of Dr. Walker from the
         age of 12 to three years before her death in 1919.

1713.   "The Soft-Spoken Fellow at NIH." Jefferson Medical Col-
         lege: Alumni Bulletin, 24:1 (Fall 1974) 17. port.
         Dr. Judith Cooper Andersen is the only female member of
         the hematology division of the National Institutes of Health
         Clinical Center.

1714.   Solomon, Barbara Miller. "Historical Determinants in In-
         dividual Life Experiences of Successful Professional Wo-
         men." Annals of the New York Academy of Sciences,
         208 (15 March 1973) 170-178.
         In 1848, when Elizabeth Cady Stanton and Lucretia Mott or-
         ganized the Women's Rights Convention in Seneca Falls, New
         York, they called for the opening of the professions, includ-
         ing medicine, to women. Women doctors made visible con-
         tributions in the Civil War and helped to popularize the fact
         that women could become M.D.s. One such example was
         Mary Frame Myers Thomas, who practiced with her husband,
         an army surgeon, and who herself later made distinguished
         contributions to public health. The intent of many of these
         first women doctors was to improve the health care of fe-
         males and children. Some women doctor pioneers include

Elizabeth Blackwell, who overcame her repugnance for the
human body and attended Geneva College in 1847 (later in
1868, she started the Women's Medical College of New York
Infirmary). Dr. Alice Hamilton became a doctor because
she perceived herself as 'scientifically-minded' and because
becoming a doctor could give her mobility to foreign lands
or city slums. As a result of her research in bacteriolog-
ical studies relating to industrial diseases, Dr. Hamilton
received an appointment as assistant professor at Harvard
Medical School. The half-sister of Mary Myers Thomas,
Hannah E. Myers Longshore, apprenticed herself to her
brother-in-law, one of the founders of the Female Medical
College of Pennsylvania which she later attended. When she
received her degree in 1851, police guarded the commencement exercises. Florence Sabin was renowned for her
studies on blood in the 1920s and 1930s. Helen Taussig
pioneered in heart research and in 1959 became the first
woman full professor at Johns Hopkins. Women doctors also
became prominent in the field of public health. In the 1920s
and 1930s, such pioneers included Josephine Baker, Connie
Guion, Leona Baumgartner and Margaret Barnard. Continuing that tradition in the 1970s were Mary Calderone, Gertrude Hunter, and Judianne Densen-Gerber.

1715.   Soriano, Victor. "The Exemplary Life of Elizabeth Black-
              well First Woman Medical Doctor in the World." In-
              ternational Journal of Neurology, 9:2 (1974) 192-197.
              illus.
          Professor Soriano describes Elizabeth Blackwell as "a weak
          woman who brought about one of the most extraordinary
          revolutions in history, without aggressiveness, without dis-
          cursive activity, no high-sounding attitudes."

1716.   Spalding, Warren F. "Resumé of Dr. Mosher's Work in
              the Massachusetts Reformatory for Women." Medical
              Woman's Journal, 32:5 (May 1925) 145-146.
          In 1877, Dr. Mosher became the first physician at the
          Massachusetts Reformatory Prison for Women. She later
          became superintendent at that institution and initiated pro-
          grams to help the prisoners develop "self-control and ...
          self-respect ... to take the place of repression."

1717.   Spillman, Ramsay. "In Memory." Medical Woman's Jour-
              nal, 51:8 (August 1944) 42.
          Ethel Leonard obtained her M.D. from the University of
          Southern California in 1902. Her career included 15 years
          of service in China. Wanting "to aid humanity even after
          her death" (in 1944), Dr. Leonard dedicated her body to
          medical research.

1718.   Stack, N. "Americans Not Everybody Knows: Elizabeth
              Blackwell." PTA Magazine, 61 (February 1967) 26-27.
          [Article not examined by editors.]

1719.   Stasny [sic], Olga. "American Women's Hospitals: Med-
          ical Service Committee." Medical Woman's Journal,
          31:5 (May 1924) 126-137. photos.
          The author provides a narrative on her experiences while
          working with the American Women's Hospitals in Greece.

1720.   Stastny, Olga. "Autobiographical Sketch." Medical Review
          of Reviews, 41:8 (August 1935) 410-423.
          Dr. Stastny relates incidents from her earliest childhood
          when she was fascinated by concerns of health and disease.
          Married at the age of 17 and the mother of two by the age
          of 21, Dr. Stastny began to consider medical school. It
          was not until her husband's death (when she was 28) how-
          ever, that she felt the need for activity, and she planned to
          enter medical school. Dr. Stastny entered the University
          of Nebraska College of Medicine, from which she graduated
          in 1913. In 1914 she opened her general practice in Omaha,
          Nebraska. Dr. Stastny's work in France with the American
          Women's Hospitals is extensively covered, as is her work in
          Czechoslovakia. For these efforts she received much recog-
          nition. In 1924 Dr. Stastny reopened her office in Omaha.

1721.   Stern, Madeleine B. So Much in a Lifetime: The Story of
          Dr. Isabel Barrows. Julian Messner, Inc., New York,
          New York, 1964, 191 pp.
          This biography of Isabel Barrows, first woman ophthalmolo-
          gist in America, is written for young adults. Daughter of
          a New England physician, she resolved to study medicine
          after a brief sojourn in India, where her husband died of
          diphtheria. She studied both at Bellevue Hospital and at
          Women's Medical College of the New York Infirmary, where
          she found the work more limited in scope than at Bellevue,
          despite Bellevue's horrors in the late 1860s. In Vienna in
          1870, at the age of 25, she obtained a degree in ophthal-
          mology, which she practiced in Washington for several
          years. Later, as an editor in Boston, she taught English
          to Catherine Breshkovsky, the Russian patriot. During
          Breshkovsky's subsequent imprisonment in Moscow, Barrows
          traveled to Russia and attempted unsuccessfully to free
          Breshkovsky by appealing to officials. The book also re-
          counts several experiences of Mary Safford, obstetrician and
          gynecologist, with whom Barrows studied in New York and
          Vienna, and tells of Barrows's years in Washington as Con-
          gress's first woman stenographer. There is no index.

1722.   Stetler, Pearl M. "Mary Edith Williams, M.D." Journal
          of the American Medical Women's Association, 11:9
          (September 1956) 329. port. (Album of Women in Med-
          icine.)
          Dr. Williams received her M.D. degree in 1917 from the
          University of Illinois. This article cites Dr. Williams' ac-
          complishments and affiliations.

1723.   Stevens, Audrey D. "Arizona's Territorial Tales." Ari-
            zona Medicine, 29:9 (September 1972) 727-728. photo.,
            ports. (ArMA Medical History.)
         Four of Arizona's pioneer women physicians, all of whom
         graduated from the Female Medical College of Pennsylvania
         [now the Medical College of Pennsylvania], are profiled. A
         physician for the Navajo and Hopi Indians, Mary H. McKee
         was the first Arizona woman to be named in Polk's Medical
         and Surgical Register of the United States (1890). While
         Anna M. Longshore-Potts was in Arizona, she probably be-
         gan writing Discourses to Women on Medical Subjects (1897)
         and Love, Courtship, and Marriage [1891]. The first wo-
         man to practice medicine in Arizona was Jennie Hildebrand
         (in 1882). Elizabeth Ryland Snyder, who worked among the
         Indians, obtained her Arizona license in 1904.

1724.   Stewart, George Walter. A Biographical Portrait of Zella
            White Stewart, M.D. Privately printed, Iowa City,
            Iowa, 1943, 139 pp.
         [Item not examined by editors.]

1725.   Stewart, Margaret R. From Dugout to Hilltop. Murray &
            Gee, Inc., Culver City, California, 1951, 223 pp.
         Margaret Stewart's autobiography covers her childhood in
         Nebraska with her pioneer family, and her personal and pro-
         fessional adult life. She graduated from a medical school
         in San Francisco in 1900 but later attended the Woman's
         Medical College of Pennsylvania, from which she graduated
         in 1906. She practiced in California until 1911, when she
         was appointed superintendent of the Washington Sanitarium.
         Dr. Stewart was called into the Public Health Service in
         1917 to serve in the Fort Worth, Texas extra cantonment
         zone. She spent 25 years of her medical career with the
         U.S. government, first with the Public Health Service, and
         then with the Veterans Administration, which was organized
         out of the Public Health Service following World War I. Her
         outstanding positions were those of chief of the tuberculosis
         section of the Veterans Administration (1918-1925), and then
         chief of the Veterans Diagnostic Center at the Cincinnati Gen-
         eral Hospital (1925-1933). In 1933 she was transferred to
         the Veterans Hospital in Asheville, North Carolina, where
         she remained until her retirement in 1943.

1726.   "Still Pioneering." Journal of the American Medical Wo-
            men's Association, 9:12 (December 1954) 403-406.
         Abstracts from letters of women physicians in Ohio are pre-
         sented as proof that the "pioneering luster" is still very
         much in evidence in the Northwest territory. Abstracts
         from letters of Dr. Barbara Hewell, Dr. Louise Du Breel,
         and Myrta M. Adams are included.

1727.   Stone, Berenice. "Anita M. Mühl, M.D." Journal of the
            American Medical Women's Association, 16:10 (October

1961) 782-783. port.
Dr. Mühl willed $20,000 to the American Medical Women's
Association (AMWA) to be incorporated into the Scholarship
Loan Fund for women in medicine. She received her M.D.
degree from Indiana University School of Medicine in 1920.
In about 1920 she summered in Iceland, where she organized
that country's first Mental Hygiene Conference. Her inter-
national orientation is witnessed by lectureships in Australia,
Iceland, and the United States, as well as by memberships
in the Medical Women's International Association and the
Pan American Medical Women's Association.

1728.   Storkan, Margaret Ann. "Elisabeth Larsson, M.D." Jour-
         nal of the American Medical Women's Association, 9:11
         (November 1954) 377. port. (Album of Women in
         Medicine.)
         Coming to America from Sweden in 1920, Dr. Larsson
         studied at the College of Medical Evangelists in Los Angeles.
         Her work in obstetrics and gynecology is complemented by
         her daily charities.

1729.   Straight, William M. "The Lady Doctor of the Grove."
         Journal of the Florida Medical Association, 56:8 (August
         1969) 615-621. facsim., illus.
         This article briefly sketches the obstacles to women in med-
         icine immediately preceding and contemporary with Eleanor
         Galt Simmons's training and period of practice. Next is
         given a brief account of her known career, the transporta-
         tion and residential conditions of and opportunities for phy-
         sicians in Coconut Grove at the time she began to practice.
         When Dr. Simmons was issued an occupational license to
         practice medicine in Dade County, Florida for the year 1893-
         1894, she became one of the first five physicians so licensed,
         and the first woman physician to practice in Dade County.

1730.   Stuart, N. G. "Mother Is a Doctor Now! Frances A. Ol-
         sen of Philadelphia." Ladies' Home Journal, 75 (May
         1958) 131-134, passim.
         [Article not examined by editors.]

1731.   "A Student Health Center Practice: Time is the Essence."
         University of New Mexico School of Medicine Alumni
         News, 1:3 (December 1974) 6. port.
         Effie Medford, the only female on the University of New
         Mexico Student Health Center's staff of seven, is the subject
         of this article.

1732.   "Student News." Medical Woman's Journal, 53:7 (July 1946)
         70.
         The first woman student in the Emory University School of
         Medicine, Winton Elizabeth Gambrell obtained her M.D. in
         March 1946. Also profiled in this article: Dr. Mary Mc-
         Daniel Richardson, who has practiced medicine in the Orient
         for 18 years.

1733. Sturgis, Katharine R. "First Woman Fellow of the College
       of Physicians of Philadelphia: Memoir of Catharine
       Macfarlane, 1877-1969." Transactions and Studies of
       the College of Physicians of Philadelphia, 38:3 (January
       1971) 157-160. (Presentation, College of Physicians of
       Philadelphia, 4 November 1970.)
       Drawing heavily on the anecdotes and personal reflections
       in Dr. Macfarlane's diary, Dr. Sturgis recalls the profes-
       sional accomplishments and the personality of "Kitty Mac."

1734. Sturgis, Margaret Castex. "Ann Preston: Physician."
       Journal of the American Medical Women's Association,
       3:12 (December 1948) 509-511. port.
       Ann Preston was one of eight members of the first graduat-
       ing class of the Female Medical College of Pennsylvania.
       Dr. Preston established a hospital for women and children
       which was under the management of women and enabled wo-
       men medical students to have clinical opportunities for in-
       struction. In 1866 she was appointed dean of the faculty of
       the Woman's Medical College and the following year was
       made a member of the Board of Corporators of the College.
       "The furtherance of the medical education of women was the
       cause to which she had dedicated her life with a true con-
       secration. It was said that she made the 'interests of the
       college her interest, its honor her honor, shrank not from
       its obloquy, shared its pecuniary embarrassments, labored
       to increase its advantages and elevate its standards of schol-
       arships.'"

1735. "Surgery Is a Way of Life." Jefferson Medical College:
       Alumni Bulletin, 24:1 (Fall 1974) 22-23. port.
       Kathleen McNicholas (M.D. 1973), a general surgery resi-
       dent at Columbia Presbyterian Medical Center, "is emphat-
       ically not a feminist." Ms. magazine's request to photo-
       graph her was "'silly,'" for sex has never been a factor
       in her career. Dr. McNicholas is the first woman in 30
       years to be accepted for Columbia Presbyterian's surgical
       residency.

1736. "Surgery Made Plain." Time, (4 November 1940). photos.
       This brief article on Dr. Bertha Van Hoosen elaborates
       upon Dr. Van Hoosen's technique of demonstrating a cesar-
       ean operation utilizing a box representing a woman's abdo-
       men. The various organs are modeled out of household
       materials (e.g., red yarn "knitted by Dr. Van Hoosen her-
       self" represents the pattern of abdominal muscles, fallopian
       tubes, and ovaries).

1737. "Susan Hayhurst." American Journal of Pharmacy, (Janu-
       ary 1911) 32-40. port.
       Susan Hayhurst, M.D., Ph.G., was, in 1883, the first wo-
       man graduate of the Philadelphia College of Pharmacy. She
       graduated from the Woman's Medical College in 1857.

1738.   "Susan M. Anderson, M.D." Medical Woman's Journal,
            50:10 (October 1943) 269. (News Notes.)
         This biography of "Doc Susie" (reprinted from Pic, May 11,
         1943) gives an episodic, narrative account of the life of
         Dr. Susan M. Anderson, the only doctor in Fraser, Colo-
         rado.

1739.   Swartz, Philip Allen; Shaw, Lillian E.; and Atkinson, Doro-
            thy Wells. "Alice Stone Woolley, M.D.: In Memoriam."
            Journal of the American Medical Women's Association,
            2:11 (November 1947) 503-505.
         A member of the editorial board of the Journal of the Amer-
         ican Medical Women's Association, president of the Amer-
         ican Medical Women's Association, and chairman of its
         Committee on International Affairs, Alice Stone Woolley was
         instrumental in advancing "social and medical activities not
         only in her own locality but throughout the nation and the
         world." In a tribute to Dr. Woolley, Philip Swartz writes,
         "Her unusual capacity for creating confidence and for includ-
         ing so many in the circle of personal friendship may be
         traced back to those days when she was associated with
         Miss Mary Ellen Reid, executive secretary of the Young
         Women's Christian Association. These two women became
         life long friends and worked together to forward many of
         the outstanding projects of Dutchess County. Their home,
         the beautiful old homestead 'Stoneridge,' was always the cen-
         ter of gracious hospitality."

1740.   Taylor, Ruth E. "M. Alice Phillips, M.D." Journal of the
            American Medical Women's Association, 10:3 (March
            1955) 96. port. (Album of Women in Medicine.)
         A gynecologist, M. Alice Phillips was a graduate of Rush
         Medical College.

1741.   Teffeau, Cleora. "Sophia Presley, M.D.: The Spinster
            Who Struggled Seven Years Against Bias of Male Doc-
            tors." Bulletin of the Camden County Historical So-
            ciety, 28 (May 1975) 36-45. port.
         A chronological recounting of Sophia Presley's efforts to
         "break through the barrier of opposition to women physi-
         cians" in Camden, New Jersey is presented. Excerpts
         from various records form the content of this article.

1742.   Tenbrinck, Margaret S. "The American Women's Hospitals
            Service." Journal of the American Medical Women's
            Association, 22:9 (September 1967) 628-629. (Presenta-
            tion, Pan American Medical Women's Alliance, Xth
            Congress, Lima, Peru, February, 1967.)
         1967 marked the 50th anniversary of the American Women's
         Hospitals Service to which Esther Pohl Lovejoy contributed
         so much of her energy and time. Dr. Lovejoy was the sec-
         ond woman to graduate from the University of Oregon Med-
         ical School. The first woman to practice in Portland, she

also was the first woman to head Portland's Department of Health. Under her direction, stricter hygienic practices and stricter methods of collecting milk were instituted. When the Medical Women's International Association was founded, Dr. Lovejoy was appointed the first president. The establishment of the American Women's Hospital resulted in a supportive atmosphere for women around the world desiring to enter the field of medicine.

1743.   Terry, Robert J. "Recalling a Famous Pupil of McDowell's Medical College: Harriet Goodhue Hosmer, Sculptor." Washington University Medical Alumni Quarterly, 7 (1944) 59-65. port.
[Article not examined by editors.]

1744.   Thelander, Hulda E. "Helen Brenton Pryor, M. D. --Pediatrician (1898-1972)." Journal of the American Medical Women's Association, 28:11 (November 1973) 595, 598-599. port.
The daughter of a woman physician, Helen Brenton Pryor served her internship at the Rockefeller Institute and Medical Center in Peking and then worked at the Nanking University Hospital until 1927 when the Chinese civil war interrupted her work. After she returned to the States, she specialized in child growth and development, making several contributions in pediatrics. After studying 6,000 girls and 6,000 boys in the San Francisco area, she established anthropometric measurement statistics to form height-weight tables. Dr. Pryor co-authored several papers with Hulda E. Thelander including several on the effect of varying degrees of microcephally on mongoloid or trisomy 23, and the intelligence of children. In addition to this work, Dr. Pryor co-authored The American Health series which had a book for every elementary school grade. She wrote the section under "Baby" in the World Book. As the Child Grows is a text she wrote in 1943 for students interested in child development.

1745.   Thelander, H[ulda] E. "Mary Elizabeth Glover, M. D." Journal of the American Medical Women's Association, 12:9 (September 1957) 307. port. (Album of Women in Medicine.)
Mary Glover practiced general medicine in San Francisco from 1906 to 1956. She was one of the founders of the Women Physicians' Club of San Francisco.

1746.   "'There Were Bets ... I Fooled Them': Loree Florence Ends 45 Years Active Practice." MCG Today, 1:4 (Spring 1971) 4-5, 29. ports.
In 1926 Dr. Florence became the first woman graduate of the Medical College of Georgia [MCG].

1747.   "These Were the First." Journal of the American Medical

Women's Association, 11:6 (June 1956) 214.
Beatrice O. Jones was the first woman president of the
Racine County Medical Society and the first woman president of a county medical society in Illinois.   Emma Moss
was the first woman president of the American Society of
Clinical Pathologists.   Jaya Luke, a physician, judge, and
lay preacher served the isolated area of Sironcha district,
India and maintained a 26 bed hospital, with six dispensaries
in outlying villages.   Ellen G. Wallace was a pioneer in
health work in New Hampshire and started practicing in Manchester in 1867.   She was the first physician to work for
the prevention of tuberculosis in that state, introduce public
nursing, and institute Health Day on the calendar.   Anna M.
Young was the first woman on the board of the Cleveland
Academy of Medicine.

1748.   Tissue, Florence. "In Memory: Florence Brown Sherbon,
          M. D., 1869-1944." _Medical Woman's Journal,_ 51:6
          (June 1944) 37-38. port.
          "Dr. Sherbon succeeded as nurse, doctor, administrator,
          teacher, mother, and writer, weaving her varied experi-
          ences into a full and complete life."   Examples of her ac-
          complishments within these fields are given.

1749.   "Too Busy for Anniversaries." _Medical Woman's Journal,_
          33:11 (November 1926) 321-322. port.
          An article that appeared in the _Brooklyn Times_ is reprinted
          on Eliza M. Mosher's fifty-first "medical birthday."   Her
          professional affiliations and accomplishments are listed.
          She became "the originator of the notion of quartering physi-
          cians in office buildings" when she entered into practice
          with her cousin, Dr. Burr Burton Mosher, in New York
          City's Galen Hall.   As founder of the New York Posture
          League, she designed subway seats which properly support
          the back.

1750.   Touff, Roselyn. "Esther C. Marting, M. D." _Journal of
          the American Medical Women's Association,_ 10:9 (Sep-
          tember 1955) 317. port. (Album of Women in Medi-
          cine.)
          Dr. Marting received her M. D. degree from the University
          of Cincinnati Medical School in 1932.   Facts of her pro-
          fessional and non-professional lives are given.

1751.   Tower, Elizabeth A. "Report From Alaska." _Case West-
          ern Reserve Medical Alumni Bulletin,_ 31:4 (Fourth
          Quarter, 1967) 7. illus.
          Dr. Tower tells of her activities in Anchorage, Alaska and
          provides generalized information on the practice patterns of
          other Alaskan women physicians.

1752.   Travell, Janet. _Office Hours: Day and Night. The Auto-
          biography of Janet Travell, M. D._ The World Publishing

Company, New York, New York, 1968, 496 pp.
In this autobiography, Janet Travell, first woman to serve
as personal physician to a president at the White House,
recounts her energetic pursuit of a career in medicine and
states that the rewards outweigh the sacrifices.   Daughter
of a physician, her independence was encouraged early in
life.   She graduated from Cornell Medical School in 1929
and taught part-time there (an unusual arrangement) until
she went to the White House with John F. Kennedy in 1961.
Dr. Travell also describes how she combined marriage and
motherhood with medicine.   (She dedicated this book "To
Jack, my husband, with love and appreciation for his words,
'Writing a book excuses everything.'")   An extensive bibliography lists Travell's many works in pharmacology and
in treatment of muscle and skeletal pain and disability, for
which she treated John Kennedy.   The book contains personal reminiscences of her treatment of Kennedy and some
of her poems, and concludes with an index.

1753.   A Tribute to Lilian Welsh.   Goucher College, Baltimore,
              Maryland, 1938, 42 pp.   port.
          Speakers at this service were Dr. Florence Rena Sabin,
          associated with Dr. Welsh in the higher education of women
          in Baltimore; Dr. Jessie L. King, Dr. Welsh's successor
          as chairman of the Department of Physiology and Hygiene
          at Goucher College; Eline von Borries, former student and
          associate of Dr. Welsh; and Dr. Gertrude C. Bussey,
          Goucher professor of philosophy and friend and colleague of
          Dr. Welsh.

1754.   "A Trio from the Woman's Medical of Pennsylvania."   Wo-
              man's Medical Journal, 1:4 (April 1893) 75.
          This article, reprinted from Woman's World, Pittsburgh,
          briefly profiles three women physicians--Dr. Emma Farrar,
          the first woman to practice medicine in Pittsburgh; Dr. Jane
          Vincent; and Dr. Margaret Forcee.

1755.   Tripp, Wendell.   "Dr. Elizabeth Blackwell's Graduation--
              An Eye-Witness Account by Margaret Munro DeLancey."
              New York History, 43:2 (April 1962) 182-185.
          Margaret Munro DeLancey was one of the Geneva, New York
          townspeople who witnessed Elizabeth Blackwell's graduation
          ceremony on January 23, 1849 from the Medical Institution
          of Geneva College (now Hobart).   Her letter, written to her
          sister-in-law, describes the ceremony from the viewpoint of
          the local citizens, who, in Dr. Blackwell's opinion, were
          unsympathetic.   But the letter also expresses a female re-
          action: while Miss DeLancey voices no strong approval,
          she is not hostile.   As Tripp says in his introduction, "Her
          tone may be one of pride or simple amazement or both."
          The letter (preserved in the Museum of the City of New
          York) apparently was not, prior to its publication here,
          known to Blackwell biographers.

1756.   Truax, Rhoda. The Doctors Jacobi. Little, Brown and
            Company, Boston, Massachusetts, 1952, 270 pp. port.
        "In the fall of 1863 when Mary Putnam became a student at
        the Female Medical College [of Pennsylvania], there were
        scarcely more than a handful of 'lady doctors' in the United
        States." The school's earliest announcements boasted that
        women could study anatomy in rooms "'kept strictly pri-
        vate.'" Hostility toward women seeking to enter the med-
        ical profession was running high, but the worst Mary ex-
        perienced were "some tobacco juice, a great many catcalls,
        and the inevitable practical jokes." As the daughter of
        George Palmer Putnam, of publishing fame, it had been as-
        sumed that Mary would have a literary career, but her par-
        ents believed in the right of women to practice medicine
        and did not prevent her. After studying pharmacy in New
        York and medicine in Philadelphia, she became the first
        woman to be admitted to the renowned Ecole de Medicine
        in Paris. In 1876 Mary won the Boylston prize for an es-
        say on modern female invalidism. Knowing from experience
        that women need not be invalids for one week of every
        month, she surveyed 286 women by questionnaire and came
        to the startling conclusions that (1) there is some connection
        between celibacy and menstrual suffering; (2) boredom can
        cause breakdowns and (3) rest can cause menstrual pain in
        healthy but indolent women. After two disappointing love
        affairs, she married the twice-widowed Abraham Jacobi,
        father of American pediatrics. Together they became an in-
        spiration to those "who were crusading for good schools
        and for hospitals better than pesthouses, and were trying to
        save the thousands of children who died of unknown causes
        every year." The author of this biography describes the
        Doctors Jacobi as "an American couple who faced happiness
        and tragedy together as they worked to benefit the country,
        the people and the science they both loved." A section of
        notes follows the text.

1757.   True, Mabelle. "Emma Linton Hill, M.D." Medical Wo-
            man's Journal, 50:8 (August 1943) 214, 218.
        This obituary retraces the life of Dr. Emma Linton Hill of
        Kansas. In 1901 (at the age of 43) she received her M.D.
        degree from Rush Medical College (Chicago). She was a
        "horse and buggy doctor" in those early days after her in-
        ternship at Woman's Hospital, Chicago, and was reputed to
        be a "keen diagnostician."

1758.   "Two 'Firsts' in the Society." Medical Missionary, 27:1
            (January-February 1953) 15. photos.
        Dr. Anna Speetjens (Sister M. Paraclita) was the first re-
        ligious in Holland to finish her medical studies since Rome
        granted permission for this purpose (1936). She was
        awarded the doctorate in medicine from the University of
        Utrecht.

1759.   Ulrich, Mabel S. "Men Are Queer That Way: Extracts
         from the Diary of an Apostate Woman Physician."
         Scribner's Magazine, 93 (June 1933) 365-369. (Life in
         the United States.)
         April 4, 1904: "S. and I have decided to get married next
         year when we get through medicine.... We are going to
         divide up the care of the children exactly as we divide the
         housework." September 23, 1905: "It is no go. We have
         given up the 50-50 housekeeping... I have to laugh when I
         think how scared I was before we married lest I might be
         the more successful at the start! Would he mind?...
         Well, you are perfectly safe, my dear S.! I have sat in
         that damned office for three months without a real call."
         June 5, 1907: "Twenty-five today--a quarter of a century
         old. A doctor, a wife and a mother--yet I don't seem to
         have learned anything. January 16, 1910: "S. could stand
         and watch me cut off a leg or make the most brilliant of
         diagnoses and remain unmoved--but let him catch me in the
         kitchen with an apron on, or sewing on a button, and he is
         dissolved in loving admiration. This I have endured with a
         'twisted smile' for two years." May 4, 1911: "Have de-
         cided to try my hand as S.'s technician since Miss Johnson
         is leaving to get married.... I should by this time be get-
         ting used to my role of giving the anaesthetics while he has
         the exciting operations." This diary ends on January 2,
         1932 and chronicles Dr. Ulrich's feelings over 28 years as
         wife, mother, and physician. [This article is reprinted in
         the "Lost Women" department of Ms. magazine, July 1972,
         11-12, 14, under the title "A Doctor's Diary, 1904-1932."]

1760.   "Utah's Oldest Doctor Is a Lady." Utah Medical Bulletin
         (March 1971) 8, 10. ports.
         Graduating from medical school in 1911, Lena Fimpel
         Schreier was, at the time this article was written, Utah's
         oldest living practicing doctor. In response to women's
         liberation, she says that nothing can take the place of chil-
         dren in a woman's life.

1761.   [Van der Vlugt, Martha.] "Living Portraits." Journal of
         the American Medical Women's Association, 16:9 (Sep-
         tember 1961) 706-707. photo. (Presentation, Midyear
         Meeting, AMWA Board of Directors, Hot Springs, Ar-
         kansas, 15 November 1959.)
         A "Who Am I" sketch of Dr. Esther Pohl Lovejoy is given
         which includes an episodic biography of Dr. Lovejoy's life.
         This vignette was part of the Sunday evening program at
         the midyear meeting. The name of the person whose life
         is portrayed is not given in the article itself, but elsewhere
         in the Journal.

1762.   Van Erp, Ymkje M. "Beulah Wells, M.D." Journal of
         the American Medical Women's Association, 16:5 (May
         1961) 397. port. (Album of Women in Medicine.)

A very brief biography of Dr. Wells is given. She received her M.D. degree from Johns Hopkins University Medical School in 1922 and practiced pediatrics in Cleveland,
Ohio.

1763.   Van Hoosen, Bertha. "Elizabeth Blackwell: The Woman
        of the Century." Journal of the American Medical Wo-
        men's Association, 4:11 (November 1949) 484-487. port.
        (Elizabeth Blackwell Memorial Address, Medical Wo-
        men's International Association, Copenhagen, Denmark,
        13 July 1949.)
This article traces Elizabeth Blackwell's journey as a pioneer woman in medicine, with emphasis on the qualities
that "seem to have a large and definite place in her make-
up." The article begins with this statement by the author:
"... I look upon Elizabeth Blackwell's accomplishments as a
manifestation in the growth of an extraordinary pattern of
chromosomes that were unusual as to kind and number."

1764.   Van Hoosen, Bertha. Petticoat Surgeon. Pellegrini &
        Cudahy, Chicago, Illinois, 1947, 324 pp.
Dr. Bertha Van Hoosen recalls impressions and events of
her life over 74 years. From her birth in 1863 in Stony
Creek, Michigan, a village settled and constructed by her
grandparents and great-grandparents, Dr. Van Hoosen traces
her heritage and the strong family ties that formed her personality. Bertha Van Hoosen's decision to enter medicine
was reached in a methodical way. Weighing the advantages
and disadvantages of a medical career, Bertha finally decides to enter the field because "I wanted to be my own
boss." Dr. Van Hoosen's training and practice revolved
around the cities of Detroit, Michigan where she attended
the University of Michigan for her medical education, and
Chicago, Illinois where she set up practice ("if I had ever
felt for any man what I had experienced for Chicago...").
The book is filled with Dr. Van Hoosen's experiences as an
obstetrician and surgeon. "I tackled a job for which I was
wholly unprepared"; "I acted at once." For Dr. Van Hoosen
efficiency was beauty, and she believed in the concept of an
inexpensive delivery for working mothers and ten days of
day care for the woman's children while she was in the hospital being delivered. When in 1918 Dr. Van Hoosen was
offered the position as Acting Head and Professor of Obstetrics in the Loyola University Medical School (the first
woman physician to hold such a position in a coeducational
medical school), she turned the Lakota Hotel into the Lewis
Maternity Hospital, her "dream fulfilled." Dr. Van Hoosen,
after working extremely hard and unceasingly to build up the
obstetrical department at Loyola and securing for the medical school a Grade A rating, was totally unprepared for
the "exhibition of sex prejudice from the American Medical
Association" which followed--the AMA recommended, now
that the school was rated Grade A, "that Loyola put a man

at the head of the Department of Obstetrics." A fervent
advocate of the use of "twilight sleep" in obstetrical cases,
Dr. Van Hoosen discusses the benefits of this form of
anesthetic. She is continually concerned about women's
health care--there are two categories of obstetricians, says
Van Hoosen, "One delivers the baby, the other attends the
woman in labor." Many incidents are recalled by Dr. Van
Hoosen which give the reader insight into her strong personality and firm grasp of things obstetrical, as well as a
glimpse of her overwhelming "medical-practice inferiority
complex" which she combated through extensive, intense
preparation combined with decisive action. A chapter is
devoted to her friend, Dr. Alice Lois Lindsay Wynekoop,
Dr. Wynekoop's murder conviction, and Dr. Van Hoosen's
efforts to exonerate her. The book concludes with Dr. Van
Hoosen's travels abroad which reveal many exciting stories
of life in China and Japan (where she was caught in the
earthquake of 1923). [This work also appeared in a Danish
edition: Kirurg I Skørter. Berlingske Forlag, Copenhagen,
Denmark, 1949, 267pp.]

1765.   Van Hoosen, Bertha. "Travel Letters through the Orient:
        Personal Observations and Experiences of Dr. Bertha
        Van Hoosen." Medical Women's Journal, 30:3 (March
        1923) 76-78.
The first of a series of journal-style observations on the
Orient, this article relates Dr. Van Hoosen's impressions
and experiences in San Francisco, California, including a
portion on Dr. Margaret Chung's medical practice (and lifestyle).

1766.   Van Hoosen, Bertha. "Traveling through the Orient: Per-
        sonal Observations and Experiences of Dr. Bertha Van
        Hoosen." Medical Woman's Journal, 30:[4] (April 1923)
        111-114.
"In this letter Dr. Van Hoosen describes her experiences in
Honolulu; the various physicians, especially the women physicians she met, and her reception by them. She tells of
her visit to and inspection of the leper colony. The hospitals of Honolulu are mentioned and brief descriptions are
given of some of the beautiful Honolulu homes where she
was a guest." [Article summary.]

1767.   Van Hoosen, Bertha. "Traveling through the Orient: Per-
        sonal Observations and Experiences of Dr. Bertha Van
        Hoosen." Medical Woman's Journal, 30:5 (May 1923)
        145-149.
Dr. Van Hoosen in New Zealand records her impressions of
the efforts in this country to "bring up the statistics regarding maternal and infant welfare." Dr. Van Hoosen
deals at length with the recommendations of the director-
general of health of New Zealand regarding puerperal mortality.

1768.   Van Hoosen, Bertha. "Traveling through the Orient: Per-
           sonal Observations and Experiences of Dr. Bertha Van
           Hoosen." Medical Woman's Journal, 30:6 (June 1923)
           175-177.
         Dr. Van Hoosen discusses her visit to New Zealand and
         Australia, the high degree of surgical skill she found, and
         the delightful personality of the surgeons there. She re-
         views interesting surgical techniques she observed and tells
         about the opportunity she had to spend time with Sir Alex-
         ander McCormick, a leading surgeon.

1769.   Van Hoosen, Bertha. "Traveling through the Orient: Per-
           sonal Observations and Experiences of Dr. Bertha Van
           Hoosen." Medical Woman's Journal, 30:7 (July 1923)
           210-214.
         In this article Dr. Van Hoosen observes the dress and
         habits of Chinese men as witnessed on a nine-hour train
         ride from Peking to Tehchow. In Tehchow Dr. Van Hoosen
         stayed with Dr. Emma Tucker and her husband. Life in
         Tehchow and the operations she saw there are described.
         An account is given of the Chinese technique of obstetrical
         delivery and the care of the newborn (of whom about 50 per
         cent die of tetanus during the first week of life).

1770.   Van Hoosen, Bertha. "Traveling through the Orient: Per-
           sonal Observations and Experiences of Dr. Bertha Van
           Hoosen." Medical Woman's Journal, 30:8 (August 1923)
           234-237.
         "This month's letter [from Dr. Van Hoosen] deals with some
         of the phases of village life, the way Chinese people travel,
         and the position women occupy." Dr. Van Hoosen discusses
         her experiences at the Peking Woman's Medical College and
         the Shantung Christian College.

1771.   Van Hoosen, Bertha. "Traveling through the Orient: Per-
           sonal Observations and Experiences of Dr. Bertha Van
           Hoosen." Medical Woman's Journal, 30:10 (October
           1923) 300-303.
         Dr. Van Hoosen describes in detail the Peking Union Med-
         ical College, a woman's medical school in existence since
         1906 and originally under the auspices of a union of six dif-
         ferent mission boards.

1772.   Van Hoosen, Bertha. "Traveling through the Orient: Per-
           sonal Observations and Experiences of Dr. Bertha Van
           Hoosen." Medical Woman's Journal, 30:11 (November
           1923) 336-345.
         This installment of Dr. Van Hoosen's journal relates inci-
         dents leading up to the 1923 earthquake in Tokyo, Japan, as
         well as her experience in Tokyo during the quake. Dr. Van
         Hoosen, the obstetrician, faithfully records in her journal
         the minutes between earth tremors, and muses: "I wondered
         if the earth or anyone on it would live through this terrible
         travail."

1773.   Van Hoosen, Bertha. "Traveling through the Orient: Per-
        sonal Observations and Experiences of Dr. Bertha Van
        Hoosen." Medical Woman's Journal, 30:12 (December
        1923) 371-375.
        In this journal segment, Dr. Van Hoosen recounts incidents
        from her China visit. Among them is her description of the
        Door of Hope, a police manned institution designed to re-
        ceive former prostitutes and to hold them until claimed by
        family (a rare occurrence) or some males who might "take
        a fancy" to them. Dr. Van Hoosen also comments upon
        the "equal ... if not superior" brain of the Chinese woman
        (to that of the man). In Peking, also, reports Dr. Van
        Hoosen, you will find midwifery, "this branch of quackery
        in all its crudeness."

1774.   Van Hoosen, Bertha; Bacon, [Dr.] and Schmidt, Otto. "Dr.
        Rachelle Yarros: Physician, Scientist, Humanitarian."
        Medical Woman's Journal, 38:1 (January 1931) 10-13,
        24. port.
        Friends and professional associates paying tribute to Dr.
        Rachelle Yarros at a banquet held in November 1930 in-
        cluded Jane Addams of Hull House, Dr. Ethel Snow of the
        National Social Hygiene League, and Dr. Yarros's husband,
        who left the audience "with the impression that although Dr.
        Yarrow had won for herself the highest of titles in the edu-
        cational world, the homage of all countries in the work of
        social reform, the privilege of pioneering in the twentieth
        century, the respect and homage of the largest and most in-
        fluential of women's clubs in Chicago, over and above it all
        was her success as a devoted and loving wife...."

1775.   Vaschak, Mathilda R. "The Elizabeth Blackwell Annual
        Award, 1974." Journal of the American Medical Wo-
        men's Association, 30:2 (February 1975) 84-85. port.
        This award was presented to Dr. Laura Ehrlich Morrow.
        A brief biography of Dr. Morrow is given, followed by her
        acceptance speech.

1776.   Vaughan, E. "The Early Days of Elizabeth Blackwell."
        Fortnightly Review, (1 November 1913) 976-985.

1777.   "Vicki Nichols Views Being Black, Female, a Physician."
        Mayovox, (September 1973) 1, 3. ports.
        Dr. Nichols feels that the discrimination she has faced as
        a female is greater than what she has had to confront as a
        black. She discusses her life in Rochester, Minnesota as
        an obstetrics-gynecology resident at the Mayo Clinic and
        gives examples of some overt racial and sexist discrimina-
        tion she has encountered.

1778.   Vietor, Agnes C., ed. A Woman's Quest: The Life of
        Marie E. Zakrzewska, M.D. D. Appleton and Company,
        New York, New York, 1924, xviii, 514 pp. illus., port.

This biography appears to be a complete treatment of the
professional and personal life of Marie Zakrzewska (Dr.
Zak), the German midwife who came to the U.S. in 1853 to
seek a medical degree. With assistance from Elizabeth
Blackwell, with whom she worked in New York, she was admitted to the Cleveland Medical School and received her
M.D. in 1856. She was resident physician of the New York
Infirmary 1857-59. In 1859 she moved to Boston to become
professor of obstetrics at the New England Female Medical
College. In 1863 she established the New England Hospital
for Women and Children. This work is based on autobiographical material given to the author. Several photographs
of Dr. Zakrzewska have been included along with an index,
bibliography, and explanatory notes.

1779.   Wagner, Wyonia. "She Wears a Magic Necklace." MD's
            Wife, (September 1972) 6-9, 14, 28, 30. photos.
         "Pat Smith, M.D., has become a legend in her own time
         as she ministers to the Montagnard tribes of South Viet-
         nam." Dr. Smith discusses in this article her motivation
         for going to Vietnam, as well as the social and working
         conditions and problems at the hospital in Montagnard.

1780.   Waite, Frederick C. "Dr. Lucinda Susannah (Capen) Hall:
            The First Woman to Receive a Medical Degree from a
            New England Institution." New England Journal of Med-
            icine, 210:12 (22 March 1934) 644-647.
         Lucinda Hall, née Capen (1815-1890), obtained a midwifery
         certificate in 1848 from the Boston Female Medical College
         --an unaccredited course sponsored by the Female Medical
         Education Society in Boston. In 1852 she graduated from
         the Worcester Medical Institution (an eclectic school or-
         ganized in 1846 in Worcester, Massachusetts), becoming the
         first woman to receive a medical degree from a New Englan
         school. In this biography of Dr. Hall, the author comments
         that hers was the only case he has ever found where the
         wife graduated first and was followed into the profession by
         her husband.

1781.   Waite, Frederick C. "Dr. Lydia Folger Fowler, The Sec-
            ond Woman to Receive the Degree of Doctor of Medicine
            in the United States." Annals of Medical History, 4:3
            (May 1932) 290-297.
         The author traces substantial documented evidence to estab-
         lish Lydia Folger as the second woman to receive the de-
         gree of Doctor of Medicine in the United States, as well as
         the first woman in America to hold a professorship in a
         medical college. Her career is also traced.

1782.   Waite, Frederick C. "Dr. Martha A. (Hayden) Sawin.
            The First Woman Graduate in Medicine to Practice in
            Boston." New England Journal of Medicine, 205:22 (26
            November 1931) 1053-1055.

1783.   Waite, Frederick C. "Dr. Nancy E. (Talbot) Clark: The
             Second Woman Graduate to Practice in Boston." New
             England Journal of Medicine, 205-25 (17 December 1931)
             1195-1198.
             The first woman to receive a medical degree from the Cleve-
             land Medical College (in 1852), Dr. Clark missed by three
             days the distinction of being the first woman medical gradu-
             ate west of the Alleghenies. She missed by three months
             being the first woman physician to practice in Boston or
             New England. That distinction was held by Dr. Martha
             Sawin, who set up practice in Boston in early 1852. Dr.
             Clark was the first woman to apply for membership in the
             Massachusetts Medical Society; her application was rejected,
             however. When she went to Paris for a year's study, Dr.
             Clark became the second American woman to go to Europe
             for medical study. The author writes that "she was cer-
             tainly the best trained woman physician in Boston at this
             time...." Following her marriage in 1856, she stopped
             medical practice, but became active again in 1874.

1784.   Waite, Frederick C. "The Three Myers Sisters--Pioneer
             Women Physicians." Medical Review of Reviews, 39:3
             (March 1933) 114-120.
             While not as well known as the Blackwell sisters, the three
             daughters of Samuel Myers who became early medical pio-
             neer practitioners deserve historical attention: Hannah E.
             Myers Longshore, Jane Viola Myers, and Mary Frame
             Myers Thomas. After studying medicine under her brother-
             in-law, Hannah E. Longshore entered the Female Medical
             College of Philadelphia, becoming one of the first matricu-
             lants there, and was graduated in 1851. In the third ses-
             sion of that school she became demonstrator of anatomy;
             this made her one of the first three women teachers on a
             United States medical school faculty. Dr. Longshore was
             the first woman graduate in medicine to enter private prac-
             tice in Philadelphia. Jane Myers studied at Penn Medical
             University and received her degree from there in 1855.
             Although she had her residence and practice next door to
             Dr. Longshore's, they practiced independently. Mary
             Thomas graduated from Penn Medical University in 1856
             and became one of the earliest women members of the In-
             diana State Medical Association. Besides editing a woman's
             journal called The Lily, she published several articles on
             the necessity of having women physicians for insane women
             in prisons. When she became president of the Wayne
             County Medical Society in 1887, she was one of the first
             women in the country so honored. [Portraits of the sisters
             are appended at the back of this issue of the journal.]

1785.   Wallin, Mathilda K. "War Service of Dr. Chard." Med-
             ical Woman's Journal, 45:4 (April 1938) 115.
             Marie Louise Chard helped establish the American Women's
             Hospitals and was active during World War I as a member

of the Medical Women's National Association's War Service
Committee.

1786.   Ward, Vera [Chance]. How to Sleep on a Windy Night.
             [Clar-Mar Press, Phillipsburg, Kansas, c 1970], 363
             pp. illus.
         This book deals with the life of Dr. Mary Townsend Glas-
         sen. [Book not examined by editors.]

1787.   Watkins, Rachel A. and Campbell, Grace. "Obituary."
             Bulletin Medical Women's Club of Chicago, 5:7 (March
             1917) 3.
         A brief biographical sketch is presented in this obituary of
         Dr. Helen R. Kellogg.

1788.   Waugh, Elizabeth S. "M. Eugenia Geib, M.D." Journal of
             the American Medical Women's Association, 12:3 (March
             1957) 80.
         A pediatrician, Dr. M. Eugenia Geib became editor of the
         Journal of the American Medical Women's Association in
         1953 and resigned c. 1957.

1789.   Waugh, Elizabeth S. "Martha Tracy, M.D." Journal of
             the American Medical Women's Association, 10:8 (Au-
             gust 1955) 283. port. (Past Presidents of AMWA.)
         Dr. Tracy received her M.D. degree in 1904 from the Wo-
         man's Medical College of Pennsylvania. She later became
         the seventh dean of the College.

1790.   Waugh, Elizabeth S. "Our New Editor." Journal of the
             American Medical Women's Association, 12:3 (March
             1957) 81.
         A biographical sketch of Dr. Frieda Baumann includes the
         fact that she was the first woman appointed chief of a med-
         ical service at the Philadelphia General Hospital.

1791.   Webster, Augusta. "Evangeline E. Stenhouse, M.D.:
             Thirty-Sixth President of the American Medical Women's
             Association." Journal of the American Medical Women's
             Association, 7:9 (September 1952) 346. port. (Album
             of Women in Medicine.)
         Dr. Stenhouse graduated from Rush Medical College in
         1931. Professional affiliations of Dr. Stenhouse are given.

1792.   Welsh, Lilian. Reminiscences of Thirty Years in Balti-
             more. The Norman, Remington Co., Baltimore, Mary-
             land, 1925, xvii, 254 pp. illus., photos., ports.
         This memoir covers the period from 1890 to 1925, when
         Lilian Welsh ended a 30-year career as founding professor
         of the Department of Physiology and Hygiene at Goucher
         College. She also recounts her work in the 1890s in the
         Evening Dispensary for Working Women and Girls, the first
         public health clinic for women in Baltimore, where several

obstetrical patients named their children after her in gratitude for her insistence on sympathetic prenatal and post-
natal care and scientific childbirth. One chapter is devoted
to Dr. Welsh's personal experiences in the suffrage campaign. The activities of Baltimore women physicians in public health work is reported. Dr. Welsh also presents a
history of educational opportunities for women in Baltimore
from 1892 to 1916 and emphasizes the city's contribution to
women's medical education. There is no index.

1793. "Wendy Stewart, M. D. , LL. B." Medical Woman's Journal,
          49:3 (March 1942) 90.
       A profile of Wendy Stewart lists her many activities as a
       lawyer and a physician.

1794. Wessel, M. A. and Blodgett, F. M. "Edith B. Jackson,
          M. D. and Yale Pediatrics." Connecticut Medicine, 26
          (July 1962) 438-441.
       [Article not examined by editors.]

1795. "Western College Writes About--Jane Merrill Ketcham,
          M. D." The Quarterly Bulletin of Indiana University
          Medical Center, 27:1 (Spring 1965) 35-36. port.
       Dr. Ketcham received her M. D. degree in 1906 from Purdue
       University. She served as a house doctor for the Sue Em-
       ma Coleman Home for unwed mothers and was professor of
       clinical medicine at the Indiana University School of Medi-
       cine.

1796. Wharton, May Cravath. Doctor Woman of the Cumberlands:
          The Autobiography of May Cravath Wharton. Uplans
          Press, Pleasant Hill, Tennessee, 1953, 208 pp. illus.
       [Book not examined by editors.]

1797. "What Medicine Means to Me." The Medical College of
          Pennsylvania: Today, 3:4 (February/March 1972) 1, 8.
          photo.
       Alumni and students of the Medical College of Pennsylvania
       affirm their dedication to medicine.

1798. Wheaton, Walter F. "Laura Marion Plantz, M. D. (1829-
          1923)." Ohio Medical Journal, 44 (1948) 1229-1231.
          port.
       [Article not examined by editors.]

1799. Wheeler, Emily C. "The Birds' Nest." Medical Woman's
          Journal, 31:10 (October 1924) 293.
       Dr. Harriet H. Parker heads the Women's Hospital in
       Madura, India. Dr. Parker cares for more than 13,000
       patients a year and is constantly being "pressed into service,"
       as the Hindu woman "still resents the entrance of a man doc-
       tor into her home."

1800.   White-Thomas, Cornelia; Hinche, Charles L. and Potter,
        Marion Craig. "Tribute to Dr. Evelyn Baldwin: Pre-
        pared by the Special Committee on Resolutions March
        28, 1917, for the Junior Staff of the Rochester General
        Hospital." Woman's Medical Journal, 27:4 (April 1917)
        91.
        A niece of Dr. Frances Hamilton, Evelyn Baldwin succeeded
        to her aunt's practice in Rochester, New York where she
        worked hard for those who were ill and suffering until her
        own death in 1917.

1801.   Whittier, Isabel. Dr. Elizabeth Blackwell: The First Wo-
        man Doctor. Brunswick Publishing Company, Bruns-
        wick, Maine, 1961.
        [Book not examined by editors.]

1802.   Wickner, Hali. "Chief Residents: New Role Models for
        Women." Stanford M.D., 13:4 (Fall 1974) 22-24.
        ports.
        Although they are not the first women to hold higher posi-
        tions in a field where standards have been largely set by
        and for men, the three women profiled in this article serve
        as role models who "offer hope of increased opportunities
        for their sex in years to come." All three are head resi-
        dents at the Stanford University Hospital. Libby Short, a
        1968 graduate of Yale Medical School and Stanford's chief
        resident in medicine, notes, "Previous social conditioning
        for 'female' roles works to the advantage of women....
        Long hours on your feet, taking care of childlike patients
        in a strange environment, making sure they get tests and
        medication on time is not unlike organizing a family or get-
        ting a five-course meal on the table." Marriage and medi-
        cine do not always mix for women, however: after seven
        years of marriage Dr. Short is divorced. Chief resident
        of psychiatry Joellen Werne, who received her M.D. from
        Yale in 1970, sees a need for women psychiatrists to relate
        more closely to other women in the field. A 1966 graduate
        of Stanford Medical School and chief of neurosurgery resi-
        dents (all men), Frances Conley married a "very understand-
        ing man" and chooses not to have children because "there is
        no way I could do my work and be a housewife at the same
        time." Women can meet the challenge of a medical career
        "in a feminine and gracious manner that is competent and
        effective," Dr. Conley asserts. The author writes that none
        of these women ever experienced "overt hostility or encoun-
        tered any obstacles in the pursuit of medicine." An inset
        compares female enrollment at Stanford Medical School with
        national figures.

1803.   Wigginton, R. M. "Obituary Sketch of Dr. Mary Reynolds
        of Milwaukee." Transactions of the State Medical So-
        ciety of Wisconsin 1889, [1889?], 270-273.
        [Article not examined by editors.]

1804.   Williams, Mary Edith. "Pearl M. Stetler, M.D." Journal
         of the American Medical Women's Association, 9:10
         (October 1954) 333. port. (Album of Women in Medi-
         cine.)

1805.   Wilson, Dorothy Clarke. Dr. Ida: The Story of Dr. Ida
         Scudder of Vellore. McGraw-Hill Book Co., Inc., New
         York, New York, 1959, 358 pp. photos., port.
         Ida Scudder was a third generation medical missionary to
         India, following in her father's and grandfather's work. She
         decided to enter medicine to serve the women of India, and
         in 1895 she enrolled in the Woman's Medical College of
         Pennsylvania. In 1899 she completed her studies at Cornell
         Medical College (which had opened to women the previous
         year) and was commissioned to raise funds for a woman's
         hospital in Vellore, near Madras. This biography recounts
         the work and personal life of Dr. Scudder in India, until
         1959. In that year, on her 88th birthday, she was given an
         award by Cornell for her contributions to medical education,
         public health, and international understanding. Sources for
         this book include the biography by Pauline Jeffery; there is
         no formal bibliography, and no index.

1806.   Wilson, Dorothy Clarke. Lone Woman: The Story of Eliza-
         beth Blackwell The First Woman Doctor. Little,
         Brown and Company, Boston, Massachusetts, 1970, 469
         pp. illus., photo., port.
         This detailed biography of Elizabeth Blackwell tells of her
         upbringing in a spirited abolitionist family, her struggles to
         obtain a medical education (she was the first woman to at-
         tend and graduate from medical college), and to obtain rele-
         vant experience in midwifery, for which she had to go to
         La Maternité in Paris, and her work in England, where she
         finally became the first woman to be certified by the Med-
         ical Council of England. The book recounts her refusal to
         be discouraged by the struggle involved in founding the New
         York Infirmary with Marie Zakrzewska, tells of her experi-
         ences in the women's rights movement, and describes her
         friendship with Sophia Jex-Blake and Elizabeth Garrett An-
         derson. The work ends with her departure for England in
         1869 to work for the medical education of women. The
         book, based on family reminiscences and Blackwell papers
         stored in many libraries, devotes several pages to Dr.
         Emily Blackwell (Elizabeth Blackwell's younger sister), her
         education, and her years at the New York Infirmary. An
         index and bibliography conclude the work.

1807.   Wilson, Mary Lena. "Dr. Norton's Experiences in the Near
         East." Medical Woman's Journal, 28:1 (January 1921)
         43-45. port.
         Dr. Norton was the first and only woman physician ever to
         receive the Greek War Cross. Dr. Norton received this
         honor for her work with the Greek refugees suffering from

trachoma. Her work in Greece is reviewed in this article.

1808.   Wissler, Robert W. "Eleanor Mary Humphreys: 1892-
                1971." Proceedings of the Institute of Medicine of Chi-
                cago, 29 (January 1972) 25-26.
           This memorial to Eleanor Mary Humphreys summarizes her
           education at Smith College, Rush Medical College (M.D.,
           1931), and the University of Chicago, where she eventually
           became professor of pathology and a popular teacher and
           counselor of students. Her scholarly work included papers
           on phosphorus poisoning, heart disease, adrenal disease,
           protein deficiency, lupus erythematosus, and carcinoma.
           Dr. Humphreys received many honors, including the presi-
           dency of the Chicago Pathological Society and an honorary
           degree from Smith College.

1809.   Withington, Alfreda. Mine Eyes Have Seen: A Woman Doc-
                tor's Saga. E. P. Dutton & Co., Inc., New York,
                New York, 1941, 311 pp.
           Alfreda Withington studied medicine at the Women's Medical
           College of the New York Infirmary in the 1880s. Following
           her graduation she traveled and studied in Europe, and in
           1891 she began a general practice in Pittsfield, Massachu-
           setts. In 1893 she was the first woman elected councilor
           to the state medical society. This reminiscent autobiography
           emphasizes the unusual events in her professional life, be-
           ginning with her service with the Deep Sea Mission of Dr.
           Wilfred Grenfell in Labrador in 1906. Dr. Withington also
           served with the Red Cross in France (1917-21), concentrat-
           ing her efforts on the treatment of tuberculosis among refu-
           gees. In 1924 she began a practice among the mountain
           people in Kentucky. No bibliography or index is included.

1810.   Withington, Alfreda. "The Mountain Doctor [Part I]." At-
                lantic Monthly, 150:3 (September 1932) 257-267.
           Dr. Withington's work during the war as a surgeon with the
           Red Cross in France "did not conduce to a resumption of
           conventional practice." So she went to the wilds of the Ken-
           tucky mountains, where she made all calls on horseback
           and where there were no other physicians within 25 miles.
           Dr. Withington describes her work there and some people
           she treated from 1924 to 1926.

1811.   Withington, Alfreda. "The Mountain Doctor [Part II]." At-
                lantic Monthly, 150:4 (October 1932) 469-477.
           Dr. Withington's continuing story of her adventures as a
           physician in the Kentucky mountains covers the years from
           1926 to 1928.

1812.   Withington, Alfreda. "The Mountain Doctor [Part III]."
                Atlantic Monthly, 150:6 (December 1932) 768-774.
           In this article, the final installment of Dr. Withington's

story of life as a physician in the Kentucky mountains, she
concentrates on the events occurring between 1928 and 1930.
In addition to descriptions of the ruggedness and simplicity
of mountain life, Dr. Withington tells of the death of her
beloved horse Billy.

1813.   Witthoff, Evelyn. "Thirty-Seven Months in Santo Tomas."
        Medical Woman's Journal, 52:7 (July 1945) 30-33.
        Dr. Witthoff recalls her 37 months as a prisoner on the
        island.

1814.   Wittke, Carl F. "Dr. Marie Elizabeth Zakrzewska--Class
        of 1856." Voice of Reserve (July 1951) 15, 37, 39.
        This article is a memorial to Dr. Zakrzewska, an early
        graduate of Western Reserve University. The memorial
        was inspired by a bequest left in her memory by Dr. Helen
        Cordelia Putnam. Dr. Zakrzewska supported a number of
        causes during her lifetime besides medical education and
        equality for women. She was active in such causes as
        lunchrooms for the working women and the poor in Boston;
        projects for Jewish children; abolition; rights of blacks.
        One of her closest friendships was with the uncompromising
        radical, Karl Heinzen, who crusaded against censorship,
        bureaucracy, militarism, slavery, and all the political,
        social, and economic evils of his day.

1815.   "Woman Consultant in Administration of Sheppard-Towner
        Maternity Act." Medical Woman's Journal, 29:6 (June
        1922) 119.
        Dr. Ethel M. Watters of San Francisco is profiled.

1816.   "A Woman Country Doctor." Medical Woman's Journal,
        38:7 (July 1931) 179.
        Anna Perkins practices in a rural New York area where the
        "country is rugged and bleak, and the people partake of the
        same characteristics. They were not so sure they were
        willing to accept the services of a woman doctor...."

1817.   "Woman Doctor." Look, (December 1949) 120-123. photos.
        A photo essay depicts the daily routine of Alice E. Shep-
        pard, the only woman physician in Pottstown, Pennsyl-
        vania.

1818.   [No entry]

1819.   "'The Woman Physician.'" Medical Woman's Journal, 30:
        3 (March 1923) 94-95. (Notes and Comments.)
        A biography of Dr. Rosalie Slaughter Morton is incorporated
        into this article, which describes the bas-relief she presented
        to the Woman's Medical College of Pennsylvania. The work,
        sculpted by Clara Hill of Washington, D.C., is an interpreta-
        tion of Dr. Morton's conception "of the maternal spirit which

especially animates woman to lessen suffering and heal the
sick."

1820.   "A Woman Physician and Counsellor-at-Law." Woman's
             Medical Journal, 13:10 (October 1903) 204.
        Mary C. Lowell, M.D., LL.B., the "only woman in the
        world" entitled to pursue both law and medicine, was the
        first woman assistant superintendent of the Maine State
        Hospital for the Insane.

1821.   "A Woman Physician in China." Medical Woman's Journal,
             46:9 (September 1939) 286. (Editorial.)
        Annie Walter Fearn's 40-year medical and diplomatic career
        in China is praised.

1822.   "A Woman Physician Is the New Chief of the U.S. Children's
             Bureau." Medical Woman's Journal, 59:1 (January 1952)
             40-41. (News Notes.)
        Dr. Martha May Eliot's qualifications for the appointment as
        chief of the Bureau are given in this article.

1823.   "Woman Superintendent of State Hospital." Woman's Med-
             ical Journal, 18:5 (May 1908) 105.
        As the superintendent of the Norristown (Pennsylvania) State
        Hospital, Dr. Mary M. Wolfe is the only woman physician
        in charge of a state institution.

1824.   "Woman Surgeon of U.S. Medical Corps." Medical Woman's
             Journal, 29:8 (August 1922) 185. port.
        Dr. Daisy M. O. Robinson was given the rank of Surgeon in
        the U.S. Medical Corps in 1920. A review of her education
        and professional activities is included. Dr. Robinson is the
        only woman who holds membership in the French Society of
        Dermatology and Syphilology, having been appointed in 1901.

1825.   "The Woman the Country Delights to Honor." Woman's
             Medical Journal, 27:9 (August 1917) 185.
        Anna Howard Shaw, honorary president of the National Amer-
        ican Woman Suffrage Association and Chairman of the Wo-
        man's Committee of the National Council of Defense, re-
        ceived several honors. She was asked to preach the bac-
        calaureate sermon at Bryn Mawr College (Pennsylvania):
        the first time that a woman was asked to do this at a large
        college. Temple University then asked her to give its bac-
        calaureate address.

1826.   "A Woman Who 'Stuck It Out.'" Literary Digest, 85 (4
             April 1925) 64-70.
        Based on an interview with Eliza M. Mosher during the year
        of her "medical golden jubilee," this article quotes Dr.
        Mosher on her memories as a "third-generation pioneer."

1827.   "Women Doctors in England." Medical Woman's Journal,

49:4 (April 1942) 123.
Brief biographies of American physicians Barbara Stimson
and Aschsa Bean focus upon their activities in England during [World War II].

1828.   Women in Medicine, 69 (July 1940) 7.   port.
        This brief biography of Dr. Elizabeth Mason-Hohl mentions
        Dr. Mason-Hohl's professional affiliations and her hobbies.

1829.   "Women in Medicine."   USC Medicine, 24:1 (1974) 7-18.
            photos. , ports.
        Biographies and portraits introduce the women physicians on
        the faculty of the University of Southern California School of
        Medicine.   This article also provides information on the
        status of women students.

1830.   "Woman Physician Honored."   Medical Woman's Journal,
            45:2 (February 1938) 54.
        Upon the fiftieth anniversary of Mary J. Kearsley's gradua-
        tion from the Women's Medical College of Chicago (in 1888),
        she was honored at a banquet, given by prominent male phy-
        sicians "who declared that no similar honor had ever been
        paid to a women [sic] by the men of the medical profession,
        and is an indication of the high regard in which she is
        held...."

1831.   "Women Warworkers' Problems Discussed."   Medical Wo-
            man's Journal, 51:7 (July 1944) 44.
        This article, reprinted from the Los Angeles Times, tells
        of "an attractive girl doctor," Marion Dakin, who investi-
        gated women workers' physical problems by working incog-
        nito among employees at Lockheed Aircraft Corporation.

1832.   "Women's and Children's Hospital: Madeline J. Algee,
            M.D. , Founder and Director."   Medical Woman's Jour-
            nal, 51:11 (November 1944) 28.   photo. , port.
        The Women's and Children's Hospital in Compton, California
        is believed to be the only hospital in the U.S. owned and
        operated by a woman physician.   Madeline J. Algee built
        the hospital, which was opened in 1943, as an addition to
        her office.   Dr. Algee obtained her M.D. from Stanford
        University School of Medicine in 1929.   The mother of two
        sons, Dr. Algee "is prouder of this achievement than of
        her medical career."

1833.   Woodbridge, Helen McFarland.   "Margaret F. Butler, M.D.:
            October 16, 1931."   Bulletin of the Woman's Medical
            College of Pennsylvania, 82:4 (March 1932) 11.
        This poem on Dr. Butler was written upon her death.

1834.   Woodward, Helen Beal.   "The Right to Wear Pants: Dr.
            Mary Walker."   In: The Bold Women.   Farrar, Straus
            and Young, New York, New York, 1953, 281-298.

"You never could slice a right too equal for Mary Walker."
The author discusses Dr. Walker and her eccentricities,
and muses "by what chemical process does a proud, ambi-
tious girl of more than average intelligence coagulate into
a freak?" Dr. Walker had two proud accomplishments in
her life: her Congressional Medal of Honor and her exchange during the Civil War for a Confederate first lieutenant. A bibliography of sources for information presented
in each chapter of this book (including this one on Mary
Walker) appears at the end of the book.

1835.   Woolley, Alice Stone. "Dr. Mary Putnam Jacobi, Path-
            finder in Medicine." Women in Medicine, 88 (April
            1945) 16-17.
        This address was delivered on the occasion of the 50th an-
        niversary of the founding of the Town Hall Forum in Town
        Hall, New York.

1836.   Woolley, Alice Stone. "Tributes to Dr. S. Josephine Bak-
            er." Women in Medicine, 89 (July 1946) 24-26.
        Dr. Baker entered the New York Department of Health in
        1901 and was shortly thereafter appointed assistant to the
        commissioner. In 1908 she founded the Bureau of Child
        Hygiene and became its director. This article consists in
        tributes by the president of AMWA, Dr. Woolley; a personal
        tribute by I. A. R. Wylie; and a reminiscence by Dr.
        Martha M. Eliot, associate chief of the U.S. Department
        of Labor's Children's Bureau.

1837.   Woolley, Alice [Stone]. "In Memoriam: Grace N. Kimball."
            Women in Medicine, 79 (January 1943) 21-22.   port.
        This article presents a sketch of the professional life of
        Grace N. Kimball, who practiced medicine in Turkey until
        the Armenia massacres forced her to return to the United
        States. She was instrumental in founding the Bowne Me-
        morial Hospital in Poughkeepsie.

1838.   Worcester, Blandina. "New AMWA President-1964: Rosa
            Lee Nemir, M.D." Journal of the American Medical
            Women's Association, 19:1 (January 1964) 44.

1839.   "Work of the Woman Health Inspector." Woman's Medical
            Journal, 5:10 (October 1896) 271-272.
        Praise is given to Dr. Susan R. Pray, an inspector with
        the health department of Brooklyn, New York.

1840.   "World War I." Medical Woman's Journal, 50:9 (September
            1943) 234.   port.   (Section on War Service.)
        A brief biographical sketch is herein given of Dr. Regina
        Flood Keyes Roberts, who headed the AWH service at Sa-
        lonica in the winter of 1917-18.

1841.   "The World's First Woman Doctor: No Seemingly Insur-

mountable Obstacle Could Stop a Woman Who Had a
Mind of Her Own." Woman's Chains, (January-Febru-
ary 1948) 10-11. (Famous Women.)
The life of Elizabeth Blackwell is the subject of this article.

1842.   Wright, Katharine W. "History of Women in Medicine; A
        Symposium: Nineteenth Century or Transitional Period."
        Bulletin of the Medical Library Association, 44:1 (Janu-
        ary 1956) 16-22.
        Dr. Wright gives brief biographies of several 19th-century
        women physicians whom she found listed in A Woman of the
        Century, edited by Frances E. Willard and Mary A. Liver-
        more.

1843.   Yakovlev, Paul I. "Dr. Naomi Raskin as Neuropathologist."
        Journal of the American Medical Women's Association,
        20:4 (April 1965) 354-356. [Testimonial, Boston State
        Hospital, 19 October 1964.]
        This testimonial to Dr. Raskin was presented on the occa-
        sion of her retirement. High points of Dr. Raskin's con-
        tribution to neuropathology and medical writing are reviewed.

1844.   Yarros, Rachelle S. "The Experiences of a Graduate of
        1893." In: 75th Anniversary Volume of the Woman's
        Medical College of Pennsylvania. Westbrook Publishing
        Company, Philadelphia, Pennsylvania, [1925?], 184-190.
        Dr. Yarros's autobiographical article focuses upon her ex-
        periences and her philosophies as an obstetrician.

1845.   Yarros, Rachelle S. "From Obstetrics to Social Hygiene."
        Medical Woman's Journal, 33:11 (November 1926) 305-
        309.
        Rachelle S. Yarros recalls her life as a woman physician
        and as one who, "if not actually a pioneer, has helped to
        extend the sphere of women in medicine." Born in Russia,
        where she was filled "with ideas of freedom and justice,"
        Dr. Yarros emigrated to the United States and obtained her
        M.D. from the Woman's Medical College of Pennsylvania.
        The teacher who inspired her most there was Dr. Anna E.
        Broomall. In 1894, after internship at the New England
        Hospital, Dr. Yarros went to Chicago. She persuaded the
        dean of the College of Physicians and Surgeons to fund a
        dispensary, which she opened in 1899--the first year the
        College admitted women. The dean doubted that a woman
        doctor could teach and hold the interest of men students, but
        Dr. Yarros "found no difficulty. In fact, they often forgot
        while at work that there was any difference between us."
        In addition, she "had ample opportunity to learn a great deal
        about masculine psychology." She observed her male pupils
        to be "most chivalrous," often protecting her "from vulgar-
        ities," "more comfort-loving than women, and mentally not
        very different, in spite of all the claims for masculine su-
        periority." Dr. Yarros believes that because of "domestic

and social distractions" a woman is less likely to keep up
with medical progress and therefore teaching positions are
great incentives for women physicians. As a specialist in
gynecology and obstetrics, Dr. Yarros became involved in
venereal diseases and sex education. In connection with
these interests, she served with several social hygiene organizations.

1846.   Zakrzewska, Marie A. "Fifty Years Ago--A Retrospect."
             Woman's Medical Journal, 1:10 (October 1893) 193-195.
         Because abortionists flourished at the time Elizabeth Black-
         well and Harriot Hunt sought medical work, society feared
         the increase of "licentious prostitutions" and ostracized the
         two women. In 1853, when Dr. Zakrzewska landed in New
         York from Berlin, the position of women physicians was "a
         really pitiable, ignominious, and despised one, only endur-
         able by the most courageous, strong natures among woman-
         kind." Women could study, but it was impossible to acquire
         patients. Obtaining practical training, Dr. Zakrzewska notes,
         was the true pioneer work done by the Drs. Blackwell and
         herself.

1847.   "Zella White Stewart, M.D." Medical Woman's Journal, 50:
             12 (December 1943) 315.
         Dr. Stewart (whose portrait appears on the front cover of
         this issue of the Journal) graduated in 1903 from Cornell
         University Medical College. Her specialty was allergy and
         she was one of 150 selected specialists in the American
         Association for the Study of Allergy. In addition to her med-
         ical interests, Dr. Stewart was active in woman suffrage
         and founded the Iowa City League of Women Voters.

1848.   Zink, Pearl L. "Mary Mitchell Henry, M.D." Journal of
             the American Medical Women's Association, 14:11 (No-
             vember 1959) 1019. port. (Album of Women in Medi-
             cine.)
         A charter member and organizer of the Academy of General
         Practice in San Antonio in 1947, Dr. Henry was the first
         woman physician to serve as its president.

1849.   "Zoe Allison Johnston, M.D." Medical Woman's Journal,
             50:5 (May 1943) 128.
         Dr. Johnston (whose portrait appears on the front cover of
         this issue of the Journal) was nominated for president-elect
         of the Allegheny County Medical Society (Pennsylvania), the
         first woman in the Society's 78-year history so honored.
         She specialized in radiology and was a member of several
         radiological societies.

RECRUITMENT

1850.   Stokvis-Cohen Stuart, N.   ["Women Doctors for the Indies"].
         Nederlandsch Tijdschrift voor Geneeskunde, 74:10 (8
         March 1930) 1268-1270.   (Dut)
         The author has served as a physician in the Indies for 18
         years and is now trying to recruit younger doctors, espe-
         cially women doctors, with ideals and a desire for hard
         work to take over.   In Europe people are accustomed to
         male doctors, even in gynecology and obstetrics.   In the
         Far East, however, in addition to the natural womanly mod-
         esty, the Moslem religion forbids treatment of women pa-
         tients by male doctors.   There is still much pioneering work
         for women doctors in the Indies, not only in caring for wo-
         men patients but also for babies, gaining the confidence of
         women, teaching them hygiene and family care, establishing
         polyclinics and hospitals.   She has included in her nursing
         courses instruction in how to deal with patients not only
         scientifically but also psychologically.   Those who consider
         volunteering for this service should be willing to learn
         something about the country and the Malay language so they
         can communicate with the nursing personnel as well as
         their patients.   From those applying, five candidates are to
         be selected by the government to be sent to this challenging
         area.

GREAT BRITAIN

1851.   Owens, Joan Llewelyn.   Hospital Careers for Girls.   Evans
         Brothers Limited, London, England, 1961, 152 pp.
         (Summit Career Guides.)
         After a general introduction, this guide breaks hospital ca-
         reers down into eight areas.   Section 5 covers medicine and

and surgery (pp. 54-82). Such concerns are discussed as
the type of work, the personal qualities necessary, educational requirements, length and cost of training, and openings for employment. Concluding the section is a list of
medical schools and their addresses, as well as "other useful addresses."

UNITED STATES

1852.   [American Medical Women's Association.] Medicine: A
          Woman's Career. American Medical Women's Associa-
          tion, New York, New York, 1973. (Pamphlet.) illus.
        This is a recruitment pamphlet to help and to encourage
        "qualified young women" to enter medicine. The study of
        medicine requires a lifetime of learning. Since "one of
        the major decisions that faces the woman medical student
        is the possibility of marriage," the young woman should
        know that "a professional practice and a homemaking career
        ARE COMPATIBLE if planned carefully." This pamphlet
        also broadly discusses planning and preparation for a med-
        ical career in secondary school and college.

1853.   Fay, Marion. "Aggressive Recruitment." Journal of the
          American Medical Women's Association, 19:5 (May 1964)
          405-406.
        "Why aren't more women going into medicine?" asks the au-
        thor. What can be done to increase the number? Dr. Fay
        suggests women physicians set a positive example, advise
        premed women what to study, speak to high school and col-
        lege groups, and invite qualified girls to visit their offices.

1854.   Fay, Marion. "Why Don't More Women Apply to Medical
          Schools?" Journal of Medical Education, 37:5 (May
          1962) 500-501. (Medical Education Forum: Editorials.)
        In 1959-1960 one out of two women applying to medical
        schools was accepted, but the distressing statistic is the
        small number of women applicants (1,026 women as com-
        pared with 13,926 men in 1959-1960). An active campaign
        to interest high school girls in medicine is needed, and stu-
        dent advisers need to be better equipped to counsel in this
        area. Young women considering a medical career should
        be realistic about marriage and family responsibilities and
        the possibilities of combining these with a career.

1855.   Fenten, D. X. Ms.--M.D. The Westminster Press, Phil-
          adelphia, Pennsylvania, 1973, 144 pp. photos.
        This book outlines the career of medicine for young high
        school and junior high school students. It covers the current
        status of women in medicine, the viability of medicine as a
        career for women, the history of women in medicine, the
        high school and college preparation necessary for medical
        study, the MCAT, the medical school course of study, and

the routine of practice. It also summarizes the various
specialties of medicine and their requirements. A chapter
on the future for medical women includes recommendations
made by the American Medical Women's Association, the
President's Study Group on Careers for Women, and the
Women's Bureau of the U.S. Department of Labor during a
conference entitled "The Fuller Utilization of the Woman
Physician." An appendix lists American medical schools,
their tuition and admission requirements. There is also an
index to the text.

1856. Grundy, Betty L. "Career Roles in Medicine." In: Ca-
       reer Guidance for Young Women: Considerations in
       Planning Professional Careers. Edited by Richard E.
       Hardy and John G. Cull. Charles C. Thomas, Spring-
       field, Illinois, 1974, 17-26.
A woman physician writes of the thrill and satisfaction a
medical career can offer a woman. Dr. Grundy discusses
the advantages women bring to medicine (compassion, gentleness, and tender understanding) and the disadvantages (nine
per cent fail to practice medicine). Discrimination and social pressure are also discussed: "On the whole, a woman
doctor must be a bit more capable than a man to achieve
like successes in the practice of medicine." Dr. Grundy
also writes about the fields of practice women physicians
may select. In conclusion, she describes her own lifestyle as a 33-year-old woman physician.

1857. Kerr, Charlotte Herman. "Medical Education and Practice."
       Journal of the American Medical Women's Association,
       18:1 (January 1963) 60-62. (Special Committee Re-
       ports.)
This is a report of the American Medical Women's Association's Committee on Medical Education and Practice.
AMWA members are concerned with ways to encourage women to consider medicine as a profession. Therefore AMWA
members take part in recruitment panels of county and state
medical societies, distribute their pamphlet, "So, you want
to be a Doctor?", make accessible their tape recording on
the increased use of medical womanpower, answer questions
and requests for information by means of telephone calls
and correspondence, grant loans to freshmen women, and
cooperate with other groups interested in recruiting for
health careers. This Committee perceives several other
needs: a pamphlet that would address college students and
another that would identify specialties that women would find
advantageous, and an attractive bulletin board that could be
loaned to schools and medical societies for their "Health
Career Day." They have been in correspondence with the
deans of 88 medical schools; 79 have written back. They
give $100 achievement awards to women who graduate at the
top of their class and citations to women who graduate in
the upper 10 per cent. Their Journal has a section to ad-

vertise job openings for women physicians, their job requirements, and their job qualifications. They are also advocating part-time employment for women physicians with
small children.

1858.   Klinefelter, Lee M. Medical Occupations for Girls: Wo-
            men in White. E. P. Dutton & Co., Inc. [New York,
            New York], 1939, 320 pp. charts, photos.
         A fictional situation--high school girls visiting a local hos-
         pital--is the method through which several allied medical
         occupations are introduced. The author (who also wrote
         Medical Occupations for Boys) devotes two chapters to ex-
         amining the activities of women holding M. D. degrees:
         "The Physician," and "The Medical Specialists." Placing
         particular emphasis on the difficulties faced by women med-
         ical students and physicians, the suitability of women for
         various specialties is also discussed. A six-page chart,
         based on data compiled from 400 questionnaires, lists U.S.
         and Canadian medical schools that accept women students,
         and provides 1938 enrollment and graduation statistics. A
         bibliography follows each chapter. The "Conclusion," dur-
         ing which the book's characters sum up their feelings to-
         wards medical careers, includes "condensed information" on
         the number of women in related health fields, training cost,
         and average income. This book contains a glossary and in-
         dex.

1859.   "A Medical Career for the Girl Graduate." Medical Wo-
            man's Journal, 29:6 (June 1922) 118. (Editorial.)
         For "remuneration, the social position and the personal
         satisfaction," few careers offer more than medicine.

1860.   Medical College of Pennsylvania. Medicine! Are You Wo-
            man Enough to Try? The Student American Medical
            Association Women in Medicine Committee of the Med-
            ical College of Pennsylvania, Philadelphia, n.d. (Pam-
            phlet.)
         Some questions and answers about medical school admissions
         and characteristics of women physicians are followed by a
         brief annotated bibliography of books to read for those wo-
         men interested in medicine as a career.

1861.   "'Medicine a Glorious Craft.'" Medical Woman's Journal,
            39:12 (December 1932) 307-308.
         In an interview at the congress of the American College of
         Surgeons, Catharine Macfarlane urges "the young woman of
         stamina and idealism" to enter medicine. "Sex has nothing
         to do with medicine. It hasn't anything to do with mental-
         ity. The field of exact science is open to both men and
         women."

1862.   Medicine as a Career for Women. American Medical Wo-
            men's Association, Inc., [New York, New York], 1968,

16 pp. illus.

Following a narrative on the qualities needed by a physician and the rewards a medical career offers women, this booklet offers advice on financial planning and educational preparation for medical school. A section titled "Combining Marriage and Medicine" assures young readers that a medical career does not mean sacrificing chances to marry; proof of this can be found in "the number of pretty, obviously feminine women students who can be seen in any medical school." To successfully combine a career with a home, women physicians need the "three essentials": an understanding husband, good health, and good household help and childcare. "The neighbors rarely criticize a physician for continuing to work while raising a family--the importance and prestige of her work are too great."

1863.   "More Women Medical Students." Woman's Medical Journal, 28:9 (September 1918) 202.
"An educational campaign is needed to induce college women to study medicine." Too little is actually known, by the average woman graduate, of medicine as a career. The American Medical Association reports only 581 women studying medicine (29 less than in 1917).

1864.   "Need for More Women Doctors." Medical and Professional Woman's Journal, 41:4 (April 1934) 115.
In an address before Goucher College (Baltimore) students, noted cancer specialist Dr. Joseph Bloodgood emphasized the need for women physicians. Asserting that "women can do certain things better than men," Dr. Bloodgood offered an example: "they [women] can, for instance, take better care of the health of the family; and preventive medicine is just a scientific care of the family."

1865.   Nemir, Rosa Lee. "Facing the Future: The Changing World and Medicine." Journal of the American Medical Women's Association, 20:8 (August 1965) 759-761.
Scientific and socioeconomic factors will have the major effect on medicine in the future, so a greater supply of well-qualified medical personnel must be found. "Women constitute the largest untapped reservoir of talent in our North American Society." In order to attract these women to medicine, women educators, modification of medical curricula, and day care centers will be needed. A clarification of the role of the private practitioner in our society is also essential. The American Medical Women's Association can play a large part in helping to formulate plans for the future.

1866.   Nemir, Rosa Lee and Brodie, Jessie Laird. "Recruitment in Health Careers: Third National Council on Health Careers, September 24-25, 1962, New York City." Journal of the American Medical Women's Association,

18:1 (January 1963) 47-48.
To attract women to health careers, retraining opportunities
must be created for people who have left the job market for
a while, especially in fields with high turnover, such as the
health fields. In addition, more publicity must be given to
ancillary health fields so that people who want to work in
health can choose a career that best suits them. Recruitment panels should be formed which are composed of a
variety of health personnel. These panels will address
meetings of parents, teachers, guidance counselors as well
as provide students with accurate information. People interested in health careers should be encouraged to take volunteer and short term positions in health jobs. Information
on health careers should also be placed in libraries (bulletin board displays, vertical file material). "So You Want
to Be a Doctor?", a booklet published for the high school
girl by the American Medical Women's Association, was
also recommended as a recruitment device.

1867.   Pierrel, Rosemary. "Medical Career Interests Among Col-
            lege Women." Journal of the American Medical Wo-
            men's Association, 19:2 (February 1964) 135-137.
         Dr. Pierrel, dean of Pembroke College at Brown University,
         discusses her experiences in career counseling of under-
         graduate women interested in medicine: "the largest pro-
         portion of questions deals with the arguments they have
         heard against women in medicine." Dr. Pierrel discusses
         the ways, "relevant to the pursuit of medicine," that women
         differ from men; the success of marriage and medicine; the
         nature and extent of discrimination against women in medi-
         cine; and prejudice exhibited by patients and by other med-
         ical students.

1868.   Potter, Ellen C. Medicine: A Supreme Service for Col-
            lege Women. Young Women's Christian Associations,
            National Board, New York, New York, 1918, 4 pp.
            (Vocational Bulletin.)

1869.   Ryder, Claire F. "President's Message." Journal of the
            American Medical Women's Association, 16:2 (February
            1961) 149-150.
         In response to the physician "man power" shortage, the
         doors to women in medicine should be opened wide. To
         double the proportion of women in all medical schools
         "should be our minimum goal for the 1960s."

1870.   Schuck, R. F.; et al. Attitudes of Guidance Counselors in
            Western Pennsylvania High Schools Toward Medicine as
            a Career Choice for Women. Division of Research in
            Medical Education, School of Medicine, University of
            Pittsburgh, Pittsburgh, Pennsylvania, 1974, 423 pp.
         "This study sought to determine the attitudes of guidance
         counselors toward the entrance of women into the profession

of medicine. In order to answer this broad question two
research methods were employed. The counselors were
given a paired comparisons task, i.e., they were asked to
make sixty-six choices among twelve high school students
to determine who they felt would be most successful in medical school. To supplement these data, both counselors and
women medical students at the University of Pittsburgh were
interviewed and their answers analyzed. One conclusion
reached by the study was that the sex of a potential medical
school applicant was not a significant variable in the perceptions of the high school counselors when taken with other
more obvious academic considerations. The data from this
study also support the conclusion that counselors do not play
an active role in the student's decision-making process;
rather, they facilitate it by providing information. A mis-
conception by most counselors was that career decisions were
not made until late in college, whereas over 50 per cent of
the women interviewed made their decisions before or during high school. Several recommendations for further study
in the area are included." [Document abstract; document
not examined by editors.]

1871. Thomas, Mary A. "Should a Girl Be Encouraged to Be-
         come a Physician?" The Woman Physician, 25:10
         (October 1970) 629-630.
         "Many young girls have never seen or been in contact with
         a woman physician.... The changing patterns of admission
         to medical schools, the freedom a medical education pro-
         vides women, the mobility it allows, the availability of part-
         time residencies, the medical specialties that permit flex-
         ible schedules, all should be made known to the young high
         school and college girl, as well as to those who mold her
         attitudes." A brief biographical inset on Mary A. Thomas
         is included.

1872. Tracy, Martha. "A Campaign of Propaganda for Recruits
         to Medical Colleges. Interesting Communication from
         the Dean of the Woman's Medical College, Philadelphia,
         Pa." Woman's Medical Journal, 28:10 (October 1918)
         226.
         Dr. Tracy's letter is written in response to a previous
         article in the Journal on "More Women Medical Students"
         [September 1918, p. 202]. Dr. Tracy reports that while the
         total number of women enrolled in medicine in the U.S.
         may be down by 29 in 1918 as compared to 1917, the en-
         rollment at the Woman's Medical College of Pennsylvania
         doubled from 1916 to 1917, and the entering class for 1918
         was one-third as large as that in 1917. Dr. Tracy next
         presents the requirements for medical school admission and
         explains the various classes of medical schools.

1873. Whitlock-Rose, Elise. "Catholic Women in Medicine."
         Catholic World, 141 (May 1935) 222-226. (The Ball

and the Cross.)
Among women physicians, less than ten per cent are Catholic; a number of the others are "weakly Protestant," and
many are pagan.   Catholic women must enter the medical
profession and combat the "menace of birth control, steril-
ization, and so-called therapeutic abortions."   The author
urges women to attend Catholic medical schools, establish
Catholic clinics, and recruit young women into the field.

1874.   "Women in Medicine ... Examining the Opportunities."
        BCM: Inside Baylor Medicine, 4:8 (October-November
        1973) 3.   photos.
Baylor College of Medicine's Women in Medicine committee
hosted a conference for women students in Houston, Texas-
area high schools and colleges.

1875.   Wulsin, John H.   "Letters from other desks: Admission of
        Women to Medical School."   Journal of the American
        Medical Women's Association, 21:8 (August 1966) 674-
        676.
A male chairman of the University of Cincinnati College of
Medicine writes that prejudice that excluded women from
attending medical school a generation ago is disappearing.
He wishes more women would consider applying.   Girl high
school students who are considering a premedical course
should avoid small colleges with poor science laboratories.
Medical school admission committees want assurance that
women who marry have their husbands' understanding and
support in order to get through.   The author fears that one
possible reason more able girls do not apply to medical
school is that families and educational advisors discourage
them from applying.   He believes the business of counter-
acting the prejudice of families against their girls attending
medical school is that of women physicians, public relations
people, and sociologists.   Medical schools should inform
high school education counselors and science teachers as
well as college premedical advisors about the need for women in medicine.   Women students "keep the males, students and faculty alike, on their toes for a variety of reasons which need no discussion in a letter such as this,"
writes Wulsin.

MEDICAL EDUCATION

Included are statistical articles on medical education, general discussions about how women should acquire that education, and material relating in a general manner to medical students, faculty, administration, and educational trends. Undergraduate and premedical education articles are cited as well. (Discussions about women's motivations for entering medicine can be found under PSYCHOSOCIAL FACTORS. General histories of medical education are located in HISTORY OF WOMEN IN MEDICINE.)

ASIA

1876. "Medical Colleges." Journal of the Association of Medical
          Women in India, 24:2 (May 1936) 68, 70-76.
          A brief description of entrance requirements, fees, courses,
          and other particulars is given for each of the medical
          schools in India which is listed.

1877. "Medical Education for Women in India." Medical Woman's
          Journal, 30:1 (January 1923) 30. (Notes and Comments.)
          The need for a separate medical school for Indian women
          is evidenced by 1920 statistics: only 135 women physicians
          were practicing in India, where the female population to-
          taled more than 21 million. A school is proposed for lo-
          cation in Madras. And Dr. Ida Scudder is currently on a
          fund-raising lecture tour of the U.S., endeavoring to raise
          two million dollars for the education of medical women.

1878. "Projects Sponsored by Medical Women." Medical Woman's
          Journal, 39:4 (April 1932) 101. photo.
          The Medical Women's Society of New York State sponsors
          medical education for women in China and Korea including
          some women medical students at the Woman's Medical In-
          stitute, Seoul, Korea.

AUSTRALIA & NEW ZEALAND

1879. Nanson, E. M. "Medical Education 100 Years After."
          New Zealand Medical Journal, 81 (12 February 1975)
          134-149.
          This article is written one hundred years after the opening
          of doors at the University of Otago Medical School in New
          Zealand. Statistics covering the 100-year period are given
          on the number of applicants for medicine and the methods
          of selection. In 1891 the University of Otago admitted its
          first woman undergraduate student. In 1975 the quota of
          women students admitted is 20 per cent. In Auckland there
          is no quota and the number of women students there has
          varied from 20 per cent to 40 per cent. The writer sug-
          gests that 20 to 25 per cent may be a "fair" quota of wo-
          men admitted to medical school, yet the final answer rests
          upon the question of whether New Zealand wants a predom-
          inantly male or female medical profession. Other aspects
          of the medical course of study are discussed with no further
          differentiation between male and female.

CANADA

1880.   Fish, C. G. and Clarke, G. G. "Medical Education; Part
             I; Medical Students in Canadian Universities: Report of
             Statistics, 1965-66." Canadian Medical Association
             Journal, 94:14 (2 April 1966) 693-700. tables.
         In 1963-64 there were 13.4 per cent women enrolled in med-
         ical schools in Canada, which is the highest percentage re-
         corded of women attending Canadian medical schools. In
         the 1965-66 freshman class, 12.7 per cent women were en-
         rolled, and 10.9 per cent were enrolled in the 1964-65
         class.

1881.   Fruen, Mary A.; Rothman, Arthur I. and Steiner, Jan W.
             "Comparison of Characteristics of Male and Female
             Medical School Applicants." Journal of Medical Educa-
             tion, 49:2 (February 1974) 137-145. tables.
         Male and female medical school applicants are compared on
         academic, biographic, and psychological factors. Compar-
         ison is based on the information gathered in an unpublished
         study by Rothman of the applications to the 1972 entering
         class of the University of Toronto Faculty of Medicine. "No
         bias on the basis of sex was found in selection, but there
         was some evidence for greater self-selection by females
         prior to application. A number of differences in psycholog-
         ical and biographic factors were observed, the implications
         of which are uncertain." Tables include differences by sex
         in academic performance among accepted applicants; com-
         parative statistics in academic performance among rejected
         applicants; sex of applicants by population of home commun-
         ity; comparison of Personality Research Form applicants;
         and sex differences among all applicants.

1882.   Grainger, R. M. "Medical Student Enrolment [sic] in Can-
             ada in 1971-72: Report of Statistics." Canadian Med-
             ical Association Journal, 107:12 (23 December 1972)
             1220-1222. tables. (Medical Education.)
         One statistical table and a brief comment in the text deal
         with women in this report of undergraduate enrollment in
         16 Canadian medical colleges. The percentage of women
         students tripled from 1957-58 to 1971-72. For the class
         of 1971-72, women numbered 332 (21.2 per cent) of a total
         of 1,568 students.

1883.   Macleod, J. W. "Medical Student Enrolment [sic] in Ca-
             nadian Universities." The Canadian Medical Association
             Journal, 88:14 (6 April 1963) 683-690. tables. (Med-
             ical Education.) (Presentation, Association of Canadian
             Medical Colleges, Vancouver, British Columbia, Octo-
             ber 22-24, 1962.)
         This statistical study was based on data for 1961-62 from
         Canada's 12 medical schools and on additional information
         from the deans' offices of these schools for the 1962-63

session. Total enrollment increased at these schools and
the percentage of women accepted increased as well from
8.6 per cent in 1957-58 to 11.3 per cent in 1962-63. In
the United States during the years 1961-62, the percentage
of women who were medical students was 6.4 per cent,
and 5.6 per cent were graduates. While the exact ratio of
men to women applicants is not known, returns from nine
of the 12 schools indicate that women made up 8.8 per cent
of the total number of applicants for the 1962-63 class.
Women now comprise ten per cent of the medical students
in Canadian universities.

1884.   Macleod, J. W.; Fish, D. G.; and Howes, Joyce. "Med-
         ical Students in Canadian Universities: Report of Sta-
         tistics, 1963-64 and 1964-65." Canadian Medical Asso-
         ciation Journal, 92:14 (3 April 1965) 689-693. tables.
         (Medical Education.)
The statistics which appear on some of the tables in this
report are based upon two different questionnaires with two
different sets of definitions. Some statistics were prepared
and published by the Council on Medical Education of the
American Medical Association in conjunction with the Association of American Medical Colleges; other data came from
the Association of Canadian Medical Colleges. Because of
this dual source, there are discrepancies in these authors'
findings. To meet the rising need in Canada for physicians,
there was an increase in admittance of the first-year class
from 946 students in 1959-60 to 1133 in 1964-5. For the
first time since 1959-60, the percentage of women among the
first-year class has shown a decrease, with an enrollment
of 10.9 per cent compared to 13.4 per cent in the previous
year.

1885.   Macleod, J. W. and Howes, J. "Medical Students in Ca-
         nadian Universities, 1962-63 and 1963-64." Canadian
         Medical Association Journal, 90:14 (4 April 1964), 809-
         813. tables. (Medical Education.)
The 12 Canadian medical schools have increased enrollment
from the low of 946 students in 1959-60 to 1086 students in
1963-64. The increase from 1962-63 of 1061 students admitted to medical school, to the 1963-64 statistics, is due
entirely to 25 additional women medical students. Male
registration declined by one. At the 1962-63 commencements, 826 people received degrees--761 men and 65 women (8.1 per cent of the total). At the time this article
was written, one in 14 medical students in the United States
was female while one out of every nine medical students in
Canada was female. Thirteen point four per cent of the
first-year students in 1963-64 were female compared with
10.3 per cent in 1960-61 and 8.6 per cent in 1957-58. In
order to learn whether medicine is recruiting its share of
university men and women, a more reliable method of count-
ing the number of students who prepare themselves seriously
for the study of medicine is needed.

1886.   Nelson-Jones, Richard and Fish, David G. "Women Stu-
            dents in Canadian Medical Schools." British Journal
            of Medical Education, 4:2 (June 1970) 97-108. tables.
         This article discusses the participation of women in Cana-
         dian medical education by providing data on the number and
         percentage of Canadian and Landed Immigrant women med-
         ical students in the entering classes at 13 medical schools
         from 1965-66 through 1968-69. Included were: (1) the par-
         ticipation rate of women in Canadian higher education, (2)
         the proportion of women in the medical school applicant
         pool, and (3) selected social characteristics of Canadian wo-
         men medical students. From 1965-66 to 1968-69, the num-
         ber of women entering medical school increased by 68 per
         cent: in 1968-69, 14 per cent of all undergraduate students
         in Canadian medical schools were women. Still, women
         constitute a much smaller proportion of medical school en-
         rollment than they constitute of total enrollment in Canadian
         universities and colleges. Of the women applicants to Ca-
         nadian medical schools, 55 per cent received acceptances as
         compared with 48 per cent acceptances of male applicants.
         MCAT scores reveal that the mean for accepted and regis-
         tered women in the 1968-69 class was 12 points higher than
         the mean for accepted and registered men; the means for
         rejected women were lower on all MCAT subtests than the
         means for rejected men. The authors feel that this fact
         "provides some evidence that for their 1968-69 entering
         classes Canadian medical schools were not discriminating
         against women applicants." Social characteristics discussed
         include community size during high school years, education-
         al level and professional qualification of parents, and occu-
         pational status of fathers of medical students. It was dis-
         covered that women medical students as compared with male
         medical students come from families where a significantly
         larger proportion of parents are university educated. The
         medical careers chosen by women differ from those chosen
         by men. The authors conclude that women will continue to
         play a significant role in the Canadian medical world, and
         their increasing numbers in medical schools "has profound
         implications for the direction, type, and quality of medicine
         practised in Canada."

EUROPE, EASTERN

1887.   Baudouin de Courtenay R[omualda]. ["On Better Education
            of Women Doctors"]. Swit., 2:18 (1885) 142-143.
            (Pol)
         Apparently this article is continued in issue number 19 (p.
         149-150), and issue number 20 (p. 155-156). [Article not
         examined by editors.]

1888.   Herzenstein, G. M. ["Medical Lectures for Women: Sta-
            tistics of Attendance"]. Vrach. (St. Petersburg), 1

(1880) 553.   (Rus)
[Article not examined by editors.]

1889.   Ostrowska, Antonina and Bejnarowica, Janusz. "Research
Report: The Decision to Become a Medical Student."
Social Science and Medicine, 4:5 (December 1970) 535-
550. tables. (Current Research.)
After lectures in medical sociology were presented to first-
year medical students at the Medical Academy in Warsaw,
a survey was made among those students. This article
makes few distinctions between the way female and male
students responded. Of those students surveyed, 65.3 per
cent were women and 34.0 per cent were men. While university hospitals and big hospitals were equally attractive
as employment possibilities for women and men, more women (14.6 per cent) than men could perceive themselves
working in small hospitals and nursing homes. More men
(27.8 per cent) than women (19.4 per cent) were interested
in surgery in this first year's class. In contrast, 10.2
per cent women and 1.0 per cent men were interested in
pediatrics. "It seems that contemporary beliefs about the
respective roles of men and women influence the division
into 'male' and 'female' specializations such as pediatrics
or surgery." Concerning salaries, women expected to earn
lower salaries than men when their training was completed.

1890.   ["The Question of the Admission of Women to Academic
Studies Before the Two State Universities in Hungary"].
Wiener Medizinische Blatter, 3:19 (6 May 1880) 489-
491. (Original Correspondence.) (Ger)
[Article not examined by editors.]

1891.   Tolstoi, K. ["Women as Physicians and Female Medical
Lecture Courses"]. Vestnik Obsh. Hig. Sudeb. i Prakt.
Med. St. Petersburg, 2: Part 7 (1889) 49-63. (Rus)
[Article not examined by editors.]

1892.   Zhbankoff, D. N. ["On Female Medical Courses"]. Trudi
V. syezda obsh. russk. vrach. v pamyat Pirogova, 2
(1894) 728-732. (Rus)
[Article not examined by editors.]

EUROPE, WESTERN

1893.   ["Admission of Women to Medical and Pharmaceutical Professions"]. Wiener Medizinische Presse, 39 (1900)
1793-1795. (Ger)
Regulations published on 15 September 1900 by the Ministry
of Education concerning the admission of women to medical
studies and to the doctorate in general medical science, as
well as to the pharmaceutical profession, were considered
a major step toward the introduction of women into the

learned professions in Austria. A regulation of March 1896 had permitted women who had completed medical studies and the doctorate in foreign countries to be admitted to "nostrification" [the administrative procedure which results in one country's recognition of a foreign medical diploma] at an Austrian medical faculty after passing stringent examinations. This procedure, however, effectively limited medical careers to a few women from economically and socially secure families. The new regulation, promulgated with the apparent approval of most medical faculties and docents, permitted women, who had passed the school-leaving examination and completed the same preparatory studies as were required of male candidates, to enroll as regular students in Austrian schools of medicine and pharmacy. This opportunity to enter two of the important professions was an advance in both equal rights and equal responsibilities for women.

1894.   Bluhm, Agnes. ["The Evolution and the Present Situation of Women in Medical Studies."] Deutsche Medicinische Wochenschrift, 21:39 (26 September 1895) 648-650. (Ger)
In this factual description of women's admission to medical studies in different countries, the author especially illustrates the situation in England, Switzerland, and Russia. She also mentions the position of women medical students and physicians in most of the other European nations. The author underlines the ready acceptance of women in medical studies and practice in these countries as opposed to their controversial situation in Germany and Austria. Her article introduces facts and objectivity into the male discussion on the topic of women and medical education. [This article also appeared in an English translation entitled "The Development and Present Status of Medical Research as Pursued by Women." Woman's Medical Journal, 5:4 (April 1896) 85-90.]

1895.   Böhmert, Victor. [Women at the Universities, with Special Regard for Medical Studies]. Leipzig, Germany, 1872, 44 pp. (Ger)
This book on university education for women concentrates on the experiences in Zurich (Switzerland). The author discusses the situation of the first medical students in Zurich and extensively quotes contemporary views on aptitudes and successes. He concludes that, despite severe opposition to women in medicine, there is no objective reason to exclude them from the field.

1896.   Bowditch, Henry Ingersoll. "The Medical Education of Women." Boston Medical and Surgical Journal, 101:2 (10 July 1879) 67-69.
This letter-to-the-editor was written in support of the cause of educating women in medicine. It is affirmed that Zurich does indeed educate women successfully, and an extract

from a letter from one woman who had earned the respect
of her teachers is presented. It is suggested that the questions are by whom and in what manner shall women be so
educated. The author prefers separate instruction for male
and females, but feels that female medical education is inevitable and should be accepted by every reasoning person.
An editorial note affirms objection to medical coeducation
and requests that the faculty at Zurich prepare a history of
their coeducation experiment.

1897.   Eulenburg, Albert. ["Women Medical Students in German
            Universities during the Summer Semester of 1901"].
            Deutsche Medicinische Wochenschrift, 27:28 (11 July
            1901) 472. chart. (Ger)
         A questionnaire designed to obtain data on female medical
         students brought replies from the deans of the medical
         faculties in 19 of the 20 German universities having med-
         ical schools. Of the 19, ten reported no women students;
         the other nine had a total of 39 German women and 56
         foreigners. Berlin had 25 women with 21 foreigners, and
         Leipzig 24 women with 22 foreigners; and Halle had nine
         Russians of a total of 12 women. The other schools re-
         ported mainly or only German students. In German-speak-
         ing Austria, Graz reported two German women medical
         students and Innsbruck none. Berne reported one German,
         six Swiss, and 180 Russians, out of 188; Zurich had 12
         Germans out of 85 women medical students. These figures
         indicate an increase of not more than 52 in the number of
         women practitioners for the coming year.

1898.   Fickert, A[uguste K]. ["The Study of Medicine by Women"].
            Wiener Klinische Rundschau, 13 (1899) 241-243. (Ger)
         [Article not examined by editors.]

1899.   Fickert, Auguste K. ["Women and Medical Studies"].
            Wiener Klinische Rundschau, 13:15 (9 April 1899) 241-
            243. (Ger)
         On February 9, 1899 the clinical students (male) at the Uni-
         versity of Halle-Wittenberg submitted a petition to the med-
         ical faculty of that school, protesting the clinical instruction
         of women and men together and demanding the exclusion of
         women from these classes, since "experience has taught us
         that simultaneous clinical instruction of men and women stu-
         dents has as little relation to thorough medical education as
         it has with the fundamentals of morality." Without waiting
         for the faculty reply, they put out a call to students of oth-
         er universities to join them in this protest. The medical
         faculty replied that it highly disapproved of the actions of
         a few students claiming to represent the whole clinical
         group, in making this local question public without waiting
         for a response from the faculty. The basic problem was
         partly due to misunderstanding and partly to tendentious dis-
         tortion of some actions of the administration and of insignifi-

cant incidents. The faculty would not take disciplinary
measures against the petition authors, believing that they
were not aware of the consequences of their actions.   The
author of this comment is less upset by the incident than
by the ambivalence shown at the previous year's medical
meeting at Wiesbaden: official endorsement of the admission of women to their ranks, while repeating all the arguments against it.   The suggestions that instead of competing
with male doctors, women should become governesses,
nurses, dentists or pharmacists, or enter commercial or
industrial careers--implying inferiority of women--anger
him.   He points out the results of an English survey of
139 universities of the world, which showed that only 12
admitted no women, while 100 (including 24 of the 28 in
North America) made no distinction between men and women.   In 1894 there were 259 women medical students in
England, 261 in the Indian colonies, 161 in Switzerland,
155 in France, and 18,000 in North America.   He says that
there were 3000 women physicians in North America in
1893 and 5000 in 1898, and the numbers are increasing
steadily in other countries.

1900.   Hjort, G.   [On the Performance of Medical Care by Women,
          and Their Education for It].   Gothenburg, Sweden, 1869,
          16 pp.   (Swe)
          Hjort's idea was that midwives should be able to get a sim-
          plified three-year medical education and become involved in
          the care of women and children in the rural districts.
          [Swedish abstract provided to the editors by Märtha Elvers-
          Hulth, retired librarian of the National Swedish Board of
          Health and Welfare Library.]

1901.   Höfstatter, Robert.   ["On Higher Education for Women in
          Austria with Special Consideration of Medical Studies"].
          Archiv fuer Frauenkunde und Konstitutions Forschung,
          16:3/4 (1929) 301-319.   tables.   (Ger)
          The first part of the article cites figures on the number of
          students, male and female, and medical students in particu-
          lar, in the University of Vienna over the years from 1888
          to 1928.   In the three Austrian universities (Vienna, Graz,
          and Innsbruck) in the academic year 1927-28, there were
          10,700 male students and 2,214 females; 473 of the latter
          were studying medicine.   Women were first admitted to the
          University of Vienna in 1897.   The number in the medical
          curriculum rose slowly to about 150 in 1910, and rose rap-
          idly to a peak of about 600 in the late war years and im-
          mediate postwar period, then dropped by about 50 per cent.
          Women medical students, as a percentage of all women stu-
          dents, dropped from around 22 per cent in 1900 to 15-20
          per cent during the period 1902-1910, peaked over 40 per
          cent in 1917, and stabilized at around 20 per cent in 1923-
          27.   The early decrease is attributed to the opening of oth-
          er professional curricula to women during these early years.

The absolute number and percentage of male medical students reached low and high levels at about the same times
as the per cent figures for women. Figures are quoted
showing that in America, where the professions had been
open to women longer than in Europe, the marriage rate
for professional women had dropped steadily from the 1840s
to 1910. The author devotes approximately half the article
to the reasons why women are not as well suited to the sciences as men, and to a dissertation on the "enormous danger" to the race or to society of having the most intelligent
women devote their talents and energies to working instead
of to raising children.

1902.   Kunn, Carl. ["On Medical Studies for Women"]. Wiener
        Klinische Rundschau, 17:30 (26 July 1903) 548-549.
        (Ger)
        In a recent issue of the Wiener Medizinisch Wochenschrift,
        Professor Ludwig Stieda, professor of anatomy at Koenigs-
        berg, noted that although women were theoretically admitted
        to medical studies at all German universities, in actuality,
        their admission to lectures was up to the individual profes-
        sors. Some took all women, some took none, some al-
        lowed them in lectures but not in practical instruction.
        Stieda himself, although in favor of women's studies, would
        not teach men and women together in anatomy because he
        did not think it suitable for delicate young women to see and
        hear embarrassing things in lectures and demonstrations,
        and because he thought it dangerous to have men and women
        live and work so closely together. Kunn disagrees heartily.
        Of all places where there should be no danger, it should be
        in the scientific atmosphere; certainly if one does not object
        to their working together in shops and factories, one should
        not expect trouble among the educated and more intelligent
        young people in medical school. Anyway, God did not make
        man the guardian of woman; they are both people and woman
        has the right to speak and decide for herself.

1903.   Lange, Helene. ["University Training Women"]. In:
        [Times of Struggle: Essays and Speeches of Four Dec-
        ades], 2 vol., Berlin, Germany, 1900. (Ger)
        Discussing the situation of women in university studies, the
        author emphasizes the situation of women medical students.
        She extensively quotes university professors who were very
        satisfied with their female students despite the strong pre-
        judice against women physicians prevalent during that peri-
        od. [This article was also published in Die Frau in 1897.]

1904.   Lange, Helene and Baumer, Gertrud. [Manual of the Wo-
        men's Movement]. 3 vol., Berlin, Germany, 1901.
        (Ger)
        This extensive manual on the history and the present situa-
        tion of the women's movement contains a series of articles
        on the state of women in universities. These articles in-

clude short but detailed accounts of the situation of women
in medical faculties in different European countries. The
structure of medical education is emphasized and the authors
discuss whether or not women are trained the same way and
in the same facilities as men. In some cases, statistics
are given.

1905.   Lion-Meitner, Gisela. ["Leopold von Schroetter and Women
            in Higher Education"]. Wiener Medizinische Wochen-
            schrift, 87:6 (1937) 163-164. (Ger)
        In commemoration of Professor Schroetter's 100th birthday,
        the author, one of his former students, expresses her ap-
        preciation of his unprejudiced assistance to female medical
        students in Vienna in the late 19th century. She emphasizes
        his objective assessment of women physicians and praises
        his defense of female studies and better education for women
        in general in a time when women's studies were a highly
        controversial issue.

1906.   "Note to the Article on 'Women Physicians.'" Macmillan's
            Magazine, 18:108 (October 1868) 528.
        The article which appeared in the September issue of Mac-
        millan's Magazine [Vol. 18, 1868] stated that Zurich was the
        only place where women had access to a complete medical
        education and university degree. This "note" announces that
        the same facilities will also be granted in Paris. Follow-
        ing a description of the educational opportunities is the warn-
        ing that because "no attempt has been made to adapt either
        the education or the examinations to the peculiarities of the
        female mind," females should be prepared for "severe" ex-
        amination.

1907.   "Progress of the Medical Education of Women in Europe."
            Medical and Surgical Reporter, 14 (1881) 550. (Edi-
            torial.)
        [Article not examined by editors.]

1908.   ["Report by Karolinska Institute Collegium of Teachers on
            Medical Instruction for Women"]. Hygeia, 31 (1869)
            476-479. (Swe)
        In response to a letter from His Royal Majesty, the chan-
        cellor, after hearings, determined that before the medical
        schools could be opened to women, those responsible for
        regulations on admission would have to establish the require-
        ments and conditions for their instruction. He therefore
        transmitted the letter to the Collegium of Instructors of the
        Karolinska Institute. They begin by assuming that women
        might be supposed to have no special aptitude except in the
        fields of obstetrics, pediatrics, and gynecology. However,
        they are opposed to the creation of restricted fields of prac-
        tice, which has been tried with regret in other countries.
        They point out that women would have the same responsibil-
        ities as men not only to be familiar with the special branches

but also with medicine in general. The issuance of death
certificates or employment certificates involves legal medicine for which the women would have to take the medico-
philosophical examination. In addition, the women would
need the same premedical preparation in the humanities,
natural science, etc. as do men. The full training of women would indubitably require changes in the course of
studies and special arrangements and would also increase
the number of students. The Institute is already in need of
additional space. The facilities are presently not available
for admission of women to the various courses. They would
need a separate location for anatomical dissection, for which
space is lacking. The obstetric clinic has room for only
eight or at most 12, but there is no extra room in the delivery room.

1909.   Sandelin, Ellen. ["A Few Words on the Position of the Fe-
         male Doctor in Sweden"]. Dagny. Tidskrift För Sociala
         Och Litterära Intressen, 4 (1901) 161-169. (Swe)
         This article presents discussion and comments on Carl
         Johan Svensen's motion in the peasants' estate No. 313 in
         the National Diet 1865-66, that "Swedish women like men
         must be entitled to be examined publicly at the national uni-
         versities not only for the complete matriculation examina-
         tion, but also for receiving the degrees of doctor of philoso-
         phy and medicine. Sandelin believes that the time has now
         arrived for women doctors to acquire general practice,
         since "the same examinations should give equal access to
         all positions where no principle forbids it" (i.e., commis-
         sion). [Swedish abstract provided to the editors by Märtha
         Elvers-Hulth, retired librarian of the National Swedish Board
         of Health and Welfare Library.]

1910.   Shaver, Phillip; French, John R. P., Jr.; and Cobb, Sid-
         ney. "Birth Order of Medical Students and the Occu-
         pational Ambitions of Their Parents." International
         Journal of Psychology, 5:3 (1970) 197-207. tables.
         In order to extend and report a cross-cultural replication of
         a study by Cobb and French (1966) to determine connections
         between parental job aspiration, birth order, and motivation
         of children to become doctors, this study was conducted
         with students in Gothenburg, Sweden. The study is an at-
         tempt to identify some of the intervening processes that ac-
         count for an overrepresentation of firstborns in high achieve-
         ment groups (including medical students). Sweden was se-
         lected because the proportion of female medical students is
         higher there than in the United States and because while
         there has been speculation about the effects of primogeni-
         ture on the birth order-achievement relationship, there had
         not yet apparently been an investigation. Approximately 50
         per cent of the students contacted (112 females and 183
         males) returned the questionnaire sent to them in the winter
         of 1967. The questions concerned parents' ages, occupations,

incomes, educational histories, and marital status, as well as relevant family structure (e. g. , number of brothers and sisters and their birth order). The findings show that first-borns were overrepresented among Swedish medical students, a finding all the more marked among daughters, and especially so for daughters in families with three children; a high proportion of students were the first children of fathers with frustrated professional ambition (high education but low in occupation status). Males seemed to be unaffected by their mothers' aspirations, while females registered a negligible trend of being so influenced. The authors suggest that more information of the intervening process would be known by interviewing parents directly and by studying firstborns as children in their interactions with their parents.

1911.   Stieda, Ludwig. ["A Comment on the Admission of Women to Medical Studies"]. Wiener Medizinische Wochenschrift, 16 (1903) 765-769. (Ger)
As a teacher in a medical school, the author explains his decision to exclude women from attending his lectures--an option faculty members had been given with regard to female students. He argues in particular that because sexually related topics could not be taught in the presence of women, male students would receive an inferior education if male and female students were taught in the same medical schools. The author favors the formation of separate medical schools for women based on the example of the St. Petersburg School of Medicine for Women. He suggests that women should be treated the same as men in their studies.

1912.   Swiss Association of University Women, ed. [Women in Swiss Universities]. Rascher & Cie., Zurich, Switzerland, 1928, 316 pp. figs., tables. (Ger, Fre)
This book contains a collection of articles by different authors, each dealing with the early stages of female students' admissions to Swiss universities. The universities described are: Zurich, Berne, Geneva, Lausanne, Basel, Neufchatel, Fribourg, and St. Galles. Each article contains extensive material on female medical students, who constituted the majority of female students in the early days of women's admission. The articles are in German or French depending on the official language of the university. Most articles are accompanied by tables or diagrams. All have a bibliography.

1913.   ["Women in Medical Sciences in Austria"]. Liecnicki Viestnik, 22:10 (1900) 371. (Ser)
By a decree of the minister of education, issued in Austria on 3 September 1900 (which included remarks of the dean of the medical faculty and the council of medical teachers), women are allowed admission to the doctorate in medical sciences and to the practice of pharmacy after they have fulfilled the conditions of being 18 years of age and taking the

prescribed preliminary courses and the usual examinations. They can then become ordinary students. If the women should succeed in finishing the courses and becoming doctors, it is possible they might become assistants to the teachers and even become teachers or professors. In such an event, their marriages would raise many questions, both practical and legal.

1914.   "Women Medical Students in Paris." Woman's Medical
        Journal, 6:7 (July 1897) 239.
        M. Charles Richet, France's most distinguished medical sci-
        entist, is quoted on the success of women as medical stu-
        dents. Words of praise include special mention of Russian
        Jewesses. He favorably compares women with men students
        but concludes, "It is early yet to say whether they will ever
        rival men in experimental and scientific medicine."

GREAT BRITAIN

1915.   Aird, L. A. and Silver, P. H. S. "Women Doctors from
        the Middlesex Hospital Medical School (University of Lon-
        don) 1947-67." British Journal of Medical Education,
        5:3 (September 1971) 232-241. figs., tables.
        Statistical data are given on women medical students at the
        Middlesex Hospital Medical School, an "exclusively male pre-
        serve" prior to 1947. Data given in areas of ability, at-
        trition, performance, and professional and non-professional
        activity were collected by examining published information
        on professional examinations and school prizes as well as
        circulating a questionnaire to all women who had qualified
        at the Middlesex. A bibliography of papers surveying wo-
        men medical students in other British medical schools con-
        cludes the article.

1916.   Beveridge, W. H. "Medical Co-Education." Medical Wo-
        men's Federation News-Letter, (March 1929) 38-47.
        tables.
        This article consists in the Report of the University of Lon-
        don on the Medical Education of Women Undergraduates.
        The curriculum of the school as well as the training hos-
        pitals' attitudes towards admitting women practitioners is
        stated. Tables represent the number of men and women in
        medicine in Great Britain and in London over the past ten
        years (and portions thereof). "The real issue is as to the
        maintenance in London on a substantial scale of facilities
        for medical co-education at the clinical stage." Arguments
        for and against medical coeducation in London are presented.
        In conclusion, while the University is in favor of medical
        coeducation, such coeducation, "... if it is to succeed, must
        be voluntary."

1917.   Buxton, R. St. J. "Medical Students Leaving Before Quali-

fication." Britain Journal of Medical Education, 7:3
(September 1973) 155-156. tables.
A study of medical students at the University of Bristol
from 1968 to 1972 showed that of 483 admitted, there were
58 withdrawals (12 per cent). Of the withdrawals (43 males
and 15 females), 39 (8 per cent) of those admitted left because of academic failure. Sex difference was found not to
be statistically significant.

1918. Drysdale, C. R. "Notes on Female Medical Education in
Ordinary Medical Schools." Medical Press and Circ.
(London), 15 (1873) 548-550.
[Article not examined by editors.]

1919. "English Women Attacked in Newspapers." Bulletin of the
Medical Women's National Association, 15 (January
1927) 10.
This article responds to an article that appeared in the American Medical Association Journal of October 30, [1926] titled,
"Fewer Women Medical Students." In fact, there are more
women entering medicine than ever before, and women physicians work hard once they earn their degrees. Impressive
indeed are the contributions [British] women physicians have
made in London and especially in India.

1920. "The Exclusion of Women Students from Medical Schools."
Medical Woman's Journal, 35:5 (May 1928) 140.
This article offers a brief comment on, and a reprint of,
a notice published in the April 21 issue of the Journal of
the AMA, which examines the trend to ban women students
from medical schools and hospitals in London, England.

1921. Forster, Emily L. B. How to Become a Woman Doctor.
Charles Griffin & Company, Ltd., London, England,
1918, xii, 138 pp.
This book is designed for the use of "girls desirous of training for the profession of Medicine and Surgery," headmis-
tresses of schools, and teachers who advise girls as to
courses of study. The book is divided into numerous short
sections which treat the history of the woman doctor: how
to enter the medical profession in the United Kingdom (i.e.,
required courses, examinations, considerations as to type
and place of study desired, expenses); the choice of a medical school; coeducation; and the making of a woman doctor.
One section is entitled "A Day in the Life of a Woman House
Physician (Charing Cross Hospital)."

1922. General Council of Medical Education and Registration (Great
Britain). Special Education for Women. Resolutions
and Report on the Education of Women in Midwifery,
Management of Medical Institutions, Dispensing Medi-
cines, and Nursing. W. J. & S. Goldbourn, London,
England, 1873, 33 pp.

Within this report, the Committee--appointed by the General
Medical Council to consider the education of women in selected branches of medicine--emphasizes that they do not
enter into the question of whether women should have special
education for "ordinary medical or surgical practice." The
case before the Council now is quite different from complete
medical education; rather, they are deciding how to respond
to a need for the "services for which women are specially
adapted."

1923.   "Increasing Demand for Women Physicians." Medical Wo-
               man's Journal, 41:11 (November 1934) 303-304. (Edi-
               torial.)
         In Great Britain during 1931-1932, the total number of den-
         tal and medical women students enrolled in medical schools
         was 1,272 (males numbered 9,107). "This indicates an un-
         usually large percentage of women medical students in coedu-
         cational schools outside of London, while the only school
         open to them in London is the London School of Medicine
         (which is confined to them)...." More than 5,000 women
         are listed on the country's medical register.

1924.   Jefferys, Margot; Gauvain, Suzette; and Gulesen, Ozdemir.
               "Comparison of Men and Women in Medical Training."
               Lancet, 1 (26 June 1965) 1381-1383. tables.
         A survey was taken of medical school deans in the United
         Kingdom and Scotland to ascertain how men and women med-
         ical students compared in a number of areas. The data
         were collected for the 1963-1964 academic year and revealed
         that although mean data, for the 24 schools who were able
         to provide application data, would indicate that women who
         applied had only slightly less chance than men of being ac-
         cepted (6.4 per cent men accepted to 4.6 per cent women),
         the proportionate acceptance of men to women at individual
         schools varied sharply. There was no statistically signifi-
         cant difference in the proportion of men and women who
         withdrew before qualifying in either the premedical and pre-
         clinical years or in the clinical years, although more men
         dropped out during the former period, more women during
         the latter. The most common reason for withdrawal for
         both sexes combined was "unsuitability": a higher propor-
         tion of men withdrew for reasons of failure in examination,
         and a higher proportion of women for health reasons. Only
         four out of 2755 women who began the year's medical work
         left for reasons of marriage or children. The results of
         the first and second MB examinations showed women to be
         more successful than men (although the difference was not
         statistically significant).

1925.   Jex-Blake, Sophia. "The Medical Education of Women in
               Great Britain and Ireland." Women's Medical Journal,
               1:6 (June 1893) 105-110.
         In this report, presented before a women's conference in

Chicago, Dr. Jex-Blake reviews the battles at the Universities of Edinburgh and London for women's admittance to medical studies, and more generally, medical women's victories in Ireland, England, and Scotland. Appended to her speech is a list of the schools and examining boards open to women of the British Isles.

1926.   Little, Ernest Gordon Graham. "Undergraduate Medical
        Education of Women in London." Nineteenth Century,
        102 (May 1928) 665-677. table.
        Universities are closing their doors to women medical undergraduate students. The motives seem to lie in the belief that schools admitting women would lose men students. The author examines the situation thoroughly.

1927.   "London Letter. Women in the Medical Schools." Woman's
        Medical Journal, 26:11 (November 1916) 268.
        The physician shortage due to [World War I] caused an influx of women into the medical profession. Prior to the war, women physicians were not admitted to most London hospitals. St. George's Hospital, however, admitted a strictly limited number of women. In case the war ended before these students were qualified, they would be allowed to continue their studies until qualification. A discussion of policies for admitting women to hospitals and medical schools in Great Britain follows.

1928.   "Medical Education of Women." British Medical Journal, 2
        (3 September 1921) 371.
        Listed are the examining bodies and medical schools in Great Britain which admit women.

1929.   "Medical Education of Women." British Medical Journal,
        2 (2 September 1922) 439-440.
        Listed for England, Ireland, and Scotland are the qualifying bodies admitting women to medical examinations and the medical schools accepting women. Due to the increased number of women students and the keen competition for medical posts, women physicians should consider the large field opening in India. The British Medical Association receives praise for its cooperation with the Federation of Medical Women and its efforts to eradicate sex distinction within the profession.

1930.   "Medical Women." Medical Times and Gazette, 1 (31
        March 1877) 338-339.
        All "extraneous obstacles" to the entrance of women into the medical profession have been overcome. Parliament has ruled that any medical licensing body may admit candidates for its degrees or licenses without regard to sex. And the London School of Medicine for Women has at last found a hospital which will furnish females with necessary practical instruction. While the perseverance of medical women de-

serves admiration, "we cannot honestly congratulate the women in their victory." For the great majority of women
physicians, "only disappointment and failure await them."
This experiment is "a pitiable mistake" that will end in
wasted years and energy.

1931.   "Medical Women and the Government Medical Bill." Med-
              ical Times and Gazette, 1 (11 May 1878) 507-509.
         This article restates an article by Elizabeth Garrett-Ander-
         son which appeared in the London Times. Garrett-Ander-
         son's article "utterly and mercilessly condemned" both the
         Duke of Richmond and Gordon's bill and the amendments to
         the bill decided on by the General Medical Council. She
         calls the bill "'a mere mockery of what is wanted, both as
         to uniformity of standards [throughout the United Kingdom]
         and as to the admission of women.'" Garrett-Anderson's
         specific objections are detailed and commented upon in this
         article.

1932.   "Medical Women; or, Qualified Female Medical Practition-
              ers." Leisure Hour, 19 (1 November 1870) 709-712.
         Following a definition of the "qualified medical practitioner,"
         this article reviews the struggle of women to obtain the
         necessary education to become physicians. Particularly ex-
         tensive is an account of the situation at the University of
         Edinburgh, complete with the examination marks won by wo-
         men in various medical courses. Concluding remarks af-
         firm the need for medical women--particularly for adminis-
         tering to women--and states that women's medical training
         should now become "simply a matter of detail."

1933.   Ministry of Health, Department of Health for Scotland, Inter-
              Departmental Committee on Medical Schools. Report of
              Inter-Departmental Committee on Medical Schools. His
              Majesty's Stationery Office, London, England, 1944,
              313 pp. tables.
         Appointed in March 1942, this committee of the Ministry of
         Health surveyed the medical schools in Great Britain, pre-
         sented their findings, and made recommendations on the
         status of medical education in Britain. This report [famili-
         arly known as the Goodenough Report] discusses women stu-
         dents in Chapter 5, pages 97-100. Under this section the
         following recommendations are made: coeducation should be-
         come the practice in every medical school in Great Britain,
         government funds to medical schools should be conditional
         upon the school being coeducational and admitting a reason-
         able proportion of women students, and all hospital appoint-
         ments for qualified practitioners should be filled by open
         competition without restrictions as to sex.

1934.   "Mixed Clinical Classes." Woman's Medical Journal, 5:11
              (November 1896) 301-302.
         In this article (apparently reprinted from Medical Press),

the announcement that "Mr. Jonathan Hutchinson has been compelled to exclude ladies from his popular clinical afternoons" is reported. The reason: "the modesty of the British workman."

1935.   Morton, Jane. "Women Doctors." New Society, 27 (28 February 1974) 517.
Without statutory sanctions, the memorandum of the Committee of Vice-Chancellors and Principals to the government on the equal opportunity of women entrants to medical school will be ineffective. According to the latest statistics available to the author, such universities as Cambridge and Wales (where five men to every woman were accepted) were still well below equal acceptance policies.

1936.   "The Scottish Universities Commission." Lancet, 1 (19 March 1892) 661.
Ordinance 18 issued by the Commission provides regulations for the graduation and instruction of women in medicine. Part of the ordinance states that "no professor whose commission is dated before the approval of the Ordinance by Her Majesty shall be required, without his consent, to conduct classes to which women are admitted."

1937.   Smith, B. "The School Education of Girl Candidates for the Profession of Medicine." Edinburgh Medical Journal, 21 (1918) 160-165.
[Article not examined by editors.]

1938.   Tait, L. "The Medical Education of Women." Birmingham Medical Review, 3 (1874) 81-94.
[Article not examined by editors.]

1939.   "Women in British Medical Schools." School and Society, 4:98 (11 November 1916) 741-742.
The wartime physician shortage caused an influx of women medical students. Several London hospitals and schools subsequently relaxed previous regulations concerning the acceptance of women.

INTERNATIONAL

1940.   Jäderholm, Axel. ["The Woman As Doctor"]. Nordiskt Medicinskt Arkiv., 3:20 (1871) 1-30. (Swe)
At the request of the editors and in connection with a royal letter of the preceding year, the author reviews recent progress in the rights of women to medical education and practice in Sweden and the status of the problem in other countries. The first half of the article consists mainly of extensive quotations from public documents from the preceding decade and from the royal decree of 1870. The latter affirms the right of women to pursue a medical career under

conditions previously set forth, and to take the school-leaving examinations and the college entrance examination in
medicine and philosophy. For the first time it opens the
medical faculty of the Karolinska Institute to women, and
instructs the Institute to provide facilities for separate instruction in anatomy for women medical students and to
make such other changes as are found necessary to permit
the women to receive instruction along with male students
in other subjects. The second half of the article is a review of the status of medical education for women in North
America and the European countries, from the United States
with its women's medical colleges to Austria, which at that
time did not recognize even foreign degrees. There is also
a discussion of European opinion on the subject and of the
implications for Sweden of the opening of the Karolinska to
women. Several women healers and physicians, both historical and contemporary, are mentioned.

1941. "Outlook for Oriental Women." Medical Woman's Journal,
          37:3 (March 1930) 78.
       Oriental women may surpass their Western sisters in educa-
       tional opportunities. Missionary medical colleges have made
       possible the training of nationals in such countries as those
       of Latin America, Mexico, China, India, and Japan. These
       women may then hold positions of leadership in their own
       countries.

1942. "Progress of the Medical Education of Women in Europe."
          Medical and Surgical Reporter, 45 (12 November 1881)
          550-551. (Editorial.)

1943. Rosenfeld, Siegfried. ["Medical Studies for Women in the
          Present: Part I. History"]. Wiener Medizinische Blät-
          ter, 19:1 (2 January 1896) 6-9. (Ger)
       This, the first part of a series of articles, presents a brief
       historical review up to the late 19th century and then de-
       scribes the recent developments and present status in indi-
       vidual countries. Switzerland was popular with Russian wo-
       men, first at Zurich and then at Berne after Zurich was
       closed to them by imperial decree. Between 1864 and 1892
       Zurich had 344 female medical students and Geneva 175,
       mostly foreigners. Russia had courses for women from
       1872-1882; they were to be reopened in 1897. Russian wo-
       men doctors are highly regarded by their male colleagues
       and are practicing in all parts of European and Asiatic
       Russia. England had one of the first medical schools for
       women, in London; 73 women graduated between 1889 and
       1893, and 32 from schools in Ireland and Scotland. In
       France, the University of Paris has been open to women
       since 1868, but most of the women students there and at
       Montpelier have been foreigners. In 1885 there were 14
       women practicing in Paris. Italy has admitted women to
       medical schools since 1876 and has women practicing in

most of the large cities; this includes one professor, at
Pisa. In Scandinavia, women have their own medical school
at Gothenburg, and the other schools are open to them.
Only Germany and Austria of the European countries do not
accept women, and Germany will probably do so in the near
future. The U.S. has admitted women since 1850, and in
1890 had 4555 practicing women physicians.

SOUTH, CENTRAL, LATIN AMERICA AND MEXICO

1944. Aguirre de Gonzales, Amelia. "The Paraguayan Medical
Woman." Journal of the American Medical Women's
Association, 11:10 (October 1956) 356.
A summary of a paper presented during a symposium on
"Women as Medical Students and Physicians in the Countries
of the Americas." In Paraguay "women and men have an
equal opportunity to study medicine": 17.31 per cent of
registrants at the School of Medicine were women. Women
physicians also have the same employment opportunities as
male physicians. Women who drop out of the medical
course do so mainly for economic reasons.

1945. Pelaez de Alvarez, Pola. "Educating Women in Medicine
in Chile." Journal of the American Medical Women's
Association, 11:10 (October 1956) 361.
Women were not admitted to the universities of Chile until
the end of the 19th century. In a thesis by Dr. Mariano
Requena of the University of Chile, it is reported that between 1932 and 1952, 816.8 men (vs. 183.2 women) were
admitted to the first year of medicine. During that period,
71.7 per cent of the total number of students admitted graduated (92.6 per cent were women, while only 70.3 per cent
were men). Women do not exclusively turn down positions
in rural areas, but do turn down geographically isolated, un-
attractive positions on the par with male physicians' rejec-
tions of such posts.

UNITED STATES

1946. AAMC Division of Student Affairs, Office of Student Records.
"U.S. Medical Student Enrollments, 1968-1969 Through
1971-1972." Journal of Medical Education, 47:2 (February 1972) 150-153. figs., tables. (Datagram.)
Women medical students comprised 1,673 (13.5 per cent) of
the 1971 freshman class, a 33.2 per cent increase over
1970. Minority-group women are responsible for high percentages within their own groups: American Indian women--
8 (36 per cent); American black women--200 (23 per cent);
American Oriental women--43 (20 per cent); non-U.S. women
--31 (17 per cent); Mexican American women--10 (12 per
cent).

1947.   "As a Matter of Record."   Medical Woman's Journal, 51:
            11 (November 1944) 34.
         An article originally published in Intern (the journal of the
         Association of Internes and Medical Students) pleads for
         government assistance to women medical students.

1948.   Beyer, M. Virginia. "Annual Opportunities Report." Med-
            ical Woman's Journal, 51:5 (May 1944) 36. (Editorial.)
         Dr. Beyer, chairman of the American Medical Women's
         Association's opportunities for medical women committee,
         reports that seven of the 86 U.S. and Canadian medical
         schools do not admit women students. Updated information
         is also provided on the Army Specialized Training Program
         (ASTP), a government plan for financing medical students.
         Due to recent changes, only enlisted men are eligible for
         the ASTP.

1949.   Blackwell, Elizabeth and Blackwell, Emily. Address on
            the Medical Education of Women. Baptist and Taylor,
            New York, New York, 1864.
         [Item not examined by editors.]

1950.   Boucot, Katharine R. "Special Problems of Women Medical
            Students." Canadian Medical Association Journal, 86:
            14 (7 April 1962) 614-617. tables.
         The author (a professor at Woman's Medical College of
         Pennsylvania) identifies the psychological, sociological, fi-
         nancial, and physical problems of women medical students.
         Mentioned are: the female conditioning that makes them
         emphasize details and have difficulty grasping broad implica-
         tions; a tendency to be hypersensitive; interference in study
         from marriage and pregnancy; and a "residual antagonism"
         towards medical women. Accompanying the article are two
         statistical tables concerning women applicants and students
         in U.S. and Canadian medical schools.

1951.   Bowen, Earl A. "The Female Family Practitioner." New
            England Journal of Medicine, 285:17 (21 October 1971)
            973. (Letter to the Editor.)
         "The U.S. Government [should] establish federal medical
         schools 'for women only' adjacent to large urban general
         hospitals ...," then women doctors, this male doctor writes,
         can become general practitioners and make initial diagnoses;
         that way only those patients who need intensive care will be
         admitted to the hospital and, by implication, to the male
         doctor specialists who have not wanted to do general prac-
         tice for quite a while.

1952.   Bowers, John Z. "Special Problems of Women Medical Stu-
            dents." Journal of Medical Education, 43:5 (May 1968)
            532-537. (Presentation, 78th Annual Meeting, Associa-
            tion of American Medical Colleges, New York, Octo-
            ber 28, 1967.)

Special problems of women in medicine include the "'anti-medical'" counseling given to women in college, "'secret'" quotas for the number of women admitted to medical school, the hostile environment in which women must pursue their medical education, the extremes of behavior women medical students are forced into (i.e., "masculine rules" or "super-femininity") in their search for identity in the male world of a medical school, problems of marriage and pregnancy, and the inflexible requirements of American boards. The "unique situation" of the Negro woman is discussed also. The utilization of women in medicine can be improved through programs designed to help women reenter the medical field, programs to provide child care for women in medicine, the assurance of greater opportunities for the women medical school graduate, and programs to subsidize women to stay in training or to return to medicine.

1953.   Bundy, Elizabeth R. "Introductory Address." Medical and Surgical Reporter (10 October 1896). (Opening exercises, Woman's Medical College, Philadelphia, Pennsylvania, 30 September 1896.)
Dr. Bundy, professor of anatomy at Woman's Medical College, draws an analogy between the student's preparation for a medical career and the soldier's preparation for war. She offers advice in tackling medical studies, emphasizing the importance of a thorough knowledge of anatomy, physiology, and chemistry. Students are warned against ignoring their personal health. Concluding remarks allude to the rewards of being a physician and of developing "unity in spirit and work."

1954.   C. B. "Public Demands and the Medical Education of Women." Nation, 50:1290 (20 March 1890) 237-238.
The current position of women in medical education offers an example of "social congestion." While the public supports employment of women physicians, especially in women's prisons and hospitals, the public has not offered women the proper academic preparation. Women must have the right to appointments in hospitals and admission to the best university medical departments. Endowments offer one hope of forcing schools to admit female students.

1955.   Campbell, Margaret A. Why Would a Girl Go Into Medicine? Medical Education in the United States: A Guide for Women. Published by the author, New York, New York, 1973, 113 pp. tables.
"This document has been assembled to assist women in selecting and surviving a medical school education." Predicated on the fact that "all medical schools exhibit some degree of discrimination against women students," this study specifically seeks to examine the discrimination and concomitant "coping, change, and concern for the health care of women." The document "is intended to encourage." In-

formation reported in the study was collected from women
medical students and from "case study" data from medical
schools via an exploratory questionnaire, between February
and September of 1973. Seventy-six questionnaires were
returned from 146 women students at 41 medical schools.
The major forms of discrimination considered are institutional discrimination, overt discrimination, and subtle discrimination. In addition, the author discusses stereotyping
of women medical students and the "'men's club' atmosphere
of medical school." Coping mechanisms are also covered,
as are constructive support, working for changes, and the
need for unity among women. [An edition of this book was
also published by the Feminist Press.]

1956.   Chapman, John E. "A Common Denominator in the Equa-
             tion toward a Medical Education." Journal of the Amer-
             ican Medical Women's Association, 24:7 (July 1969) 561-
             565. (Presentation, Josiah Macy, Jr. Foundation Con-
             ference, "The Future of Women in Medicine," Williams-
             burg, Va., 8-11 December 1968.)
Medical schools are going to have to broaden their means
of financial support, and the federal government is the only
organization able to support such expensive operations. The
Health Professions Act of 1963 made loans and some limited
scholarships available to not only medical students but also
other medically-related specialists. Women medical students
are discriminated against in a variety of financial ways:
families tend to give less support to a daughter than to a
son; a woman bringing a debt from an expensive medical
education is less attractive on the marriage market than one
bringing a dowry; living facilities and other paraeducational-
related conditions have not been accessible to women; traditional scholarship support is more available to men than to
women; women incur special expenses "to retain their feminine role"; a man may be supported by a working wife and
still assume access to financial aid, a woman, on the other
hand may not qualify for financial aid for herself, no less
if she's married; childbearing can increase the time a woman spends in school thereby making school more expensive;
women who attend medical school and who still want "to retain their femininity," are "less members of the class" and
have "less accessibility to class resources." If medical
schools intend to accept minority students like women, they
should plan on additional space and more students.

1957.   "Co-Education in Medical Colleges." Woman's Medical Jour-
             nal, 11:1 (January 1901) 13-14. (Editorial.)
The question of the appropriateness of coeducation will be
decided in the near future. If it is found right and proper,
however, coeducation should extend to faculty appointments
also.

1958.   "Co-Education in Medical Study: Editorial in American

Medicine (Selected)." <u>Woman's Medical Journal</u>, 12:
3 (March 1902) 54.

1959. Crawford, Susan A.; Crowley, Anne E.; Egan, Richard L.;
Hillis, William C.; Leymaster, Glen R.; Mason, Henry
R.; Petersen, Edward S.; and Uzemack, Edward A.
"Undergraduate Medical Education." <u>Journal of the</u>
<u>American Medical Association Supplement</u>, 231 (January
1975) 6-33. figs., tables.
Under the section of this article on medical students, statistics are given for the number of women applicants, admissions, and graduates of U.S. medical schools from 1939-
1974. The attrition rate for women and men for 1971-1972,
1972-1973, and 1973-1974 shows what appears to be a re-
versal in 1973-1974 from previous years: in 1973-1974,
1.4 per cent of the women students dropped out as compared
to 1.7 per cent of the men.

1960. Crowley, Anne E., ed. <u>Medical Education in the United</u>
<u>States: 1973-1974</u>. 74th Annual Report. American
Medical Association, Chicago, Illinois, 1975, 139 pp.
charts, tables. (Annual supplement to the <u>Journal of</u>
<u>the American Medical Association</u>.)
The first report on medical education in the United States
was published on 21 September 1901 in the <u>Journal of the</u>
<u>American Medical Association</u> (<u>JAMA</u>). This annual report
came to be known as the "Education Number" of <u>JAMA</u>.
This year, because of the scope and complexity of the subject, the "Education Number" was published as a Supplement to <u>JAMA</u>. [A bound, five-volume set of all "Education
Numbers" is available. We have cited in this bibliography
only the most recent annual report. Previous annual reports
contain similar information for their respective years, and
beginning in 1910, the data on medical schools was broken
down by sex. This supplement consists in a number of
articles on medical education by various contributors. These
articles (one by Susan A. Crawford, et al., and one by
Leonard D. Fenninger, et al.) are listed in this bibliography
under the names of the respective authors.] In addition to
the individual articles on medical education, statistical data
on medical schools in the U.S. and Canada are given in two
concluding appendixes. U.S. and Canadian medical school
enrollment by sex (and by school) is given for 1973-1974.

1961. "The Deplorable London Situation." <u>Medical Woman's Jour-</u>
<u>nal</u>, 35:10 (October 1928) 290.
This article's title refers to the British woman's struggle
to maintain the co-educational privileges in medical schools
that they enjoyed during the world war, and compares that
conflict with the situation of colleagues in the United States.

1962. Dubé, W. F. "Applicants for the 1973-74 Medical School
Entering Class." <u>Journal of Medical Education</u>, 49:11

(November 1974) 1070-1072. tables. (Datagram.)
Women accounted for approximately 18 per cent of all applicants and about 20 per cent of all 1973 acceptances to
U.S. medical schools. The acceptance rate for women exceeded that of men (39 per cent vs. 34 per cent). This
article compares, in narrative form and statistical tables,
application activity from 1969-70 through 1973-74.

1963.   Dubé, W. F. "Applicants for the 1974-75 First-Year Med-
             ical School Class." Journal of Medical Education, 50
             (December 1975) 1134-1136. tables. (Datagram.)
         For both men and women, slightly lower acceptance rates
         were recorded for 1974-75 than for the previous year: 38.9
         per cent for women (39.5 in 1973-74) and 34.4 per cent for
         men (34.5 in 1973-74). Women obtained 23 per cent of all
         acceptances--a slight increase from the comparable per-
         centage of 20 in 1973-74 and "a spectacular doubling of the
         11 per cent of all acceptances for women in 1970-71." One
         of the tables included in this article provides statistics on
         women applicants and first-year women students from 1970-
         71 through 1974-75.

1964.   Dubé, W. F. "Undergraduate Origins of U.S. Medical Stu-
             dents." Journal of Medical Education, 49:10 (October
             1974) 1005-1010. tables. (Datagram.)
         Tables list the 100 undergraduate institutions providing the
         largest number of first-year U.S. medical students for
         1973-74. The figures are broken down by sex.

1965.   Dubé, W. F. "U.S. Medical School Enrollment, 1969-70
             Through 1973-74." Journal of Medical Education, 49:
             3 (March 1974) 302-307. fig., tables. (Datagram.)
         There are 2,786 (19.7 per cent) women in U.S. medical
         school 1973-74 first-year classes. This figure includes
         449 minority women and 41 non-U.S. women [the minority
         enrollment tables are not broken down by sex]. For all
         but three schools, women made up at least ten per cent of
         the entering class, with 42 (of the 114) medical schools re-
         porting 20 per cent or more. This increase (between 1972
         and 1973) is smaller than the gain between 1971 and 1972.

1966.   Dubé, W. F. "U.S. Medical Student Enrollment, 1970-71
             Through 1974-75." Journal of Medical Education, 50:3
             (March 1975) 303-306. tables. (Datagram.)
         "The participation of women in first-year medical classes
         was greater in 1974-1975 than ever before in the history of
         U.S. medical education." Women represented 22 per cent
         (3,275) of all entering classes and 20 per cent of the 1974-
         1975 applicants. Of these 3,275 first-year women, 563
         (17.2 per cent) were minority group members. During 1973,
         the minority-group women represent the following percentages
         with their own groups: American Indian women--24 per cent;
         American black women--34 per cent; Mexican American wo-

men--21 per cent; and mainland Puerto Rican women--29 per cent. All of the 114 medical schools in the U.S. report at least ten per cent first-year enrollment for women. In only 42 schools do women constitute at least 20 per cent of the freshman class.

1967. Dubé, W. F. "Woman Students in U.S. Medical Schools: Past and Present Trends." Journal of Medical Education, 48:2 (February 1973) 186-189. tables. (Datagram.)

The number of women students enrolled in medical schools rose gradually from four per cent in 1914 to nine per cent in 1969 (except for 1949-1950 when medical enrollments were affected by special military training programs as a result of World War II). In 1972-1973, women represented 12.8 per cent of all medical students and 16.8 per cent of the 1972 fall freshman class. In 1964 only 14 medical schools out of 87 enrolled women students as ten per cent or more of their student body. Since 1964, the number of medical schools enrolling ten per cent or more women students gradually increased: 1969-1970, 25 schools out of 101; 1970-1971, 31 schools out of 102; in 1971-1972, 56 schools out of 108; and in 1972-1973, 84 schools out of 114 enrolled ten per cent or more women students.

1968. Dubé, W. F. and Johnson, Davis G. "Study of U.S. Medical School Applicants, 1972-73." Journal of Medical Education, 49:9 (September 1974) 849-869. tables.

Applicant, applications, and enrollment data for the 1972 entering class of 112 U.S. medical schools highlights rises in the number of women applicants, and in women minority students. In 1972, the "largest annual increase in the number of women applicants ever recorded" occurred, when 5,480 women (15.2 per cent of the applicants) competed for first-year places. "Despite the seemingly high accompanying increase in applications over 1971 (14,597 or 60.5 per cent), women filed only 7.1 applications per individual while men applicants filed 7.5 each. Moreover, 43.0 per cent of the women applicants were accepted (compared with 37.2 per cent for men) and thus achieved higher acceptance percentages than men for the fourth consecutive year." One-fourth (24.9 per cent) of the 1,437 minority students in the 1972 class were women.

1969. Dubé, W. F. and Johnson, Davis G. "Study of U.S. Medical School Applicants, 1973-74." Journal of Medical Education, 50:11 (November 1975) 1015-1032. tables.

"This annual study reports applicant, application, and enrollment statistics for the 1973-74 entering class of the 114 U.S. medical schools in comparison with previous years." Women comprised 18 per cent (7,202) of all applicants and 40 per cent (2,726) of all who were accepted. In 1972-73 women had constituted 17 per cent of the entering class, while in 1973-74 women constituted 19.6 per cent (2,726) of the entering class. Women applicants had higher acceptance rates than men in every age category except in the 38-year-and-older age group, where only eight per cent women and men were accepted. "Considering underrepresented minorities only, 381 women were enrolled, an increase of 78 (26 per cent) over 1972. The highest numerical gain (55) was achieved by black women, while the highest percentage gain (150) was recorded for the small number of U.S. mainland Puerto Rican women. Of 114 medical schools, 98 enrolled minority women; but only 25 schools (including Howard and Meharry) reported five or more each."

1970.   Dubé, W. F.; Johnson, Davis G.; and Nelson, Bonnie C. "Study of U.S. Medical School Applicants, 1971-72." Journal of Medical Education, 48:5 (May 1973) 395-420. figs., tables.

Summarizing applicant, application, and enrollment activities of the 1971-72 entering class of all U.S. medical schools, this study contains a section on women applicants. Women represented 12.8 per cent of the total applicant pool, an increase of 36.7 per cent over 1970. In 1971, 45.1 per cent of all women applying received acceptance offers. This study provides historical data, including MCAT scores, for the preceding five years. Tables of related applicant characteristics are also presented.

1971.   Dubé, W. F.; Stritter, Frank T.; and Nelson, Bonnie C. "Study of U.S. Medical School Applicants, 1970-71." Journal of Medical Education, 46:10 (October 1971) 837-857. tables.

In this study, applicant data is arranged chronologically for four decades (1929 to 1959) and for the past five years (1966-1970). Information on women applicants includes the following: Of the 2,734 women applying to medical school in 1970, 1,297 (47.4 per cent) were accepted--11.3 per cent of all acceptances that year.

1972.   Dykman, Roscoe A. and Stalnaker, John M. "The History of the 1949-50 Freshman Class." Journal of Medical Education, 30:11 (November 1955) 611-621. charts, tables.

Based upon the 79 medical schools in operation during 1949-1950, this article is a statistical study of that freshman class to consider the factors believed to be related to regularity in attending medical school. For the purpose of this study, students were categorized as follows: regulars (people who complete their medical training in four years without interruption); irregulars (people who complete their medical education but do so with at least one form of interruption; or who vary their training from the expected sequence); dropouts or withdrawals (those who do not earn degrees). In this study, 86.9 per cent of the students were regulars,

4.6 per cent irregulars, and 8.5 per cent dropouts. Regular students earned better grades than irregular or dropout students, on the average. In the Medical College Admission Test (MCAT), which consists of four sections (verbal, quantitative, understanding modern society, and science), students' scores varied most in the science section, with the regular group scoring higher (as the regular group did in the other areas as well). The MCAT was first introduced in 1948 and has been used to anticipate who the poor students would be and therefore reject ahead of time those people who score low. At the time this survey was made, not every student had taken the exam, but those who had taken this exam were better students than those who had not. By 1955, 95 per cent of the applicants admitted to medical school had taken this test. Residence requirements or other medical school restrictions may lower the correlation between those who get accepted and their scores on the MCATs, with their actual performance in school. Thirteen per cent of the students who were 27 years or older dropped out. Older students earned higher verbal and modern society scores, but their quantitative and science scores were much lower. Exactly 5.6 per cent of the total was female: 13.5 per cent women and 8.2 per cent men withdrew; 81 per cent women and 87 per cent men finished as regulars. Women medical students had slightly lower average grades than men. Women earned higher average verbal scores and lower quantitative scores (which, for women, are not important in predicting medical school grades). It was shown that 58.5 per cent of the freshmen who drop out do so because of failure, while 16.3 per cent do so because of lack of interest. More women than men drop out because of illness, environmental difficulties, accident, and death.

1973.   [No entry]

1974.   "Editorial." Medical Woman's Journal, 51:11 (November 1944) 31.
Reprinted is the text of a resolution submitted to the American Medical Association (AMA) by Dr. Emily Barringer, on behalf of the American Medical Women's Association. The resolution requests the AMA to "go on record as lifting sex discrimination from young women desiring to study medicine" and to "request the government to give aid to these young women ... commensurate with that granted to the young men." The subsequent report, from the AMA Reference Committee on Medical Education, replies in part: "It is the belief ... that there is no large reservoir of qualified premedical women from which schools could select substantially increased numbers of women medical students." The committee recommended that the resolution not be approved.

1975.   "Education of Women Physicians." Medical Woman's Jour-

nal, 51:6 (June 1944) 30, 31. (Editorial.)
This editorial expresses concern for the subsidization of
women medical students by government funds.

1976.   Flexner, Abraham. Medical Education in the United States
            and Canada: A Report to the Carnegie Foundation for
            the Advancement of Teaching. Carnegie Foundation,
            New York, New York, 1910, xvii, 346 pp.
        Chapter twelve of this report consists of two pages (178-
        179) covering the medical education of women. "Woman has
        so apparent a function in certain medical specialties and
        seemingly so assured a place in general medicine under
        some obvious limitations that the struggle for wider educa-
        tional opportunities for the sex was predestined to an early
        success in medicine." The number of coeducational schools
        in the U.S., as well as the total number of women students
        in them and the total number of women graduates from them
        is given for the six-year period, 1904 to 1909. The figures
        are construed by Dr. Flexner to indicate that "now that wo-
        men are freely admitted to the medical profession, it is
        clear that they show a decreasing inclination to enter it."
        Flexner favors spending money on coeducational schools rath-
        er than on the development of separate women's medical col-
        leges, with the condition that intern privileges be granted to
        women graduates on the same terms as to men.

1977.   [Franklin, C. L.] "Women and Medicine." Nation, 52:
            1337 (12 February 1891) 131.
        The decision by Johns Hopkins Medical School to open its
        doors to women--under pressure of a gift of a hundred
        thousand dollars from the women of the country--may be a
        turning point for women physicians. The trustees still hesi-
        tate over undergraduate coeducation, however. This editorial
        wonders whether women have to organize and raise money to
        gain entrance into every university or whether trustees will
        ever take such an action on their own. This article also men-
        tions the medical education of women in Switzerland and other
        countries. A discussion of women's "peculiar adaptedness" to
        medicine quotes Dr. Susan Dimock concerning female sympa-
        thy; she is profiled as having led a professional life that, by its
        example, settled the question of women's intellectual suitabil-
        ity for medical careers.

1978.   Gross, Wendy and Crovitz, Elaine. "A Comparison of Med-
            ical Students' Attitudes Toward Women and Women Med-
            ical Students." Journal of Medical Education, 50 (April
            1975) 392-394. tables.
        The authors enumerate and document the various findings
        that give rise to the idea of discrepancy between women's
        professional and feminine identities. In order to "shed some
        light on [this] discrepancy," the authors have undertaken a
        comparison which comprises this article. The study groups
        consisted of Duke University medical students enrolled in

February 1974. A questionnaire (a modified Personality
Record Form by Jackson) designed to reflect attitudes towards women medical students and towards women was sent
to each student. This questionnaire focused on the eight
factors of aggression, cognitive structure, endurance, desire for social recognition, achievement orientation, nurturance, understanding, and dominance. "The factors were
chosen because they measured masculine and feminine traits
as identified by Broverman." Twenty per cent of the student body responded (26 per cent of the males and 43 per
cent of the females). Results indicated that the student population saw women medical students as exhibiting traits defined as masculine by Broverman (aggression, dominance,
achievement-orientation, and intellectual understanding).
These traits are also those necessary for students to become successful physicians. Because they are opposite
traits to those which define a "feminine identity," however,
a great deal of stress and anxiety may be generated in the
female medical students. The "common bond" between women physicians and women in general revealed by this survey was that of nurturance. It was also shown that "male
and female students do not significantly differ except for
dominance," in their responses: women medical students
perceive themselves as more dominant.

1979. Hannett, Frances. "Report on the Survey of Female Phy-
        sicians Graduating from Medical School between 1925
        and 1940." Journal of the American Medical Women's
        Association, 13:3 (March 1958) 80-85.
The author reviews the Dykman and Stalnaker "Survey of
Women Physicians Graduating from Medical School: 1925-
1950." [This survey appears elsewhere in the GENERAL
classification of this bibliography.] Dr. Hannett submits
that "the question posed by these findings is: should not our
efforts be directed toward interesting women undergraduates
in the career of medicine who are best suited for the rigors
of this type of education and professional life rather than
trying to influence the medical schools to admit more women
in general?"

1980. Helz, Mary K. "Medical Education: AMWA Preceptorship
        Program." Journal of the American Medical Women's
        Association, 15:9 (September 1960) 876. (Reports from
        Committees: Presentation, Annual Meeting, American
        Medical Women's Association, Miami Beach, 10 June
        1960.)
The American Medical Women's Association has been trying
to arrange for practicing physicians to accept medical students for preceptorships. One hundred and forty-six (eight
per cent) of the membership polled responded. Fifty-six of
those answering were willing and able to participate in this
program.

1981.   Helz, Mary K. "Proposed Preceptorship Program of the
        American Medical Women's Association." Journal of
        the American Medical Women's Association, 14:4 (April
        1959) 317-318. (Report from Committee on Medical
        Education: Presentation, 1958 Midyear Meeting, Board
        of Directors, AMWA, Washington, D.C., 14 November
        1959.)
        "(Editor's Note: This report by Dr. Helz is a preliminary
        outline of the preceptorship program of the AMWA, which
        was authorized by action of the Annual Meeting in June,
        1958. Since the matter will be brought up for discussion
        and action at the 1959 Annual Meeting, it has been presented
        in full.)" Preceptorship programs, which are low-cost ex-
        perimental educational programs, have been very successful.
        They provide school administration with improved care and
        students with a working knowledge of business and medical
        procedures that are easier to learn and to understand in
        practice than in the classroom. AMWA is sponsoring a
        preceptorship program. Preceptors will be members of
        AMWA and meet requirements of that organization and of
        the deans of the medical schools. Preceptors will share
        with the preceptees "the peculiar role of the woman physi-
        cian in her professional, civic, community, and home life,
        as well as the social and economic problems imposed be-
        cause of her sex." She will provide maintenance, room,
        board, and laundry. Preceptees will be women medical stu-
        dents who have finished the third year of medical school and
        meet requirements of AMWA and the deans of medical
        schools. Preceptees will pay their own travel expenses and
        will not receive financial reimbursement but will take part
        in all aspects of professional activities under close super-
        vision.

1982.   Hilberman, Elaine; Konanc, Judy; Perez-Reyes, Maria;
        Hunter, Rosemary; Scagnelli, Joan; and Sanders, Shir-
        ley. "Support Groups for Women in Medical School:
        A First-Year Program." Journal of Medical Education,
        50 (September 1975) 867-875. table.
        A model support system for first-year women medical stu-
        dents at the University of North Carolina School of Medicine
        is presented. Under the assumption that women entering
        medical school are "products of traditional sex-role social-
        ization" and that successful medical student behavior "is at
        odds with the usual definitions of femininity," the support
        group was formed to provide a place where students could
        meet in small groups at weekly intervals throughout the aca-
        demic year with women faculty members from the Depart-
        ment of Psychiatry. Factors are identified which either
        help or hinder successful conflict resolutions between pro-
        fessional and female identity. Faculty and student year-end
        assessment is included.

1983.   Howell, Mary C. "Sounding Board: What Medical Schools

Teach About Women." The New England Journal of
Medicine, 291:6 (August 8, 1974) 304-307.
The adoption of approved professional attitudes relating to
patients, colleagues, and one's work, brings the novitiate
into full membership in a profession. In our society, demeaning attitudes toward women are expressed in a variety
of ways which some term "trivial" but which, accumulated,
amass to an aggregate whose message is "that women are
regarded as of little value, and that message is not trivial
for women." Because women (51 per cent of the population)
are involved in so many physician-patient encounters, "medical-school teaching of attitudes about women is of major importance in determining the quality of health-care services
delivered." In addition, these demeaning attitudes have a
direct and personal effect on women medical students. The
article discusses discrimination against women as patients
and women as student physicians, the use of humor as a device in the instillation of attitudes during professionalization,
and the origins of these discriminatory attitudes. The author submits that harmful behaviors can and should be dis-
couraged now, without waiting for attitudes to change. If
appeals to faculty and administrative offices do not effect
the desired change, there is recourse to legal action: Title
IX of the Higher Education Amendments of 1972 forbids discrimination in educational facilities.

1984. Howell, Mary C. "A Women's Health School?" Social
Policy, 6:2 (September/October 1975) 50-53.
Mary Howell outlines her vision of a women's health school
that would train women physicians to give health care in an
atmosphere of mutual support, and reaffirm the values of
service and respect for patients and coworkers alike. Such
health care and training would be more human and more effective for both patients and health care providers.

1985. Hutchins, Edwin B. "The Study of Applicants, 1961-62."
Journal of Medical Education, 38:9 (September 1963)
707-717. tables.
Statistical tables compare data on men and women medical
school applicants for selected years from 1929 to 1961,
MCAT scores for men and women, and applications to U.S.
medical schools in 1961-1962. It is noted that currently
women make up 8.5 per cent of all applicants accepted to
medical school, in contrast to 4.5 per cent 32 years ago.
The actual numbers of women applying doubled from 1940
to 1950, and the number accepted doubled in the last decade.

1986. Jarecky, Roy K.; Johnson, Davis G.; and Mattson, Dale E.
"The Study of Applicants, 1967-68." Journal of Medical
Education, 43:12 (December 1968) 1215-1228. tables.
This study presents and discusses "the current status and
trends of medical school applicant activity," and suggests
"some implications of these data for recruiting and admissions

programs." Information presented in this study was "provided
by medical school officials." Non-comparative statistics
[not broken down by men and women] are presented in the
areas of applications made, applicants accepted, nonmatricu-
lants, MCAT scores (broken down by areas tested) of applicants accepted and those not accepted, and geographic data
on applicants. The only comparative data for men and women are in the areas of number of applicants, number accepted, and percentage accepted for each of the eight years
from 1960 to 1968. These figures reveal the lowest percentage of women physicians (of total) accepted to have occurred in the 1960-61 class (7 per cent), and the highest
percentage in 1967-68 (10.1 per cent). Comparative data
are also presented by name of medical school as to the
number of applicants and the number of new entrants (1967-
68). A final comparative breakdown is done by "state of
residence" for applicants receiving one or more acceptances
and applicants not accepted (for 1967-68).

1987.   Johnson, Davis G. and Hutchins, Edwin B. "Doctor or
        Dropout? A Study of Medical Student Attrition." Jour-
        nal of Medical Education, 41:12 (December 1966) 1097-
        1260. figs., tables.
        This detailed report on attrition in medical schools between
        1949 and 1958 is divided into eight chapters concerning the
        attrition problems, etiology of the dropout, the national at-
        trition picture, the student, school characteristics, student
        and school in interaction, and what can be done; the final
        section is a summary. In "The Student," chapter 4, the
        discussion and statistics are broken down by sex. Figures
        indicate that of all students who entered medical school from
        1949 to 1958, 16 per cent of the females and 8 per cent of
        the males failed to graduate. There were almost 2.5 times
        as many nonacademic dropouts among women as men.
        These statistics represent the only discussion of women med-
        ical students, per se, in the report.

1988.   Johnson, Davis G. and Sedlacek, William E. "Retraining by
        Sex and Race of 1968-1972 U.S. Medical School En-
        trants." Journal of Medical Education, 50 (October
        1975) 925-933. tables.
        This report on a national Association of American Medical
        Colleges (AAMC) study reveals that recent attrition rates
        are only about half that of the 9 per cent reported in the
        last AAMC study of 1949-1958 entrants. "Although the re-
        tention rate for women and for underrepresented minorities
        is still slightly less than that for white males, the gap ap-
        pears to be narrowing." In this report, "underrepresented
        minorities" refers to black Americans, American Indians,
        Mexican Americans, and mainland Puerto Ricans. "Sugges-
        tions for optimum retention include: (a) enlarging the pool of
        minority applicants, (b) improving the techniques of student
        selection, and (c) increasing the flexibility of academic pro-
        grams in the medical schools."

1989.   Kaplan, Harold I. "Half of Us Will Soon Be Women--Phy-
              sicians, That Is." Medical Opinion, 6 (May 1971) 62-
              64. illus.
         Ten years from now women will make up 40 to 50 per cent
         of the medical profession. Dr. Kaplan discusses his involve-
         ment in the training of women physicians and the flexible
         schedule program developed at the New York Medical Col-
         lege, psychiatry department.

1990.   Kaplan, Harold I. "Women Physicians: The More Effec-
              tive Recruitment and Utilization of Their Talents and
              the Resistance to It--The Final Conclusions of a Seven-
              Year Study." The Woman Physician, 25:9 (September
              1970) 561-570.
         Given in this article is a sample of responses by medical
         school administrators to five standardized questions on wo-
         men in medicine. The questions deal with children in re-
         lation to mothers' medical schooling and professional assign-
         ments, special provisions in work schedules of pregnant and
         postpartum medical students, special provisions for children
         of women medical students and physicians, and a fifth ques-
         tion invites explanations for the increasing percentage of wo-
         men doctors. A summary of conclusions is given, based
         upon answers to these questions. Findings reveal that there
         is still prejudice against women in medicine in the United
         States. A list of seven recommendations is included, rang-
         ing from flexible training schedules for women to "financial
         help during periods of need and/or stress such as preg-
         nancy, or the post-partum period when adequate domestic
         mother-surrogate help is needed." [This article also ap-
         pears in the New Physician, (January 1971) 11-19.]

1991.   Keyes, Joseph A.; Wilson, Marjorie P.; and Becker, Jane.
              "The Future of Medical Education: Forecast of the
              Council of Deans." Journal of Medical Education, 50
              (April 1975) 319-327. tables.
         The Delphi approach was used to survey medical school
         deans regarding their perceptions as to the most significant
         changes they see occurring in medical education (and in the
         health care system that would influence medical education)
         over the next 20 years. Among other findings, it was pre-
         dicted that "women will comprise at least 30 per cent of
         medical school enrollment," and "women have a somewhat
         greater than even chance of reaching 24 to 30 per cent
         representation on the faculty and staff."

1992.   Lambson, Roger O. "Medical School Admissions: A
              Glimpse at the Future by Looking Back." Journal of
              Medical Education, 50:9 (September 1975) 912-915. fig.,
              table. (Datagram.)
         In 1929 women comprised only 3.5 per cent of the total ap-
         plicants to medical school, and 4.5 per cent of entering
         freshmen. In 1974 women comprised 20.4 per cent of all
         applicants and 22.2 per cent of first-year medical students.

1993.   Leymaster, Glen R. "An Answer: A National Center for
         Medical Education for Women--Forecast or Fantasy?"
         Journal of the American Medical Women's Association,
         20:4 (April 1965) 346-348.
         The battle for acceptance of women into medical schools
         being won, the author suggests women "regroup" to attack
         the problem of the physician shortage: "Since there seems
         to be no limit to the needs of our society for the gifted,
         and the best are in demand in every field in medicine, it
         is unlikely that enough men are going to be available to
         meet all the needs." Greater flexibility of schedules, both
         in medical school and in postgraduate and professional work,
         is necessary. The Woman's Medical College of Pennsyl-
         vania can play a key role in these developments.

1994.   Leymaster, Glen R. "Tomorrow's Target." Journal of the
         American Medical Women's Association, 19:10 (October
         1964) 874-877. (Inaugural Address, Woman's Medical
         College of Pennsylvania, Philadelphia, 6 March 1964.)
         Women physicians have achieved their place in the medical
         profession by diligence, intelligence, and stubbornness. A
         medical school oriented to the training of women physicians
         may be a better place for women to study. Women need a
         flexible curriculum in order to take time off to become
         homemakers if they want to, or to return to school after
         they have been homemakers. They should have the option
         of being mobile so that they can follow their husband's ca-
         reers and the option of having access to continuing education.
         Society will benefit if the skills young women acquire pre-
         pare them to fulfill themselves and be gainfully employed.

1995.   Linde, Harry W. "Admissions Committees Not Misogynis-
         tic." New England Journal of Medicine, 282:11 (12
         March 1970) 634.   (Correspondence.)
         Women applicants to medical schools suffer no discrimina-
         tion, asserts this letter-writer. He, a member of the ad-
         missions committee at Northwestern University Medical
         School, quotes admissions statistics and notes that only four
         of 101 American medical schools discriminate because of
         sex--"one of these is Woman's Medical College."

1996.   Macfarlane, Catharine. "A Challenge: Cherchez les
         Femmes." Journal of the American Medical Women's
         Association, 20:4 (April 1965) 345.
         Women physicians should consider training other women
         physicians to succeed them; such training is as important a
         contribution as anything else they do. For 97 years, from
         1866 to 1963, the dean of the Woman's Medical College of
         Pennsylvania was a woman. After 1963 men held this im-
         portant position and women lost the opportunities, responsi-
         bilities, and honors of this office. The Infirmary for Wo-
         men and Children in New York City, founded by Drs. Eliza-
         beth and Emily Blackwell, had women as approximately 50

per cent of its officers of instruction; in 1963, 39 per cent
of the officers of instruction were women.

1997.   McGrew, Elizabeth A. "More on Dropouts." Journal of
          the American Medical Women's Association, 22:3
          (March 1967) 194. (AMWA President's Message.)
        After D. G. Johnson's and E. G. Hutchins's report "Doctor
        or Dropout?" appeared in the Journal of Medical Education,
        December, 1966, Elizabeth A. McGrew, president of the
        American Medical Women's Association, expresses concern
        that the Johnson and Hutchins conclusions, that women med-
        ical students drop out at double the percentage of men, will
        adversely affect male medical school administrators' atti-
        tudes toward women medical students. She suggests that
        studies be initiated that examine the reasons women drop
        out. She further suggests that medical school curriculum,
        internship, and residency schedules become more flexible so
        as not to discriminate against women.

1998.   McGrew, Elizabeth A. "Women Medical Dropouts." Jour-
          nal of the American Medical Women's Association, 22:2
          (February 1967) 128. (AMWA President's Message.)
        D. G. Johnson and E. G. Hutchins, with the Association of
        American Medical Colleges, published a study in the Journal
        of Medical Education, December 1966. Their findings are
        significant to women physicians and medical school faculty
        in that the dropout rate for women is twice as high as that
        for men.

1999.   Maher, Irene E. "The Education of a Woman Physician."
          Pi Lambda Theta Journal, 28:2 (December 1949) 108-
          109.
        In 1948-1949, women totaled 2,109 (8.9 per cent) of the med-
        ical students in the United States. That same year, 12.1
        per cent of all medical graduates were women (an increase
        over 5.1 per cent in 1939 and 4.8 per cent in 1929). Only
        three medical schools (Dartmouth, Jefferson, and North Da-
        kota), of the 71 U.S. medical institutions approved by the
        American Medical Association, admitted no women in 1948-
        1949. This article goes on to list requirements for admis-
        sion to medical schools and internships.

2000.   "Medical Education of Women Has Proved Worth While."
          Journal of the American Medical Women's Association,
          10:3 (March 1955) 84-86. tables.
        A review of contemporary studies on women physicians being
        carried out by various groups is presented. This material
        is reprinted from Admissions Requirements of American
        Medical Colleges-1955. In 1954-1955 "only" six medical
        schools "estimat[ed]" they would not have any women in the
        freshman class. "The absence of women ... does not imply
        a change in policy [as four of the six schools previously ad-
        mitted women]," submits the author. Rather, "it is likely

that they received no applications this year from women
properly qualified to study medicine."

2001.   "Medical Students Speak Out!" Journal of the American
            Medical Women's Association, 23:10 (October 1968) 925.
        This article summarizes the way women medical school stu-
        dents feel about their medical education and their role con-
        flict of physician and mother. They feel "frustration and
        disappointment with the curriculum and the disinterest of
        professors [in medical school]." Too often the professor
        is one who emphasizes scientific detail without regard for
        interpersonal relationships and patient contact. As a result,
        the emphasis is on memorization rather than individual and
        creative thinking, and although the students concede that
        learning by rote is inevitable, it leaves little time for appli-
        cation and consideration of knowledge acquired. All of the
        students agreed that women were accepted in medical schools
        on an equal footing, and no difficulties arose, no extra
        pressure was brought to bear, and no demands were made
        because they were women. The married women found that
        marriage and studies were compatible and that the "secur-
        ity of marriage was an asset in medical school." Some are
        married to classmates while others benefit from the knowl-
        edge of husbands who are upperclassmen. However, some
        have found that compromises have to be made in schooling
        and the selection of an internship in order to have time to
        devote to a husband and children. Praise was voiced for
        the Journal [of the American Medical Women's Association],
        which the students found informative and useful.

2002.   Men and Women Medical Students, and the Woman Move-
            ment. [Philadelphia, Pennsylvania], 1869.
        [Item not examined by editors.]

2003.   Men and Women Medical Students: The Hospital Clinics
            and The Woman Movement. No. 2. [Philadelphia,
            Pennsylvania, 1870], 20 pp.
        [Item not examined by editors.]

2004.   "More Women Go into Medical Jobs as Career Work."
            Medical Woman's Journal, 54:12 (December 1947) 23.
        Although a record number of women are expected to grad-
        uate from medical school in the next few years, fewer are
        expected to enter medical training in 1947 than in 1946.
        Dr. Donald G. Anderson, secretary of the American Med-
        ical Association (AMA) Council on Education, "has denied
        charges that this was because crowded universities and col-
        leges have reduced quotas for women medical students."
        Figures on women in medicine for the AMA survey are
        cited.

2005.   "More Women in Medicine." Medical Woman's Journal,
            52:12 (December 1945) 34.

A jump in the enrollment of women students at the University of Illinois College of Medicine indicates the increased interest among women in the medical profession. In 1945, seven to eight times as many women applied as in previous years. The average age for the 36 "girls" enrolled as freshmen in 1945, is 25 years.

2006.   Morgan, Beverly C. "Admission of Women into Medical Schools in the United States: Current Status." The Woman Physician, 26:6 (June 1971) 305-309.

This article proposes to investigate the current status of admission of women into medical schools in the United States, and discern whether or not discrimination on the basis of sex does exist. Such an investigation of prejudice is difficult because of the many factors upon which admission is based. In the area of MCAT scores, women do not seem to be the victims of discrimination; "available data" fail to confirm any "definite" prejudice toward women at the time of application to medical school. The author suggests that discrimination begins very early, and she quotes Catharine Macfarlane's statement that "'college vocational counselors are the single most potent force steering women away from medicine.'" Lack of funds may also be a factor. A high attrition rate for women who do get accepted into medical school, the author suggests, may play a part in denying women admission to medical school. Various studies are cited in support of the statements in this article.

2007.   Nadelson, Carol and Notman, Malka[h]. "Success or Failure: Women as Medical School Applicants." Journal of the American Medical Women's Association, 29:4 (April 1974) 167-172. tables. (Panel presentation, "Feminine Career Goals," American Psychological Association, Montreal, August 1973.)

Exploring the reasons for the relatively low number of women physicians, the authors discuss the masculine/feminine role conflict, the inflexibility of medical school schedules, and the rigidity of schedules at medical institutions in general. The authors submit that "since doctors are traditionally men they often think of and act toward patients as they would toward women and children, expecting passivity and compliance, assuming the role of the authoritarian and protective parent with a dependent child who cannot participate actively in the process of getting well." There is a benefit in the patient being able to choose a doctor of either sex, depending on the patient's prior experiences and orientation toward the model presented by the physician. Medical school admissions committees often use quantitative and science MCAT scores as criteria--scores which have generally been lower for women than for men, and despite the fact that "ability in the basic sciences has no clear relationship to performance as a physician." The fact that women have been admitted to medical school in proportion to the numbers

who apply is deceptive "since women represent a preselected
group of gifted and perhaps more highly motivated people by
virtue of the counter pressures they encounter at each step
in the process of making career decisions." The backgrounds from which women medical students come is examined. Medical school experience and ultimate career
choice at the end of medical school is discussed.

2008.   Nelson, Bonnie C. "Medical College Admission Test."
         Journal of Medical Education, 49:7 (July 1974) 712-714.
         tables. (Datagram.)
         Women usually obtain higher mean scores than do men on
         the Verbal Ability and General Information subtests, while
         men have scored higher on the Quantitative Ability and Sci-
         ence subtests.

2009.   Pondrom, Cyrena N. "Setting Priorities in Developing an
         Affirmative Action Program." Journal of Medical Edu-
         cation, 50:5 (May 1975) 427-434. (Presentation, Spring
         Meeting, AAMC Council of Deans, Phoenix, Arizona,
         26 April 1974.)
         "'Affirmative action' programs call for special activities to
         ensure that women and minorities participate in employment
         and educational opportunities in the numbers in which quali-
         fied members of these groups are represented in the nation
         or community. Six kinds of activities should receive pri-
         ority in establishing a medical school affirmative action pro-
         gram: (a) review of salaries for equity, (b) establishing
         goals for hiring in both faculty and nonfaculty jobs, (c) re-
         view of admissions criteria to assure that women and minor-
         ities are not required to meet a higher standard than white
         males and to include accurate predictors of the success of
         applicants from these groups, (d) survey of physical facil-
         ities to assure that lounges and facilities for women are
         equivalent to quality and convenience to those available to
         men, (e) examination of employment and instructional poli-
         cies to identify any which have a 'disparate effect' on the
         success of women and minorities and modification of such
         policies wherever alternatives are possible, (f) review of
         staff, student, and administrative attitudes to assure that
         the institutional atmosphere conveys support of equal oppor-
         tunity. Success in accomplishing each of these priorities
         will build a basis for success in other aspects of the equal
         opportunity program." [Article abstract.]

2010.   "Record Number of Women Seek Careers as Doctors."
         Medical Woman's Journal, 53:10 (October 1946) 35.
         A record number of women--864--completed their freshman
         terms in U.S. medical schools, compared with 5,991 men.
         The incoming freshman class is expected to have 700 wo-
         men, including 18 former WACs and WAVEs.

2011.   Remonstrance Against Clinical Instruction Being Given to

Classes Composed of Both Sexes. Collins, Printer, [Philadelphia, Pennsylvania], 15 November 1869, 8 pp. Published in both pamphlet and "broadside" form, this "remonstrance" was signed by professors of the University of Pennsylvania, Jefferson Medical College [Philadelphia], members of major Philadelphia hospitals, and many "physicians at large in the city of Philadelphia." The undersigned, "out of respect for their profession, and for the interests of the public," express opposition to mixed classes of male and female medical students. The judgment is based upon the fact that clinical instruction demands "personal exposure" of "all the organs and parts of the body": "It cannot be assumed, by any right-minded person, that Male patients should be subjected to inspection before a class of Females, although this inspection may, without impropriety, be submitted to before those of their own sex." Also, in the medical lecture room, there occurs "an inevitable and positive demoralization of the individuals concerned"; womanly qualities are lost.

2012.   Renshaw, Josephine E. "AMWA President's Message: Progress in Medical School Acceptance of Women." The Woman Physician, 25:3 (March 1970) 188-189.
Medical schools restricted the admission of women to 4.5 to five per cent of the total acceptances. Currently, seven per cent of the total physician population of this country are women: about one-third of that number are foreign medical graduates.

2013.   Sachs, Bernice C. "President's Message." Journal of the American Medical Women's Association, 20:10 (October 1965) 959. port.
Currently, 8.6 per cent of the people entering the 88 American medical schools are women. "This is the first major increase in the number of women entering medical school from the static six per cent of medical graduates that has represented the percentage of medical woman power in America for the past 20 years."

2014.   Saul, Ezra V. and Kass, Joan S. "Study of Anticipated Anxiety in a Medical School Setting." Journal of Medical Education, 44:6 (June 1969) 526-532. tables. (Presentation, Conference on Research in Medical Education, 79th Annual Meeting, Association of American Medical Colleges, Houston, Texas, 1 November 1968.)
In order to examine the specific situations which create anxiety in medical students, the S-R Inventory of Anxiousness was adapted to the variety of situations likely to be encountered in medical school. It was administered on the first day of school and again at the end of the school year to the freshman class at Tufts University School of Medicine. For the class in general, the stress of entering a final exam was higher, but not significantly so, than either dis-

cussing a fatal illness with a patient or telling a relative
that a patient had died. Freshmen were most exhilarated
by watching their first surgical operation. Of the 18 female students who were compared with 98 male students,
two-thirds of the women registered Total Anxiety scores
above the mean Total Anxiety score for the entire sample.
Tests of mean differences between situation scores of male
versus female students indicated that females exhibit more
anxiety than males in all situations except examining a female patient and participating in an experiment. Females
showed statistically significant higher stress when examining
a male patient, watching an operation, drawing blood, and
entering an examination.

2015.   Scharlieb, Mary Ann Dacomb Bird. "The Medical Educa-
             tion for Women." Nineteenth Century and After, 92
             (August 1922) 317-329.
        [Article not examined by editors.]

2016.   Schwartz, Barry J. and Snow, Laurence H. "On Getting
             Kicked Out of Medical School." American Journal of
             Psychotherapy, 28:4 (October 1974) 574-583.
        Two psychiatrists at a predominantly female medical school
        [The Medical College of Pennsylvania] describe the kind of
        personality patterns found in medical students who fail.
        They identify a number of personality types that appear to
        have in common the fact that they all take themselves too
        seriously, not that they suffer from lack of motivation, and
        that in taking themselves so seriously they adhere tenacious-
        ly to a role they are playing and are devoid of the flexibil-
        ity necessary to meet the academic situation. The types
        they identify include, for example, the "princess" who has a
        difficult time working as a member of a team and who
        makes requests that people grant yet after they have granted
        them, are left with a vague feeling of resentment; the "peas-
        ant," an overachiever who comes from such a poor family
        that to be in medical school makes that person feel like a
        socioeconomic Atlas holding the family's world, present and
        future, upon her shoulders; the "caretaker," whose major
        sense of identity comes not from her own worth but from
        having been responsible for the physical and psychologic
        well-being of some other person. Furthermore, the authors
        observe the difference in the patterns of rearing girls and
        boys. American culture assumes that it is all right to test
        a boy by a certain amount of humiliation and even beatings
        without his breaking down, while a girl may break down and
        cry, which is an inappropriate response in the medical
        school rites of passage training.

2017.   Sedlacek, William E. "Study of Applicants, 1965-66."
             Journal of Medical Education, 42:1 (January 1967) 28-
             45. figs., tables.
        A brief narrative section and two statistical tables in this

article deal with women applicants. Of the 1,676 women who applied to medical school in 1965-66 from a total of 18,703 applicants, 799 were accepted for admission (47.7 per cent compared with male applicants' 48.2 per cent acceptance rate). Women comprised 9.0 per cent of all applicants, provided 8.0 per cent of the applications, and were offered 8.9 per cent of the acceptances. The 8.9 per cent figure for 1965-66 compares with 9.1 per cent for 1964-65, 8.4 per cent for 1963-64, and 8.0 per cent for 1962-63. Comparative figures for male and female applicants are broken down by individual medical schools and state of residency.

2018.   Sheehan, Donal. "Medical Education of the Future." Medical Woman's Journal, 51:12 (December 1944) 17-23. (Address, Women's Medical Association of New York City, 14 November 1944.)
Following a lengthy, generalized discussion of changes that should occur within medical education, Dr. Sheehan, acting dean of the New York University College of Medicine, states: "I had not intended to discuss the problems of women in medicine, believing firmly, as I do, that it is our duty to select students and train physicians, irrespective of whether they may be men or women." He admits that before this particular audience, however, such an omission "might appear rude and even sinister." He goes on to explore the charge that a "substantial proportion" of women abandon their medical careers when they marry. Noting that the number of women medical students in Great Britain exceeds the number studying in the United States, Dr. Sheehan concludes that in America there is not "a large enough reservoir of women students interested and qualified to study medicine." He further believes that sex discrimination in medicine does not exist.

2019.   "Slight Increase in Number of Women Medical Students." Medical Woman's Journal, 52:10 (October 1945) 44. According to the Women's Bureau of the U.S. Department of Labor, there were 1,146 women students in approved medical schools in 1943, and 1,176 in 1944.

2020.   Stalnaker, John M. "The Study of Applicants, 1954-1955." Journal of Medical Education, 30:11 (November 1955) 625-636. tables.
An analysis of the applicants to the 1954-1955 freshman medical school class is made by the director of studies of the AAMC. For the fifth consecutive year, the total number of students applying for admission to medical schools decreased. Comparative data for men and women are given in all areas of this study except for MCAT scores, where only collective data for both men and women are reported, and the total number of individuals applying to medical school for eight consecutive years [from which figures the

above comment regarding total decrease in applications is
extrapolated]. Although statistics are discussed and analyzed for each area, there is no discussion of the male/
female breakdowns.

2021.   Stevenson, Sarah Hackett. "Co-Education of the Sexes in
         Medicine." Medical Woman's Journal, 36:1 (January
         1929) 12-15. port.
         Dr. Stevenson likens the situation of women who have been
         granted a taste of the study of medicine unto the slaves
         whose masters placed "the cups of knowledge" to their lips,
         and the slaves were thereafter unsatisfied with the "A, B,
         C." Women who aspire to be physicians, "granted the
         right to study ... must also [be granted] the right to study
         in the best possible way." In conclusion, Dr. Stevenson
         asks "why is peerage more unbecoming to women than vas-
         salage? If it is indelicate for a woman to be a physician,
         much more is it indelicate for her to be a nurse and thrice
         over is it indelicate for her to be a patient." A biograph-
         ical inset on the author is included.

2022.   Storrie, V. Marie. "Supply." Journal of the American
         Medical Women's Association, 21:10 (October 1966)
         837-839. (Report, First Scientific Session, Xth Inter-
         national Congress.)
         Since there is a shortage of doctors around the world, we
         should consider the potential of medical womanpower. If
         there were increased training facilities for women doctors,
         many more women could utilize their talents and increase
         the supply of doctors.

2023.   Stritter, Frank T.; Hutton, Jack G.; and Dubé, W. F.
         "Study of U.S. Medical School Applicants, 1968-69."
         Journal of Medical Education, 45:4 (April 1970) 195-
         209. tables.
         This study's information on female applicants to medical
         schools notes that of the 2,091 women applying, 976 (46.7
         per cent) were admitted. Nine per cent of all applicants
         were women, while ten per cent of the total accepted were
         women.

2024.   Stritter, Frank T.; Hutton, Jack.; and Dubé, W. F.
         "Study of U.S. Medical School Applicants, 1969-70."
         Journal of Medical Education, 46:1 (January 1971) 25-
         40. fig., tables.
         In 1969-70, 2,289 women constituted 9.4 per cent of the
         medical school applicant pool; 1,011 women, or 9.6 per
         cent of the total accepted group were offered one or more
         admissions; 929 actually matriculated. Women constituted
         9.1 per cent of all entering students.

2025.   Thomas, Mary F. "The Influence of the Medical Colleges
         of the Regular School, of Indianapolis, on the Medical

Education of the Women of the State." Transactions of
the Indiana Medical Society, 33 (1883) 228-238.
[Article not examined by editors.]

2026. "Urge College Women to Study Medicine Where?" Medical
Woman's Journal, 51:6 (June 1944) 30, 31. (Editorial.)
Quoting from a New York Times article, this editorial laments the U.S. armed services' refusal to subsidize the
medical education of women.

2027. [Van Hoosen, Bertha]. "The Modern Pioneer." Medical
Woman's Journal, 37:4 (April 1930) 102-103.
"One has only to study the catalogues of our medical schools
to realize that the modern medical woman is doing more
pioneer work than her sisters did forty years ago." Dr.
Van Hoosen discusses the quotas in medical schools and the
psychological effect that only "one girl in a class" has on
other women who might apply. "The modern medical woman is having as much or perhaps more direct contact with
sex prejudice [as her pioneer medical sisters had], but it
is so camouflaged that she cannot even acquire the strength
that she would have if she were able to fight it face to face
and hand to hand as the women doctor did forty years ago."
Dr. Van Hoosen concludes with the call for mass support
of the few women who do get into medical school.

2028. Van Hoosen, Bertha. "Report of the National Committee
on Medical Opportunities for Women." Medical Woman's
Journal, 37:7 (July 1930) 200-202.
Mrs. Lester Bartlett wrote a Ph.D. thesis entitled "The
Present Status of the Woman Physician," upon which Bertha
Van Hoosen bases the majority of her remarks. Most medical schools severely restricted admission of women (if they
accept any at all) despite an increasing number of applicants.
Therefore the percentage of women enrolled in medical
schools had decreased sharply for the previous decade:
"... it appears that under the present practice women are
not being replaced at the rate which their persistency and
higher scholarship would warrant." Furthermore, if a woman were the only female accepted at a school, she was
likely to decline to go at all if her presence meant being
the "'only woman' in the class." Another possible reason
for this exclusion of qualified women in medical schools
includes the fact that there are no medical women on any of
the co-educational medical school admissions committees.
Mrs. Bartlett concludes, "In view of the practices in medical schools, which have been outlined above, it appears that
the present method of selection of students discriminates
against women. The most democratically American method
of determining the number of medical women would seem to
be (1) the desire of women to study and practice medicine;
(2) the ability to meet medical standards which are applied
equally to men and women; (3) demand for their professional

services." Dr. Van Hoosen proposes several courses of action among which are that the Medical Women's National Association send resolutions to the Council on Medical Education and Hospitals of the American Medical Association; and that to assist women in getting internships, hospitals accepting women interns be asked to notify the Medical Women's National Association when there are vacancies.

2029. Wainer, Robert A.; Ratzan, R. Judith; and Lansdown, Frances S. "Female Feldshers Fusilladed." New England Journal of Medicine, 285:26 (23 December 1971) 1490. (Correspondence.)
In separate letters, three physicians take strong exception to the ideas on women physicians expressed in a letter by Earl A. Bowen [New England Journal of Medicine, 285:17 (21 October 1971) 973].

2030. Warren, Fidelia. "Medical Education of Women." Syracuse Medical and Surgical Journal, 6 (November 1854) 293-295.
[Article not examined by editors.]

2031. Weinberg, Ethel and Rooney, James F. "The Academic Performance of Women Students in Medical School." Journal of Medical Education, 48:3 (March 1973) 240-247. tables.
"A survey of major measures of academic performance of men and women in medical school reveals that although women's performance in the early years is slightly but consistently lower than that of men, overall academic performance is equal by the senior year. Women students achieve an average score on the freshman-year subjects in the National Board examinations of 1.93 points less than male students. On the second-year subjects, the difference has decreased to 0.68 point. The Science subtest scores of the Medical College Admission Test predict these differences in that women students, whether science majors or humanity majors, score lower than their male counterparts. The differences in total scores on Part II of the National Board examinations are virtually zero. Women lead in three sections and men lead in three sections. With certain exceptions, National Board examination scores of women tend to vary less than those of men. Although attrition for academic reasons is slightly higher for women than for men, the likelihood of their being selected for membership in Alpha Omega Alpha National Honor Medical Society is at least equal to or slightly greater than that of their male counterparts." [Article abstract.]

2032. Wilson, Jno. Stainback. "Female Medical Education." Southern Medical and Surgical Journal, 10:1 (January 1854) 1-17. (Original and Eclectic: Article I.)
Females should be educated in obstetrics and gynecology be-

cause: women's "sexual idiosyncrasies" would aid in diagnosis and therapeutics; some women need employment; "re-
fined and lovely women, (in the South particularly)" demand
female practitioners; and, the physician welcomes relief
from what is "one of the most disagreeable and irksome
branches of his profession." Acknowledging the absurdity
of conferring on women the comprehensive degree of Doctor
of Medicine, Dr. Wilson suggests special limited courses
in obstetrics for women within established medical schools.
Such an arrangement assures that female medical education
would remain "untainted by the heteroclitical errors which
are likely to creep into those independent institutions that
are surrounded by the external forces of Bloomerism and
Woman's Rights." As for the "difficulty of confining female physicians to their proper sphere of practice," Dr.
Wilson advocates reserving the power to revoke licenses if
the "prescribed limits should be transcended."

2033.   Woman's Work in the Field of Medicine. College of Mid-
           wifery of the City of New York, 1883, 54 pp. facsims.
        Medical schools for women usually prove unsuccessful: take
        for example the Woman's Medical College of the New York
        Infirmary, where a low number of women have graduated;
        they undertook "too much in compelling women to go through
        the whole curriculum of surgery, pharmacy, materia medica,
        jurisprudence, etc." On the other hand, the College of Mid-
        wifery owes success to the fact that it teaches what "by ex-
        perience, has been found to cover the sphere of woman's
        usefulness in medicine ... the intention being not to make
        regular practitioners of medicine, but to educate women in
        those special duties of the profession for which they are
        peculiarly adapted." This book reprints comments about the
        school published in the medical press, describes duties of
        the midwife, and concludes with dietary articles (recipes
        for the sick).

2034.   "Women and Medicine." Nation, 52 (21 February 1891)
           131.
        Johns Hopkins Medical School, "under the pressure of a
        gift of a hundred thousand dollars from the women of the
        country," will admit women students. This opening marks
        a turning point for women physicians because only through
        medical coeducation can women prove their ability to hold
        their own with the men in the profession. This article goes
        on to review the status of medical education for women in
        several countries, and the prevalent attitudes towards women
        as medical practitioners.

2035.   "Women in Medical Schools." Journal of Medical Education,
           41:2 (February 1966) 184-185. fig., tables. (Data-
           gram.)
        Over the years there has been a slow but steady increase
        in the numbers of women applying to and being accepted by

U.S. medical schools. From 1929 to 1964, the proportion
of women accepted to medical schools has increased from
4.5 per cent to 9.1 per cent. Between 1949 and 1958, a
higher percentage of males completed their medical education (91 per cent males vs. 84 per cent women). The majority of men drop out because of academic problems, while
the majority of women leave for reasons other than academic difficulty. The number of women graduates has increased
from 4.5 per cent in 1930 to 7.3 per cent in 1965.

2036.   "Women in Medicine." Journal of Medical Education, 38:
             6 (June 1963) 518-519. tables. (Datagram.)
         Comparative tables between women and men are presented
         showing that women tend to score higher than men on the
         verbal tests but lower on the quantitative and science tests;
         that the number of men accepted in medical schools has re-
         mained fairly stable while the number of women has in-
         creased from 4.5 per cent in 1929 to 8.5 per cent in 1961-
         62 with the major increase occurring in 1950-51 and im-
         mediately following the post World War II years; that while
         35 per cent of all bachelors degrees conferred over the
         past nine years go to women, yet only five per cent of
         medical degrees conferred in the United States go to wo-
         men. By comparison, the percentage of all women medical
         graduates in Canada is 12 per cent and in Great Britain,
         24 per cent.

2037.   "Women in Medicine." New England Journal of Medicine,
             291:21 (21 November 1974) 1138-1142. (Correspon-
             dence.)
         This series of letters comments upon Dr. Mary C. Howell's
         article "What Medical Schools Teach About Women" [New
         England Journal of Medicine, 291 (1974) 304-307]. Dr.
         Christian V. Cimmino from the Medical College of Virginia
         writes, "I simply don't recognize the paranoic medical
         milieu that Dr. Howell describes." Dr. Cimmino "readily
         admit[s] the female's academic superiority, her more highly
         developed intuitive sense, her greater moral courage and
         her stamina." Dr. Susan Kilgore Aoki feels that although
         many of Dr. Howell's conclusions were valid, discrimina-
         tory practices in the medical field should be documented
         with "carefully collected statistics." Dr. Phillip L. Grait-
         cer, D.D.S. draws a parallel situation of discrimination in
         dental schools. Several women physicians who read Dr.
         Howell's article with "progressing disbelief" wonder if they
         may not have been "thoroughly sublimating" their feelings
         to not have realized the discriminating behavior that exists.
         In conclusion Dr. Howell responds to these letters.

2038.   "Women in Medicine." Saturday Evening Post, 200 (21
             January 1928) 22.
         Women physicians should be afforded adequate training.
         There are not enough facilities to meet the growing numbers

of women seeking a medical education, and those facilities
there are (such as the Woman's Medical College of Pennsylvania) are woefully underfunded.

2039.   "Women Medical Students." Woman's Medical Journal, 19:
        12 (December 1909) 258. (Editorial.)
        In 1849 the first medical degree was granted to a woman.
        In 1899, 162 women graduated in medicine.   Currently,
        three women's medical colleges exist, and 91 of the re-
        maining 141 U.S. medical schools are coeducational.   Four-
        fifths of the women graduating last spring studied at the co-
        educational institutions.   While the number of women med-
        ical students decreased since 1904, in 1909 the number of
        women medical graduates rose again--to 4.2 per cent.

GRADUATE MEDICAL EDUCATION

Material concentrates on internships, residencies, fellowships, retraining programs, and continuing education programs.

2040. Van Hoosen, Bertha. "Opportunities for Medical Women Internes." Medical Woman's Journal, 33:11 (November
   1926) 311-318.
   A survey of hospitals which admit women interns proved,
   to Dr. Van Hoosen, that the Philippine General Hospital's
   rules governing interns more nearly approached perfection
   than any other hospital.

AUSTRALIA & NEW ZEALAND

2041. Gill, P. F. "Recycling Doctors." Medical Journal of
   Australia, 2:14 (4 October 1975) 562-565. (Retiring
   President's Address, Annual General Meeting, Tasman-
   ian Branch, Australian Medical Association, March 22,
   1975.)
   Dr. Gill lists four major factors affecting decreasing productivity of Australian medical manpower. The first reason
   is an increasing enrollment of women in medical school; in
   1974 they comprised 22.5 per cent of all students in all
   Australian medical faculties. He claims the net productivity of women physicians is 65 per cent that of their male
   counterparts. Other causes for productivity decline are
   decreasing hours of practice, increasing early retirement,
   and professional obsolescence. The Family Medicine Pro-
   gramme, cited as a pilot project to retrain women physicians
   out of training for a number of years, is also used by other
   physicians changing from specialties to general practice.
   The thrust of the address was directed at overcoming professional obsolescence.

2042. Howqua, June L. "Refresher Course at Queen Victoria
   Hospital, Melbourne, for Married Women Wishing to Return to Medical Practice." British Medical Journal, 1
   (25 March 1967) 752-753. (Medical Education.)

2043. Nelson, Selwyn. "Women in Medicine." Medical Journal of
   Australia, 1:13 (27 March 1971) 717. (Letters to the
   Editor.)
   The postgraduate committee in medicine at the University
   of Sydney in Australia, in conjunction with the Medical Women's Society, has conducted two retraining programs to
   enable women physicians to reenter the work force: one in
   1967; one in 1970. After the first course, which was held
   every morning for four weeks, many of the 40 women who
   attended entered full-time or part-time employment, some
   in private practice and others in salaried positions. Many

students gained from further instruction either from formal
courses organized by the postgraduate committee or by attending public hospital clinics with chosen preceptors.   Such
courses are tailored to meet the requirements of students.

CANADA

2044.   Godden, J. O.   "Reactivation of the Inactive Physician: A
          Participant's View."   Canadian Medical Association Jour
          nal, 113:11/12 (13 December 1975) 1091-1092, 1094.
          photo.
        The views are given of learning participants in the retrain-
        ing program sponsored by the Toronto Chapter of the Fed-
        eration of Medical Women of Canada in 1973 (held at the
        University of Toronto's Sunnybrook Medical Center) for
        which ten women and five men registered.   The average
        ages of the trainees was 48.5 years.   Less than half the
        course was devoted to a didactic review of most of the
        subjects needed in family medicine (except obstetrics); the
        remainder of the time was spent in active practice in a
        preceptor's office.   One participant would have preferred
        a teaching clinic to the lecture method that was used in the
        course.   Other criticisms include the need to have refresh-
        er material emphasize the practical everyday problems rath-
        er than the extraordinary problems, which might be better
        dealt with by means of "handouts."

EUROPE, WESTERN

2045.   Macy, Mary Sutton.   "Post-Graduate Medical Work for Wo-
          men in Europe."   Woman's Medical Journal, 20:3
          (March 1910) 59-61.
        Dr. Macy confines her discussion to the requirements for
        postgraduate study in England and in Vienna, Austria.

GREAT BRITAIN

2046.   "The Annual Meeting of the Medical Women's Federation,
          London, May 7th, 1931."   Medical Women's Federation
          News-Letter, (July 1931) 47-57.
        This article presents a summary of the proceedings of the
        annual meeting.   A major topic of discussion was the dif-
        ficulties women have in obtaining graduate posts in hospitals
        because of discriminating practices.

2047.   Arie, Tom.   "Married Women Doctors as Part-time Train-
          ees."   British Medical Journal, 3:5984 (13 September
          1975) 641-643.   (Medical Education.)
        In six years Goodmayes Hospital in Essex, England has en-
        abled ten part-time trainees to learn in their psychiatric

unit. While the author, representing the staff, feels the program is successful, he also identifies the problems involved in employing part-time people. As married women and mothers, many of them bring qualities that are relevant to their work, e.g., practical good sense and conscientiousness. On the other hand, the kinds of problems involved in such a program include such pragmatic considerations as continuity in effective handover and communications, and having to miss certain events (such as ward rounds) to attend courses.

2048.   Eskin, Frada. "Review of the Women Doctors' Retainer Scheme in the Sheffield Region 1972-73." British Journal of Medical Education, 8:2 (June 1974) 141-144. tables.
"This paper describes the first year of the Women Doctors' Retainer Scheme in the Sheffield Regional Hospital Board area. It gives an outline of the scheme and discusses the applicants in relation to age, marital status numbers of children, and employment status at the time of application. Other aspects considered include the type of employment desired and the specialty chosen. Reasons for non-acceptance into the schemes are discussed." [Article summary.]

2049.   Rue, Rosemary. "Employment of Married Women Doctors in Hospitals in the Oxford Region." Lancet, 1:7502 (10 June 1967) 1267-1268. (Special Article.)
This article is a result of the Lawrie, Newhouse, Elliott article (British Medical Journal, 1 [1966] 409) on the survey carried out by the Medical Women's Federation which revealed that approximately 150 women doctors living in the Oxford region were doing less than full-time work. The author of this article made personal contact with as many of these women as possible to discover the reason why they were not doing full-time work. Three main groups emerged. A "scheme" was developed to provide part-time residency training for these women. The progress and future of this program are reviewed: "Reports received during the first year of the scheme have been overwhelmingly favorable."

UNITED STATES

2050.   Buzek, Joanna and McNamara, Mary. "Communications: A Partial Solution to the Manpower Problem." Journal of Medical Education, 43:11 (November 1968) 1197-1199. tables.
Since 1963 there have been more than 13,000 inactive physicians in the United States and of these, 18 per cent have been under 55 years of age. To encourage these people, especially women, to return to practice, the Bureau of Health Manpower of the U.S. Public Health Service initiated 6-12 month retraining programs they call "preceptorships-

residency" programs. In 1967 questionnaires were sent to
these people inquiring about their reasons for not practicing
and if they would be interested in retraining programs.
Nearly 25 per cent showed an interest in such a program.

2051.   "Can Medicine Win Back the Retired Woman Doctor? Short-
         ages Spur U.S. Refresher Plans Despite Poor Response
         in Britain." Medical World News, 7:35 (23 September
         1966) 94-95.

2052.   Coulter, Molly P. "Residency Programs for Women."
         Journal of Medical Education, 47:10 (October 1972) 836-
         837.
         The greatest obstacle for women with children to serve
         residencies is working a 70 to 80 hour week and having to
         care for their children besides. Strong Memorial Hospital
         has tried to solve this conflict in the following ways: by
         allowing two women to serve part-time for two years, en-
         abling them to fulfill both their residency requirement as
         well as provide coverage at the hospital; dividing a female
         resident's time between the hospital one half-day and the
         community health center the other half-day; another woman
         works one half-day for two years at the community health
         center and at the hospital.

2053.   "'Cultural Turn-Off' Blamed for Shortage of Female MDs."
         House Physician Reporter, (June 1972).
         Included in this article are a description and discussion of
         a retraining program at the Medical College of Pennsylvania,
         and the part-time residency program in psychiatry for phy-
         sician-mothers at the New York Medical College. [Article
         not examined by editors.]

2054.   Fenninger, Leonard D. and Tracy, Rose H. "Graduate
         Medical Education: Annual Report on Graduate Medical
         Education in the United States." Journal of the Ameri-
         can Medical Association Supplement, 231 (January 1975)
         34-62. tables. (Section III.)
         Under the Special Studies in Graduate Medical Education sec-
         tion of this article, women are discussed. A table gives
         the number of U.S. and foreign women in internship posi-
         tions (as of 1 September 1973) in each state in the U.S.
         Of the U.S. and Canadian graduate women interns, 74 per
         cent receive appointments in major teaching hospitals, while
         only 34 per cent of the foreign women graduates receive
         such appointments. Another table indicates the number of
         U.S., Canadian, and foreign women physician graduates seek-
         ing residencies as of 1 September 1973. The numbers are
         listed by specialty. Women physicians on teaching staffs of
         hospitals, women employed full-time in hospitals, and re-
         fresher courses for women physicians are also briefly cov-
         ered.

2055.   Fernandez-Fox, Eva. "Graduate Medical Education at Wo-
         man's Medical College of Pennsylvania." Journal of the
         American Medical Women's Association, 5:9 (September
         1950) 368-370. photos., ports.
         This article is a brief description of the program and or-
         ganization of the Woman's Medical College of Pennsylvania.
         Because this College is both a medical school and hospital,
         the students have access to lectures as well as to pre-clin-
         ical faculty "consultations." Psychiatric problems and con-
         tagious diseases are the only kinds of cases that were not
         dealt with by the hospital at the time this article was writ-
         ten. The programs for each medical area's residency or
         fellowship are given: anesthesia, gynecology and obstetrics,
         medicine, pathology, pediatrics, surgery. Portraits of Ann
         Preston and Rachel L. Bodley are included.

2056.   Fried, Frederick E. "Women in Medicine--The Training
         Years." Journal of Operational Psychiatry, 5:2 (Spring-
         Summer 1974) 101-102. (Commentary.)
         Because of the nature of the medical profession (i.e., its
         character as a "calling" requiring strong commitment and
         continual education), the choice open to most married wo-
         men physicians is a severely restricted one, and role con-
         flicts in the U.S. are particularly intense for women prac-
         titioners. The situation in other countries is reviewed,
         especially in Sweden and the USSR wherein women are given
         differential treatment in the professions in recognition of
         their childbearing function. The author concludes that more
         innovative and flexible training programs are needed in the
         U.S.

2057.   Gabrielson, Ira W. and Burkett, Gary L. "Part-time Resi-
         dency Study." Alumnae News [Medical College of Penn-
         sylvania], 26:1 (February 1975) 18-19. port.
         Described is the Medical College of Pennsylvania's four-
         year contract to study problems in operating part-time resi-
         dency programs.

2058.   Gardner, Mabel E. "Keeping Abreast with Progress."
         Medical Woman's Journal, 36:3 (March 1929) 78.
         In order to keep abreast with progress in the medical field,
         one must associate with "people and books," attend clinics
         and medical societies, travel and take postgraduate courses
         in one's specialty. The woman physician should also join
         the local medical society and attend meetings. Finally, wo-
         men are still in the minority in medicine and have problems
         to face as women; therefore women "should co-operate with
         each other as individuals or ... lose out on the onward
         march of progress."

2059.   Gregory Society of Boston. "The Woman Interne: A Re-
         port." Journal of the Association of Medical Students,
         2 (January 1938) 110-112, 127. photo.

Out of 690 hospitals approved for internship in the U.S. in 1936, 531 (77 per cent) take no women. And out of 6,900 internship positions, 96.4 per cent are closed to women. This article seeks to uncover the reasons for exclusion of women physicians from hospital internships. One major reason for excluding women had nothing to do with "any prejudice against women, not any distrust of women's competence which lay back of their exclusion, but a single material lack of facilities for having them." Another reason was found in the opposition of "'old-fashioned'" board members: "'Women are not accepted because they menstruate.'" In summary, the case of a "typical girl student" is reviewed.

2060.   "Hospital Opportunities for Women." Woman's Medical
         Journal, 20:1 (January 1910) 17. (Editorial.)
Medical women are urged to make repeated applications for internships--"repeat the process until continued hammering shall arouse the hospital authorities ... to the realization that a woman interne in a general hospital is not an anomaly...."

2061.   "Interneships for Women." Woman's Medical Journal, 21:5
         (May 1911) 106-107.
Hospitals which accept only women as interns, and those which accept both women and men interns, are listed.

2062.   Kaplan, Harold I. "Part-Time Residency Training: An Ap-
         proach to the Graduate Training of Some Women Phy-
         sicians." Journal of the American Medical Women's
         Association, 27:12 (December 1972) 648-650.
"Part-time residency training in psychiatry for physician mothers was introduced at the New York Medical College in 1962. Since that time 64 resident mothers have been graduated from this training program. Key aspects characterizing this program are that it is 9 months in length during each calendar year so that it requires four 9 month periods to become qualified in psychiatry--requiring 4 instead of 3 years for completion. Additionally, night duty and weekend duty are less frequent. This program was established because of the unique needs of women doctors with children who must be available at hours during key vacation periods (summer, Christmas) and most evenings and weekends. It has been readily accepted by male residents on the staff." [Journal abstract.]

2063.   Kaplan, Harold I.; Kaplan, Helen S. and Freedman, Alfred
         M. "Psychiatric Residency Training Program for Phy-
         sician Mothers: A Progress Report." Journal of the
         American Medical Women's Association, 19:4 (April
         1964) 285-289.
Recognizing the "multifaceted problems arising from the professional education for women who have young children," the

New York Medical College began a program of psychiatric
training for physician mothers. A modification of the traditional training allows for "flexibility in scheduling, time sequence changes, and certain curriculum enrichments." At
the time of this article, eight residents were enrolled in
this program: each stated that it was only because of this
program that she could continue with psychiatric training.
Their performance was rated as "progressing most satis-
factorily."

2064.   Kaplan, Harold I.; Kaplan, Helen S. and Freedman, Alfred
              M. "Residency Training in Psychiatry for Physician
              Mothers." Journal of the American Medical Association,
              189:1 (6 July 1964) 11-14.
A report is presented on the modifications of the psychiatric
residency training program at New York Medical College.
Modifications were designed for mother-physicians in order
"to increase the number of women physicians entering graduate training in psychiatry" and to increase these residents'
functioning by minimizing role conflicts. Modifications include a three-year residency spread over four nine-month
periods, supplementary educational programs where necessary, and the cooperation and understanding of male residents.

2065.   Kaplan, Helen Singer. "A New Concept of Graduate Train-
              ing for Women Physicians." Journal of the American
              Medical Women's Association, 17:10 (October 1962) 820-
              821.
This article provides an explanation of the need for and development of the part-time residency training program in
psychiatry at the New York Medical College.

2066.   "List of Hospitals Approved by the American Medical Asso-
              ciation for the Training of Women Internes." Medical
              Woman's Journal, 48:5 (May 1941) 139-147, 158.

2067.   "List of Hospitals Approved by the American Medical Asso-
              ciation for the Training of Women Internes: Information
              Received in Response to Questionnaire Sent Out." Med-
              ical Woman's Journal, 47:5 (May 1940) 147-153, 162.
This state-by-state list, obtained by Dr. Elise S. L'Esperance, includes the number of women interns serving at specific hospitals, the kinds of openings available, and, in
some cases, institutional policies regarding women interns.

2068.   Lowenstein, Leah M. "Who Wants Lady Interns?" New
              England Journal of Medicine, 284:13 (1 April 1971) 735.
              (Letters to Editor.)
Excellent internship programs usually do not include women. Such discrimination is all the more ironic because
women comprising the five to 20 per cent quota of women
in medical schools were chosen with great care and had to
be superior to begin with.

2069.   Lowenstein, Leah M. "Women Interns and Residents."
         Boston University Medical Center Centerscope, (July/
         August 1971) 8-9. (Women in Medicine.)
         Dr. Lowenstein identifies problems faced by women interns
         and residents and suggests alterations be made within post-
         graduate training programs.

2070.   "MD-Mothers Retrain for Comeback to Practice." Medical
         World News, 6:48 (31 December 1965) 134-135, 139.
         photos.
         Although it costs $8,000 to $10,000 per year to retrain
         each student, the cost is modest in comparison to the loss
         to the country when a trained doctor does not return to
         practice. The retraining program at the Woman's Medical
         College of Pennsylvania is not yet fully established, but
         several women are taking refresher courses.

2071.   Maffett, Minnie L.; Fay, Marion; Severinghaus, A. E.;
         and Miller, George. "The Intern and Resident Situa-
         tion in the Voluntary Hospitals: A Panel Discussion
         Before the Members of the American Medical Women's
         Association at the Annual Meeting in Atlantic City, June
         4, 1949." Journal of the American Medical Women's
         Association, 4:9 (September 1949) 359-373. (Introduc-
         tory remarks by Elise S. L'Esperance and postscript
         remarks by Emerson Day.)
         In this panel discussion of conditions for women as interns
         and residents, a number of examples of discrimination
         against women are mentioned. Examples of discrimination
         include the fact that less than 4 per cent of the residencies
         at the 107 hospitals approved by the American Medical
         Association go to women. Co-educational medical schools
         still had a quota in accepting women students so that, "Yes,
         indeed, we take women, and we do not want one woman we
         take to be lonesome, so we take two per class." While
         some schools will accept two women, others will accept
         four. Coeducational medical schools will err in the other
         direction of a quota system by accepting women who are
         improperly qualified to study medicine and who drop out.
         The reason given against accepting women by male medical
         faculty is that women marry and drop out of practice. In
         fact, 91 to 93.5 per cent of the women who have had medi-
         cal training practice medicine. Associate Dean of the Col-
         lege of Physicians and Surgeons, Columbia University, Dr.
         Severinghaus was proud that his school had the largest num-
         ber of women medical graduates ever: 22 in a class of 108.

2072   Mann, Kristine. "Medical Women's Handicap." Harper's
         Weekly, 58 (28 February 1914) 32.
         The public erroneously believes women physicians are now
         on equal footing with men. While women have access to a
         medical education equal to men, women have a severe handi-
         cap in sex in gaining hospital appointments as interns.

2073.   "Mothers 'Liberate' Specialty Training."   Medical World
         News, (13 July 1973) 68-69.
         A "Mother's Program" for residents means shorter hours
         and take five years rather than four to complete.   A psy-
         chiatry residency program is given as an example.   [Article
         not examined by editors.]

2074.   "New Program to Retrain Inactive Women Physicians at
         WMCP."   Journal of the American Medical Women's
         Association, 23:3 (March 1968) 285.
         The Woman's Medical College of Pennsylvania (WMCP) re-
         ceived a $30,000 grant from the Josiah Macy Jr. Founda-
         tion in October 1968 to retrain women physicians.   At the
         time this article was written, 250 women physicians were
         not in full-time practice within a 100-mile radius of Phila-
         delphia.   Ethel Weinberg will assist the president of WMCP,
         Dr. Leymaster, in establishing this program, which will
         include a systematic and comprehensive review of diseases
         including basic mechanisms, pathophysiology, diagnosis,
         and management.   This program will emphasize new tech-
         niques and knowledge and give trainees an opportunity to
         work in clinics, accident wards, and with inpatient care.
         The program will be tailored to the needs of each partici-
         pant.   Each student will have the opportunity to study for
         six months full-time, or 12 months half-time.

2075.   "Opportunities for Medical Women--1942."   Medical Woman's
         Journal, 49:6 (June 1942) 167-180.
         The Opportunities Committee of the American Medical Wo-
         men's Association sent questionnaires to hospitals approved
         by the AMA for internships.   Of the 866 replies, 463 hos-
         pitals take or are willing to take women graduate students.
         The text of the questionnaire and a state-by-state listing of
         replies are included.

2076.   "Part-Time Internship Program Designed to Salvage Moth-
         ers with MD Degrees."   Medical Post, (7 May 1968) 11.
         [Article not examined by editors.]

2077.   Paterson, Susanne J.   "Post-Graduate Study in the United
         States."   Medical Women's Federation News-Letter,
         (April 1933) 45-48.
         Dr. Paterson speaks of opportunities for study at the Mayo
         Clinic (Rochester, Minnesota).

2078.   Reardon, Rosalie M.   "Dear Colleagues."   Medical Woman's
         Journal, 56:10 (October 1949) 29.
         This article, the first in a proposed monthly feature of the
         Journal, offers information on opportunities for women in
         internships and residencies.   The appointments of several
         specific women are mentioned.

2079.   Reardon, Rosalie [M].   "Dear Colleagues."   Medical Wo-

man's Journal, 56:12 (December 1949) 45, 50.
Information on opportunities for women in internships and
residencies includes the recent appointments of several specific women.

2080.   Scanlan, Theresa; Pierce, Clara M.; Beyer, M. Virginia;
         Koeneke, Irene A.; and Woolley, Alice Stone. "Oppor-
         tunities for Medical Women." Medical Woman's Jour-
         nal, 50:5 (May 1943) 127. (Editorial.)
One thousand and thirty-two questionnaires were sent in
1941 to the superintendents of hospitals approved for the
training of interns and residents, by the Council on Medical
Education and the American Medical Association: 866 replies were received. Of these 866, 463 were taking or
willing to take women interns and residents. Since the
questionnaire was sent, war had broken out and changed the
complexion of the medical field. The American Medical Women's Association had received requests for women physicians to fill hospital posts but, due to the inavailability of
a list of applicants, was not able to be of much help. Other requests have come from communities with openings.
In general, the field is opening up for women physicians.

2081.   Smart, Isabelle Thompson. "Report on Internships." Wo-
         man's Medical Journal, 27:6 (June 1917) 142-146. (Pre-
         sentation, Second Annual Meeting, Medical Women's Na-
         tional Association, 6 June 1917.)
As chairman of the committee on interneships, Dr. Smith
sent letters to 752 hospitals in an effort to gain data concerning internship opportunities for women. Of those responding (293 hospitals "did not have the courtesy to reply"),
132 hospitals claimed to favor women interns; 240 were
either not in favor of, or lacked suitable accommodations
for women; 87 were indefinite, i.e., either never had women interns or never received application from women.
Dr. Smart's report includes the responses of specific institutions and offers suggestions for what the Association can
do to increase graduate medical openings for women.

2082.   Smart, Isabelle T[hompson]. "Report on Interneships for
         Women." Woman's Medical Journal, 27:2 (February
         1917) 37-38. charts.
This report lists hospitals that are known to accept women
as interns, what the entrance requirements are, and what
the hospital does and does not supply in the way of compensation.

2083.   Smart, Isabelle T[hompson]. "Report on Interneships for
         Women." Woman's Medical Journal, 27:3 (March 1917)
         58-59. chart.
A list of hospitals that will accept women as interns is
given.

2084.   Smart, Isabelle T[hompson]. "Report on Interneships for
        Women." Woman's Medical Journal, 27:4 (April 1917)
        88-89. table.
        A table provides data on several general hospitals, and a
        "note" offers information on New York's state hospitals.

2085.   Smart, Isabelle T[hompson]. "Report on Interneships for
        Women." Woman's Medical Journal, 27:7 (July 1917)
        162-163. table.
        Data is provided on internship opportunities at general hos-
        pitals in several states.

2086.   South, Virginia. "Internships for Women." Medical Wo-
        man's Journal, 43:8 (August 1936) 217.
        A medical student outlines the difficulties of locating hos-
        pitals that accept women interns.

2087.   "Special Studies in Graduate Medical Education." Journal
        of the American Medical Association, 210:8 (24 Novem-
        ber 1969) 1542-1555. tables. (Special Studies.)
        This article includes a section on women physicians serving
        in graduate education as of September 1, 1968. (Data pro-
        vided is the result of a questionnaire sent to hospitals to
        obtain information for the 1969-1970 Directory.) Findings
        show that 657 women graduates filled nine per cent of the
        positions filled by all U.S. and Canadian graduates in in-
        ternship programs, while women comprised only eight per
        cent of the 1968 graduating class; women make up 18 per
        cent of positions filled by foreign graduates. Women held
        12 per cent of all filled positions. Part-time internships
        for women were offered by 62 (7 per cent) of the 857 hos-
        pitals. Six per cent of U.S. graduates serving residencies
        were women; women comprised 16 per cent of the residen-
        cies filled by foreign graduates. Of all filled resident posi-
        tions, nine per cent were women. Of the 1,023 hospitals
        responding to the question of part-time residencies, 61 per
        cent answered affirmatively. The largest proportion of wo-
        men filled pediatric residencies, making up 27 per cent of
        the total. Only 53 out of 1,035 hospitals offered refresher
        courses to women who have been out of practice. Data on
        women physicians on teaching staffs indicate that 2,991 wo-
        men teach in graduate programs (1,770 as part-timers).

2088.   "Statistical Report on Women Physicians in Illinois Hospitals."
        Bulletin Medical Women's Club of Chicago, 13:4 (De-
        cember 1924) (unpaged). table.
        The information offered in this report was obtained through
        a questionnaire sent out by the Medical Women's Club of
        Chicago to hospitals throughout the state of Illinois. A
        table lists these hospitals by name and indicates for each
        institution whether women interns are accepted, whether wo-
        men are staff members, whether there are medical clinics
        in the hospital, whether there are sufficient nurses in train-

ing school, and whether the hospital has difficulty in securing help.

2089.   Thomas, Mary A. "Is There a Need for Postgraduate Part-
            Time Training Programs?" The Woman Physician, 26:
            11 (November 1971) 551-552.
         There are some medical school graduates who, after gradua-
         tion, must postpone further training because of various ob-
         ligations which prevent a full time internship or residency.
         AMWA receives many letters requesting the names of schools
         offering part-time or flexible training programs. In hopes
         of assessing the specific needs of women physicians for
         these programs, AMWA sent out questionnaires to 1500
         junior members: 428 responses were received. Of these,
         275 indicated an interest in such programs. Seventy-nine
         per cent (178) of 224 married women indicated an interest.
         Seventy-four of 174 single women responded in the affirma-
         tive. One respondent felt that "'part-time internships and
         residency programs should be available for election by phy-
         sicians of either sex and without a demand for explanation
         of reasons.'"

2090.   Van Hoosen, Bertha. "Correspondence Consultation Depart-
            ment." Medical Woman's Journal, 35:8 (August 1928)
            235-236.
         Several distinguished women physicians wrote replies to the
         following inquiry received by the Journal: Is it desirable
         for young women graduates in medicine to take their turn,
         when interning, in the male genito-urinary service?" S.
         Josephine Baker, seeing no "real reason" for women to
         avoid the service, draws the analogy of a gynecological ser-
         vice for men.

2091.   Van Hoosen, Bertha. "Opportunities for Medical Women as
            Interns." Medical Woman's Journal, 33:3 (March 1926)
            65-66.
         Currently, 127 American hospitals offering accommodations
         for 1,407 interns accept women applicants for internships.
         Hospitals open to men number 527, with 3,832 internships
         available. "The worst feature in the statistics are that,
         when actually put to the test, many of these hospitals will
         not consider a woman intern unless it is impossible to get
         a desirable man." Appended to the article is a list of in-
         stitutions willing to receive women interns.

2092.   Van Hoosen, Bertha. "Opportunities for Medical Women as
            Internes." Medical Woman's Journals, 34:4 (April 1927)
            106-108.
         Very few of the nearly 25 hospitals under Jewish manage-
         ment in the U.S. admit women as interns, the main reason
         cited being lack of proper accommodations. An explanation
         of Jewish customs precedes descriptions of notable Jewish
         hospitals.

2093.   Van Hoosen, Bertha. "Opportunities for Medical Women as
        Internes." Medical Woman's Journal, 34:5 (May 1927)
        138-139.
        Making a plea for equal opportunities for black medical wo-
        men, Dr. Van Hoosen lists the hospitals that accept black
        interns. "... only 21 out of the 1,696 hospitals having ac-
        credited schools for nurses ... used colored internes, and
        of these 14 were hospitals for colored patients." "[White]
        women who have themselves suffered accusations of mental
        inferiority--who have been denied educational opportunities--
        who have only recently obtained the vote, and who are still
        only half-heartedly given opportunities for advancement ...
        should shake themselves free from mean prejudice and as-
        sist the Negro in getting education and contact."

2094.   Van Hoosen, Bertha. "Opportunities for Medical Women In-
        terns: A Series of Articles on this Interesting and Im-
        portant Subject (Continued)." Medical Woman's Journal,
        33:4 (April 1926) 102-105.
        Correspondence with the superintendents of the hospitals
        listed in the American Medical Association directory as
        being approved for internships, revealed that the "most out-
        standing difficulty in women being appointed to internships
        on an equality with men seems to be the lack of housing ac-
        commodations for the two sexes." The author lists those
        hospitals that would consider admitting women interns, those
        that would accept women when "proper housing facilities"
        are found, and those that are "lukewarm" on the subject.
        Many hospitals report dissatisfaction with the service of the
        woman intern. One hospital official wrote that one woman
        "unfortunately used her good looks to win favor with the
        [chief residents] when her work was not properly finished."
        Also, women interns "are not so popular with the genito-
        urinary service as the men interns."

2095.   Van Hoosen, Bertha. "Opportunities for Medical Women
        Interns." Medical Woman's Journal, 33:5 (May 1926)
        126-128.
        The superintendents of 41 hospitals report that the work of
        women interns was not as satisfactory as that of men; 81
        hospitals say the services of women interns has equalled
        that of the men's. One objection to women interns is in
        reference to ambulance duty, though it is not clear whether
        institutions are unwilling to give ambulance service to wo-
        men or whether women refuse to accept the responsibility.
        Another complaint is that women interns cannot handle male
        genito-urinary services. Institutions must be convinced that
        women interns do not want "sex privileges." Bertha Van
        Hoosen urges the young medical student to "understand that
        she is not only making a reputation for herself, but that her
        success in hospital work makes a great difference with the
        rapidity with which all women may be received in all hos-
        pitals on an equality with the male students." Recalling the

pioneer women physicians who "would risk their lives rather
than not be equal to the performance of their duty," Dr.
Van Hoosen says, "this is no time for the medical woman
to dare lag behind or to look for special favors.... 'No
man liveth to himself,' and this perhaps is nowhere more
significant than in the life of the present-day woman intern."

2096.   Van Hoosen, Bertha. "Opportunities for Medical Women In-
            terns." Medical Woman's Journal, 33:7 (July 1926)
            194-195.
         Unless the hospitals for women and children offer general
         services, the AMA cannot approve those hospitals for intern-
         ship. Therefore, all women's hospitals should affiliate with
         medical schools or see that all branches of medical work
         are well represented in their own hospitals. Women's hos-
         pitals should offer opportunities to women interns that can-
         not be obtained in hospitals staffed by men. At present,
         Bellevue Hospital in New York City gives opportunities for
         more women than any other institution in the world. Other
         hospitals in which large numbers of women intern are listed.

2097.   Van Hoosen, Bertha. "Opportunities for Medical Women In-
            terns." Medical Woman's Journal, 33:8 (August 1926)
            228-230.
         Dr. Van Hoosen emphasizes the importance of carefully se-
         lecting the hospital where the medical woman serves her in-
         ternship.

2098.   Van Hoosen, Bertha. "Opportunities for Medical Women In-
            terns." Medical Woman's Journal, 33:9 (September
            1926) 257-258.
         This general discussion of the decisions a woman should
         make before entering the fifth year of medical work advises
         young physicians to question whether to teach or practice,
         what specialty to follow, and where to locate.

2099.   Van Hoosen, Bertha. "Opportunities for Medical Women
            Interns." Medical Woman's Journal, 33:10 (October
            1926) 281-284.
         The history of medical women is divided into three eras:
         the establishment of women's medical schools and hospitals;
         the opening of schools and hospitals previously closed to
         women; and the representation of women on medical school
         faculties in proportion to the number of women students en-
         rolled, and also the representation of women on hospital
         staffs in proportion to the number of women practicing in
         the hospital's community. "Until the medical woman has
         passed through all these phases of development, we have no
         right to judge her as a success or failure in the medical
         profession." The difficulties that women encountered at
         Chicago's Cook County Hospital are recounted. In 1881,
         Mary Bates became its first woman intern, and among her
         struggles was the attempt to hold her own with fellow in-

terns. In one especially vivid incident, the male interns
burst into her room at night, and "like real cave men, carried her off ... to the gynecological ward to be entered as
an interesting case ... the affair ended by a nurse bringing
her her clothes...." The conditions under which Dr. Bates
interned is contrasted with the much improved conditions
under which women interns work presently at Cook County.

2100.   Van Hoosen, Bertha. "Opportunities for Medical Women
            Interns." Medical Woman's Journal, 33:12 (December
            1926) 341-343.
         In 1913 Dr. Frank Billings, dean of Rush Medical College,
         addressed a gathering of medical women, Bertha Van Hoosen
         among them. "Women medical students ... make good
         grades and are faithful in every way, but after they gradu-
         ate who hears of them? Where do they go?" he asked.
         Dr. Van Hoosen and the others "were shocked at Dr. Bill-
         ings' rude, and ... unwarranted, attack...." After men-
         tioning the accomplishments of notable women physicians,
         Dr. Van Hoosen compares the views of the women physi-
         cian with the attitudes towards the Negro. She suggests
         that "men taught" schools and male-staffed hospitals de-
         velop an inferiority complex in the woman student. Seventy-
         five per cent of women who are members of the American
         College of Surgeons attended women's colleges or interned
         at hospitals staffed by women.

2101.   Van Hoosen, Bertha. "Opportunities for Medical Women
            Internes." Medical Woman's Journal, 34:3 (March
            1927) 68-70.
         Of the 6,694 hospitals in the U.S., 520 are maintained by
         the Roman Catholic Church, and 25 of those hospitals are
         AMA-approved for internship. The opportunities for wo-
         men interns in Catholic hospitals are examined.

2102.   Wallace, Joyce. "Part-Time Internships and Residencies:
            Programs to Be Encouraged." Journal of the Ameri-
            can Medical Women's Association, 24:7 (July 1969) 566-
            570. photos.
         In 1964 the American Medical Association committee on
         graduate medical education issued a statement which in ef-
         fect "allows" and does not "discourage" alternatives to the
         traditional internship schedule for physician mothers. Dr.
         Wallace gives an account of her seeking a part-time intern-
         ship and her consequent experience in this half-time pro-
         gram at St. Vincent's Hospital in New York's Greenwich
         Village. She concludes her article with advice on "How to
         Get a Part-Time Program."

2103.   Weinberg, Ethel. "Part-time Residency Training." Journal
            of the American Medical Association, 210:8 (24 Novem-
            ber 1969) 1435-1437. table.
         "In order to make medicine a more feasible career choice

for women and in order to increase the level of training
and, therefore, the quality of practice, it is important to
decrease the scheduling rigidity of standard residency training programs. The steadily increasing numbers of women
in medical school makes the problem more pressing at this
time. This communication reports the result of a survey
of the specialty boards concerning the acceptability of part-
time training. [All boards will consider part-time training
on an individual basis except pathology.]... Part-time
specialty training does merit a trial." [Article abstract.]

2104.   Weinberg, Ethel. "Retraining Physicians." Journal of Med-
         ical Education, 47:8 (August 1972) 625-630. table.
         At the time this article was written, there were 2,000 phy-
         sicians in the United States under the age of 55 not in med-
         ical practice. The Medical College of Pennsylvania estab-
         lished a three-day-a-week, 9 A.M. to 4 P.M. retraining
         program which included lectures by clinicians, inpatient and
         outpatient rotations in areas of interest, patient work-ups,
         rounds, and conferences. A six-week program, offered to
         physicians who could not commute from where they lived,
         included a review of general medicine, and training in his-
         tory-taking and physical examination. The spirit of cama-
         raderie in this program has been invaluable. Forty-nine
         physicians have finished this program. Some participants
         had practiced in specialties intermittently, others had been
         uprooted several times because of their husbands' careers.
         Several men participated in the program. Some had been
         inactive for personal reasons, others because they wanted
         to change their specialty. Fifteen years of inactivity seems
         to be the maximum absence from the field of medicine to
         enable one to return to practice.

2105.   Willard, L. "Campaigning for More Opportunities in Medi-
         cine: Internships for Women." Independent Woman,
         18 (June 1939) 174.
         [Article not examined by editors.]

2106.   "The Woman Intern Problem." Medical Woman's Journal,
         45:10 (October 1938) 309. (Editorial.)
         An investigation conducted by the Internship Committee of
         Alpha Epsilon Iota (a national women's medical fraternity)
         reveals that of the 725 hospitals approved by the American
         Medical Association for internship training, only 23 per cent
         accept women. The remaining 77 per cent refuse women
         interns due to supposed housing problems or definite an-
         tipathy toward women physicians. Notes Dr. Luvia Willard,
         the report's author, "Many of these were publicly owned
         hospitals supported by the very women taxpayers who were
         refused admission."

2107.   "The Woman Interne." Interne, 4:1 (January 1938) 31-32.
         (Letters to the Editor.)

An unidentified woman intern attacks the justifications given by hospital officials for refusing to accept women interns. "Against these arguments we are weak because prejudice rather than reason is an almost insurmountable wall."

2108.   "A Woman Interne." Woman's Medical Journal, 6:2 (February 1897) 37-38.
Despite a two-year-old mandatory law providing for women interns in various state hospitals, no woman has yet been appointed to the Ohio State Hospital for the Insane. Officials at the Toledo, Ohio institution say no funds are available to pay a woman.

2109.   "Women Internes." Medical Woman's Journal, 39:10 (October 1932) 259.
Of the 696 accredited hospitals for internships in the United States, only 99 accept women as interns.

2110.   "Women Interns." Medical Woman's Journal, 42:10 (October 1935) 277. (Editorial.)
"Of the 697 hospitals approved for internship training in the United States and its possessions, 127 accept women."

2111.   "Women Physicians Eligible." Medical Woman's Journal, 47:10 (October 1940) 311.
The U.S. Civil Service Commission announced examinations to fill an internship and a residency position at Washington, D.C.'s St. Elizabeth Hospital. The Civil Service reported that the exam is open to both men and women, but that "the department or office requesting certification of eligibles has the legal right to specify the sex desired."

MEDICAL ACTIVITY

Statistical and narrative material covers
practice patterns, specialties, teaching,
and administration. (Material discussing
societal attitudes or cultural patterns which
ultimately affect medical activity is cited
in the PSYCHOSOCIAL FACTORS classification.)

2112.   Klempman, Sarah; Naudé, Anneke te Water; and Rennie,
        Joan. "Women Doctors." <u>South African Medical Jour-
        nal</u>, 44 (11 April 1970) 460. (Letters to the Editor.)
These letters are reactions to an editorial which stated
that women physicians may be expected to be out of active
practice for over a year of their professional life. Klempman feels that male physicians represent a permanent loss
to medicine in South Africa because of their annual exodus
to other countries. Anneke te Water Naudé cites the reasons women doctors are a good risk and feels that the editorial represents another attempt to limit the number of women medical students. Joan Rennie states that cold statistics are necessary to substantiate the editorial claim. In
a footnote, the editor declares correspondence on the subject
closed and regrets that "unfortunately, virtually all our cor-
respondents have misunderstood the article."

2113.   Klenerman, Pauline. "Medical Women in South Africa."
        <u>Medical Women's Federation Quarterly Review</u>, (July
        1936) 64-65. (Correspondence.)
Dr. Klenerman discusses conditions in South Africa for the
benefit of those women physicians who feel they might wish
to practice there. "The idea of a woman doctor was stag-
gering to the inhabitants" but ultimately the women and children were joyous, and occasionally a male patient would express approval.

2114.   Naudé, Anneke te Water. "Women Doctors." <u>South African
        Medical Journal</u>, 44:15 (11 April 1970) 460. (Letters
        to the Editor.)
Training women to be doctors is a good risk for the following reasons: women outlive men and therefore are able
to give more years of service; men change their occupations; women physicians made a significant contribution
during World War II when they replaced their male colleagues in giving medical care to the civilian population;
and, when women doctors are able to hold low-paying part-
time jobs, they not only repay society for the investment
it has made in them but they also help to keep the tax structure from spiralling higher.

2115.   Péraud, J. M. [The Woman Physician in North Africa and
        <u>Her Role in Education</u>]. Bordeaux, France, 1932.
        90 pp. (Fre)
[Book not examined by editors.]

ASIA

2116.   Balfour, Margaret I.; Young, Ruth; and Scharlieb, Mary.
         The Work of Medical Women in India. Humphrey Mil-
         ford, Oxford University Press, London, England, 1929,
         xiv, 201 pp. map, photos., ports.
         This book reviews the role of women in medical service to
         India, from the arrival in 1869 of the first woman physician
         (Clara Swain of the U.S.) to 1929. At the end of the 60-
         year period, 183 hospitals were staffed by women, and
         there were 698 women studying medicine. This history
         covers the work of missionaries, the Women's Medical Ser-
         vice for India, and women physicians independently employed
         in various government situations. Women physicians worked
         principally in the fields of maternity and child welfare; data
         on the condition of Indian women are detailed and health
         statistics taken from Dufferin Fund annual reports are given.
         References to the various English, American, and Indian wo-
         men who served in India are numerous and listed in the in-
         dex. The foreword is written by Dame Mary Scharlieb, one
         of the earliest medical pioneers; her portrait is included, as
         are pictures of Clara Swain, Elizabeth Bielby, and Edith
         Pechey Phipson. The principal author, Margaret Balfour,
         was chief medical officer of the Women's Medical Service;
         Ruth Young was her assistant.

2117.   "British Medical Women in India." British Medical Journal,
         (27 June 1925) 1195. (Correspondence.)
         A medical woman questions whether there is really unlimited
         scope for women in India. Her doubts are predicated upon
         advertisements for physicians in newspapers and the natu-
         ralizing of the medical population in India, in addition to
         the lack of ads for physicians for state service in British
         India.

2118.   Brodie, Jessie Laird. "President's Message." Journal of
         the American Medical Women's Association, 15:2 (Febru-
         ary 1960) 175.
         In Pakistan, it is reported that for the ten years before this
         article was written, there were on the average 30 women to
         70 men in a medical class. Few of these women could
         practice, however, because in Pakistan, "no husband will
         allow his wife to work." Jessie Brodie inquires of her
         Pakistan informant, "there surely must be some way you
         could continue to practice medicine without renouncing mar-
         riage and the possibility of a home and family." "Not un-
         less I stay an old maid." In the United States, physician-
         mothers with small children continue to contribute as "ex-
         tremely valuable and influential consultants on P.T.A. com-
         mittees and in voluntary community organizations such as
         heart, allergy, poliomyelitis, muscular dystrophy and other
         associations." Because many physician-mothers anticipate
         reentering practice, they need part-time medical work dur-

ing these years to "stimulate and enhance the alertness, judgment, and skill that makes them valuable community leaders among mothers with less preparation."

2119.   Fischer, Golda. "Medical Women in Israel: Their Fields
of Work." Journal of the American Medical Women's
Association, 7:6 (June 1952) 215-217. photos.
At the time of this article (Part III in a series of three
articles), nearly half of the women physicians in Israel
were over 50 years of age, and less than one-fifth were
under 40. General practice, pediatrics, and obstetrics and
gynecology head the list of specialties. How these women
live and how and where they practice is discussed. [Part
I in this series deals with historical perspectives, and Part
II considers biographical data.]

2120.   Hoggan, Frances Elizabeth. "Medical Women for India."
Contemporary Review, 42 (August 1882) 267-275.
"Reason, propriety, and that tolerance of national usage
which has been the rule followed by [the British] Government in all dealings with our Indian fellow-subjects, point
to the substitution of medical women for medical men in
all the institutions subsidized by Government for the treatment of native women." This article thoroughly documents,
through historical background and current information, India's need for women physicians. The article further offers advice to the British woman physician who wishes to
serve in India, suggests funding proposals, and makes
procedure suggestions for achieving medical care for women
by women.

2121.   Jhirad, J. "Careers for Medical Women in India." World
Medical Journal, 11:1 (January 1964) 29-30.
The number of women physicians in India is on the increase.
Women are being attracted to various specialties other than
obstetrics and gynecology. Marriage has not been a hin-
drance to women in medicine, and 60 per cent of the women
physicians in practice are married.

2122.   MacCorquodale, Donald W. "Sex Differentials Among Family Planning Physicians in the Philippines." Health
Services Reports, 88:10 (December 1973) 963-967.
tables.
The author concludes that there are few differences between
men and women physicians who work in family planning in
the Philippines. More men physicians than women physicians
would recommend tubal ligation as a contraceptive method,
while more women than men would recommend a vasectomy.
While neither female nor male physicians differ on preference for intrauterine devices (IUDs), women physicians have
a higher percentage of IUD acceptors than men physicians
do.

2123.   "Medical Women in India." The Doctor and Od Quarterly,
            48:1 (January 1938) 1-2.
         In 1870, Clara Swain became the first woman physician to
         go to India. Anandibai Joshi was one of the first Indian
         women to study medicine. Another Indian woman, Anni
         Jaganadhan, was appointed house surgeon to Cama Hospital
         in 1892. Rukhmabai, a graduate of the London School of
         Medicine (1895), took charge of first the Women's Hospital
         at Surat, then the Zanana State Hospital, Rajkot. Currently
         there are about 200 hospitals in India staffed by women.
         There is an Association of Medical Women in India, a med-
         ical college at Delhi staffed by women, and 12 provincial
         centers of the Countess of Dufferin's Fund. Many Indian wo-
         men physicians engage in private practice.

2124.   "The Power of Team Work." Medical Woman's Journal,
            39:9 (September 1932) 229-230.
         In response to the "Semi-Jubilee" issue of the Journal of
         the Association of Medical Women in India, this editorial
         reiterates the benefits that medical women are able to
         realize when they work closely together, in terms of pro-
         fessional support, professional research, and professional
         patient care of women's health problems--not only in India
         but other countries as well.

2125.   Stinson, Mary H. Work of Women Physicians in Asia, by
            Mary H. Stinson, M.D., of Norristown, Pa., Read be-
            fore the State Medical Society of Pennsylvania, at Its
            Meeting in Philadelphia, 1884. J. H. Brandt, Norris-
            town, Pennsylvania, 1884, 30 pp.
         [Item not examined by editors.]

2126.   Szkop-Frankiel, Susana. "Supply." Journal of the Ameri-
            can Medical Women's Association, 22:5 (May 1967) 339-
            340.
         This article gives a regional report for the Medical Women's
         International Association on the countries of Madagascar,
         India, and Israel. Madagascar has 4.6 per cent women phy-
         sicians (3 per cent actually practicing; the rest are still stu-
         dents). Of these, 45 per cent are in hospitals and general
         practice, 50 per cent are in public health, and only one wo-
         man is in the private practice of internal medicine. In In-
         dia, two per cent of the physicians are women, with 42 per
         cent of them in general practice. Israel had, in 1963 (the
         latest figures available), 24 per cent women physicians with
         26.3 per cent in pediatrics and 20 per cent in general medi-
         cine.

2127.   Thomson, Bertha M. "Opportunities for Medical Women in
            India." Medical Woman's Journal, 39:10 (October 1932)
            251-254. (Presentation, Nebraska Women's Medical
            Association, Lincoln, Nebraska, May 24, 1932.)
         Because of the cultural customs of high caste Hindus and

Mohammedans, women in these families may only be seen by the men in their families. Hence, there is great need for women physicians in India. At the time this article was written, American and British Missionary women physicians were involved in direct patient care in mission hospitals. India needed native women physicians. Because there was no co-educational schooling, there was a great need for women physicians to serve on the faculties of the two existing women's medical colleges. The Government also has hospitals and dispensaries. "Some of these hospitals are very well equipped and staffed by English surgeons and Indian assistant surgeons. In a large number of these, women physicians are employed as well as English nurses for hospital superintendents."

AUSTRALIA & NEW ZEALAND

2128.   Alexander, W. S. "Women in Medicine." New Zealand
        Medical Journal, 73 (April 1971) 238. (Letters to the
        Editor.)
        This letter corrects the minutes of the Central Education
        Committee council meeting of December 1970 (published in
        February 1971 in the New Zealand Medical Journal) in which
        it was stated that women do not return to medical work after
        they have dropped out to raise their families. The author
        responds that overseas surveys indicate that 20-25 per cent
        women graduates are not working at any given time; 50 per
        cent are working full-time, and the balance work part-time.
        The author offers to cooperate with the New Zealand Medical Women's Association when they attempt to ascertain the
        situation in New Zealand.

2129.   Battersby, Cameron. "Fifteen Years On." Medical Journal
        of Australia, 2:8 (23 August 1975) 314-316. table.
        (Presentation, Australasian Association for Medical Education, Canberra, Australia, August, 1973.)
        "Sixty students who graduated from the University of Queensland in 1958 were traced 15 years later. Sixty per cent
        were in private practice and 40 per cent were in full-time
        salaried jobs. Those who ultimately became physicians had
        the best average course performance. [There was no difference in course performance between male and female students.] After specialization, there appeared to be a tendency for the less academically able students to take on full-time salaried jobs rather than to enter private practice.
        Seventy per cent of women were still in substantially full-time practice." [Article abstract.]

2130.   Constable, Judith A. "Women in Medicine." The Medical
        Journal of Australia, 1:9 (27 February 1971) 500-501.
        (Letters to the Editor.)
        Regardless of the United Nations Charter on Human Rights

that states there should be no discrimination because of
sex, the medical profession in practice does discriminate
against women. For a woman physician to want marriage
and children means she has to give up practice of her profession because of: the unavailability and/or unsatisfactory
aspects of part-time and full-time work; the disadvantage of
having had to take time off during the early years of her
career and attempting to return to practice without enough
professional experience; the lack of child care centers at
hospitals for all women employees so that if they want to
breast feed their babies, they can, and time is not lost
delivering the babies and children elsewhere; and the lack
of tax relief for babysitting expenses.

2131.   Dixon, C. W. and Manley, D. C. E.   "Medical Council of
         New Zealand: Report on the 1973 and 1974 Question-
         naires, with Particular Reference to House Surgeons
         and Registrars."   New Zealand Medical Journal, 82:547
         (10 September 1975) 173-174.
In this annual survey of the medical profession, data are
reported on women practitioners. Fourteen per cent of
New Zealand graduate house surgeons and registrars are
women; their proportion is expected to increase rapidly in
the near future. Career specialization choices for women
as compared with men are also reported.

2132.   Fett, [M]. Ione.   "Australian Medical Graduates in 1972."
         Medical Journal of Australia, 1:18 (4 May 1974) 689-
         698.   figs., tables.   (Original Articles.)
"This paper reports findings from a survey of Australian
medical graduates carried out in 1972. An account is given
of trends in practice from 1920 to 1969, of present distribution in occupational areas, and sex differentials in medical practice. A general trend is shown from individual to
group practice, from longer to shorter hours of medical
work, from non-salaried to salaried forms of practice, and
from medical to non-medical work. Exceptions are that the
participation of women graduates in both medical and nonmedical work is increasing. The effect of marriage and
parenthood on practice by graduates of both sexes is shown."
[Article abstract.]

2133.   Fett, M. Ione.   "The Monash University Survey of Austra-
         lian Women Medical Graduates."   Medical Journal of
         Australia, 1:17 (24 April 1971) 920-922.   tables.
This article is a response to an editorial that appeared in
The Medical Journal of Australia titled, "Women in Medicine," January 9, 1971, that erroneously reported that 60
per cent of Australia's women doctors are not practicing
medicine. This author's statistical research as of December
1970 found that 14.7 women were not practicing; nearly 56
per cent were engaged in full-time work (35 hours or more
per week), and of these 22.5 per cent had children under 16,

another 7.5 per cent are working part-time (20-34 hours per week), and 10 per cent are doing no medical work at the present time.

2134.   Fett, [M]. Ione. "Women in Medicine." Medical Journal of Australia, 1:12 (20 March 1971) 660-661. tables. (Letters to the Editor.)
In response to a previous correspondent's "perturbation" about the number of women doctors not practicing, the author cites data from the survey of women doctors. The percentage of women physicians married, those married to medical men, the hours per week worked, and the husbands' attitudes about their wives' employment are discussed.

2135.   Greenslade, N. F. "The Medical Profession in New Zealand: Answers to the Medical Council Questionnaire of 1972." New Zealand Medical Journal, 77 (February 1973) 107-108. (Report.)
This article reports physicians' practice patterns in New Zealand, gathered from responses to a questionnaire sent in 1972 to doctors holding practicing certificates in 1971. A total of 82 per cent returned the questionnaire. The increased number of women students accepted at New Zealand medical schools is not reflected in the findings of this report because these women had not commenced practice. Therefore the ratio of 88 per cent men and 11 per cent women recorded by this report is the same as the ratio of male and female doctors qualifying for certificates in 1930, and the same as that in the 1967 and 1968 survey. Of those physicians polled, 60 per cent had additional medical and nonmedical qualifications--67 per cent men and 49 per cent women, which is virtually the same as existed before 1930. Identical with the 1967 and 1968 surveys is the percentage of female and male physicians in general practice: 8 per cent women and 92 per cent men.

2136.   Heslop, Barbara F.; Molloy, Robyn J.; Waal-Manning, Hendrika J.; and Walsh, Ngaire M. "Women in Medicine in New Zealand." New Zealand Medical Journal, 77:491 (April 1973) 219-229. tables.
"Professional activity and factors influencing it were investigated in 313 out of the 374 women graduates of the University of Otago Medical School who were living in 1970-71, and in 118 out of 141 registered women doctors from overseas medical schools who were resident in New Zealand. The total professional activity of each doctor was expressed as a percentage of the maximum work possible during the time which had elapsed since graduation (i.e., continuous full-time work or postgraduate study). New Zealand-trained women doctors showed a median professional activity of 87 per cent ... while the corresponding figure for graduates of overseas medical schools was 70 per cent.... Only two women had not worked since graduation. Those Otago grad-

uates who lived overseas (22 per cent) showed greater professional activity than the 78 per cent residing in this country, but the composition of the sample partly accounted for
this.   In general specialists were professionally more active
than non-specialists.   Among New Zealand-trained doctors,
undergraduate excellence was unrelated to subsequent professional activity.   Motherhood was the main reason for reducing medical work; marriage without children was associated with a relatively small work reduction.   Not all of
the 280 women doctors with children gave up professional
work; 19 per cent worked full-time apart from maternity
leave, 22 per cent merely reduced their professional commitments, 41 per cent stopped working for varying periods
of time but subsequently resumed, and 18 per cent were not
working at the time of the survey.   A number of doctors returned to medicine after long absences--ten after 16-20
years of professional inactivity, 14 after 11-15 years and
29 after 6-10 years.   Loss of confidence was the main difficulty associated with the return to professional work.
Domestic considerations influenced job selection for approximately one out of two women doctors.   Of 220 doctors who
employed domestic help 40 per cent never had trouble finding suitable staff and 35 per cent experienced difficulty only
occasionally.   There were in this country in 1971 seven medical women under the age of 65 who were not working and
who intended to resume professional work, and 60 who were
working part-time but intended ultimately to increase their
professional commitments.   The small number of potential
candidates raised some doubts about the feasibility of retraining courses.   With few exceptions medical women were
enthusiastic about medicine as a career for women, although
the majority expressed reservations which were mainly related to the difficulty in combining marriage and children
with professional work to the detriment of neither.   There
was a noticeable absence of women from the top professional
and administrative positions in New Zealand, a situation at
last partly attributable to lack of interest." [Article abstract.]

2137.   Holland, R. "Women in Medicine." Medical Journal of
          Australia, 1:6 (6 February 1971) 349. (Correspondence.)
        Referring to an editorial (Medical Journal of Australia, 9
        January 1971) which stated that 60 per cent of Australian
        women doctors are not practicing, this writer reasons that
        grave doctor shortages will not be the only serious conse-
        quence.   Due to medical school quota systems, "competent,
        well-motivated males" will never get the opportunity to
        study medicine; they will be "'redirected' to other occupa-
        tions, which may, for them, carry much less job satisfac-
        tion."   Restrictions on female enrollment "may well be a
        social necessity."

2138.   McEwan, Lena E. "Medical Women in Victoria." The

Medical Journal of Australia, 1:20 (May 20, 1967) 1042-
1045. figs., tables. (Address, Annual Meeting, Victorian Medical Women's Society, Melbourne, November
15, 1965.)

Of the 4,667 registered medical practitioners known to be
resident in Victoria, Australia in May, 1965, 598 of them
were women and of these, 262 were members of the Victorian Medical Women's Society. Questionnaires prepared
by the Medical Women's Federation and by the Medical
Practitioners' Union were sent to women who qualified as
physicians to find out their employment and domestic patterns in Victoria. Some of the findings include that there
is difficulty in finding suitable part-time work, especially
in the country, and there is a small but definite interest
in postgraduate study. Women who were single and women
who married but had no children were working full time.
The women with children responded that if they were not
working currently, they intended to work at least part-time
as soon as their domestic duties permitted. "It is evident
that the medical women in Victoria who answered this
questionnaire are interested in and aware of their responsibilities to their profession, and it is obvious that they
make very real efforts to fulfill them, especially when one
considers the dearth of good reliable domestic help in this
country." There is need to re-equip medical personnel
after prolonged absence or to encourage them to proceed
to more specialized studies.

2139.   "Medical Council of New Zealand Questionnaire." New
         Zealand Medical Journal, 65:401 (January 1966) 1-3.
         tables.

Responses to a questionnaire sent by the New Zealand Medical Council to all registered doctors showed women numbered 289 of a total of 2725 physicians. Of those women
living in New Zealand, 23 were in general practice, 39 in
specialist practice, and 21 in full-time administration; no
women did teaching or research (as opposed to 55 men).
Percentages of women retired or partly retired seemed
comparable with men. Women physicians were most commonly institutional doctors, anesthetists, obstetricians and
gynecologists, pathologists, or psychiatrists. Women practicing overseas included five general practitioners, 21 specialists, five administrators, and three teachers or researchers. Eleven women practiced in institutions, five
were psychiatrists, four were anesthetists, four were pathologists, and three were pediatricians. A survey of the
time women spent on professional duties showed 144 spent
90-100 per cent, 63 spent between 0-49 per cent, 23 spent
50-59 per cent, 37 spent between 60 and 90 per cent, and
74 were retired.

2140.   Salmond, G. C. "Medical Manpower Planning." New Zea-
         land Medical Journal, 80:528 (27 November 1974) 459-

462. fig., tables. (Report.)
A statistical model to assist in medical manpower planning
for New Zealand was devised. The model does not differ-
entiate between male and female graduates, although women
account for close to 20 per cent of all recent medical
school graduates. The article cites an Australian study by
Fett (1974), which suggested that the productivity of medical
women as a group might be equivalent to about two-thirds
of their male counterparts. This and related factors will
be taken into account in the model, states the author.

2141.   Saunders, Ida B.; Clarke, Ann D.; and Vautin, Joy M.
        "Women in Medicine." Medical Journal of Australia,
        1:15 (10 April 1971) 825-826. tables. (Letters to the
        Editor.)
        These authors are responding to what they perceive as an
        inaccuracy in a previous article in this journal (January 9,
        1971) when a book entitled A Short History of Medical Wo-
        men in Australia by Dr. E. Sandford Morgan was quoted
        saying that 1,767 women doctors were registered in Aus-
        tralia and that only 40 per cent were estimated to be in
        active practice. What is inaccurate about this statistic of
        40 per cent is that this percentage only accounts for full-
        time practice and not part-time. In fact nearly two-thirds
        of the medical women were working and "about half of
        those not working were anxious to do more, or to resume
        practice respectively."

2142.   "Women Doctors." New Zealand Medical Journal, 80:519
        (10 July 1974) 23-24. (Editorial.)
        This article examines two surveys comparing women doctors
        to men in Australia and New Zealand. In Australia, a ques-
        tionnaire administered to men and women who graduated
        from medical school between 1920 and 1969 showed women
        made up 13 per cent of all physicians, and that they tended
        to work full time for five years, then drop out during early
        childbearing years. Fifteen per cent did not resume prac-
        tice (but five per cent of males also dropped out). Women
        doctors worked an average of 39.9 hours per week--64 per
        cent of the hours worked by men. A New Zealand survey
        showed women physicians, all considered, to be about 60
        per cent as productive as men. However, women preferred
        specialties where there are shortages: psychiatry, anes-
        thetics, and pathology. New four- or five-year full-time
        courses for specialties exclude married women from quali-
        fication unless they postpone childbearing to the medically
        dangerous age of 30. The author recommends part-time
        training programs during childbearing years in order not to
        waste a valuable resource.

2143.   "Women in Medicine." Medical Journal of Australia, 1:18
        (4 May 1974) 685-686.
        This paper consists of a discussion of Ione Fett's article

"Australian Medical Graduates in 1972" which appeared in the Journal.

CANADA

2144.   Buck, Carol; Scoffield, Mary; and Warwick, O. H.   "A
        Survey of Women Graduates from a Canadian Medical
        School."   Canadian Medical Association Journal, 94
        (2 April 1966) 712-716.   tables.
        Britain has a higher percentage of women doing medical
        work than either Canada or the United States; these latter
        two countries have about the same percentage of practicing
        women physicians.   Of the 104 surviving and cooperating
        women physicians studied out of 110 who graduated from the
        University of Western Ontario Medical School between 1924
        and 1963, 85 per cent were engaged in medical work (66
        per cent full-time and 19 per cent part-time).   The fields
        of practice most frequently entered include general practice,
        psychiatry, and preventive medicine.   The most important
        determinant for women not to practice was childbearing and
        correlated reasons.

2145.   "Canada Trying to Get Nonpracticing Woman Doctors Back
        to Work."   American Family Physician/GP, 1:2 (Feb-
        ruary 1970) 147.
        The Canadian Medical Association wants to channel non-
        practicing women physicians back into practice.   Canadian
        Medical Association officers admit they do not know how
        many women are inactive.

2146.   MacDonald, Eva Mader and Webb, Elizabeth M.   "Survey
        of Women Physicians in Canada, 1883-1964."   Canadian
        Medical Association Journal, 94:23 (4 June 1966) 1223-
        1227.   tables.
        This survey, made in 1963-64, was the first attempt to
        undertake a comprehensive study of women physicians in
        Canada.   Prior to this study, Canadian medical schools
        were obliged to use statistics on medical women in other
        countries.   As far as could be determined, there were
        1753 women physicians living in Canada in 1964 compared
        to 21,452 male physicians.   At the time of the survey, 18
        per cent were in postgraduate training, 61 per cent were in
        active medical practice, nine per cent had retired after
        practice, and four per cent were not in practice.   Forty-
        eight point five per cent of the married women were work-
        ing full-time and 17.6 per cent were working part-time.
        Of the single women, 59 per cent were working full-time
        and 35.7 per cent were in postgraduate training.   The more
        recent the graduation period, the higher the percentage of
        women doing full-time medical work: from 15 per cent of
        all graduates between 1910 and 1919, to 60 per cent of all
        graduates between 1930 and 1939, to 71 per cent for gradu-

ates between 1950 and 1959. The percentage doing part-time work was fairly constant at about eight per cent for all age groups graduating between 1930 and 1960. The women who were temporarily retired or had never practiced numbered 61, and most of them (75 per cent) were young married doctors who graduated after 1950. There is a higher percentage of women in public health, pediatrics, anesthesiology, pathology, and radiology. The percentage of graduates from Canadian universities who are doing full-time medical work is higher than that for graduates from schools elsewhere (59 per cent vs. 47 per cent); the percentage of graduates from other countries who are working part-time is higher than that for graduates from Canadian schools (eight per cent vs. five per cent). The more specialized the training of medical women, the less likely they are to be dropouts at an early age from active medical work. One of the concerns for the authors of this study is that ways and means of preventing the complete dropout of medical women following periods of enforced medical inactivity be found.

2147. Moffatt, Agnes K. "Medical Women and Group Practice: As Seen by a Canadian." Journal of the American Medical Women's Association, 5:7 (July 1950) 287-290.
This article was written "to illustrate the trend ... of unsocialized medicine in Canada, to point out some of the advantages of such a trend, and to show the part a medical woman plays in this type of practice." The author discusses the advantages of organized group medicine for the doctor, the woman doctor, the married woman doctor, and the patient, emphasizing for the woman doctor (married and unmarried) the advantage of "male companionship which is necessary to keep a woman's perspective true." Such acceptance by males will also elevate the woman physician's status in the eyes of the community.

2148. Nicholson, J. Fraser. "Dalhousie's Medical Women: A Survey of Graduates 1964-1973." Nova Scotia Medical Bulletin, (August-October 1975) 138-139. table.
This study examines the question of women physicians' utilization of their education. Sixty female graduates of Dalhousie University Faculty of Medicine, who graduated between the years 1964 to 1973 inclusive, were asked to fill out a questionnaire concerning their "marital and maternity status, occupational history since graduation, income, and future plans." Fifty-six out of 60 responded. Of these 56, 33 were married, 19 single, four divorced or separated. Thirty-three were in general practice. "55 of the 56 indicated that their future plans are for full-time medical work" (one out of the 56 was engaged in nonmedical work). At the time of the survey, 80 per cent were employed full-time, 18 per cent part-time, and 2 per cent (the one woman) in nonmedical work. Nine of the 30 doc-

tors with children (56 children total) had taken no time
from medical work (except vacations). Of the 37 doctors
employed full time (excluding those in residency), 11 earned
between $20,000 and $30,000 per year; 16 earned over
$30,000. In 1973, 8.4 per cent of the total physician pop-
ulation in Nova Scotia were women as compared with 6.3
per cent in 1967 (U.S. figures show a similar ratio of
8.4 per cent women physicians in 1973 as compared with
6.3 per cent in 1963). The author concludes that the study
demonstrates that "the present policy of the Admissions
Committee [at Dalhousie University Faculty of Medicine]
regarding admission of female medical students is justified."

2149.   "Nonpracticing Women MDs May Be Recruited in Canada."
         Medical Tribune, (23 October 1969) 8.
         [Article not examined by editors.]

2150.   R. R. "Québec Study Shows Women Physicians Have Loy-
         alties to Medicine and Family." Canadian Medical
         Association Journal, 113:10 (22 November 1975) 1000.
         Published here are the results of a study of women phy-
         sicians by the Professional Corporation of Physicians and
         Surgeons of Québec. In addition to giving the percentage
         of women entrants to Canadian medical schools, the article
         notes that women physicians average 30 per cent fewer ser-
         vices to patients than do men, and work 20 to 30 per cent
         fewer hours. Statistics on specialty choice and geograph-
         ical location are also provided. Comments on the study
         are made by the Corporation's president, the president of
         the Federation of Residents and Interns of Québec, and the
         president of the Québec Medical Association.

EUROPE, EASTERN

2151.   ["District Physicians in Poland"]. Zeitschrift fur All-
         gemeinmedizin; der Landarzt, 51:5 (20 February 1975)
         236. (Ger)
         [Article not examined by editors.]

2152.   Kubankova, V. and Vysohlid, J. ["Demography of Physi-
         cians in Czechoslovakia and Some Aspects of Postgrad-
         uate Education"]. Ceskoslovenske zdravotnictvi, 23:7
         (1975) 260-267. (Cze)
         A survey of doctors of the Czech Republic shows that the
         number of women in the profession doubled between 1960
         and 1973; the percentage of women increased from 31 to
         45 per cent of the present total of 25,887 physicians. Six-
         ty per cent of the women specialists are grade I and 11 per
         cent were grade II, compared with 57 and 28 per cent of
         the males. The proportion of women in most fields who
         have reached grade II is notably lower than the proportion
         in grade I, while the reverse is true for the men in ob-

stetrics-gynecology, hygiene-epidemiology, surgery, and internal medicine. Younger physicians predominate in anesthesiology, stomatology, pathology, internal medicine, surgery, theoretical medicine, and psychiatry, while physicians
over 39 predominate in public health administration, rehabilitation, respiratory diseases, and rural and industrial
medicine.

2153.   Wlodarska, H. ["The Women's Hospital Camp at Brzeziny"].
        Przeglad Lekarski, 26 (1970) 213-216.
        [Article not examined by editors.]

EUROPE, WESTERN

2154.   Bastman, A. E. ["The Admission of Women Doctors to
        Regular Positions on the Medical Staffs of Hospitals"].
        Hygiea, 81 (1919) 547-572. (Swe)
        At the request of His Majesty, in connection with the es-
        tablishment of new salary scales for personnel in state hos-
        pitals for the mentally ill, the Royal Medical Commission
        reviewed the question of women doctors on hospital staffs
        and makes recommendations concerning appointments and
        salaries. The first portion of this article reviews various
        petitions, recommendations, and pronouncements during the
        years 1901 to 1919, during which time the options open to
        women physicians in the official service gradually increased,
        although women were still not permitted to hold high-level
        staff positions in certain hospitals. The present recommen-
        dations would give women a reasonable equality with men in
        starting positions, pension rights, advancement, and certain
        other areas. A table of recommended salaries, however,
        shows a differential at all levels--full-time or substitute--
        of about 15 per cent. This is justified, as men usually are
        supporting families.

2155.   "Belgium." La Semaine Médicale, (1890) 48. (News.)
        (Fre)
        "In its session of last Wednesday, the House of Representa-
        tives has consecrated the right of women to practice medi-
        cine and pharmacy, in a general manner and without dis-
        tinguishing, as was done in the law of 1876, among the vari-
        ous branches of the art of healing."

2156.   Borrino, Angiola. "Medical Women's Work in Pediatrics."
        Medical Woman's Journal, 29:10 (October 1922) 240-242.
        The work of women physicians in Italy is discussed. In
        addition, the author suggests areas in which medical women
        can be of substantial benefit, particularly through participa-
        tion in the reform of early infancy assistance.

2157.   Bui-dang-ha-doan, J. "The Feminization of French Medi-
        cine." World Medical Journal, 11:1 (January 1964) 33.

Difficulties arise when trying to do comparative studies on women and men physicians in France because the sex of the physician is never mentioned in directories, etc. The medical universe can be broken down into total medical profession, and practicing medical profession (which can be further broken down to nonsalaried or " 'liberal' " doctors and practicing doctors. There are no figures on the "feminization" of the total medical profession, but estimates for practising doctors set the "degree of feminization" at nine per cent. Feminization is expressed by the number of women per 100 persons of both sexes. Among nonsalaried doctors the figure drops to 7.3 per cent (30 June 1962). The proportion of women in medicine in France is low in comparison to other professions: 14.5 per cent among accountants, 25 per cent among practicing dentists, and over 44 per cent among practicing pharmacists. There is a correlation between youth and feminization.

2158.   ["Careers of Female Physicians"]. Osterreichische
          Arztezeltung, 30:20 (25 October 1975) 1261. (Ger)
    Facing a physician shortage, the Austrian Institute for Urban Research investigated the number of female physicians who did not practice but would possibly be willing to return to work. They expected a large percentage of female doctors in this situation. Reviewing the careers of female physicians graduated from the University of Vienna, Graz, and Innsbruck in 1950/51, 1955/56, and 1960/61, they found that only 10.2 per cent were not practicing. Sixty-two point five per cent of practicing female physicians are specialists and the trend is rising. Preferred specialties are dental medicine, anesthesiology, internal medicine, and pediatrics. More than half work in the city where they studied and obtained their M.D. Forty-three per cent are in private practice; 40.5 per cent work in hospitals.

2159.   ["The Female Doctors' Petition"]. Dagny. Tidskrift för
          Sociala Och Litterära Intressen, 1 (1901) 82-85. (Swe)
    This petition for the right to receive public office was submitted to the king on 28 January 1901. The document was signed by Karolina Widerström, Hedda Anderson, Maria Folkeson, Anna Stecksen (Sweden's first doctor of medicine), Ellen Sandelin, Sofia Holmgren, Hanna Christer Nilsson, Sigrid Engstrom, Alma Sundquist, and 14 female medical candidates and nine medical students. [Swedish summary provided to the editors by Mårtha Elvers-Hulth, retired librarian of the National Swedish Board to Health and Welfare Library.]

2160.   ["Female Service Doctors"]. Allmänna Svenska Läkartid-
          ningen, 14 (1917) 246-254. table. (Swe)
    The journal reprints a petition dated 19 December 1916, signed by Karin [sic] Widerström, Ada Nilsson, Lilly Paykull, Elin Odenkrantz, and Andres Andren-Svedberg. It was

presented to the medical board after meetings between the
petitioners and the board to discuss admitting women to
more equal opportunities in the government service.   The
petition reviews previous progress in opening hospital positions and obtaining better pay, and requests: (1) that unmarried women doctors have the same chance as men at
provincial physician or assistant physician jobs, the railway
service, district, town and city services, assistant hospital
physician posts and supervisory posts in tuberculosis hospitals, all at the same pay scale as men; (2) that married
women be appointed to these positions and to those included
in the decree of 1903; and (3) that His Majesty instruct the
board to order that women doctors, married or unmarried,
have equal opportunity with men for temporary or full-time
positions as described above.   An attachment to the petition
is a statement of the medical superintendent of the St.
Goerens tuberculosis hospital that he thinks women are capable of filling positions in these hospitals.

2161.   "French Medical Women."   Medical Woman's Journal, 45:4
           (April 1938) 112-113.   (Editorial.)
         There are approximately 1,000 women physicians in France
         and its colonies (compared to 27,000 medical men).   About
         30 per cent of the women enter general practice; the re-
         mainder "either specialize or marry."   Few women stay
         in practice after marriage.   The effects of current political
         conditions upon German and Austrian women physicians are
         also alluded to.

2162.   "French Women in Medicine."   Journal of the American
           Medical Association, 214:3 (19 October 1970) 606.
           (International Comments.)
         Women medical graduates in France for the years 1937-
         1938 and 1957-1958 indicate that the percentage of women
         physicians has risen from 13.3 per cent to 21 per cent.
         This brief article also provides data on French women phy-
         sicians' age at graduation, specialty choice, marital status,
         and spouse occupation.

2163.   Gingras, Rosaire. ["The Situation of the Woman in Medi-
           cine"].   Laval Médical, 39 (June 1968) 512-524.   (Fre)
         The results of a study of graduates of the University of
         Laval are shown in 20 statistical tables.   This article in-
         cludes a bibliography. [Article not examined by editors.]

2164.   ["His Majesty's Gracious Letter to the Royal College of
           Health Concerning the Procedure in the Cause of Rikets
           Ständers' Humble Representation on Extending Women's
           Civil Rights"].   Hygiea, 31 (1869) 206-207.   (Swe)
         Ständers had petitioned in June 1866 that women be given
         the right to become doctors or scholars the same as men,
         and requested that the medical or academic faculties be in-
         structed to comply with her demands.   The royal reply

cites previous actions concerning the right of women to become teachers. Women should receive the right to the private practice of medicine, but the question must be resolved individually, depending on the outcome of the unavoidable and necessary theoretical and practical education and examinations. This reply does not immediately open the way, but says that the problem will receive more consideration.

2165.   Holmberg, Anton. ["The Competency of Female Doctors for Medical Service: Part I"]. Hygiea, 63 (1901) 756-770. (Swe)
The first part of these two papers contains a petition to the king of Sweden from all of the women in Sweden who were licensed to practice or who were studying for this purpose, and an answer to the petition by the Royal Medical Council. Since the answer involved statements affecting other bodies, their advice was also sought and is printed in part II, which contains the replies of the Council for Prisons, the State Railroad Commission, and the medical faculties of the three medical schools, the Karolinska Institute in Stockholm, the University of Uppsala, and the University of Lund. I. A petition to the king of Sweden from above mentioned women led by Karolina Widerström, dated January 28, 1901, requests full equality with men in the practice of medicine for women, since they have undergone completely equal training to that provided for men. They assert their complete competence but are denied complete equality. (This refers to the restrictions supplied by the government decree number 28 of the Code of Laws restricting the practice of women doctors to exclude positions as chiefs and members of the Royal Medical Council together with certain chief, legal, and faculty positions.) The women describe the expanded opportunities for women physicians in Denmark, Finland, Russia, and Berlin. They request the king to declare that women are fully competent to exercise the full duties of medical service. The king referred this petition to the Medical Council, who comment that many of the matters are within the competence of the faculties of medicine. There are certain positions now open, such as that of quarantine officer at Kaensoe, for which an obligation of five years service is required. This seems unsuitable for women. The administrative duties connected with teaching post positions on the state railroads, etc., require abilities not included in the education of women. In mental hospitals there are inmates with sexual deviations, and positions in such places would be disagreeable to women. The teaching positions also require long training and experience which the women lack. However, there are certain subordinate posts which would be suitable for unmarried women, such as assistantships to city district Medical Board of Health physicians. For the position of women physicians in state prisons, there are questions of some delicacy. There seems no reason why women could not fill

posts in prisons for women. The choice of male physicians exclusively for male prisoners might be suitable.
These matters lie within the choice of Your Majesty's
Prison Council, who can doubtless choose which sex of doctors would be suitable for the posts. Concerning the choice
of physicians in the army and navy, the women physicians
have not made any claims, and we can leave the matter to
one side. Many of the other posts presently denied to women could possibly be occupied by unmarried women, although posts involving administrative decision, including in-
structorships and professorships in the medical schools,
the School of Midwifery, or the Institute for Swedish Physical Health, are not suitable for women, nor are they suited
to be councillors in chemistry, prosectors in anatomy, or
to hold laboratory or teaching posts of subordinate character in the medical schools.

2166.   Holmberg, Anton. ["Competency of Female Doctors for
         Medical Service: Part II"]. Hygiea, 65 (1903) 293-
         300. (Swe)
         Part II of the report by Anton Holmberg gives the delayed
         responses of the Prison Council, the Railroad Council, and
         the medical faculties of the Universities of Uppsala and
         Lund and the Karolinska Institute for Medicine and Surgery
         in Stockholm concerning the petition of the women physicians.
         The Prison Council agrees with the Medical Council. The
         Railroad Council replies that railroad physicians must be
         available at all times, must be on duty for a definite term
         of five years, must care for men who are usually single
         and require visits to their private dwelling places, often
         remote from the railroad line. The railroad doctors must
         also travel to remote places even in the far north and care
         for the sick along the lines. Not only does this require
         the strength and hardness of men, but if women undertook
         the tasks the railroad cars used would have to be modified
         at considerable expense. The Railroad Council thus re-
         plies to the petition of Karolina Widerstroem, Hedda An-
         dersson, etc., that women are not suitable for posts as
         physicians of the state railroads. The replies of the three
         faculties generally agree with the Medical Council, pointing
         out in addition that the lectureships and preceptorships are
         steps to the professorships, and the reasoning applied to
         the professors applies also to them. They also point out
         that the posts are not to be chosen by those who want them,
         but to be acceptable to the professors, or the qualifications
         might deteriorate. The medical faculty in Lund merely
         agrees with that in Uppsala. The latter seems to rely on
         the validity of the state law number 28. However, the pro-
         fessor of otorhinolaryngology apparently sees no reason
         why women should not engage in this field. Finally, the
         chancellor, having inspected the reports of the councils and
         faculties concerned, discusses certain positions which appear
         to be open at the time, i.e., the associate professorship in

anatomy at the University of Uppsala and Lund, a lecture-
ship in legal medicine at the Karolinska Institute, and certain positions as prosectors in anatomy which the faculties
concerned have been agreed were not in the area where women are competent. He then comments on the opinions
admitting that women might be competent in otology, rhin-
ology, and laryngoscopy.

2167. Holmstrom, Marta. "Optimal Utilization of Medical Woman-
          power." Journal of the American Medical Women's
          Association, 22:5 (May 1967) 336-337.
       Covering a specific region of the MWIA, the author briefly
       discusses similarities and differences among women physi-
       cians in Norway, Finland, Denmark, Sweden, the Nether-
       lands, United Kingdom, and Germany. The Republic of
       South Africa is also mentioned.

2168. Joyce, Nessa M.; Bourke, Geoffrey J.; and Wilson-Davis,
          Keith. "The Careers of Some Women Graduates of
          Medical Schools in the Republic of Ireland." Journal
          of the Irish Medical Association, 68:16 (13 September
          1975) 389-394. tables.
       "The careers of a sample of women graduates of all med-
       ical schools in the Republic of Ireland, and now living in
       Ireland or Great Britain, were ascertained by questionnaire.
       The sample was composed of graduates of the class of 1943
       and classes at five yearly intervals thereafter up to and in-
       cluding 1968. Questionnaires were sent to 297 women and
       242 (81.5 per cent) replied. Fifty-seven per cent of the
       women graduates are working full-time, 25 per cent part-
       time, and 18 per cent are not working in medical posts.
       Fifty-five per cent hold a postgraduate qualification. The
       four most common specialties in which those working are
       engaged are general practice, community medicine, psy-
       chiatry, and anaesthesia. The views of these women doc-
       tors were obtained on many topics which included job
       satisfaction, discrimination, and marriage and career."
       [Article summary.]

2169. Montreuil-Straus, G. "Foreign Letters." Medical Wo-
          man's Journal, 47:1 (January 1940) 33. (Letters to
          the Editor.)
       Dr. Montreuil-Straus, a member of the Journal's editorial
       board, mentions the war conditions and the major concerns
       it has imposed upon French women physicians. She also
       details the activities of the "Comité d'Education Feminine
       de la Société Française de Prophylaxie Sanitaire et Morale."
       That organization (of which she is president) prepares young
       girls for their future roles as wives and mothers, and safe-
       guards them from venereal diseases.

2170. Murphy, Thomas and Joyce, Nessa M. "Structure of the
          Medical Profession in Ireland." Journal of the Irish

Medical Association, 61:373 (July 1968) 233-238.
tables.

The major portion of this article explains the data-gather-
ing methodology used for this study, which was begun in
1966.   The authors, who confined their analysis to doctors
permanently established in practice, identify a number of
difficulties encountered.   (For example, in compiling their
list of physicians' names, there was a problem with women
who practiced under married names but were still registered under maiden names.)   The study showed that approximately 14 per cent of all practicing physicians in Ireland are women.   About the same proportion of women are
in general practice.   Women are unevenly distributed over
the specialties.   Of all specialists in anesthetics, pediatrics,
psychiatry, and ophthalmology, the percentages of women
are 32, 30, 23, 23, respectively.   Very few women are
represented in obstetrics and gynecology (only three out of
57 specialists), radiology, and internal medicine.   No women are registered as surgeons.   Only two tables provide
comparative data on male and female physicians: table I
breaks down specialties by sex and by geographical residence, table IV sets out medical school by sex and specialty.

2171.   Nilsson, Carl-Axel.   ["1500 Female Doctors Jobless in
        1980?"]   Läkartidningen, 68:52 (1971) 6078-6084.
        tables.   (Swe)

The author suggests that the Swedish Medical Federation
overestimated the available positions as full-time working
doctors for female doctors in its health plan of 1961 and
should now make a better estimate.   At present there are
2000 female doctors, and if they are produced at the present
rate there would be 5000 by 1980.   Table I shows that women are very unequally divided by specialty fields.   It also
shows that the available women specialists outside of the
supervisory positions at official hospitals are very differently distributed by specialties from the women with official
positions.   Of the women with official posts, 50 per cent
are engaged in child psychiatry and 27 per cent in psychiatry, while there are only three women surgeons and one
orthopedic specialist, and only five gynecologists and 16
pediatricians.   Part of the problem lies in the tendency of
women over the age of 40 to seek appointments after intervening years in family and social responsibilities.   However, there is great competition for hospital posts, especially in fields where women are underrepresented (including gynecology, internal medicine, and pediatrics), and
supervisory posts require long and continuous experience.
There are unfilled specialist opportunities for women in
the "open ward," and women are underrepresented in official posts as district and provincial physicians.   A brighter
outlook is opened by the scheme of General Director Bror
Rexed (in Läkartidningen, 68:48 [1971]) for an improvement
of the program for the allotment of official posts, and to

this should be added the change in the plan of 1961 which
does not correspond with existing realities. The plan anticipated that 75 per cent of female doctors would be in
full-time work, but 65 per cent would be closer to the
mark. Other tables show that women are increasing in the
field of long-term care and in ophthalmology, while there
are only two women as city public health officers and 26 as
provincial district health officers.

2172.   Nilsson, Carl-Axel. ["Only Small Advancement Possibil-
         ities for Surgeons and Female Physicians"]. Läkartid-
         ningen, 68:44 (27 October 1971) 4985-4990. figs.,
         tables. (Swe)
         The author cites figures and shows graphs on the number
         of men and women who have achieved various ranks in the
         hospital service in several specialties, showing that there is
         usually a smaller percentage of women in the higher ranks
         in all duration-of-service classes. In specialties where
         progress is normally slow, such as gynecology, the situa-
         tion is even worse for women. Most specialties are heavily
         weighted with young doctors. Putting these two observations
         together seems to indicate that the outlook for advancement
         for women doctors in the future is not good. [Translators
         note: The conclusions concerning rank achieved by age are
         based on very small numbers of women, e.g., a total of
         26 women in internal medicine, 26 in gynecology, 22 in
         pediatrics.]

2173.   Pirami, Edmea. "Supply." Journal of the American Med-
         ical Women's Association, 22:5 (May 1967) 338-339.
         A report for the MWIA on the five countries of Austria,
         France, Italy, Spain, and Switzerland shows that the per-
         centage of women physicians in each of these countries as
         of this report is Austria, 17.4 per cent; France, 12.8 per
         cent; Italy, 21.06 per cent; Spain, 2.5 per cent; and Swit-
         zerland, 13.5 per cent. Pediatrics claimed the highest
         comparative percentage of women physicians in each coun-
         try with the exception of Austria where, although the larg-
         est number of women were pediatricians, the greatest per-
         centage of women to men could be found in anesthesia
         (51.1 per cent women physicians in this specialty). Com-
         parative data on women medical students are also given.

2174.   Pouzin, Yvonne. "Women Doctors Among the Professors
         in Hospitals." Medical Woman's Journal, 29:10 (Octo-
         ber 1922) 248-250. port. (Presentation, Convention,
         Medical Women's International Association, Geneva,
         Switzerland, 4-7 September 1922.)
         A brief discussion of official positions held by women phy-
         sicians as teachers, professors, and lecturers in the med-
         ical schools of France is followed by the accomplishments
         of women physicians in hospitals.

2175.   Rosdahl, Nils and Plum, Gunnar.   ["A Study of Interest in
        Work as a Physician in Foreign Countries"].   Ugeskrift
        for Laeger, 132:25 (18 June 1970) 1206-1209.   tables.
        (Dan)
        Answers to a questionnaire on interest in foreign practice
        were received from 154 young Danish physicians--39 women
        and 115 men.   The survey also included questions on age,
        sex, civil status, number and age of children, foreign ex-
        perience as a student or locum tenens, and intent to take
        the ECFMG, as well as on preferred type and location of
        foreign service.   About two-thirds of the women and three-
        fourths of the men were married; the married women usual-
        ly had more and older children than the married men.
        About a third of the women expressed interest in practicing
        in a foreign country, the proportion ranging from four of
        16 married women with children to six of 15 unmarried wo-
        men, compared to just over half of the men, among whom
        the greatest interest was expressed by married men without
        children.   Figures are given for interest by age for each
        sex, but the numbers in each age group are too small to
        have much significance.   Data on foreign experience and
        preferred service are not broken down by sex.

2176.   Schondel, A.; Frolund, A.; and Alsing, I.   ["Survey Con-
        cerning Positions of Women Doctors in Denmark"].
        Fra Sundhedsstyr, 4:17 (May 1967) 668-677.   (Dan)
        [Article not examined by editors.]

2177.   ["Women Physicians"].   Wiener Medizinische Wochenschrift,
        76:27 (1926) 837-838.   (Ger)
        This short notice describes the geographical distribution,
        choice of specialty, type of activity, and hospital affiliation
        of female physicians in Austria for the year 1926.

GERMANY

2178.   Bauknecht, Ruth.   "Optimal Utilization of Medical Woman-
        power."   Journal of the American Medical Women's
        Association, 22:6 (June 1967) 407-410.
        The situation of women physicians in Germany is discussed.
        Twenty-five per cent of all approbated women doctors do
        not work as such in the Federal Republic of West Germany.
        The League of Women Doctors sent questionnaires to their
        colleagues and, according to the responses, deduced that
        family ties play a major, although not the sole, role in the
        noncontinuance of medical activities by women.   Finances
        did not seem to be a problem.   Only five per cent of all
        women doctors (as compared with 5.5 per cent of all male
        doctors) achieve preeminent positions in medicine.   Most
        doctors in West Germany are "nonpolitical, and indifferent
        to the party, race, or religion to which they belong."   Very
        few women are to be found in professional organizations.

2179.   Beske, Fritz. [Future Physicians: Medical Students Be-
         tween 1947 and 1959]. Deutscher Aerzte Verlag GNBH,
         Koeln-Berlin, Germany, 1960, 94 pp. tables. (Ger)
    This extensive statistical survey of medical students in
    Germany contains data on the social background, training,
    choice of specialty, and place of work--mostly separated
    for male and female students. The book contains numer-
    ous statistical tables but no index or bibliography.

2180.   Fehling, Hermann. ["On Women in Medicine"]. Deutsche
         Medizinische Wochenschrift, 44:11 (14 March 1918) 301-
         302. (Ger)
    In the controversy on women in medicine, the author, a
    medical school professor, was asked to state his experi-
    ence with women students and physicians. Although he must
    admit to their excellent performance as students, he does
    not employ female residents routinely. However, when he
    did so during the world war, he was very satisfied with
    their work in obstetrics. In the author's view, married
    women doctors should not work--and marry they will by
    nature's laws. Forced by the changing social values to ad-
    mit women into academe, he maintains that they will con-
    tribute little to scientific and social progress, which he
    predicts will be shaped by male minds.

2181.   "German Medical Women." Medical Woman's Journal, 37:
         10 (October 1930) 287.
    The enrollment of women medical students in the United
    States and Germany decreased in comparison to the enroll-
    ment during the decade previous to when this article was
    written. In Germany, the statistics include 555 women en-
    rolled in 1911; 3,428 in 1929-1930; and only about 17 per
    cent of all medical students in Germany when this article
    was written. Most of the women who choose medicine
    come from the middle class. Women physicians tend to
    practice in large cities rather than in rural districts in
    Germany.

2182.   Lattin, Cora Billings. "The Woman Physician in Foreign
         Clinics." Woman's Medical Journal, 20:4 (April 1910)
         81-83. (Presentation, Fourth Annual Meeting, Wo-
         men's Medical Society of New York State, New York,
         New York, 11 March 1910.)
    Dr. Lattin draws upon her own experiences as a physician
    in and visitor to German and Austrian clinics and univer-
    sities, to outline opportunities for medical women.

2183.   "Medical Women in Germany." British Medical Journal,
         (14 September 1912) 654.
    Data collected from 125 of the reported 175 women physi-
    cians in Germany showed that of the 47 women who married,
    34 gave up practice. Figures on geographic distribution
    are provided as well.

2184.   "Medical Women in Germany." Medical Woman's Journal,
             43:7 (July 1936) 189-190. (Editorial.)
         Despite "the recent unsettled conditions of the country,"
         figures received from the League of German Women Phy-
         sicians show that the number of women physicians in Ger-
         many has increased eight per cent over the 1932 statistics.
         Figures reflect geographic distribution, specialties selected,
         and the number of women in independent practice.

2185.   "Medical Women in Germany." Medical Woman's Journal,
             44:9 (September 1937) 258. (Editorial.)
         As of 1935, there were 3,675 women physicians in Ger-
         many. Most of the women practitioners in independent prac-
         tice are in general practice; 28.5 per cent are specialists.
         Of the total 52,000 German physicians, seven per cent are
         women.

2186.   Moll, Albert. ["Statistics on the Activity of Women Phy-
             sicians"]. In: Manual of Sex Sciences; With Special
             Consideration of the Cultural-Historical Relationships.
             Edited by Albert Moll. F. C. W. Vogel, Leipzig, Ger-
             many, 1912, 1001-1011. tables. (Ger)
         This is an appendix to a chapter on the women's movement,
         in a section titled "The Social Forms of Sexual Relation-
         ships: The Place of Women." It contains a series of
         tables and a discussion on the activity of women doctors in
         the medical insurance plans in Berlin in the years 1907 to
         1911. In plans allowing a free choice of doctors, and tak-
         ing the proportion of fees paid to women doctors as equiva-
         lent to the proportion of patients treated by them, Moll finds
         that the latter figure is unrelated to the changes in the pro-
         portion of women doctors on the plan panel. He concludes
         that the "demand" of women for treatment by women, often
         cited as a reason for training more women doctors, does
         not exist, since when women doctors are available they do
         not attract their share of patients. Even in the plans with
         a high proportion of women members, such as the dress-
         makers and tailors and the hotel workers, the women doc-
         tors had smaller case loads than the men.

2187.   Rath, F. ["The Tax Status of Women Physicians Employed
             as Assistants"]. Therapie de Gegenwart (Berlin), 102
             (March 1963) 358-362. (Ger)
         [Article not examined by editors.]

2188.   Rath, F. ["The Wife (a Woman Physician) of a Specialist
             as Her Husband's Substitute"]. Deutsches Medizinisches
             Journal (Berlin), 14 (20 September 1963) 581-583.
             (Ger)
         [Article not examined by editors.]

2189.   Stelzner, Helene Friderike. ["Female Physicians (Part I)"].
             Deutsche Medizinische Wochenschrift, 38:26 (27 June

1912) 1243-1244. (Ger)
This article is the first of two parts of a statistical survey
of women physicians in Germany at the beginning of the
20th century. Based on answers to 125 questionnaires, the
article computes the data concerning the following areas:
geographic distribution, place of study, number of transfers
during medical school, previous training and experience,
marital status, and husband's profession.

2190. Stelzner, Helene Friderike. ["Female Physicians (Part
II)"]. Deutsche Medizinische Wochenschrift, 38:2 (27
July 1912) 1290-1292. (Ger)
This is the second and last part of a statistical survey of
female physicians in Germany at the beginning of the 20th
century. It contains data on the following areas: choice of
specialty, duration of studies including specialty training,
choice of place of specialty training and work, and income.
The author concludes that on the basis of these data, women are readily accepted by the public and find no particular difficulty in withstanding the stresses of medical training and practice.

2191. ["The Woman Physician and Her Relation to Nursing Care"].
Veska, 28 (January 1964) 64. (Ger)
[Article not examined by editors.]

2192. "Women Physicians in Germany." Medical Woman's Journal, 38:3 (March 1931) 70-71.
In Germany in 1909 there were only 82 women physicians,
or 0.27 per cent of the total number of physicians. In
1930 there were 2,807 women doctors, comprising 5.95
per cent of the profession.

GREAT BRITAIN

2193. Bennett, A. H. English Medical Women: Glimpses of
Their Work in Peace and War. Sir Isaac Pitman &
Sons, Ltd., London, England, 1915, 159 pp. ports.
Following a mention of women healers in ancient times, a
history of the entrance of modern women into the medical
profession is presented; particular attention is given to
events affecting women in Edinburgh University and at the
London School of Medicine for Women. The major portion
of this book describes the work performed by British women physicians in various hospitals, before and during the
World War. Biographies are given of several specific women physicians. The author, noting in the foreword that
a medical woman's point of view and method of work differs from a man's, explains that in her descriptions of women physicians' work, she "emphasized the little womanly
touches that are noticeable in the hospitals officered and
carried on by them." A preface by Stephen Paget explains

why women are just as suited to practice medicine as are
men.

2194.   Berry, (Lady) F. M. Dickinson. "The Work Done by the
         Standing Committee of the Medical Women's Federa-
         tion." Medical Women's Federation News-Letter, (July
         1931) 19-27.
This article discusses the history of attempts by various
organizations to prevent married medical women from holding paid positions under the government or local authorities.
The situation is then viewed from the standpoint of the employer, the individual herself, and the community.

2195.   Bewley, Beulah R. and Bewley, Thomas H. "Hospital Doc-
         tors' Career Structure and Misuse of Medical Woman-
         power." Lancet, 2:7928 (9 August 1975) 270-272.
         (Hospital Practice.)
"Biological and cultural differences between men and women
lead to severe discrimination against women doctors who
bear the burdens of pregnancy, child-rearing, and housework. These lead, from equality within medical school and
at qualification, to increasing failure to obtain posts commensurate with their innate abilities. Women doctors who
temporarily and partially drop out of full-time practice have
been studied frequently, but men (who are equally expensive
to train) have not, despite their disappearing from National
Health Service practice through emigration, death, alcoholism, suicide, or removal from the Medical Register. In
a working lifetime of forty years, a woman doctor with an
average family is likely to do seven-eighths of the work of
a doctor who has not had to carry the primary responsibility of bearing and rearing children. Doctors with de-
pendants are handicapped, and a separate career structure
might be set up for them. Supernumerary consultant posts
are proposed." [Article summary.]

2196.   Black, Dora. "Women Doctors in the N.H.S." British
         Medical Journal, 1:5954 (15 February 1975) 393-394.
         (Letters to the Editor.)
Dr. Black refers to an article titled "State of Health"
(British Medical Journal, 28 December 1974, p. 732), which
stated that while women form 32 per cent of medical school
entrants in England and Wales, they constitute only 11.8
per cent of principals in general practice and 7.9 per cent
of consultants. She describes her own situation as a consultant child psychiatrist and a clinical assistant. In addition to spending 53 hours a week in professional activities,
Dr. Black performs "some of the activities conventionally
left to mothers." She details her annual expenditures in-
curred only because of her professional work (totalling
£1,980) and asks: "If one-third or so of British-trained
women doctors have to face these expenses in order to pursue their chosen career, is it surprising that they drop out?"

2197.   Carter, Mary. "Notes on Married Women in the Medical
               Profession." Journal of the Medical Women's Federa-
               tion, 44:4 (October 1962) 159-162.
         The author discusses professional activity for married wo-
         men with and without children as well as the place of moth-
         ers in the medical profession. "I am convinced that pro-
         fessional activities can, under the right circumstances, be
         of benefit to the mother, the family and the state."

2198.   Collins, A. Dorothy. "Married Women in Medicine."
               Journal of the Medical Women's Federation, 43:4 (Octo-
               ber 1961) 202-203.
         In response to two articles that had appeared in the July
         1961 issue of the Journal of the Medical Women's Federa-
         tion (Monica Holmes-Siedle's "Problems facing the young
         married woman doctor," and Mabel L. V. Andrews' "Rem-
         iniscences of my return to medical work"), a married wo-
         man doctor writes of her own experiences. Because Dr.
         Collins works in the same hospital as her husband, oppor-
         tunities for her seem more restricted. She observes that
         one's sex limits one, that the World Health Organization
         will not employ married couples, that it is imperative for
         a woman to amplify her experience and qualifications in
         order to advance, and that married women--irrespective
         of qualifications--seem to be eliminated from employment
         lists.

2199.   Curran, A. P. "Public Health in the University of Glas-
               gow; A Historical Review of Female Diplomates: 1925-
               1959." The Medical Officer, 107:2 (12 January 1962)
               17-22. tables.
         Reviewed are the subsequent academic, civil, and profes-
         sional achievements of the 140 women doctors who took pub-
         lic health diplomas (D. P. H. s) at Glasgow between 1925 and
         1959. The majority of the women are in the Public Health
         Service in Great Britain. Data is given on marital status,
         spouse occupation, and practice patterns (and its relation
         to family commitments). The results are compared with a
         parallel study of the 405 male diplomates of the same time
         span.

2200.   "The Dean's Dilemma." Lancet, 1:7845 (5 January 1974)
               21.
         Proposed legislation to increase the proportion of women
         medical students may also increase the medical school
         dean's dilemma. His problem: as more women enter
         medicine, "a reduction in the doctor-years available to the
         community is more than likely." Women doctors must re-
         ceive better employment opportunities and home-help pro-
         visions. Otherwise, as a result of the legislation, "the
         nation may find itself with more unfilled posts and an army
         of doctors inappropriately employed in British kitchens."

2201.   "Editorial Comment."   Medical Woman's Journal, 42:5
             (May 1935) 135.
         "There are 5,971 women on the medical register in Great
         Britain." Of these, 996 are "insurance practitioners."
         [The insurance practitioner practices under the National
         Health Insurance Act.] Since World War I, the attitude of
         the public has completely changed "and women are quickly
         realizing the advantages of being treated by women doctors."

2202.   Edmunds, J. "Female Medical Society, and Mortality in
             Childbirth." Medical Times and Gazette, 2 (1866) 207-
             209.
         [Article not examined by editors.]

2203.   Edwards, Sally; Essex, Nina; Jack, Bridget; and Smith,
             Isabel. "Women Doctors' Retainer Scheme." Lancet,
             1:7913 (26 April 1975) 974. (Letters to the Editor.)
         Commenting upon the Scheme, the letter-writers urge that
         all part-time posts be graded and approved in the same way
         as full-time ones.

2204.   "English Women Protest Against Sex Distinction in Medical
             Appointments." Medical Woman's Journal, 27:9 (Sep-
             tember 1920) 232.
         The sex distinction, against which the Medical Women's
         Federation and the British Medical Association protested,
         was the inequity in the bonus paid to women assistant med-
         ical officers of the Metropolitan Asylums Board. The situa-
         tion has been altered to provide equal bonus. The Federa-
         tion has not yet been so successful in removing the in-
         equity in salaries paid to male and female medical faculty.

2205.   Eskin, Frada. "A Survey of Medical Women in Lincoln-
             shire 1971." British Journal of Medical Education, 6:3
             (September 1972) 196-200. tables.
         "In a survey of Lincolnshire done in 1971, 15 married wo-
         men doctors stated that they were available for training for
         hospital employment on a sessional basis. Thirteen out of
         15 were willing to travel 10 or more miles for retraining.
         At the time of the survey, five out of 15 were unemployed,
         seven out of 15 were employed part time, and three out of
         15 were employed whole-time outside the hospital service.
         Six out of 15 had higher qualifications in the specialty in
         which they expressed interest in further training. All
         were willing to be employed after training completion."
         [Article summary.]

2206.   Essex, Nina and Holt, Mary C. "Misuse of Medical Wo-
             manpower." Lancet, 2:7930 (23 August 1975) 362-363.
             (Letters to the Editor.)
         These letters respond to an article by Drs. Beulah Bewley
         and Thomas Bewley on the misuse of medical womanpower
         (The Lancet, August 9, 1975, p. 270). Of special concern

to these letter writers is the difficulty women have in obtaining the status of consultant when they cannot work full time.

2207.   Essex-Lopresti, Michael. "Recruitment of Women Doctors for Hospital Service." Lancet, 2:7665 (25 July 1970) 204-206. charts.
To encourage women doctors to seek part-time employment and return to hospital service, it is important to make clear to them that they have other options for employment than junior training grades in full-time resident appointments. Women who have had to take time off to fulfill domestic commitments respond very well and take advantage of schedules tailored to their needs which will enable them to have a career in a senior grade in the hospital service.

2208.   "Exclusion of Married Women Physicians by London County Council." Medical Woman's Journal, 32:1 (January 1925) 22.
Before 1916 women physicians who married had to resign their professional medical appointments with the London County Council. Because of World War I and the shortage of physicians, this injunction was suspended. This article reports that the London County Council voted to once again exclude married women physicians but retain the married women still on the staff from the war.

2209.   "Female Doctors Afield." New England Journal of Medicine, 270:18 (30 April 1964) 960.
This brief article reviews British surveys of the practice patterns of married women physicians.

2210.   "The Flexible Employer." Lancet, 1:7222 (27 January 1962) 201. (Annotations.)
Hospital administrators should be more flexible concerning employment of married women physicians.

2211.   Flynn, Ann C. and Gardner, Frances. "The Careers of Women Graduates from the Royal Free Hospital School of Medicine, London." British Journal of Medical Education, 3:1 (March 1969) 28-42. figs., tables.
A detailed follow-up study was made of the graduates of the Royal Free Hospital School of Medicine from 1945 to 1964, which had a particularly high output of women doctors. Eighty-seven per cent completed a questionnaire sent to them between April and December 1966. They were divided into four groups according to the five-year period in which they qualified as graduates: Group I (1945-1949), Group II (1950-1954), Group III (1955-1959), Group IV (1960-1964). When married women alone are studied it is seen that when one or more diplomas or degrees are held, the percentage working full-time is higher and the percentage not working is lower, but that these figures of 37 per cent and 17 per

cent respectively are not very different from the average
for all married women of 32.2 per cent and 21.4 per cent.
Ninety-three point six per cent of the single women were
working full-time and 4.7 per cent were working part-time
and 1.7 per cent were not working. Over a 20-year period,
95 per cent of the single women have worked throughout the
period, and the percentage is usually between 97 and 98.5:
80.2 per cent of formerly married women were working
full-time, 17.4 per cent were working part-time and
12.4 per cent not working. A higher percentage of women with preschool children are working. There is not
much difference between the work situation of wives of
doctors and wives of nonmedical men. The main difference between the work of married and single full-
timers is that public health and research are considerably
more frequently selected by the former. No relationship
could be found between under-employment and area of
residence. The commonest main reason for not working
is the presence of small children, and this is frequently
combined with difficulty in running the home and looking
after older children in the school holidays. Lack of reliable domestic help is more a problem than complete
absence, and the cost of help becomes heavy if small
children have to be cared for over long hours. Only a
small minority of respondents were unemployed because
it was not financially worthwhile, but many stated in
cover letters that the rewards were very small or even
that they had to pay for the pleasure of working, especially when a second car was necessary.

2212.   Fox, Ida E. "Women on Hospital Staffs and Boards of
            Management." Medical Women's Federation News-Let-
            ter, (March 1925) 18-23.
Questionnaires were sent to 581 London and provincial hospitals to determine the number of hospitals in which women
were serving either on the medical staff or as lay members on boards of management. There were 423 replies.
Results showed that 308 of these had women on the board
of management, the house committee, or both. There were
321 hospitals with medical women serving or eligible in
professional capacity. Statistics are further broken down
geographically and by type of hospital.

2213.   Gillie, Annis. "The Scope of General Practice for Medical
            Women." Journal of the Medical Women's Federation,
            42:2 (April 1960) 74-78. tables. (Address, General
            Practice Section, Scientific Meeting, British Medical
            Association, July 1958.)
This article gives 1957 statistics on women in general practice in Great Britain. These figures are compared with
statistics for 1951 which were obtained from a questionnaire
circulated by the Medical Women's Federation to all women

physicians on the British Medical Register in 1933 and
1948. In 1957 it was estimated that of the 12,000-13,000
women's names on the Register, 20 per cent were in general practice. Out of the 95 women physicians who entered
general practice in 1957, 64 favored mixed partnership.
Few 'all-women' partnerships existed. Solo practice for
women also appeared to be on the wane.

2214. Holmes-Siedle, Monica. "Problems Facing the Young Married Woman Doctor." Journal of the Medical Women's
Federation, 43:3 (July 1961) 123-126.
Ninety-five per cent of women qualifying in medicine marry within a few years of graduating: 45 per cent of these
are no longer practicing. The question is asked: "how
[does one] combine the practice of medicine with marriage
and founding a family"? A part-time practice may be the
answer, but first, several obstacles must be overcome:
prejudice, scarcity of jobs, and the "domestic problem."
Each of these obstacles is dealt with in this article.

2215. Hurdon, Elizabeth. "Foreign Letters: London." Medical
Woman's Journal, 47:12 (December 1940) 373.
Dr. Hurdon, a member of the Journal's Editorial Board in
London, writes that "there is very little doing" for medical
women in England. She briefly discusses the work to which
most women physicians are assigned.

2216. Jefferys, Margot and Elliott, Patricia M. Women in Medicine: The Results of an Inquiry Conducted by the
Medical Practitioners' Union in 1962-63. Office of
Health Economics, London, England, 1966, 47 pp.
tables.
This study was undertaken to explore the efficient use of
medical personnel in Great Britain through examining the
effects of marriage and maternity on women physicians.
The study focuses on: (1) the relationship among the age,
marital status, place of residence, and qualifications of
women doctors and their work, (2) the obstacles to employing women on a full- or part-time basis, (3) the trends in
marriage rates, age, and maternity of women doctors, and
(4) the implications of the findings for the future employment of women physicians. The findings are based on
8,209 questionnaires returned by women listed in the medical directory for 1960 who were also on registration lists
of 1960-62. This was a 75 per cent return rate. The
questionnaire, appended to this report, asked for: (1) marital status, (2) date of marriage, (3) number of children,
(4) whether or not married to a doctor, (5) date of qualification, (6) advanced degrees or diplomas, (7) desire to
work if not practicing, (8) absence of suitable work opportunities, (9) length of time worked since qualification, and
(10) the utility of a postgraduate course in returning to
work. Statistical data are displayed on 25 tables. Some

of the conclusions included the following items: (1) over
85 per cent of the qualifying women physicians may be expected to marry and most will be married by their 30th
birthday, (2) of those doctors age 30-34, 85 per cent had
at least one child, (3) only 54 per cent of the married
childless women worked full-time compared with 82 per
cent of the single women physicians, (4) only one in six
of the respondents with a preschool child worked full-time,
and a third were not working at all, (5) eighty per cent of
the respondents with school age children worked, but less
than a third worked full-time, (6) two-thirds of the unem-
ployment among the respondents was involuntary and one-
third of the part-time practitioners felt they could work
more, (7) there is an unmet demand among young women
doctors with families for regular part-time work, which
could be met through easing childcare problems and providing part-time work in hospitals and local health services, and (8) women who temporarily withdraw from service for child rearing should be offered opportunities for
continuing professional participation in scientific meetings
and postgraduate course work.

2217.   Kahan, J. and Macfaul, M. "Medical Women Graduates,
            1947-1961. A Survey of Their Careers." Middlesex
            Hospital Journal, 62 (1962) 192-194.
        Of the participants in this survey, 100 per cent of the un-
        married women physicians were employed fulltime; 60 per
        cent of those with children were working full time. [In-
        formation derived from secondary source; article not ex-
        amined by editors.]

2218.   Kettle, M. H. "The Fate of the Population of Women Med-
            ical Students." Lancet, 1 (13 June 1936) 1370-1374.
            tables. (Special Articles.)
        Between 1916 and 1924 inclusive, St. Mary's Hospital Med-
        ical School was open to both women and men. Two hundred
        and fifty-five women entered St. Mary's during the nine
        years (222 of these came for the medical course only).
        This study presents an "analysis of the subsequent careers
        of those women who qualified from St. Mary's and of their
        distribution through various branches of the profession."

2219.   Lawrie, Jean E. and Newhouse, Muriel L. "Working Wo-
            men Doctors." British Medical Journal, 1 (20 Febru-
            ary 1965) 524. tables. (Letters to the Editor.)
        These two authors made a survey for the Medical Women's
        Federation of all the medically qualified women in the
        United Kingdom to ascertain how many are working and to
        what capacity. They found over half were working either
        full-time or for more than half the working week. Many
        women felt underemployed; those not working wished some
        professional work. Only 9.7 per cent of those who replied
        were neither working nor wanting work.

2220.   Lawrie, Jean E.; Newhouse, Muriel L.; and Elliott, Pa-
        tricia M. "Opportunities in Medicine: Working Capa-
        city of Women Doctors." British Medical Journal, 1:
        5484 (12 February 1966) 409-412. tables.
        This article is a correlation of the Medical Women's Fed-
        eration (1963) and the Medical Practitioners Union (1962)
        survey about medically qualified women in the United King-
        dom. Of the women who responded, nearly 50 per cent
        were in full-time work, 30 per cent in part-time work, and
        20 per cent not working. Twenty years after qualification,
        more women practice than they do immediately after quali-
        fication. "About 30 per cent of the women doctors were
        single, working predominantly in full-time jobs, but among
        recently qualified married women, with presumably young
        children, 60 per cent were without professional work. Ap-
        proximately 1,200, a third of those not fully employed,
        wished for some or more medical work. Factors which
        exerted a favorable influence on the careers of women
        were possession of a postgraduate qualification and resi-
        dence in a large town. It is suggested that the health ser-
        vices should adopt a more flexible attitude to part-time
        workers, and, as well as at the consultant level, opportun-
        ities for part-time employment and study should be avail-
        able in all grades."

2221.   Lister, John. "By the London Post. There Is No Use
        Chasing an Illusion." New England Journal of Medi-
        cine, 293:5 (31 July 1975) 245-247. (Medical Intelli-
        gence.)
        Discussing problems within the British medical profession,
        this article's author focuses specifically on the "attack on
        private practice" within the National Health Service by Mrs.
        Barbara Castle, secretary of state for social services.
        The author also describes an "unnerving diversion" that
        occurred while he was surveying the medical politics in
        the United States. He was accused of making "a discrim-
        inatory remark" when he stated that the current 33 per cent
        intake of women medical students in Britain "seemed fair
        in view of the proportion of their lives that they are likely
        to spend in professional practice."

2222.   Lister, John. "By the London Post: Women in Medicine
        ...." New England Journal of Medicine, 293:18 (30
        October 1975) 919-920.
        As the quota restrictions for admittance of women to med-
        ical schools are being dropped in Britain, as much as 50
        per cent of the students enrolled in future medical classes
        may be women. Since Britain is currently seriously defi-
        cient in British-trained doctors, it is presently dependent
        upon foreign medical graduates. To rectify this deficit,
        the National Health Service should offer equal career oppor-
        tunities to all British medical graduates, women and men
        alike. Besides the restrictions which childbearing and child

rearing place on one's time and energy, women also find
it difficult to establish themselves in a profession that is
still male dominated. British medicine should help recruit
women physicians who have lost contact with the profession
because of domestic responsibilities and make it possible
for fewer women physicians to lose contact with medicine
during the years they are bearing and rearing children.

2223.   Lister, John. "Changing Patterns of Medical Care--Women
         in Medicine--A Tribute to Long Service." New England
         Journal of Medicine, 290:5 (31 January 1974) 271-272.
         (By The London Post.)
Of the approximately 17,000 women on the British medical
register, 15 per cent are retired, 15 per cent are not
working, and of the remaining 70 per cent, many work only
part time. Yet one in every three medical school entrants
is a woman. "If this high proportion of women in the student intake is to be justified" many more women should
take full-time posts in the National Health Service where
there is a shortage of doctors. The considerable problems
of married medical women especially require review.

2224.   Lunn, John E. "A Survey of Sheffield Medical Women
         Graduating over the years 1930-1952." Medical Care,
         2 (1964) 197-202. figs., tables.
Investigating medical women who graduated from Sheffield
University with ten or more years of postgraduate experience, this survey examines the work and family patterns of
those women who graduated between 1930-52 and what they
were doing through the end of 1962. "Nearly one half of
the medical women were in full-time employment, and nearly one-quarter in part-time employment at the end of 1962.
The majority of the single women were working full-time.
About one-third of the married women were working full-
time and about one-quarter part-time.... The hospital and
general practice services were the most popular among the
single graduates.... Medical women with three or more
children tended to work part-time rather than full-time,
but the proportions not working were the same for both the
larger and the smaller families.... Whereas the single
graduates worked in full-time posts for over 90 per cent
of the period from graduation, the married graduates held
full-time posts for only 50 per cent of this time.... Fifteen years after marriage over 60 per cent are working
full-time.... Some of the younger women gave up their
work before completing their pre-registration posts. These
women may require special facilities in the future if they
are to return to medicine.... The ability of the wives of
general practitioners to work full-time and also have relatively large families was presumably related to the special
conditions of employment many of them enjoyed."

2225.   McIntyre, A. D. and Parry, K. M. "Career Attainment--

ment--Chance or Choice: Survey of Career Experience
of Doctors Graduating in Scottish Medical Schools in
1962." British Journal of Medical Education, 9:2
(June 1975) 70-77. tables.

The Scottish Council for Postgraduate Medical Education
sent questionnaires on training and career experience to
338 graduates from Scottish medical schools in 1962 who
were on the Medical Register at the end of August 1973.
There was an 89 per cent return rate from the 254 physicians resident in the United Kingdom and a 59 per cent return rate from the 84 physicians living abroad. "Few of
those in general practice in the United Kingdom had undergone the minimal period of vocational training now considered necessary for new entrants to practice." One hundred four of the sample were women; their response rate
was 80 per cent. Of the 67 women physicians in the United
Kingdom, 17 were not married and practiced full-time.
Four were in general practice, four were hospital consultants (anesthetics 2, general medicine 1, psychiatry 1),
four were senior registrars (anesthetics 1, obstetrics and
gynecology 2, pediatric surgery 1), and five were in varied
posts outside the hospital. Their career patterns were
similar to those of their male colleagues in the same specialties. Twelve of the 50 married women worked full-
time (general practice 6, consultants in hospital anesthetics
and bacteriology 2, clinical assistant in anesthetics 1, non-
clinical university lecturers 2, and local authority doctor 1).
Many of the remaining 38 were doing only occasional part-
time work; nine were unemployed. There was a tendency
(among the married women) to choose posts with office
hours or which permitted maximum flexibility. Of the sev-
en married women working overseas, two worked full-time
(microbiology and renal dialysis), four were in part-time
work, and one was temporarily unemployed. It was concluded that many married women physicians were under-
employed. Statistical tables illustrated the general survey
findings but did not always separate women from total
counts.

2226.   Mackenzie, Joan. "Factors Affecting Part-Time Work for
        Married Medical Women." Journal of the Medical Wo-
        men's Federation, 40:4 (October 1958) 283-284. (Sym-
        posium on Part Time Work: Part 2.)

Domestic and financial factors, as well as place of residence, and the character of the woman physician are briefly
discussed in relation to part-time work for married women
physicians.

2227.   "Marriage and Matrimony." Lancet, 1:7450 (11 June 1966)
        1308-1309. (Annotations.)

"If matrimony among women doctors is inevitable, consequent waste of their training is not." So concludes a report by the Medical Practitioners' Union (Jefferys, Margot;

Elliott, Patricia M. Women in Medicine: The Results of an Inquiry Conducted by the Medical Practioners' Union in 1962-63. Office of Health Economics, London, England, 1966, 47 pp.). This article reviews that report.

2228.   "The Married Woman Physician." Medical Woman's Journal, 38:5 (May 1931) 126-127.
The chairman of the management board of England's Birmingham General Hospital--a woman--raised the point that "the duties of marriage and motherhood unfit a woman for active public life." The opposition, advocating that married women physicians are capable of holding hospital positions, was led by Dr. Barnes, F.R.S., "a modernist" and a man. The Federation of Medical Women also rallied to support the rights of married women physicians.

2229.   "The Medical Woman and the Hospitals." Woman's Medical Journal, 12:1 (January 1902) 8.
With the appointment of Miss Murdoch Clark as junior house surgeon to the Macclesfield Infirmary in Macclesfield, England, six honorary surgeons resigned. Dr. Clark refused to resign, stating that the matter was not her cause alone but that of all medical women. Seven months after her appointment, Dr. Clark was finally prevailed upon to resign, as the hospital could not carry on without the male staff.

2230.   "Memorandum of Evidence Presented to the Interdepartmental Committee on the Remuneration of Medical Practitioners." Medical Woman's Federation Quarterly Review, (October 1945) 11-18.
Various statistics regarding British medical women (age distribution, experience before general practice, distribution in various types of practice, income, hours worked per week, time off-duty, part-time work, sickness rate) are given in tabular form, with explanations. Results are based on questionnaires sent to all women on the British Medical Register (over 7,000), of which 3,856 replies were received. Some of the results were: 1,172 had taken pregnancy leave; almost 2,000 were engaged in general practice; the age group 40-50 showed the largest number of women in general practice; 82.6 per cent had held resident hospital posts; 55 per cent purchased their own practices: showing that women doctors go where there is a need for a doctor, not a woman doctor; their average work week is 40 to 60 hours; those working part-time usually have young children or are older and cannot afford to fully retire; and women doctors do not seem more susceptible to illness than their male counterparts.

2231.   Murray, Flora. "The Position of Women in Medicine and Surgery." New Statesman, Special Supplement (1 November 1913) xvi-xvii.
[Article not examined by editors.]

2232.   "Oxoniennes in Medicine." New England Journal of Medi-
        cine, 268:9 (28 February 1963) 504-505.
        A survey of the practice patterns of women physicians by
        A. H. T. Robb-Smith ["The Fate of Oxford Medical Wo-
        men," Lancet, 1 December 1962] is reviewed. This arti-
        cle's writer comments that while efforts should be made to
        make available the services of inactive women physicians,
        the necessary domestic arrangements will be difficult--
        "especially in view of the right of children to enjoy a moth-
        er's care and affection, partly in order that they, too, may
        develop an appreciation of the accustomed roles in life of
        each sex, which are not easily interchangeable."

2233.   Paulin, L. Estelle. "Our Paris Letter." Woman's Med-
        ical Journal, 10:7 (July 1900) 299-304.
        An American woman physician writes about her observations
        of medical facilities and personnel on her trip from Edin-
        burgh to Paris. In London she notes that women physicians
        may get training at the Woman's Medical School founded by
        Dr. Garrett-Anderson, but that there are many areas to
        which women physicians still could not assume access. One
        such disappointing place was the New Woman's Hospital
        where women interns were not allowed, although this hos-
        pital is where the students from the Woman's Medical
        School acquire hospital training. The Soho Square Hospital
        for Women did not allow women students or physicians any
        professional training or appointments, short-staffed as it
        was. She concludes that "perhaps ... they are trying to
        'protect' women from themselves...." In France she ob-
        served that women may work hard as street cleaners and
        in other hard work non-decision-making positions.

2234.   "Requirements Necessary to Practice Medicine in England."
        Woman's Medical Journal, 26:2 (February 1916) 47.
        As a result of the War, the Royal Army Medical Corps
        has needed the services of many thousands of medical men
        in the field, and therefore the civilian population of England
        sorely needs doctors. If American medical women want to
        go to England to practice, they have to take a British quali-
        fication. The requirements for such qualification are given.

2235.   "Retaining Women Doctors." Lancet, 2:7771 (5 August
        1972) 268.
        Because so many women do not practice medicine once they
        marry and acquire domestic commitments, the National
        Health Service has devised a Women Doctors' Retainer
        Scheme. To encourage women to practice their professional
        skills and training, this program pays participants £50 a
        year under the stipulation they retain their medical registra-
        tion and membership in a medical defense organization, read
        a professional journal, attend at least seven "education"
        sessions a year, and do at least 12 "service" sessions a
        year.

2236.   Robb-Smith, A. H. T. "The Fate of Oxford Medical Wo-
          men." Lancet, 2:7266 (1 December 1962) 1158-1161.
          Questionnaires were sent to 139 pre-1951 women graduates
          of Oxford University who had received the B.M. degree
          since 1922 (when the first four women received this degree
          from Oxford). The questionnaires inquired as to "civil
          state, number of children, husband's occupation, whether
          they were, or had been, practicing medicine, and if so in
          what branch of the profession. If they had given up prac-
          tice they were asked why and whether they would like to
          resume." Responses were received from 138 women. The
          graduates were divided into three groups: those who quali-
          fied in 1922-30, 1931-40, and 1941-50. Of those who re-
          mained single, 60 per cent were in the 1922-30 group, 27
          per cent in the 1931-40 group, and 19 per cent in the 1941-
          50 group. Of the single women (40), nearly half were con-
          sultants, six were not in practice (three of six because of
          ill health), and four had died. Of the 71 married graduates,
          the greatest number (14) were in public health, followed by
          general practice (13). Twenty-eight graduates were not in
          practice. Those who were in practice said "'they had been
          blessed with an adequate supply of nannies and domestic
          staff.'" In the discussion that follows, the author submits
          that "if the lack of clinical opportunities of the Oxford med-
          ical women graduating between 1941 and 1950 applies to all
          medical women, it deserves the serious attention of the
          Ministry of Health, the University Grants Committee, and
          the medical schools; it would seem a waste to give a large
          number of women a lengthy and expensive training, and then
          ensure that their professional activities were restricted to
          40 per cent."

2237.   Rue, Rosemary. "Women in Medicine: Great Britain."
          British Medical Journal, 4 (17 November 1973) 404.
          About one-fifth of the doctors in Britain are women. They
          account for 7.6 per cent of hospital consultants and 11.6
          per cent of general practice principals. Despite these
          figures, women are still experiencing difficulties in achiev-
          ing careers in medicine. A 1970 National Health Service
          study revealed that "women doctors follow the same career
          patterns as men until they have commitments to children--
          or elderly relatives." The degree to which the woman doc-
          tor participates in the medical field thereafter depends on
          how much extra help she can muster. The author suggests
          appropriate career counseling for women medical students
          and young women doctors.

2238.   Savage, Anne. "Part-Time Work." Journal of the Med-
          ical Women's Federation, 44:1 (January 1962) 39-40.
          A personal account is given by the author of her experience
          in reentering medicine after her second child was born.
          Her eventual part-time employment consisted in managing
          the practices of vacationing physicians.

2239.   Shore, E. "Women in Medicine." Health Trends, 1:2
           (1969) 2-3.
         [Article not examined by editors.]

2240.   Stanley, Gillian R. and Last, John M. "Careers of Young
           Medical Women." British Journal of Medical Educa-
           tion, 2 (1968) 204-209. tables.
         In 1961 a survey for the Association for the Study of Med-
         ical Education was made by a team in the department of
         Social Medicine at the University of Edinburgh. The study
         was made of the approximately 9,500 students attending
         medical schools in Great Britain. In 1966 these authors
         made a follow-up investigation of those who had since com-
         pleted their training. Some of those previously questioned
         were excluded because their "numbers were small, and
         these students were in some ways atypical." In the 1961
         survey, almost 25 per cent of the respondants were fe-
         male and in the 1966 survey 24.6 per cent were women.
         "Significantly higher proportions of women than men had
         completed the undergraduate course without failing any ex-
         aminations, and fewer women than men failed on two or
         more occasions." Of both the women who had married and
         those who had remained single, approximately 70 per cent
         had not gained any additional professional qualification at
         the time of this survey. Married doctors of both sexes con-
         stituted a higher proportion not continuing their training
         than single doctors. "Proportionately twice as many mar-
         ried women as married men felt that they were no longer
         in training; this no doubt reflects where the burden of prac-
         tical domestic responsibility lies heaviest." The survey
         included a section on the reading habits of these doctors
         and found that three-fifths of the married women read an
         hour a week and that three-fifths of the married men read
         seven hours a week or more. The authors conclude "that
         married men are more strongly oriented professionally.
         It may be that their lives and ambitions are more sys-
         tematically ordered, by necessity if not by choice, and
         that steady working habits are part of a pattern of domes-
         tic life for married men but not for married women col-
         leagues." Married men had a much higher participation
         rate in postgraduate courses than married women. Single
         women and men attended such courses in the same pro-
         portion. One interpretation the authors give their findings
         is that "behavioral and attitude differences ... appear to be
         more directly related to marital status than to sex." Nine-
         ty-five per cent of the recent male graduates were employed
         full-time while 62 per cent of the recent female graduates
         were employed full-time. The authors quote one of the wo-
         men who participated in the survey as saying, "I went into
         dermatology because ... I felt that I would progress in my
         chosen career without subjugating my husband and children
         by having to undertake full-time employment. It is dis-
         tressing to find that outside London it is well-nigh impos-

sible to get people to accept part-time workers even when faced with difficulty in getting full-time workers.... The tragedy is that experience is being wasted in the face of administrative intransigence."

2241.   Timbury, Morag C. and Ratzer, Maria A. "Glasgow Med-
             ical Women 1951-4: Their Contribution and Attitude to
             Medical Work." British Medical Journal, 2 (10 May
             1969) 372-374. tables. (Medical Education.)
"This survey was undertaken to find out how a group of medical women in early middle age had coped with the conflict between career and family and what their attitude was to continuing work after marriage." Postal questionnaires were sent to 137 women who had graduated from the University of Glasgow Medical Department during 1951-4; there were 106 responses. Most single women were in full-time posts and had worked full-time for more than twice as many years as their married colleagues. When this group of women was compared with a group of 137 men practicing medicine, a higher proportion of women were in public health and the proportion of women in general practice was considerably lower. Surgery was the most popular specialty among men; no women were recorded as being in surgery. If married women did practice, there seemed to be some correlation to whether or not a member of their family was in medicine. In addition, those women who married tended to practice medicine if they wanted to become doctors at a "relatively" early age. Part-time medical people, while satisfied with their posts, would have liked improved promotion possibilities. "Less than a fifth [of married women] were prepared to do night duty, thereby limiting their usefulness in most hospital specialties and general practice." "The attitude of married women to work is determined largely by the attitude of the community where they live towards working mothers, the ease with which domestic arrangements can be made during working hours, and the availability of suitable and congenial work." The authors conclude that if full employment of women physicians "was considered necessary, new incentives to work would have to be found. These might include provision of secure posts with flexible hours, child-minding services, tax allowances and planned postgraduate training. The appointment in each region of the country of a person whose primary task would be to act as a postgraduate advisor for women doctors might be a prerequisite of any major increase in the working contribution of the married women doctors in that area."

2242.   "U.K. Hospitals Urged to Lure Women MDs to Resume
             Practice." Medical Tribune, (6 March 1969) 2.
This brief article notes that 28 per cent of the women doctors in the United Kingdom are inactive. [Article not examined by editors.]

2243.   Whitfield, A. G. W. "Current Work of Birmingham Med-
              ical Graduates 1948-58." Lancet, 1 (15 February
              1964) 374-375. figs., tables.
         This article reports a survey that was made among the
         men and women who have graduated from the University of
         Birmingham medical program since the advent of the Na-
         tional Health Service. The survey was limited to graduates
         of the years 1948-58. Of the 976 graduates, 229 were wo-
         men. At the time of the survey, 58 (or 25.3 per cent)
         were not working medically. All 58 were married and had
         the responsibility for raising children and running a house.
         A handful had other problems finding employment: three
         were unable to get jobs for which they qualified; two were
         living overseas where their British qualifications did not
         make them eligible to practice; "one felt she was not fitted
         for the practice of medicine." Sixty women of the 229
         were unmarried and were all working full-time. The au-
         thor says that there has been a loss to medicine of 35.8
         per cent of all the women graduates and 8.4 per cent of
         the eleven-year output of the Birmingham Medical School.
         "Undoubtedly some of those not working medically at the
         time of the survey will resume work when their children
         are older, and others at present working part-time may get
         back to full-time work; but the loss to medicine is formid-
         able, and universities might well consider reducing their
         intake of women medical students now that the 'bulge' is
         producing more candidates than medical schools can ac-
         commodate."

2244.   Whitfield, A. G. W. "Emigration of Birmingham Medical
              Graduates: 1959-63." Lancet, 1:7596 (29 March 1969)
              667-669. fig., tables. (Medical Education.)
         A 1968 survey of 419 graduates of the University of Bir-
         mingham Medical School (classes of 1959-63) revealed the
         following: "48 were abroad, and all but six of these had
         emigrated permanently"; dissatisfaction with general prac-
         tice under the National Health Service was the most com-
         mon reason for emigrating. Data given are not analyzed
         by sex. However, the author notes that 96 of the survey's
         subjects are women, that three of the six physicians still
         abroad but intending to return are women, and that two
         married women emigrants are not working in medicine.

2245.   Whitfield, A. G. W. "Women Medical Graduates of the
              University of Birmingham 1948-58." Postgraduate Med-
              ical Journal, 40 (April 1964) 175-178. figs., tables.
         All those graduating from the University of Birmingham
         from 1948-58 were surveyed in order to obtain information
         about medical emigration. Since the information about med-
         ical emigration has been published elsewhere, this article
         is concerned with additional information the survey col-
         lected on women graduates. During 1948-58, 747 men and
         229 women graduated in medicine from the University of

Birmingham. Over the eleven year period, the male/fe-
male ratio was a little over three to one although in 1948,
1949, and 1950 there was a greater proportion of women
because so many men who would have qualified were serving in the armed forces. The author observes "that a
greater degree of selection is exercised in respect of female applications as compared with male and this is commonly thought to result in female medical students being intellectually superior to male." On the other hand, the author notes little difference between the intellectual capacity
of men and women medical students because while a proportion of female students received honors degrees, men
students received the same proportion of distinctions. Ninety-four of the 229 women graduates received higher medical
qualifications--a smaller proportion than the men. The author observes that marriage with resultant domestic and
family commitments could be the chief factor and adds that
ambition and necessity play a considerable part in the men
acquiring additional qualifications. Of the 229 women graduates, 168 are married, 60 are unmarried and one is dead.
Sixty-one of the married graduates and all the single graduates work full-time. Another 48 of the married women
graduates work part-time while 58 are not doing any medical work. During the training years, seven men and four
women withdrew from the medical course: "While the numbers were small, the wastage is appreciable and is proportionately a little greater among women students than male,
though the number involved is too small for this to be statistically significant." Because of the 58 married women
who do not work at all and the 48 married women who
work part-time, there is a 36.9 per cent loss to medicine
among the 233 women who were accepted as medical students, and an 8.4 per cent loss of the total 11-year output
of the Birmingham Medical School. Because of this loss,
the author observes, "Universities may well think it prudent
to reduce their intake of women medical students during the
'bulge' years when there will undoubtedly be many more
candidates with the requisite 'A' levels in the General Certificate of Education than there are places available." Of
the 229 women graduates, 36 (15.7 per cent) live abroad.

2246. Winner, Albertine. "The Changing Numbers of Women Stu-
       dents." Proceedings of the Royal Society of Medicine,
       68:8 (August 1975) 499-502. figs., tables.
This article reviews the findings of selected recent surveys
in Great Britain on the number of women in medical practice. Since 1944 all medical schools in Great Britain have
been coeducational, and recent data from the Department
of Health indicate that women comprise about one third of
the total qualifying physicians in any one year. In 1968
the Royal Commission on Medical Education established that
there were about 13,360 women in active medical practice
in Great Britain. In 1974 the Department of Health and

Social Security found the hospital service in England and
Wales employed about 4,100 women (1973 data). In general practice there were 2,864 women in England only.
Other surveys were conducted from 1962-69 by various organizations. In a 1962 survey, 47.5 per cent of women
physicians were in full-time practice; 18.7 per cent were
not working at the time of the study. The age distribution
shows a decline in full-time work over age 29 with a rise
following to age 64; the trend for part-time work was opposite. It appeared that the presence of young children
was a deterrent to full-time work. A retainer scheme,
promulgated in 1972, provides an annual payment of £50 a
year in return for registration, membership in a defense
society, and a declaration of intent to return to medicine;
this has attracted about 250 women. Another system introduced in 1969 provides for part-time training for doctors
on every level from house officer to senior registrar.
These programs are among the efforts to keep women in
the field. Tables and graphs illustrating data are included,
as is a bibliography of data sources.

2247.   "Women Doctors." British Medical Journal, 1 (10 March
         1962) 734. (Commons Questions.)
Due to the physician shortage, married women doctors would
be welcome in the "total doctor force." A spokesman for
the Minister of Health sees "no reason why a married woman should not be taken on as an assistant or partner in
general practice, or, apart from restricted areas, set up
single-handed in certain areas."

2248.   "Women Doctors in London. Many Obstacles Are Placed
         in Their Way, But Three Qualify." Woman's Medical
         Journal, 27:2 (February 1917) 40.
With the staff of London Hospital greatly reduced because
of the war, three women physicians were hired to serve on
that staff. Now five hospitals in London allow women physicians to practice, and a military hospital for wounded
soldiers is run by women.

2249.   "Women Doctors' Retainer Scheme." Lancet, 1:7911 (12
         April 1975) 850. (Special Article.)
The terms of the Scheme, which was introduced in 1972
to "encourage women to continue working in medicine,"
are outlined.

2250.   "Women in Medicine." Lancet, 2:7368 (14 November 1964)
         1055-1056. (Annotations.)
The major obstacle to making use of married medical women is "unwillingness and lack of imagination" on the part
of employers. This article examines the problem of training new women doctors "(each at a cost of some £5000)
even though qualified women are left, at least professionally, idle."

2251.   "Women in Medicine: The Avoidance of Wastage." British
         Journal of Medical Education, 7:3 (September 1973)
         143-145. (Editorials.)
         This editorial speaks of the obligations women who enter
         the medical profession have to the State, which often paid
         for their education, and the obligations of the medical
         schools and governments not to mislead women by admitting
         them to medical schools "unless we are satisfied that there
         are opportunities for them to acquire the necessary con-
         tinued training in a way that is compatible with family re-
         sponsibilities." Women physicians' practice patterns, as
         presented in various other sources, are reviewed. Recom-
         mendations on how to cut down on undue wastage of med-
         ical womanpower are summarized in conclusion.

2252.   "Women in the British Colonial Service." Medical Woman's
         Journal, [28]:1 (January [1921]) 22-23.
         Although few in number, the appointments of women phy-
         sicians to serve in British colonies are examples of wo-
         man's advancement.

INTERNATIONAL

2253.   Balfour, Margaret. "The Role of Medical Women in Ex-
                otic Countries." Medical Woman's Journal, 39:1 (Jan-
                uary 1932) 1-6. (Presentation, Sixth Convention, In-
                ternational Association of Medical Women, Vienna,
                Austria, September 15-20, 1931.)
         Medical women are needed in many parts of Africa and the
         Orient because the cultures there prohibit men who are not
         close relatives to see women for any purpose, including
         medical care. Where medical women have served the lo-
         cal populations, there has been a positive effect on health
         care and hygiene. Only in towns is it possible to find
         people with enough money to reimburse a doctor so that
         she might have a private practice. The villages are too
         poor to support a doctor in private practice. Many more
         medical women are needed because health care of women
         in these areas is inadequate.

2254.   Gracey, J. T. Woman's Medical Work in Foreign Lands.
                Boston, Massachusetts, [n. d.].
         [Book not examined by editors.]

2255.   MacMurchy, Helen. "Hospital Appointments. Are They
                Open to Women?" New York Medical Journal, (27
                April 1901) 1-16.
         This article discusses the hospital appointments for women
         by reproducing a list compiled by the Woman's Medical Col-
         lege, Toronto, Canada. The list shows a total of 559 med-
         ical appointments (government, municipal, and hospital) held
         by women physicians. Hospitals are listed (by name) in

various states of the U.S., in England, Scotland, Ireland, Australia, Egypt, Ceylon, India, France, Germany, Russia, Holland, Switzerland, and Korea. Positions held by women physicians at each hospital are given.

2256.   Macy, Mary Sutton. "The Field for Women of Today in Medicine." Woman's Medical Journal, 27:3 (March 1917) 49-58. tables.
In order to establish the opportunities available for medical women, the author sent a questionnaire through the Woman's Medical Journal to state medical societies, medical colleges, etc. in the United States and Canada in 1916. The questionnaire is reproduced. The 41 questionnaires returned represent 28 states of the United States, the Panama Canal Zone, and one province of Canada. The approximate proportion of women physicians to men physicians in each state is given. State medical societies where women hold positions as officers or as chairmen of standing committees are mentioned, as are states that have coeducational medical colleges and states where women hold positions on medical faculties. To verify her findings and to enlarge her scope, Dr. Macy checked the 1916 Directory of the American Medical Association (Fifth Edition) for the numbers of medical women in the United States and Canada. She found that in the continental United States, of the 145,240 physicians, 5,518 were women; in the territories and island possessions, of the 1,372 physicians, 33 were women; and in Canada, of the 7,707 physicians, 107 were women. (The author acknowledges that when uncertain about whether or not a name were that of a man or a woman, she assumed that the name was probably a man's.) Included is a table based on this data from the directory showing, by geographical location, the percentages of physicians to the estimated population, the percentages of physicians who were women, the percentages of the women members and men members of the state medical societies, and the percentages of all medical women who were also members of state medical societies. When these percentages, based on information from the directory, were compared to the information based upon the returned questionnaires, some discrepancies were found. A chart based on Directory of the American Medical Association list shows the number of women in the respective medical specialties. Thirty-four colored women were numbered among the active medical women. Because of the unavailability of statistics showing the representation of medical women on hospital staffs, the author suspects that women are discriminated against in such appointments. Dr. Macy also observes that she did not find that any colored medical women belong to state medical societies and, therefore, suspects that these societies exclude colored women from membership.

2257.   Martindale, Louisa. "The Hospitals We Run." Medical

Women's Federation News-Letter, (July 1930) 18-25.
photos., port.
Dr. Martindale discusses facts and figures relating to hospitals run and staffed by women. Her statistics relate to
hospitals in Great Britain (where 164 women physicians and
surgeons have sole charge of 838 inpatient beds in women-
run hospitals alone), India, Australia, and Yugoslavia.

2258. "Medical Women in Mental Hospitals." Medical Women's
International Journal, 1:5 (November 1927) 40-44.
A questionnaire designed to ascertain the position of women
physicians employed in mental hospitals was sent by the
Medical Women's International Association to its representatives in various countries. The questionnaire is reproduced
in this article. Replies from Canada, Denmark, Germany,
and India are summarized.

2259. "The Medical Women's International Association." Medical
Woman's Journal, 41:11 (November 1934) 303. (Edi-
torial.)
Given is a summary of major issues considered at the
Third Quinquennial Congress of the Medical Women's Inter-
national Association, held in Stockholm, August 7-12, 1934.

2260. "Notes and Comments." Medical Woman's Journal, 29:8
(August 1922) 194-196.
"Dr. Josephine Baker, of the U.S. Department for Child
Hygiene, has been nominated to the Health Committee of
the League of Nations." She will be the first woman identified with the League of Nations in a professional capacity;
however, as the U.S. does not belong, she cannot represent the government. Another news note announces that on
June 4, the first woman graduates in medicine received
their degrees from McGill University in Montreal, Quebec.

2261. Nuysink-Steinbuch, D. C. ["Women Doctors in the Netherlands and in the Netherlands Indies"]. Nederlandsch
Tijdschrift voor Geneeskunde, 70 (6 November 1926)
2091-2096. photos., port. (Dut)
This is a transcript of a lecture given before the Congress
of the International Federation of University Women in
Amsterdam, 31 July 1926, in which the speaker summarizes
the situation of women doctors in the Netherlands and its
Eastern colony. Of the 216 women physicians in the home
country, 175 are performing medical work, 16 are not practicing, and the status of 25 could not be determined. Of
those in practice, 47 are general practitioners, 25 pediatricians, 21 in government service (school physicians, health
inspectors, infant welfare, etc.), 11 are gynecologists, 10
are neurologists/psychiatrists, 28 are hospital assistants,
18 are practicing part-time, and the others are in other
special fields. A hundred and two are married, 59 to doctors; of these 102, 56 are in full-time practice and 19 work-

ing part-time. Brief notes on the first few women physicians in the country are given, including Aletta Jacobs,
Catherine van Tussenbroek, Cornelia de Lange, and Marianne van Herwerden. There are seven women practicing
in South Africa and 35 in the Netherlands East Indies. Of
the latter, 19 are in government service, 11 are in general practice, four are specialists, and one is a missionary;
17 are married. One of the outstanding pioneers in the
Indies is Mevrou Stokvis-Cohen Stuart, who started a school
for nurses and midwives and a clinic in Semarang, originally for women and infants, which is now open to all. These
women are an inspiration to all who will come after them.

2262. "Woman Physicians and Woman's Health, the Y.W.C.A.
          Conference." Survey, 43 (15 November 1919) 110-111.
       [Article not examined by editors.]

2263. "Women in Medicine." New York State Journal of Medi-
          cine, (1 October 1963) 2771. (Editorial.)
       Included in this editorial are percentages on the numbers
       of women physicians in the United States, Great Britain,
       and Canada. [Article not examined by editors.]

2264. Woodside, Nina B. "Women Too Often on the Fringes."
          Annals of Internal Medicine, 82:3 (March 1975) 418-
          420. table. (Editorial.)
       After commenting upon the paper by Ione Fett entitled "Out-
       standing Medical Graduates in 1972" [Medical Journal of
       Australia, 1 (1974) 689-698], Dr. Woodside compares the
       findings on Australian women physicians, as presented in
       Fett's study, to the situation in the United States, especial-
       ly with reference to the inactive women physicians; the
       choice of specialties by women in Australia, the United
       Kingdom, and the U.S.; and the lack of support women phy-
       sicians experience in problem situations.

SOUTH, CENTRAL, LATIN AMERICA
AND MEXICO

2265. Franke, Meta E. "South American Medical Women." Med-
          ical Woman's Journal, 32:11 (November 1925) 306-307.
       After touring South America and meeting medical women
       there, Dr. Franke observes, "Officially women work in the
       hospitals and laboratories on the same basis as medical
       men and have their respect and cooperation." While some
       women have large private practices, others do not practice
       after they marry.

USSR

2266. Antipenko, E. S. ["Increasing Interest of the District

Therapeutists in Their Work"].   Zdravookhranenie
Rossiiskoi Federatsii, 1 (January 1975) 22-25.   table.
(Rus)

A survey was carried out confirming the tendency of district therapeutists toward specialization in the three major
fields of medicine: cardiology, pulmonology, and gastroenterology, and less often in rheumatology, endocrinology,
and other specialties.   Of 100 physicians working in 25
outpatient clinics in different districts of Moscow, 87 were
women and 13 were men; 65 had five to six years of experience; 74 said they had better knowledge and experience
in some fields of medicine than others; 64 said they turn to
specialists for consultation on their patients.   One of every
three considered himself more specialized in some one
field.   The author recommends advanced training of doctors
in fields of medicine they show the most interest in.

2267.   Chikin, S. Y. and Alexeyev, Y. A.   ["Problems of Med-
            ical Personnel Training in the Russian Soviet Federated
            Socialist Republic (1959-1966)"].   Sovetskoe Zdravookh-
            ranenie, 29 (1970) 9-14.   tables.   (Rus)

Statistical data presented in seven tables compare conditions of medical personnel practicing in 1958 and 1965-66
in the Russian Soviet Federated Socialist Republic (RSFSR)
as an example of changes occurring during the realization
of the 1959-1966 seven-year plan.   A number of trends
emerge and are commented on in the text.   The tables deal
with MD age bracket percentages, percentages of female
MDs by age group and by specialty, percentages of MDs
aged 30 and under, nationalities of MDs staffing RSFSR
Health Ministry Establishments, indigenous MDs working in
their native autonomous republics or elsewhere in the
RSFSR, and a breakdown by length of general medical service in urban as against rural areas.   While the number of
physicians increased by 37 per cent, the proportion of
males increased owing to active government efforts to attract younger students (presumably males) into the medical
institutes, and by 1966 predominance of women in the 40-
plus age bracket was already noticeable, with the reverse
true for those under 25, i.e., the newly graduated.   While
there was an increase in numbers of specialists in the ob-
stetrical-gynecological field (which was consistently dominated by women), this specialty and also the public health
field showed a percentage decline in consequence of the
greater gains in the therapeutic and surgical categories.
There were significant increases in numbers of MDs in
more highly specialized fields: urology, neuropathology,
cancer, and lung disease--especially the latter in view of
a government campaign against tuberculosis initiated in
1960.   References are made to efforts to ensure equitable
distribution of medical personnel through establishment of
medical institutes in the industrial regions of Siberia and
the Far East, training of national minorities, and greater

opportunities for clinical internship. The authors make
reference to two negative trends: physicians practicing outside the specialized fields in which they were trained and
rural physicians moving into the industrialized population
centers.

2268. Daniels, Robert S. "A Comparison of Physician Education
         in the USSR and the United States." American Journal
         of Psychiatry, 131:3 (March 1974) 315-317.
       Drawing contrasts between medicine in the USSR and the
       U.S., the author describes the influence of public policy on
       Soviet medicine, the emphasis in training and practice, and
       the role of women. Women, who comprise 73 per cent of
       the total number of physicians in the USSR, frequently staff
       primary care sites. Noting that the U.S.'s weakest area
       of medical service is primary care, the author suggests
       that the U.S. might "do well to shift the proportion of [its]
       physicians in the direction of more women, particularly in
       family medicine, obstetrics, pediatrics, and psychiatry."

2269. Field, Mark G. "American and Soviet Medical Manpower:
         Growth and Evolution, 1910-1970." International Jour-
         nal of Health Services, 5:3 (1975) 455-474. tables.
         (Articles on International Health and Comparisons of
         Health Care.)
       "Between 1910 and 1970 the number of physicians in the
       United States increased 2.5 times, in Soviet Russia almost
       25 times. The number of physicians per constant unit of
       population remained fairly stable in the United States, ris-
       ing slightly in the last few years. In the USSR that num-
       ber increased 16 to 18 times, and now stands about 50 per
       cent higher than in the United States. About ten per cent
       of American physicians are women; in the USSR it is about
       70 per cent." Under a section entitled "Feminization of the
       Medical Profession" it is reported that under Czarism, less
       than ten per cent of the medical profession in Russia was
       comprised of women. Since the revolution, the figure has
       climbed to 85 per cent in the 1960s. It appears, however,
       that the government is reducing the percentage in recent
       years. The situation is compared with that in the U.S.,
       where less than ten per cent of the profession are women.
       "Neither society has resolved the problem of deploying
       physicians to the rural areas. American physicians are
       more specialized than their Soviet colleagues. The article
       concludes with general remarks about the two health sys-
       tems, pointing out resemblances and divergences. The
       hypothesis of a possible 'convergence' is entertained."
       [Article summary adapted.]

2270. Kritskii, E. I. ["Nature of Work Absenteeism and Amount
         of Lost Time of Physicians--Male and Female--in the
         Course of a Year"]. Sovetskoe Zdravookhranenie, 29
         (1970) 62-67. tables. (Rus)

"Factual duration of a physician's working year is of great significance for planning the public health service. The article presents the materials of investigations of the work of 5,000 physicians in four regions of the RSFSR. The causes of distraction from the primary occupation and the number of working day losses during a year in physicians of different sex, age, specialty, and position are studied. The materials of investigations may be used to better and rational employment of medical workers." [Journal summary.]

2271. Kritskii, E. I. ["Part-time Employment of Physicians in Various Specialties (Based on Data of Studies Conducted in 4 Districts of the RSFSR)"]. Sovetskoe Zdravookhranenie, 29 (1970) 32-36. tables. (Rus)
"The results of studying the problems of holding more than one job are given according to the materials of four regions of the RSFSR. The investigation defined the extent of this factor in physicians of different sex, age, and specialty, the nature of holding several jobs, as well as dependence of such physicians' work on certain social-hygienic factors." [Journal summary.]

2272. Parrish, John B. "Women in Medicine: What Can International Comparisons Tell Us?" The Woman Physician, 26:7 (July 1971) 352-353, 356-357, 360-361. tables.
The United States registers the lowest percentage of women as physicians of almost any other country. Whereas only 7 per cent of United States' doctors are women, the percentage ranges between 12 to 25 per cent in some Far Eastern countries, from 13 to 20 per cent in Western Europe, to 30 per cent in Eastern Europe and up to 65 per cent in the Soviet Union. The author identifies three temporary demographic, socio-economic, and political factors that are the probable causes for the higher percentage of women physicians in the Soviet Union: the general necessity for self-support and independent careers because of the acute shortage of male marriage partners (in 1959 over one-half of all Soviet women, 50 to 59 years of age, were single); the necessity for life-long work, even if married, because of the low real family income levels (Soviet women doctors do not escape "poverty" since they are paid at or below "blue collar wage levels"); and the desire for Soviet women to rise out of the lowest manual class and obtain the perquisites of professional status (in the Soviet Union men opt for and are given preference in the nonmedical sciences which pay the highest salaries and carry the highest prestige). Women comprise less than five per cent of the membership in the Soviet Academy of Medical Sciences, which means that few top-level Soviet medical positions are held by women. In contrast to the United States, if a woman opts to compete with men for a medical education, she enters one of the highest paid and one of the most

prestigious professions in the country. "The decimation of
the U.S. eligible bachelor male population, as a way of
compelling more young women to seek medical careers,
vis-a-vis the Soviet Union, is hardly an attractive or practical proposition (although the more militant leaders of the
Woman's Lib Movement might just go for it). Nor does it
appear desirable that a free society should institute rigid
allocation of openings in higher institutions so as to force
more women into medicine. Having achieved the highest
level of living in world history, it doesn't appear reason-
able to give it up as a way of forcing more women to
work at something. Nor would we want to reduce levels
of living for manual workers in order to force more women students into the professions as an escape route from
the manual class." The author concludes that the utilization of women in medicine could change to create more
"in between jobs" as physician's assistant, anesthetic assistant, clinical associate, etc. "This would open up other
professional areas for more talented women who wish to
combine work and home responsibilities."

2273.   Petrov, B. D. ["The Role of Women in the Health Ser-
            vice of the USSR"]. Concours Medical (Paris), 87
            (13 March 1965) 1889-1890. (Fre)
        [Article not examined by editors.]

2274.   Petrov, B. D. "Women in the Health Services of the
            Soviet Union." World Medical Journal, 11:1 (January
            1964) 30.
        Complete equality of rights to men and women is guaran-
        teed under the constitution of the Soviet Union. Three-
        quarters of the physicians are women, and the proportion
        is even greater "at the lower level in the Health Services."
        The editor of the national Medical Journal is also a wo-
        man, highly esteemed.

2275.   Ryan, T. M. "Primary Medical Care in the Soviet Union."
            International Journal of Health Service, 2:2 (May 1972)
            243-253. tables.
        An examination of the problems of overspecialization within
        the Soviet medical profession prompts the suggestion that
        the Soviet Union would do well to consider the example of
        the British general practitioner. While this report does
        not deal with physicians as women, readers are reminded
        that women constitute nearly 75 per cent of the medical
        work force within the Soviet Union; the author attributes a
        high turnover rate among district doctors to this fact.

2276.   "Thirty Thousand Women Physicians in Russia." Medical
            and Professional Woman's Journal, 40:9 (September
            1933) 276. (Editorial.)
        Of the total of 68,000 physicians in Soviet Russia, more
        than 30,000 are women. "The average income of the phy-

sician is less than that of the expert factory worker.
There is almost no private practice, and there are practically no rural physicians." The ratio of doctors to population in the cities is 17.6:10,000. Three per cent of
the total number of physicians belong to the communist
party.

2277.   Toropoff, D. I. ["Statistics of Woman Physicians in Rus-
         sia"]. Vestnik obsh. hig., sudeb. i prakt. med., 50
         (1914) 852-885. (Rus)
         [Article not examined by editors.]

2278.   Vlasenko, V. I. ["Incidence and Character of Morbidity
         Among Physicians with Temporary Disability According
         to Data of Personal Estimation"]. Vrach Delo, 7
         (1974) 143-146. tables. (Rus)
         The paper summarizes data obtained in Kiev during the
         years 1969-1971. A table gives data for men, women, and
         all physicians combined (according to specialty of practice)
         for number of illnesses, total number of days lost, average
         number of days per case. For women the average time
         lost per illness was 13.3 days, and for men 11.6. The
         types of diseases most common among the men were those
         of the circulatory system, the nervous system, and infec-
         tions. Among the women, the most frequent diseases were
         those of the circulatory system, the genito-urinary system,
         the nervous system, and musculo-skeletal diseases.

2279.   "Women Doctors in Russia Have Distinguished Themselves
         at Front in Country's Wars." Woman's Medical Jour-
         nal, 26:10 (October 1916) 244.
         Women in Russia have been determined enough to learn
         medicine to go to Switzerland and other foreign countries
         before women were accepted at Russian medical schools.
         Since then, women physicians have been active practitioners
         in the Serbian-Turkish War, the Russo-Japanese War, and
         World War I.

UNITED STATES

2280.   Ballintine, Eveline P. "Women Physicians in Public Insti-
         tutions." Woman's Medical Journal, 18:4 (April 1908)
         79-80.
         Women are on the medical staffs of 61 of the 131 hospitals
         for the insane in the United States. The laws in various
         states requiring women to be on the staffs of these hos-
         pitals are discussed.

2281.   Barringer, Emily Dunning; and Wakefield, Alice E. "Sen-
         ate Bill 2507: An Insult to Medical Women." Medical
         Woman's Journal, 27:1 (January 1920) 23.
         Women physicians are opposed to U.S. Senate Bill 2507 on

public health and national quarantine as it provides for employment of all males (with the exception of a female nurse
or doctor as third assistant secretary of public health).
The resolution adopted by the Women's Medical Association
of New York City in regard to the bill is reprinted.

2282.   Birch, Carol L.; Galbraith, Maurice J.; and Moon, George
        R. "Women Physicians Graduating from University of
        Illinois." Illinois Medical Journal, 105 (May 1954) 268-
        269.
        In 1951 a survey was made of the women who graduated
        from the College of Medicine of the University of Illinois
        from 1921-1945. Of the 151 women who had graduated,
        117 returned their questionnaires. Of those who responded,
        90 per cent were making use of their medical education,
        and the 12 who were not practicing were married with
        children. Questionnaires were sent to the men who gradu-
        ated in June of the years 1928, 1933, and 1935; 54 per cent
        responded. Of the men who responded, two per cent had
        left medicine, 56 per cent of the men were specializing in
        their practice as compared with 83 per cent of the women,
        40 per cent of the men have board certificates compared
        with 33 per cent of the women, 31 per cent of the men
        compared with 35 per cent of the women hold teaching ap-
        pointments.

2283.   "Bi-yearly Cancer Examinations." Medical Woman's Jour-
        nal, 49:5 (May 1942) 151. (Editorial.)
        Drs. Catharine Macfarlane, Margaret C. Sturgis, and Faith
        Fetterman of Philadelphia have been conducting biyearly can-
        cer examinations of 1200 women volunteers since 1938.
        The results of this research are given.

2284.   Bodley, Rachel L. Valedictory Address to the Twenty-
        Ninth Graduating Class of the Woman's Medical College
        of Pennsylvania: March 17th, 1881. Grant, Faires &
        Rogers, Printers, Philadelphia, Pennsylvania, 1881,
        16 pp.
        Dr. Bodley presents statistics on work accomplished by
        graduates of the Medical College of Pennsylvania over the
        preceding 30 years. She had gathered these statistics by
        means of a questionnaire sent to the 244 living graduates
        of the College. A total of 189 responded by mail (a further
        55 nonresident alumnae responded in person or by letter
        after this lecture was prepared. The statistics in the ad-
        dress have been revised to the date of publication--April
        6th, 1881). Of the 189 respondents, 166 are in active med-
        ical practice. Of the 23 who are not in active practice,
        six give ill health as the reason; three are retired; and
        eight list domestic duties as the cause. Of the specialties
        engaged in, gynecology practice predominates (32 respond-
        ents). Gynecology in conjunction with other specialties
        (e.g., gynecology and obstetrics, gynecology and surgery,

gynecology and medicine) total another 68 responses. One hundred and fifty of the 157 who responded to the "social status" question, report cordial social recognition in the community. A fourth question deals with the woman practitioner as resident or visiting physician in various institutions. The average income of each of 76 respondents is $2,907.30, with 24 women reporting between $1,000 and $2,000 annual income and four reporting between $15,000 and $20,000 per year. Women graduates as medical faculty total seven professors and 14 instructors and lecturers. Seventy-eight women are members of county, state, or other local medical societies. Of the 61 answering the inquiry as to what effect the study and practice of medicine has had upon their domestic relations as wife and mother, 45 answer "favorable." Eleven strike the words "as wife and mother" from the question and then respond, and one woman states "definitely" that she has "'remained single for reasons entirely distinct from her profession.'"

2285.   Downes, Helen R. and Lowther, Florence deL. "Reflections
        on a Study of the Performance of a Group of Women
        Physicians." Medical Woman's Journal, 53:2 (Febru-
        ary 1946) 39-41. ports., table.
        [This article is a sequel to a study that appeared in the
        Journal of the American Medical Association, October 13,
        1945 with the additional returns of the graduates of the
        Woman's Medical College.] Of those responding to a sur-
        vey of graduates of the Woman's Medical College, 93.5 per
        cent are eligible to practice medicine. Of those who are
        married, 88 per cent are engaged in full-time practice.
        Altogether, 91.5 per cent of the women surveyed at eastern
        medical schools practice medicine full-time. Twenty-five
        per cent are engaged as specialists in a wide variety of
        fields. If the percentage of women who leave medicine
        could be compared to the percentage of men who leave,
        the proportion would be similar. Class rank, perhaps a
        better criterion of ability, would indicate that a higher per-
        centage of women than men are in the upper half of their
        class.

2286.   Dykman, Roscoe A. and Stalnaker, John M. "Survey of
        Women Physicians Graduating from Medical School:
        1925-1940." Journal of Medical Education, 32:3 (March
        1957 Part 2) 3-38. figs., tables.
        This comprehensive survey has as its main objective the
        appraisal of the extent to which women physicians utilize
        their education. Initially, similar "utilization" studies are
        discussed: their inadequacies are pointed out. The physi-
        cian sample studied for this survey included 1,040 women
        physicians and 697 male physicians, educated in the United
        States and graduating from medical school between the peri-
        od 1925-1940 (inclusive). These figures represent the re-
        turned questionnaires sent to a group of 1,548 women, and

1,000 men--representing a 67.2 per cent response for women and a 69.7 per cent response for men. The names
were systematically selected from files of the American
Medical Association. Results indicate that 93 per cent of
the men and 82 per cent of the women were under the age
of 55 when they answered the questionnaire. A slightly
higher proportion of women practiced in very large (over
500,000 population) metropolitan areas. Ninety-five point
one per cent of the men and 57.1 per cent of the women
physicians were married. Seven per cent of the men compared with 5.1 per cent of the women physicians were divorced. Three point two per cent of the men and 31.4 per
cent of the women were single. Most of the men and women who married, married after completion of their medical education (73.2 per cent men; 49.8 per cent women).
There was an average of 1.8 children per woman who was
or had been married, as compared with 2.3 children per
man. Forty-eight per cent women and 14.1 per cent men
had no children. While 51.9 per cent of the women married men in medicine, 1.4 per cent of the men married
women in medicine. And while no women were married to
"housewives," 90.9 per cent of the men were; however, 1
per cent of the women physicians were married to men who
were unemployed, while no male physician was married to
an unemployed woman. A greater proportion of the women
physicians than men had college degrees (66.4 per cent:
58.1 per cent). Women also had a greater percentage of
master's and Ph.D. degrees than men (15.4 per cent: 6.6
per cent). Seven point five per cent of the men and 2.6
per cent of the women reported no additional training beyond the internships. A greater percentage of men than
women indicated private practice as their major type of
practice (85.2 per cent: 61.4 per cent), while the percentage of women was higher in local and state government
and hospital salaried employment (24 per cent women; 7.3
per cent men). An unexpected finding showed a higher
proportion of the younger than the older physicians (both
men and women) were in general, rather than specialty,
practices. Self-declared areas of specialization reveal
pediatrics as the most popular specialty for women (17.5
per cent), and surgery the most popular specialty for men
(17.1 per cent), while certification data support women's
most popular specialty (7.9 per cent certified in pediatrics);
men had the highest percentage of certification in internal
medicine (6.9 per cent) followed by 5.3 per cent in surgery.
Twenty-eight per cent of the women and 37.9 per cent of
the men were not certified at all. While 99 per cent of
the women had spent some part of their medical career in
full time practice, it was revealed that women practice
less than men. Forty-nine point one per cent of the women
and 88.9 per cent of the men had been in full time practice
exclusively. Fifty-two point two per cent of the women had
to curtail their employment sometime, while 9.8 per cent

of the men had to (however, only 25.7 per cent of the
single women physicians found it necessary to curtail their
medical activity and that mainly for reasons of physical
disability). Thirty eight point one per cent of the women
curtailed their medical activity because of "pregnancy and
family problems," while 0.1 per cent of the men gave this
reason for curtailment. Men on the average worked a
greater number of hours than did the women, and also
spent more time in income-producing work. Women earned
less than men. The greatest percentage of men, 34.8 per
cent, earned over $20,000 (compared to 7.7 per cent wo-
men), while the greatest percentage of women, 36.3,
earned between $8,000 to $9,999 (compared to 13.3 per
cent of the men). Six point four per cent of the women
and 1.1 per cent of the men expected to be inactive in ten
years. A greater percentage of men hold more prestigious
positions than do women, while a greater proportion of
women hold memberships in honorary societies than do men.
Attitudes of men and women physicians toward medicine
were also measured. Sixty-three point nine per cent of the
women would recommend medicine as a career for their
daughter while 75.4 per cent would encourage their son to
enter the field (as compared with 34.7 per cent of the men
encouraging their daughter to study medicine, and 74.7 per
cent encouraging their sons). A related finding shows the
greatest percentage of women encouraging their children to
enter medicine primarily for reasons of "intellectual advantage," while the largest percentage of men encourage
their children for reasons of "spiritual advantage and altruism." A sample of the questionnaire used for the survey
is included.

2287.   Eisenberg, Leon. "Medical Womanpower: A Statistic Goes
             Astray." American Journal of Orthopsychiatry, 41:3
             (April 1971) 348-349.
        The report of the Carnegie Commission on Higher Educa-
        tion, entitled "Higher Education and the Nation's Health:
        Policies for Medical and Dental Education" has the follow-
        ing serious error in citation: "'Among female medical
        school graduates active from 1931 to 1956, 45 per cent
        were working full time or part time in 1964.'" The cor-
        rect figure for full-time and part-time practice is 91.1
        per cent. [This information from Dr. Eisenberg also ap-
        pears in letter form in a number of other medical journals
        at this same time. See, for example, New England Journal
        of Medicine, 284:13 (1 April 1971) 734-735; Science, 172:
        3980 (16 April 1971) 218-219; American Journal of Psychia-
        try, 127:11 (May 1971) 145-146.]

2288.   Elkin, Edward M. "Male Thought of the Female Doctor's
             Dilemma." New England Journal of Medicine, 284:19
             (13 May 1971) 1106. (Correspondence.)
        Dr. Elkin refers to the paper by Powers, et al. ("Practice

Patterns of Women and Men Physicians," Journal of Medical Education, Vol. 44, 1969, pp. 481-491), in which it was pointed out that 46.1 per cent of women physicians practiced only part-time. He urges women physicians to delay maternity, and medical schools to modify programs to permit women to become doctors, wives, and mothers.

2289.   "The Employment of Women Physicians in State Hospitals." Woman's Medical Journal, 22:5 (May 1912) 116-117. (Communication.)

2290.   Everitt, Ella B. "Timely Suggestions to the Recent Graduate. Address Before the Medical Society of the Woman's Medical College of Pennsylvania." Woman's Medical Journal, 10:7 (July 1900) 283-288. (Original Articles.)
In this address to a class of women medical students who were about to graduate at the Woman's Medical College of Pennsylvania, Dr. Everitt gives advice regarding location of future medical practice, scheduling of office hours, fee schedules, and dress. As for locale, she advises that women may have more independence and social influence if they practice in inland towns and smaller cities. Regarding office and residence requirements, Dr. Everitt warns that acquiring cheap quarters will immediately affect one's "social standing in the community." Professional etiquette requires that a new physician in the area visit the other doctors already in practice there. "An invitation to return the call, and the business card left as a reminder, will usually win a courteous, if not a cordial response." For as little confusion as possible and to facilitate consultations and co-operative work, Dr. Everitt advises that the doctors in the same area keep uniform office hours. She knows "of no valid reason why a woman should not ask the same remuneration for her service that a man would under the same circumstances." Furthermore, she feels the "art of dressing well" to be most important. "Let us not forget that we are women first, (or should be,) and physicians second. It is a woman's life we each shall lead, therefore let us hold to that which is distinctively womanly. Our influence upon the community will be correspondingly greater and sweeter and truer."

2291.   "First Jury of Medical Women in the World's History." Bulletin Medical Women's Club of Chicago, 3:3 (November 1914) 3.
A list of the women doctors to serve on the first jury of medical women in the world is given. They were jurors in the court for the insane at the [Cook County] psychopathic hospital [Chicago, Illinois].

2292.   Fishbein, Morris. "More About Women in Medicine." Postgraduate Medicine, 37:3 (March 1965) 372. (Editorial.)

Fishbein surveys medical women's situation in Russia
(where women's medical school enrollment is declining)
and in England (where the Ministry of Health has recommended an increase in admittance of women medical students). Noting that men are more likely to practice medicine once they have graduated, Fishbein suggests that women can relieve a physician shortage. Part-time employment, day nurseries, and "more automation in the home"
will help women accomplish this task."

2293.   "Flexibility for Doctor-Mothers." Medical World News,
         (3 March 1972) 60.
         [Article not examined by editors.]

2294.   Gaffin, Ben, et al. "1 Out of 20 MDs in Private Practice
         Is a Woman." New Medical Materia, (October 1959)
         14-15.
         Statistics (1958) regarding specialties of women physicians
         and geographical distributions of women physicians are
         presented pictorially. There is no text.

2295.   Gardner, Mabel E. "The Danger of Isolation." Medical
         Woman's Journal, 31:10 (October 1924) 290-291.
         While the first wave of pioneer medical women have helped
         to "elevate the standard of the practice of medical women,"
         women physicians should be aware of the current second
         wave of pioneer medical women: the specialists. If it is
         possible to refer patients to a "well-qualified woman spe-
         cialist" such women deserve "the confidence of their con-
         freres."

2296.   G[ardner], M[able] E. "The Reason Why." Medical Wo-
         man's Journal, 39:10 (October 1932) 258.
         Women physicians have professional responsibility to help
         women with the efficient detection and care of health prob-
         lems that face women.

2297.   Glick, Ruth. Practitioners and Non-Practitioners in a
         Group of Women Physicians. Western Reserve Uni-
         versity, [Cleveland, Ohio], 1965, v, 105, 3 pp. tables.
         (Ph. D. thesis.)
         The purpose of this study was to identify personal interest
         differences (measured by the Strong Vocational Interest
         Blank) and attitudinal and background differences (measured
         by a questionnaire) between women practitioners and non-
         practitioners. One hundred and forty-six women who grad-
         uated from Western Reserve University School of Medicine
         between 1923 and 1963 responded (out of a total sample of
         180 women). Comparisons were drawn among six groups:
         practicing, part-time practicing and nonpracticing mothers,
         single women, married but childless women, and recent
         school graduates. No significant differences were found
         among the pre-1958 classes. However, several trends re-

lating extent and intensiveness of practice to factors such
as socioeconomic status and husband's occupation might
have reached significance had the number of nonpracticing
women surveyed been larger. Some significant differences
existed between the pre- and post-1958 groups. These differences, concludes the author, "provide some evidence for
the observations presented by a number of contemporary
social historians that the educated middle-class young women of today are to a marked extent rejecting the professional and career world in favor or marriage and full-time
motherhood. The decline of the feminist orientation is
linked to the pervasive influence of psychoanalytic doctrine
in our culture today." This thesis contains a review of
relevant literature, a list of references, and appendixes.

2298.   Groff, Margaret T. "The Story of a Thousand Volunteers:
         By One of Them." Medical Woman's Journal, 51:1
         (January 1944) 26-27.
         The author, who participated in Dr. Catharine Macfarlane's
         five-year experiment in cancer research, describes the pro-
         gram and the volunteers' admiration for Dr. Macfarlane.

2299.   Harding, Frances Keller. "The Interface Between the Wo-
         man Physician and the Family: Inaugural Address."
         The Woman Physician, 27:1 (January 1972) 9-11.
         The author discusses the concept of "family" and its
         threatened disintegration in American society. She touches
         upon such concepts as 25 years of "marital stability,"
         three-year renewable marriage contracts, and "bizarre, so
         called 'meaningful relationships' ... as ... new family pat-
         terns ... the marriage of homosexuals with subsequent
         adoption of children, the commune where a group of men
         and women live indiscriminately with each other, serial
         monogamy, adoption of children by unmarried men or wo-
         men...." "As women physicians," adds Dr. Keller, "we
         must be flexible in our attitudes to cope with the emotional
         as well as the physical symptoms generated by these
         changes." The physician "must make the value judgement
         of what is good and what is not acceptable." Women phy-
         sicians will be called upon to diagnose family problems,
         and "the nature of feminine psychology with its maternal
         instinct and understanding associated with the scientific
         knowledge and insight of a physician, male or female" equips
         them to be involved deeply.

2300.   Hendrickson, Robert M. "Women Physicians: Where They
         Rank on the Money Tree." Prism, (July-August 1975)
         20-21. illus., tables.
         Although more women are entering medicine, their incomes
         are still well below those of male physicians. This brief
         article discusses this situation in relation to specialties
         chosen, hours worked, and board certification.

2301.   "In Lieu of American Medical Association Convention."
            Medical Woman's Journal, 49:11 (November 1942) 348.
            (Editorial.)
        Because of the heavy demands of the war on physicians'
        time, the American Medical Association did not meet in
        1942.   One result of not having such a meeting is that doc-
        tors will have to keep each other informed about late find-
        ings, methods and treatments, by writing articles.   At this
        time, women have never had a greater opportunity to get
        articles published.

2302.   "Increasing Demand for Women Physicians."   Medical and
            Professional Woman's Journal, 41:3 (March 1934) 86.
            (Editorial.)
        Medicine today is one of the best-paid professions open to
        women: the annual income of 50 per cent of all women
        physicians is $5,000 and over.   In the lower income
        brackets, women physicians' incomes compare favorably
        with the incomes of men physicians.

2303.   "International Conference of Women Physicians Still in
            Session: 'Prevention Rather than Cure' the Slogan."
            Woman's Medical Journal, 29 [19]:9 (October 1919)
            214.

2304.   Jacobi, Mary Putnam.   "Female Physicians for Insane Wo-
            men."   Medical Record, 37 (10 May 1890) 543-544.
            (Letters to the Editor.)
        Dr. Jacobi takes issue with a Medical Record editorial (3
        May 1890), which stated that "women do not want to be at-
        tended by women doctors, and it is hardly fair to take ad-
        vantage of their lunacy to impose such upon them by the
        law."   The bill under discussion finds its justification in
        the belief in women's "superior kindness" and on the exist-
        ence of "erotic manias" among insane women.   Another
        reason for appointing women physicians to insane asylums:
        the necessity for gynecological treatment, and the fact that
        "for poorly paid physicians a relatively higher grade of wo-
        men is usually obtainable than of men."

2305.   Jolly, H. Paul and Larson, Thomas A.   "Women Physicians
            on U.S. Medical School Faculties."   Journal of Medical
            Education, 50:8 (August 1975) 825-828.   figs., table.
            (Datagram.)
        While proportionately far fewer women graduate from med-
        ical school (in 1940 4,844 men were graduated, 253 women;
        in 1950 4,958 men, 595 women; in 1960 6,676 men, 405
        women; in 1970 7,667 men, 700 women), "a greater propor-
        tion of the women than of the men for every class since
        1940 except in 1945 and 1946 are now serving on faculties."

2306.   Jussim, Judith and Muller, Charlotte.   "Medical Education
            for Women: How Good an Investment?"   Journal of

Medical Education, 50:6 (June 1975) 571-580. table.
The authors qualify their findings by stating at the beginning of this article that "substantial methodological difficulties were experienced in making [a cost] estimate [for physician training]." Women physicians practice on the average fewer total hours than men do primarily because of
household responsibilities. Recent medical school graduates
lose less time from professional activity than their predecessors did. More women would be in a position to apply
their medical education if part-time graduate training programs did not have the stigma of being second-class, and
if other factors like retraining programs, tax deductions,
and more equitable division of household responsibilities
existed. "It must be recognized," the authors conclude,
"that social equity, like other good things, is obtained at
a price."

2307.   Kahler, Elizabeth S. "President's Message." Journal of
         the American Medical Women's Association, 13:3
         (March 1958) 106.
         Ideally there should be no difference between scholarships
         available for women and men in the sciences. Employment
         opportunities and salary scales favor men. Better qualified
         women may not get jobs because men with dependents have
         greater need for work. As industry begins to appreciate
         womanpower, more businesses may make available part-
         time positions, maternity leaves, and emergency absence
         provisions. Part-time and limited medical practice offers
         flexible hours for women. Women doctors in a vicinity
         might consider pooling their available time to create the
         equivalent of full-time practice. Even if a woman doctor
         is not practicing, she may be serving the community in
         ways that surveys and statistics do not record. High school
         and college vocational counselors must have a difficult time
         making years of graduate study attractive when job oppor-
         tunities are limited.

2308.   Kehrer, Barbara H. "Women in Medicine." In: Profile
         of Medical Practice. Edited by R. J. Walsh, et al.
         Center for Health Services Research and Development,
         American Medical Association, Chicago, Illinois, 1972,
         102-109.
         This section of the American Medical Association's Profile
         deals with practice patterns of women physicians. [Article
         not examined by editors.]

2309.   Kehrer, Barbara H. "Professional and Practice Charac-
         teristics of Men and Women Physicians." In: Profile
         of Medical Practice. Compiled and edited by Judith
         Warner and Phil Aherne. Center for Health Services
         Research and Development, American Medical Associa-
         tion, Chicago, Illinois, 1974, 38-44. tables.
         "Current trends in medical school enrollments suggest that

the participation of women in the medical profession will
increase dramatically in the coming years. Such projec-
tions focus attention on differences in the professional and
practice characteristics of male and female physicians.
Data obtained from AMA's Eighth Periodic Survey of Physicians supplemented by an 'oversample' of women physicians
show that female physicians are distributed differently from
male physicians among specialties, with heavy concentra-
tions in psychiatry and pediatrics compared to the male
preference of surgery and general practice. Male physicians
are most likely to be board certified, and this may contribute to their higher net incomes from their medical practices: on average, women physicians earned only 57 per
cent as much as men physicians in 1972. Other factors
which may contribute to the lower incomes of women physicians are the smaller number of hours which they work
during a week and their greater tendency to work for salaries rather than in entrepreneurial situations." [Author
summary.]

2310.   Kennedy, Melanie. "Facilitating Woman's Medical Work."
        New England Journal of Medicine, 285:3 (15 July 1971)
        182-183. (Letters to the Editor.)
        In the Woman Physician (26:187, 1971) the statistics pre-
        sented from the "AMA 'physician master file'" on women
        physicians state that "84.3 per cent of all women physicians
        were active in 1969," while the author's calculations show
        83.4 per cent. "Those considered 'inactive' included 2.2
        per cent whose address was unknown to the AMA. Of the
        male physicians 93.2 per cent were active, not including
        0.7 per cent whose address was unknown." A total of 8.1
        per cent of all women physicians are retired, semiretired,
        or disabled--a higher percentage than all inactive males
        (6.8 per cent). This is logical since women live longer.
        This leaves just 8.5 per cent of all women physicians in-
        active because of reasons other than health and retirement."
        Dr. Kennedy calls for comparative statistics of "the aver-
        age male physician's years spent in medical practice versus
        the average female's years spent."

2311.   Kirkpatrick, Martha J. "A Report on a Consciousness
        Raising Group for Women Psychiatrists." Journal of
        the American Medical Women's Association, 30:5 (May
        1975) 206-212. (Presentation, Panel on Women in
        Psychiatry, Annual Meeting, American Psychiatric As-
        sociation, Detroit, May 9, 1974.)
        Women physicians "did not at first respond eagerly to the
        Women's Movement." Women psychiatrists were especially
        dismayed over the accusation "that women psychiatrists
        themselves have not only failed to escape the bondage of
        male chauvinists but have embraced the philosophy that
        justifies the bonds, namely confusing mental health with con-
        formity to the status quo." Local branches of the American

Psychiatric Association have begun consciousness raising
(CR) groups for women psychiatrists. Their goal is for
the members to "develop first an awareness and second an
ability to question and challenge social processes which
have limited their freedom of expression and behavior."
In 1972, 98 women members of the Southern California
Psychiatric Society were sent questionnaires concerning
personal experiences in their professional lives. Those
who expressed an interest in getting together meet in January 1973 to form a women psychiatrist CR group. The history of this group is followed; it was discovered that "being
a good doctor provided no relief from guilt if domestic
duties were shirked.... We experienced anxiety in situations where we felt ourselves to be seen as openly competing with men--for position, for money, for the right to
speak, for 'room at the top.'" The CR group "offers women physicians, who are often isolated and insulated, a
unique opportunity for peer group feedback and support as
well as a better understanding of themselves and other women."

2312.   Kral J. J., trans. "A Woman Surgeon." Woman's Med-
          ical Journal, 26:12 (December 1916) 288-290.
        In this article--originally published in Čas, February 2,
        1908, in Prague, Bohemia--a Bohemian describes a visit
        to the United States, during which he observed a difficult
        childbirth operation performed by Bertha Van Hoosen on a
        woman for whom having a child meant more than her own
        life. Reflecting on Dr. Van Hoosen's surgical skills, the
        author remarks, "I feel pity and resentment when I re-
        member that, in Austria, we have had and still do have
        idiots who would not admit a woman to the study of medi-
        cine."

2313.   Lakeman, Mary R. "Cancer Control." Medical Woman's
          Journal, 50:4 (April 1943) 100.
        Cancer prevention clinics and the work of Dr. Catharine
        Macfarlane in this area are discussed herein.

2314.   Lathrop, Ruth Webster. "Women Physicians as Teachers."
          Woman's Medical Journal, 18:4 (April 1908) 70-72.
          (Presentation, Annual Meeting, Women's Medical Soci-
          ety of the State of New York, Rochester, New York,
          11 March 1908.)

2315.   Lewis, Margaret C. "Let's Help the Girl Scouts." Med-
          ical Woman's Journal, 50:3 (March 1943) 83-84. (Let-
          ters to the Editor.)
        Dr. Lewis requests the assistance of the American Medical
        Women's Association in carrying on a drive for health ex-
        aminations for the Girl Scout organization. The desire to
        provide checkups for all girl scouts is handicapped by the
        decreasing numbers of civilian physicians during these war
        years.

2316.   Lowther, Florence deL. and Downes, Helen R.   "Women
            in Medicine."   Journal of the American Medical Asso-
            ciation, 129:7 (13 October 1945) 512-514.   tables.
        For the 20-year period previous to when this article was
        written, only five per cent of those allowed to enroll in
        American medical colleges were women, while English med-
        ical schools allowed women to comprise 20 per cent of the
        enrollment.   The chief arguments against accepting more
        women in medical schools in the United States is that wo-
        men physicians marry and stop practicing.   To examine the
        validity of these charges, a survey was made in 1942-43
        of the women medical graduates of Eastern medical colleges.
        Of the women responding, 90 per cent were engaged in full-
        time medical work, which includes not only medical practice
        but also public health work, medical research, teaching in
        medical colleges and institutional medicine.   Twenty-two
        other women responded that they were engaged in part-
        time work, which is often voluntary, such as at clinics,
        Red Cross blood banks, research projects, and school and
        public health activities.

2317.   Macy, Mary Sutton.   "The Field for Women of Today in
            Medicine: College, Hospital, Laboratory and Practice.
            Opportunities and Comparisons."   Woman's Medical
            Journal, 26:4 (April 1916) 94-96.   table.
        Based on the 1901 United States census, there are 7,387
        women physicians in the country.   This article is a geo-
        graphical analysis of the locations in which these women
        practice and how receptive the county and state medical
        societies are to women in the five states of Connecticut,
        New York, South Carolina, Georgia, and Ohio.

2318.   Macy, May [sic] Sutton.   "American Medical Women and
            the World War."   American Medicine, 23 (May 1917)
            322-328.   tables.   (Original Articles.)
        Tables give the total number of physicians and total num-
        ber of women physicians in the U.S. and Canada; the per-
        centage of women physicians in each state; the percentage
        of women in each state who are members of that state's
        medical society; and the number of women licensed to prac-
        tice medicine in each state.

2319.   "Make It Worth Their While."   World Medicine, (23 Sep-
            tember 1970) 7.   (Editorial.)
        There is little incentive for a woman physician to be active.
        The reasons: their earnings are lumped with their husband's
        and therefore are heavily taxed, and housekeepers have to
        be hired.   [Article not examined by editors.]

2320.   Marble, Ella S.   "Woman's Contribution to Medical Litera-
            ture."   Woman's Medical Journal, 5:3 (March 1896) 59-
            63.   port.   (Original Articles.)
        Dr. Marble prefaces her subject with a short sketch of what

women underwent in order to contribute to medical literature. Mentioned in her historical overview are Harriot
Hunt, the Blackwell sisters, Sophia Jex-Blake, and Elizabeth Garrett-Anderson. She further discusses the closing,
in 1892, of Columbia University (Washington, D.C.) to women medical students. Turning to women physicians as
writers of medical literature, Dr. Marble focuses on the
work of Trotula, Elizabeth Blackwell, and several contemporary physicians.

2321. Mason-Hohl, Elizabeth. "Women Doctors and the Cancer
Campaign." Medical Woman's Journal, 49:2 (February
1942) 53. (Editorial.)

2322. Matlin, Margaret W. "Sex Ratios in Authorship and Acknowledgments for Medical Journal Articles." Journal
of the American Medical Women's Association, 29:4
(April 1974) 173-174. table.
Sampling articles which appeared in the prestigious New
England Journal of Medicine for 1967-1972, the author concludes that although women constitute a small percentage of
authors of medical journal articles and receive only a
small percentage of high status acknowledgments, the percentage in both these areas was not significantly different
from the percentage of women in the medical population.

2323. "Medical Woman Honored." Medical Woman's Journal, 33:
10 (October 1926) 298. (Editorial.)
It does not necessarily follow that because the 33rd annual
meeting of the American Association of Obstetricians, Gynaecologists and Abdominal Surgeons sponsored a program
of more than 30 papers, and not one by a medical woman,
that women physicians are without recognition. The evidence: Rachelle Yarros was just elected social hygiene professor at the University of Illinois Medical School, and
Eliza M. Mosher and Charlotte Baker both hold positions
in city government. "It is only necessary to prove intellectual ability and individual fitness to win distinction in
any field, regardless of sex."

2324. "Medical Womanpower." Massachusetts Physician, 140 (February 1962). (Editorial.)
[Article not examined by editors.]

2325. "Medical Women and Their Recorded Work." Woman's
Medical Journal, 11:4 (April 1901) 139-140. (Editorial.)
Women physicians should record their experiences and make
contributions to medical literature.

2326. Mermod, Camille. "Doctors Are Teachers." Journal of
the American Medical Women's Association, 9:9 (September 1954) 290-292. (Inaugural Address, American
Medical Women's Association, San Francisco, June 20,
1954.)

Physicians serve as teachers of their patients, of other
physicians, and of the community.

2327.   "Michigan's Women in Medicine--Their 'Vital Statistics.'"
            Michigan Medicine, 74:2 (January 1975) 18.
         There are 1,087 women physicians in Michigan (or ten per
         cent of the total). The largest number of women (197) are
         in pediatrics, with approximately 90 per cent of women
         physicians in patient care. The article breaks down the
         number of women by kind of practice. Less than half (or
         505) of Michigan's women physicians are graduates of U.S.
         medical schools; a geographical breakdown by county and
         state is given.

2328.   "More Women Physicians Needed." Medical and Profession-
            al Woman's Journal, 40:8 (August 1933) 235. (Editorial.)
         Questionnaires sent out [presumably by the American Med-
         ical Women's Association] reveal than there are more posi-
         tions open for medical women that there are applications.
         The average yearly income for a woman physician in the
         United States was approximately $5,000: eight per cent
         earn over $10,000. Over 50 per cent are married.

2329.   "Opportunities for Medical Women." Medical Woman's
            Journal, 39:2 (February 1932) 41.
         Burton D. Myers, dean of the School of Medicine at Bloom-
         ington, Indiana, said in a speech, "there is no longer dis-
         crimination shown against women in medical schools be-
         cause women are better prepared than men in their pre-
         medic work." He identifies several medical specialties
         "for which the medical woman was particularly well fitted":
         psychiatry, health officers in schools and universities,
         specialization in children's diseases, in anesthetics, in
         laboratory work, and in departments of education for back-
         ward children. The Dean also stated that the results of a
         four-year study showed that "about one-fourth of the men
         and less than one-half of the women" who applied to med-
         ical school were accepted.

2330.   "Opportunities for Women in Medicine." Woman's Medical
            Journal, 21:5 (May 1911) 105-106.

2331.   Oreman, Jennie G. "The Medical Woman's Temptation and
            How to Meet It." Woman's Medical Journal, 11:3
            (March 1901) 87-88.
         "For some reason or other" women who try to escape the
         duties of maternity seek out women physicians to procure
         criminal abortions. Medical women must refuse these re-
         quests and show these women that abortion is murder.
         "Practical moral sympathy is what the world needs, and
         not a flimsy sensual sympathy which has not altruism in
         view."

2332.   Parke, Davis & Company. <u>Women in Health Professions:</u>
        <u>Part I: Physicians.</u> Park, Davis & Company, Detroit,
        <u>Michigan, 1968,</u> 5 pp. charts. (Patterns of Disease
        series.)
        Data from a variety of other sources is presented. Main
        points include: women are likely to practice in large cities,
        the U.S. ranks low in comparison with other nations, pedi-
        atrics is the number one specialty for women, women phy-
        sicians work fewer hours and see fewer patients than do
        men physicians, medical schools are accepting more women,
        23.3 per cent of women physicians stay single, and many
        women physicians marry other physicians.

2333.   Pennell, Maryland Y. and Renshaw, Josephine E. "Distri-
        bution of Women Physicians, 1970." <u>Journal of the</u>
        <u>American Medical Women's Association,</u> 27:4 (April
        1972) 197-199, 201-203. tables.
        Because there was such widespread misinformation and a
        lack of factual information about the use women physicians
        make of their professional training, the American Medical
        Women's Association initiated a study of the distribution of
        women physicians in 1970. Women physicians at that time
        comprised 6.9 per cent of all active M.D.s in the United
        States. Of the total number of physicians (male and fe-
        male) whose major professional activity is patient care,
        6.6 per cent are women. Women provide 9.1 per cent of
        the work force for such medical activities not directly in-
        volving patient care as teaching, administration, medical
        research, and others. The top seven specialties that 75
        per cent women physicians primarily practice include pedi-
        atrics, psychiatry, general practice, internal medicine,
        anesthesiology, obstetrics-gynecology, and pathology. The
        federal government employs 5.8 per cent of active women
        physicians in contrast to 9.8 per cent of active men phy-
        sicians. Thus women account for 4.2 per cent of federal
        physicians and as much as 7.1 per cent of the nonfederal
        supply. Of federal women physicians, 78.1 per cent are
        engaged in patient care, and 86.6 per cent of the nonfederal
        females have patient care as their major professional ac-
        tivity. Three-fifths of the active non-federal women phy-
        sicians practice in seven states: New York, California,
        Pennsylvania, Illinois, Ohio, Massachusetts and New Jersey.
        Between 1969 and 1970 the number of women physicians
        was increased by 1,313 of whom 1,014 were in active prac-
        tice. The rate of increase of active physicians was great-
        er for women than for men.

2334.   Pennell, Maryland Y. and Renshaw, Josephine E. "Distri-
        bution of Women Physicians, 1971." <u>Journal of the</u>
        <u>American Medical Women's Association,</u> 28:4 (April
        1973) 181-186. tables.
        Because of widespread misinformation and lack of facts
        about the use women physicians make of their professional

training, the American Medical Women's Association sponsored this study of practice patterns of women physicians.
Women physicians accounted for 7.1 per cent of all active
M.D.s in the United States at the time this study was made.
"Of the total number of physicians (male and female) whose
major professional activity is patient care, 6.9 per cent
are women.... Women account for 5.1 per cent of all
office-based practitioners and 10.8 per cent of all those
hospital-based." Women provide nine per cent of the work
force for other medical activities such as teaching in hospitals and educational institutions, administration as a staff
member or executive of a health facility or agency, and
medical research. More than 75 per cent of the active
women physicians specialize in pediatrics, psychiatry, internal medicine, general practice, anesthesiology, pathology
and obstetrics-gynecology. The federal government employs
5.8 per cent of the women physicians and 9.4 per cent of the
men physicians. "Thus women account for 4.5 per cent of
Federal physicians in 1971 but as much as 7.3 per cent of
the nonFederal supply." Three-fifths of all women physicians are concentrated in New York State, California,
Pennsylvania, Illinois, Ohio, Massachusetts, and New Jersey. Between 1970 and 1971 there was an increase of 7.4
per cent women physicians engaged in patient care. The
rate of increase of active physicians was greater for women than for men.

2335.   Platt, Lois Irene. "Women Doctors in Washington Today:
        A Statistical Survey." Journal of the American Med-
        ical Women's Association, 6:11 (November 1951) 446-
        449. tables.
        The questionnaire that Branch One of the American Medical
        Women's Association distributed to known women doctors in
        the Washington, D.C. metropolitan area was completed by
        73.2 per cent of those who received them; 189 answers were
        tabulated. Respondents included 172 white women physicians,
        13 Negro women, and four other (Chinese, Filipino). Six-
        ty-three of these women were under 35 years old, 107
        ranged in age from 35 to 60, and 19 women were over 60.
        Ninety-five point four per cent of these women doctors re-
        ceived their medical schooling in coeducational institutions.
        Of the three local medical schools, Howard graduated the
        first woman physician, Mary Dora Spackman, from its sec-
        ond medical class in 1872; George Washington University,
        then the Columbian University Medical Department, gradu-
        ated its first woman doctor, Clara Bliss Hinds, in 1887;
        Georgetown University did not accept women students until
        1949. Of the women polled, 157 were in active full-time
        medical practice (82.6 per cent); 18 in part-time practice;
        14 were not in practice. Of those not in practice, three
        were married and had children; two of these did active
        medical work for five or more years, and only one woman
        out of the 189 never practiced. The two largest recorded

specialties were psychiatry and pediatrics. Sixty-six per cent were married and only 13 of the 91 doctors with children had been out of practice five or more years. There were 426 hospital affiliations listed by 104 of the women surveyed. The 71 others without listed hospital affiliations were employed by the government or were active in research. Sixty-one women held teaching appointments and the professorial rank had been attained by 13 (or 6.7 per cent).

2336.   Powers, Lee; Parmelee, Rexford D.; and Wisenfelder, Harry. "Practice Patterns of Women and Men Physicians." Journal of Medical Education, 44:6 (June 1969) 481-491. tables.

A survey undertaken in 1965 concerned all women and a random sample of men who graduated from medical schools in the years 1931, 1936, 1946, 1951, and 1956. This survey's findings are compared in detail with the findings of the 1953 Dykman and Stalnaker survey of physicians who obtained degrees from 1925 to 1940. Among the study's conclusions: "1) Approximately twice as many subjects in the present study reported being married before graduation from medical school as did those who participated in the Dykman-Stalnaker study. Two to three times as many children were born to the former physicians when they were in medical school as compared with the latter. Over 50 per cent of the female respondents in both studies were married to physicians. 2) About 12 per cent fewer women than men in the present study reported certification in a specialty.... Two-thirds of the women who were certified as specialists chose pediatrics, psychiatry, internal medicine, and anesthesiology, in descending order by number listing the specialty; there is much greater diversification in the specialties reported by the men respondents. 3) Forty-five per cent of the women respondents report full-time medical activity since completion of training in contrast to 95 per cent of the men.... When all of the hours of professional activity were totaled for 1964 and divided by all respondents (including those who reported no activity), it was found that a woman graduate contributed an average of 1,932 hours and a man 2,831. From the data presented it would appear that in 1964 men practiced about 30 per cent more hours than women and attended about one-third more patients. 4) The number of hours of medical activity reported by women respondents is directly related to the size of their families...." In their concluding remarks, the authors point to the increased number of women accepted in medical school (from "5 to 8 per cent over the past few years"), and warn that "it is important that medical school attrition be kept to an absolute minimum and that graduates accept their responsibility to society to continue throughout their lives in a contributing professional capacity."

2337.   "The Reason Why." Woman's Medical Journal, 5:4 (April
              1896) 100.
          The woman physician, in applying for positions in state
          hospitals, faces many difficulties. Those problems are
          defined.

2338.   Renshaw, Josephine E. and Pennell, Maryland Y. "Dis-
              tribution of Women Physicians, 1969." The Woman
              Physician, 26:4 (April 1971) 187-195. tables.
          "The AMA 'physician master file' shows that at the end of
          1969, 84.3 per cent of the [24,000] women physicians in
          the United States were professionally active. Their distri-
          bution by field of practice and by geographic location is
          analyzed." [Article abstract.]

2339.   "Resignation of Dr. Amy Stannard." Medical Woman's
              Journal, 42:9 (September 1935) 251. (Editorial.)
          This article briefly discusses the "forced resignation of
          Dr. Amy Stannard from the United States Board of Parole,"
          with a warning that women were being excluded from civic
          and governmental positions. "The Attorney-General quite
          frankly asked her to resign in order to create a vacancy
          on the Board, while highly praising her intelligence, ability,
          and devotion to duty."

2340.   Roberts, Sheila M. H. "Demand." Journal of the Amer-
              ican Medical Women's Association, 22:7 (July 1967)
              482-484.
          From the premise that today there is "very little" preju-
          dice against women doctors, the author discusses what wo-
          men must do if they expect equal opportunities and equal
          pay to men, e.g., do the job well, practice in areas for
          which they are best suited as women.

2341.   Rodgerson, Eleanor B. "Questions." Journal of the Amer-
              ican Medical Women's Association, 21:8 (August 1966)
              673-674. (Forum.)
          Part-time practice poses a number of financial problems
          for women physicians, i.e., the necessity of paying full
          rates for malpractice insurance and full rates for profes-
          sional organization dues.

2342.   Rosenlund, Mary Loretta and Oski, Frank A. "Women
              in Medicine." Annals of Internal Medicine, 66:5 (May
              1967) 1008-1012. tables. (Special Article.)
          "The present report presents recently accumulated facts
          that pertain to the situation in the United States." The
          87 female graduates of the University of Pennsylvania
          School of Medicine between the years 1943 and 1956 were
          sent questionnaires: 174 male graduates were also sur-
          veyed. Seventy-two women (82.7 per cent) responded and
          141 (81 per cent) men. Seventy-seven point seven per cent
          of the women and 92.2 per cent of the males were married.

Eighty-three per cent of the women took some form of residency training as compared with 84.3 per cent of the males. Women engaged in medicine 36.4 hours per week and earned as an average annual income $11,789, while men worked an average of 58.2 hours per week earning $31,602 annually. Women working 40 or more hours per week have as many children as those women devoting 20 hours or less to medicine. The leading initial specialties for women physicians were pediatrics (23.4 per cent), anesthesia (16.7 per cent), and psychiatry (11.1 per cent). "Present area of practice" at the time of the survey, showed pediatrics still the leader (15.3 per cent), public health second (13.9 per cent), followed by psychiatry (12.5 per cent).

2343.   Ryder, Claire F. "The Doctor's Dilemma-Updated." Journal of the American Medical Women's Association, 16: 12 (December 1961) 933-938. (Commencement Address, Woman's Medical College of Pennsylvania, Philadelphia, 13 June 1961.)
"What will your role be as physicians in this rapidly changing world of ours?" Dimensions of the dilemma are presented which touch upon the areas of geriatrics, research, and continuing education.

2344.   Schneider, Margaret Jane. "Survey of Women Graduates from Cincinnati Medical Colleges 1879 to 1953." Journal of the American Medical Women's Association, 9: 12 (December 1954) 400-401. charts.
Through searching alumnae files in addition to sending out questionnaires to graduates of Cincinnati medical colleges, the question of utilization of medical education by women physicians was explored. Between 1879 and 1953, 212 women completed their medical course at eight medical schools in the Cincinnati area [eight schools over a period of 75 years]. Questionnaires were sent to the 153 living graduates and replies were received from 133. Of the 133, 95 have married and 38 have remained single. "In spite of their busy schedules, 68 of the women doctors have had a total of 157 children, an average of 2.3 children per mother or 1.6 children per married woman doctor." Of the 133, 6 have never done anything in the field of medicine. Thirty-eight are in general practice; 18 in pediatrics; 13 in internal medicine; 11 in psychiatry; and under ten in each of several other specialties. Seventy-five women are working full time and 47 part time. The author concludes "the number of married women who have reared families, managed homes, and continued their medical work proclaims the well-rounded, efficient, capable woman of today."

2345.   Shane, Jessie F. "The Woman Physician in the Country." Woman's Medical Journal, 12:1 (January 1902) 4.

2346.   Shapiro, Carol S.; Stibler, Barbara-Jean; Zelkovic, Audrey
            A.; and Mausner, Judith S. "Careers of Women Phy-
            sicians: A Survey of Women Graduates from Seven
            Medical Schools, 1945-1951." Journal of Medical Edu-
            cation, 43:10 (October 1968) 1033-1040. tables.
        Women who attend six coeducational medical schools in the
        Middle Atlantic States from 1945-1951 were compared with
        graduates of the Woman's Medical College of Pennsylvania
        during this period. After a postal mailing to 310 women,
        269 responded. Ninety per cent of the respondents were
        active professionally. Using as a criterion for "full time"
        individuals those who worked more than a forty-hour week,
        the proportion of women working full time was 66 per cent;
        95 per cent of single women were working full time. All
        the women who responded shared strong similarities in
        specialization: pediatrics was the most popular, with in-
        ternal medicine, psychiatry, and anesthesiology being the
        next most common choices. The authors found that pro-
        fessional activity and number of children were related.
        "An understanding and helpful husband and adequate house-
        hold help were repeatedly mentioned as factors essential to
        the success of a combined personal and professional career."

2347.   Shea, Petrena Abbe and Pincock, Caroline S. "A Census
            of Women Physicians in Washington, D.C. Metropolitan
            Area." Journal of the American Medical Women's
            Association, 21:6 (June 1966) 503-505. photo., tables.
        "This is a comparative study of women physicians and total
        number of physicians in the Metropolitan Area and their
        distribution in types of practice." According to the AMA
        Directory, there were 6,656 physicians in the Metropolitan
        Area in 1964: 594 of these were women (8.9 per cent).
        "The percentage of retired women physicians and those not
        working is under nine per cent of the total area women
        physicians."

2348.   Silver, George A. "Women in Medicine." The Nation,
            220:24 (21 June 1975) 741-742.
        In response to the United States government sponsorship of
        the conference celebrating International Women's Year in
        Washington, June 16-18, this article makes the point that
        while women comprise 75 per cent of the work force in the
        health industry, they do not hold policy-making positions--
        neither in the United States nor in the socialist countries,
        where there are far more women physicians. If women
        physicians were to hold policy-making jobs in the health
        care professions, perhaps some of the problems of medical
        practice would be solved, e.g., impersonality, lack of hu-
        manity in the treatment of patients, and the inflation due to
        competitive practice.

2349.   Stastny, Olga. "The President's Address." Medical Wo-
            man's Journal, 37:7 (July 1930) 198-199. (Address,

Annual Meeting, Medical Women's National Association,
Detroit, Michigan, June 22-24, 1930.)
The 7,000 women physicians in the United States should
join the men physicians "to purge the statute books of the
grossly inhumane laws that cripple our high service to
mankind and compromise our all-too-sensitive self-respect.
As members of an austerely honorable profession we have
abhorred political alignments; yet our viciously ignorant ad-
versaries have resorted to every political weapon that
chanced to be at hand, and it is time for us to show the
strength that is born of truth." Dr. Stastny further suggests that United States physicians "should co-operate with
our less persecuted colleagues of Europe" in compiling a
comprehensive bibliography on the subject of sex-pathology.
So that medical knowledge will have the distribution it
should instead of being distributed by "such self-appointed
guardians of virtue as the Watch and Ward Society and the
United States Bureau of Immigration, and other medical
inquisitors who presume to dictate to an intelligent person
what he may read."

2350.   "Statistics." Woman's Medical Journal, 18:7 (July 1908)
        153.
        Given are the results of a survey conducted by the State
        Society of Iowa Medical Women. The survey covered num-
        bers of women physicians in Iowa, their locality, and the
        nature of their work.

2351.   "Statistics on Women in Medicine and Addendum to Publici-
        ty and Public Relations: 1972 Annual Report." Journal
        of the American Medical Women's Association, 28:11
        (November 1973) 600-602. tables.
        This article publishes statistics on women physicians in the
        United States, reflecting conditions between 27 April and 3
        May 1973. The statistics were compiled for the Fisher-
        Stevens Report. Of the 29,745 women physicians in the
        country, 25,803 (86.7 per cent) are active. 3,942 of the
        29,745 women physicians are inactive, a percentage com-
        parable to that of male M.D.s of whom 18,564 are inactive
        out of a total of 344,384. Women constitute nearly 22 per
        cent of the pediatric field; 25 per cent of the child psy-
        chiatry field; and 20 per cent of the public health field.
        A geographical breakdown by specialty is included.

2352.   Stenhouse, Evangeline E. "Women in Medicine." Journal
        of the American Medical Women's Association, 1:7
        (October 1946) 201-202. (Editorial.)
        Basing her remarks on a study of seven medical schools'
        alumnae, done by Dr. Florence DeL. Lowther, associate
        professor of zoology, and Dr. Helen R. Downes, professor
        of chemistry, Evangeline Stenhouse editorializes that most
        women physicians remain in full-time medical work, that
        they have made use of their opportunities for training, and

that the present limitations on opportunities for women is
unjustified.

2353.   Thelander, H. E. "Opportunities for Medical Women:
             The Myth of a Wasted Medical Education." Journal of
             the American Medical Women's Association, 3:2 (Feb-
             ruary 1948) 67.
The statement that women waste their medical education is
a myth, as has been proven by the Lowther and Downes
statistics in "Women in Medicine," Journal of the American
Medical Association, 129 (October 13, 1945) 512-514. This
myth has often had "a distinctly detrimental effect" on some
women. Women with children and a family can often utilize their training by organizing and/or assisting in community health programs.

2354.   Thelander, Hulda E. and Weyrauch, Helen B. "Women in
             Medicine." Journal of the American Medical Associa-
             tion, 148:7 (16 February 1952) 531-535. tables.
This article proposes that a married professional woman,
i.e., a physician, cannot justly be compared to a professional man. "The married woman has two jobs, but the
primary one should be the maintenance of a family unit
and the rearing of the young. The woman is the integral
part in homemaking. No matter how great recognition a
professional married woman attains, she will not be considered a success if she has failed in her home.... Lo-
cating herself is secondary to the establishment of her husband in his career. She must create her opportunity in the
environment in which she finds herself, which may limit
her as to the type of work available, the time that can be
devoted to it, and the remuneration. In other words, she
does not have full choice in deciding what she is best
fitted to do." Other problems for the married woman physician include finding competent household help and the at-
tendant expenses (which are not tax-deductible), maintaining
knowledge of the field while performing household responsibilities, or finding a program to update and refresh herself after a period of inactivity. There are also biological
differences adjusting to menstruation and the problems accompanying childbearing and child rearing which include the
adjustment to it and the adjustment when it is over and
there is a "void."

2354a.   Thompson, Theodis. "Selected Characteristics of Black
             Physicians in the United States, 1972." Journal of the
             American Medical Association, 229:13 (23 September
             1974) 1758-1761. tables. (Special Communications.)
"The profile of black physicians in the United States has
not changed appreciably since 1967. A sample of 3,405
black physicians (91 per cent male, 9 per cent female) who
responded to a mailed questionnaire survey shows that black
physicians are more likely to concentrate in the fields of

general practice, medical and surgical specialties, and solo
practice as opposed to group practice than the universe of
U.S. physicians.   Black male physicians are twice as likely
to be in solo practice as self employed than are black female physicians.   Fee-for-service is reported as the pursuing source of income." [Article abstract.]

2354b.   Tracy, Martha. "Women Graduates in Medicine." Asso-
         ciation of American Medical Colleges Bulletin, 2 (Janu-
         ary 1927) 21-28.   charts. (Presentation, 37th Annual
         Meeting, American Association of Medical Colleges,
         25, 26 October 1926.)
The results of a questionnaire sent to 471 women physicians
are reported in this article.   The questionnaire was sent to
women graduates in medicine in the years 1905-1910, and
1912-1921.   Areas of survey were qualification, marriage,
types of practice, areas of specialization, and income.

2354c.   [Van Hoosen, Bertha]. "A Closer Relation Between the Wo-
         man Physician and the Woman in Pure Science." Med-
         ical Woman's Journal, 36:9 (September 1929) 249.
Women in pure science are "giving a striking demonstration
of the great importance of the co-operation of the sexes in
scientific medical research...."   Dr. Van Hoosen in this
article calls for recognition of their contribution in overcoming sex prejudice as well as a closer relationship with
them.

2354d.   Van Hoosen, Bertha. "Medical Opportunities for Women."
         Medical Woman's Journal, 32:7 (July 1925) 188-189.
         (Presentation, Annual Meeting, Medical Women's Na-
         tional Association, Atlantic City, New Jersey, May,
         1925.)
Job situations where medical women are likely to be employed include state institutions for the insane, public health
departments, and laboratories, as well as the Women's
Board of Foreign Missions.   Geographically, women physicians on the West Coast are better recognized than they are
in the Atlantic Coast states or in the South.   Indeed, there
still remain hospitals in the North, like the University
of Michigan's University Hospital which, while it has accepted women as students, has never had a woman intern.
This committee has acquired such information on opportunities for medical women as where women are accepted for
internships, scholarships, public health positions, and positions for resident physicians.

2354e.   Van Hoosen, Bertha. "Medical Opportunities for Women."
         Medical Woman's Journal, 34:6 (June 1927) 173-175.
         (Report, Thirteenth Annual Convention, Medical Wo-
         man's National Association, Washington, D.C., May 15-
         17, 1927.)
An investigation of the opportunities for medical women to

teach in medical schools revealed that the highest position
given to a woman in the U.S. was at Loyola University
Medical School (Chicago): a full professor and department
head.   Most of the 198 medical women teaching in medical
schools, however, are instructors or assistant professors.
The only eastern U.S. medical school with women as full
professors is the Woman's Medical College (Philadelphia).
Out of an 81-member faculty, 50 of whom are women, ten
women have full professorships.   Of the college's 20 departments of teaching, nine are headed by women.   "There are,
however, five departments that are not only headed by men,
but they have no women teachers in the department."   While
praising the Woman's Medical College for the opportunities
it does offer women, Dr. Van Hoosen comments: "so long
as it is not possible to have all the heads of departments
and the teaching force made up entirely of women in a woman's medical school, we can hardly push the matter of
having more teachers and more rapid promotion in the so-
called men's medical schools."   A state-by-state report is
also given of the women physicians employed under the
Sheppard-Towner Act.

2354f.   V[an] H[oosen], B[ertha].   "Medical Women Not Represented
              on Scientific Programs."   Medical Woman's Journal,
              35:5 (May 1928) 139-140.
         Lamenting that on medical society programs, the woman
         physician "is conspicuous by her absence," Dr. Van Hoosen
         urges her peers to emulate the pioneer spirit of early med-
         ical women: "Our pioneers were not satisfied with getting
         an opportunity for studying medicine, nor were they satis-
         fied with giving unselfish service to humanity.   They felt
         that they must put their stamp upon the medical world by
         founding institutions, writing articles, occupying positions
         that would make them stand out as having met with suc-
         cess."

2354g.   Van Hoosen, R. [sic].   "Future Position of the Woman Doc-
              tor."   Medical Woman's Journal, 35:9 (September 1928)
              262-263.
         "... women physicians are the poorest advertised class ...
         in America."   For women physicians to make significant
         advances, they must utilize publicity, and obtain universal
         loyalty from lay women.   In addition, "it is absolutely im-
         perative for men and women to work together if women are
         to receive recognition and inspire confidence in the public."

2354h.   Van Liere, Edward J. and Dodds, Gideon S.   "Women in
              Medicine in West Virginia University."   Journal of
              Medical Education, 34:9 (September 1959) 911-915.
              table.
         Since the formation of the University's two-year medical
         curriculum in 1902, qualified women have been accepted.
         This article represents the results of a study of living

women graduates of the school.   Questionnaires were sent
in 1951 and 1957 to the 59 living women graduates who
had later received the M.D. degree from another institution:
41 women replied.   Questions covered such areas as locality of practice, marriage and children, fields of practice,
and women's feelings about their place in practice.   It was
concluded from the study that women "have made a definite
and useful contribution to the practice of medicine."

2355.   Vaschak, Mathilda R.   "Household Help--The Woman Doc-
          tor's Gordian Knot."   The Woman Physician, 25:6
          (June 1970) 383-385.
A partial solution to the shortage of doctors in the United
States and other countries would be found if women physicians could obtain tax deductible and competent household
help.   When a survey was made of approximately 1,000 doctors, 788 made identifiable reference to the problem; 514
of these replied that household help problems interfere with
their medical practice.   The 274 doctors who claim to have
no household help problem were unmarried, childless, or
"lucky" (in that they had "'an understanding husband and
housekeeper' or a mother or maiden aunt who acts as a substitute in the home.")   Dr. Vaschak points out that one of
the resources in the past--maids from Europe--is no longer
as easily accessible due to the change of immigration service regulations.   One woman physician is quoted as saying, "A woman doctor needs a wife."

2356.   Vaschak, Mathilda R.   "Special Report of the Medical Edu-
          cation and Research Committee of the American Med-
          ical Women's Association: Results of Pilot Survey of
          Household Help Problems of Women Physicians in the
          United States."   Journal of the American Medical Wo-
          men's Association, 27:6 (June 1972) 324-327.   table.
Family responsibilities, child care, food preparation, chauf-
feuring, and the lack of household help are serious problem areas for women physicians, especially those between
the ages of 30 and 59.   Such extraneous obligations affect
the time and energy of these women and their chances for
professional improvement.   Of the 673 questionnaires sent
to women, 271 were returned: on the average, 12 months
during their years of practice were lost per doctor for various reasons.   One-third of the women physicians not practicing said that they would return to work if they could
have competent substitutes caring for children, dependent
parents, and other household duties.

2357.   "Wages and Hours Bill."   Medical Woman's Journal, 45:1
          (January 1938) 18-19.   (Editorial.)
The potential passage of the Wages and Hours Bill may
profoundly affect the economic life of women physicians.
Noting that the Bill could impose limitations on women of
the wage-earning class, this editorial states that "any at-

tack on the freedom of any class of women adversely affects the freedom of all women." Medical women are urged to oppose this legislation.

2358. Walker, Emma E. "Professional By-Ways Open to Medical Women." Medical Record, 65 (28 May 1904) 864-868.
Following a review of medical women's history, Dr. Walker offers advice to the young woman physician whose practice is not yet lucrative enough for self-support. Dr. Walker suggests editing and writing for medical journals, and even ghost-writing for other physicians. She examines employment possibilities for women in insurance companies as medical examiners, in hospital posts, within charity organizations, and within the New York City Board of Health, as medical book and drug company agents, as expert witnesses in court cases, and as lecturers. General advice on how women physicians can gain success includes a reminder that "no one cares for a 'manly woman'." Dr. Walker considers the consequences of male opposition to medical women, as well as the failure of women to seek women physicians.

2359. Westling-Wikstrand, Helena; Monk, Mary A.; and Thomas, Caroline Bedell. "Some Characteristics Related to the Career Status of Women Physicians." Johns Hopkins Medical Journal, 127 (November 1970) 273-286. tables.
This study reveals that 69 out of 81 women who graduated from Johns Hopkins Medical School between 1948 and 1958 were in active practice in 1967; 78 per cent had married; marital status and family size were closely related to career; the most successful women (i.e., professors) were more likely to be single; and daughters of physicians seem to have low professional ambitions. "It is suggested that part of the reason women medical graduates do not realize their full potential in later careers lies in the views and practices of society and medical institutions."

2360. "What's a Provost?" MCG Today, 5:1 (Fall 1975) 7-10. photos., port.
Dr. Ellison, recently appointed provost at the Medical College of Georgia, is interviewed by a staff member of MCG Today regarding her new position.

2361. "Who May Attend Physical Examination of Female Plaintiff." Woman's Medical Journal, 6:8 (August 1897) 250.
Section 873 of the New York Code of Civil Procedure provides that female plaintiffs in personal injury cases are entitled to physical examinations by women physicians.

2362. "Why This Muteness?" Woman's Medical Journal, 5:8 (August 1896) 201-202. (Editorial.)
Women physicians should publish reports of their work.

2363. Williams, Marjorie J. "Underemployment of Women Physicians." <u>Annals of Internal Medicine,</u> 71:4 (October 1969) 862. (Editorial.)

While society now agrees that both men and women belong in medicine, it "has failed to evolve and maintain an epicene environment," writes Dr. Williams. Her conclusion follows a review of several studies of the professional activity of women physicians.

2364.   Wilson, Marjorie P. "Women in Medicine: Improving Prospects?" <u>Journal of Medical Education,</u> 47:4 (April 1972) 303-304. (Editorial.)

Admissions of women to medical school appear to be on the increase. But the statistics--showing, for example, that 13 per cent of the 1971-1972 admissions were women, compared with 11.1 per cent in 1970-1971--fail to impress everyone. Charges of condoning discrimination in medical schools' admissions policies were recently filed by the Women's Equity Action League (WEAL) against the Liaison Committee on Medical Education. In addition to taking action on the issue of equal educational opportunity, WEAL and other women's groups are concerned with women's rights to medical school faculty appointments (e.g., of full-time faculty with M.D.s listed in the Faculty Roster Study for 1969-1970, only 8.6 per cent were women). Executive Order 11246, prohibiting sex discrimination by federal contractors, is one legal tool used extensively by women. This editorial's author (director of the Association of American Medical Colleges' Department of Institutional Development) concludes with affirmation of women's rights to medical careers and concern over the continuing conflict women have to face between career and family.

2365.   Wolfe, Mary M. "The Present Status of Women Physicians in the Hospitals for the Insane." <u>Proceedings of the American Medical-Psychological Association,</u> 16 (1909) 349-356.

[Article not examined by editors.]

2366.   "A Woman's Clinic in Washington, D.C., Attended Only by Women Physicians." <u>Woman's Medical Journal,</u> 27:1 (January 1917) 16.

The Woman's Evening Clinic of Washington, D.C. is three years old and has the largest white female service of any dispensary clinic in Washington. It was founded by Dr. Eleanor Folkmar.

2367.   "The Woman's Hospital and Infants' Home, Detroit, Michigan. Established by Women in 1869--Continuously Conducted by Women for Forty-seven Years--Internes are Women Physicians--Medical Women on Medical and Surgical Staffs." <u>Medical Woman's Journal,</u> 26:5 (May 1916) 128-130. photo., port., tables.

The Woman's Hospital and Infants' Home has several func-

tions: it serves as a hospital and shelter for foundlings
and other children; it helps to provide for adoption; it
helps to provide hospital services and shelter for women
who are about to (or have) become mothers; and it helps
to provide for the temporal, mental, moral, and spiritual
welfare of women and girls who have been in reformatories,
and other such females who need protection. No unmarried mother will be helped twice. This hospital also has
large, airy, and well-furnished rooms for private patients
where they can be secluded and comfortable. The kinds of
cases the hospital handled from January 1, 1915 to January
1, 1916 are listed in accompanying tables.

2368.   "The Woman's Hospital of Detroit." Medical Woman's
           Journal, 39:2 (February 1932) 40-41.
         The Woman's Hospital of Detroit, originally founded 60
         years before this article was written, had opened a new
         million-dollar building three years previously which demon-
         strates "that an institution can be successfully carried on
         by a management composed entirely of women." The De-
         troit Free Press is quoted as saying that "... Detroiters
         may again scan proofs that womenfolk of this city are as
         capable of managing a large public institution, well and
         thriftily as any one of them, individually, is able to run
         her own home."

2369.   "Women Doctors." Medical Woman's Journal, 56:7 (July
           1949) 30.
         A survey, published in the June issue of Medical Economics
         provides the following facts: women physicians net an an-
         nual average income of $7,929 (male physicians average
         $11,036); work nine hours a day (one hour less than men);
         vacation 25 days a year (to men's 16 days); and only 12
         per cent specialize (as against 31 per cent men specialists).

2370.   "Women in Medicine." Medical Woman's Journal, 48:4
           (April 1941) 118.
         Since 1917, 55 women have graduated from the Long Island
         College of Medicine [New York]. A questionnaire was sent
         to the 34 women graduates between 1920-1935. Thirteen
         replied. Of these 13, all took internships and were in
         active practice.

2371.   "Women in Texas Medicine." Texas Medicine, 71 (January
           1975) 88-90. photo.
         Women physicians comprise 5.2 per cent (681) of the active
         and classified non-federal physician population in Texas.
         There was an increase of women admitted to medical school,
         from 112 in 1973 to 152 in 1974. Most women physicians
         practice in large cities. Women physicians in Texas who
         have earned honors and titles of distinction are listed.

2372.   "Women or Doctors?" Newsweek, 26 (12 November 1945)
           84.

The most common reason for limiting female registrations
in American medical colleges to approximately 5 per cent
of the total enrollment (British medical schools limit women to 20 per cent) is that "at least 50 per cent" of these
women leave the profession. Recently, two Barnard professors, Drs. Florence deL. Lowther and Helen R. Downes
(both Ph. D. s) presented documented defense of women's
"seriousness of purpose." Of 1,240 women surveyed,
1,115 or 90 per cent were full-time practitioners. "As
might be expected," pediatrics lead as the specialty most
often selected by women (24 per cent).

2373.   "Women's Medical Association of New York." Medical Wo-
            man's Journal, 50:7 (July 1943) 184.
The subject of this meeting of the Association was a panel
discussion of the socioeconomic future of medical practice.
Dr. Ernst Boas said the future "lies in group practice centered around large institutions." He felt that voluntary
prepayment health insurance was a limited field, and some
form of compulsory health insurance on the part of the federal government was in the future. Dr. William B. Rawls
took the opposite stand. Dr. Mary Crawford spoke of her
experiences in industrial medicine. Dr. Howard Taylor
summarized the points of the discussion by stressing, among
other things, that "brotherhood within the profession of medicine" must be maintained.

2374.   "Your Economic Weather Vane: A Report on the Seventh
            Medical Economics Survey." Medical Economics, 30:5
            (May 1953) 117-125, 225. illus., tables.
Some of the results of a survey of about 5,000 "private"
American physicians are presented in this article. The
data, gathered in 1952, cover group practice, salaried
practice, and the woman doctor. Women comprised only
1.5 per cent of the survey respondents. Their average
gross income was $16,243 (compared with $25,014 for men),
and netted an average of $9,006 ($15,327 for men). Women worked an average of 51 hours per week (devoting
eight hours to charity patients) while men worked 59 hours
(giving seven hours to charity patients). Income for specialists and general practitioners are also given. From
1947 to 1951, the net income of women physicians increased 13 per cent; income of men physicians rose 28 per
cent.

2375.   [Zapoleon, Marguerite Wykoff]. The Outlook for Women in
            Occupations in the Medical Services: Women Physi-
            cians. Bulletin 203, Number 7. United States Depart-
            ment of Labor, Women's Bureau, Washington, D.C.,
            1945, vii, 28 pp. photos., tables.
Part of a series prepared by Marguerite Zapoleon of the
Women's Bureau, this pamphlet--"a dynamic study as dis-
tinct from a static description"--discusses the prewar situ-

ation, the wartime changes, and the postwar outlook for women physicians.   Included are statistics and discussion on
geographical and age distribution, specialty selections, earnings, and opportunities for women with special employment
problems (older, married, Negro, and physically handicapped physicians).   An appendix gives information on medical school and state licensure requirements and qualifications for service in the armed forces.   An extensive bibliography concludes the work.

SPECIALTIES

Articles discuss specific specialties--careers
in, difficulties encountered, dangers, rewards,
and opportunities, as well as historical aspects of women's involvement in specific specialties.

CANADA

2376.   McDade, Dorothy. "G. P. Not for Women Claims Lady
            Doctor--Nor Surgery--Too Slow in Decision-Making for
            This. --Should Specialize in Pediatrics, Dermatology,
            Anesthesiology and Gynecology." Canadian Doctor,
            (July 1964) 15.
         [Article not examined by editors.]

2377.   Trenholme, Marilyn. "Women Doctors in Family Practice
            [Part I]." Canadian Family Physician, (September
            1967) 45-47, passim.
         [Article not examined by editors.]

2378.   Trenholme, Marilyn. "Women Doctors in Family Practice
            [Part II]." Canadian Family Physician, (October 1967).
         [Article not examined by editors.]

EUROPE, EASTERN

2379.   Glinsky, B. B. ["Women Physicians in Social Service"].
            Istoricheskii Vestnik, 60 (June 1895) 827. (Rus)
         [Article not examined by editors.]

EUROPE, WESTERN

2380.   Bader, Christine. "The Work of Dutch Medical Women in
            Pediatrics." Medical Woman's Journal, 30:3 (March
            1923) 73-75. (Presentation, Convention, Medical Wo-
            men's International Association, Geneva, Switzerland,
            September 1922.)

2381.   Becker-Manheimer, Olga. "Utilization of Medical Woman-
            power in the Specialty of Radiology." Journal of the
            American Medical Women's Association, 22:7 (July
            1967) 480-482.
         Women need not fear physics and mathematics to be radi-
         ologists because a radiologist is judged on her ability to
         interpret pictures, not on her technical facility in producing
         them, especially since modern equipment makes the tech-
         nical side easy. "Since women are supposed to be more
         sentimental than men, they should have a better understand-
         ing of suffering. Therefore, this is one reason to consider
         radiology a suitable specialty for women." Her other rea-
         sons why women would like the specialty of radiology in-
         clude: it is clean work limited to specified office hours
         without home calls; one makes appointments convenient to

oneself; interpretation of the pictures can be done at the
convenience of one's own schedule and adapted to family
and household duties; and the nature of the job is conducive to part-time work.

2382.   Blechmann, Jane. "The Position of French Women Physi-
        cians in Pediatrics." Medical Woman's Journal, 29:11
        (November 1922) 281-284. (Presentation, Convention,
        Medical Women's International Association, Geneva,
        Switzerland, 6 September 1922.)
About half of the 300 women physicians named in the 1922
Year Book of French Physicians specialize in children's
diseases. A discussion of the progress made by French
women pediatricians considers women associated with charitable agencies, women concerned with the child's preschool
and school years, and women working with social agencies.
Noting that "the more a woman physician has specialized
the better will she be received by her masculine confrere,"
Dr. Blechmann accounts for women's success as pediatricians, e.g., the motivation of the maternal instinct. The
author also discusses the degrees of acceptance shown women physicians by the bourgeoisie and by the lower classes.

2383.   Borrino, Angiola. "Medical Women's Work in Pediatrics."
        Medical Woman's Journal, 29:10 (October 1922) 240-
        242. (Presentation, Convention, Medical Women's In-
        ternational Association, Geneva, Switzerland, 4-7 Sep-
        tember 1922.)
Women are making progress in the medical profession in
Italy, yet "it would seem that with us, feminine activity
succeeds best in the care of women and children." A
discussion of the reform of early infancy assistance in
Italy, and woman's participation in it, follows.

2384.   Dohrn, R. ["On the Admission of Female Physicians, Es-
        pecially to the Practice of Obstetrics"]. Deutsche
        Medizinische Wochenschrift, 8 (23 February 1893) 179-
        180. (Ger)
A professor of gynecology states his opinions concerning
the most frequently advanced argument for allowing women
to practice gynecology and obstetrics, i.e., the offense to
the modesty of women being treated for reproductive tract
problems by a male person. He objects to the implication
that men doctors lack the necessary sensitivity to treat women. A woman in labor is more concerned with getting
assistance in her hour of need than with protecting her
modesty. "The people think very differently of the value
of [male obstetricians] than one would presume from the
oratory of the ladies agitating for emancipation of women
or from the tirades of sentimental writers." In addition,
women are not equipped with the physical strength or with
the understanding and strength of will to cope with deliveries.
The thought of a fragile woman trying to conduct a difficult

forceps extraction would be comical if it were not so serious. Women do not have the strength of character to
stand up to the pressures of husbands and families for
operative intervention in a slow or difficult delivery which
should be allowed to proceed without interference. It was
only when men took over obstetrics from the midwives that
it became a discipline on a par with the rest of medicine;
neither the women doctors recently trained in Switzerland
nor modern midwives have contributed any significant advances. No matter how one looks at it, the interests of
the sick would not be served by the admission of women to
the practice of obstetrics.

2385.   Fischer-Hofmann, Hedwig. "The Need for Women Police
         Surgeons: Austria and Juvenile Delinquents." Medical
         Women's International Journal, 1:4 (February 1927) 48-
         49.

2386.   Schönfeld, W. ["Women Specialists in the Treatment of
         Syphilis in the 18th Century"]. Medizinische Welt,
         39/40 (September 1944) 552-553. (Ger)
         When syphilis appeared in Europe, the treatment was left
         to charlatans and "surgeons" as the university-trained
         "medicus purus" would refuse to treat it. In this article,
         the author describes two women charlatans who practiced
         as syphilis specialists in the 18th century. Franziska
         Maria Charlotte Gering advertised her cure in a newspaper
         and called herself a "doctor by royal privilege," but there
         is no proof of her title. She is, however, mentioned as a
         physician in the List of Physicians in Frankfurt. Antonia
         Elisabeth de Held, married to Muellerin, was another
         syphilis specialist. The author describes a controversy
         where she is by mistake named as the midwife who assisted
         at the birth of Johann Wolfgang von Goethe. Though it is
         probable that numerous charlatans practiced in this manner,
         there are no documents to indicate where and when they
         worked.

2387.   Svendsen, H. J. ["New Methods in School Health Care"].
         Ugeskrif for Laeger, 131:32 (7 August 1969) 1371-1372.
         (Dan)
         The author describes some facets of school health care as
         he saw it during a trip to France and Holland in May of
         1969. He notes that in the southern part of France, 72 per
         cent of the school physicians are married women, for whom
         the pay is not the most important part of the job. In the
         Versailles area he visited some village schools with a wo-
         man doctor who was responsible for 11,000 schoolchildren.
         She would have preferred half that number, because she was
         able to examine most of them only every other year instead
         of yearly.

GREAT BRITAIN

2388.   "Assistants in General Practice." Medical Women's Fed-
                eration News-Letter, (July 1928) 85-86.
         This article refers to and comments upon a letter published
         in the British Medical Journal. The letter expressed con-
         cern for women physicians who accept assistantships for
         general practice at extremely low salaries, or even for
         room and board only. The Federation's stand on this is-
         sue is reiterated.

2389.   Balfour, Andrew. "The Tropical Field: Its Possibilities
                for Medical Women." Lancet, 2 (6 October 1928) 721-
                723. (Address, London School of Medicine for Women,
                1 October 1928.)
         Dr. Balfour, director of the London School of Hygiene and
         Tropical Medicine, outlines the opportunities for women in
         India, Africa, and several Far Eastern countries. In ad-
         dition to urging women to learn how to diagnose and treat
         tropical diseases, he discusses the possibilities for doing
         research in tropical medicine.

2390.   Butlin, Henry T. "Introductory Address on Research in
                Medicine and Women in Research. Delivered at the
                London School of Medicine for Women." British Med-
                ical Journal, (7 October 1911) 835-837.
         After discussing research in general and the characteristics
         a physician needs in order to do medical research, Sir
         Henry Butlin submits that women possess these qualities to
         a higher degree than do men: humanity, dexterity in
         manipulation, cleanly habits, continued industry, patience,
         perseverance, and attention to detail. Since this is so,
         Butlin wonders why the British Medical Association has not
         given any awards to women researchers. Julia Brinck,
         the first woman recipient of the British Medical Association's
         research award (1890), and Janet Lane-Claypon (1904) are
         mentioned. Sir Henry concludes by saying that whether wo-
         men have the breadth of mind necessary for such work re-
         mains to be seen.

2391.   Byers. "Address on Medical Women and Public-Health
                Questions." British Medical Journal, 2 (1906) 823-
                828.
         [Article not examined by editors.]

2392.   Campbell, Janet. "Opportunities for Medical Women in
                Public Health Work." Medical Women's Federation
                Quarterly Review, (October 1935) 42-48.

2393.   Crawford, Margaret D. "Part-Time Work in Social Medi-
                cine." Journal of the Medical Women's Federation,
                40:4 (October 1958) 273-275. (Symposium on Part-
                Time Work: Part 2.)

Social medicine is defined by Dr. Crawford who also discusses the problems of medical women who are married, have children, and wish to return to work. [Part 1 of this Symposium appeared in the April, 1958 issue of the Journal.]

2394.   Daly, Flora M. "Part-Time Work in General Practice." Journal of the Medical Women's Federation, 40:4 (October 1958) 278-280. (Symposium on Part-time Work: Part 2.)
The advantages of general practice for married women physicians are discussed. [Part 1 of this Symposium appeared in the April, 1958 issue of the Journal.]

2395.   Fairfield, Letitia. "Medical Practice and the Criminal Law." Medical Women's Federation News-Letter, (November 1927) 21-24.
The author, an attorney and an M.D., advises women physicians in performing as "expert witnesses" before criminal courts. Among the problems identified by the author: the poor carrying power and resonance of the unpracticed female voice.

2396.   Hall, Winifred S. "My Work as a Police Surgeon." Journal of the Medical Women's Federation, 43:2 (April 1961) 71-72.
Dr. Hall, a police surgeon in Manchester, England, the first city to appoint a woman police surgeon (in 1927), discusses the types of cases with which she deals, as well as the work involved. Ninety per cent of the cases (women and children) seen by Dr. Hall involved sexual assault, and one-half of these cases are of small girls.

2397.   Henry, Lydia M. "British Medical Women and Public Health Work." Medical Woman's Journal, 29:4 (April 1922) 74-75.
There is plenty of room in public health for women physicians of sympathetic character, "provided they are content to work hard in spheres other than Harley Street and Rodney Street." Women medical officers can be especially useful in carrying out schemes for the welfare of women and children in different towns where superstitions often still exist.

2398.   Knill-Jones, R. P.; Moir, D.D.; Rodriques, L. V.; and Spence, A. A. "Anaesthetic Practice and Pregnancy: Controlled Survey of Women Anaesthetists in the United Kingdom." Lancet, 1:7764 (17 June 1972) 1326-1328. tables.
"Obstetric histories from 563 married women anaesthetists and 828 women doctor control subjects were analyzed for the frequency of congenital abnormality, spontaneous abortion, and involuntary infertility. Anaesthetists working

during pregnancy had a significantly higher frequency of
congenital abnormality (6.5%) than those not at work (2.5%)
but not significantly different from the control frequency
(4.9%).   They had a frequency of spontaneous abortions
(18.2%) which was significantly higher than in the control
group but not significantly different from anaesthetists not
at work.   Involuntary infertility among anaesthetists (12%)
was twice as frequent as in the control group." [Journal
summary.]

2399.   Lawrie, Jean. "Women Doctors and Family Planning."
         British Medical Journal, 3 (4 August 1973) 296.
         Dr. Lawrie, as Secretary of the Medical Women's Federa-
         tion, expresses the concern of the Federation for the job
         security of women physicians in family planning after April
         1974, when it is open as to where family planning advice
         will be given to patients (in hospitals? G.P. surgery? sep-
         arate clinics?).   Dr. Lawrie suggests the Family Planning
         Association seek the advice and collaboration of its employ-
         ees in outlining future services.

2400.   McGill, M. Isabel. "Women Police Surgeons." Journal of
         the Medical Women's Federation, 43:1 (January 1961)
         70-71.
         Women should be available for "those aspects of police
         work where women and children are involved." Dr. Mc-
         Gill briefly discusses the need for a training of such police
         surgeons.

2401.   Mackenzie, Marion E. "Women Doctors and Pediatrics."
         British Medical Journal, 2 (1921) 171.
         [Article not examined by editors.]

2402.   Maynard, Edith L. Women in the Public Health Service.
         Scientific Press Limited, London, England, 1915,
         128 pp.
         A minor portion (three pages) of this guide deals specifical-
         ly with the appointment of medical women as public health
         officials.   The required training, opportunities, salaries,
         and duties of women physician health officers are discussed.
         The remainder of the book deals generally with preparation
         for public health work, the work itself, midwives, and the
         regulations concerning the appointment of women to public
         health posts.

2403.   "Medical Women in Public Health Posts--a Good Example
         for American Medical Women in Great Britain." Med-
         ical Woman's Journal, 28:12 (December 1921) 307.
         Inequality of payment and treatment of medical women as
         compared with men in public health posts has brought pro-
         test (from in one case the Medical Women's Federation and
         the British Medical Association).   Instances of discrimination
         should be brought promptly before the "Council."

2404.   Parbrook, G. D. and Norris, W. "Anaesthesia in the
          Western Region of Scotland." British Journal of Anaes-
          thesia, 44 (August 1972) 887-892. figs., tables.
        "A comparison of consultant anaesthetic staffing in the West-
        ern Region with that of [all] Scotland shows that the West
        has its proportionate shortage of anaesthetists. This short-
        age is exacerbated by an inadequate supply of trained anaes-
        thetists in the region. Training programmes are success-
        ful, but there is an inadequate number of junior staff when
        allowance is made for the special factors applying in the
        region. [Mention is made of the changing proportion of fe-
        male medical graduates and trainees in anesthesiology.]"
        [Article summary.]

2405.   "The Place of Women in Medicine." Saturday Review,
          137 (31 May 1924) 556-557.
        Women can play an important role in the "gradual produc-
        tion of a healthier stock and in the elimination of compli-
        cations and disease" by going into the practice of obstetrics.

2406.   Roberts, E. Louise; Spiller, Violet; and Cullum, Iris M.
          "Women in the Public Health Service." Medical Wo-
          men's Federation Quarterly Review, (July 1941) 45-52.
          (Correspondence.)
        Three women physicians respond to Dr. Violet Russell's
        letter regarding women in public health which appeared in
        the April 1941 issue of the Quarterly Review. Dr. Roberts
        sees Dr. Russell's recommendation--that women concentrate
        on certain aspects of public health work--as a division of
        work along sex lines and "a most retrograde step." Dr.
        Roberts also disagrees that women in public health must
        remain unmarried. Dr. Spiller focuses her comments on
        the prerequisites for work in the field. Regarding the re-
        striction of public health appointments to women over 30
        years old to preclude women taking appointments and then
        marrying (hence being barred from practicing), Dr. Spiller
        feels "this may be sound under present conditions, but in
        my humble opinion present conditions are deplorably wrong."
        Dr. Spiller also disagrees with Dr. Russell that men pos-
        sess superior ability to be medical officers of health, as
        opposed to women. Dr. Cullum in general agrees "whole-
        heartedly" with Dr. Russell, with the exception of Dr.
        Russell's feelings that public health workers do not neces-
        sarily enjoy opportunities for social activity emanating from
        this work.

2407.   Russell, Violet. "Women in the Public Health Services."
          Medical Women's Federation Quarterly Review, (April
          1941) 63-67. (Correspondence.)
        Dr. Russell gives her personal viewpoint on the place of
        women in the "service of preventive medicine." Public
        health offers security and a wide variety of areas in which
        to subspecialize. Dr. Russell would dissuade a woman from

trying to become a medical officer of health, however, as
the job requires the type of brain "... rarely found at its
best in a woman." Dr. Russell feels a woman should specialize in an area in which her "feminine cast of mind will
be an asset," and such work (dealing exclusively with women
and children) should be reserved for medical women over
the age of 30.

2408. Sutherland, Joan. "Married Women Doctors--Particularly
in General Practice." Journal of the Medical Women's
Federation, 45:3 (July 1963) 216-219.
Dr. Sutherland explores the subject of work for married
women doctors, and especially the area of general practice.
She feels that such work should be encouraged.

2409. Tattersall, Joan. "Part-Time Work in Student Health."
Journal of the Medical Women's Federation, 40:4 (October 1958) 275-278. (Symposium on Part-Time Work:
Part 2.)
This "comparatively new branch of medicine" is examined
in detail and presented as an option for women physicians
who desire part-time work.

2410. Wattie, Nora I. "Employment of Medical Women Part-
Time in the Public Health Services." Journal of the
Medical Women's Federation, 45:4 (October 1963) 220-
221.

2411. Williams, Ethel. "Thirty Odd Years in General Practice."
Medical Woman's Journal, 33:10 (October 1926) 284-
286.
Ethel Williams, a general practitioner--or, as she describes herself, "mother's help and chief cook and bottle
washer to families in distress"--contends that general practice is fitted to women, since "their peculiar cast of mind
... fits them to deal with individuals, specially with the
helpless or infirm. They can be infinitely patient with a
fretful child or a sick and irritable man, while humanity
in the mass or some annoying mechanical contrivance quickly wears their endurance thin." Entering into partnership
with other women physicians helps combat the tendency to
get "amateurish in our presentment if not in our thinking"
as a result of men who are "principally occupied in trying
to keep us in what they hoped would be our place." [This
article also appears in the Medical Women's Federation
News-Letter (July 1926) 52-57.]

2412. "Women Police Surgeons." Medical Women's International
Journal, 1:5 (November 1927) 45-46. (Current Topics.)
Nesta H. Wells, M.B., Ch.B., reports on the appoint-
ment of a woman police surgeon in Manchester.

INTERNATIONAL

2413.   G[ardner], M[abel] E.   "Greater Opportunities for Medical
             Women Than Ever Before."   Medical Woman's Journal,
             39:1 (January 1932) 14.   (Editorial.)
        Medical women, through their ability to serve and inspire
        confidence, are called upon more and more for such posi-
        tions as physical advisors for high schools, gymnasium
        classes and colleges, as specialists of children's diseases,
        as consultants in women's diseases, and as doctors in
        countries such as India where women may not be seen by
        men [outside their families].

2414.   Spence, A. A.; Knill-Jones, R. P.; and Newman, Barbara
             J.   "Studies of Morbidity in Anaesthetists with Special
             Reference to Obstetric History."   Proceedings of the
             Royal Society of Medicine, 67:10 (October 1974) 989-
             990.   (Section on Anaesthetics.)
        This article briefly reviews several studies dealing with the
        frequency of congenital abnormality and spontaneous abortion
        among women anesthesiologists.   A recent study was ex-
        tended to include questions relating to morbidity other than
        that associated with childbearing; its preliminary findings
        are outlined.

SOUTH, CENTRAL, LATIN AMERICA
AND MEXICO

2415.   Tichauer, Ruth W.   "A Rewarding Activity for Women
             Physicians ... The Family Clinic."   Medical Woman's
             Journal, 57:8 (August 1950) 34-39.
        Dr. Tichauer notes a "certain onesidedness" to the activ-
        ities of women physicians: limiting their work to the care
        of women and children (those who are not engaged in re-
        search or administration).   Even JAMWA's ads are aimed
        mainly at these two fields.   Dr. Tichauer suggests women
        physicians should return to general practice.   She examines
        the case for women in general practice, the scope of such
        a practice as well as its history.   Case histories are used
        to illustrate the desirable aspects of this "approach" to the
        profession (i.e., treating the individual as a whole).   In
        addition, Dr. Tichauer discusses drawbacks to general
        practice, office location, equipment and staff, and relations
        with colleagues.   In general practice "a woman physician
        is always regarded as a woman.   She is liked as one or
        disliked, and in fact seems to arouse stronger emotional
        response both ways.   You will be surprised by unusual at-
        tachment, and also by violent hostility, both unwarranted."

UNITED STATES

2416.   Anthony, Catherine W.   "Careers in Pathology."   The Wo-

man Physician, 25:6 (June 1970) 390-391.
Oriented to recruit women to the field of pathology, the
relevance of this article lies in the reasons that are given
for women (especially) to consider pathology as a career.
According to Dr. Anthony, women are welcomed in the
field of pathology, especially in research. A woman may
take a leave of absence and return to work after having a
family. Since pathologists do not rely on a private practice, "a married woman pathologist can move readily with
her husband if the occasion should arise." Also, pathologists work more predictable hours than most other medical
specialists do, and night calls are less likely. While pathologists do not enjoy warm personal relationships that attending physicians may assume they can have with patients,
there is satisfaction in knowing one has helped to diagnose
other people's patients, and in dealing oneself with tangible
and demonstrable facts.

2417.   Apgar, Virginia. "Careers in Anesthesiology." Journal
        of the American Medical Women's Association, 24:9
        (September 1969) 720-724, 741. (Careers.)
This article, an "updated version" of the same article published in the Journal of the American Medical Women's
Association, 19:8 (August 1964) 675-680, gives an abbreviated history of anesthesiology, and answers the questions "What
is an anesthesiologist?" and "Who should be one?" A few
of the requisites for the person considering anesthesiology
are: "He must work with people well.... He must be
sensitive to the over-all situation.... He must have a
capacity for keen observation, quick decision and action....
He [must handle a needle with minimal discomfort and with
dexterity]." "Residency and requirements" and "Opportunities," are given mention. The article concludes with a
section on "Anesthesiology as a Career for Women." The
author can see "no reason why [the unmarried woman physi-
cian] should not be as expert and as successful in anesthesiology ... as her male counterpart." Although not a
"mechanical gadgeteer," a woman can learn easily enough
the simple tasks involved in the profession. Manual dexterity, being a "by-product of ... sewing or knitting,"
especially fits the woman for this specialty, as well as the
tact and diplomacy which are part of woman's nature "(with
a few exceptions)." A married woman, however, may find
it difficult to do justice to her small children as well as
to her patients and, of course, "an understanding husband
is invaluable for he must be indeed unusual to be tolerant
of so little family life." Eleven per cent of members in
the 1963 American Society of Anesthesiology directory are
women, while "the average for all types of practice is just
under six per cent."

2418.   Apter, Julia T. "Number of Women Pathologists." Ar-
        chives of Pathology, 94 (October 1972) 371-372. (Let-

ters to the Editor.)
Contrary to inaccurate information given to secretary of
health, education, and welfare, Elliot Richardson, there
are women pathologists--536 of them who are board certified and many more who are not board certified and who
practice pathology. Therefore the National Institutes of
Health is discriminatory in its selection of male pathologists
for public advisory groups to the exclusion of women. "It
probably should also be pointed out that the selective processes now in practice in academic institutions, medical
schools, and hospitals have produced women pathologists
with a better natural endowment and stronger drives than
the male pathologists."

2419.   "Are Women Physicians Good Surgeons?" Medical Woman's
         Journal, 34:10 (October 1927) 308-309.
         A report by the American Automobile Association proves
         that women score higher averages than men on reaction
         time, variability, and "innate conception of mechanics."
         The writer draws an analogy between good automobile driv-
         ing and surgery, concluding that women may be better sur-
         geons than "the masculine portion of the profession."

2420.   Balsam, Rosemary Marshall and Balsam, Alan. "The
         Pregnant Therapist." In: Becoming a Psychotherapist:
         A Clinical Primer. Little, Brown and Company, Bos-
         ton, Massachusetts, 1974, 265-288.
         Pregnancy "may exaggerate aspects of [the] interaction be-
         tween patient and therapist." This chapter discusses such
         aspects as whether or not the pregnant therapist should
         work; feelings of therapists during, and reactions of pa-
         tients to, pregnancy; returning to work after the birth of a
         baby. "A therapist even in early pregnancy, may want to
         relinquish too much of her work in the interests of proving
         herself a better mother, or she may take on too much
         work to prove herself a reliable professional woman, thus
         draining off time needed to care for herself and her fam-
         ily." Case examples of patients' responses to the pregnant
         therapist are given and discussed.

2421.   Baum, O. Eugene and Herring, Christina. "The Pregnant
         Psychotherapist in Training: Some Preliminary Find-
         ings and Impressions." American Journal of Psychia-
         try, 132:4 (April 1975) 419-422. (Panel, 127th Annual
         Meeting, American Psychiatric Association, Detroit,
         Michigan, May 6-10, 1974.)
         A male M.D. training and supervising analyst and a fe-
         male medical student who conducted interviews, write their
         observations about pregnant psychotherapists based on the
         Medical College of Pennsylvania's residency program in adult
         basic psychiatry begun in 1967. For women to become preg-
         nant in their first year of the three required years of resi-
         dency training mobilized more defensive reactions on the

part of the pregnant resident than it did in the other two
years of training. The authors observed that there was a
conflict in the pregnant therapist of denying any impact of
the pregnancy on the patient, staff, and the learning experience: at the same time, she desired more acceptance
and understanding. The authors conclude that one area requiring further study and information is the area of role
conflict between professional identity and that of being wife
and mother. The therapist seemed more comfortable with
her pregnancy by its middle phase--probably because by
that time she had adjusted to it. Analytic students seemed
to adjust best to the late phases of pregnancy which was the
most difficult period marked by fatigue, mobilization of
fears concerning delivery, a gradual withdrawal of libido
from patients and work, and conflict about professional
identity, all of which must have mobilized guilt and anxiety,
the authors conclude.

2422.   Benedek, Elissa P. "The Fourth World of the Pregnant
        Therapist." Journal of the American Medical Women's
        Association, 28:7 (July 1973) 365-368.
"The therapist works in four worlds. Her own world of
reality; the world of countertransference; the world of her
patient; i.e., the world of transference, and the world of
the staff and organization that she works in. Any event
in the therapist's life has its own implications in these
four worlds and must be dealt with in them. An event so
obvious, critical, and personal as a pregnancy must be
worked through by the therapist in each of the worlds.
Previous literature has described reactions of the patients
to a therapist's pregnancy and the therapist's own reactions
to her pregnancy. The paper attempts to explore some of
the staff's feelings about a therapist's pregnancy and ways
of dealing with these feelings." [Author's summary.]

2423.   Benedek, Elissa P. "Training the Woman Resident to be
        a Psychiatrist." American Journal of Psychiatry, 130:
        10 (October 1973) 1131-1135.
This woman psychiatrist observes that women who wish to
enter the field of psychiatry experience unique problems
that men generally do not have to face. Her examples include: the unwritten quota systems that seem to exist at
most medical schools and psychiatry residency programs
which limit women; her own experience that while there
might be women psychiatrists, only men ever interviewed
her; her experiences of having to account for her intentions
of combining a career with married life while relatively few
men ever have to account for this (potential) conflict; her
observation that while people who manage these programs
might be "geared" to handle the problems of other minority
groups, they are not geared to be sensitive to the problems
of women and so the problems of the woman resident are
ignored, e.g., "on call" time, rooming arrangements, vaca-

tions and holidays, pregnancy; the lack of a woman peer
group and the isolation a lone woman feels; dealing with
sexual feelings as a result of the closeness that is necessary in the peer group; from her experience, the inability
of women in the field to be models or give peer group support because they have been so worn out by, or so identified with, the system; and the special problems of being a
maternal transfer object.

2424.   Berman, Ellen. "Acting Out as a Response to the Psychi-
           atrist's Pregnancy." Journal of the American Medical
           Women's Association, 30:11 (November 1975) 456-458.
           tables. (Panel presentation, "The Pregnant Therapist,"
           American Psychiatric Association, Detroit, Michigan,
           1974.)
         The author undertook an investigation of destructive be-
         havior and "acting out" exhibited by patients during the
         pregnancy of therapists. The purpose was to determine if
         a therapist's pregnancy constitutes risks to the patient's
         well-being or progress in therapy. Data were obtained on
         129 patients in therapy during the last six months of nine
         women psychiatrists' pregnancies, and on 130 patients in
         therapy during a six-month period with the same nine psy-
         chiatrists when they were not pregnant. The study showed
         an increase in patient "acting out" and behavioral distur-
         bance during the therapist's pregnancy as compared with
         during nonpregnancy. "The most common major disturbance
         was dropping out of therapy (six patients). There were
         two suicide attempts (one successful), and two unplanned
         pregnancies. Minor disturbances included alcohol and drug
         intoxication, stopping contraceptives briefly, and brief per-
         iods of homosexual contacts." The author concludes that
         the effects of pregnancy on the patient population are not
         serious enough to warrant therapists stopping practice dur-
         ing pregnancy. She does warn, however, that "special
         dangers" may exist where an "impulsive borderline patient"
         is concerned.

2425.   Berman, Ellen. "The Woman Psychiatrist As Therapist
           and Academician." Journal of Medical Education, 47:
           11 (November 1972) 890-893.
         Women psychiatrists "bring to their work different attitudes
         and are perceived by patients in very different ways. Wo-
         men therapists provide badly needed role models for women
         testing the old stereotypes of the housebound and subser-
         vient woman. For male patients, they can offer proof that
         not all women are like the dreaded mother of his
         childhood." Advantages of working with a female therapist
         are illustrated in two case histories. The woman physician
         in the academic setting must refute both the "illogical, un-
         intellectual" as well as the castrating "bitch" stereotypes
         and prove that she is "competent but not dangerous."

2426.   Blain, Daniel. "Women in Psychiatry." In: <u>Careers in</u>
         <u>Psychiatry.</u> Macmillan Company, New York, New
         <u>York, 1968,</u> pp. 111-127. chart, illus.
         While women comprise only about seven per cent of all phy-
         sicians, they make up almost 12 per cent of all psychia-
         trists. Citing statistics and quoting leaders in the medical
         field, the author examines the factors that attract women to
         this branch of medicine and looks at the reasons that women
         remain a minority among psychiatrists (and among physi-
         cians).

2427.   Bliss, Barbara E. "A Thousand Men and I." In: <u>The</u>
         <u>Crumbling Walls: Treatment and Counseling of Prison-</u>
         <u>ers.</u> Edited by Ray E. Hosford and C. Scott Moss.
         <u>University of Illinois Press, Urbana, Illinois, 1975,</u>
         72-87.
         Dr. Bliss describes her experiences as a psychiatrist work-
         ing in an all-male prison in California: "It's an unusual
         and exhilarating experience to be a woman in a prison of
         almost a thousand young men." The interactions that de-
         velop depend upon the personality and orientation of the
         therapist, as well as on the setting. One factor in the
         setting which made a difference for Dr. Bliss was the
         fact that she was 20-30 years older than the men: "there
         is no inmate who could not be my son." Because of the
         facilities, geared toward men (open toilets and showers),
         and the preparation they necessitate before she can walk
         through an area, Dr. Bliss feels her femininity is accentua-
         ted and she is seen not only as a physician, but as a wo-
         man also. Incidents which reflect the author's sense of be-
         longing--being one of the staff--are related, as well as the
         rumors she had to deal with regarding her motives for
         working in that prison. Dr. Bliss believes that "psycho-
         therapy is an interaction between two basically equal human
         beings; that it may be ... one of the most intimate inter-
         actions that we can experience." She feels anyone has the
         right to ask her about herself as a person. She follows
         this statement with background material on her professional
         activities and choices. Because Dr. Bliss feels she is
         often seen as a sexual object, she has accentuated her ma-
         ternal features and she is referred to by several inmates
         as "mom." Dr. Bliss also discusses the importance of
         language within prison and how one is addressed by both
         staff and inmates. In conclusion Dr. Bliss notes that "no-
         where in our society, in my experience, is the double
         standard so strong as in a prison, and nowhere is it more
         imperative to 'act like a lady.'"

2428.   Bluestone, Naomi. "Careers in Medical Care Administra-
         tion." <u>Journal of the American Medical Women's Asso-</u>
         <u>ciation,</u> 24:9 (September 1969) 725, 728-731.
         Because most of the bourgeois benefits are available in med-
         ical administration jobs, the "regularity" of this kind of job

"blends delightfully with marriage." These benefits include:
excellent working hours, i.e., nine-to-five five-day week,
liberal vacations, short training period, early earning capacity, mobility in seeing the country, "and attitudes toward women doctors are far more liberal than those in the
masculine recesses of clinical medicine." A short inset
about Naomi Bluestone is included.

2429. Bouzarth, William F. "The Role of Women Physicians in
         Disaster Medicine." Journal of the American Medical
         Women's Association, 20:9 (September 1965) 872-874.
         (Presentation, Meeting of Branch Twenty-Five of the
         American Medical Women's Association, Eastern Penn-
         sylvania, February 24, 1965.)
The primary emphasis of this article by a male doctor who
coordinated Medical Education for National Defense at the
Woman's Medical College of Pennsylvania is that women
medical students as well as women faculty are interested
in participating fully in disaster medicine and training for
the specialized practice of certain aspects of it like atomic
radiation and aviation pathology. "... although more effort may be required to initiate the interest of the women
physicians in disaster medicine, once the interest is aroused
they are equal to and may even surpass men in their response. Those women physicians who serve their primary
role as mother and secondary role as physician will, during
disaster conditions, represent a reserve pool of medical
manpower."

2430. Brindley, Clare Evalyn. "Careers in the Pharmaceutical
         Industry." The Woman Physician, 26:7 (July 1971)
         364-365.
The advantage of women physicians considering a professional career working for the drug industry is that one
"can keep a regular 8-hour day schedule, five days a week,
with free nights and weekends, no emergency calls to the
hospital and no house calls." A brief inset about Clare
Evalyn Brindley is included.

2431. Brown, Caree Rozen and Hellinger, Marilyn Levitt.
         "Therapists' Attitudes Toward Women." Social Work,
         20:4 (July 1975) 266-270. tables.
In order to discover therapists' attitudes towards women,
the authors designed a 42-item questionnaire and distributed
it to 274 psychiatrists, residents in psychiatry, psychologists, social workers, and psychiatric nurses. Sixty-six
per cent of the questionnaires were returned. The findings
reveal that male therapists' attitudes were normally distributed across the total sample, and female therapists tend
to have more contemporary attitudes toward women than
those of other therapists. In addition, female therapists attained a significantly higher contemporary score on items
related to female-male roles during sexual intercourse, the

maternal instinct, and childrearing. The authors conclude
that there is a need for therapists to investigate the changing notions of women and men and possible new concepts
of family and community life.

2432.   Cabot, Richard C. "Women in Medicine." Journal of the
          American Medical Association, 65:11 (11 September
          1915) 947-948.
        Obtaining a medical education is no longer a great problem
        for women, but obstacles to a full career present them-
        selves after graduation. A doctor may choose medical sci-
        ence (investigation and teaching), medical practice (the
        most competitive choice), or social medicine. Because of
        the prejudice against women practitioners and because of
        women's natural dislike of competition, the article suggests
        that social medicine is an appropriate area for women.
        Medical colleges, especially women's medical colleges,
        should provide thorough courses of study in social medicine.

2433.   Carter, Charlene A. "Advantages of Being a Woman Thera-
          pist." Psychotherapy: Theory, Research and Practice,
          8:4 (Winter 1971) 297-300.
        Because helping others emotionally is more often a feminine
        than a masculine activity (as a result of different role ex-
        pectations for boys and girls in our society), "being a
        therapist is more natural for a woman." Male therapists,
        consequently, must learn to be more "womanly." Female
        and male therapists bring different approaches to their pa-
        tients. One crucial difference in approach is that "men
        work from a cognitive framework and women operate on
        the basis of feelings." The one exception to the male
        therapist's ability to quickly "grasp concrete difficulties of
        the patient's dilemma, and ... begin to formulate coping
        alternatives" is the hysterical patient "who will be difficult
        for a male therapist to work with because her central prob-
        lems are with her mother." Three types of patients with
        whom the woman therapists work exceedingly well are (1)
        severely disturbed patients, (2) female delinquents and post-
        adolescent women experiencing developmental crises, and
        (3) female hysterical patients. In conclusion, a multiple
        approach is recommended which "combines the unique per-
        ceptions" of both male and female therapists and is espe-
        cially desirable in working with male and female neurotic
        patients.

2434.   Clower, Virginia Lawson. "Careers in Psychiatry." The
          Woman Physician, 26:5 (May 1971) 251, 254-57, 260-
          63.
        Virginia Lawson Clower became a psychiatrist herself "be-
        cause it was so frustrating to recognize emotional factors
        in illness but not know what to do about them." Male col-
        leagues and teachers in the field of psychiatry recognize
        the competence of women. Indeed, "in psychiatry femininity

is not only tolerated, it is a positive advantage." Successful men in psychiatry "have a capacity for intuitive understanding, empathetic identification, and a kind of tolerant
patience and willingness to let situations and people develop [which are] outstanding characteristics of women in
general." Because psychiatry does not usually demand
night and weekend duty or have crises common in other
medical specialties, the medical coverage on a "psychiatric
service does not have to be so extensive to be adequate."
Therefore, a woman who wants to combine training with
keeping a house and raising children might well consider
psychiatry. Because there is a need to increase the number of women psychiatrists, there has been experimentation
in residency programs. To minimize the conflict for women between the role of mother and the role of resident,
the traditional one-year residency program is spread over
four nine-month periods so that mothers can be home with
their children during summer vacations, Christmas, and
Easter. Furthermore, with a sound-proofed office and private entrance, one can work at home at one's convenience.
"The fact that mother is on the premises and accessible if
necessary can be a great comfort to mother herself as well
as to children and household help." Psychoanalysis is also
a field women might consider. She concludes by referring
to Erik Erikson, "... women in professions may find themselves in conflict because some professions highly satisfying to intellectual strivings and drives toward activity, do
not satisfy the feminine need to use ... 'woman's productive inner space.'"

2435. Cole, Helen Grady. "Careers in Ophthalmology and Eye
        Surgery." Journal of the American Medical Women's
        Association, 24:9 (September 1969) 732-734.
        Unlike other areas of medicine, the ophthalmologist can
        practice anywhere. Because kindness and gentleness are
        peculiarly womanly characteristics, and because these
        qualities are especially suitable to the practice of ophthal-
        mology, this medical specialty is appropriate to a woman's
        "nature and ability." Because most of one's work in this
        field is by appointment, a woman physician will not find
        her work interfering "with her vocations as wife, mother,
        and homemaker...." Also, emergencies are relatively
        rare. "The delicacy of the eye and the small size of the
        organ seem to suit a woman's capacity for detail work and
        for accuracy and attention." She advises that when planning
        a residency, it is a good idea to plan to have one's chil-
        dren before or after it.

2436. Copple, Peggy J. "Careers in Pediatric Neurology." The
        Woman Physician, 26:12 (December 1971) 626-627.
        The practice of pediatric neurology is not conducive to
        regular hours because children do not get sick on schedule.
        Because the physician is working directly with parents and

children, one has the rewards of seeing a child recover
and the parents happy or, in terminal cases, the sorrow
of having to convey that news. Therefore "pediatric neurology is not specifically a 'good field for a woman.'" It is
a good specialty for a physician "whose interests and abilities
lie in the diagnosis and treatment of disorders of the nervous system in children."

2437.   Corcoran, Paul J. Journal of the American Medical Wo-
           men's Association, 24:2 (February 1969) 176-177.
           (Open Forum.)
         Physical medicine and rehabilitation is a field of medical
         specialty that is short of personnel, a male doctor writes,
         and therefore a good field for women physicians to consider
         entering. A career in this area is not incompatible with
         family life because of the minimum number of emergency
         calls and light amount of night work. "The emphasis on
         the whole patient in his social and community setting also
         has special appeal for many women physicians. In addi-
         tion, this is one field where no prejudice exists against
         women ... 10.4 per cent of [physicians in this specialty]
         are women."

2438.   Coryllos, Elizabeth. "Careers in Pediatric Surgery."
           The Woman Physician, 26:2 (February 1971) 100-103.
         Pediatric surgery is probably most efficiently practiced by
         teaming up with other pediatric surgeons or else working
         in a hospital and perhaps in association with a teaching
         position at a medical school. As a result, one has ready
         access to other people who can take responsibility and with
         whom one can share professional expertise. With such a
         practice, one can expect more regular hours, which lends
         itself to home and family life. Because the woman "usual-
         ly has more facility and ease than does the man" with chil-
         dren, the woman's characteristics "of patience and per-
         severance, which are more part of the feminine than of the
         masculine personality" will enable her to fulfill "the meticu-
         lous attention to detail, which again is more suited to the
         female disposition." The patient is small and therefore
         one does not need physical strength as much as one needs
         stamina, and "this again fits in with the woman's make-up.
         The work demands a high degree of manual dexterity and
         delicate handling of tissues--neither of which presents too
         great a problem to the average woman." "The woman in
         pediatric surgery needs no special qualifications, except
         that she must be just a bit better than the average man in
         the same specialty...." "the choice of a husband is most
         important, and he can be a great asset to his wife's career
         as well as on the home front." A biographical sketch of
         the author is included as an inset.

2439.   Coveny, Mary A. "Women Physicians in Care of the State
           Insane." Woman's Medical Journal, 11:7 (July 1901)
           262-263.

The first appointments of women physicians in hospitals
for the insane were made in 1870 (at Worcester, Massachusetts and Augusta, Maine). The names of women presently filling such posts (as well as the number in various
states) are given.

2440.   Ducker, Dalia Golan. The Effects of Two Sources of Role
        Strain on Women Physicians. City University of New
        York, New York, New York, 1974, x, 138 pp. figs.,
        tables. (Ph.D. thesis.)
        This thesis is based on interviews conducted with 93 wo-
        men and 82 men physicians (selected from the 1970 Direc-
        tory of Medical Specialists) in four specialties--psychiatry,
        pediatrics, otolaryngology, and surgery. These specialties
        represent the various combinations of the two main sources
        of role strain investigated by the study: believed unsuitabil-
        ity of a field for women and specialty time demands. Be-
        liefs about women's suitability for certain specialties "were
        established empirically through questionnaires administered
        to male physicians," all of whom were faculty members of
        Mount Sinai School of Medicine. Time demands were de-
        termined from literature. Neither of these two variables
        were found to have the expected results on the behavior
        and feelings of women physicians. However, an important
        factor related to professional activity level and feeling that
        personal life suffers was whether or not a woman had ever
        been married or had children. This factor was concep-
        tualized in terms of degree of family and/or career com-
        mitment, rather than merely time allocation.

2441.   Esterly, Nancy B.; Arak, Gladys; Furey, Nancy; Ginsberg,
        Michele; Howell, Sarah E.; Kirschner, Barbara S.; Miller,
        Marilyn; and Zurbrugg, Jo. "The Obstetrician and
        Breast Feeding: Some Views of Women Physicians."
        Journal of Reproductive Medicine, 14:3 (March 1975)
        89-97.
        The participants of this symposium presented their opinions
        on the obstetrician's role in a woman's decision to breast
        feed, and the advantages and disadvantages of breast feed-
        ing. All of the participants were physician-mothers who
        breast fed their own children and found the experience re-
        warding. As Dr. Esterly put it, "The joy and intimacy of
        nursing one's infant is an experience equalled by few others
        in life." Dr. Esterly wrote the introduction and the con-
        clusion to this article.

2442.   Gardner, Mabel E. "How May a Medical Woman Secure
        Surgical Training?" Medical Woman's Journal, 36:11
        (November 1929) 301.
        Mabel Gardner relates her experience in discovering that
        there is, indeed, prejudice against women desirous of en-
        tering the field of surgery.

2443. Gillette, Harriet E. "Careers ... in Physical Medicine and Rehabilitation." Journal of the American Medical Women's Association, 19:7 (July 1964) 582-585.
The relatively high percentage of women in the specialties of physical medicine and rehabilitation compared to other medical specialties is indicative of how well suited the specialty is to women either with or without family responsibilities. "Personality characteristics peculiar to a woman do not make her a better psychiatrist, neither do they detract from her qualifications for this field." Included is a biographic inset about Harriet E. Gillette.

2444. Gough, Harrison G. "Specialty Preferences of Physicians and Medical Students." Journal of Medical Education, 50:6 (June 1975) 581-588. tables.
"In 1970 approximately 81 per cent of the nation's physicians were in specialty practice, and by 1990 this figure is projected to rise to 94 per cent. A phenomenon of this magnitude clearly warrants intensive study. In this inquiry preference ratings for 40 specialties were obtained from 140 male and 20 female physicians and from 71 male and 18 female third-year medical students. Although significant differences were noted, there was a common hierarchy of preference observable in all four groups. For example, family and internal medicine were rated high by all four groups, whereas neurological and colon-rectal surgery were rated low. Males, and particularly male physicians, gave significantly higher ratings to surgical specialties, whereas females expressed stronger preferences for obstetrics and gynecology. Students gave lower ratings than physicians to surgical and eye, ear, nose, and throat specialties." [Article abstract.]

2445. Goz, R. "Women Patients and Women Therapists: Some Issues that Come Up in Psychotherapy." International Journal of Psychoanalytical Psychotherapy, 2 (1973) 298-319.
[Article not examined by editors.]

2446. Haycock, Christine E. "Careers in General Surgery." The Woman Physician, 25:11 (November 1970) 732-733.
The general surgeon, in this age of specialization, is vanishing. Today, general surgery is usually restricted to abdominal surgery. Requirements and opportunities for women in general surgery are discussed. "Surgery would be a difficult field for a woman with a growing family and I would not advise it unless the woman physician is employed by an agency, such as the VA." A short biographical inset on the author is included.

2447. Jakoby, Ruth Kerr. "Careers in Neurosurgery." The Woman Physician, 25:10 (October 1970) 655-657.
The history of, and training for, careers in neurosurgery

are discussed, as well as the nature of the practice. Women in neurosurgery are mentioned briefly and by way of a personal account of concerns for the author whose biggest problem "was that of obtaining residency after completing surgical internships" [in the mid-1950s]. Biographical information about the author is included in an inset.

2448.   Jones, Vera Heinly. "Child Welfare and Public Health: The Role of the Woman School Physician." Medical Woman's Journal, 41:11 (November 1934) 296-300. port.
"In our school system, where the physical examinations are optional, there would probably be no girls to examine if the examinations were conducted by a man physician." Women school physicians, however, have a better rapport with the adolescent girl, who is "quite reticent about her body, self-conscious, and shy." In addition to providing health care, women physicians can instruct adolescents in social hygiene.

2449.   Kanof, Naomi M. "Careers in Dermatology." The Woman Physician, 26:10 (October 1971) 506a, 522a.
Dermatology is presented as a challenging specialty and a medical discipline which affords "a great variety and a large number of opportunities for fulfilling an interest in medicine." The author put no special emphasis on the sex of the physician choosing this specialty. Biographical information about the author is given in an inset.

2450.   Kavinoky, Nadine R. "Women Physicians and Social Hygiene." Medical Woman's Journal, 46:6 (June 1939) 184. (Editorial.)
"Women physicians who themselves are normal in their attitudes towards this subject ..." should consider specializing in social hygiene, the objective of which "is the stabilization of family life."

2451.   Kearney, Elizabeth F. "The Woman Physician in Official Positions." Woman's Medical Journal, [8]:7 (July 1899) 229-231. (Original Articles.)
Dr. Kearney, assistant physician to Cook County Insane Asylum, emphasizes the need for management by women physicians in municipalities and institutions. Women should serve as school inspectors, on boards of education, as factory inspectors, and as supervisors in insane asylums.

2452.   Kosa, John and Coker, Robert E. "The Female Physician in Public Health Conflict and Reconciliation of the Sex and Professional Roles." Sociology and Social Research, 49:3 (1965) 294-305. tables.
"The female physicians, representing about 5 per cent of the practitioners in a predominantly male profession, tend to face three types of role conflicts: (1) The professional

role restricts the full realization of the sex role, and female physicians defer marriage more frequently than male physicians. (2) The sex role restricts the full continuous performance of the professional role, and female physicians are more likely to interrupt their work career, take part-time positions and stay in any position for a shorter time than men doctors. (3) Female physicians face difficulty in accepting those aspects of the professional role which are noncompatible with the female role such as entrepreneurship in medical practice. As an institutionalized way to reducing role conflict, female physicians tend to take up practice in those fields of medicine (pediatrics, public health, psychiatry) where the sex and professional roles can be expected to be most compatible." [Author abstract.] These conclusions were based upon the results of a survey of a nationwide sample of 525 male and female physicians who at one point in their careers worked in public health. Comparative data, presented in tables and commented upon within the text, provide information on income, attitudes, and factors affecting specialty selection.

2453.   "Laboratory Research--A Career for Women." Medical Woman's Journal, 44:5 (May 1937) 138. (Editorial.) Careers in research laboratories "offer a most promising career to women." The author laments the scarcity of women physicians who attend meetings such as those of the American Association of Pathologists and Bacteriologists, the American Association of Immunologists, the American Association for Cancer Research, and the International Association of Medical Museums.

2454.   Lax, Ruth F. "Some Considerations About Transference and Countertransference Manifestations Evoked by the Analyst's Pregnancy." International Journal of Psycho-Analysis, 50:3 (1969) 363-372. The author details patient reaction to her pregnancy and also discusses the experiences of other pregnant analysts. She concludes that an analyst's pregnancy "may interfere with the sequence of the transference neurosis but need not necessarily interfere with the unfolding of a pattern of infantile conflicts characteristic for a given patient."

2455.   McCombs, A. Parks. "Careers in Internal Medicine." Journal of the American Medical Women's Association, 24:12 (December 1969) 972-973, 976-978. (Careers.) A woman who wants to enter medicine should know from the beginning of her training in undergraduate school that she will have to "develop into a well-integrated individual." While the average man can assume that "at some stage in his training or work he will marry and be able to raise a family without any interruption of his career ... this is not always true for the woman." Medical schools are reluctant to accept women because "they drop out to have

their children and thus deprive a man of the opportunity
to study." The author warns that "the woman considering
a career in medicine should give careful thought to these
hazards and to the long wait which may be necessary before she can start a family. If she is unwilling to face the
added tasks ahead of her, and fears that she will be
cheated in her feminine role in life she may be well advised to seek her career in another less arduous field."
"There are many ways married women can find employment.
Substituting for other physicians during vacations, holidays,
or periods of illness, as well as taking on part-time work
in the local hospitals to cover the emergency wards during
certain hours or to provide time off for the house staff, are
but a few suggestions for short-term or regular work,
which can be done either to supplement the income or on
a voluntary basis." An inset about A. Parks McCombs is
included.

2456.   Meyer, Blanche M. "The Unique Role of Women As Thera-
             pists in Psychiatry." Medical Woman's Journal, 57:6
             (June 1950) 18-23. (Presentation, Second Congress,
             Pan American Medical Women's Alliance, Los Angeles,
             California, November 1949.)
Because psychological problems originate in the home, and
mothers or substitutes are usually responsible, women are
peculiarly fitted for treating the maladjusted: "... what
women have failed to do, only women can rectify." Women
psychiatrists should help develop a "positive feminine idealism" and foster an "idealized feminine symbol such as the
Virgin Mary...." Women psychiatrists can help women
become aware of "the quiet power of acceptance, receptiv-
ity, the use of silence and of diplomacy, with a willingness
to receive--be it ideas or sperm...." Dr. Meyer outlines
how her own methods of therapy accomplish these objectives.

2457.   Morton, Rosalie Slaughter. "Woman's Place in the Public
             Health Movement [Part I]." Woman's Medical Journal,
             22:4 (April 1912) 83-87. (Presentation, American Med-
             ical Association Section on Preventive Medicine and
             Public Health, Los Angeles, California, June 29, 1911.)

2458.   Morton, Rosalie Slaughter. "Woman's Place in the Public
             Health Movement [Part II]." Woman's Medical Journal,
             22:5 (May 1912) 99-104. (Presentation, American Med-
             ical Association Section on Preventive Medicine and
             Public Health, Los Angeles, California, June 29, 1911.)
Suggestions are given as to what women physicians can and
should do in the public health movement.

2459.   Nadelson, Carol C. "Women in Surgery." Archives of
             Surgery, 102:3 (March 1971) 234-235. (Editorial.)
Quoting figures from a recent government survey (Facts

on Prospective and Practicing Women in Medicine. Women's
Bureau, Wage and Labor Standards Administration, U.S.
Department of Labor, 1968), the author reveals that of the
total number of women physicians active in 1965, only 17.4
per cent were in surgical specialties, while 25.4 per cent
of women physicians went into general practice. Arguments against women in surgery "are in the direction of
the rigors of training and the physical strength and stamina
required to meet tasks in the operating room." The ag-
gressiveness necessary to pursue such a surgical career is
also said to be lacking in females. Women do not apply
for surgical residencies for many reasons. One reason
relates to predominant male attitudes toward women applicants. Women are made to feel that their sexuality is
being called into question and that they and their sex are
continuously on trial. Women, also, are made to feel that
surgery is a man's domain. "If a female surgeon is allowed to act as a woman and still be a surgeon, she could
possibly bring to the healing art more of the gentleness and
compassion with which the hand of a woman is historically
linked."

2460.   Nadelson, Carol [C].; Notman, Malkah; Arons, Elissa; and
         Feldman, Judith. "The Pregnant Therapist." Ameri-
         can Journal of Psychiatry, 131:10 (October 1974) 1107-
         1111. (Presented in part at a panel, 127th Annual
         Meeting, American Psychiatric Association, Detroit,
         Michigan, 6-10 May 1974.)
The authors' assumption in this article is that when a woman who is a therapist becomes obviously pregnant, this
pregnancy affects her as well as affecting her relationships
with her patients, her colleagues, and her supervisors.
Such effects are manifested in a heightened awareness and
change of the therapists' own fantasies, moods, attention
span, fears, and the subsequent "physical or emotional"
limitations in her work. The recognition of these limitations may be a challenge to her fantasies of omnipotence.
Physicians often use counterdependent mechanisms to handle
stress, particularly that resulting from illness or disability. This may be even more of a problem for the woman
physician, who is preselected for traits traditionally considered 'unfeminine,' such as strength, assertiveness, and
independence. "Instead of acknowledging a change of need
for a more flexible work schedule, the pregnant therapist
may perceive limiting her activity ... to be an admission
of weakness." The colleagues of the pregnant therapist,
both men and women, "may feel envious of her pregnancy
and angry about having to assume extra work. The extended training period postpones parenthood for many, and
they may resent the woman who seems ready to handle a
family as well as a career. To defend against their anger
and guilt, they often become over-solicitous of their pregnant colleague." Patients of the pregnant therapist may

experience a variety of reactions to her pregnancy. "Male
patients may experience the reawakening of fears about
sexual competence, or competitive feelings toward the
therapist's husband ... [and] increased awareness of direct
sexual feelings toward the therapist." "The female patient
may envy her therapist's apparent personal fulfillment,
since the pregnancy may remind her of what she herself
has lost or never experienced." A female patient may get
pregnant herself as "an expression of hostile feelings toward the therapist." Both male and female patients "may
be threatened by the idea that the therapist will be more
committed to her own family than to them." Other patients
may fear that the pregnant therapist is abandoning them,
while still others perceive the baby as a sibling rival or
as a sibling with whom to identify. The authors give special consideration to lesbian patients' responses to the
therapist's pregnancy. "Lesbian patients sometimes experience a particular sense of betrayal with the realization
of a therapist's pregnancy. For some, the fantasy exists
that the therapist is also homosexual. The pregnancy,
representing a confirmation of the therapist's heterosexuality, is a rejection of the patient's transference wishes.
It may also be seen as an implicit criticism of the patient
for what she may feel to be the depreciated choice of homosexuality. In some cases this aspect of a highly sexualized
transference is extremely difficult for the patient to tolerate
or to disclose.... Other lesbian patients may envy the
baby's intimacy with the therapist." If the pregnant therapist is aware of the changes she goes through and what the
people with whom she has to interact professionally go
through in response to her pregnancy, then she may be productive during this time. "She may find that there are certain situations within which she is less effective, such as
working with violent patients or doing abortion consultations."

2461.   Nemeth, Magdalene C. "Single Women in Psychiatry."
        American Journal of Psychiatry, 131:3 (March 1974)
        329-330. (Letters to the Editor.)
        The author hypothesizes that there are probably more
        single women among physicians than there are single wo-
        men among the general population. She suspects that there
        are several reasons for women physicians' reluctance to
        marry: some women chose medicine over marriage; a
        woman's value on the marriage market decreases propor-
        tionately with her increased professional status and age; a
        woman cannot marry below her social status; and, once past
        a certain age and unmarried, a woman physician is driven
        deeper and deeper into social isolation.

2462.   Paluszny, Maria and Poznanski, Elva. "Reactions of Pa-
        tients during Pregnancy of the Psychotherapist." Child
        Psychiatry and Human Development, 1:4 (Summer 1971)
        266-274.

The reactions of both patients and therapists to the pregnancies of the psychiatrists who wrote this article were
observed and recorded. The patients were observed responding in the following ways: feeling rejected, feeling
sibling rivalry with the fetus and then the babies, and feeling oedipal conflict. Some patients identified with the baby
and in doing so reenacted patterns of their own childhood
conflicts in relation to the therapist; othere were defensive;
and still others were stimulated into pregnancy labor symptoms. The therapists themselves recorded that during
their pregnancies they experienced "a heightened awareness"
of their physiological changes and an awareness of the baby.
Therefore, some of the patients' feelings of rejection in the
sense of competing with the baby for the therapists' attention had a basis in reality.

2463.   Renshaw, Josephine E. "Careers in Obstetrics and Gyne-
            cology." The Woman Physician, 26:3 (March 1971)
            160-162.
        The specialty is defined and its "suitability for women" dis-
        cussed. The woman physician "will find that marriage and
        a family of her own are completely compatible with a career
        in obstetrics and gynecology provided she chooses her hus-
        band wisely and keeps her plans flexible." Opportunities,
        income, and challenges for the future in this field are also
        discussed.

2464.   Roeske, Nancy A. "Women in Psychiatry: Past and Pres-
            ent Areas of Concern." American Journal of Psychi-
            atry, 130:10 (October 1973) 1127-1131.
        In 1972 the American Psychiatric Association created a
        Task Force on Women to examine 1) special issues and
        problems of women in general, as those problems arise in
        the practice of psychiatry, and 2) collect data on men and
        women psychiatrists that would delineate pertinent problems
        and conflict areas and to offer suggestions and recommenda-
        tions for solving problems. Projects initiated include:
        1) communication with psychiatry journals for information
        about women on editorial boards and policies on acceptance
        of articles by and about women; 2) questioning NIMH and
        AMA about their utilization of women psychiatrists; 3) es-
        tablishing a talent bank of women psychiatrists at APA
        headquarters; 4) suggestion to include a course on the
        psychology of women during residency training, and a re-
        view of curricula in such courses to make material avail-
        able; 5) planning a monograph summarizing literature about
        women in psychiatry and the psychology of women; 6) de-
        velopment of questionnaires for department chairmen and
        training directors exploring the role of women psychiatrists
        in education. Other suggestions are: placement of women
        on admissions committees, counseling of women by women,
        taking of an active role by women in revising medical train-
        ing programs to reduce career-family conflicts, interviewing

by a man and a woman and exploration of potential conflicts
when applying for residency training programs. The Task
Force, in a pilot study regarding the characteristics of men
and women in psychiatry, found that the major difference
centered on the family-career conflict. The data supported
other studies which recommended that women should have
the option of flexibility in professional training programs
and that child care facilities should be available.

2465. Romm, May E. "Women and Psychiatry." Journal of the
       American Medical Women's Association, 24:8 (August
       1969) 629-636. port. (Presentation, Meeting of Amer-
       ican Psychiatric Association, Boston, Massachusetts,
       16 May 1968.)
The author reviews the prevalent attitude toward women,
women as physicians, and women physicians as psychiatrists. She submits that "women physicians appear to be
better suited to some specialties, especially psychiatry.
Their talents and empathy enables them to deal more easily
with patients though treatment by both men and women psychiatrists often produce good results. The practice of
psychiatry can be fitted into a schedule allowing the woman
to encompass adequately the roles of wife and mother, as
well as physician."

2466. Root, Eliza H. "The Medical Woman as Teacher in Med-
       ical Schools." Woman's Medical Journal, 11:9 (Sep-
       tember 1901) 325-330. (Original Articles.) (Presenta-
       tion, Iowa Medical Women's Social Society, 14 May
       1901.)
Dr. Root offers information on women faculty members of
the nation's medical colleges.

2467. Ruland, Dora. "Hospital Administration as a Field for
       Women." Journal of the American Medical Women's
       Association, 7:12 (December 1952) 460-461.
A history is given of hospital administration as a career.
Dr. Mary R. Lewis was one of the pioneers in establishing this field. She was formerly superintendent and medical director of the Woman's Hospital of Philadelphia. At
the time of this article, the American Hospital Association
Directory listed 6,832 hospitals and "it has been estimated
that more than 200 new administrators are required each
year."

2468. Ryder, Claire F. "Careers in Public Health." Journal of
       the American Medical Women's Association, 24:6 (June
       1969) 514-519.
Dr. Ryder discusses "natural aptitudes of women physicians
in public health," "preparation for a career in public
health," "public health opportunities at the local level,"
"careers in federal service," "community health," and "international opportunities," among other aspects of the profession.

2469.   Samilowitz, Hazel. "Women in Psychiatry: Report on a
         Conference." Psychiatric Communications, 8:1 (1966)
         11-15. graphs, tables.
         This article consists of a summary of the proceedings of
         the 1966 Philadelphia conference on "Women in Psychiatry."
         Panel discussions are summarized and graphs and tables
         represent the age distribution of residents, interruption in
         training, and marital status and number of children of the
         women psychiatric residents.

2470.   Scher, Maryonda. "Women Psychiatrists in the United
         States." American Journal of Psychiatry, 130:10 (Octo-
         ber 1973) 1118-1122. tables. (Special Section: Women
         in Psychiatry and Medicine.) (Revised version of a pre-
         sentation meeting, Group Without a Name, Seattle,
         Washington, 8-10 September 1972.)
         Of the women graduating from medical school in the United
         States, between 10 and 20 per cent enter psychiatric train-
         ing. "The statistics show that women complete their psy-
         chiatric training as often as men--indeed, U.S.-trained wo-
         men complete it more often than men,"--even though it
         takes women longer to complete training than it does men.
         There are approximately 3,000 women psychiatrists, or
         12.5 per cent of the total in the United States. Twenty-
         two per cent women practice child and/or adolescent psy-
         chiatry which is over twice the percentage of men in this
         specialty. Seventy-three women and 81 per cent men were
         working, sixty-two per cent men in contrast to 53 per cent
         of the women worked in two or more locations; women are
         more often employed in salaried positions like state mental
         institutions and educational institutions than men are; wo-
         men average direct patient contact for 25 hours a week
         while men averaged 32 hours; both women and men donated
         on the average 8 hours a week; the average woman psychi-
         atrist's professional work week had approximately 80 per
         cent of the number of hours that the average man's did.
         "Considering the fact that most [of the women] function in
         the roles of wife and mother in addition to their profes-
         sional work, they are not only highly productive people but
         in addition must be efficient and well organized." Women
         psychiatrists cost their employers less because fewer are
         board certified. A former surgeon general, Dr. Luther
         Terry, of the U.S. Public Health Service, is quoted as
         saying, "Women are good for psychiatry. First, I think
         that from a biological standpoint, the evidence has indi-
         cated that they tend to adapt better to many of the seden-
         tary requirements of psychiatry, particularly of psychother-
         apy, and that in many respects they have less need of some
         of the action orientation which is often so important to, and
         on occasion impairs the effectiveness of, men as psycho-
         therapists. Even more important, I think, from a psycho-
         logical and sociological standpoint ... women as a group
         tend to be more intuitive than men and to function better in

a nurturing capacity which is often required in psychotherapy." Dr. Scher concludes, "Perhaps women in greater
numbers could alter the image that the American public
has of the doctor, i.e., the cold, impersonal, scientific
man on a gluttonous quest for riches at the expense of his
helpless and suffering patients.... The absurd phallocen-
tric theme has dominated the lore of medicine and psychiatry."

2471. Schurter, Maxine. "Careers in Plastic Surgery." The Wo-
       man Physician, 26:6 (June 1971) 312-313.
       Plastic surgery as a career is discussed in terms of its
       definition, scope, history, training requirements, and as
       a specialty for women. "It is a field in which there is lit-
       tle, if any, prejudice against women, either by colleagues
       or by patients." A brief discussion of Catherine Stephenson,
       a pioneer in plastic surgery in the United States, is in-
       cluded.

2472. Seaman, Barbara. "Pelvic Autonomy: Four Proposals."
       Social Policy, 6:2 (September/October 1975) 43-47.
       illus.
       Following a discussion of the attitudes and practices preva-
       lent in the male-dominated field of obstetrics and gynecol-
       ogy, and predicated on the fact that "the individuals who
       determine health-care policies are not responsive to the
       demands of feminists," four demands (originally issued at
       a Women's Health Conference in Boston on 7 April 1975)
       are listed: "(1) Effective immediately, only women shall
       be admitted to obstetrics and gynecology residencies. Males
       who are currently in training may remain, as may those
       who are in practice.... (2) Effective immediately, no
       more foundation monies will be awarded to men for any
       kind of research into the female reproductive system....
       (3) Effective immediately, the establishment and adminis-
       tration of laws concerning female reproduction, abortion,
       and sterilization shall be removed from the court and
       legislative systems. An agency modeled after the NLRB,
       FCC, FTC, or Atomic Energy Commission shall handle
       all such matters.... (4) Effective immediately, the United
       Nations and the United States will not sponsor nor partici-
       pate in any international population activity or conference
       unless women are represented in proportion to their num-
       bers in the population of every participating nation."

2473. Shainess, Natalie. "Is Anatomy Destiny? Panel: The
       Changing Role of Women Psychiatrists." Journal of
       the American Medical Women's Association, 28:6 (June
       1973) 293-295. (Presentation, Tenth Divisional West-
       ern Branch Meetings, American Psychiatric Associa-
       tion, October, 1972.)
       Anatomy is "sexual and reproductive" destiny. The mother-
       ing aspect of the reproductive factors is "not necessarily"

destiny. A professional woman "with a sense of social responsibility and/or love for her offspring [is] hampered to
some extent," but she can be helped by the husband "who
has, until recently, refused to recognize, or else ignored,
the significance of his role as husband and father, as well
as by the society which has refused to offer the necessary
solutions." The author cites several studies on women in
psychiatry and concludes by listing six changes she feels
are necessary: (1) male attitudes, "in the direction of
seeing women as people rather than as life-support systems
for themselves"; (2) "medical schools and residency programs should allow a year's leave for each child, with a
guarantee of a place to return to"; (3) male attitudes--"to
a more collaborative approach to marriage"; (4) "some way
of opening doors [social and political] in the exclusive male-
bonding structure"; (5) "women's exclusion from the world's
affairs [which] until very recently has left them to cope
with problems that arise on an individual basis"; and (6)
"perhaps the only change I see necessary in women generally, and especially in medicine and psychiatry, is that they
internalize their superegos. This means giving up male
standards, judgments, and views of what is permissible for
them."

2474.   Simon, William E. "Age, Sex, and Title of Therapist as
           Determinants of Patients' Preferences." Journal of
           Psychology, 83:1 (January 1973) 145-149. tables.
         This study was done to determine the basis of patients'
         preferences for psychotherapists and to see what effects
         age, sex, or title might have on such preferences. Two
         subject groups were used: 102 females whose mean age
         was 25.36 and who attended a Roman Catholic college for
         women; 34 female and 33 male students in an adult educa-
         tion psychology class whose mean age was 36.85 years.
         They were asked to assume that they were patients and
         would consult a therapist according to title, sex, and age.
         In general, the findings include that male therapists were
         generally preferred to female therapists and that 40-year-
         old therapists were generally preferred to 55-year-old
         therapists who, in turn, were preferred to 25-year-old
         therapists. The preferences of females and males and of
         younger and older respondents were also compared. The
         authors conclude that additional research is needed to find
         out the specific reasons as to why age, sex, and title of
         therapist have an effect upon patients' preferences.

2475.   Smith, Myrtle Lee. "Rural County Health Work in the
           South: As Viewed by 'The Human Guinea Pig'--a Wo-
           man County Health Officer." Medical Woman's Journal,
           49:6 (June 1942) 181-183, 193. (Public Health Section.)
         The first woman county health officer in a rural Alabama
         county, Dr. Smith tells of her experiences and the cases
         she encountered there and in Tennessee. She stresses the
         need for more women to serve in rural districts.

2476.   Smith, Olive W.   "Opportunities for Women in Medical Re-
            search."   Harvard Medical Alumni Bulletin, 4:4 (1969)
            6-7.   (Adaptation of Address to Seniors, Wellesley Col-
            lege, Wellesley, Massachusetts, 5 October 1966.)
         Dr. Smith, after outlining the history of women's education
         in the medical sciences at Harvard University (Cambridge,
         Massachusetts), discusses the rewards of research as a
         career for women.   To cope with the difficulty of combin-
         ing marriage and a career, Dr. Smith advises these Welles-
         ley College seniors to be sure and marry a man who is
         "in sympathy with your objective," and get "good and
         permanent domestic help when the children begin to arrive."

2477.   Snyder, Ruth E.   "Careers in Radiology."   The Woman
            Physician, 26:9 (September 1971) 460-461.
         In a look at radiology as a career for women physicians,
         Dr. Snyder suggests "... it is an ideal specialty for a wo-
         man inasmuch as it offers a wide choice as to type of
         practice, hospital, industrial, and private practice, each
         full or part time.   It can be fitted into family life with lit-
         tle disruption of one's private activities after hours, and
         there is usually good financial reward."   In conclusion, Dr.
         Snyder says: "Although we would like to think that the sex
         of a physician makes no difference, it is inescapable that
         the frailties and errors of a woman seem to count more
         against her than the same weaknesses in the male" and
         therefore, "as holds with all fields of medicine, a woman
         must be a better than average radiologist to maintain her
         position."

2478.   Solomon, Rebecca Z.   "Women in Psychiatry."   American
            Journal of Psychiatry, 130:10 (October 1973) 1136-1137.
            (Editorial.)
         This editorial introduces a special section on women in
         psychiatry in this issue of the Journal.   "... it is essen-
         tial to refine our ideas about gender-linked attitudes in
         order to provide an atmosphere in which women can be
         most productive.   Our concepts of activity, passivity, and
         receptivity require clarification."

2479.   Tayson, Juyne M.   "General Practice: Advantages and Dis-
            advantages."   Journal of the American Medical Wo-
            men's Association, 13:6 (June 1958) 242-243.
         The advantages of general practice include working with and
         helping families as well as individuals, and seeing a num-
         ber of patients with a variety of problems so that one sel-
         dom has monotonous days.   The disadvantages of general
         practice include: a 24-hour call schedule, house calls,
         hospital calls with resulting irregular hours, and seeing old
         people who have multiple problems.   The qualifications for
         being a good general practitioner include: being an extro-
         verted person and one who is able to meet emergencies as
         well as being warm and able to work with a variety of peo-
         ple.

2480. Thelberg, Elizabeth. "Report of Chairman of Public Health
      Committee National Council of Women Given in Phila-
      delphia, November 15, 1921." Medical Woman's Jour-
      nal, 28:12 (December 1921) 310-312.
      Dr. Thelberg reiterates the report on public health work
      which she gave at the Christiania (now Oslo) meeting in
      Norway. Resolutions passed by the council concern vene-
      real disease, prostitution, and sex hygiene.

2481. Uzman, Betty Geren. "Reply to Dr. Apter." Archives of
      Pathology, 95:2 (February 1973) 142. (Letters to the
      Editor.)
      This letter is a response to an article by Dr. Julian T.
      Apter "about discrimination in the appointment of patholo-
      gists to serve on federal advisory councils" in which she
      suggested that the Directory of Medical Specialists be used
      to remedy "the inadequate procedures being used by the Na-
      tional Institutes of Health in its selection of pathologists for
      public advisory groups." Dr. Uzman responds saying that
      many highly qualified women research pathologists do not
      list themselves in the Directory, that they are too busy to
      serve, and that the rewards for serving in this time-con-
      suming work are limited.

2482. Van Hoosen, Bertha. "Opportunities for Women to Do Re-
      search in Medicine." Medical Woman's Journal, 37:6
      (June 1930) 162-164. (Read at Sigma Delta Epsilon
      Breakfast, Des Moines, Iowa, December 30, 1929.)
      Nowhere (not even in transportation) has progress been
      more marked and more important to the welfare of the hu-
      man kind than the field of medicine. To determine the con-
      tributions of women to research, the Women's Bureau of
      the United States Department of Labor sent out question-
      naires to assess the professional activity of women in med-
      icine. Women in research are primarily women who have
      their training and degrees in pure science. Women in sci-
      ence "are succeeding in getting equal opportunities for posi-
      tions on medical faculties in far greater numbers than med-
      ical women." A greater percentage of women applying to
      medical schools get rejected than accepted. Indeed, more
      than a dozen and a half of the medical schools in the United
      States accepted only one woman medical student in the year
      this article was written, which "is putting co-education on
      a trap door basis, with every expectation of its falling
      through."

2483. Van Hoosen, Bertha. "Report of the Committee on Medical
      Opportunities for Women." Medical Woman's Journal,
      35:7 (July 1928) 198-199. (Report, Meeting, Medical
      Women's National Association, June 10-12, 1928.)
      A survey intended to discover the status of women in the
      public health service revealed that state insane hospitals
      "are very inadequately staffed with women physicians."

Vacancies in public health positions are often not announced to the public. The Committee on Medical Opportunities will keep in touch with public health departments to facilitate the appointments of women. Women are also under-represented in medical societies. Out of 50 meetings of societies held in 1928, 35 had no women at all represented on their programs.

2484.   [Van Hoosen, Bertha]. "The Woman Surgeon." Medical
          Woman's Journal, 37:1 (January 1930) 13-14. (Editor-
          ial.)
This editorial was written in response to an inaccurate article in the New York Sun about women in surgery, which claimed that Connie Guion was one of the first women surgeons. In fact, Emily Barringer was the first woman ambulance surgeon in the world; Lillian K. Farrar was the only woman member of the National Association of Gynecology and Obstetrics at the time this article was written; Marie L. Chard had been doing major surgery in New York City for more than 30 years. More than in surgery, the medical field continues to discriminate against women in faculty positions where women primarily hold titles of assistant and instructor rather than professor and associate professor. "The present method of selecting medical students [on account of 'personality'] gives room for great injustice, but considering that for some time to come the woman physician must rise or fall according to her ability to please the men in the profession, the apparent injustice may become a means of making her pathway more pleasant in climbing."

2485.   Van Leeuwen, Kato. "Pregnancy Envy in the Male." In-
          ternational Journal of Psycho-Analysis, 47 (Parts 2-3,
          1966) 319-324. (Read at the 24th International Psycho-
          Analytical Congress, Amsterdam, July 1965.)
While Freud's theory that feminine psychology includes and is manifested in penis envy, little research has been done on man's envy of the female sex and child-bearing function. This article includes a review of the literature on men's envy of women's biological functioning, a case study of a male patient who exhibited such envy, the course of therapy the analyst used with the patient, as well as a discussion and case summary.

2486.   Vaschak, Mathilda R., comp. Career Choices for Women
          in Medicine: Volume I. American Medical Women's
          Association, New York, New York, [1965?].
Both Volume I and Volume II of this work are a compilation of the "Career Choices" articles which appeared individually in the Journal of the American Medical Women's Association. [These items appear as individual citations in this bibliography.]

2487.   Vaschak, Mathilda R., comp. Career Choices for Women
        in Medicine: Volume II. American Medican Women's
        Association, New York, New York, 1971.
        [See annotation for Volume I of this compilation.]

2488.   Vietor, Agnes C. "The Making of a Woman Surgeon."
        Woman's Medical Journal, 10:1 (January 1900) 19-22.
        Dr. Vietor speaks to the questions: What is the field for
        a women surgeon--present and future? How does one go
        about studying to become a surgeon? Is a woman capable
        of the position--has she the judgment? Is she incapacitated
        by her natural sympathy? Will she break down early? and,
        Why are women not admitted to the staffs of general hos-
        pitals? The author feels that "the limitations of sex do
        not exist" (neither mental nor physical), but that society
        has forced men and women into classes with certain pre-
        scribed characteristics for each.

2489.   von Sholly, Anna I. "Women in Preventive Medicine."
        Columbia University Quarterly, 17 (June 1915) 236-240.
        This article presents a historic overview of the field of
        preventive medicine and the woman physician's role in that
        field.

2490.   Wassertheil-Smoller, Sylvia; Arnold, Charles B.; Lerner,
        Raymond C.; and Heimrath, Susan L. "Woman Ob-
        stetricians in New York and the State Abortion Law."
        Health Services Reports, 87:4 (April 1972) 328-335.
        chart, tables.
        This article reports part of a survey funded by the Popula-
        tion Council and the New York Foundation, which investi-
        gated physicians attitudes toward abortion, including tech-
        niques and fees charged. This paper focuses on demograph-
        ic differences between men and women obstetricians and
        the differences in their attitudes towards the New York
        abortion law. Two questionnaires were filled out by 1,146
        physicians listed in the AMA tape-file. The profile of the
        11.1 per cent of obstetricians who are women showed they
        were less likely than men to be U.S. trained, board certi-
        fied, or engaged in private practice (they were more likely
        to be in institutional practice). They were more likely to
        be Catholic than the men, who were more likely to be Jew-
        ish, while the percentage of Protestants was about the same.
        Racially, 63 per cent of the women were white compared
        with 89 per cent of men; 66 per cent of female medical
        residents were Oriental or Indians vs. 39 per cent of men.
        Only 62 per cent of the women were married as compared
        with 90 per cent of men. Of the married women, 76 per
        cent had children. Attitudes to abortion revealed that 56
        per cent of women (vs. 68 per cent of men) favored the
        law. It appeared that the Catholic and foreign women were
        opposed; a breakdown by religion showed those in the "other"
        group--mainly foreign women residents--were opposed to

the law.   There was no statistical difference between Catholic men and women.   Questions on willingness to perform
abortions again showed foreign women to be most opposed.
Catholics, both male and female, declined to perform abortions in 83 per cent of the cases, while Protestants declined in only about 30 per cent.   For contraception following abortion, 61 per cent of men preferred the pill, while
57 per cent of women were flexible.   Men tended to perform more abortions than women and had more experience
with different techniques.

2491.   Weinstein, Morton R.   "Psychiatric Manpower and Women
          in Psychiatry."   Journal of Nervous and Mental Disease,
          145:5 (November 1967) 364-370.   tables.
         In order to determine to what extent women utilize psychi-
         atric training in comparison with males in the same resi-
         dency program, a study was made of the residents trained
         at Langley Porter Neuropsychiatric Institute.   Results were
         based on 22 completed questionnaires for women and 27 for
         men.   The study showed that "male graduates work up to
         half again as much as the women, and that the women are
         only 60 per cent as likely to be certified in psychiatry."
         The author concludes that training centers should not ac-
         cept women if the programs can be regularly filled by
         males.   Centers that decide to solicit applications from
         women should redesign programs to accommodate special
         needs of women residents.   Although males practice more
         energetically than females, however, the same percentage
         of women as men complete training, and women do make
         professional contributions.

2492.   Weyman, Else Krug.   "Careers in Family Practice."
          Journal of the American Medical Women's Association,
          24:12 (December 1969) 981-983.
         This article discusses family practice as a career in terms
         of training required and opportunities for women.   "Women
         are especially family minded" and this fact works for their
         benefit.   The woman who selects family practice rather than
         a specialty for a career will have a shorter training period
         and a more flexible and varied practice.   A brief inset on
         the author is included.

2493.   "What Is Being Done in Boston to Secure Medical Women
          as School Inspectors."   Woman's Medical Journal, 22:
          2 (February 1912) 41.   (Communication.)

2494.   Williams, Anna W.   "Group Work in Public Health Labora-
          tories."   Medical Woman's Journal, 43:6 (June 1936)
          151-153.   (Presentation, 30th Annual Meeting, Women's
          Medical Society of New York State, New York City,
          April 27, 1936.)
         Dr. Williams illustrates the benefits of group work with
         anecdotes of her own career in public health and examples

of the achievements of other women physicians in public
health laboratories.

2495. Williams, Marjorie J. "Women Physicians as a Source of
          Recruitment for Pathology." Archives of Pathology,
          88 (July 1969) 42-45. tables.
       Statistical data charts for the 1960s are included to support
       the contention that women physicians are more attracted to
       the specialty of pathology than are men, and that a certain
       percentage of women physicians are professionally inactive.

2496. Wojcik, Ladislas D.; Bain, Katherine; and Smith, Margaret
          H. D. "Pediatrics as a Career for a Woman Physi-
          cian." New Physician, 11 (July 1962) 228-231. ports.
       Drawing from her own experiences, Dr. Ladislas D. Wojcik
       writes about the satisfactions for women pediatricians in
       private practice. Dr. Katherine Bain (deputy chief of the
       Children's Bureau, U.S. Department of Health, Education,
       and Welfare) addresses herself to the role of women pedi-
       atricians in public health work. Dr. Margaret H. D. Smith,
       a professor at Tulane University, discusses women in aca-
       demic pediatrics.

2497. Wolfe, Claire V. "M.D.? MRS.? .... PM&R!" Journal
          of the American Medical Women's Association, 28:1
          (January 1973) 16-18. (Presentation, Annual Meeting,
          American Medical Women's Association, Columbus,
          Ohio, November 13, 1972.)
       "One of the major challenges to a professional woman is
       the organization of, and balance between, her professional
       career and private life. Especially when children are in-
       volved, major determinants in the woman physician's choice
       of a specialty become flexibility of training programs and
       adaptability of an active practice to a growing family.
       Physical medicine and rehabilitation (PM&R) ... [offers]
       flexibility, ... direct doctor-to-patient contact, ... a wide
       range of patients."

2498. "Women As Examiners for Life Insurance Companies."
          Woman's Medical Journal, 26:4 (April 1916) 98.
       Not all life insurance companies employ women physicians
       and yet women physicians are taking out life insurance
       policies. Women physicians should be circumspect when
       taking out insurance and take out policies with those com-
       panies that do employ women.

2499. "The Woman 'Family Physician.'" Medical Woman's Jour-
          nal, 29:11 (November 1922) 299-300. (Editorial.)
       Stressing the need for women physicians to enter family
       practice, this editorial mentions the special attributes that
       make women especially suited for this specialty.

2500. "Women in Industrial Medicine." Medical Woman's Journal,

44:1 (January 1937) 18-19. (Editorial.)
A brief general history is given of the rise of industrial
medicine in the United States. "Curiously enough," women
physicians do very well in this type of work: they adapt
well to the medical-social service-counselor viewpoint, and
are more businesslike than men physicians.

2501.   "Women Physicians and Public Hygiene." Woman's Med-
            ical Journal, 19:11 (November 1909) 236. (Editorial.)

2502.   "Women Physicians--Public Health Boards." Woman's Med-
            ical Journal, 9:8 (August 1899) 283-284.
More women physicians should serve on public health boards.
A woman is not only naturally neat and clean, but an "energetic women physician could, with her woman's keenness of
vision, see more need for improvement, more filth and
squalor in a moment, than the average man could in a day
...." Furthermore, women would undoubtedly make more
practical, economical suggestions for improvements.

2503.   Woodruff, Kay H. "Equal Opportunities for Women in Path-
            ology." American Journal of Clinical Pathology, 64:2
            (August 1975) 284. (Letters to the Editor.)
A letter from Kay H. Woodruff, M.D., assistant clinical
professor of pathology at the University of California, San
Francisco, complains about the lack of distinguished women pathologists on the boards of pathology, as officers of
societies, chairmen of university departments, and editorial
boards of pathology journals. The editor replies that his
journal will act affirmatively to correct this situation in its
own operations, hopes that others will do likewise, and reminds readers that academic appointments are subject to review under the following antidiscrimination laws: the Civil
Rights Act of 1964 Equal Employment Opportunities Commission, the Equal Pay Act of 1963, the Age Discrimination in Employment Act of 1967, Executive Order 11246,
Office of Federal Contract Compliance, title IX of the education amendments of 1972, and titles VII and VIII of the
Public Health Service Act.

2504.   Woodruff, Kay H. "Women in Academic Pathology." Hu-
            man Pathology, 6:5 (September 1975) 640. (Letters to
            the Editor.)
The lack of women in the decision-making levels of pathology such as academic and policy making positions, editor-
ships and memberships of the editorial board of the major
journals, is a real pathological condition.

MISSIONARY ACTIVITY

Along with material on missionary organizations, this section contains material which
focuses on the missionary work of individual
physicians

AFRICA

2505. Breeze, Gabrielle. "Women's Medical Mission and Hospital, Tangier." Double Cross and Medical Missionary Record, 12:1 (January 1897) 21-23.
Dr. Breeze describes her hospital and the types of medical cases she treats.

2506. Cushman, Mary Floyd. Missionary Doctor: The Story of Twenty Years in Africa. Harper & Brothers, New York, New York, 1944, viii, 279 pp. photos., ports.
Mary Floyd Cushman became a missionary doctor at the age of 52. She was sent to Ocileso, Angola in 1922 by the American Board of Foreign Missions. During her 20 years of service, she opened a hospital and trained many native paramedicals. This autobiography recalls highlights of her practice in Angola and includes photographs of the Ocileso mission, its staff, and many patients.

2507. Cuthbert, Sister M. "Sister--Doctor--Missionary--to South Africa." Medical Missionary, 31:1 (January-February 1957) 28-29.
[Article not examined by editors.]

2508. "'Left Alone.'" Medical Missionary Record, 7:7 (July 1892) 151.
Dr. Alice Harris, a graduate of the Homeopathic Medical College of Cleveland, first studied medicine for the purpose of knowing how to care for herself as a missionary. She now works in Sierra Leone, West Africa.

2509. Taylor, William. "A Heroine's Resting Place: Mary Myers Davenport, M.D." Medical Missionary Record, 5:5 (May 1890) 101-102.
Bishop Taylor recounts Dr. Davenport's decision to become a missionary and her consequent medical work in Africa.

ASIA

2510. Allen, Belle Jane. "The Preparation of Women for Medical Mission Service and How It Should Be Differentiated if at All, from That of Men." Woman's Medical Journal, 26:8 (August 1916) 194-196.
In this article [reprinted from American Medicine, May 1916], Dr. Allen concludes that differentiation must exist, "not in preparation so much as in practice," and illustrates the necessity for medical care for women by women in the Occident as well as the Orient. Dr. Allen outlines in detail

582

the preparation needed for effective missionary service and
reminds readers that the medical missionary "has no time
to fight for her rights as a woman nor gesticulate wildly
for political or any other power but that power of Christ-
like service...."

2511.   Angela, Sister M. "Doctor's Dream." Medical Missionary,
             37:4 (July-August 1963) 100-104. photos.
         Sister Angela recounts Mother M. Benedict's efforts as
         chief medical officer and surgeon in St. Michael's Hospital,
         Mymensingh, East Pakistan.

2512.   Benedict, Sister M. "Surgeon for Six Million." Medical
             Missionary, 24:6 (November-December 1950) 100-102.
             illus.
         Sister Benedict describes her medical work as a physician
         at St. Michael's Hospital, "the only place in the Mymen-
         singh district [a community of six million people in East
         Pakistan] where surgery is available."

2513.   Benedict, Sister M. "Surgeon in East Pakistan." Medical
             Missionary, 30:2 (March-April 1956) 40-43. photos.

2514.   Buckley, Olive B. "Life in Papua." Medical Woman's
             Journal, 56:10 (October 1949) 45-46. (Letters to the
             Editor.)
         Dr. Buckley tells of the life and customs of natives on the
         northeast coast of New Guinea and the medical cases she
         treats at the Anglican Mission dispensary in Dewade, Papua.

2515.   Carr, J. Walter. "Who Will Go?" Medical Women's Fed-
             eration News-Letter, (March 1925) 39-40.
         A call is issued to qualified medical women to consider
         serving as medical missionaries in needy hospitals in the
         Far East. Interested parties are urged to write to the
         Zenana Bible and Medical Mission.

2516.   "Catholic Medical Mission Sisters." Medical Woman's Jour-
             nal, 57:6 (June 1950) 29-30. (News Notes.)
         One of the projects of the Roman Catholic Order's Medical
         Mission Sisters, founded by Mother Anna Dengel, M.D.,
         was establishing the Holy Family Hospital in Rawalpindi,
         Pakistan; construction was completed on March 25th, 1950,
         after much adversity.

2517.   Christian Medical Service in India, Burma and Ceylon.
             "Women's Hospitals." In: Tales From the Inns of
             Healing of Christian Medical Service in India, Burma
             and Ceylon. Christian Medical Association of India,
             Burma and Ceylon, Wesley Press and Publishing House,
             Mysore City, India, 1942, 30-47. photos.
         This brief history of women's health care and women's hos-
         pitals that foreign women missionaries established in India
         includes description of the variety of medical cases treated.

2518.   Cote, Marie M.   "Heathen Medicine."   Medical Mission-
        ary Record, 4:3 (July 1889) 71.
        In writing of her work in Rangoon, Burmah [sic], Dr. Cote
        notes that she is the only woman doctor in the area and
        wishes she had a female companion.

2519.   "Dr. Anna Barbara Grey in Burma and India."   Medical
        Woman's Journal, 49:9 (September 1942) 292-294.
        Dr. Anna Barbara Grey describes her experiences in Burma
        during the World War II Japanese offensive, and her subse-
        quent flight to India.   She headed the Ellen Mitchell Memo-
        rial Hospital in Moulmein, Burma until it was bombed by
        the Japanese.

2520.   "Dr. Lillias Horton, of Korea."   Medical Missionary Rec-
        ord, 3:12 (April 1889) 285.

2521.   "Dr. Mary E. Bradford, the Heroine of Tabriz."   Medical
        Missionary Record, 8:2 (February 1893) 28-29.
        Dr. Bradford (whose portrait appears on page 26 of this
        issue) deserves praise for her work during a cholera epi-
        demic in Tabriz, where she has been stationed for five
        years.

2522.   Dowkonitt, Mrs. George D.   "Woman's Need and Woman's
        Work."   Medical Missionary Record, 4:7 (November
        1889) 157-160.
        This article paints a picture of death and suffering in Asia
        and Africa before missionaries brought medical advances.
        A contrast is drawn between these former times and the
        present situation.

2523.   Eddy, Mary Pierson.   "Medical Work in Syria and America
        Contrasted."   Double Cross and Medical Missionary
        Record, 11:12 (December 1896) 253-255.
        Dr. Eddy tells of her encounters with robbers, lepers, and
        patients who pay for her services with hedgehogs and fos-
        sils, and of her opportunity to "freely preach Christ to per-
        ishing souls" in Syria.

2524.   Eddy, Mary Pierson.   "Notes from the Diary of a Medical
        Missionary."   Double Cross and Medical Missionary
        Record, 12:2 (February 1897) 33-34.
        Dr. Eddy describes a few episodes of her life in Beirut,
        Syria.

2525.   Ernst, Alice L.   "My Patients Block the Road."   Medical
        Missionary Record, 8:10 (October 1893) 229-230.   (Wo-
        man's Needs and Woman's Works.)
        Dr. Ernst treats so many patients in her missionary work
        with the Mohammedans, that they sometimes block the road
        to her house, waiting to see her.   This article relates one
        of the many incidents which happen to her in connection with
        her work.

2526.   Grace, Sr. M. "Is There a Doctor on Board?" Medical
             Missionary, 28:5 (September-October 1954) 226-228.
             photo.
         Sister M. Grace describes her experiences in Beirut, Alex-
         andria, Jeddah, and Djibouti, where she saw and treated
         many medical cases.

2527.   Gracey, Mrs. J. T. Medical Work of the Woman's Foreign
             Missionary Society: Methodist Episcopal Church. A. O.
             Bunnell, Printer, Dansville, New York, 1881, 191 pp.
             illus.
         This book gives an account of the first decade (1870-80) of
         medical missionary work in India and China sponsored by
         the Woman's Foreign Missionary Society of the Methodist
         Episcopal Church in the U.S. This society sent the first
         women physicians to both countries, beginning with Clara
         Swain who went to India in 1870. Brief summaries are
         given of the work of Clara Swain, Nancy Monelle, Julia
         Lore, Lucilla Green (Cheney), and Henrietta Woolston in
         India, and of Lucinda Combs, Sigourney Trask, Letitia
         Mason, Leonora Howard, Julia Span, and Kate Bushnell in
         China.

2528.   Hall, Rosetta Sherwood. "Foreign Medical Women in Ko-
             rea." Journal of the American Medical Women's Asso-
             ciation, 5:10 (October 1950) 404-405.
         Dr. Meta Howard went to Korea in 1887 and under her di-
         rection, the first women's hospital in Korea was inaugurated,
         the Po Ku Nyo Kwan or "Caring for and Saving Women's
         Hospital." After Dr. Howard returned to the U.S., Dr.
         Lillias Horton was sent out to Korea and became the phy-
         sician to Queen Min. Several other women physicians who
         practiced in Korea are discussed.

2529.   Hall, Rosetta Sherwood. "Woman's Medical Mission Work
             in Korea." Medical Missionary Record, 8:5 (May
             1893) 111-114. (Woman's Needs and Woman's Works.)
         Dr. Hall refers to social customs and the "awful practices
         pursued by the native doctor" in this report of her work
         among "the poor suffering bodies and sin-sick souls" of
         Korea.

2530.   Howard, Meta. "A Woman's Medical Mission for Korea."
             Medical Missionary Record, 6:4 (April 1891) 91-92.

2531.   Hurd-Mead, Kate Campbell. "Women in Medical Missions
             in Foreign Lands." Medical Review of Reviews, 41:7
             (July 1935) 348-361.
         Following a discussion of mission work in general and its
         history in India, Dr. Hurd-Mead follows the history of med-
         ical missionaries through the personalities of the women
         who chose this field. The second half of the article deals
         with medical missionaries in China, listing names and ac-

complishments of several women physicians. The organization of institutes to prepare physicians for the mission
fields is also discussed.

2532.   Millican, Edith F. "Medical Women in Foreign Missions."
         Journal of the American Medical Women's Association,
         6:12 (December 1951) 478-480. port.
         The author begins her account with Dr. Clara Swain, the
         first woman medical missionary in the world, and touches
         upon the work in China of both Drs. Eleanor Chestnut and
         Mary Fulton.

2533.   Scharlieb, Mary. "The Health of Married Women Mis-
             sionaries." China Medical Journal (Shanghai), 29
             (1915) 385-393.
         [Article not examined by editors.]

2534.   Selmon, Bertha. "Medical Opportunity for Women Spreads
             Abroad (Continued)." Medical Woman's Journal, 54:5
             (May 1947) 40-42. photos., ports. (History of Wo-
             men in Medicine.)
         This article continues the discussion of specific medical
         missionaries in China and India. Quotes from the writings
         of J. T. Gracey and Frances J. Baker support the article.

2535.   Selmon, Bertha. "Pioneer Women in Medicine: Early Ser-
             vice in Missions (Continued)." Medical Woman's Jour-
             nal, 54:7 (July 1947) 46, 48-52. ports. (History of
             Women in Medicine.)
         This article continues the installments on medical mission-
         ary work from 1885 to 1890. The profiles of individual wo-
         men are taken from the works of J. T. Gracey and Fran-
         ces J. Baker on medical missionary work outside the
         United States.

2536.   Selmon, Bertha. "Women in Medicine Early Service in
             Missions (Continued)." Medical Woman's Journal, 54:
             8 (August 1947) 43-46. photo., port. (History of Wo-
             men in Medicine.)
         Dr. Selmon picks up the thread of this series of articles
         on medical missionaries in 1891 with an account of the
         work of Dr. M. Ida Stevenson. Profiles of women appear-
         ing in this article are taken from publications on medical
         missionary work outside the U.S., written by J. T. Gracey
         and Frances J. Baker.

2537.   Selmon, Bertha. "Women in Medicine Early Service in
             Missions (Continued)." Medical Woman's Journal, 54:
             9 (September 1947) 40-44, [64]. photo., ports. (His-
             tory of Women in Medicine.)
         Continuing with this series of articles on medical mission-
         aries, Dr. Selmon profiles women in mission work from
         1894 to 1900. Information on these women is quoted from

the publication of J. T. Gracey and Frances J. Baker on medical missionary work outside the U.S.

2538.   Sharp, Helen Carmeleta. "Careers in Medical Missionary Work." Journal of the American Medical Women's Association, 24:12 (December 1969) 979-980.
The author illustrates the life of a foreign medical missionary through relating incidents from her own experience in Pakistan. A biographical inset on the author is included.

2539.   "Womans' [sic] Work and Worth in Medical Missions." Medical Missionary Record, 5:7 (July 1890) 147-149.
Testimony is given to the work of Christian women physicians in India and China.

CHINA

2540.   Brown, Mary. "'The Only Thing That Reminds One of the Home Land.'" Medical Missionary Record, 9:4 (April 1894) 75.
Dr. Brown writes about her mission in Wei Hien, China, where telegraph posts are the only local features that remind her of home.

2541.   Cunningham, Gladys Story. "Medical Women in West China." Journal of the American Medical Women's Association, 1:6 (September 1946) 188-192. photo., port.
This article describes medical training and practice in Chengtu, Szechuan, China by American medical women missionaries who opened a hospital for women and children there in 1896. Because there were not enough foreign personnel, these women opened a nurses' training school in 1902 to train women who were willing to become nurses which was considered to be "a degrading and humiliating task" at that time. "Since 1933 no male nurses have been trained in Chengtu. Women nurse men, women and children." In 1912, The West China Union University in Chengtu was opened, and a Faculty of Medicine and Dentistry opened soon after: Chinese doctors and dentists were trained there. The first woman to be graduated from there was Dr. Helen Yoh in 1930 who specialized in obstetrics and gynecology. When Japan attacked China in 1937, many hardships were endured: inflation, shortage of supplies, inadequate hospital conditions, fire, air raids, etc.

2542.   "Englishwomen as Doctors in China." British Medical Journal, 1 (1880) 983.
[Article not examined by editors.]

2543.   Fielde, Adele M. "Medical Missionary Ladies in China." Medical Missionary Record, 1:1 (May 1886) 15-16.

(The Ladies' Department.)
The work of several American women physicians is mentioned.

2544.   Hemenway, Ruth. "Dawn Brings New Courage." Medical
         Woman's Journal, 53:6 (June 1946) 59-60.
         Subheaded "Two Blue-Eyed Children," this article [one in
         a series by Ruth Hemenway on her experiences as a phy-
         sician in China] supplies description of a visit from "Mr.
         Stockwell" and his family.

2545.   Hemenway, Ruth. "Dawn Brings New Courage." Medical
         Woman's Journal, 53:7 (July 1946) 64-65.
         In this article [one in a series by Ruth Hemenway on her
         experiences as a physician in China], Dr. Hemenway writes
         of her desire to develop preventive medicine throughout the
         country.   In 1932 she assembled a staff capable of such
         work and began a health program which illustrated health
         topics through skits, songs, lectures, and charts.

2546.   Hemenway, Ruth. "Dawn Brings New Courage." Medical
         Woman's Journal, 53:8 (August 1946) 55-58.
         Anecdotes of medical cases make up the major portion of
         this installment [one in a series of articles by Ruth Hemen-
         way on her experiences as a physician in China].

2547.   Hemenway, Ruth. "Dawn Brings New Courage." Medical
         Woman's Journal, 53:9 (September 1946) 52-55, 66.
         In addition to describing several patients and their physical
         problems, Dr. Hemenway writes of her personal spiritual
         struggle in this installment [one in a series of articles by
         Ruth Hemenway on her experiences as a physician in China].

2548.   Hemenway, Ruth. "Dawn Brings New Courage." Medical
         Woman's Journal, 53:10 (October 1946) 56-57.
         Dr. Hemenway tells of her treatment of lepers in this in-
         stallment [one in a series of articles by Ruth Hemenway on
         her experiences as a physician in China].

2549.   Hemenway, Ruth. "Dawn Brings New Courage." Medical
         Woman's Journal, 53:11 (November 1946) 54-55.
         The summer "medley of dysentery, abscesses, tumors, in-
         juries, new babies, tragedies and humorous episodes" is
         described in this brief article [one in a series of articles
         by Ruth Hemenway on her experiences as a physician in
         China].

2550.   Hemenway, Ruth. "Dawn Brings New Courage." Medical
         Woman's Journal, 53:12 (December 1946) 66-68, 70.
         The author recalls malaria cases in this installment [one
         in a series of articles by Ruth Hemenway on her experi-
         ences as a physician in China].

2551. Hemenway, Ruth. "Dawn Brings New Courage." Medical
            Woman's Journal, 54:1 (January 1947) 54, 56, 58.
       This article [one in a series of articles by Ruth Hemenway
       on her experiences as a physician in China] consists in
       journal-style entries in which Dr. Hemenway describes the
       acceptance by a Chinese man of his child's death, a case
       of smallpox, and the birth of a baby.

2552. Hemenway, Ruth. "Dawn Brings New Courage." Medical
            Woman's Journal, 54:2 (February 1947) 54-56.
       A description of Nanchang constitutes this article [one in a
       series of articles by Ruth Hemenway on her experiences as
       a physician in China]. Foot-binding is also discussed.

2553. Hemenway, Ruth. "Dawn Brings New Courage." Medical
            Woman's Journal, 54:3 (March 1947) 60-61, 63.
       In this installment [one in a series of articles by Ruth
       Hemenway on her experiences as a physician in China] Liu
       Tai Ching, the new social worker at Mintsing hospital, is
       introduced.

2554. Hemenway, Ruth. "Dawn Brings New Courage." Medical
            Woman's Journal, 54:5 (May 1947) 54-56, 61.
       A uterine inversion repair and the removal of a 40-pound
       tumor are among the operations discussed in this article
       [one in a series of articles by Ruth Hemenway on her ex-
       periences as a physician in China].

2555. Hemenway, Ruth. "Dawn Brings New Courage." Medical
            Woman's Journal, 54:7 (July 1947) 60, 62, 64.
       In this article [one in a series of articles by Ruth Hemen-
       way on her experiences as a physician in China] Dr. Hemen-
       way describes casualties of a storm which killed many peo-
       ple in the village. The opening of a dispensary in the vil-
       lage of South Den (near Nanchang) is also covered, as well
       as events of the Christmas of 1936.

2556. Hemenway, Ruth. "Dawn Brings New Courage." Medical
            Woman's Journal, 54:8 (August 1947) 52-55.
       Medicine in Nanchang, a medical conference in Shanghai,
       and various incidents of everyday life as a woman physician
       in China constitute this article [one in a series of articles
       by Ruth Hemenway on her experiences as physician in
       China].

2557. Hemenway, Ruth. "Dawn Brings New Courage." Medical
            Woman's Journal, 54:9 (September 1947) 52, 54-56.
       War has begun--Dr. Hemenway's year in Nanchang is over
       and she prepares to leave for Kuliang where she will study
       until she receives orders to leave. The excitement and
       fear of being in a country at war is captured as Dr. Hemen-
       way recounts her preparation to leave and actual trip out of
       Nanchang.

2558.   Hemenway, Ruth. "Dawn Brings New Courage." Medical
                Woman's Journal, 54:10 (October 1947) 60-61.
           Individual obstetrical cases Dr. Hemenway dealt with in
           Chungking at the Syracuse-in-China Hospital are presented
           in this article [one in a series of articles by Ruth Hemen-
           way on her experiences as a physician in China].

2559.   Hemenway, Ruth. "Dawn Brings New Courage." Medical
                Woman's Journal, 54:11 (November 1947) 50-51, 62.
           Experiences with various people during her work in Chung-
           king constitute this article [one in a series of articles by
           Ruth Hemenway on her experiences as a physician in China].

2560.   Hemenway, Ruth. "Dawn Brings New Courage." Medical
                Woman's Journal, 54:12 (December 1947) 52-55.
           Dualism, Yin and Yang, and Shang Ti are subjects of this
           article.   Interesting obstetrical cases seen by Dr. Hemen-
           way while she worked in Chungking are also discussed in
           the article [one in a series of articles by Ruth Hemenway
           on her experiences as a physician in China].

2561.   Hemenway, Ruth. "Dawn Brings New Courage." Medical
                Woman's Journal, 55:2 (February 1948) 46-48, 67.
           The horrors of the Japanese invasion are described in this
           article [one in a series of articles by Ruth Hemenway on
           her experiences as a physician in China].

2562.   Hemenway, Ruth V. "Dawn Brings New Courage." Med-
                ical Woman's Journal, 55:9 (September 1948) 49-54.
           Medical cases and procedures are detailed in this install-
           ment [one in a series of articles by Ruth Hemenway on her
           experiences as a physician in China].

2563.   Hemenway, Ruth. "Dawn Brings New Courage (In China--
                The Story of a Medical Missionary)." Medical Woman's
                Journal, 52:6 (June 1945) 43-48.
           This article [one in a series of articles by Ruth Hemenway
           on her experiences as a physician in China] covers various
           incidents in the everyday life of a medical missionary in
           China.   Various Chinese customs are also explained.

2564.   Hemenway, Ruth. "Dawn Brings New Courage (In China--
                The Story of a Medical Missionary)." Medical Woman's
                Journal, 52:7 (July 1945) 51-53.
           The Chinese New Year festivities are described in detail in
           this installment [one in a series of articles by Ruth Hemen-
           way on her experiences as a physician in China].

2565.   Hemenway, Ruth. "Dawn Brings New Courage (In China--
                The Story of a Medical Missionary)." Medical Woman's
                Journal, 52:8 (August 1945) 45-50. photo.
           A description of the countryside over which Dr. Hemenway
           travels on her way to the clinic constitutes the first portion

of this article. Experiences at the clinic and patients to
whom she ministered comprise the remainder of the article
[one in a series of articles by Ruth Hemenway on her experiences as a physician in China].

2566. Hemenway, Ruth. "Dawn Brings New Courage (In China--
        The Story of a Medical Missionary)." Medical Woman's
        Journal, 52:9 (September 1945) 49-51.
In this installment [one in a series of articles by Ruth
Hemenway on her experiences as a physician in China] Dr.
Hemenway relates the adventure of her trip to Kuliang dur-
ing a period of anti-foreign demonstrations in Foochow.
Medical experiences are interspersed throughout the article.

2567. Hemenway, Ruth. "Dawn Brings New Courage (In China--
        The Story of a Medical Missionary)." Medical Woman's
        Journal, 52:10 (October 1945) 47-49, 51.
This article [one in a series of articles by Ruth Hemenway
on her experiences as a physician in China] gives insight
into the social customs of China and how they are changing.
Dr. Hemenway also expresses her vague feeling of dissatis-
faction with her life: "I began to realize more and more
clearly that one's goal in life and one's security must some-
how be based on something more than work, something
more than a child."

2568. Hemenway, Ruth. "Dawn Brings New Courage (In China--
        The Story of a Medical Missionary)." Medical Woman's
        Journal, 52:11 (November 1945) 52-54.
This installment [one in a series of articles by Ruth Hemen-
way on her experiences as a physician in China] covers Dr.
Hemenway's trip to the northern part of Mintsing County.
The patients seen along the route are recalled.

2569. Hemenway, Ruth. "Dawn Brings New Courage (In China--
        The Story of a Medical Missionary)." Medical Woman's
        Journal, 52:12 (December 1945) 50-53.
A variety of medical cases seen by Dr. Hemenway are de-
scribed in this article [one in a series of articles by Ruth
Hemenway on her experiences as a physician in China].

2570. Hemenway, Ruth. "Dawn Brings New Courage (In China--
        The Story of a Medical Missionary)." Medical Woman's
        Journal, 53:1 (January 1946) 49-50.
In this installment [one in a series of articles by Ruth
Hemenway on her experiences as a physician in China], Dr.
Hemenway describes how she took a Chinese girl baby from
its parents, who had offered it for adoption. Although the
mother wept as the child was carried away, Dr. Hemenway
told herself, "She can get another if she really wants one."
Dr. Hemenway's adopted daughter was renamed Huia Sing--
Star of China.

2571.   Hemenway, Ruth.   "Dawn Brings New Courage (In China--
              The Story of a Medical Missionary)."   Medical Woman's
              Journal, 53:2 (February 1946) 60, 62.
          An adventure with bandits is recalled in this article [one
          in a series by Ruth Hemenway on her experiences as a
          physician in China].

2572.   Hemenway, Ruth.   "Dawn Brings New Courage (In China--
              The Story of a Medical Missionary."   Medical Woman's
              Journal, 53:3 (March 1946) 51-54.
          More adventures with bandits and a few interesting medical
          cases are described in this installment [one in a series of
          articles by Ruth Hemenway on her experiences as a phy-
          sician in China].

2573.   Hemenway, Ruth.   "Dawn Brings New Courage (In China--
              The Story of a Medical Missionary)."   Medical Woman's
              Journal, 53:4 (April 1946) 54-57, 70.
          In this installment [one in a series of articles by Ruth
          Hemenway on her experiences as a physician in China],
          bandit raids and the resulting injuries to the village in-
          habitants are described.

2574.   Hemenway, Ruth.   "Dawn Brings New Courage (In China--
              The Story of a Medical Missionary)."   Medical Woman's
              Journal, 53:5 (May 1946) 57-60.
          More atrocities committed by bandits are the subject of
          this installment [one in a series of articles by Ruth Hemen-
          way on her experiences as a physician in China].

2575.   Hemenway, Ruth.   "In China ... (The Story of a Medical
              Missionary)."   Medical Woman's Journal, 52:2 (Febru-
              ary 1945) 34-38, 40.
          This first installment in a series of articles by Ruth Hem-
          enway on her experiences as a physician in China describes
          her return to Foochow, China, in 1927 and the experiences
          with bandits at the Mintsing hospital, where she worked.
          Women's place and the traditions of China are discussed.
          In addition, the types of patients seen at the hospital are
          reviewed in anecdotes.

2576.   Hemenway, Ruth.   "'In China' ... (The Story of a Medical
              Missionary)."   Medical Woman's Journal, 52:3 (March
              1945) 45-49, 52.
          This article [one in a series of articles by Ruth Hemenway
          on her experiences as a physician in China] begins by re-
          viewing Dr. Hemenway's efforts to learn the Chinese lan-
          guage.   The march of the northern troops through the vil-
          lage and incidents of life at the Mintsing Hospital are dis-
          cussed.

2577.   Hemenway, Ruth.   "'In China' ... (The Story of a Medical
              Missionary)."   Medical Woman's Journal, 52:4 (April

1945) 43-47.
Common diseases among Chinese people in Fukien Province
is the topic of this installment [in a series of articles by
Ruth Hemenway on her experiences as a physician in China].

2578.   Hemenway, Ruth. "'In China' ... (The Story of a Medical
             Missionary)." Medical Woman's Journal, 52:5 (May
             1945) 47-51.
         This article [one in a series of articles by Ruth Hemenway
         on her experiences as a physician in China] relates an
         evening of medical care of severely ill patients and a
         Chinese wedding ceremony.

2579.   Hemenway, Ruth V. "Medicine in China." Medical Wo-
             man's Journal, 56:3 (March 1949) 49-51.
         Dr. Hemenway relates her experiences as the administrator
         of a small hospital in Tzechow, China.

2580.   Killain, Maud. "'It Is Such a Privilege.'" Double Cross
             and Medical Missionary Record, 14 (September 1899)
             145-146.
         Dr. Maud Killain, serving under the Canadian Methodist
         Board, writes of her work in Chentu, China.

2581.   Kittredge, Elizabeth. "News of Medical Women." Journal
             of the American Medical Women's Association, 2:5
             (May 1947) 270-271. port.
         Dr. Mary Latimer James went to China first under an ap-
         pointment from the Chinese government as Staff Physician
         in Pei-Yang Woman's Hospital in Tientsin in 1912. She
         then found it easy to become appointed a medical mission-
         ary (her life-long dream). Her work in China is briefly
         reviewed.

2582.   "Medical Missionary Work in China." British Medical
             Journal, 2 (1878) 228.
         [Article not examined by editors.]

2583.   "Medical Work for Women in Foochow." Medical Mission-
             ary Record, 6:7 (July 1891) 161.
         Dr. Kate C. Woodhull, who has been in Foochow, China
         for five years, built a hospital there.

2584.   Murdoch, Virginia C. "'The Best Way of Reaching the
             People.'" Medical Missionary Record, 8:12 (Decem-
             ber 1893) 278-279.
         Dr. Murdoch tells of work near Peking.

2585.   Niles, Mary W. "The Handmaid of Missions." Medical
             Missionary Record, 7:10 (October 1892) 222-224.
         Dr. Niles takes an informal look at the medical education
         of Chinese women and relates a few of her experiences in
         and near Canton, China.

2586.   Niles, Mary W. "What One Noble Woman Is Doing." Med-
              ical Missionary Record, 7:7 (July 1892) 157.
         Dr. Niles writes about her life as a physician and a mis-
         sionary in Canton, China.

2587.   Rankin, Hattie Love. I Saw It Happen to China: 1913-
              1949. J. Horace McFarland Company, Harrisburg,
              Pennsylvania, 1960, vii, 235 pp. map, photos., ports.
         This book presents the diary of Hattie Love Rankin, which
         covers her 36 eventful years as a physician-missionary in
         China. A 1911 graduate of Woman's Medical College of
         Pennsylvania, Dr. Rankin joined the Methodist Church's
         missionary program in 1913. She served on the staffs of
         the Woman's Medical School and Hospital (Soochow) and the
         Mission Hospital (Changchow), and supervised the Margaret
         Williamson Hospital (Shanghai). Following marriage to a
         lawyer-turned-missionary, she established a clinic in Chen-
         ju, and later, a hospital in Shanghai. Dr. Rankin describes
         her difficulties in learning the Chinese language and cus-
         toms and in combatting "ignorance and malpractice." She
         details her harrowing 30-month stay in a Japanese concen-
         tration camp. While much attention is devoted to the so-
         cial status of women, a major portion of the book explores
         political events and the philosophies of Sun Yat-sen, Chiang
         Kai-shek, and Mao Tse-Tung. Dr. Rankin expresses bit-
         terness towards communism (especially its atheistic aspect).
         Eventually, she tired of fighting against it. Shortly before
         fleeing China, Dr. Rankin wrote, "Today I am sixty-five
         years old, just a plain, old, good-for-nothing, kau-feh-zu
         (unreliable), worn-out missionary." She concludes the book
         with a warning to Americans who are apathetic about com-
         munism. The book contains a biographical foreword by
         Dr. Rankin's nephew.

2588.   "Reports of Medical Missionary Ladies in China." Chinese
              Recorder, 17 (1886) 16-23.
         [Article not examined by editors.]

2589.   Selmon, Bertha L. They Do Meet; Cross-Trails of Amer-
              ican Physicians and Chinese People. Froben Press,
              New York, New York, 1942, xvii, 254 pp. facsims.,
              photos., ports.
         Dr. Selmon tells of her experiences, beginning in 1903, as
         a missionary physician in China. Even though her work
         seems to take second place to her missionary-husband's in
         the discussion, the book describes how she developed a suc-
         cessful clinic for women in a time when one foreigner of
         their acquaintance was stoned by a mob. She developed her
         own "Chinese" proverb for courage: "Within the circle of
         the four seas all are brethren." Kate Campbell Hurd-Mead
         wrote the foreword to this book.

2590.   Sugden, Louisa Grace. "Medical Mission Work--By Women

Amongst Women." Medical Missionary Record, 9:12
(December 1894) 255-257.
The author speaks of the need for women medical mission-
aries in China.

2591.   Sydenstricker, (Mrs.). "Medical Lady Missionaries."
Medical Missionary Record, 3:6 (October 1888) 156.
Medical lady missionaries are needed in China for "relieving and enlightening the blind, satan bound souls among
our own sex," writes Mrs. Sydenstricker.

2592.   Van Hoosen, Bertha. "A Lay Contributor to the History
of Women in Medicine." Medical Woman's Journal,
37:3 (March 1930) 61-63.   photo.
An evangelist, Howe Kai Po went to China as a young girl
to serve in Nanchang. Miss Howe adopted Ida Kahn when
she was a baby and saw to it that she received a medical
education. She sent her to the University of Michigan with
the daughter of a Chinese Christian missionary, Mary Stone.
The two women were the first women to be given diplomas
at the Medical Department there and the second two to practice in China. With Dr. Hoag, Dr. Kahn, and Dr. Mary
Stone, Miss Howe founded 4 hospitals staffed with Chinese
women doctors and nurses.

2593.   Young, T. K. "Women Medical Missionaries." American
Journal of Psychiatry, 131:3 (March 1974) 328. (Letters to the Editor.)
Contrary to the belief that women have been "left out of
medicine's hall of fame," women medical missionaries were
doing responsible work in foreign lands. Dr. Young cites
the examples of several medical missionaries, including Dr.
Lucinda Combs, whom he calls the first woman medical
missionary.

INDIA

2594.   Allen, Maud. "A Lady Doctor's Experience in India."
Double Cross and Medical Missionary Record, 11:11
(November 1896) 233-234.
Dr. Allen offers, in journal form, examples of her daily
work at a dispensary.

2595.   "Association of Medical Women in India: Constitution."
Journal of the Association of Medical Women in India,
37:3 (November 1949) 61-64.
[Article not examined by editors.]

2596.   Baksh, Ilahi. "Medical Women Needed in India." Woman's
Medical Journal, 20:5 (May 1910) 109.

2597.   Brown, Edith M. "Making Doctors of India's Daughters."

Medical Woman's Journal, 36:12 (December 1929) 328-329.

Dr. Brown relates how she came to the conclusion, through her work as a medical missionary in India, that a school should be started to train Indian women to be doctors and nurses. The Medical School for Indian Girls was open in 1894 in Ludhiana, Punjab. The author describes the realization of this school and a consequent hospital.

2598.   Brown, Edith M. "Medical Training for Women in India." Double Cross and Medical Missionary Record, 11:5 (May 1896) 97-100.

This article [apparently reprinted from The Missionary Review] reviews the results of a conference of women medical missionaries, held in Ludhiana, in 1893. It was proposed that a nondenominational Christian medical school for Eurasian and native Christian girls be established. It was felt that such a school was needed because medical missionaries are among the most useful agents in the evangelization of a country. A sexually segregated school is necessary because at a young age, association with male students presents moral dangers. Propositions for the establishment of the school are summarized.

2599.   Carr, J. Walter and Warren, Elsie. "Women Medical Missionaries for India." British Medical Journal, (17 January 1925) 144. (Letters, Notes, Etc.)

In a letter, Dr. Carr laments that mission hospitals in India are being closed because no women doctors can be found to staff them. This development causes surprise, considering the fact that one of the chief appeals for training early medical women was that they could render service to women in the East. Dr. Carr urges women to carry out their responsibilities to the millions "we [the British] have been called to rule" and remember that "our Empire in the East will last only so long as we use it...." Appended to Dr. Carr's letter is a note by Dr. Elsie Warren, acting medical secretary to the Zenana Bible and Medical Mission, apologizing for the inadequate salaries given medical missionaries; she further tells women how to apply for mission work.

2600.   Condict, Alice B. "Dr. Alice Condict in Bombay." Medical Missionary Record, 2:6 (October 1887) 147.

2601.   Cummings, Emma J. "Enjoying the Pure Delight of Relieving Suffering." Medical Missionary Record, 4:4 (August 1889) 88-89.

Dr. Cummings tells about her day-to-day work as a missionary in Ramapatam, India.

2602.   Cummings, Emma J. "Medical Missions in India." Medical Missionary Record, 4:4 (August 1889) 76-77.

2603.   D. R. L.   "Pundita Ramabai and Medical Work for Wo-
         men."   Medical Missionary Record, 5:10 (October 1890)
         212.
         A socially tinged religious justification for the existence of
         women doctors in India is given.

2604.   Dengel, Anna.   "The Work of Medical Women in India."
         Medical Woman's Journal, 37:5 (May 1930) 132-135.
         ports.
         Because of the purdah system, Indian women in Moham-
         medan and Hindu families could not be seen by any men
         other than their nearest relatives.   While there had been in
         India a hereditary dai (native nurse) class to care for such
         women, the Zenana missionaries, who instructed women
         isolated by the purdah system, felt such care was inade-
         quate because their pupils, young mothers, would die of
         childbirth, and their babies would die of dysentery.   The
         women missionaries often spent their furloughs at home
         learning medical information that would help such women.
         Several women who had received their training as M. D. s
         specifically came to India to practice medicine: Clara
         Swain (the first qualified medical woman missionary from
         the United States), Sarah C. Seward, Sarah Norris, Fanny
         Butler (the first qualified medical woman from England),
         Rose Greenfield, and Elizabeth Bielby.   The first Indian
         woman to study medicine was Anandibai Joshi, who gradu-
         ated from the Woman's Medical College of Pennsylvania in
         1886 but contracted tuberculosis and died in 1887.

2605.   Dengel, Anna.   "The Work of the Medical Mission Sisters
         in India."   Medical Woman's Journal, 49:9 (September
         1942) 263-267.
         Anna Dengel, a native of Austria, took a British medical
         degree in order to go to India to take charge of St. Cath-
         erine's Hospital for Women and Children, Rawalpindi, In-
         dia.   In this reminiscence, Dr. Dengel describes some of
         the diseases she treated in infants and women when they
         came to the hospital dispensary, as well as some of the
         medical problems she encountered when she traveled in In-
         dia.   In 1924, Dr. Dengel went to America and founded The
         Society of Catholic Medical Missionaries which was the first
         Catholic sisterhood to combine the practice of medicine
         with life in a religious community.   This Society was a
         vehicle for American Catholic women to help Indian women
         obtain health care, and to train medical women mission-
         aries.

2606.   "Dr. Margaret McKeelar."   Medical Woman's Journal, 37:
         2 (February 1930) 51.
         A missionary to India for 40 years, Margaret McKeelar
         helped to found a hospital with a contemporary operating
         room in Neemuch.

2607.   "Dr. Mary McGeorge." Medical Missionary Record, 8:3
           (March 1893) 51-52. port.
         A medical missionary to India, Dr. McGeorge (M.D., 1885)
         died in the wreck of the Romania.

2608.   "Dr. Susan Campbell." Medical Woman's Journal, 37:12
           (December 1930) 349.
         In 1894 Susan Campbell went to India as a medical mis-
         sionary. For 35 years she worked in and around Ajmer,
         Rajputana at the Ajmer Women's Hospital, except for two
         years which she spent organizing a tuberculosis sanatorium
         for girls.

2609.   Francis, Sr. M. "Sister Doctor on an Island." Medical
           Missionary, 32:1 (January-February 1958) 22-24. pho-
           tos.
         In 1954, the Medical Mission Society opened the Archbishop
         Attipetty Jubilee Memorial Hospital in Thuruthipuram, South
         India. Here, Sister M. Francis, M.D. is medical director.
         Her work is described herein.

2610.   Frederic, Sr. M. "The Doctor's Diary." Medical Mission-
           ary, 30:4 (July-August 1956) 105-107. photos.
         Sister M. Frederic's diary covers her work as a physician
         in India from June 1955 to March 1956.

2611.   Frederic, Sr. M. "Sister Surgeon in a Village Hospital."
           Medical Missionary, 32:1 (January-February 1958) 16-
           18. photos.
         Sister M. Frederic describes life and work at Holy Family
         Hospital in Mandar, India.

2612.   H. "The Woman's Medical Mission at Allahabad." Med-
           ical Missionary Record, 6:7 (July 1891) 181-182. (Wo-
           man's Needs and Woman's Work.)

2613.   Johnson, Sophie E. "Medical Work in Jhelum and Bhera,
           India." Medical Missionary Record, 9:10 (October
           1894) 220.
         The effects of a devastating flood on Dr. Johnson's work
         is the topic of this report.

2614.   Johnson, Sophie E. "They Came in Crowds." Medical
           Missionary Record, 6:10 (October 1891) 228-230.
           (Woman's Needs and Woman's Work.)
         Dr. Johnson tells of her work in Jhelum and Bhera, India.

2615.   Kugler, A. "Medical Work for Women in India." Mission-
           ary Review of the World, 42 (October 1919) 788-792.
         [Article not examined by editors.]

2616.   Kugler, Anna S. "Medical Work in India." Medical Wo-
           man's Journal, 31:12 (December 1925) 330-331.

Anna S. Kugler reviews the medical work of women medical missionaries in India, including her own in Guntur
where she helped to found a hospital dispensary. Women
who want to receive medical training may attend the Medical College of Madras which was founded in the early
1880s and was helped financially by the Dufferin Fund,
which was started in 1885. In 1918, a Union Medical Missionary School for Women was opened in Vellore, South
India.

2617.   Lamont, Margaret. Catholic Medical Missions and Women
            Doctors. Catholic Truth Society, India, 1949.
        [Item not examined by editors.]

2618.   "Life in an Himalaya Village." Medical Missionary Record,
            3:5 (September 1888) 127. (India.)
        Dr. Jessica Carleton describes her work in Ani, India.

2619.   "Medical Mission Work Among the Telugus." Medical Mis-
            sionary Record, 5:10 (October 1890) 213.
        This reprint from the seventy-sixth annual report of the
        Baptist Missionary Union highlights the work of Dr. Emma
        J. Cummings.

2620.   M'George, Mary. "Our Medical Mission. Ahmedabad."
            Medical Missionary Record, 7:9 (September 1892) 195-
            196. (Woman's Needs and Woman's Works.)

2621.   "Miss Clara Swain, M. D.: The First Woman Medical Mis-
        sionary Sent to the Foreign Field from America."
        Double Cross and Medical Missionary Record, 12:10
        (October 1897) 215.

2622.   Munson, Arley. Jungle Days: Being the Experiences of an
            American Woman Doctor in India. D. Appleton and
        Company, New York, New York, 1913, viii, 298 pp.
        photos., port.
        Dr. Arley Munson spent five years as a medical mission-
        ary in Medak, India. This is an autobiographical reminis-
        cence of her work and travel experiences. It is illustrated
        with many photographs of her staff, patients, and scenes
        representative of India in the early 20th century. There is
        little information with respect to date, her education and
        training, and there is no bibliography or index.

2623.   O'Hara, Margaret. "A Grand Record." Double Cross and
            Medical Missionary Record, 14 (December 1899) 215-
            217.
        Dr. O'Hara writes of her new dispensary and the work she
        performs in Dhar, India.

2624.   Pailthorpe, Mary E. "What Women Are Doing for Women."
            Medical Missionary Record, 4:3 (July 1889) 63-64.

An account of the good work being done in Benares, India by "Dr. Maxwell" is taken from her journal.

2625.   Reardon, Rosalie M. "Dear Colleagues." Medical Woman's
            Journal, 59:1 (January 1952) 48.
         Sister Frances Webster, M.D. writes of her experiences in
         India at the Holy Family Hospital at Mandar.

2626.   Scudder, Dorothy Jealous. A Thousand Years in Thy Sight:
            The Story of the Scudders of India. [Published by the
            author, Shelter Island, New York, 1970], vii, 418 pp.
            chart, maps, photos., port.
         Characterized by "persistent unity of purpose," four genera-
         tions of the Scudder family devoted themselves to medical
         missionary work. This family chronicle begins with the
         pioneer "Dr. John" of 1819, and concludes with his great-
         grandson. Much of this group biography is focused on Ida
         S. Scudder. Born in 1870, Ida grew up under the "ruth-
         less discipline" of five older brothers and the deprivations
         experienced by missionary children. "Dr. Ida" attended
         Woman's Medical College of Pennsylvania for three years
         and graduated from Cornell Medical College in 1898. Al-
         though in love with a young male medical student, she re-
         jected romance in order to "embrace thousands of women
         and children of India." She opened, in 1918, the Vellore
         Medical School. Dr. Ida's niece, Ida Belle Scudder, came
         to work at Vellore in the 1930s. The accomplishments of
         Ida B., a graduate of Woman's Medical College in Phila-
         delphia, are detailed. This book contains several ap-
         pendices, a glossary, a bibliography, and a genealogical
         chart; there is no index.

2627.   Seward, S. C. "Female Medical Missions in India." Med-
            ical Missionary Record, 1:4 (August 1886) 99. (The
            Ladies' Department.)
         Dr. Seward offers statistics from her dispensary report
         and describes how she attempts to provide Christian knowl-
         edge to the Indian female patients. "I sometimes hear it
         asserted that the natives of India do not wish Christianity
         thrust upon them," she writes, but adds that patients show
         an eagerness to learn religious doctrines and that "as phy-
         sicians, we often gain access to those whom no other mis-
         sionary can reach." Dr. Seward further addresses those
         who throw glamour upon the subject of female medical mis-
         sionaries: the actual work "is laborious and wearing, often
         thankless and discouraging, and I sincerely pity those who
         take it up in any spirit of mere enthusiasm or ambition."

2628.   "Sister Alma Lalinsky, M.D." Medical Woman's Journal,
            49:9 (September 1942) 287.
         Alma Lalinsky joined the Society of Catholic Medical Mis-
         sionaries in 1927 and is believed to be the first woman to
         have studied medicine as a member of a religious order.

At the time this article was written, she was the medical
officer in charge of the Society's Holy Family Hospital for
Women and Children in Rawalpindi, India. Her portrait
appears on the front cover of this issue of the Journal.

2629.   Stewart, Eleanor Wolf. "A Day in an India Hospital." In:
        75th Anniversary Volume of the Woman's Medical Col-
        lege of Pennsylvania. Westbrook Publishing Company,
        Philadelphia, Pennsylvania, [1925?], 393-397. port.
        Dr. Stewart's story about a day in the life of a missionary
        physician is apparently based on the experiences of Dr.
        Anna S. Kugler of Guntur, India.

2630.   "The Story of Vellore." Medical Woman's Journal, 49:11
        (November 1942) 352. (News Notes.)
        In this fund-raising appeal for the Medical School for Wo-
        men in Vellore, India (founded in 1918), the history of Dr.
        Ida Scudder's commitment to her vision of medical care for
        Indian women forbidden male contact is reviewed. Working
        with [Lucy Whitehead McGill Waterburg] Peabody [a pioneer
        in ecumenical foreign missions programs], Dr. Scudder
        helped to establish a medical college that would train Indian
        women to become doctors and serve the medical needs of
        women in countries where purdah is custom. Not only did
        they establish a college, but also a hospital which set up
        roadside clinics to which doctors and nurses traveled in
        automobiles.

2631.   Swain, Clara A. A Glimpse of India: Being a Collection
        of Extracts from the Letters of Dr. Clara A. Swain,
        First Medical Missionary to India of the Woman's
        Foreign Missionary Society of the Methodist Episcopal
        Church in America. James Pott and Company, New
        York, New York, 1909, ix, 366 pp. photos., ports.
        These letters from Dr. Swain, medical missionary to In-
        dia, are arranged in three sections covering first her work
        in Bareilly (1870 to 1875), then her service in Khetri (1885
        to 1896), and finally her return to India from America
        (1906 to 1908). Dr. Swain's principal correspondent was
        her sister; many of the names of others to whom the let-
        ters were addressed were deleted in the editing. [Persons
        responsible for the collection, selection, and editing are
        not mentioned in the foreword.]

2632.   "'A Terrible Sight.'" Medical Missionary Record, 7:9
        (September 1892) 197.
        It was "a terrible sight" to see the way women in Kashmir,
        seeking relief from suffering, pressed upon Dr. Fanny But-
        ler's dispensary door. "The evil odours, the heat, the un-
        sanitary conditions" in which Dr. Butler worked contributed
        to her death.

2633.   "Three Noble Women." Double Cross and Medical Mission-

ary Record, 12:7 (July 1897) 147-148.
The lives of medical missionaries Drs. Sophie Johnson,
Mary Platter, and Maria White (whose portraits appear
elsewhere in this issue) are briefly sketched, with emphasis on their spiritual strengths.

2634.   The Union Missionary Medical School for Women: Vellore,
        India.   Insurance Press, Inc., Boston, Massachusetts,
        [n.d.], 19 pp.   photos.
        This pamphlet describes Vellore and the work of Dr. Ida
        Scudder.   It is written by an unnamed woman who travelled
        with another woman and their two daughters (identified only
        as "Wellesley" and "Vassar") to India.   The group visited
        the Mary Taber Schell Hospital in Vellore.   A biography of
        Dr. Scudder is also given in this article.   The booklet ends
        with a section devoted to the "medical needs" which must be
        met in order to carry on the work in Vellore (e.g., X-ray
        equipment, ambulance, doctors, nurses, dormitories), and
        the cost of those necessities.

2635.   Vines, Charlotte S.   A Woman Doctor on the Frontier.
        Church of England Zenana Missionary Society, London,
        England, 1926, 78 pp.
        Dr. Janet M. C. Gray writes of this book: "This little
        book brings back vividly the good times I have had on the
        Frontier and have spent in the Mission Stations at Amrit-
        zar, Dera Ismail Khan, Jhelum, Mardan and Peshawar.
        From what I have seen, known and heard I can testify how
        true to life are these vivid little sketches."   [Book not ex-
        amined by editors.]

2636.   "Well Done!--Noble Women."   Medical Missionary Record,
        4:11 (November 1889) 162.
        Dr. Maria White reports on the building of the Women's
        Memorial Hospital in Sialkot, India and pleads for more
        financial support.   One woman, converted from heathenism,
        is quoted as saying, "'Tell your people how fast we are
        dying, and ask if they cannot send the Gospel a little fast-
        er.'"

2637.   White, Maria.   "Correspondence."   Medical Woman's Jour-
        nal, 37:5 (May 1930) 145-146.   (Letters to the Editor.)
        A medical missionary who went into Punjab, India to open
        a hospital for women and children in 1887, Maria White
        was sponsored by the American United Presbyterian Mis-
        sion.   Before she left the United States, she was the first
        woman doctor admitted to the New York Post Graduate
        School.

2638.   White, Maria.   "A Devoted Lady Doctor."   Medical Mis-
        sionary Record, 5:7 (July 1890) 144-145.
        Dr. White rejoices in the completion of the Memorial Hos-
        pital in Sialkot, India.

2639. White, Maria. "Medical Work Among the Women and Children of India." Double Cross and Medical Missionary
Record, 12:7 (July 1897) 148-151.
Dr. White gives readers "a glimpse into the sorrows of
the heathen women" of Punjab, India, women to whom she
has ministered for eight years. To illustrate the success
of women medical missionaries in India, Dr. White quotes
a "high-caste Hindu" who said that while "we do not fear
the usual method of mission work ... we dread your lady
doctors; they enter our homes, win the hearts of our women, threatening the foundation of our religion."

2640. White, Maria. "Sick Women Coming in Large Numbers."
Medical Missionary Record, 2:11 (March 1889) 269.
Dr. White writes of her medical missionary work in Sialkot,
India.

2641. White, Maria. "A Terrible Effort, but a Sufficient Reward." Double Cross and Medical Missionary Record,
10:7 (July 1895) 146-150.
Dr. White tells of her experiences as a medical missionary in India. She recalls specific medical cases on which
she operated and the many hardships she endured.

2642. White, Martha [sic]. "For the Young." Medical Missionary Record, 3:7 (November 1888) 179-180.
Dr. White, stationed in Sialkot, India, outlines her daily
routine and details an interesting medical case. She urges
Christian children to send contributions towards a hospital
she hopes to build.

2643. Wilson, Dorothy Clarke. Palace of Healing: The Story
of Dr. Clara Swain, First Woman Missionary Doctor,
and the Hospital She Founded. McGraw-Hill Book Company, New York, New York, 1968, x, 245 pp. photos.
Clara Swain went to India as the first woman missionary
doctor in 1869. Strict caste taboos and the seclusion of
women prevented their treatment by male doctors, so there
was a desperate need for women doctors and for training
in medicine for Indian women. Dr. Swain opened the first
women's hospital in India. For nearly 30 years she combined education, evangelism, and medical care for Christian,
Hindu, and Mohammedan women. The hospital at Bareilly,
now called the Clara Swain Hospital, retained its Christian
character and grew under the direction of Drs. Charles and
Wilma Perril, who established a family planning clinic and
began treating male patients in the 1940s. The greatly expanded hospital has continued to play an important role in
Indian health care, with a growing nursing school, innovations in dental care and occupational therapy, and a large
increase in Indian medical personnel in the 1960s.

2644. Wylie, A. M. McElroy. "Women in Medical Missions."

Medical Missionary Record, 6:4 (April 1891) 88-90.
Reverend Wylie praises the delicacy, sympathy, patience,
endurance, and pluck of women medical missionaries in
India.

2645.   Wyne, Sister M. Elise. "Recollections of a Sister Doctor."
         Medical Missionary, 32:1 (January-February 1958) 13-
         15. photos.
         Dr. Wyne (Sister M. Elise) records in this article remi-
         niscences of her 16 years work as a physician in India.
         Primarily working in Rawalpindi and Patna, Dr. Wyne con-
         cludes her recollections with the question: "Now I ask
         you, where in the world would one doctor see so many in-
         teresting patients in such a short time, except in the mis-
         sions?"

INTERNATIONAL

2646.   Butavand, Arlette. [Women Medical Missionaries]. Edi-
         tions de l'Aucam, Louvwain, France, 1933, 142 pp.
         (Fre)
         Based largely on information gathered directly from mis-
         sionary societies and congregations and from the mission-
         aries themselves, this study explains the tasks performed
         by women physicians in missions. The book reviews prob-
         lems of women physicians in Africa, the Islamic countries,
         and in China--where women "find themselves in a pitiable
         material and moral situation," and where the role of the
         woman physician consists in "elevating her mind while tak-
         ing care of her body, and through her, spreading more
         hygiene as well as religion into the population at large."
         The author then reviews the history of women physicians in
         Protestant missions, from Miss Beilby's 1876 dispensary
         in Lucknow through the development of missions in India,
         Turkey, Egypt, and China, to the Scottish mission in Man-
         churia in 1894. The author reports that by 1925, of 1157
         missionary physicians, 356 were women. Detailed reports
         are included from Madura, India and Foumban, Africa. A
         brief history of Catholic missionaries follows, from Saint
         Theodosia and Fabiola to Dr. Agnes McLaren. Hospitals
         run by medical nuns, such as Les Soeurs du Bon Pasteur,
         are listed along with those sponsored by the Society of
         Catholic Medical Missionaries. The book includes a bibli-
         ography as well as statistics on missionary physicians.

2647.   Dengel, Anna. "Medical Mission Sisters." Medical Mis-
         sionary, 31:5 (September-October 1957) 130-131.
         [Article not examined by editors.]

2648.   Dengel, Anna. Mission for Samaritans: A Survey of
         Achievements and Opportunities in the Field of Catholic
         Medical Missions. The Bruce Publishing Company,

Milwaukee, Wisconsin, 1945, 126 pp. photos.
Dr. Dengel's book defines medical missions, sets the historical background, and discusses Catholic medical mission
work in Africa, India, China, the Pacific Islands, Latin
America, and North America. Special attention is given to
work with the American Negro and underprivileged white
groups in the United States. The book concludes with a
bibliography and index.

2649.   Fay, Marion. "Alumnae Serve as Medical Missionaries in
        Many Parts of World." Alumnae News [Woman's Med-
        ical College of Pennsylvania], 26:1 (February 1975) 16-
        17.
        Since 1869, when Clara Swain (newly graduated from the
        Woman's Medical College of Pennsylvania) became the
        world's first woman medical missionary, 230 graduates of
        the College have served as missionaries. Several of the
        women are mentioned and their accomplishments highlighted.

2650.   Ferrier, (Miss). "Female Medical Missions." Medical
        Missionary Record, 7:11 (November 1892) 241-243.
        (Woman's Needs and Woman's Works.)

2651.   Griffith, G. de Gorrequer. "Medical Mission Women."
        Medical Missionary Record, 8:2 (February 1893) 38-
        39.
        This short article in praise of medical women on the mis-
        sion field defends the shortened, more practical curriculum
        at Zenana Medical College on the basis of "the terribly ur-
        gent needs" of so many in Eastern lands.

2652.   Hume, Edward H. Doctors Courageous. Harper & Broth-
        ers, New York, New York, 1950, xiv, 297 pp. maps,
        photos., ports.
        Women physicians take a prominent part in this book, a
        narrative of Christian medical missionaries and the social
        changes that accompany their ministry. Anecdotes dominate
        brief biographies of specific personalities, both foreign and
        native women who converted to Christianity and studied
        "Western" medicine. The book is divided into four parts,
        covering Africa, India and Pakistan, the Near and Middle
        East, and China. Portraits of women are included. There
        is an extensive bibliography as well as an index.

2653.   McLean, Mary H. "Responsibility of Medical Women of
        the United States to Women of Non-Christian Lands,
        and How We Are Meeting It." Woman's Medical Jour-
        nal, 21:11 (November 1911) 245-249. (Presentation,
        Alumnae Association, Woman's Medical College of
        Pennsylvania, 1 June 1911.)
        Because Jesus Christ "died for us ... we medical women
        of the United States have the privileges which we accept to-
        day as our birthright." Under other religions in other

countries, women live in degradation and ignorance, at the mercy of native doctors who--as in China--thrust needles into suffering bodies, and practice other dangerous treat-ments. "We owe it to Jesus Christ ... to pass on to others the blessings we so richly enjoy," says Dr. McLean. In addition to spelling out the dire need for women medical missionaries, she tells of the work of several specific Christian women physicians, many of whom graduated from the Woman's Medical College of Pennsylvania.

2654.   Root, Pauline. "Young Women as Medical Missionaries." Medical Missionary Record, 9:6 (June 1894) 133-134.

2655.   Selmon, Bertha. "Pioneer Women in Medicine: Early Service in Missions." Medical Woman's Journal, 54:4 (April 1947) 51-57. ports. (History of Women in Medicine.)
         Dr. Selmon's discussion of medical missionaries is undergirded with quotes from the works of two authors, J. T. Gracey and Frances J. Baker, who wrote on women physicians' work outside the United States. Several women medical missionaries are mentioned.

2656.   Selmon, Bertha. "Women in Medicine Early Service in Missions (Continued)." Medical Woman's Journal, 54: 6 (June 1947) 44-46, 48-49, 57. photo., port. (History of Women in Medicine.)
         This continuation of the discussion of medical missionaries begins with the women sent out in 1881 and continues through 1884. J. T. Gracey and Frances J. Baker are quoted from their publication on medical missionary work outside the United States.

2657.   "The Training of Women for Medical Mission Work." Double Cross and Medical Missionary Record, 13:6 (June 1898) 92-94.
         [Article not examined by editors.]

UNITED STATES

2658.   Beck, Sister M. Bonaventure. The Society of Catholic Medical Missionaries, Origin and Development. Washington, D.C., 1955.
         [Item not examined by editors.]

2659.   Dengel, Anna. "The Medical Mission Sisters." Medical Woman's Journal, 52:11 (November 1945) 40-43. photo. In 1936 the Catholic Church clearly expressed the desire for sisters to obtain their medical degrees as doctors and nurses. This expression gave confirmation to the work of the Society of Catholic Medical Missionaries, a religious community established in 1925. A history of this religious community is given.

2660.   Dengel, Anna. "A Practical Effort to Reduce Maternal and
             Infant Mortality in New Mexico." Medical Woman's
             Journal, 55:5 (May 1948) 23-26.
         Because the war made it impossible for the women of the
         Society of Catholic Medical Missionaries to continue their
         work in many Asian and African nations, some of the Sis-
         ters were free to undertake work in New Mexico. In 1944
         the Society opened the Catholic Maternity Institute in Santa
         Fe. Its services--the nurse-midwifery school--as well as
         its medical care are described.

2661.   F. W. "The Role of a Sister Doctor." Medical Mission-
             ary, 32:1 (January-February 1958) 10-12. photos.
         The Medical Mission Sisters, founded in 1925, were to be
         a "test case" in the Catholic Church to prove that it was
         possible to combine the religious life with the medical.
         After thorough training, the religious sisters' field of la-
         bor will be in an underdeveloped country. Some of the
         problems associated with such work are outlined.

2662.   "First Medical Mission Sisterhood." Medical Woman's
             Journal, 57:10 (October 1950) 9-12, 14-18. photos.
         The Medical Mission Sisters of Philadelphia was the first
         religious society of women founded to bring professional
         medical care to the sick (1925). This article presents a
         history of the founding and first 25 years of service of the
         organization [later renamed the Society of Catholic Medical
         Missionaries].

2663.   Latham, V. A. Suggestions in Special Lines of Research
             Work for Women. E. G. Swift, Publisher, Philadelphia,
             Pennsylvania, 1906, 36 pp. photo. (Address, Alumnae
             Association, Woman's Medical College of Pennsylvania,
             Philadelphia, Pennsylvania, 25 May 1906.)
         The author suggests that women physicians research the
         physiological study of foods, tropical medicine, and, in gen-
         eral, better preparation for medical missionaries. Spe-
         cific organisms encountered in foreign climates are dis-
         cussed, and personal tips for people who expect to become
         foreign residents are given.

2664.   "Medical Sisters Ease the World's Pain." Medical Pocket
             Quarterly, 21 (1 March 1941) 10-11. photo.
         This article discusses the work of the Philadelphia, Penn-
         sylvania-based Society of Catholic Medical Missionaries,
         and its founder Dr. Anna Dengel.

2665.   Polcino, Sister M. Regis. "The Medical Mission Sisters:
             Their Founder, Mother Anna Dengel, M.D., and Their
             Role in the Historical Evolution of the Medical Mission
             Apostolate." Transactions & Studies: The College of
             Physicians of Philadelphia, 35:1 (July 1967) 1-25. pho-
             tos., ports.

Dr. Polcino begins her article with an analysis of the history and philosophy of Protestant medical missions; included are statistics on the number of missions and personnel. Following an historical discussion of the Roman Catholic attitude towards missionary work and medical care, the author provides background information on the Society of Catholic Medical Missionaries. Among the early pioneers profiled are two Scottish physicians who converted to Catholicism, Agnes McLaren and Margaret Lamont. Dr. Anna Dengel's campaign to establish medical missions is detailed, as is Dr. Joanna Lyon's role in starting the Society. In 1936 the Society's work was formally approved by a change in canon law, so that Catholic women could combine religious life with that of medicine. The article concludes with an accounting of the work of the Society in Asia, Africa, and South America. An extensive bibliography is included.

2666.   ["The Sacred Experiment of a Tirolese Woman: In Honor of the Founder of the Medical Missionary Sisters"].
         Die Presse, 5433 (24 May 1966) 5. (Ger)
In a public session of the state legislature recently, the Tyrolian state honored Dr. Anna Dengel, founder and Mother General of the Medical Mission Sisters, with its highest decoration, the Circle of Honor of the State of Tyrol (Ehrenring des Landes Tyrol). Dr. Dengel received her medical education in Ireland and spent three years in Rawalpindi. Shocked by the desperate need for medical care of the Mohammedan women, she returned to America to work for the organization of Catholic doctors and the establishment of a congregation dedicated to filling that need. The Medical Mission Sisters was founded in 1925, became a congregation in 1941, and was recognized by the papal court in 1959. It now has about 800 sisters--doctors, dentists, pharmacists, and all types of medical auxilliaries. It runs 48 hospitals, clinics, maternity stations, and tropical disease clinics in Asia, Africa, and South America, with study houses and novitiates in America, Europe, and Asia. The founding of the Medical Mission Sisters has been called a great and successful "holy experiment."

2667.   Schrattenbach, Vilma. ["Mother Dr. Anna Dengel: Austrian Pioneer for Medical Missionary Work"]. Religion, Wissenschart, Kultur, 8 (1957) 237-245. (Ger)
The world-wide activity of the Society of Catholic Medical Missionaries results from the pioneer work of two women physicians: Agnes McLaren and Anna Dengel. Their training and their efforts in preparing and finally creating the Society are described in this article. The author underlines the serious medical problems in Asia that prompted the interest of these women, and later of the Catholic Church, in medical and missionary work in the late 19th and early 20th century. She describes the difficulties encountered by the Medical Mission Sisters in building hospitals and medical dispensaries.

2668.   "Women's Rightful Place in Medicine: Women Graduates
         Have Dedicated Their Lives to Overseas Mission Ser-
         vice." Alumni Journal [Loma Linda University, School
         of Medicine], 44:3 (May 1973) 17.   ports.
The article is a brief outline of Seventh-Day Adventist medical women who have chosen to serve at various mission
outposts, from 1900 to the present. Names, locations, and
dates of graduation (from College of Medical Evangelists or
American Medical Missionary College) are given for several dozen women.

WAR TIME ACTIVITY

Covered are the activities of specific organizations during times of war, which directly
related to war. Material on specific women
emphasize work in war situations or in the
military service.

CANADA

2669.   Guest, Edna M. "Medical Women in Canada." Journal of
            the American Medical Women's Association, 1:8 (No-
            vember 1946) 254-255.
         In 1939, when war was declared by Canada, an invitation
         went out to British women physicians to seek harbor in
         Canada for the duration. British women physicians were
         welcomed and granted temporary license to practice in Can-
         ada. Women physicians in Canada tried unsuccessfully in
         1939 to offer their services in the armed forces. In 1942
         came the Order-in-Council giving authority for women phy-
         sicians to be legally commissioned, which they were, on the
         basis of equal rank and equal pay with men physicians.
         Now the plans are to demobilize women physicians as there
         are no plans for retaining their services in the permanent
         forces of Canada. "In Canada," concludes Guest, "the wo-
         man physician has no frustration," and she cites the recent
         election of Dr. Ethlyn Trapp to the presidency of the Pro-
         vincial Medical Association.

2670.   Mugan, Monica. "Women Doctors at Camp Borden, On-
            tario." Women in Medicine, 80 (April 1943) 14-15.
         A reprint of a Canadian Broadcasting Company broadcast of
         November 16, 1942, this article gives a personal account
         of life as a woman physician in the Royal Canadian Army
         Medical Corps at Camp Borden, Ontario. The emphasis is
         placed on how "well integrated socially" the men and wo-
         men are. The article gives some insight into the fashions
         and foods at the camp.

EUROPE, EASTERN

2671.   Glasgow, Maude. "Women in the Medical Corps of the Red
            Army." Medical Woman's Journal, 51:11 (November
            1944) 17-22.
         Primarily because Russia's Red Army Medical Corps is
         currently staffed almost entirely by women, "in the Russian
         medical world the revolution is as complete as it is in the
         political or domestic branches." Dr. Glasgow's discussion
         of Russian medical women includes relevant statistics (e.g.,
         90 per cent of Russian medical students in 1943 were wo-
         men). A major portion of the article mentions the accom-
         plishments of specific women physicians and describes sev-
         eral heroic acts performed by medical women in the Red
         Army. "Part II" of this article contrasts the status of
         American medical women with that of her Russian counter-
         parts. Lamenting the relatively small number of U.S. wo-

men physicians, the medical schools' discriminatory quota
systems, and the woman physician's inferior status in the
U.S. armed services, Dr. Glasgow writes that these conditions are "insulting to every American woman citizen
who possesses even a vestige of self-respect."

2672.   Gorinevskaya, Valentina. "Soviet Women Doctors in War."
        Women in Medicine, 86 (October 1944) 18.
        In 1877, during the Turkish campaign, Russian women doc-
        tors appeared for the first time on the military front.   Dur-
        ing World War I, however, the tsarist government did not
        allow women doctors in the army, with the exception of the
        author (who was at that time Professor Kalyan), who went
        to the front as a senior surgeon.   The October Revolution
        gave women the same rights as men and now they serve in
        equal work with men in the defense of their country.

2673.   Grigoréva, N. N.   ["Glory Undimmed Through the Cen-
        turies"].   Voprosy Okhrany Materinstva i Detstva, 20:
        5 (May 1975) 4-8.   (Rus)
        Soviet women in medicine contributed greatly to the fight
        against fascism during World War II.   Many of them
        fought and died on the battlefields, trying to save the lives
        of the wounded soldiers, and immortalized their names.
        One of them, E. V. Bakhireva, a pediatrician, volunteered
        to help in evacuation of the wounded to the other side of
        the Volga but was badly wounded herself and died heroical-
        ly.   Feldschers and nurses also died in battle.   Twenty-
        three young women graduates of the 4th Moscow Medical
        Institute in 1941, with Liza Katysheva at their head, made
        their triumphant way from Moscow to Berlin saving soldiers'
        lives.   A young physician, E. F. Murav'eva, donated blood
        100 times.   In the Soviet Union at present 72 per cent of
        physicians are women, many of them holding high administra-
        tive positions.

2674.   Hanson, H. B.   "Serbia as Seen by a Red Cross Worker
        [Part I]."   Woman's Medical Journal, 26:4 (April 1916)
        88-93.
        The crowded medical facilities and over-worked medical
        staff at the plague, typhoid, scarlet fever, small pox, and
        diphtheria-ridden location in Serbia where this British phy-
        sician/author worked for six months, are described.

2675.   Hanson, H. B.   "Serbia as Seen by a Red Cross Worker
        [Part II]."   Woman's Medical Journal, 26:6 (June 1916)
        149-153.
        An English woman physician describes her experiences
        serving in the midst of war-torn Serbia where a team of
        British women doctors was giving medical care to the
        soldiers and civilian population.

2676.   Lesnikova, R. V.   ["Women Physicians on the Battlefields in the Russian-Turkish War 1877-1878 (on the Centenary of Women's Medical Education)"]. Sovetskoe Zdravookhranenie, 31 (1972) 74-77. (Rus)

The article lists Russian women physicians who took part in the wars of 1876 and 1877-78. During the Serbo-Turkish War (1876), five women served as physicians in Serbian hospitals. Sofia Ivanovna Bolibot (1850-1918) was the first military surgeon and took part in both wars. She was highly praised for her amputation surgery and was awarded a Russian decoration. After the war she worked as a physician in Siberia and various parts of Russia. Vera Petrovna Matveeva (1851-1916) took part in both wars, apparently as a surgeon, then worked as a physician in various parts of Russia. Vera Michailovna Dmitrieva (died 1901) worked in Petersburg after the war as a physician and as a school doctor. Raisa Samoilovna Svyatlovskaya, nee Frenkel (1853-1914), was at the head of military hospitals in both wars and, after that, worked in Moscow. Maria Alexandrovna Zibold also took part in both wars as head of a military hospital. Forty women took part in the Russian-Turkish war in 1877-78. Not much is known about them. Besides those mentioned above, others included: Sofia Ivanovna Bestuzheva (1840-1912), who worked in various hospitals, took part in the outbreak of plague in Veluanka in 1879, then worked in Paris in the clinic of Sharko; Maria Pavlovna Mardvinova (1846-1882); Maria Michailovna Melnicova; Nadezhda Bontle; Elena Solovjeva; Nadezhda Ostrogorskaya; Varvara Stepanovna Nekrasova (died 1877); Bronislava Pashkevitch; Ekaterina Cristofovna Malyarskaya (1852-1904), who worked at Petersburg in a pediatric clinic and then, with her physician husband U. V. Malyarovsky, took a special interest in retarded children. Alexandra Vasylievna Dileva worked as a physician in Bulgaria.

2677.   Lovejoy, Esther. "A Thrilling Letter from Turkey." Medical Woman's Journal, 28:11 (November 1921) 277-280. (Hospitals & Colleges.)

Dr. Lovejoy writes about conditions in the war-torn city of Ismid, Turkey and how Dr. Mabel Elliott and the other women stationed at the American Women's Hospitals there were affected. The text of a letter by Dr. Elliott is included.

2678.   MacRobert, Rachel N. "Greetings from the Russian Medical Women Serving in a Military Hospital in Leningrad." Medical Women's Federation Quarterly Review, (October 1942) 55-58.

This article consists of a letter to Lady MacRobert from the women doctors in Leningrad Military Hospital, and Lady MacRobert's reply. The letter from the Soviet women expresses sorrow upon the loss of Lady MacRobert's sons: "the hearts of Soviet mother doctors whose sons have also fallen in battle as yours did" share her sorrow. The letter

also discusses the war and eventual victory. Lady Mac-
Robert's reply thanks the women and also expresses admiration for the "amazing people of [Stalingrad] and the
heroic Red Army fighting there."

2679.   ["Self-Sacrifice and Heroism of Women Military Medical
               Doctors: In Honor of the International Women's Day
               of March 8"].   Voenno-Meditsinskii Zhurnal, 3 (March
               1975) 10-13. (Rus)
         During the war of 1941-1945 women made up 46 per cent
         of the military medical personnel (57 per cent of paramed-
         ics, 59 per cent of pharmacists, 62 per cent of dentists,
         42 per cent of field hospital personnel, and 54 per cent of
         evacuation hospitals staff). Seventeen women were declared
         Heroes of the Soviet Union, of a total of 44 so honored.
         The article describes in detail the work and heroism of a
         number of women in different types of medical work during
         that period. Two medical doctors are mentioned: V. V.
         Gorinevskaya, a well-known traumatologist, worked in the
         main military sanitation administration; and Lidia Stepanovna
         Dmitrienko, a graduate of the Military-Medical Academy,
         took part in the Soviet-Finnish War and in the war of 1941-
         45, and now works in the Kiev Military Hospital.

2680.   "Soviet Medical Women."   Medical Woman's Journal, 51:7
               (July 1944) 32.
         The information in this article, extracted from a Russian
         embassy information bulletin, includes descriptions of
         heroic deeds at the front by several specific women sur-
         geons. Over 150 women doctors, nurses, and stretcher
         bearers have received the Order of Lenin, and some 15,000
         Soviet medical women have received other decorations for
         heroism.

EUROPE, WESTERN

2681.   "Dr. Louise Hurrell, of Rochester, N.Y., Writes Most
               Interestingly of Experiences in French Villages." Wo-
               man's Medical Journal, 28:11 (November 1918) 243.
         Given is a report of one of the women physicians who com-
         prised the first hospital of the American Women's Hos-
         pitals in France.

2682.   "Interesting Letters from Women Physicians at the Front."
               Woman's Medical Journal, 28:1 (January 1918) 15-19.
         Among other letters, Dr. Alice Barlow-Brown writes of the
         Ambulance Fund contributed by her hometown. She gives
         details of day-to-day life and living conditions in Paris,
         where she is stationed. In a later letter, she discusses
         the opening of dispensaries in France. The specifics of
         women physicians' military positions in working within
         France are discussed by Dr. Regina Flood Keyes in her

letter, while Dr. Mabel H. F. Bancroft tells also of her
work in Paris.   An unsigned letter offers "Practical Suggestions to Medical Women Going to France."

2683.   Kilham, Eleanor B.   Letters from France: 1915-1919.
          Salem, Massachusetts, 1941, 81 pp.   port.
        Dr. Kilham spent three and one-half years in France dur-
        ing World War I, working part of the time at a French
        military hospital.   Her observations about the progress of
        the war and her continuing efforts to relieve wartime suf-
        fering are chronicled in letters written to her sisters in
        America.

2684.   "Little Tales of Real Life: From Letters from Members
          of the Staff of American Women's Hospitals Number
          One."   Woman's Medical Journal, 28:12 (December
          1918) 260-262.
        Drs. Margaret E. V. Fraser, Helen Woodroffe, and Jean
        H. Pattison, among others, give their impressions of and
        experiences in France, serving with the American Women's
        Hospitals during the war.

2685.   McIlroy, A. Louise.   "The Work of a Unit of the Scottish
          Women's Hospitals in France, Serbia, and Salonica."
          Glasgow Medical Journal, 88 (November 1917) 277-287.

2686.   Medical Women's International Association.   Women Doc-
          tors at Work During the Second World War.   Albert
          Bonniers, Stockholm, Sweden, 1948, 88 pp.
        The book consists in a collection of papers presented at
        the September 1946 meeting of the Medical Women's Inter-
        national Association held at the Royal Society of Medicine,
        London, England.   The papers survey the work of women
        physicians during World War II (e.g., in France, Holland,
        London, and Denmark).   In addition, articles appear on the
        physical health of persons in German occupied territory,
        the psychological effects of war on children in France, and
        a report "On the Question of Frenchmen Deported for Po-
        litical and Racial Reasons."

2687.   "Women Doctors' Wonderful Work Amid War's Horrors."
          Literary Digest, 56 (16 February 1918) 40-41, 43.
        Described are the heroic acts of women physicians during
        wartime and especially the work of those associated with
        the Scottish Women's Hospitals.

GREAT BRITAIN

2688.   Aitken, Janet K.   "British Medical Women."   Journal of
          the American Medical Women's Association, 1:8 (No-
          vember 1946) 253.
        A brief description of British women physicians' contribu-

tion to the war effort and a general belief that because of
the positive feeling about women physicians during this
period, "it would appear ... that any disabilities from
which women doctors suffered are to be at an end."

2689.   "British Medical Women and War Services." Medical Wo-
         man's Journal, 49:4 (April 1942) 121. (Editorial.)

2690.   Campbell, Janet. "Medical Women and War Services."
         Medical Women's Federation Quarterly Review, (Janu-
         ary 1941) 31-35.
         Dr. Campbell discusses the situation in the British armed
         forces which finds medical women granted "relative rank"
         in the R. A. M. C. instead of commissions. The history of
         the medical women's struggle with the war office is re-
         viewed.

2691.   Campbell, Janet M. "Medical Women in the Bombing of
         Britain." Journal of the American Medical Women's
         Association, 1:9 (December 1946) 309-318. photos.
         Given is an accounting of how American women physicians,
         under the auspices of the War Service Committee of the
         American Medical Women's Association, worked with Brit-
         ish women in rendering aid during the Battle of Britain,
         1940-1945.

2692.   "Demand for More Women Physicians in the Army." Wo-
         man's Medical Journal, 27:1 (January 1917) 17.
         The work of women physicians attached to the army medical
         corps in England has been so successful that the demand
         for more women physicians has increased.

2693.   Fairfield, Letitia. "Women Doctors and the Services."
         Medical Women's Federation Quarterly Review, (Octo-
         ber 1939) 43-45.
         The Medical Women's Federation, supported by the British
         Medical Association, sought to improve the unsatisfactory
         position of medical women during wartime. It has been
         learned that the army council has not seen fit to grant
         commissions to women. They have, however, granted com-
         plete equality of pay and enrollments plus a definite rank.
         The question of disability pension is still under considera-
         tion by the Treasury. Women wishing to serve in the mili-
         tary under these conditions should submit their names to
         their local war emergency committee.

2694.   Fairfield, Letitia; Knowles, Frances Ivens; Hutton, Isabel
         Emslie; Adamson, R. H. B.; and Ramsay, Mabel L.
         "Medical Women's Service in the Great War, 1914-
         1919." Medical Women's Federation Quarterly Review,
         (January 1939) 26-43.
         Many medical women made meaningful contributions during
         the Great War, often under difficult conditions of prejudice.

Letitia Fairfield, who served at the Southern Command Headquarters at Salisbury, describes her work with the "uniformed women's services." Frances Ivens Knowles describes her work with the Scottish Women's Hospitals of Royaumont and Villers Cotterets. Isabel Emslie Hutton discusses the courageous work undertaken by the Scottish Women's Hospitals in France, Belgium, Serbia, and Russia, while the privilege of serving in their own country was withheld. R. H. B. Adamson discusses her medical work in the munitions factories. And Mabel Ramsey describes her work as a civilian medical practitioner. All agree that women are able to endure war conditions to an unlimited extent--"It was all a matter of grit and heart"--and if their services should be required in wartime in the future, arrangements must be made for them to receive adequate remuneration and to have the same status as the noncombatant RAMC officers.

2695.   Fenwick, Dorothy. "The Work of Medical Women in the Royal Air Force." Journal of the American Medical Women's Association, 1:8 (November 1946) 252-253. This history of women in the Royal Air Force (RAF) begins with the March 1940 acceptance of women into the RAF as W. A. A. F. s (Women's Auxiliary Air Force). Although the women felt this title was discriminating, there was no differentiation in privileges, obligations, rank, and rate of pay between women and men in this service.

2696.   Glasgow, Maude. "Women Physicians and War Service." Medical Record, (6 July 1918) 26-27. (Correspondence.)

2697.   Hanson, Helen B. "Women Doctors with the Army in the Field." Bristol Medico-Chirurgical Journal, 33:128 (June 1915) 88-94.

2698.   Haskins, Grace. "Report on British Emergency Medical Service." Medical Woman's Journal, 52:3 (March 1945) 32-33. port. Approximately two-thirds of the doctors sent to Great Britain during World War II worked for the Emergency Medical Service (EMS). Facilities at the EMS and work done there by the physicians are reviewed.

2699.   Ivens, Mary H. Frances. "The Part Played by British Medical Women in the War." British Medical Journal, (18 August 1917) 203-208. photos. Dr. Ivens describes the work of women physicians in the French Red Cross at the Abbaye de Royaumont. She then covers the activities of the Scottish Women's Hospitals during the war and concludes the article with a section on the work of women physicians under the British War Office. [Dr. Ivens' article, with the same title, also appears in Woman's Medical Journal, 28:3 (March 1918) 53.]

2700.   Lovejoy, Esther P. "American Women's Hospitals Over-
            seas Service (Medical Service Committee of the Amer-
            ican Medical Women's Association)." Medical Woman's
            Journal, 51:10 (October 1944) 20-22. facsim.
         The American Women's Hospitals' work within war-torn
         countries and its cooperation with the British Medical Wo-
         men's Federation and other medical organizations are de-
         scribed.

2701.   "Major Bean of the Royal Army Medical Corps." Medical
            Woman's Journal, 49:10 (October 1942) 322. (News
            Notes.)
         Ascha Bean went to Britain in 1941 in order to give med-
         ical care to victims of bombings. Dr. Bean thinks the re-
         fusal of the American medical corps to offer commissions
         to women is "unreasonable and based on silly misconcep-
         tions."

2702.   Martindale, Louisa. "Women Doctors in the British Army."
            Medical Woman's Journal, 50:1 (January 1943) 6-7.
         This article outlines the requirements for, and work of,
         women doctors in the British army.

2703.   "Medical Women and National Defense." Medical Women's
            Federation Quarterly Review, (July 1939) 47-51.
         The contributions of medical women during World War I
         are recounted as a prelude to opening the case for equality
         with male physicians during wartime. Although women
         served meritoriously without complaint during the war, it
         was obvious that "lack of a commissioned rank placed them
         at a serious disadvantage." Also, there was no provision
         for promotion, and pay and emoluments were inadequate.
         Worst of all, even the unsatisfactory position they achieved
         required a struggle. The basic request of commissions for
         women has been turned down because "medical women could
         not perform all tasks which are at present undertaken by
         medical officers." The Federation believes this may be a
         good reason for not employing women in war service at all,
         but certainly not for refusing them commissions, which are
         not rewards for nobility of service, but an authorization
         given "to anyone thought worthy to serve according to his
         ability with the forces of the Crown."

2704.   "Medical Women and War Services." Medical Women's
            Federation Quarterly Review, (January 1942) 47-48.
         In 1939, medical women in England were offered "relative
         rank" without commissions but with similar status to those
         of men in the armed forces. The offer was accepted.
         When the women were finally offered commissions they were
         offered a commission in the Women's Forces, not in the
         medical services on equal terms with men. While the fi-
         nancial arrangements were equal to that of the men, the
         proposed status of medical women was inferior. As a

result of negotiations, the medical woman was given the choice to retain "relative rank" or to accept the commission in the Women's Forces. The Medical Women's Federation will continue to press for commissions for medical women in the medical service: "Medical women volunteered to serve as doctors, not as women."

2705.   Murray, Flora. Women As Army Surgeons: Being the History of the Women's Hospital Corps in Paris, Wimereux and Endell Street: September 1914-October 1919. Hodder and Stoughton Ltd., London, England, [1920]. 263 pp. photos.
This history of the Women's Hospital Corps, formed in England in 1914 to assist with the medical and surgical care of military casualties, was written by the only woman lieutenant-colonel in the British army, Flora Murray. Dr. Murray was doctor-in-charge of the Military Hospital, Endell Street (London). The Corps first established a hospital in the Hôtel Claridge, Paris, in cooperation with the French Red Cross. They later expanded to facilities near Boulogne at Wimereux. In 1915 the Corps staffed and operated the Military Hospital, Endell Street, a facility with 573 beds. Endell Street remained in operation until 1919. This history and memoir includes the names of many women physicians and surgeons affiliated with the Corps and its services; however, the work is not indexed. Anecdotes illustrating the reaction of military and government authorities to these enterprises of women physicians are recalled throughout the text.

2706.   Robertson, Elizabeth E. "A Woman Doctor's Work in Britain's Army." Medical Woman's Journal, 51:8 (August 1944) 20-21, 30.
Providing background on James Miranda Stewart Barry (the male impersonator who became in 1813 the first woman in Britain's Army Medical Service), the author (a captain in Great Britain's Army Medical Corps) wonders if James Barry would have envied modern women army doctors their "unequivocal acceptance by their male colleagues." Captain Robertson goes on to describe life in the armed services, comparing the duties of a military medical woman to those of a civilian practitioner. Among the difficulties faced by women physicians in the military service are low morale, brought on by boredom, and the demanding responsibility of "woman management." Whereas men have learned to handle other men "by force, by fear, by personality ... [or by] a great ideal ... the handling of large masses of women has only become a problem since their emancipation, and so far much is yet unknown about mass female psychology."

2707.   Stewart, Clara. "Medical Women in British Forces." Medical Woman's Journal, 49:7 (July 1942) 203.

The president of the Medical Women's Federation writes to
clarify the differences in terms and conditions offered to
medical women and men serving with His Majesty's Forces,
and what strategies might be taken to rectify the inequali-
ties of rank and salary.

2708.   Stewart, Clara and Campbell, Janet M.   "Medical Women
            and War Services."   Medical Women's Federation Quar-
            terly Review, (October 1941) 77-79.
         A memorandum is reprinted which was submitted to the di-
         rector general, Army Medical Services from the Medical
         Women's Federation.   The memorandum urges the army
         council to reconsider its decision not to grant medical wo-
         men commissions in the medical service, but rather to
         commission men in the women's forces.   "Women doctors
         volunteer to serve with the army as doctors and not as
         women, and they consider that any arrangement which places
         them in a separate category from their professional col-
         leagues infringes this fundamental principle."

2709.   Stimson, Barbara B.   "Three-and-a-Half Years in the
            Royal Army Medical Corps."   Journal of the Ameri-
            can Medical Women's Association, 1:2 (May 1946) 47-
            49.
         Dr. Stimson relates her experiences while serving in Eng-
         land during World War II under the auspices of the Amer-
         ican Women's Hospitals.

2710.   Toland, Gertrude M. B.   "War Surgery at Dover, England."
            Medical Woman's Journal, 51:3 (March 1944) 25-27.
            photo.
         Dr. Toland, a staff surgeon at the Dover Emergency Med-
         ical Service Hospital, outlines the hospital routine, details
         a few of the medical cases, and describes daily life in
         wartime Dover.

2711.   Walker, Jane.   "How Is Medicine as a Profession for Wo-
            men Affected by the War?"   Practitioner, 95 (Septem-
            ber 1915) 288-292.
         The war has increased the demand for medical women to
         take the place of medical men.   However, an examination
         of advertisements for hospital staff members shows that
         practically none of the posts offered to women are for old-
         er, experienced doctors.   The most hopeful possibility is
         that the war will assist in creating equal medical education
         opportunities for women.

2712.   Walsh, James J.   "The War and Women Physicians."   In-
            dependent, 84 (27 December 1915) 520.
         Dr. Walsh lists reasons the war will bring new opportun-
         ities for women to study and to practice medicine.   Statis-
         tics cited concern the high number of young male physicians
         in military service; the subsequent need for women physi-
         cians to administer to civilians is discussed.

2713.   White, Marguerite. "An English Woman Surgeon's Message
            to Her American Sisters." Bulletin Medical Woman's
            Club of Chicago, 6:3 (November 1917) 3-4.
        Dr. White, who is with the British Expeditionary Forces in
        Malta, writes of her experiences there and expresses the
        hope that after the war, men and women will pursue the
        "better understanding and sympathy" which the war has
        fostered between them.

2714.   Winner, Albertine. "Six Hundred Women Doctors in Brit-
            ain's Army." Women in Medicine, 91 (January 1946)
            7-13.   photos.
        "The story of medical women's service with the British
        Army" is told in this article, beginning in 1865 when the
        inspector-general of Britain's Army Medical Department,
        Dr. James Barry, died and was discovered at the post-
        mortem to be a woman; through World War I and the forma-
        tion of the Women's Hospital Corps and the Queen Mary's
        Army Auxiliary Corps; to World War II and establishment
        of the Auxiliary Territorial Service (ATS).   The author re-
        calls her own service in the ATS with the Army Blood Sup-
        ply Depot.   A brief tribute is also paid to two American
        women physicians serving in England.   The article con-
        cludes with a description of the life and work of women
        physicians in the British army.

2715.   "Women and Emergency Services, 1939." Medical Women's
            Federation Quarterly Review, (July 1939) 51.
        A brief notice describes openings for women doctors in
        emergency services, both in preparation for emergencies
        and for duty after the outbreak of hostilities, and tells
        where to apply.

2716.   "Women and War." Lancet, 2 (17 July 1915) 134-135.
        This article praises the activity of women physicians in
        France, Serbia, and England, and further asserts that the
        scope of women's work in medicine--and in all occupations
        --will expand immensely after the war.   Speculating on
        the consequences of women's increased work activity (i.e.,
        low birthrate), the writer predicts "great social readjust-
        ments."

INTERNATIONAL

2717.   Bass, Elizabeth. "Wars and Women Doctors." Medical
            Woman's Journal, 51:7 (July 1944) 22-24.
        This article (reprinted from the January 1944 issue of New
        Orleans Medical and Surgical Journal) provides mythological
        and historical examples of medical women who served in
        time of war.   Among the women mentioned are Lady Anne
        Halkett (1622-1699) of Scotland, a surgeon in the Royal
        Army; James Barry, the male impersonator who was in-

spector general of all British hospitals; and Mary Walker,
the U.S. Civil War surgeon. The first woman contract
surgeon in the U.S. Army was Anita McGee, who served
during the Spanish War. The military medical women who
served during World War I, and those currently serving,
are discussed in a generalized manner.

2718.   Ellsworth, Adelaide. "The Woman Doctor in War." Penn-
          sylvania Medical Journal, 22 (October 1918) 23-25.
          (Presentation, Warren County Medical Society, 22 July
          1918.)
          "It is no longer necessary for woman to plead her own
          cause. Every government is doing that for her," asserts
          Dr. Ellsworth, who illustrates how the war has opened up
          opportunities for women to work on an equal basis with
          men "from the fireside to the firing line." Dr. Ellsworth
          overviews the wartime activities of French and British
          women. Turning to the work of American women physi-
          cians, she discusses the American Women's Hospitals, the
          "wide field of usefulness at home" in civilian health care,
          and resolutions recently introduced that would provide med-
          ical women in government service the same rank and pay
          as men.

2719.   Lovejoy, Esther Pohl. "Medical Women's War Work."
          Medical Woman's Journal, 50:3 (March 1943) 65-66.
          An international look at the work of women physicians in
          military service constitutes this article.

2720.   Smith, Frederick C. "The Woman Doctor." Medical Wo-
          man's Journal, 50:4 (April 1943) 102.
          This article, written by the editor of The Medical World,
          compares England's and Canada's progressive attitudes to-
          wards women in the armed services to the "curious situa-
          tion" in the United States, where women are denied military
          rating.

UNITED STATES

2721.   "American Legion Bill Commissioning Women Physicians
          Introduced February 15th." Medical Woman's Journal,
          50:3 (March 1943) 83. (Editorial.)
          This article consists in letters relating to the introduction
          (by Senator Johnson and Representative Sparkman) of a bill
          drafted by the American Legion. The bill, which "provides
          for the appointment of female physicians and surgeons in
          the Medical Corps of the Army and Navy," is presented
          herein.

2722.   American Medical Women's Association. "We Request Ad-
          mission to the Medical Reserve Corps." Women in
          Medicine, 75 (January 1942) 8-9.

This reprint of the letter sent to the President of the
United States sets forth the resolution, adopted by the
Board of Directors of the American Medical Women's Association in 1942, requesting admittance of women physicians to the Medical Reserve Corps of the United States
Army "upon the same terms as all the rest of its members...."

2723.   "American Women's Hospitals." Woman's Medical Journal,
        27:9 (September 1917) 205.
        As part of the medical and surgical service of the Ameri-
        can Red Cross, women physicians will be able to give
        maternity service and perform village practice in the devas-
        tated parts of the Allies' countries; in the United States
        they will be able to care for soldiers' dependents, interned
        alien enemies, and take over the hospital service and pri-
        vate practice of physicians who have gone to the front.
        The War Service Committee of the Medical Women's Na-
        tional Association has organized the American Women's
        Hospitals to enable women physicians to do this patient
        care.

2724.   "An Executive Order Might Cut the Gordian Knot." Wo-
        man's Medical Journal, 27:10 (October 1917) 226.
        (Editorial.)
        If President Wilson would pass an executive order, women
        physicians could serve in the army with the same rank and
        salary as men physicians.

2725.   "The Army and the Navy Need Women Physicians." Wo-
        men in Medicine, 82 (October 1943) 7.
        This article represents a listing of members of the Ameri-
        can Medical Women's Association who are serving in the
        armed forces.

2726.   "Army Nursing Bill. An Expression from Medical Women."
        Woman's Medical Journal, 10:6 (June 1900) 267-268.
        A meeting of the alumnae association of the Laura Memorial
        Woman's Medical College (Cincinnati, Ohio) passed a reso-
        lution requiring alumnae of the College to write to their
        congressmen to vote against section 2 of bill H. R. 6879.
        The bill provides for the employment of women nurses in
        the army; section 2 of the bill states that a nurse shall be
        the superintendent of women nurses. The women physicians
        feel a woman physician, with the rank of assistant surgeon,
        can better perform these duties.

2727.   "Army's Women Physicians Serving in Various Assignments
        Around the World." Journal of the American Medical
        Women's Association, 8:3 (March 1953) 103-104.
        There are 21 women physicians in the Army Medical Corps.
        A paragraph about each woman is included, giving each
        one's home town, specialty and rank. Major General Ray-

mond W. Bliss, Surgeon General of the Army in 1950 said:
"There has never been any question in my mind that the
duties incumbent upon care of military sick and injured
can be performed equally well by qualified women as by
men in various medical specialties.   Women doctors served
with distinction in the Army during World War II.   We look
forward to welcoming them again."

2728.   Baker, S. Josephine; Speer, Alma Jane; Parmelee, Ruth;
               Schrack, Helen; and Barringer, Emily Dunning.   "Com-
               missions for Women Physicians in the Medical Reserve
               Corps of the United States Army."   Women in Medi-
               cine, 79 (January 1943) 7-9.
          A year after Pearl Harbor, women physicians were still
          only offered positions with the military as contract surgeons
          and then later promised that they would receive commis-
          sions in the WAACS.   This article describes the strategy
          of women physicians to organize women's clubs, congress-
          men, newspapers, the American Legion, and the President, to
          assure that women physicians might serve in the armed
          services with commissions and pay commensurate with what
          male physicians could expect to receive.

2729.   Barringer, Emily Dunning.   "The American Woman Physi-
               cian and War Time Rating."   Medical Woman's Journal,
               49:12 (December 1942) 361-365, 371.   (Address, Wo-
               men's Medical Association, Town Hall Club, New York
               City, 4 November 1942.)
          Contrary to a ruling of the Comptroller General of the
          United States, the woman physician is a person and her
          medical degree means that she is as prepared to be "sub-
          ject to the same rules, regulations, fines and penalties as
          the male physician."   Women physicians are not being al-
          lowed commissions to practice medicine for the men in the
          armed services.   One firm repercussion this non-status of
          women physicians had was at patriotic schools like the Uni-
          versity of Arkansas Medical School which up to that time
          had been co-educational but since there was a war on and
          since doctors were needed for the war and since women
          were not as acceptable as male physicians in the armed
          services, the University only accepted male students in
          their Fall 1942 class.   The male dean was quoted at the
          time as saying, "We felt that our duty in wartime, since
          medical students are deferred, is to turn out as many med-
          ical officers as possible.   A woman applicant as yet can-
          not become an officer in the Medical Corps."   The Ameri-
          can Medical Association did not support the women physi-
          cians' resolution to serve.   Perhaps they believed that
          equality did exist or more likely the woman physician is
          "such a negligible problem that she was not worth mention-
          ing."   On the other hand, women physicians received com-
          missions in the WAVES and after some legal rulings, in the
          WAACS where they had only been allowed to be contract

surgeons previously. While women physicians are a minority "let us be so on a truly democratic basis."

2730. Barringer, Emily Dunning. "Commissions for Women Phy-
           sicians: Report of Special Committees." Women in
           Medicine, 81 (July 1943) 11-14.
This report concerns the research and lobbying effort of
the American Medical Women's Association to guarantee
women physicians commissions in the Medical Reserve
Corps of the United States Army and Navy. At the time
this Committee was formed, the American Medical Association was still not supporting the commissioning of women
physicians. The army was willing to offer women contract
surgeon jobs (for fewer working and personal benefits than
a permanent position) for working in the WAACs. Eventually permanent appointments became accessible in the WAACs
but the navy continued to retain its disqualifying "MALE"
ruling. This Committee decided to focus its energies to
change the army's appointments of women physicians as
contract surgeons to being commissioned. They found out
"that even if commissioned, it would be in only the lower
ranks and that women physicians' work would be limited to
service in the WAACs. These women physicians would be
debarred from the bigger privileges of the medical corps
in regard to medical opportunity, rank, pay, and veteran's
privileges." The reason for this is that "the word 'person'
in the requirements for entrance to the Medical Corps did
not include women physicians." Finally, Emanuel Celler,
congressional representative from New York, introduced a
bill to amend the existing law "so as to substitute 'men and
women' for the word 'person'." Finally women physicians
were allowed full appointments to the Medical Corps of the
Army and Navy, and their practice need not be limited
solely to hospitals and stations where female nurses are
employed.

2731. Barringer, Emily Dunning. "Hearing on Commissions for
           Women Physicians on March 10th Before Sub-Committee
           Military Affairs Committee, with Congressman Matthew
           Merritt Presiding." Medical Woman's Journal, 50:3
           (March 1943) 80. (News Notes.)

2732. Barringer, Emily Dunning. "Report of Progress on 'Com-
           missions for Women Physicians in the Army and
           Navy.'" Medical Woman's Journal, 50:4 (April 1943)
           99-100.

2733. Barringer, Emily Dunning. "The Sparkman-Johnson Bill
           Passed by Congress." Medical Woman's Journal, 50:6
           (June 1943) 141-142.

2734. Barringer, Emily Dunning. "Special Notice: January 1,
           1943." Medical Woman's Journal, 50:1 (January 1943)

26. (News Notes.)
This notice announces that the Celler bill, on the commissioning of women physicians in the Medical Reserve Corps
of the U.S. Army, will be introduced at the opening of the
new Congress.

2735.   Barringer, Emily Dunning. "Temporary Appointment of
            Officers in the Army of the United States--H.R. 824
            (78th Congress, First Session): In the House of Repre-
            sentatives January 7, 1943. Notice to All Women Phy-
            sicians!" Medical Woman's Journal, 50:2 (February
            1943) 53-54.
The bill is presented in this article. A list of members
of the Military Affairs Committee, U.S. House of Representatives, is also included.

2736.   Barringer, Emily Dunning. "War and the Woman Physi-
            cian." New York State Journal of Medicine, 42:2 (15
            January 1942) 118-120.
This article discusses the woman physician's ineligibility
for the Medical Reserve Corps of the U.S. Navy.

2737.   Barringer, Emily D.; Speer, Alma Jane; Whitten, Kathryn
            M.; Parmelee, Ruth; and Schrack, Helen F. "Com-
            missions for Women Physicians in Army and Navy."
            Journal of the American Medical Women's Association,
            1:4 (July 1946) 128-131. (Report, Annual Meeting,
            American Medical Women's Association, San Francisco,
            June 1946.)
There were numerous ways in which women physicians,
medical students, and premedical students were discriminated against in favor of men in the medical profession
during and after World War II. Discrimination occurred
in two primary categories: women physicians who were
commissioned in the Medical Corps of the United States
Army, Navy, and Public Health; and the problems the woman medical student faces as a result of the war. Such
discrimination took the following forms: while men were
automatically eligible for the medical reserve corps, women who had given medical service with the army had their
service terminated; women physicians who held civilian positions such as public health service terminated when the
male physicians returned from the war; the government
allotted male medical students rank, tuition, and salary
while studying medicine but did nothing for women medical
students at all; when men returned on the GI Bill to attend
medical school, the percentage of women accepted at medical school dropped from the already low ten per cent to
six per cent; women's problems were subordinated to the
problems of returning men; women's concerns were of secondary interest. Emily Barringer concludes this address
by proposing a resolution that the "American Medical Association go on record as approving the removal of sex dis-

crimination from the medical student and that henceforth a woman medical student be judged purely by her individual qualifications."

2738.   "Bill Signed." Medical Woman's Journal, 50:9 (September 1943) 234. (Section on War Service.)
"On April 16 [1943] the President signed a bill enabling the commissioning of women in the Medical Corps for duty as physicians." The logistics of putting this bill into practice are briefly reviewed.

2739.   "Commissioned War Jobs for Women Doctors." Monthly Labor Review, 57 (July 1943) 33.
[Article not examined by editors.]

2740.   "Constructive War Service." Medical Woman's Journal, 47:9 (September 1940) 278. (Editorial.)
Although women physicians should continue efforts to achieve equal rank with men in the military, medical women should strengthen plans for assuming increased responsibility in civilian health care.

2741.   "Contract Surgeon: Esther Cumberland Kratz. World War I." Medical Woman's Journal, 50:3 (March 1943) 67-68.
An autobiographical account is given of Dr. Kratz's work as a contract surgeon during World War I.

2742.   "Contract Surgeons: The Record of Agnes Scholl Ruddock, M.D." Medical Woman's Journal, 49:2 (February 1942) 34-36.
The names of contract surgeons during World War I are listed in the order in which they were hired. "Most of them were hired at First Lieutenant's pay, without rank, pension, bonus, or regulation uniform." Agnes Scholl Ruddock's experiences are herein recorded as given in a personal interview.

2743.   DeVore, Louise. "Letters to the Editor." Medical Woman's Journal, 49:6 (June 1942) 193.
Dr. DeVore happened to be in Hawaii when war was declared and volunteered to work in a military hospital although women doctors are not provided for in the military organization. She urges medical women to support the bill before Congress for a Women's Army Auxiliary.

2744.   "Dr. Coolidge Goes to France." Woman's Medical Journal, 28:3 (March 1918) 65. port.

2745.   "Enters U.S. Army Medical Corps as Contract Surgeon." Medical Woman's Journal, 50:9 (September 1943) 233. photo. (Section on War Service.)
Dr. Poe-Eng Yu, "believing she can best further the free-

dom of China by joining the women of America," entered
the U.S. Army Medical Corps.

2746.   "Equality for Women Doctors." Time, 41 (26 April 1943)
         46. (Medicine.)
         With last week's presidential signing of a bill giving wo-
         men physicians equal status with men in the military, the
         U.S. moves closer to the practices prevalent in Russia and
         Britain.   American women, however, will not go to the
         front; the navy plans to use only 60 of the WAVEs, and the
         army will use only one medical woman for every 500 WAAC
         Though 3,000 of the 8,000 U.S. women doctors could quali-
         fy for service, "most of them are content to work at home.
         What gets their dander up is to see an outstanding woman
         specialist hampered...." Such a case is Dr. Alice Mc-
         Neal of Chicago's Presbyterian Hospital.   When her entire
         operating team went to Camp Robinson in Arkansas, Dr.
         McNeal was left behind.

2747.   "Excluding Women Physicians." Woman's Medical Journal,
         9[8]:4 (April 1899) 112-113.
         The author feels that the superintendent of women nurses in
         the U.S. army should be a woman physician, not a woman
         nurse.

2748.   "First Women Physicians Report for Active Duty in the
         Army." Journal of the American Medical Women's
         Association, 6:5 (May 1951) 195.   photo.   (Medical
         Women in the News.)
         After World War II, the authorization to commission women
         physicians in the army was rescinded.   In 1950 the surgeon
         general reestablished the authorization, and Drs. Ruth E.
         Church and Theresa T. Woo were the first women physi-
         cians to be accepted for service with the army since the
         end of the war.   Dr. Dorothy Armstrong Elias was the
         first woman physician commissioned in the air force (1951).

2749.   Furtos, Norma C.   "The Navy Is My Career." Journal of
         the American Medical Women's Association, 14:4
         (April 1959) 516-517.
         During World War II, women physicians were commissioned
         under WAVE legislation "to care for the female members
         of the Navy and Marine Corps as well as dependent women
         and children."   Dr. Furtos began her military service in
         this capacity but was transferred in an emergency situation
         to care for males.   She recounts her medical career there-
         after.

2750.   Gillmore, Emma Wheat.   "Classification of Women Physi-
         cians Available for Military Service." Women's Med-
         ical Journal, 28:9 (September 1918) 196-198.
         A discussion of the comparative lack of available informa-
         tion (relating to professional fitness) on women physicians

as compared to men physicians, is the subject of this article. The Medical Women's National Association has recently completed a classification of "every female licentiate
in the United States," which is designed to provide ready
information to the war department in order that it might
select qualified women when it so desires women to fill
certain posts.

2751.   Gillmore, Emma Wheat. "Lest We Forget!" Woman's
         Medical Journal, 27:9 (September 1917) 200-201. (Med-
         ical War Notes.)
         "Co-operation is the sure foundation upon which the new
         democracy must rest." Women physicians should seek co-
         operation with their male colleagues, not equality. "It is
         not equal rights that [the woman of today] desires, but the
         right to do unhampered that work which is distinctively
         hers." The woman physician must not stand outside her
         duty in this time of war--demanding equality with men--but
         should be willing to serve her country as a contract sur-
         geon "only," "going where we are sent, doing what we are
         asked to do ... regardless of how humble the medical
         duties assigned to us may be."

2752.   Gillmore, Emma Wheat. "Medical War Notes: Medical
         Women At Attention (Special Article)." Woman's Med-
         ical Journal, 27:7 (July 1917) 159-161.
         Dr. Gillmore, who relates her reaction to the war, writes
         that "these personal reflections would be unpardonable in a
         medical journal if it were not for the fact that I believe I
         am speaking for the woman physician in general...." She
         details her attempt to offer the services of herself and her
         husband to the Allies through the English or French Red
         Cross; her offer was rejected, but her husband--a nurse--
         was accepted for medical war duty. She concludes her
         article with a call for medical women to organize and "stand
         at attention, waiting earnestly and expectantly for an oppor-
         tunity to salute and obey."

2753.   Gillmore, Emma Wheat. "The Rallying of the American
         Medical Woman." Woman's Medical Journal, 28:10
         (October 1918) 222-223.
         A letter by U.S. President Woodrow Wilson is reprinted
         in this article. In the letter [and in the article] the Volun-
         teer Medical Service Corps is praised. This Corps is con-
         stituted of men and women who have sent in their qualifi-
         cations to the Medical Division of the Council of National
         Defense. The qualifications were coded and tabulated, and
         the file is used as a clearinghouse for the army, navy,
         public health service, and for similar needs in times of
         emergency.

2754.   Gilmore, [sic] Emma Wheat. "An Unprecedented Opportun-
         ity for Women." Detroit Medical Journal, 19 (Septem-

ber 1918) 333-334.
The Volunteer Medical Service Corps, Council of National
Defense, has invited women physicians to membership on
an equal basis with men; yet, only one third of the qualified women have registered. Here is an opportunity for
women physicians to "register their qualifications and place
them in an identical coded class system with men physicians."

2755.   Greenbie, Marjorie Barstow. Lincoln's Daughters of Mercy.
         G. P. Putnam's Sons, New York, New York, x, 211
         pp.
         "This is the story of the United States Sanitary Commission,
         the great relief organization of the Civil War, which was
         the ancestor of the American Red Cross ... The WACS,
         the WAVES, the SPARS, and other women's military ser-
         vices find it the first great example of the enlistment of
         women for war." The heroines of this story include Flor-
         ence Nightingale, Dorothea Dix, and Clara Barton. The
         medical work of women physicians is told as well; detailed
         are the activities of Elizabeth Blackwell at the New York
         Infirmary (who met with Dix and other women to form a
         central aid society, and interviewed candidates for army
         nurses). It is also noted that Dr. Emeline Horton Cleve-
         land, who became the first resident woman physician of
         Woman's Hospital in Philadelphia, was one of the sanitary
         corps sent to the Gettysburg battlefield. The book contains
         a preface and a bibliography in narrative form. There is
         no index.

2756.   Haines, Frances E. "Army Service." Medical Wo-
         man's Journal, 49:8 (August 1942) 239-240. port.
         Dr. Haines recounts her struggles to serve in the army
         during World War I. She was appointed contract surgeon
         in the U.S. Army in 1918. This article recaptures the
         conditions under which she practiced her anesthesiology
         while serving in the army.

2757.   "Half-Century Crusade Puts Medical Women in Service."
         Medical Woman's Journal, 50:7 (July 1943) 166-167.
         Reprinted from the 27 June 1943 Los Angeles Times, this
         article observes the culmination of a 50-year crusade to
         gain for women in the armed services of the United States,
         "appointments [and] rank, commensurate with their pro-
         fessional qualifications." Examples are given of how war
         has affected the practice of women physicians.

2758.   Hocker, Elizabeth Van Cortlandt. "The Personal Experi-
         ence of a Contract Surgeon in the United States Army."
         Medical Woman's Journal, 49:1 (January 1942) 9-11.
         The author writes that two times in her life she had wished
         she was a man: first, when admiring her family's physi-
         cian; and second, when men were called into World War I.
         She partially fulfilled those wishes by obtaining her M.D.

at the Woman's Medical College of Pennsylvania and, later, by becoming an army contract surgeon. Dr. Hocker describes her adventures and service in the U.S. Army.

2759. "How Women Doctors Can Help Preparedness. (From the Boston Herald.)" Woman's Medical Journal, 26:12 (December 1916) 296.
Medical inspector of the United States Navy, Dr. N. J. Blackwood, addressed a meeting of the New England Hospital Society to discuss preliminary steps for organizing a unit of women doctors for service in case of war. Women should be prepared to take the places of men and learn "from the great manufacturing houses how drugs are made," organize classes for first aid, become familiar with dietetics, and join the Red Cross.

2760. "In the Service of Their Country." Medical Woman's Journal, 47:6 (June 1940) 183. (Editorial.)
The Journal urges leaders of the American Medical Association Convention (held in June 1940) to plan how best to serve the country in case of war. The editors also call for women physicians to be officially incorporated into the Army Medical Corps.

2761. Josephi, Marion G. "Medical Preparedness For National Emergency." Medical Woman's Journal, 47:8 (August 1940) 255-256.
The Medical Preparedness Committee of the American Medical Association, and the Medical Service Committee of the American Medical Women's Association have both dispatched questionnaires to physicians to determine their preparedness to assume military duty. Although women are included in both surveys, it is legally impossible for them to be commissioned in the U.S. armed forces.

2762. Josephi, Marion G. "Medical Women in the Navy." Women in Medicine, 81 (July 1943) 9-10.
"A short outline of the composition of the Naval Forces" is given by the author, a lieutenant in the U.S. Naval Reserve. Presently, 600 women physicians are desired by the Bureau of Medicine and Surgery. The qualifications for rank and the training period required are discussed. The motto of the Medical Corps is "'To keep as many men at as many guns, as many days as possible.'" Women physicians may be assigned to procurement offices, training schools, Naval hospitals (to provide care for families), naval dispensaries, air stations, naval yard dispensaries (to care for women employees), and marines. A woman physician should consider joining the service if she is willing to obey the regulations. Satisfaction will be gained in the gratitude of patients and in the knowledge that one is helping "'to keep as many men at as many guns as many days as possible.'"

2763.   Josephi, Marion G. "Medical Women of the Navy." Med-
            ical Woman's Journal, 50:8 (August 1943) 198-200.
        The structure, qualifications, training, and medical duties
        in the Medical Corps of the U.S. Naval Reserve are here-
        in given.

2764.   Josephi, Marion. "War Services for Women Physicians."
            Medical Woman's Journal, 49:11 (November 1942) 333-
            334, 344.
        In June 1940, the American Medical Women's Association
        appointed a committee to register, analyze, and to put to
        use American medical woman power in anticipation of the
        country's needs in case of a world war. This report in-
        cludes a discussion of the areas of medical work in which
        women physicians are especially needed: hospital service,
        evacuation units, private practice, industrial medicine,
        United States Department of Labor Maternal and Child
        Health programs, and care of women employed by the
        armed forces.

2765.   Kenyon, Dorothy. "Legal Opinion." Medical Woman's
            Journal, 49:9 (September 1942) 285. (Editorial.)
        Reproduced here is a legal interpretation of the flaw in
        the Surgeon-General's arguments to keep women from being
        appointed to the United States Army Medical Reserve Corps:
        namely that the word "person" is used instead of "male"
        in the United States Army Code.

2766.   Kenyon, Dorothy. "Women Doctors in the Army." Women
            in Medicine, 79 (January 1943) 9-11.
        The author, a judge, discusses the legalisms used by the
        Surgeon General to resist all efforts to put women physi-
        cians on an equal basis with their male colleagues in the
        army.

2767.   "Let Women Doctors Serve Too." Saturday Evening Post,
            215 (20 February 1943) 100.
        [Article not examined by editors.]

2768.   Lobdeli, Effie L. "Conservation--the Keynote of the Plans
            of the Medical Woman's Military Reserve." Woman's
            Medical Journal, 27:9 (September 1917) 202.
        Women physicians should not confuse patriotism and ser-
        vice on the front lines with that which their training has
        prepared them to do. They should conserve their energies
        and take care of people in their home towns. While every
        woman is willing to serve, women physicians should not
        forget that their training entitles them to the same salary
        and rank as men. Neither should women forget that it is
        not the women of the world who are at war with each oth-
        er--it is the men who are at war, and women around
        the world suffer regardless of who is identified as friend
        or foe.

2769.   Lull, George F.   "Opportunity for Women Physicians to
             Contribute to War Effort."   Medical Woman's Journal,
             50:3 (March 1943) 76.   (Editorial.)

2770.   McGee, Anita Newcombe.   "Can Women Physicians Serve
             in the Army?"   Woman's Medical Journal, 28:2 (Febru-
             ary 1918) 26-28.
         Two legal decisions placed before the U.S. Secretary of
         War are reprinted under the heading "Women Unfit for
         Medical Reserve Corps."   Dr. McGee then explains what
         a contract surgeon is and whether or not women can obtain
         commissions in the army.

2771.   McLaughlin, Kathleen.   "Professional Services."   Made-
             moiselle, (May 1943) 94, passim.   illus.
         The impact of World War II is multiplying the number of
         women within many professions--especially within medicine.
         The information contained in this article about opportunities
         for women to study and practice medicine is based on an
         interview with Dr. Margaret D. Craighill, dean of Woman's
         Medical College of Pennsylvania.

2772.   Macy, Mary Sutton.   "Available Means of Organization for
             National Service Among Medical Women of the United
             States."   Medical Record, 91 (21 April 1917) 681-683.
             tables.   (Military Medicine.)
         Dr. Macy presents statistics, delineated by state and ter-
         ritories, on the number of women physicians, their special-
         ties and practice patterns.   [The results of this study were
         also published in Woman's Medical Journal, 27 (1917) 49.]
         Of the 146,612 physicians in the United States and its de-
         pendencies, 5,551 (3.78 per cent) are women.   An examina-
         tion of women's specialties indicates that about 8.82 per
         cent of the women (34.42 per cent of those specializing)
         are equipped for active service on the front.   The remain-
         ing women should be able to carry forward civilian care.
         In her concluding remarks, Dr. Macy points out to her med-
         ical sisters that many opportunities await them in civilian
         practice; they should assume these responsibilities in a
         spirit of cooperation and "sincere appreciation of the great-
         er definite, military value of our medical brothers."

2773.   Maher, Irene E.   "Opportunities for Medical Women: The
             Status of Women Physicians in the Services."   Journal
             of the American Medical Women's Association, 6:1
             (January 1951) 41.
         This article announces that women are now allowed to be
         commissioned in the Medical Corps of the United States
         Army Reserve.   The Air Force also accepts women for re-
         serve and active duty "with the exception that women with
         dependents under the age of 18 years will not be accepted."
         In the navy, a woman is "commissioned as a WAVE and
         then assigned to appropriate medical duties."   The highest

rank a woman physician WAVE may obtain is the rank of
lieutenant commander. She may not be commissioned as
a medical officer.

2774.   "Major Craighill Reports on Health of Army Women Over-
              seas." Medical Woman's Journal, 52:9 (September
              1945) 55.
         Dr. Craighill, consultant to the Surgeon General for wo-
         men's health and welfare, reports that the health of army
         women is "even better than that of the men in many places
         because they have been given a better break in living con-
         ditions."

2775.   [Mason-Hohl, Elizabeth]. "Here's Opportunity: Medical
              Personnel." Medical Woman's Journal, 50:9 (Septem-
              ber 1943) 242. (Editorial.)
         This admonition to sign up for Naval Medical Reserve
         Corps service comes in the wake of the announcement by
         the U.S. Bureau of Naval Personnel that women physicians
         will be recruited into the service. The author urges women
         to shelve their individual ambitions in the name of this
         greater cause. Their medical practice will still be there
         when peace is declared because the patients who come to
         them do so in preference for a woman doctor.

2776.   [Mason-Hohl, Elizabeth]. "List for Service with Auxiliary
              Forces." Medical Woman's Journal, 50:3 (March 1943)
              76-77. (Editorial.)
         Of the over 7,000 women physicians in the country, 4,700
         are in practice; and 2,146 of those 4,700 are within the
         army's age limit. Women who are not eligible for com-
         missions may do part-time work in industries or schools,
         or "special work" in hospitals to aid the war effort. They
         may take over their "doctor husband's work." There are
         only 300 women graduating from medical school each year
         --a wholly inadequate number to meet the medical emer-
         gency.

2777.   [Mason-Hohl, Elizabeth]. "Women Physicians Win Medical
              Corps Status." Medical Woman's Journal, 50:4 (April
              1943) 115-116.
         A history of women physicians' fight for medical corps
         status is presented, as well as an explanation of the areas
         the Sparkman Bill (U.S. Bill H.R. 1857) will affect.
         Credit is given to those women physicians who worked for
         passage of this bill.

2778.   "Medical Corps Commissions Opened to Women Physicians."
              Medical Woman's Journal, 51:1 (January 1944) 25.
              (Section on War Service.)
         Under Public Law 38, women physicians are accepted in the
         navy medical corps on the "same status as men doctors."
         Women will serve within the U.S. continent and will not be

accepted if married to navy men or if they have children
under 18 years old. In addition, women physicians must
be approved for military duty by the Procurement and Assignment Service for Physicians "to prevent undue deple-
tion" of civilian medical services.

2779.   "The Medical Women's Club in War Time." Bulletin Med-
            ical Women's Club of Chicago, 6:7 (March 1918) 2-3.
        War-related activities of the members of the Medical Wo-
        man's Club of Chicago are given in this article.

2780.   "Medical Women's National Association: Report of the Sec-
            ond Annual Meeting, New York City, June 5th and 6th."
            Woman's Medical Journal, 27:6 (June 1917) 140-142.
        This report includes a full account of the meeting's adoption
        of the "California Resolution," which resolved that the As-
        sociation urge the United States War Department to fully
        utilize women physicians, and grant women the same rank,
        title, and pay given to men in equivalent positions.

2781.   "Military Service." Medical Woman's Journal, 49:8 (Au-
            gust 1942) 252-253. (Editorial.)
        While men doctors with families are being drafted for mili-
        tary service, bachelor women doctors are not permitted to
        serve in the medical corps. The American Medical Wo-
        men's Association presented two resolutions to the American
        Medical Association: (1) that the AMA help women physi-
        cians obtain commissions in the medical reserve corps of
        the United States Army and Navy, and (2) that the editor of
        the Journal of the American Medical Association print in
        the Journal a report furnished him by the American Medical
        Women's Association. Neither resolution was adopted by
        the House of Delegates of the AMA. In the meantime, wo-
        men physicians are needed in hospitals, defense plants,
        public health departments, and nondefense practice.

2782.   Mitchell, Elsie Reed and Deal, Louise B. "California Med-
            ical Women Urge Federal Recognition." Woman's Med-
            ical Journal, 27:10 (October 1917) 227-228.
        Because the word "male" or "men" qualifies who may be-
        come an army or navy physician for the U.S. government,
        women are excluded. Two women from the California Or-
        ganization of Women Physicians for Federal Recognition
        write a protest.

2783.   Morton, Rosalie Slaughter. "American Women's Hospitals:
            Organized by War Service Committee of the Medical
            Women's National Association. Headquarters, 637 Mad-
            ison Ave., New York." Woman's Medical Journal, 27:
            6 (June 1917) 136-139.
        An open letter from Dr. Morton, chairman of the American
        Women's Hospitals, precedes questionnaires designed to as-
        certain the number of women physicians who wish to render
        war service and what their preference would be.

2784.   Morton, Rosalie Slaughter. "War Work." In: 75th Anniversary Volume of the Woman's Medical College of Pennsylvania. Westbrook Publishing Company, Philadelphia, Pennsylvania, [1925?], 360-369.
Dr. Morton (M.D., 1897) tells of her activities in France and Serbia during the war, and reviews her part in reconstruction work.

2785.   Morton, Rosalie Slaughter; Barringer, Emily Dunning; Crawford, Mary Merritt; Cohen, Frances; Thomas, Belle; Radcliff, Sue; and Jenison, Nancy. "Report of Work June to October, 1917: War Service Committee of the Medical Women's National Ass'n." Woman's Medical Journal, 27:10 (October 1917) 218-225.
Women physicians of the United States should register their patriotism by engaging in the many opportunities there are to serve their country during the war--both by giving medical service at home and abroad, and by contributing money to the War Service Committee of the Medical Women's National Association.

2786.   Mosher, Eliza M. "California Medical Women Have Splendid State Organization for War Work: Thrilling Campaign Report." Woman's Medical Journal, 28:5 (May 1918) 115.
A letter from Dr. Etta Gray, state chairman of the California medical women's association, tells of the work of a woman ambulance driver and also of a $50,000 campaign to raise money for the American Women's Hospitals.

2787.   Mosher, Eliza M. "War Work for Women Physicians and Surgeons." International Journal of Surgery, 30 (December 1917) 392-394. (Editorial Department.)
Dr. Mosher informs Journal readers of the contributions being made to the war effort by organized women physicians. Specifically, Dr. Mosher outlines the work of the Medical Women's National Association: the establishment in June 1917 of its War Service Committee, and the activities of the American Women's Hospitals.

2788.   Mosher, Eliza M. "War Work of American Medical Women." Boston Medical and Surgical Journal, 177 (29 November 1917) 782-784. (Miscellany.)
Dr. Mosher details the meeting of the Medical Women's National Association, held in June 1917, during which the War Service Committee was established. Her report of the current extensive activities of the American Women's Hospitals (AWH) includes mention of the adoption of an AWH flag and insignia, designed by the niece of Mary Putnam Jacobi. The recent decisions of the Committee on Army Hospitals and the Women's Committee of the General Medical Board are outlined. Dr. Mosher concludes with a list of regulations regarding contract practice in the armed

services. [This article also appears in the Maryland Medical Journal, 60:12 (December 1917) 289-293.]

2789. "Navy Calls for Women Physicians." Medical Woman's Journal, 50:2 (February 1943) 57. (News Notes.)
Requirements are given for women physicians desiring to be commissioned in the U.S. Navy.

2790. Noble, Nellie S. "The Work of Women Physicians During the War." Journal of Iowa State Medical Society, 11: 2 (February 1921) 44-47. (Presentation, Sixty-Ninth Annual Session, Iowa State Medical Society, Des Moines, Iowa, 12-14 May 1920.)
American women physicians followed the lead of Dr. Elsie Inglis who established the Scottish Women's Hospitals in 1914 to offer medical care to soldiers and civilians in the first world war. The first Americans to serve were sponsored by the National Women [sic] Suffrage Association. They established a hospital unit in France in 1918. The Women's National Medical Association [which later became the American Medical Women's Association] formed the American Women's Hospitals which sent 128 women physicians abroad from 1918 to 1920. Their first unit was established in northern France. Other units went to Greece, Serbia, Turkey, and Armenia. This article gives names of some of the numerous physicians who served in both the Scottish and American Women's Hospitals, as well as summaries of the type of work they undertook. It includes data such as locations of hospitals, numbers of beds, size of staff, and number of cases served for many of the units.

2791. "Opportunity and Responsibility." Medical Woman's Journal, 48:4 (April 1941) 117. (Editorial.)
The editor discusses the opportunities for medical women to fill posts vacated by the male physicians going off to war. Medical women now have the chance to demonstrate their ability to fill any medical position and perform any medical job. She advises the women to keep in mind also how the doors of opportunity had swung wide open for women physicians during World War I and had just as surely slammed shut after the war, "when the world took up its usual occupations."

2792. "Our Cause in Congress." Women in Medicine, 80 (April 1943) 8-9.
This article is an account of the author's experience at a congressional subcommittee hearing on the Celler Bill which "provides for a re-definition of the word 'person' to mean 'men and women,'" and the Sparkman bill "to permit women physicians to be commissioned in the Medical Corps of the Army and Navy." The author reviews the testimony given by various witnesses. At one point, the committee chairman read a letter from Secretary of War Stimpson in

which he said the army did not object to the Sparkman
bill: "... every woman who would serve would mean one
less man drawn from civilian practice." The main questions, states the author, regarded care of the civilian population. "Women should stay home to care for women and
children." The bill passed the House by unanimous consent.

2793.   "Pay Allowances for Women Medical Officers." Medical
              Woman's Journal, 51:12 (December 1944) 24.
          New legislation entitles women officers of the Army Med-
          ical Corps to receive the same pay allowances for their de-
          pendents as other commissioned army personnel. Approxi-
          mately 75 women are affected.

2794.   Raven, Clara. "Achievements of Women in Medicine, Past
              and Present--Women in the Medical Corps of the Army."
              Military Medicine, 125:2 (February 1960) 105-111.
              (Presentation, Meeting, Business and Professional Wo-
              men's Club, Lawton, Oklahoma, 12 February 1958.)
          Along with a brief and general summary of the history of
          women in medicine in modern times, women physicians who
          worked in the military in various capacities and their con-
          tributions are mentioned in this article. Mary Edwards
          Walker helped to organize nursing services for the northern
          armies during the Civil War. She also became the first
          woman commissioned as an assistant surgeon. Anita New-
          comb-McGee organized a nursing corps for the army at the
          time of the Spanish-American War. This nursing corps
          served in United States conflicts through World War II.
          When the American Women's Medical Association or-
          ganized the War Service Committee (later the American Wo-
          men's Hospitals), Rosalie Slaughter-Morton became chair-
          man and was commissioned in 1917 to take supplies to
          Serbia. Regardless of women physicians' contributions to
          the military, they still could not obtain commissions at the
          beginning of World War II--only appointments to serve as
          contract surgeons. Clara Raven, who eventually became
          one of the first to receive a commission, helped to gather
          factual data for the legislation committee of the American
          Women's Medical Association. In April 1943 Congress
          passed a bill effective for the duration of the war plus six
          months, authorizing a temporary commission in the med-
          ical corps to qualified women physicians. In 1952 perma-
          nent legislation was passed that enabled women physicians
          to enter the service with the same rights and privileges as
          men.

2795.   "Red Cross Heartily Approves Work of American Women's
              Hospitals, and Will Work with Them." Woman's Med-
              ical Journal, 28:4 (April 1918) 83. port.

2796.   "Red Cross Sanitary Service." Woman's Medical Journal,

27:10 (October 1917) 226-227.
A recruitment letter is reproduced for women bacteriologists and laboratory workers to fill positions for the American Red Cross Department of Military Relief. R. H. Frost, surgeon of the United States Public Health Service, regrets the small proportion of women they are able to accept. Most women applicants placed restrictions on locality and the amount of notice needed to take such jobs, when the public health service needs these positions filled immediately.

2797. Reid, Ada Chree. "Requirements for Commissions." Women in Medicine, 82 (October 1943) 9-10.
The requirements for women physicians who want medical commissions in the army and navy are given in general terms. The army prefers women under 45. The navy specifies that "women physicians appointed in the Medical Corps of the U.S. Naval Reserve may not be married to an officer or enlisted man in the Navy or have children under 18 years of age."

2798. "Resolution on Military Service by Women Physicians." Medical Woman's Journal, 47:7 (July 1940) 224. (News of the Month.)
A resolution from the American Medical Women's Association requested the American Medical Association (AMA) to help women physicians in the military obtain the same rating and benefits as men. The AMA referred that resolution to its Reference Committee on Miscellaneous Business.

2799. "Section on War Service." Medical Woman's Journal, 50:8 (August 1943) 201. port.
This article presents a biography of Dr. Dollie Morgans, who became a contract surgeon with the U.S. Army Medical Corps. Both Dr. Morgans's mother and father, as well as her grandmother and grandfather, were physicians. Dr. Morgans received her degree in medicine from the University of Vienna.

2800. "Seek Rank for Women Doctors in War Zone: Patriotic Society to Request Recognition at Washington." Woman's Medical Journal, 28:3 (March 1918) 68.
The National Society of Patriotic Women of America will request Washington to secure rank, title, and commissions for American women serving as doctors and nurses in European war zones.

2801. "Services Held Cool to Women Doctors." Medical Woman's Journal, 50:10 (October 1943) 266. (Editorial.)
At the same time that the U.S. Army and Navy intend to take more than 80 per cent of the enrollment of all medical schools, women, to be eligible for the military medical corps, must have first received their M.D. degrees. This

places women medical students in the same 20 per cent as
male medical students who cannot qualify for military service. "The woman physician must then pay thousands of
dollars for her education before she can qualify for a commission in the medical corps ... while her brother colleague has his tuition and general expenses paid for him
during his college pre-med course."

2802.   "Shall We Enlist in the Volunteer Medical Service Corps,
            and to What Does that Enlistment Commit Us?" Wo-
            man's Medical Journal, 28:10 (October 1918) 225.
         "Pertinent facts" are presented to help women physicians
         decide whether or not to join the corps. Among the rea-
         sons given is that such a corps is the only chance for wo-
         men physicians "to be listed for military service under ex-
         isting conditions."

2803.   "Share Responsibilities." Medical Woman's Journal, 49:7
            (July 1942) 220.
         Since medical men have had to leave their civilian practice
         in order to care for those injured in the war, all medical
         women should offer their services and, if necessary, take
         refresher courses.

2804.   "Some Interesting Data Regarding the Physicians of the His-
            toric First Hospital Sent to France by the American
            Women's Hospitals." Woman's Medical Journal, 28:6
            (June 1918) 142-144.   photo.
         Personal, individual biographies of the women who went to
         France as the first "hospital" sent by the American Wo-
         men's Hospitals constitute this article. Autobiographical
         sketches are given of Dr. Barbara Hunt, Dr. Margaret E.
         V. Fraser, Dr. Mary Getty, Dr. Kate C. Doherty, as well
         as Miss Lillian Pettingill, R.N., Miss E. Pauline Whitaker,
         R.N., Mrs. Lida M. Tauzalin, housekeeper, and Mrs. Vic-
         tor M. Braschi, ambulance chauffeur.

2805.   Spencer, R. B. "Opportunities for Women in War Medi-
            cine." Medical Woman's Journal, 50:5 (May 1943) 127.
            (Editorial.)
         Trained women physicians may aid the war effort by step-
         ping into medical positions in order to free men for the
         military service. College women "of strong physique who
         have the will to serve humanity and who have special apti-
         tudes" will be encouraged to take courses preparatory for
         medical study. [This article was apparently reprinted from
         War Medicine, July 1942.]

2806.   Starbird, Adele C. "That Forelock Again: The Profes-
            sional Woman's Opportunities." Medical Woman's Jour-
            nal, 50:1 (January 1943) 9-12. (Address, Twenty-First
            Annual Convention, Association of Women in Public
            Health, St. Louis, Missouri, 26 October 1942.)

Only as the result of war were the medical schools' doors opened to women students and women faculty. As a result of war the hospitals have admitted women interns. Will medical women be able to consolidate their gains and hold their positions after the war, or will they lose them as happened in the 1930s after World War I? Women physicians must not spread themselves too thin, they must be selective as to what they devote their energies to. They must guard their leisure and insist upon the public respecting that leisure, also. Women physicians must not settle for "secondary successes"; they must not underestimate their abilities. Dr. Starbird concludes her address with a discussion of the obligations of women physicians in the war effort.

2807.   Strawn, Julia C. "Sanitary Training Detachments for Women." Woman's Medical Journal, 27:9 (September 1917) 202-203.
Looking for a loophole that would enable women physicians to serve in military service, a committee was formed to see if it would be possible for women physicians to serve through the American Red Cross sanitary training detachments.

2808.   Strott, George G. "Women Physicians Desiring Appointments in the Medical Corps of the United States Naval Reserve." Medical Woman's Journal, 50:6 (June 1943) 139, 147.
The professional requirements for appointment in the Medical Corps of the U.S. Naval Reserve are quoted from the Bureau of Naval Personnel manual.

2809.   Thelander, H. E. "Opportunities for Medical Women: Present Status of Medical Women in the Armed Services." Journal of the American Medical Women's Association, 3:6 (June 1948) 255.
"The commissioning of women physicians in the Army and Navy during World War II was a war act, and therefore, was automatically repealed when certain aspects of the war were officially declared over in July, 1947. At that time there were four women physicians on duty in the Army. The Army continued their services but the paymaster stated he was unable to pay them, for which reason two women were ordered home from abroad. The Judge Advocate's office ruled that women physicians could be commissioned in the Women's Medical Specialists Corps Reserve (usually meaning dietitians, physiotherapists, etc., which group was not affected by the repeal) and then apply for active duty and be recalled. This would mean they could not receive the extra $100 per month allowed the male physicians. I have been informed that in order to alleviate this loss in pay these women would not have their rank reduced as was generally done at the end of the fighting war." After this,

there was general agitation to have women integrated into
the regular armed forces, and various legislation was introduced to enable women physicians to receive commissions on the same basis as male physicians in the medical
reserve corps.

2810.   Thelander, H. E. "Women and War." Journal of the
           American Medical Women's Association, 4:2 (February
           1949) 82-83.
         This article presents a discussion of the psychological basis
         of discrimination against women in the armed forces based
         on the book by Dorothy Schaffter entitled What Comes of
         Training Women for War.

2811.   "The Time of Fruition." Woman's Medical Journal, 27:9
           (September 1917) 204. (Editorial.)
         The war and the consequent departure by male physicians
         to the front has opened opportunities previously unavailable
         to medical women: hospitals that had not accepted women
         as interns in the past are now requesting them, and med-
         ical schools are accepting more women students.

2812.   "Uniforms for Women Staff Corps Officers." Medical Wo-
           man's Journal, 50:10 (October 1943) 257. (Section on
           War Service.)
         This article describes in detail the style and design of the
         uniform worn by U.S. Navy women.

2813.   U.S. Congress. Public Law 408--82d Congress, Chapter
           457--2d Session, S. 2552. An Act: To Authorize the
         Appointment of Qualified Women as Physicians and
         Specialists in the Medical Services of the Army, Navy,
         and Air Force. Government Printing Office, Washing-
         ton, D.C., 1952, 1 p.
         This Act in essence states that all laws which authorize
         appointment of male commissioned officers and all laws
         which apply to them, also authorize and apply to commis-
         sioned female officers.

2814.   United States Congressional House Committee on Military
           Affairs. Appointment of Female Physicians and Sur-
           geons in the Medical Corps of the Army and Navy.
           Hearings Before Subcommittee No. 3 of the Committee
           on Military Affairs, House of Representatives, Seventy-
           Eight Congress, First Session on H.R. 824, a Bill to
           Amend the Act of September 22, 1941 (Public Law 252,
           77th Cong.), with Relation to the Temporary Appoint-
           ments of Officers in the Army of the United States and
           H.R. 1857, a Bill to Provide for the Appointment of
           Female Physicians and Surgeons in the Medical Corps
           of the Army and Navy. March 10, 11, and 18, 1943.
         Government Printing Office, Washington, D.C., 1943,
         iii, 101 pp.

Women physicians who testified before the House Commit-
tee, and whose statements are printed in full, include:
Emily Dunning Barringer, Sara Jordon (chairman, Women's
Physicians Committee of Federal Committee of Procure-
ment and Assignment of War Manpower Commission), Helena
T. Ratterman (president, American Medical Women's Asso-
ciation), Anita Muhl, Elaine P. Ralli, Zoe A. Johnston,
Marguerite McCarthy, Kathryn Whitten, Ruth Ewing, Minnie
L. Maffett (president, National Federation of Business and
Professional Women's Clubs, Inc.), Margaret D. Craighill
(dean, Woman's Medical College of Pennsylvania), and Ollie
Josephine Prescott Bairs-Bennett.   Other prominent wo-
men--president of the New York Infirmary for Women and
Children, and representatives of the National Woman's Party
and the National Woman's Christian Temperance Union--
spoke on behalf of women physicians.   Also entered into
the record were reprints of various publications advocating
wartime rating for women physicians and names of signers
of petitions in support of H. R. 824.

2815. "Value of Women's Work." Medical Woman's Journal, 48:
          5 (May 1941) 155. (Editorial.)
        This article consists of a discussion of two "items of inter-
        est" from Great Britain. "The first item recorded the de-
        cision of the British Government to conscript 500,000 wo-
        men for all sorts of work connected with national defense.
        The second item a few days later announced that in this
        conscription all women studying engineering and those study-
        ing medicine were to be exempted." The author suggests
        that the United States could take a lesson from this British
        example of valuing the work of medical personnel in gen-
        eral, and medical women specifically.

2816. Van Gasken, Frances C. "Introductory Address, Woman's
          Medical College, Session 1917-18. September 19,
          1917." Woman's Medical Journal, 27:10 (October 1917)
          216-217.
        Dr. Van Gasken observes that because of the war, there
        are more opportunities for women in medicine than there
        had ever been before. Hospitals, including those that
        never wanted women before, want women as residents and
        staff. Medical schools, like Harvard, which never accepted
        women before are now coeducational, and the General Med-
        ical Board of the Council of National Defense had recently
        appointed a woman physician.

2817. Van Hoosen, Bertha. "The American Press and Medical
          Woman in War Work." Woman's Medical Journal, 28:7
          (July 1918) 154-157.
        "No medical woman, however much she may complain as
        to the injustice of conditions brought to her by the war,
        can say that she has not been treated as a favorite sister
        by the American press." Dr. Van Hoosen follows this in-

troduction with excerpts from the press which substantiate
this statement.

2818.   "Victory Long Overdue: Commissioning Women Physicians
          in Medical Corps of Army and Navy." Independent Wo-
          man, 22 (May 1943) 132.
          [Article not examined by editors.]

2819.   "Victory Luncheon." Medical Woman's Journal, 50:8 (Au-
          gust 1943) 214. (Editorial.)
          A luncheon was held on 26 June 1943 in New York City to
          honor those who assisted during the American Medical Wo-
          men's Association's campaign for commissions for women
          physicians in the army and navy medical corps. A list of
          those in attendance is given.

2820.   "War Doctors." Medical Woman's Journal, 51:4 (April
          1944) 37.
          The army and navy need 6,000 more doctors. To recruit
          women physicians into the medical corps of the armed
          forces, the American Medical Women's Association created
          the Enlistment Committee.

2821.   "War or Peace." Medical Woman's Journal, 47:8 (August
          1940) 255. (Editorial.)
          What would happen to the status of women physicians if
          America were taken over by "totalitarian influence"?
          Readers are encouraged to ponder that possibility when de-
          ciding what influence medical women may exert on the
          question of war and peace.

2822.   "War Ratings Sought for Women Doctors." Medical Wo-
          man's Journal, 49:9 (September 1942) 285. (Editorial.)

2823.   "War Service." Medical Woman's Journal, 52:2 (February
          1945) 39-40.
          The names of women physicians serving in the U.S. Army
          and Navy in various stations constitute this article.

2824.   Willey, Florence E. "An Address on War and the Med-
          ical Education of Women. Delivered at the London
          (Royal Free Hospital) School of Medicine for Women
          on Oct. 1st, 1915." Lancet, 2 (9 October 1915) 802-
          805.
          The war has brought with it many opportunities for women
          in the field of medicine. Young men who would normally
          be training for the professions are enlisting in the armed
          services. With male enrollment down in the medical
          schools, women must make good the deficiency--and this is
          being done, as shown by the "doubling the usual entry of
          this school to-day." Questions of coeducation in medicine
          must now be faced by all medical schools. Even after the
          war there will be a demand for physicians, not only to

treat "invalided soldiers and sailors," but to develop a
thorough system of preventive medicine. Especially needful
branches of preventive medicine will be: (1) the study and
care of pregnancy, (2) the art of obstetrics, including relief of pain, (3) infant and child care, including lowering
the mortality rate, and (4) "the prevention of such diseases
as hinder conception, kill the unborn, maim childhood, and
produce chronic invalidism in women."

2825. "Woman Doctor Asks Equality in Army Duty." Medical
         Woman's Journal, 48:6 (June 1941) 183. (Editorial.)
       Dr. Emily Dunning Barringer submitted to the American
       Medical Association (AMA) a resolution asking the AMA to
       recommend to the U.S. government "that the women of the
       medical profession be given recognition and that the Sur-
       geon-General be requested to make women eligible to the
       reserve corps of the army and navy."

2826. "Woman Medical Corps Captain to Fort Riley." Medical
         Woman's Journal, 50:12 (December 1943) 314.
       This announcement was made on the occasion of Dr. Jessie
       Read's appointment to Fort Riley Station Hospital. Dr.
       Read was one of the first women doctors commissioned in
       the U.S. Army Medical Corps. A brief sketch of her previ-
       ous medical experiences is given.

2827. "Women Doctors Are Needed Now in the U.S. Naval Re-
         serve." Medical Woman's Journal, 50:2 (February
         1943) 54.
       Qualifications for the Woman's Reserve of the U.S. Navy
       are listed. [This article is reprinted from the Los Angeles
       County Medical Association Bulletin, 21 January 1943.]

2828. "Women Doctors at War." Medical Woman's Journal, 50:6
         (June 1943) 156.
       This brief commentary, reprinted from the Woman's Home
       Companion (June 1943), expresses the hope that one good
       thing the war will bring about is the end of prejudice and
       discrimination against women physicians.

2829. "Women Doctors at War." Woman's Home Companion, 70
         (June 1943) 4.
       [Article not examined by editors.]

2830. "Women Doctors Seek Army Rank." Medical Woman's
         Journal, 48:4 (April 1941) 117. (Editorial.)
       The New York women doctors make a continued effort to
       gain military status in the United States armed services.

2831. "Women Doctors Seek War Tasks." Medical Woman's Jour-
         nal, 49:1 (January 1942) 28-29. (News of the Month.)

2832. "Women Doctors to Intern in Navy Hospitals." Medical

Woman's Journal, 56:10 (October 1949) 48.
For the first time in the history of the navy's medical department, women have been assigned to navy hospitals as
interns. The first three women to receive assigned appointments, and 17 others assigned to civilian hospitals under
the navy's Civilian Intern Training Program, are mentioned.

2833.   "Women in the Medical Reserve Corps." Bulletin Medical
         Women's Club of Chicago, 6:1 (September 1917) 5.

2834.   "Women Physicians." Medical Woman's Journal, 50:11
         (November 1943) 280. (Section on War Service.)
"It is the present policy of the [U.S.] Navy Department to
assign women physicians to duties 'ashore in the continental
limits of the United States,' and they are not eligible for
duties in hospital ships or at foreign medical department
activities." Statistics on the number of women physicians
in the U.S. Naval Reserve Medical Corps, as well as their
appointments, are given. This article is followed by a section entitled "Status of Women Doctors in the Navy as of
October 16, 1943" which lists the name, commission, address, and medical college attended of the seven women
who had been commissioned in the medical corps.

2835.   "Women Physicians and National Defense." Medical Wo-
         man's Journal, 47:7 (July 1940) 222. (Editorial.)
The Journal editors observe that it is not too early for arrangements to be made concerning women physicians and
military service.

2836.   "Women Physicians Are Urged to Enlist with the Govern-
         ment in Social Hygiene Division for Fight on Social
         Diseases." Woman's Medical Journal, 28:6 (June 1918)
         146-147.
The Social Hygiene Division was formed by the U.S. War
and Navy Departments' Commissions on Training Camps.
Dr. Katherine Davis heads the section on the education of
women and girls: women physicians are being asked to
give lectures.

2837.   "Women Physicians Desiring Appointments in the Medical
         Corps of the United States Naval Reserve." Medical
         Woman's Journal, 50:12 (December 1943) 305-306.
         port. (Section on War Service.)
In this article, the announcement is made that women physicians are invited to join the U.S. Naval Reserve Medical
Corps. "The requirements for appointment ... for women
physicians will be identical to those established for male
candidates." These requirements are listed in the article.
In addition to these requirements, women physicians who
are appointed to the medical corps "may not be married to
an officer or enlisted man in the navy or have children
under 18 years of age." Following this article is a list of

the names, ranks, and stations of women physicians in the
corps. A more extensive biography of Dr. Cornelia Jane
Gaskill is given, as well as a photograph of Dr. Gaskill.

2838. "Women Physicians in the Army of the United States."
          Women in Medicine, 90 (October 1945) 7-9.
       A rundown on the 75 women physicians commissioned in
       the United States Army as of the date of this article.
       Areas covered include medical schools attended, rank,
       areas of service, and training received in the service. A
       history of women physicians' struggles to be commissioned
       in the armed services is included.

2839. "Women Physicians Medical Department of the U.S. Navy."
          Women in Medicine, 90 (October 1945) 10.

2840. "Women Seek Equality as War Doctors." Medical Woman's
          Journal, 47:12 (December 1940) 377. (News of the
          Month.)
       Speaking before the annual convention of the California Busi-
       ness Women's Council, Dr. Elizabeth Mason-Hohl described
       the barriers women physicians face in seeking equal rights
       with men in military service. Dr. Mason-Hohl also dis-
       cussed discrimination against women students at the Univer-
       sity of Southern California Medical School.

2841. "Women Wanted for the Armed Services." Women in Medi-
          cine, 83 (January 1944) 9.
       Wording of naval commissions (using as an example that
       of Dr. Marion Gertrude Josephi) is given as well as a gen-
       eral recruitment announcement.

2842. "World War I." Medical Woman's Journal, 50:8 (August
          1943) 202. photo.
       This article lists the names of the women physicians (and
       two women dentists) who joined the Red Cross unit in the
       Balkans. Dr. Mary Elliott, one of the women, is singled
       out and her war service highlighted. A group portrait is
       included.

PSYCHOSOCIAL FACTORS

Literature cited in this section examines social
and cultural attitudes affecting women in medicine: the suitability of women for medical
study and practice, motivations for entering
medicine, the need for women's influence in
health care, the problems faced by women physicians, and the attitudes they hold. (Attitudinal material on medical students will be found
in MEDICAL EDUCATION. Reports of the debates over women physicians by specific medical institutions or societies are listed under
MEDICAL INSTITUTIONS, SOCIETIES, AND
THEIR JOURNALS. Material discussing psychosocial factors from a historical perspective
are located in HISTORY OF WOMEN IN MEDI-
CINE.)

AFRICA

2843.   Redaksie, Van Die. "Women Doctors." South African
           Medical Journal, 44:8 (21 February 1970) 201. (Edi-
           torial.)
        "Women are in no way discriminated against in the med-
        ical profession," states the author, and yet can the train-
        ing of women physicians be justified since there are insuf-
        ficient facilities to train doctors and since "a woman is a
        high-risk employee"? A woman physician who is pregnant
        will have to drop out of academic activities for at least a
        year. Since an employer cannot stipulate that a woman be
        hired on the contingency that she not become pregnant, "the
        employer can be reasonably sure that, on the average, each
        of his female medical staff members will at least once or
        twice during her most active professional life be out of
        action for a year or longer." A woman physician is also
        subject to her husband's situation. "It would be a very
        serious step to debar women from entering the medical
        profession ... [however] it might be necessary ... to give
        preference to male applicants for medical studentships."

ASIA

2844.   Brown, Edith M. "Women's Medical Education in India."
           Journal of Sociologic Medicine, 16 (April 1915) 79-82.
        The need for training women physicians in India is dis-
        cussed in this article.

2845.   "Medical Women and Marriage." Journal of the Associa-
           tion of Medical Women in India, 33:1 (February 1945)
           13-14. (Editorial.)
        One solution to the problem of conflict between marriage
        and medicine might be legislating and recognizing the dif-
        ferences between married and unmarried medical women,
        and establishing two "cadres" in any medical women's ser-
        vices: "one for those free from family responsibilities,
        and one for those who are liable to require temporary re-
        lief from active professional work, and who require con-
        sideration in appointments on account of their husbands'
        work."

2846.   Wijnen, M. Elise. "Letter to a Colleague." Medical Wo-
           man's Journal, 50:7 (July 1943) 168-169.
        This letter from Sister M. Elise Wijnen (stationed in In-
        dia) to a medical colleague in Philadelphia, discusses so-
        cial factors of life in India as they relate to the practice
        of medicine there.

AUSTRALIA & NEW ZEALAND

2847.   Thomas, Laurel. "Women in Medicine." Medical Journal
            of Australia, 1:7 (13 February 1971) 405. (Correspon-
            dence.)
         This correspondent notes the practice in the business world
         of warning men of the danger of choosing "the wrong sort
         of wife" and expresses relief that women are not admon-
         ished to marry so cold-bloodedly. Thomas suggests the
         answer to the children and career problem is either that
         society accept the childless marriage as the norm and ap-
         prove of the casual affair, or change its notions about who
         is to be the traditional breadwinner.

CANADA

2848.   Schidler, K. "The Role of Women in Medicine." Cana-
            dian Doctor, (June 1972) 46-49.
         [Article not examined by editors.]

2849.   "Women's Role Vital in Modern Medicine." Canadian Fam-
            ily Physician, (February 1970) 68.
         [Article not examined by editors.]

EUROPE, EASTERN

2850.   Cybulski, N[apoleon]. ["A Response to Prof. Rydygiera's
            Article on 'Admission of Women to Medical Studies'"].
            Przeglad Lekarski, 34:8 (1875) 114-117. (Pol)
         [Article not examined by editors.]

2851.   Dobrzycki, H[enryk]. ["Response to the Articles of Prof.
            Rydygiera and Prof. Cybulskiego, on the Admission
            of Women to Medical Studies"]. Nowiny Lekarskie, 7:
            3 (1895) 226-235. (Pol)
         [Article not examined by editors.]

2852.   Jancovicova, J. ["Problems of Feminization of the Med-
            ical Profession in Slovakia"]. Ceskoslovenské Zdravot-
            nictvi 20:6 (June 1972) 218-222. (Cze)
         "The purpose of the present investigation is to provide in-
         formation on the basic objects of research into problems
         of feminization of the medical profession in the system of
         health services in Slovakia and on the motivation of its de-
         velopment. The latter is based on accumulated problems
         which are the consequence of the expanding feminization of
         the medical profession in Slovakia, in the conflict between
         intra- and extrafamilial duties of women which lead to ob-
         jective differences in the professional and functional posi-
         tion of male and female doctors in the present system of
         health services in Slovakia. The investigation is moreover

focused on assessing the means by which women doctors
try to master equally both parts and the defense mechanisms they create to this end.   The research is also concerned with defining the social role of doctors in general,
the prestige of the medical profession, values which guide
their lives, how they spend their leisure time and what is
the style of living of the investigated medical population.
The investigation was conducted by means of a questionnaire
which was sent at random to 1500 men and women doctors
in Slovakia.   Seventy-six per cent of the questionnaires
were returned and the investigation is thus representative.
In addition to the questionnaire five other research methods
were used." [Journal summary.]

2853.   Janosik, J. ["Popularity and Preference of Men and Wo-
             men Physicians Among Patients"].   Ceskoslovenské
             Zdravotnictvi, 19 (July 1971) 288-294.   (Cze)
"A survey among 82 hospitalized and 72 out-patients of the
Municipal Hospital and Polyclinic in Bratislava gave different results as regards the popularity and preference of men
and women doctors among patients.   In view of the methodical limitations of the ... survey the results are not representative.   They provide, however, material for further
elaboration of the investigated problems.   The majority of
hospitalized patients, as was revealed, prefers men doctors
which on the one hand is due to the assumed or actual
greater experience, knowledge, and skill of men doctors
the patients were in contact with, on the other hand to a
not more closely defined 'confidence' in the work of male
doctors which probably is a residue of the traditional under-
rating of the work of women.   In the survey among out-
patients of the polyclinic the respondents, mostly university
graduates, prefer women doctors.   The popularity of women doctors in this survey is also much greater than of
men.   Even if we take into account the limitations of these
data it is obvious that the positive personal experience of
respondents with the diagnostic and therapeutic experience
with female doctors markedly influences their popularity
as well as their preference.   From the results, however,
it cannot be concluded that there exists a preference of
male doctors among hospitalized patients and a preference
of female doctors among out-patients." [Journal English
summary.]

2854.   Kroslakova, E. ["Views on Professional Knowledge and
             Work of Physicians and Women Physicians"].   Cesko-
             slovenské Zdravotnictvi, 20:4-5 (April-May 1972) 190-
             192.   (Cze)
"By means of questionnaires the author assessed the views
on professional knowledge of doctors among chairmen of
attestation medical commissions in Slovakia and the views
on the specialized work of doctors among heads of the basic
medical departments in Bratislava.   The results revealed

that the professional knowledge of female doctors is evaluated less favorably than the knowledge of men. Evaluation
of professional activities was again in favor of men doctors who displayed more interest in their work, were more
successful and responsible. The majority of respondents of
both groups feels that medical work is not sufficiently ap-
preciated by the public and that the increasing percentage
of women doctors in Slovakia has a negative influence on
the provision of medical care. The respondents feel that
the reasons of the less satisfactory professional development of women doctors are mostly objective ones (professional work and home work) and to a smaller extent are
associated with the women doctors themselves (less concentration on medical work, less willingness to appear in public and avoidance of responsibility)." [Journal summary.]

2855.   Mirek, Roman. ["Feminization of the Medical and Pharma-
         ceutical Professions"]. Przeglad Lekarski, 23:3 (1967)
         356-358. (Pol)
         In the last 20 years there has been a great influx of wo-
         men into medicine and pharmacy until they now make up
         65 per cent of the students in the Polish medical and dental
         schools and 90 per cent in the pharmacy schools. This
         has come about as women in general have won the fight for
         full equality. They are now free to use their talents fully
         in helping the sick and needy through medical care. The
         author attempts to analyze some of the causes for this
         "feminization" of the professions and finds them a complex
         mixture of psychological and economic factors. Many men
         are discouraged from entering the medical profession be-
         cause doctors are the poorest paid and the most restricted
         of all the professions. A large proportion of physicians
         must work at second jobs to earn an adequate income.
         The pharmacists have a little more independence and have
         the possibility of working in the pharmaceutical industry.
         Women seem to be able to organize their lives to fit in
         both professional and family obligations and are equally as
         capable as men. However, the author does not think they
         will completely replace men, many of whom will continue
         to choose a degree of security and a sense of duty over in-
         dependence and higher income.

2856.   Semenoff, A. M. [The Merits of Women with Regard to
         Medico-Pharmaceutical Courses of Instruction]. Mos-
         cow, USSR, 1892. (Rus)
         [Item not examined by editors.]

2857.   "Women Doctors in Russia." Woman's Medical Journal,
         [8]:11 (November 1899) 396.
         Provided is a brief overview of the struggle for medical
         education and public acceptance by Russian women.

EUROPE, WESTERN

2858.   Alvarez Ricart, Maria Del Carmen. ["Some Views on
         Medical Studies for Women in 19th Century Spain"].
         Asclepio, 21 (1969) 49-54. (Spa)
         Spanish publications responded with considerable heat to
         news of women studying and practicing medicine in other
         countries.   Language was used that was "generally ironic,
         indelicate and often offensive."   This article consists of a
         number of quotations, most of them from one medical jour-
         nal, from the years 1865 to 1887, on the subject of women
         in medicine.   A few are favorable, some express confi-
         dence that it could not happen in Spain, some fear that it
         might be possible, and others think women in medicine are
         inevitable but highly undesirable.   The opponents generally
         speak of womanly modesty, loss of innocence, abandonment
         of the family to the ministrations of paid help, and even
         worse possible effects on the medical woman and her fam-
         ily.   The viewpoint was not exclusively Spanish, of course;
         some other countries had made it impossible for women to
         study medicine at home and they had to travel to foreign
         universities to pursue their goal.

2859.   Barbosa y Sabater, Antonio. ["A Word of Advice to Future
         Doctors in Skirts"]. El Siglo Medico, 25:1268 (14
         April 1878) 238-239. (Spa)
         The author raises the familiar arguments against women
         studying or practicing medicine, citing, for example, the
         dreadful things they will go through in school, such as the
         sights and smells of the dissecting room.   Women have no
         idea how difficult it will be to compete for jobs, nor do
         they realize the hazards of practice; one cannot refuse to
         go to a patient just because it is the middle of the night.
         The law does not permit women to serve as experts, so
         they cannot testify in court or make legal reports.   There
         are many other arguments--from their ridiculous appear-
         ance wearing the robe and carrying the staff of office to
         the mere thought of women learning about and treating
         venereal disease.   In the writer's opinion, woman's destiny
         is as the angel of the home, and the closest she should be
         allowed to get to medicine is helping out as a midwife.

2860.   Deschamps, (Mlle.). ["The Role of the Woman Physician
         in Society"].   In: [2nd International Congress of the
         Works of the Women's Institutes, held at the Palace
         of Congresses of the Universal Exposition of 1900.
         Vol. 4].   Charles Blat, Paris, France, 1902, 318-320.
         (Fre)
         The author notes that there are many aspects of this topic,
         but she will consider only the doctor's role as benefactor
         of the poor, the disinherited, the unfortunate of all kinds,
         and try to show the salutary influence which she can exer-
         cise for the relieving of misery and the raising of the fallen.

Briefly she considers the various groups whom the woman doctor can help, especially the woman of "the world" who needs medical care and will accept it from a woman; the working class woman, to whom she can be a friend and teacher as well as a doctor, making life more bearable for the whole family; the woman unable to cope with the world alone, to whom the doctor can be a counselor and friend; to those in prisons and other refuges, to whom she is an inspiration to find their way out of their problems. One does not have to be a doctor to do this kind of work and many lay women have devoted their lives to it, but the doctor brings something more to it and can often open doors closed to others. This is a calling for the woman of love and devotion, who is not afraid of sacrifice and suffering, who looks higher than the misery at her feet to a greater inspiration.

2861.   Dethan, G. ["Advantages and Disadvantages of the Admission of Women to the Professions of Medicine and Pharmacology"]. Journal de Pharm. (Anvers), 53 (1897) 441-445. (Fre)
[Article not examined by editors.]

2862.   Fiessinger, C. ["The Medical Inaptitude of Women"]. Méd. mod. (Paris), 11 (1900) 81. (Fre)
[Article not examined by editors.]

2863.   "Finland." Medical Woman's Journal, 47:12 (December 1940) 377. (News of the Month.)
Dr. Oetiker, the only woman surgeon who served on the battlefield and in the hospital of Finland, reports that the status of women is far better in Finland than in her native Switzerland.

2864.   Gael, A. [The Woman Doctor: Her Raison d'Etre, from the Viewpoint of Right, of Morals, and of Humanity]. E. Dentu, Paris, France, 1868, 103 pp. (Fre)
This is a collection of letters and articles published in l'Economiste Francais between 30 August 1866 and 31 January 1867, plus explanatory notes and a biography of Elizabeth Blackwell. The exchange started with an editorial note that a young woman had been authorized to attend medical preparatory courses in Algiers, where male doctors could not attend women patients. Mme. Gael pointed out that Western women do not like to consult male doctors, especially for female problems, and advocated medical practice by women, for women and children. The Economiste and some of its subscribers raised the usual counter-arguments about the moral, physical, and esthetic dangers to women doctors and their families, as well as interference with the rights and authority of the medical establishment. Mme. Gael answered each objection, frequently citing the experience of American and English women, such as Eliza-

beth Blackwell, Mary Walker, and Elizabeth Garrett.   The
book concludes with a summary of the current status of
the struggle and the biography of Dr. Blackwell, taken from
the English Woman's Journal (April 1, 1858, p. 92.)

2865.   Giraud-Teulon.   ["Women Physicians"].   Gazette Médicale
de Paris, 13:5 (30 January 1858) 57-62.   (Fre)
The author is inspired by a recent article in the North
American Review on the occasion of the graduation of the
first class of seven from the women's medical college in
Harrisburg [sic], Pennsylvania to question the qualifications
of women for medicine.   He doubts their physical strength,
their moral or emotional strength, and their intellectual
capacity, as well as the constancy of their judgment during
the physiological fluctuations imposed on them by nature.
He quotes two letters by the editors of the North American
Review, purporting to be addressed to a woman doctor and
pointing up the problems she faces during pregnancy.   His
recommendation is that these women replace the suture
needle with the knitting needle and return to the role nature
intended for them.

2866.   Holsti and Rosqvist, Ina.   ["Are Limitations Necessary in
Regard to the Right of Female Physicians to Practice
Medicine and Perform the Service of a Physician, and
What Are They, If So?"].   Förh. v. Finska Läk.-
Sällsk. 1899 (Helsingfors), (1900) 14-71.   (Dan)
[Article not examined by editors.]

2867.   Isambert, Emilié.   [The Medical Role of Women].   Joël
Cherbuliez, Paris, France, 1871, 96 pp.   (Fre)
This book consists of the text of a lecture given in 1870 by
the author, a professor of the Faculty of Medicine at Paris.
He states that women have been given by nature a remarkable talent for caring for the sick, but this aptitude needs
to be developed by special instruction.   Women could be
trained to do minor surgery, dressings, and first aid, along
with their more traditional roles as household and neighbor-
hood "doctors" and nurses.   He does not, however, fore-
see the time when French women will be educated and qualified as physicians.   The argument that women physicians
are necessary to cater to the modesty of women patients is
not acceptable.   In the first place, men doctors are sufficiently sensitive and honorable that there is no need for
women to avoid them.   If women doctors are to be restricted to women's diseases, they become superspecialists,
and he believes that the more specialized a doctor becomes
the poorer he is as a doctor.   Women are not physically
capable of doing major surgery or of the long training in
anatomy required for it.   And French women are different
from Americans, who are accustomed to sharing the activities of young men from an early age.   It would require too
great a change in French attitudes and customs for women
to cope with medical education.

2868.   Kirchhoff, Arthur. [Women in Academe: Expert Views on
         Women's Aptitude for Scientific Studies and Professions
         by Famous University Professors, Women's Teachers
         and Writers]. Berlin, Germany, 1897. (Ger)
         This collection of essays on women in academe contains 39
         articles on women in medicine. Written by university pro-
         fessors, they relate their views and experiences in working
         with women students and physicians. The articles offer a
         representative survey of the opinions in the then-raging con-
         troversy concerning women in medicine. While most of the
         articles are by German professors, there are a few views
         from abroad, especially Russia and Switzerland. The book
         contains statistics on women medical students in Switzerland
         and has an index of authors.

2869.   Kronfeld, M. [Women and Medicine: An Answer to Pro-
         fessor Albert and a Formulation of the Problem].
         Konegen, Vienna, Austria, 1895, 54 pp. (Ger)
         The author denies the value of Professor Albert's statement
         by describing him as a misanthrope whose prejudice against
         women interfered with his medical practice. Kronfeld then
         describes the position of women in medicine in Europe, the
         United States, and Russia, naming several female physi-
         cians and their particular achievements. He underlines the
         difficulties female doctors encounter in seeking Austrian
         licensure after studying abroad. Wary of the consequences
         of generalized university studies for women, he proposes
         that only those who are forced to seek a career outside the
         home for financial reasons should be allowed to study.

2870.   ["The Medical Woman"]. El Siglo Medico, 22:1125 (18
         July 1875) 478-479. (Spa)
         The anonymous author notes that the French are awarding
         M.D. degrees to women (in the absence of laws specifical-
         ly forbidding it), while the British Parliament has prohib-
         ited both the granting of degrees to women and admission
         of women to medical studies. And the Belgian government,
         although not approving of women in certain branches of
         medicine, allows them to take examinations without special
         privileges compared to men. He quotes at some length
         from an unnamed proponent of women doctors on the subject
         of womanly modesty and how it should not be a bar to med-
         ical studies, and from an opponent on the inevitability of
         loss of womanly characteristics--"a woman doctor is with-
         out doubt a hermaphrodite or sexless, and in any case a
         monster." The author does not commit himself to any con-
         clusion except to say that there will probably never be any
         great number of women in these unlikely studies.

2871.   Montanier, Henri. ["The Woman Physician"]. Lancette
         Francaise Gazette des Hôpitaux Civils et Militaires,
         41 (21 March 1868) 133-134. (Fre)
         This is an answer to Mme. Gael's recent booklet concerning

women doctors [La Femme Médecin, 1868].   The author
agrees with her noble sentiments on the plight of women
in general, but says that allowing the qualified few to take
up medical careers will not improve this situation much.
As has been pointed out by others, a woman doctor would
have to forego marriage and family since her career would
not allow time for maternal duties.   Mme. Gael says only
a few exceptional women would have sufficient drive to pay
this price; if this is so, they could do little to alleviate
the claimed great need for women doctors to care for women and children.   Nature has established woman's role
and given her the temperament suited to it.   These feminine characteristics would have to be completely changed
for her to face the "ugly spectacles" in medical training
and practice--dissections, autopsies, major surgery, and
patients slowly and painfully dying.   Montanier recognizes
that women could probably learn the necessary sciences as
well as men, and that by French law they cannot be denied
the opportunity, but he thinks the law is a misguided bit of
idealism.

2872.   Moreno, Ldo. Bonifacio Ramirez.   ["Medical Women"].
        El Siglo Medico, 25:1274 (26 May 1878) 334.   (Spa)
The writer says it is most deplorable that persons respected
for their importance in science should have such impossible,
such repugnant ideas as that woman, the most exquisite
work of creation, the loving mother, the delicate angel of
the world, should be allowed to enter a calling so completely
out of character as medicine.   He finds ridiculous, repugnant, and odious the thought of a woman, "armed with a
knife or scalpel, with her delicate hand stained with blood,
amputating a limb or removing a tumor."   The idea of
leaving one's infant at home while one answers a call from
a patient is incredible to him.   In short, modern woman
should take as her ideal Queen Isabella, whose husband
King Ferdinand never wore a shirt that she herself had not
spun and sewn.

2873.   Neumann, Isidor.   ["Should Women Be Allowed to Study
        Medicine?"].   Wiener Klinische Wochenschrift, 27
        (1894) 238-240.   (Ger)
In the controversy regarding women and medical studies,
the author gives a short historic overview of women practicing medicine and especially midwifery, and mentions
some female physicians of modern times.   He describes
the possibilities for women to study medicine in different
countries, mentioning in particular that female physicians
are of importance for Great Britain because Muslim women in India will not accept male doctors.   He uses a similar argument to plead for women's admission to medical
studies in Austria: they must treat female Muslims in occupied Bosnia and Herzegovina.   Moreover, female physicians
might be used to relieve the physician shortage in poor areas

where the male doctors fail to settle. Therefore they
should be allowed to study medicine and then be sent to
predetermined areas to prove that they are of sufficient
benefit to the community to warrant their admission to medical studies as a permanent solution.

2874. Palmieri, Vincenzo Mario. ["Women Doctors and Patients"].
       Riforma Medica, 51 (24 August 1935) 1300-1301. (Ita)
The number of women medical students in Italy has been
decreasing recently, even without restrictive measures such
as those adopted in Germany. The author believes there
are two causes for this: psychological and practical. First,
the drive to compete everywhere and in any way with men
in traditionally male professional, social and political activities has decreased. He likens this development to the
child who no longer wants something he cried for while it
was forbidden. Also, women have paid a high price for
their equality in the loss of their feminine appeal. Men
have come to regard their female colleagues as partners or
pals, not as desirable women. Economically, women have
found that the rewards of their new status were poor. A
few have made it into high academic positions or a good
practice, but most have been limited almost exclusively to
pediatrics, to low-level positions in welfare institutions, or
to volunteer work in clinics. Patients, even women patients, have been reluctant to be treated by women doctors.
There are undoubtedly some good women physicians, but the
great majority are not succeeding in the profession.

2875. Pulido, (Dr.). ["A Little of Everything"]. El Anfiteatro
       Anatomico Español y el Pabellon Médico, (1878) 46-
       47. (Spa)
The author reviews the development of a running argument
in the preceding few years between his journal and La Independencia Medica over whether women should be allowed
to study and practice medicine. He quotes from a pair of
letters in favor, written by a priest, and makes sarcastic
comments on each paragraph. The qualities cited by his
opponent show only that women are suited by nature to be
nurses, but not surgeons or doctors. The main question
is whether women have the intellect necessary for studying
science. The priest says they are better qualified than
men; Pulido says absolutely not. Women have contributed
nothing to science or medicine; in fact, only a few have
contributed anything outstanding even to literature or art.

2876. Pulido, (Dr.). ["Women Doctors"]. El Anfiteatro Anatom-
       ico Español y el Pabellon Médico, (1878) 57-59. (Spa)
In this segment of his argument, Pulido dissects a recent
communication in La Independencia by a Dr. J. La Garriga
concerning the ability of women to absorb a medical-surgical course of instruction. La Garriga believes they could
succeed, even though their intelligence is inferior to that

of men.   Pulido disagrees, repeating the arguments about
the delicacy and spiritual character of women and the damage that would be done to that character by the study of
anatomy.   He then returns to the argument that the mother's
presence in the home is essential to the well-being and
moral welfare of the family and that it and medical practice
are totally incompatible.

2877.   Spaeth, Joseph.   ["Medical Studies and Women"].   Wiener
        Medizinische Presse, 13 (1872) 1109-1118.   (Ger)
In his inaugural speech as president of the University of
Vienna, Professor Spaeth comments on women in medicine.
Arguing that women are inferior because of lower brain
weights, he admits that there are exceptions but is in general opposed to their studying and practicing medicine.   His
main points are that women are superficial and incapable of
profound thought, that they are predestined to procreate,
that medical studies would interfere with the social development of the young female to the point of compromising her
future health, that they are physically too weak.   Women
would be unsuited as gynecologists as they are indiscreet
by nature.   Their admission to lectures together with men
would lead to moral problems.   Concluding, he suggests
that women should receive an education to make them better suited for their natural purpose: the education of their
offspring.

2878.   Wagner, Marianne.   "Medical Women."   World Medical
        Journal, 12:3 (May-June 1965) 88-89.
To illustrate that medical women are not a modern phenomenon, Dr. Wagner recalls the women healers of Scandinavian folklore, of medieval Italy, and of 18th-century Germany.   She then focuses upon the advantages and disadvantages of women doctors.   Female physique (i.e., inferior
strength) accounts for the fact that few women specialize
in orthopedics and surgery.   Demands of marriage and
maternity take its toll on women's professional activity.
And some patients prefer "the authoritative and concise way
of the male physician."   However, women physicians possess the compassion and motherliness needed by some patients.   These womanly qualities "add a touch of the healing art to medical technology."

2879.   "Women-Doctors in Switzerland and Melbourne."   Medical
        Times and Gazette, 2 (27 July 1872) 111.   (Medical
        News.)
"It is pretty clear that if women-doctors really come generally into vogue we must be prepared for a kind of epicene
being 'neither fish nor foul.'"   Accounts of women medical
students from Zurich and Melbourne are cited to substantiate this opinion as well as to underscore the undesirabil-
ity of permitting women to obtain a medical education.

660 Psychosocial Factors

GERMANY

2880. Adam, H. B. ["Women at Universities and Women's Capabilities"]. Deutsche Medizinische Wochenschrift, 22 (1898) 28. (Ger)
The author, a female physician, criticizes male objections to women in medicine based on alleged physical weakness. She argues that the bad health of girls and women is the responsibility of male physicians who fail to instruct them in healthy living. Women are ignorant of their potential because the medical profession does not help them to fully develop their physical and emotional strength. At the same time, this weakness is used as an argument against their admission to medical training and practice.

2881. Albert, Edouard. [Women and the Study of Medicine]. Alfred Hölder, Vienna, Austria, 1895, 38 pp. (Ger)
In his paper, Professor Albert vehemently attacks the admission of women to university studies in general and to medical studies in particular. He bases his ideas on his "observation of thousands of women" as surgeons. His arguments are that women are intellectually and physically inferior to men, that they want children, that they cannot think logically, and that nothing, least of all a university training, could change this situation. His proposal for letting women enter the medical profession is to make them "female physicians' assistants." Women who want to study medicine should do so abroad and not in Austria.

2882. Binder, Sidonie. [Female Physicians: A Study]. Stuttgart, Germany, 1892, 80 pp. (Ger)
This study of women in higher education, especially in medicine, retraces the controversy on the subject that raged during the second half of the 19th century. The author concentrates on the problems of women in medicine and quotes the various arguments against them proposed by men. She feels that women physicians are necessary--especially in gynecology, where social and ethical barriers prevent women from seeking medical advice. She also feels that female physicians should remain unmarried, as the dual charge of profession and family would be detrimental to their professional quality.

2883. Bishoff, Theodor L. W. von. [Women in the Study of the Practice of Medicine]. München, Germany, 1872, 56 pp. (Ger)
In this article the author violently argues against the admission of women to medical education. After exposing the difficulties and the hardships of the medical profession and the high degree of scientific and clinical acumen required by a good physician, the author proceeds to a series of arguments which show that women are unsuited for medicine. His points are mainly based on a qualitative comparison of

male and female anatomy: size of the skull and brain, size
of the digestive tract and the musculoskeletal apparatus,
etc. He concludes that women are closer to the child in
their development, never reaching the height of male evolution. He also argues that their sexual functions make
them unsuitable for higher training in science and medicine.
Admitting women to medicine would, in this view, degrade
the profession to a mere trade and misguide the public,
which would no longer be receiving adequate care.

2884.   Bluhm, Agnes. [The Racial Hygiene Tasks of Women Phy-
         sicians: Writings on the Science of Heredity and Ra-
         cial Hygiene]. Alfred Metzner, Berlin, Germany, 1936,
         99 pp. (Ger)
The author, according to the editor's foreword, was known
for her work on the status of woman, especially as wife
and mother, and the German racial movement. She was the
third woman physician to set up practice in Berlin (in 1890),
and had also done research in genetics at the Kaiser Wilhelm Institute. She received the silver Leibnitz medal in
1931 for her work on the hereditary effects of alcohol.
This book describes the theoretical background of the racial
movement, the political implications of Darwinism, and the
hereditary basis of racial improvement. The physician has
the duty not only to treat disease but also to see that the
genetic material of the populace does not suffer thereby.
The woman doctor is in a special position since women,
who bear much of the burden for preserving and improving
the race, have more confidence in another woman who has
also borne children. She has the responsibility for laying
the groundwork in her patients for accepting and understanding the necessity for measures serving the race, even at
the cost of individual sacrifice. She has the opportunity to
advise individual patients on selection of the best mate and
prevention of genetic damage by avoiding such things as alcohol, drugs, and tobacco, as well as on proper rearing of
children. She should support the efforts of the state on the
basis of her knowledge of individual families and should
contribute to the advancement of genetics by observations
in her work.

2885.   Boerner, F. [Should Women Practice Medicine]. Leipzig,
         Germany, 1750, 16 pp. (Ger)
[Pamphlet not examined by editors.]

2886.   Brupbacher, Fritz. [Obstetrician Runge and the Emancipa-
         tion of Women. A Reply]. E. Speidel, Zurich, Swit-
         zerland, 1899, 16 pp. (Ger)
Professor Runge, a gynecologist from Goettingen, has just
put out a third edition of his booklet on "Woman in Her
Sexual Peculiarities." Brupbacher considers this "product
of pseudoscientific activity" an example of how little honesty
some learned men have and how they "poison the fountain of

knowledge with tendentious rubbish." Runge thinks that because of his long experience as a gynecologist he is one of
the few qualified to speak on the question of women's position.   Brupbacher quotes many statements from the booklet
and counters many with quotes from other authors.   In
discussing the barriers to higher education for women, he
notes that the young male doctor, having passed his state
examinations, goes to any hospital to become an assistant.
"It makes one wonder whether women wouldn't shine at least
as brightly in the gynecologic heavens as Runge, if they had
the opportunity to study with the leading teachers."

2887.   Buchheim, L. ["Against Women Studying at Universities.
          An 'Enraged Opponent' of Female Education Speaks"].
          Münchener Medizinische Wochenschrift, 103 (29 Sep-
          tember 1961) 1885-1888. (Ger)
          [Article not examined by editors.]

2888.   Feilchenfeld, Wilhelm. ["The Need for Women Physicians"]
          Deutsche Medizinische Wochenschrift, 45:47 (20 Novem-
          ber 1919) 1309-1310. tables. (Ger)
          In answer to statements at a recent meeting on the need
          for women doctors to treat the female population, the au-
          thor states his opinion that there is a need but not as great
          as claimed.   For one thing, really sick women who need
          specialist examination and treatment show much less shy-
          ness toward male doctors than the general run of women
          with milder diseases.   He gives statistics from the Char-
          lottenburg and Berlin sickness insurance offices for the
          previous decade (1910-1918), covering numbers of patients
          treated by male and female physicians, which he says show
          that the demand for more women doctors is not as wide-
          spread or as urgent as claimed.   In the Charlottenburg in-
          surance system there was one woman doctor in 1910 two
          in 1911, three in 1912, and four thereafter, compared to
          616 and 717 males (except during the war years).   In Ber-
          lin the number of male insurance physicians ranged from
          around 850 to 1050 between 1910 and 1918, while the num-
          ber of women insurance physicians grew from three in 1910
          to eleven in 1916-18.   The figures also do not indicate
          that women doctors are superfluous; their competition with
          males should benefit mankind.   However, he warns that
          while the early women physicians were a special group se-
          lected by the struggle necessary to get into medical studies
          and into practice, some professors are now beginning to
          complain that the present crop do not perform as well be-
          cause they do not have to fight for their right to an educa-
          tion.

2889.   Gnauck-Kühne, Elisabeth. [University Studies for Women:
          A Contribution to the Feminist Problem]. Schulzesche
          Hof-Buchhandlung und Hof-Buchdruckerei, Leipzig,
          Germany, 1891, 60 pp. (Ger)

Written for the information of the German Parliament, this article on the aims of the women's movement discusses the social and historical background of women's role in society. The author argues that women should be admitted to university studies as they are entitled to the same rights as men, given that they fulfill the same duties in society. Although dealing with the problem of women in higher education in general, the article contains extensive references to the particular problems of women in medicine.

2890. Graetz-Menzel, Charlotte. ["The Racial-Biological Effects of the Academic Careers for Women, with Special Regard to Women Doctors and Dentists"]. Archiv für Rassen- und Gesellschaftsbiologie, 27:2 (1933) 129-150. tables. (Ger)

The author has done a survey on the marital status of 860 women doctors and 140 dentists in six of the larger German cities. Results are presented here in 13 tables, giving age at qualification, marital status, numbers divorced or widowed, occupation of husband of those presently married or divorced, years married, age at marriage, number of children per marriage, number of children by duration of marriage, and the number of children of those married more than eight years. It is obvious that these women are much less likely to marry (50 per cent compared to 73 per cent of the total population over 30), and have fewer children (mean about one per marriage; 43 per cent of marriages are childless) than women in the general population. The article discusses possible reasons for the situation and concludes that it is the duty of educated women, who generally come from the higher levels of society, to see that their heritage is continued, i.e., that they marry earlier and have more children. There must be changes in the form of family life that will enable these women to practice their careers and also do their racial duty.

2891. Hannak, Emannel. [Women and the Study of Medicine: A Critical Review of Professor E. Albert's Essay]. Alfred Holder, Vienna, Austria, 1895, 42 pp. (Ger)

The author refutes point by point Professor E. Albert's condemnation of women's admission to university studies. He underlines the social influences shaping female behavior and denies any anatomic cause for a different intellectual development of men and women. He demands public schools for women to prepare them for university careers and points out the financial necessities forcing many women to provide for themselves. He also pleads for better education for women in general.

2892. Henius, Dr. von. ["On the Admission of Women to Medical Studies"]. Deutsche Medicinische Wochenschrift, 21:37 (12 September 1895) 613-615. (Ger)

In the controversy over women's admission to medical

studies, the author expresses his opposition to women in
medicine or in any other profession. He argues that women are limited by physical weakness and especially psychological and intellectual inabilities: "Women were made
to reproduce not to produce." Moreover, he fears sepsis
if women practice medicine during their menses as they can
not possibly be sufficiently clean on those days. As women
will need a replacement during their menstruation they will
have to practice in the bigger cities where the competition
is hard and they might not be able to make a living, especially as men are much stronger in the existential strife
and women will necessarily succumb. Women should therefore stay with their honored task as mothers and wives.

2893.   Hirsch, Max. [On Women's Education: A Sociological and
            Biological Study]. Wuerzburg, Germany, 1920. figs.,
            tables. (Ger)
         This well-documented study on women in higher education
         contains extensive passages on women in medicine. The
         author examines in detail the various aspects of medical
         study, giving statistical data on choice of specialty, place
         of study, matrimonial state, etc. He concludes that woman
         is capable of scientific endeavor, although her biological
         role seems to be a determinant in her life more than in
         the male. He also examines the effect of medical and oth-
         er university studies on women's physical and psychological
         well-being; he bases his remarks on a survey among fe-
         male medical students and physicians. The book contains
         an index and numerous tables and diagrams.

2894.   Lassar, O. [Medical Education of Women]. Karger, Ber-
            lin, Germany, 1897, 27 pp. (Ger)
         After an introduction on women's education in general, the
         author pleads in favor of women in medicine, with some
         reservations as to their capabilities. He feels that they
         should be given time to adjust to intellectual work and ar-
         gues that the best woman would probably do as well as the
         average male. Women doctors would be an advantage to
         their husbands or fathers, as they could help with their
         work or continue the medical practice after their death and
         thus earn a living. Despite some doubts whether women
         should be independent, the author clearly favors equal edu-
         cational and professional possibilities for women.

2895.   Müller, P. [On the Admission of Women to Medical
            Studies]. Hamburg, Germany, 1894, 43 pp. (Sammg.
            gemeinverständlicher wiss. Vorträge. Series 9, no.
            195). (Ger)
         Part of a series of conferences held by the faculty of Bern
         University, this article concerns the debate on women med-
         ical students. As an increasing number of women remain
         unmarried, they seek new ways to serve society. Medical
         studies and practice are one of their choices. Women are

mentally and with some restrictions physically capable of
becoming physicians.   They should receive the same training as their male colleagues.   In the actual practice of
medicine, the author recommends specialties like pediatrics,
gynecology, and pharmacy, which he deems particularly
suited for women.   He somewhat restricts his approval of
female professionals to those women who are not or cannot
get married.

2896.   Penzoldt, Franz.   ["Medical Studies for Women.   (Part I)"].
         Wiener Medizinische Presse, 40:1 (1 January 1899) 25-
         31.   table.   (Ger)
         This is the first part of a two-part report of a lecture
         given by Professor Penzoldt (Erlangen) at the German Med-
         ical Meeting in Wiesbaden the previous autumn.   He admits
         that he has had little direct experience related to the ques-
         tion of allowing women to study and practice medicine, but
         he has consulted with university professors who have dealt
         with women in medical school and in practice, especially in
         the Swiss schools.   Although there are some 5,000 women
         physicians in America and a large number in Russia, the
         system is different in the U.S., and Russia desperately
         needs doctors, so the experience in these countries is not
         applicable to Germany, where there are already plenty of
         doctors.   If the result in Germany is anything like that in
         Switzerland, where the relatively few women students are
         mostly foreigners, there should be no problem; only about
         300 can be expected in the next 30 years.   Because there
         is no shortage of doctors in Germany, because women
         achieve only average results in school, and because of their
         lesser bodily strength and creative energy, he can not fore-
         see that patients will have any great use for women doctors
         either in general practice or as specialists.   If the same
         conditions are set for women students as for men, there
         should not be any real flood of women to the medical
         schools.

2897.   Penzoldt, Franz.   ["Medical Studies for Women.   (Conclu-
         sion)"].   Wiener Medizinische Presse, 40:2 (8 January
         1899) 71-75.   (Ger)
         The second part of Professor Penzoldt's lecture considers
         four questions: Will any benefit arise for women them-
         selves from their admission to medicine?   Will the admis-
         sion of women have any beneficial results for the univer-
         sities?   Will the status of medicine be advanced?   Will
         there be any benefit to society in general or to the state?
         On the basis of his reasoning and his discussions with col-
         leagues, he concludes that the answer to all these is no.
         The medical profession is already overcrowded, and, al-
         though he agrees that women should have a wider choice of
         occupations, medicine should not be one of them.   If they
         must compete with men, let it be in the professions already
         opened to them--dentistry, pharmacy, nursing--or in indus-

try or business. If they want to help people, let them become trained medical helpers working under the control of
doctors, doing the necessary but time-consuming things such
as dressings, massage, electrical treatments--especially for
female patients.

2898.   Rosenfeld, Siegfried. ["Medical Studies for Women in the
        Present: Part II. Motives and Arguments"]. Wiener
        Medizinische Blätter, 19:4 (23 January 1896) 54-57.
        (Ger)
A large part of the agitation for women doctors has come
from women who do not want to be doctors themselves but
say that sick women should be treated only by members of
their own sex. Being treated by a man offends a woman's
modesty and not only leaves a spiritual scar but may prevent many from consulting any doctor until it is too late for
successful treatment. This view is held by many doctors
as well. However, there is every indication that this is
often not the true reason why women do not consult doctors.
They delay going to the midwife because they fear they may
hear that they have cancer, or because of carelessness, or
because they do not want any stranger to pry into their
secrets, or because they know that often the first symptoms
come too late. Noting that the whole question of "modesty"
is greatly influenced by cultural factors, the author makes
the distinction between innate purity and learned modesty.
Female "modesty" in connection with seeking medical treatment may sometimes be traced to the misplaced jealousy
of husbands. If feminine modesty is as important as is
claimed, similar arguments should apply to mixed classes
in medical schools. But professors at schools with mixed
instruction say they have seen no evidence of offended sensitivity or moral injury in their students. Separate instruction is more likely to turn out half-educated women
than to benefit them.

2899.   Rosenfeld, Siegfried. ["Medical Studies for Women in the
        Present. Part II. Motives and Arguments. (Conclu-
        sion.)"]. Wiener Medizinische Blätter, 19:5 (30 Janu-
        ary 1896) 70-72. (Ger)
Opponents of education for women say woman's place is in
the home; this may be true, but those who do not marry
should have access to all possible ways of making a living.
In any event, experience in other countries has shown that
marriage and medicine are not completely incompatible.
Fear of spinsterhood and poverty is a poor reason for opening education only to unmarried women, considering that
husbands do not always support wives adequately and wives
often have to support husbands. Fundamentally, there is
no work suited exclusively to men. In primitive societies
such as the German tribes, men did nothing except make
war, hunt, and drink while the women did all the work. In
early civilizations, women were the working, conserving

half of the society--often the pioneer discoverers and cre-
ators. Many find the reason women want to study medicine in the female nature itself. It is only a step from
nursing (a traditional occupation for women) to medicine,
and some fear a shortage of nurses if women are allowed
to become doctors. Such a development, however, is very
unlikely: just as not every good smith would make a good
mechanical engineer, not every nurse would make a good
doctor, or want to try. It is not a matter of emancipation
of women, either. Women do not study medicine to become equal to men, but because they are human beings,
already equal to men. As human beings they do not have
to give reasons for wanting to study medicine; it is the men
who must explain why they have deprived women of this
right.

2900. Rosenfeld, Siegfried. ["Medical Studies for Women in the
Present. [Part] III. Qualifications"]. Wiener Medizinische Blätter, 19:6 (6 February 1896) 86-88. (Ger)
The author continues his series countering the arguments
against the admission of women to medical schools and practice. Enough studies have been done to convince him that
women are capable of the work. Unbelievers may say that
the results apply only to individuals, not to women in general, but if only a few are able, the many should be given
an opportunity to see if they qualify. The point is proved
if women meet all the conditions for college study, pass
the tests in medicine as successfully and under the same
conditions as men, and are well regarded in practice.
Most of the arguments can be applied to men as well:
some drop out of school, and some discontinue practice for
one reason or another. It is true that some women are
not suited to become physicians--neither are some men. In
fact, so far there have been relatively few failures among
the women because under present circumstances those with
enough drive to study medicine are an intellectual elite.
Likewise, there have been too few women doctors for us
to be surprised that no scientific geniuses have appeared.
Theorizing about the mental and physical qualifications of
women for medicine is not convincing, since one eyewit-
ness can outweigh a thousand votes that it could not be.
The present "intellectual inferiority" of women is a type
of disuse atrophy resulting from lack of education and stimulation. Lack of physical strength is hardly a valid argument against women practicing medicine, for they do much
harder work by the thousands in factories, on farms, and
as household servants. Most of the characteristics put forward as unfitting women for medical study and practice
are cultural, not inherent sex differences.

2901. Rosenfeld, Siegfried. ["Medical Studies for Women in the
Present. Conclusion"]. Wiener Medizinische Blätter,
19:7 (13 February 1896) 102-103. (Ger)

The final paper of this series attacks the thesis that the
mental differences between men and women, that make the
latter unsuited to the study and practice of medicine, are
the result of differences in the brain itself. True, there
is a difference in cranial capacity, but it is not great. It
cannot be used to prove anything until we can know how
much of the brain is devoted to body function (motor activity) and whether there are differences in fine structure between the sexes. Various authors have listed characteristics they think are essential for the physician, but we all
know male doctors who lack one or more of them, and women in whom some are prominent. In fact, some, such
as well-developed sensory perception and memory, are undoubtedly more characteristic of women as a whole than of
men. Women may not be so well endowed in logical thinking, but if that were essential in a high degree for doctors,
many successful males would have to renounce their profession. The quick perception and comprehension that make
up much of "woman's intuition" are probably more useful
in diagnosis than is logic. The idea that medicine attracts
only superior men is as absurd as the opinion of one teacher that the only person suited to medicine is one who under-
stands four languages and is a good musician. The author
concludes that the arguments against women in medicine
rest on very weak evidence and become weaker every day.
Many learned men who were firm opponents have changed
their minds after first-hand experience: the performance
of women surgeons in the Russo-Turkish war was also
strong evidence of female strength and ability.

2902.   Runge, Max. ["The Sexual Individuality of Women"].
          Deutsche Medizinische Wochenschrift, 23 (1897) 205.
          (Ger)
          Max Runge, a professor of gynecology, wrote a book with
          the same title as this article. In this brief article, he re-
          sponds to criticism of his book and reiterates his claim
          that women are determined by their biological functions.
          Women are subject to physiological cycles that strongly in-
          fluence their psyche. Therefore women must be protected
          by society. Women who want to work should concentrate
          on work aimed at improving the social and medical condi-
          tion of women; however, they themselves should not at-
          tempt to become physicians.

2903.   Rydygier, (Ludwig Ritter v. Ruediger). ["A Propos the
          Admission of Women to Medical Studies"]. Wiener
          Klinische Wochenschrift, 15 (1896) 275-278. (Ger)
          Joining the controversy on women's medical education, the
          author points out that despite the large number of female
          physicians and midwives in the past, women have not con-
          tributed to scientific progress the way barber-surgeons
          furthered medicine. He quotes data proving that only a
          very low percentage of female medical students ever gradu-

ate or practice. Women should, therefore, not be admitted
to medical schools, especially as their different anatomical
and physiological characteristics make them unsuited for
hard work and scientific thinking. Moreover, if women
learn male professions, there will be fewer males who can
provide for a family and thus fewer women in their natural
roles as wives and mothers--as a complement to man.

2904. Schreiter, Anneliese. [Modern Medical Studies for Wo-
        men]. Düsseldorf Academy of Medicine, Düsseldorf,
        Germany, 1957, 40 pp. (Medical Thesis.) (Ger)
        After a short review of the beginnings of the women's move-
        ment, the author surveys the situation of women in medi-
        cine from the early 19th century to our times. The author
        extensively quotes contemporary sources in the controversy
        on women in medicine and discusses the social and political
        forces determining their difficulties in gaining access to
        the medical profession. The thesis contains a bibliography.

2905. Schwalbe, Julius. [On Women in Medical Studies in Ger-
        many]. G. Thieme, Leipzig, Germany, 1918, 63 pp.
        (Ger)
        This essay summarizes the controversy on women in medi-
        cine, presenting arguments for both sides of the question.
        The discussion is based on a survey among university pro-
        fessors and clinicians who were asked to express their
        views on female students and physicians.

2906. Schwerin, Ludwig. ["On the Admission of Women to Med-
        ical Practice"]. Deutsche Zeit und Streitfrage, 131
        (1880) 77-116. (Ger)
        In the controversy on women's medical studies, the author
        pleads in favor of female doctors not only out of justice
        and fairness, but because he feels that they are necessary
        for three reasons: to safeguard social ethics by treating
        women who must otherwise expose themselves to male doc-
        tors, to supply medical care in rural areas, and to guaran-
        tee health services during wars when men are at the front.
        He then explains the educational background required for
        women physicians and gives a short overview of the history
        of women in science and medicine, mentioning some fe-
        male physicians, especially Christiane Erxleben.

2907. Stoll. ["On Female Doctors in the State"]. Jahrbuch der
        Staatsarzneikunde, 5 (1815) 67-90. (Ger)
        In the controversy on women physicians for female patients
        the author argues forcefully against training female physi-
        cians. He pleads that any scientific training would adul-
        terate female morality and ethics and make women into
        lowly copies of their male superiors without the redeeming
        feature of maidenly and wifely submissiveness. Not only
        would female physicians be inferior professionally, they
        would also be inferior as human beings as they forsake fe-

male virtues without acquiring male intellectual prowess.
The historical examples of outstanding women scientists,
rulers, and physicians are not to be taken seriously and,
in the author's view, closer inspection of these women and
their work will show their inferiority.

2908.   Stötzer, F. and Gautsch, H. ["Sociological Investigation on
          Female Medical Students Regarding Their Concepts of
          Their Future Professional Activity"]. Zeitschrift fur
          die Gesamte Hygiene und Ihre Grenzgebiete, (December
          1970) 933-937. tables. (Ger)
The purpose of the study was to examine some problems
of working women--in this instance women physicians--in
a socialistic society. This field is pertinent because a
large number of physicians are women. The investigation
was conducted at the Medical Academy "Carl Gustav Carus,"
Dresden, in 1968. The total number of students at that
time was 591, of whom 277 (46.6 per cent) were women.
Interviews were conducted with 263 women students (95 per
cent). Of those interviewed, 102 (38.8 per cent) stated that
they wanted to practice their profession full-time, six (2.3
per cent) wanted to work part-time. The majority (154, or
58.5 per cent) planned to work part-time occasionally. The
reply depended partly on present or prospective family
status. The women students were also asked how they
plan to specialize. General practice (27.1 per cent), pediatrics (19.2 per cent), and internal medicine (13.0 per
cent) were the most popular specialties. The authors express surprise that only 4.3 per cent chose theoretic-ex-
perimental studies; some guidance in this direction might
be desirable. They express satisfaction that so many women students choose general practice and credit that choice
to the high status given general practice in East Germany,
while in West Germany only 5 per cent of the students
choose this field. The selection of general practice is
largely due to availability of positions and the provision of
living quarters. Only 32.1 per cent of the respondents
want to work in hospitals, and 4.5 per cent in administration. Only 16 per cent are willing to work in rural districts; 84 per cent want to stay in the city. Based on the
survey results, the authors concluded that women medical
students, in light of the complex problems facing them,
need to be better guided vocationally so that they might become more aware of the alternatives open to them, and the
areas and types of professional employment best suited to
their personal needs. Also, the authors agree that flexible employment opportunities (i.e., for part-time employment) in all areas of medical specialization need to be
created so that the talents of these women will not go to
waste because their situations preclude full-time employment.

2909.   Weber, Mathilde. [Women Doctors for Women's Diseases:

An Ethical and Sanitary Necessity].   Tuebingen, Germany, 1888, 46 pp. (Ger)
This article stresses the need for women doctors as a
means of improving the health of women.   The author argues that for reasons of modesty many women fail to see a
male physician until late in the disease process when cure
is impossible.   The existence of trained women physicians
would encourage women to seek medical advice at an earlier
stage.   The author is in favor of separate training facilities
for women in anatomy and in clinical training.

2910.   Zehender, Wilhelm von. [On Women's Vocation for the
Study and Practice of Medicine: A Speech Made in the
University of Rostock on February 15, 1875].   Rostock,
Germany, 1875, 37 pp. (Ger)
The speaker, a professor of medicine, maintains that women are inherently incapable of scientific endeavor.   They
should be excluded from medical study because of intellectual and ethical reasons.   Professional training for women
would undermine the foundations of German womanhood.

GREAT BRITAIN

2911.   Aitken, Janet K. and Lawrie, Jean Eileen. "The Career
of the Married Medical Woman with Children." World
Medical Journal, 11:1 (January 1964) 23-24.
This study discusses the problems of women physicians in
England.   Married women with children are obliged to find
part-time work that enables them to fulfill their household
commitments.   Part-time work all too often is temporary
or of such an insecure nature that it makes many women
feel unwanted and/or like failures.   It is easier for women
physicians to practice when domestic help is available.
The psychiatric profession creates further problems by
making mothers and husbands feel that unless the mother
is devoting herself to the child, she is doing an inadequate
job.   Since women are the ones who bear and rear children,
the state should make some adjustments for women lest the
world lose their talents.   At the time women apply to medical school, they should be told about the time and energy
they must devote to medicine and the problems this is going
to cause their marriage, and if they are not prepared for
such sacrifices, they should not enter medicine.   Postgraduate refresher courses followed by part-time and full-time
appointments available all over the country and not just at
university centers would help women reenter the field of
medicine.   Hospital staffing problems could complement the
needs of married women for part-time jobs.   There could
be part-time training programs in specialties so that married women could fill some of the shortages there.   There
could be more secure part-time training programs.   There
could be more comprehensive information about the medical

needs and opportunities in different parts of the country and in different specialties.

2912.   Blackwell, Elizabeth. "The Influence of Women in the Pro-
         fession of Medicine." In: Essays in Medical Sociology.
         Vol. II. Ernest Bell, London, England, 1902, 1-32.
         (Address, Opening of the Winter Session, London School
         of Medicine for Women, October 1889.)
         In summing up her speech, Dr. Blackwell says that she
         tried to show: "(1) That women, from their constitutional
         adaptation to creation and guardianship, are thus fitted for
         a special and noble part in the advancement of the healing
         art. (2) That the cultivation of the intellectual faculties
         necessary to secure their moral influence requires a long
         and patient training by methods that do not injure morality.
         (3) That the noblest department of medicine to which we
         can devote our energies, will be through that guardianship
         of the rising generation which is the especial privilege of
         the family physician."

2913.   Burt, Charles. "London School of Medicine for Women."
         British Medical Journal, 2 (4 October 1902) 1017.
         (Opening lecture, London School of Medicine for Wo-
         men, London, England, 1902.)
         In his speech, "Medicine as a Profession for Women," the
         treasurer chairman of the board of the Royal Free Hospital
         discusses the increased opportunities for and recognition of
         women physicians. Reminding the students that "medical
         women must be the brightest, purest, and most gracious
         of their sex," Burt urges the women to refrain from ciga-
         rettes, observe Sundays, and lead a "humble Christian
         life."

2914.   "Dismissal of a Married Medical Woman in England."
         Medical Woman's Journal, 28:11 (November 1921) 287.
         The St. Pancras Borough Council dismissed Dr. Gladys
         Miall-Smith as a maternity medical officer on the grounds
         that she has married. This editorial calls the move a
         "mischievous doctrine ... ancient and musty and in re-
         spects an economic fallacy."

2915.   Drysdale, C. R. Medicine as a Profession for Women.
         London, England, 1870.
         [Item not examined by editors.]

2916.   Elmes, Margaret and Shrubshall, Nancy K. "Women Doc-
         tors in the N.H.S." British Medical Journal, 1:5957
         (8 March 1975) 572-573. (Letters to the Editor.)
         Two women [physicians?] reply in separate letters to Dr.
         Dora Black's article "State of Health" (which appeared in
         the 28 December 1974 issue of the Journal, on page 732).
         Elmes feels the problem of the married woman doctor's
         child-care expenses could be solved if the present system

of personal taxation were revised. Shrubshall is tired of
hearing these mothers demand preferential treatment, as
it was their choice to "gratify their maternal instincts."

2917.   Fawcett, Millicent Garrett. "The Medical and General Edu-
            cation of Women." Fortnightly Review, 10 (1 Novem-
            ber 1868) 554-571.
        More has been done for the medical education of women
        than for their general education. Both subjects are con-
        sidered at length in this article. Those who advocate ad-
        mitting women to medical education are divided on the ques-
        tion of whether to subject women to the same training as
        men. Treating women as "a class apart" is a way of per-
        petuating the defective education of women. American wo-
        men have done a great deal of pioneer work, but their ef-
        forts toward achieving equal status with men in the pro-
        fession have been disappointing. A large section of this
        article discusses six reasons for the inferior general edu-
        cation of women, and a closing section discusses the idea
        of a new college for women as opposed to opening the ex-
        aminations to women at the University of London.

2918.   Female Doctors; or, Advice to Married Men. Contained in
            Letters Which Appeared in the Public Press and Are
            Now Compiled by B. A. Cantab. Manchester, England,
            [1861].
        [Item not examined by editors.]

2919.   Fletcher, Walter. "The Future of Women in Medicine."
            British Medical Journal, 2 (9 October 1926) 653-654.
            (Address, London School of Medicine for Women, Lon-
            don, England.)
        This article discusses the general problems of medical
        education, the problems of women's medical education,
        fields of work suitable for women physicians, and the prob-
        lem of combining marriage and a medical career.

2920.   [Gardner, Mabel E.] "English Women and Marriage."
            Medical Woman's Journal, 37:2 (February 1930) 49.
        When a woman physician in Birmingham, England applied
        to be reinstated in her annual appointment at the General
        Hospital, she also asked for four months' leave of absence
        to have a baby. This action precipitated the committee to
        advise the Board of Governors "that married women should
        not be appointed to the hospital, and that when women phy-
        sicians marry they should be asked to resign. This step
        was taken, so they reported, purely in the interest of the
        hospital services, so that they should not be interrupted."
        Lady Florence Barrett, dean of the London School of Medi-
        cine, responded by saying, "Either the character of the in-
        dividual or the quality of the work done should be the only
        reasons for dismissal." The newspapers called this inci-
        dent "another hospital sex war."

2921.   Hutchison, Robert. "'To Match the Men.' An Address at
            the Opening of the Winter Session of the London School
            of Medicine for Women at Exeter." British Medical
            Journal, 2 (1 November 1941) 623-62$\overline{5}$.
         Sir Robert Hutchison, M.D. acknowledges the pitfalls of
         generalizing about sex differences. His own experience
         proves, however, that the woman doctor is like "the little
         girl who had a curl ... when she is good she is very very
         good, and when she is bad she is horrid--even horrider
         than a bad man doctor." Sir Hutchison holds definite opin-
         ions on the subject of medical women. On coeducational
         medical schools: "Nymphs and shepherds may play togeth-
         er, but if they work together there is apt to be a good deal
         of time lost in dalliance." On studying medicine: women
         are more conscientious, greater worriers, and tend to over-
         work (this can lead to "staleness"). On applying for resi-
         dent posts: "if you paint your nails you are infallibly and
         rightly damned" (he wishes women doctors wore a uniform).
         On choosing a specialty: many women cannot stand the
         strain of general practice; public health jobs lack adventure
         but are "useful and safe." And, on matrimony: medical
         education is not really wasted on women, for they "make
         excellent wives, while their qualification is always a second
         string to their bow."

2922.   Ivens, Frances and Ramsay, Mabel L. "Women Doctors."
            British Medical Journal, (24 January 1925) 192. (Cor-
            respondence.)
         Dr. Ivens laments the limited number of resident appoint-
         ments available for women. Dr. Ramsay discusses the
         situation of discrimination against women in hospital ap-
         pointments. Why are women physicians not put in charge
         of beds or in chief positions in hospitals when the number
         of women and children patients are triple the number of
         male patients? "Pure prejudice on the part of the male
         colleague, I fear, must be the answer."

2923.   Ligertwood, Laura M. "The Things That Matter." Med-
            ical Women's Federation News-Letter, (March 1930)
            46-54. (Inaugural Address, Women's Medical Society,
            Women's University Union, Edinburgh, Scotland, 17
            October 1929.)
         Dr. Ligertwood discusses love, religion, art and nature as
         "things that matter to ourselves." In the medical profes-
         sion, remember that you are a marked woman--marked
         with the seal of your profession, your school, and your
         country; and "above all" a woman. "... be as womanly
         as you can ... make it an especial prayer that you may be
         kept a soft, loving, gracious woman to the end. Do not
         ape masculinity in your dress or your behaviour. You can
         never be a man and so you only become a neuter gender,
         than which there is no more objectionable object in this
         world."

2924.   "London Letter (From Our Own Correspondent): London,
              November 1, 1921." Medical Woman's Journal, 28:11
              (November 1921) 282-283.
         The opening section of this letter, titled "Women and Med-
         icine," deals with the refusal of several London medical
         schools to admit women. While granting that sex antagon-
         ism may be a factor, the action is attributed to overcrowd-
         ing: "There is scarcely room for the men." The situa-
         tion at the University of Cambridge is reviewed. Serving
         as an example of one London institution where women dom-
         inate is the Royal Free Hospital. Lamentably, research
         work at the hospital is hampered by a funding shortage.
         The author regrets that situation, since women's patience
         especially suits them for specializing in research.

2925.   "Manchester Medical School: An Analysis of the Entries
              of Women Students, 1899 to 1923." Medical Women's
              Federation News-Letter, (March 1931) 37-39.
         The statistics and remarks in this article were excerpted
         from an address by Professor John Stopford, given before
         the Manchester and District Association in November 1930.
         Among the survey findings: of the total women who had
         qualified, about 44 per cent were married, and more than
         half of these had retired from medical practice. While af-
         firming that marriage and medicine were not incompatible,
         Professor Stopford "felt that marriage stood for something
         much greater and more fundamental than medicine or a
         medical career."

2926.   "The Medical Education of Women in London." Medical
              Woman's Journal, 35:6 (June 1928) 157-159. (Feature
              Article.)
         Although the University of London was the first British uni-
         versity to admit women medical students, certain of its 12
         medical colleges now declare intentions to no longer admit
         women. Reasons for the desire to close their doors to
         women are: women are unable to contribute to the school's
         athletic life; women embarrass male students and lecturers
         by being present when "delicate" matters are discussed;
         and women marry and give up their profession and there-
         fore clinical opportunities are wasted upon them. The ar-
         ticle's author, identified only as someone "high in the
         councils of the British Medical Women's Federation," dis-
         misses the first two reasons as too petty to discuss. She
         responds to the third reason by quoting from a survey which
         found that 77.48 per cent of the 1000-member Federation
         were actively practicing medicine. The writer adds: "...
         there must be some truth in the contention that the real
         underlying objection to the medical education of women is
         in reality due to a sex antagonism ... which is probably
         due not to a lack of faith in the mental, physical, and in-
         tellectual abilities of women ... but rather to the fear that
         competition may be still keener in the future than it has

been in the past, and that this competition may result in a
falling off of earning capacity in men, if they do not 'watch
their step.'" It is recommended that the University of
London induce all of its schools to take a quota of medical
women students.

2927.   Murrell, Christine M. "Presidential Address." Medical
         Women's Federation News-Letter, (November 1926) 19-
         26. table. (Presentation, Council of the Medical Wo-
         men's Federation, Leeds, England, 22 October 1926.)
         Dr. Murrell feels the two greatest problems facing women
         physicians are "those connected with marriage, and those
         connected with lack of cohesion." In this address, Dr.
         Murrell concentrates on the latter problem. Discrimination
         against women in the profession is still present and active
         and several examples of such are given. Dr. Murrell dis-
         cusses the benefits of separate education for women physi-
         cians, women's obligations as members of the British Med-
         ical Association, and the need for solidarity and support
         among women physicians in general.

2928.   "Restrictions Against Married Women." Medical Woman's
         Journal, 38:9 (September 1931) 233-234.
         "The prejudice and antagonism so rampant during suffrage
         days, now pent up and rendered inarticulate owing to the
         great change in the position of women, has been concen-
         trating itself on an attempt to keep married women out of
         wage-earning and salaried posts," declared Lady F. M.
         Dickinson-Berry at the annual meeting of the British Med-
         ical Women's Federation.

2929.   Rolleston, Sir Humphry. "An Address on the Problem of
         Success for Medical Women." British Medical Journal,
         (6 October 1923) 591-594.
         The problem of success for medical women lies in the fact
         that "variability, both in body and mind, is more frequent
         in the male than in the female sex, so that genius, orig-
         inality, and initiative, as well as idiocy and crime, are
         more frequent in men than in women, who tend to preserve
         a more equable level; men have a greater aptitude for ab-
         stract problems, women for concrete subjects." This ac-
         counts for the fact that there are no women doctors of out-
         standing ability on the order of a Lister, Koch, or Osler.
         Sir Humphrey feels, in addition, that it "seems improbable"
         that a woman doctor "would consciously abstain from re-
         search and striking out a new line because it is commonly
         regarded as peculiarly a man's sphere." Sir Humphrey re-
         views the various opinions on the difference between the
         sexes. It is a generally accepted view that "genius is even
         rarer in women than in men." Whether this is due to in-
         herent sex peculiarities or is the result of long-continued
         dominance of the male sex, or to both these factors, Sir
         Humphrey feels is an academic though "interesting" question.

2930. Roughton, E. W. "An Address on Woman's Sphere in Med-
          icine." British Medical Journal, (8 October 1910) 1027-
          1029.
       This address was delivered at the London School of Medi-
       cine for Women. The author, a surgeon to the Royal Free
       Hospital, submits that owing to the inventions of anesthesia
       and antiseptics, surgery has been made a gentle art and
       therefore suitable to "the most tender hearted man or wo-
       man." Medicine is not only a suitable profession for a wo-
       man, but it is also a desirable one in that "everybody ...
       would agree that ... women should be attended by persons
       of their own sex." Mr. Roughton feels strongly that "the
       more the sexes are separated in medical matters the bet-
       ter." He is opposed to mixed classes of medical students
       and advocates separate hospitals for the sexes. Tertiary
       sexual characteristics, capable of being influenced by edu-
       cation and discipline, are important in deciding the suita-
       bility of a sex for medical work. Women, as a result of
       the necessary division of labor between the sexes, have
       developed a sense of dependence upon the male. There are,
       however, some independent, self-reliant women, and these
       women seek medical careers: "Take every opportunity of
       increasing your self-reliance by doing things for yourself
       as much as possible." While men have the muscular ad-
       vantage, women are more "mentally adaptable" and there-
       fore more tactful. However, they also have a greater capa-
       city for dissembling and must guard against this practice
       in medicine. "Another result of the primordial differences
       in the male and female environments is that the woman's
       mind retains more of its child-like characters than does
       that of the man." Brain size and woman's intellectual ad-
       vantage is also discussed. Pediatrics, obstetrics, and hy-
       giene, Mr. Roughton concludes, are suitable medical fields
       for women.

2931. Savage, Anne and Griffiths, Sheila M. "Women Doctors."
          British Medical Journal, 1 (23 June 1962) 1763-1764.
          (Correspondence.)
       In two separate letters, Savage and Griffiths suggest how
       married women doctors can become established in regular
       work.

2932. Summerfield, G. P. "Women in Medicine." British Med-
          ical Journal, 3:5934 (28 September 1974) 802. (Letter
          to the Editor.)
       The writer states that before equality between the sexes in
       medicine can occur, there must be "a change in the pattern
       of child-rearing in society as a whole."

2933. Swayne, Walter C.; Naish, A. E.; and McCall, Eva. "Wo-
          men Doctors." British Medical Journal, (7 February
          1925) 283. (Correspondence.)
       Dr. Swayne writes that during the past 10 years, 20 women

have obtained their medical degrees from the University of
Bristol. "I may also mention that two of the senior assistants to the full-time medical professors in the University are women. This does not appear to indicate that
there is any prejudice in this school against women as
such." A. E. Naish examines the question of prejudice
against women in hospital positions and feels that "when women as a body have shown themselves capable of shoulder-
ing the responsibility and worries of practice it will not be
long before they are admitted as readily as men to hospital
posts."

2934.   Timbury, Morag C. and Timbury, G. C. "Glasgow Wo-
            men Medical Students: Some Facts and Figures."
            British Medical Journal, 2 (24 April 1971) 216-218.
            tables. (Contemporary Themes.)
This study attempted to find possible connections between
the married medical woman's decision to practice full time
and her background. For this purpose a postal questionnaire
was sent to the 343 women studying medicine at the University of Glasgow during the academic years 1968-69, and
1969-70. Of the 317 women who responded, 14 were married (4.4 per cent) and five had a child. When the students
were asked if they had any doubts about their choice of medicine, "the incidence of doubts was about the same among
the girls in the early years of their study but increased
sharply in those who were nearing the end of their training."
Girls at the start of their course attributed doubts to difficulty with examinations, and the length of the course; in
later years, the difficulty of combining a medical career
with family life was cited as reason for doubt. "Relatively
more girls with doubts had a working mother" (51.3 per
cent). "The significant association of doubts about medicine
and having a working mother may indicate a more realistic
attitude among the girls whose mothers were working to
the difficulties of combining a career with family responsibilities.... This suggests that having a working mother may
be the main factor which determines whether or not a woman continues working after marriage." Pediatrics was
the most popular specialty with obstetrics, medicine, psychiatry, surgery, and anaesthetics being other main choices.
"... over a third of the girls said that they thought that
women were not so good at science as men but that they were
sympathetic as doctors and more suited to work with female
and child patients than men. Fifty-four of the girls believed that women were better at repetitive work than work
requiring initiative and 11 thought that men made better doctors." Two-thirds (98) of the women identified as the most
important aspect of a doctor's work as giving advice and
reassurance; 20 women thought that the primary task of a
doctor was to advance scientific knowledge about disease.

2935.   Ulyatt, Kenneth and Ulyatt, Frances Margaret. "Attitudes of Women Medical Students Compared with Those of Women Doctors." British Journal of Medical Education, 7:3 (September 1973) 152-154. tables.

This study was prompted by the authors' suspicion that early retirement among women physicians is not entirely due to "circumstances," but rather to "personal qualities." An attitude survey previously shown to distinguish between women physicians known to have practiced medicine for the greater part of their lives and physicians who performed only minimally was completed by female medical students at the Royal Free Hospital School and at Nottingham University. The results indicate that attitudes conducive to working or retiring after marriage are already present among women students as early as the first year of their studies. The authors suggest that this attitude survey or other "indirect" methods would reveal "under-lying feelings" of women applying to medical school: "If this could be done it would be possible to accept girls who are discovered to have no fear of neglecting and so harming their families, rather than girls who regard constant personal maternal care as the only safeguard against abnormality or delinquency in their children."

2936. Ulyatt, K[enneth] W. and Ulyatt, F[rances] M[argaret]. "Field and Training Performance of a Group of Women Doctors." Medical Officer, 124 (1970) 33-34.
[Article not examined by editors.]

2937. Ulyatt, Kenneth and Ulyatt, Frances Margaret. "Some Attitudes of a Group of Women Doctors Related to Their Field Performance." British Journal of Medical Education, 5:3 (September 1971) 242-245. table.

An attitude survey attempted to understand the differences between practicing and semi-retired married women physicians in England. Fifty-four statements on the position of married women in society, their relationships with husbands and children, professional education and responsibilities, and the effect of a working wife upon the home, were framed. The instrument was sent to 50 married women who practiced 90 per cent of the time and 50 women who worked the shortest time based on a previous study. There were 36 returns from each group. Scoring was done on a five-point scale (-2 to +2) with positives used when professional concerns predominated. The women who had been most in practice produced more positive scores. The same test was administered to a population of 62 girls in sixth form (from whom medical students are drawn). The schoolgirl scores were more directly related to those of the semiretired women physicians. It was found that the greatest differences between the working and semiretired physicians were in 14 statements related to child care and domestic responsibilities. These were extracted and sent for amplification to the 12 highest working scorers and the 12

lowest semiretired scorers. The returns were given to 16
doctors and social scientists who assigned them to either
working or semiretired classifications with a significant
degree of correct assignment. Sixteen statements producing the least difference on the initial survey were sent to
the next 13 high and low scorers in the initial survey. The
same judges correctly determined the working women but
had difficulty identifying the semiretired physicians. The
results suggested that spending a large part of life in medical practice altered the working women's perceptions. The
practicing physicians appeared able to maintain a feminine
role without the passivity or inner-directedness characteristic of female socialization. The authors compared their
findings with a study conducted by Ginzberg in 1966. They
suggested that the work performance of women graduates
in medicine might improve if it were possible to more adequately explore the self image of girls applying for university entrance.

2938.   Walton, H. J. "Sex Differences in Ability and Outlook of
         Senior Medical Students." British Journal of Medical
         Education, 2:2 (June 1968) 156-162. fig., tables.
"Many of the differences found between men and women may
be explicable on the basis of the admission procedure utilized by the medical school. Women applicants are less acceptable than men, and fewer gain entry (Bowers, 1966).
The smaller quota admitted will usually be more competent
and possibly more intelligent than their male counterpart.
However, this explanation is likely to be a partial one. The
selection of women for medicine is probably a process
which starts earlier during school education. For a girl
to plan a medical career, and to seek to enter medical
school, perhaps requires greater intellectual ability than is
the case with boys. Qualities of personality are also likely
to be important. The women among fifth-year medical students are more competent at their medical school studies
than men, taking professional examination performance as
the criterion. In the specialty of psychiatry they also performed better, both in acquiring factual knowledge and in
film tests of clinical skill. Women had higher Neuroticism
--that is, a greater level of anxiety. In addition, they
were less extroverted--they were more withdrawn socially
and less impulsive. They had less need from teachers for
guidance with their studies than male students. While they
were more censorious of the psychiatrists who taught them,
they were less moralistic towards patients than the men
students. Women are less technical, more practical, and
more patient-centered in professional orientation. They are
not prone, as men are, to consider the psychiatry instruction gave them greater understanding of their own personality. Women become more aware than men of the limitations of advice-giving as a method for helping patients.
Men are rather less committed to their psychiatry training,

less critical, and more inclined to take a detached view of the instruction provided for them." [Article summary.]

2939.   West, Charles. Medical Women: A Statement and an Argument. J. & A. Churchill, London, England, 1878, 32 pp.
The author of this publication is a fellow of the Royal College of Physicians of London. [Item not examined by editors.]

2940.   Wilks, Samuel. "The Admission of Women to the University of London." Lancet, 1 (19 May 1877) 738-739. (Correspondence.)
A professed "liberal" (his friends even call him a "radical"), the writer addresses himself to the question of the fitness of women for medical study. He notes that while the objections to women's medical education find basis in "physiological laws," the women's advocates' arguments are based on political laws of liberty, equality, and justice. Women's advocates thus "ignore the rights of nature ... they will scatter natural laws to the winds and replace them by any number of artificial ones."

2941.   Wilks, Samuel. "The Admission of Women to the University of London." Lancet, (2 June 1877) 818. (Correspondence.)
Those who would admit women to the study of medicine at the University of London are largely nonmedical people who are ignorant of the vigorous scientific training needed for a medical career. They argue that women are particularly suited to "the administration of medical solace and relief," but is this different from saying that women make excellent nurses? The writer maintains that women are physically and intellectually unsuited to a career in medicine.

2942.   "Women and the Medical Profession in Great Britain." Medical Woman's Journal, [28]:1 (January [1921]) 20.
When "Mrs. Simon, Lady Mayoress of Manchester" refused to visit a local hospital because no women were associated with its management, a lively debate ensued in the British press. Among the published comments were "clichés about women disliking to serve under women ... [and] nonsense about women and the home...."

2943.   "Women in Medical and Other Professions." Medical Woman's Journal, 37:8 (August 1930) 231.
Even though women physicians distinguished themselves during World War I, the number of women accepted to train in medicine in England has declined as has the number accepted in allied professions like dentistry. One possible reason for this decline is that families are more likely to support the education of boys rather than girls during economically pressing times. Women doctors are needed in the British colonies to care for native women and children.

2944.   "Women Physicians." Medical Woman's Journal, 46:2
             (February 1939) 58. (Editorial.)
         In an address at the opening session of the London School
         of Medicine for Women, Lord Horder said that "a good
         man physician has a little more of the feminine in him
         than the average man, and that a like statement applies to
         a good woman physician." Although originality may be
         more common in men, women have more intuition, con-
         science, curiosity, industry, and spiritual sensitivity.
         Lord Horder concluded that "it is the woman in the phy-
         sician that medicine wants just as much as the physician
         in the woman."

INTERNATIONAL

2945.   Bickel, Beatrix A. "Medical Non-Missionaries." Medical
             Woman's Journal, 52:12 (December 1945) 41-44.
         This article provides autobiographical insight into the ex-
         perience of being raised in a missionary home. Dr. Bick-
         el's father had given permission for her to study medicine
         in the hopes that his daughter would become a medical
         missionary. These hopes were frustrated, as Dr. Bickel
         did not go into missionary work but settled into a medical
         practice for a time in Hamburg, Germany. The author
         does include a variety of incidents from the reports of
         medical women missionaries. Many women doctors, at the
         close of the 19th century, were considered sexually ab-
         normal due to their choice of work. At this time the
         book, The Third Sex, was repeatedly sent to women physi-
         cians. Dr. Bickel illustrates, through various cases,
         some of the difficulties of dealing with sexual variations in
         women patients, working in rough neighborhoods, quieting
         irate male patients, and dealing with female Russian spies.

2946.   V[an] H[oosen], B[ertha]. "The Woman Physician and the
             Training Nurse." Medical Woman's Journal, 37:8
             (August 1930) 230-231.
         When [women] nurses are trained by women physicians rath-
         er than by men physicians, there is more sympathy and
         less antagonism between women physicians and nurses and
         better patient care. The army considers the woman nurse
         as "essential" as a male army surgeon but a woman sur-
         geon is an "interloper" in peace or war. "If the woman
         physician can succeed in gaining recognition from the army,
         she can only hope to do so by demanding an equality with
         the trained nurse."

2947.   Zenil, Sara. "The Woman Doctor Is a Social Necessity."
             Medical Woman's Journal, 55:7 (July 1948) 22-24.
             (Presentation, First Congress, Pan American Medical
             Women's Alliance, November 1947.)
         In this speech (published in both Spanish and English), Dr.

Zenil discusses the woman physician's "natural gift for relieving suffering humanity, not only physically, but also spiritually." She proposes that the Pan American Medical Women's Alliance honor the memory of Matilde P. Montoya, Mexico's first woman physician. She also proposes that the Alliance encourage an international confederation of women doctors.

SOUTH, CENTRAL, LATIN AMERICA AND MEXICO

2948.   Garcia Arroyo, Maria Luisa; Procel, Matilda Hidalgo de; Bermudez, Laura Contreras de; and Amat, Ana. "Problems Confronting Medical Women in Ecuador." Journal of the American Medical Women's Association, 11:10 (October 1956) 357-359.

Although legally there are no restrictions to obtaining a university education, the Ecuadorian women live under heavy cultural, prejudicial constraints. Dr. Matilda H. de Procel was the first woman in Ecuador to get her Bachelor's degree (in 1913). Social pressures exerted in the home constitute "the most serious problem confronting the woman physician" in Ecuador.

UNITED STATES

2949.   Abramowitz, Stephen I.; Weitz, Lawrence J.; Schwartz, Joseph M.; Amira, Stephen; Gomes, Beverly; and Abramowitz, Christine V. "Comparative Counselor Inferences Toward Women with Medical School Aspirations." Journal of College Student Personnel, 16:2 (March 1975) 128-130. table.

This study was conducted to amass additional data on the bias exhibited by vocational counselors in regards to women "who excell in traditionally masculine occupational areas, such as medicine." It was hypothesized that traditional counselors would be more likely than untraditional counselors to regard as psychologically maladjusted, women who were motivated toward and had the aptitude for medical studies. Ten counselors and 12 graduate students with counseling interests were the subjects. One-half of this group were women. Results show that a "medical-school aspiring (i.e., sex-role transgressing) female evoked more stern judgments from morally traditional assessors than from liberal ones...." The female counselors were more lenient in their judgments. There is evidence also that the more experienced counselor will exhibit more prejudice against the unconventional woman than will the less experienced counselor. Professionals should be sensitized to value-encroachments on applied activities, suggest the authors.

2950.   "Aiken Heart, M.D." The "Doctor Woman." How I Was
        Cured by a Female Physician. Detroit, Michigan,
        [n.d.].
        [Item not examined by editors.]

2951.   Alpert, H. "Women Doctors Preferred?" Harvest Years,
        11 (August 1971) 36-40. illus.
        [Article not examined by editors.]

2952.   "Alumnae Discuss Roles As More Women Enter Medical
        Profession." Downstate Reporter, 4:3 (Summer 1973)
        1-13. chart., photos., ports.
        At Downstate Medical Center 21.8 per cent of the 1973-1974
        entering class are women. The situation for women med-
        ical students at Downstate is discussed. In an interview,
        Dr. Iris Slater, a 1961 graduate, says that women's libera-
        tion movement is "ridiculous" because women are very
        pampered in America. She speculates that as the status
        of medicine declines in this country, more women and few-
        er men will be attracted. Dr. Marie Zeterberg feels the
        biggest problem for women in medicine is finding adequate
        household help. Dr. Barbara Delano states that "women are
        not encouraged by society to think that it's possible for them
        to become physicians." Several other women physicians'
        opinions are also given.

2953.   "American Pioneer...." Medical Woman's Journal, 51:7
        (July 1944) 32.
        Along with some historical background on the ways in which
        the New York Infirmary for Women and Children has been
        a pioneering hospital, this article compares medical wo-
        men's status at the time of the hospital's founding (in 1857)
        to the present [1944]. Following are some of the ways in
        which "the anti-feminist attitude toward women doctors still
        flourishes." Of New York City's 58 hospitals approved for
        intern training, 14 still refuse to accept women interns;
        and, unlike male students, women are denied army- and
        navy-paid medical educations.

2954.   Anthony, Catherine W. "Is There a Prejudice Against Wo-
        men in the United States?" Journal of the American
        Medical Women's Association, 24:10 (October 1969)
        787-788.
        Since the 1848 Women's Rights Convention in Seneca Falls,
        New York, there has been "a vigorous attack on men's
        domination of women ... and ... women have continually
        sought to break down barriers for equality." Of working
        women in the United States, 75 per cent are working at
        routine jobs and seven per cent are doctors. Women com-
        prise 2.5 per cent to 24 per cent of students who are ad-
        mitted to medical schools around the country, which average
        out to ten women per medical class. Of all the countries
        in the world, the United States is the fourth from the lowest

in its percentage of women physicians. On medical school faculties, women are only three per cent of the full professors. To change this discrimination, admissions should be integrated on the basis of qualifications. Since women share equally in the financial responsibilities, they should share equally in the educational facilities as well. Recruitment should change. Educators and members of the medical profession should change their attitudes that women are not a good investment and tend to be less productive than men. Women physicians should band together and keep communications open to help advance women to the status for which all women must strive.

2955. Applebaum, Ann Halsell. "Motivational Factors in the Choice of Medicine as a Profession by Women." Journal of the American Medical Women's Association, 15:4 (April 1960) 355-361.
Motivational factors based on psychoanalytic theory are presented. The author discusses the psychodynamics of femininity and its relationship to career choice.

2956. Arnold, Anna W. "Women in Medicine--50 Years of Progress." Medical Affairs, (Fall 1971) 2-7. illus., port.
Dr. Arnold looks back a half-century, when she was one of nine women of the Class of 1921 at the University of Pennsylvania School of Medicine. Quoting from a variety of other sources, she traces the increased opportunities for women to the present, and highlights the existing problems for medical women. She calls for more retraining programs and part-time residencies, flexible working hours, and increased opportunity for professional advancement.

2957. "As Others See Us." Woman's Medical Journal, 1:4 (April 1893) 63-64.
An editorial on women entering the profession of medicine is reprinted from the Philadelphia Times and Register. The writer stresses that the woman who insists upon being independent must be willing to fight the battles previously fought for her by men, be self-supporting, and weather the storms from which she was heretofore shielded by her "strong-armed protector." "With her feeble frame, her physical encumbrances, her mental organization warped and misdeveloped by the inheritance of ages of irresponsibility, she steps into the arena to contend ... in the struggle for existence." In short, her liberated position means to her what it did to the disenthralled slave. And of course the effect of such freedom is the abrogation of motherhood.

2958. Austin, Grace Baliunas; Maher, Margaret M.; and LoMonaco, Carmine J. "Women in Dentistry and Medicine: Attitudinal Survey of Educational Experience." Journal of Dental Education, 37 (November 1973) 11-17. tables.

Alumnae and students from the classes of 1966 through
1976 of the New Jersey Dental School, New Jersey Medical
School, and Rutgers Medical School were surveyed to determine how they felt their educational experience was affected by the fact that they were women. Of 196 questionnaires sent out, 97 were returned. Most women, according to the survey, did not feel there was overt discrimination in their educational experience. Many of the respondents did perceive subtle prejudice, however. Overall, 77
per cent felt that they had encountered no more difficulties
than their male counterparts.

2959.   Barclay, William R. "The Future for Medical Education
         and Women in Medicine." Journal of the American
         Medical Women's Association, 28:2 (February 1973) 69-
         70. (Address, Annual Meeting, American Medical Wo-
         men's Association, Columbus, Ohio, 14 November
         1972.)
         The author, a vice-president of the American Medical As-
         sociation, says that medical schools favor admitting women
         because women's credentials are often better than those of
         male applicants. He anticipates that the function of the
         physician will change from that of being a person in direct
         contact with the patient and to whom the patient feels "def-
         erence," to that of being a decision maker, coordinator,
         and administrator for other health personnel who will have
         direct care of the patients. Because medical knowledge
         has a half-life of five years, what has been traditional in
         medical curriculum has changed. Medical education has
         become a life-long continuum rather than a succession of
         formal education experiences. When the function of the
         physician changes, women may be better equipped than men
         to fill the role of physician--when they "will not receive
         the direct and warm gratitude patients have customarily
         given"--because "the traditional roles which women have ha
         to play in society" have prepared them [to do thankless
         work]. More women may find the practice of medicine a
         viable career because of the changes taking place in the
         amount of time spent in training and practice, i.e., that
         undergraduate premedical majors may enter medical school
         after three years of college, that medical education itself
         may take less time, that peer review is more conducive to
         the work of part-time physicians than for those engaged in
         full-time medical care, that physicians will no longer have
         to work sixty-hour weeks but will be able to adjust their
         working hours to the complex systems they will direct.
         Women physicians will find these flexible schedules more
         conducive to the "privilege of raising a family."

2960.   "The Bars Against Women." Time, (11 January 1971) 31.
         (Medicine.)
         Despite the great need for physicians, women make up only
         seven per cent of the country's 300,000 doctors. There is

a need for more flexible scheduling for women with family
obligations. Schools which have begun to meet these needs
are Boston's Children's Medical Center and New York Medical College. More changes are expected as the Department of Health, Education, and Welfare begins to take an
active part in sex discrimination charges.

2961.   Bass, Elizabeth. "Longevity...." Journal of the Ameri-
           can Medical Women's Association, 1:9 (December 1946)
           329.
         "Statistics show that women physicians are remarkably long
         lived." In a search of the obituary columns of women's
         medical journals, the author compiled these statistics: of
         1,776 women physicians, more than 180 lived beyond the
         age of 70; more than 112 lived to 80 years and over; more
         than 65 lived beyond 90 years; and "a few" reached 100.

2962.   Batt, Roberta. "Creating a Professional Identity." Amer-
           ican Journal of Psychoanalysis, 32:2 (1972) 156-162.
         Potential women physicians need models to emulate. Pro-
         fessionals, however, are "socialized" into their roles by the
         medical community, and in the process often they acquire
         the prejudices and biases of the community. Two processes
         that make socialization of a woman physician difficult are
         distortion of language and unexamined prejudice. Language
         is used to evaluate and control (e.g., use of words like
         "assertive" for the male and "aggressive" for the female
         in the same situation), and women soon learn to become
         what they are labeled. "The destruction of certain attributes
         of women's character by selective use of language ... leads
         to the self-fulfilling fact in many cases of dull, passive, in-
         secure women professionals." Unexamined prejudice may
         be described in the words of Philip Goldberg: "'women do
         consider their own sex inferior, and even when the facts
         give no support to this belief, they will persist in down-
         grading the competence--in particular, the intellectual and
         professional competence--of their fellow females.'" The
         author also points out that men and women are different,
         and these differences do not imply female inferiority. Con-
         firmation by others of these differences is necessary.
         Some of the more overt prejudices against women physicians
         are dismissed in conclusion (i.e., fraternities refusing ad-
         mission to women; lack of financial support for women
         medical students, etc.).

2963.   Bennett, Alice G. "Would You Let Your Daughter Study
           Medicine?" Woman's Medical Journal, 25:6 (June 1915)
           128-129. (Presentation, Ninth Annual Meeting, Women's
           Medical Society of New York State, Buffalo, New York,
           April 1915.)
         Dr. Bennett describes events leading up to her daughter
         Emma's decision to study medicine and her own reactions
         to that intention. In a more general vein, Dr. Bennett

discusses the increased opportunities for women physicians
and the compatibility of marriage with a medical career.

2964.   Bennett, Laura B. "The Prophecy of the Ephah and a
         Prophecy by a Medical Woman." Woman's Medical
         Journal, 29[19]:3 (March 1919) 41-43. (Original Arti-
         cles.)
         Dr. Bennett uses a story from the prophecies of Zachariah
         to illustrate how women are rising up on the wings of wis-
         dom elevating earth's standards to a place "between earth
         and heaven." The author speaks of the advancement of
         women in medicine and of their ideals.

2965.   Blackwell, Elizabeth and Blackwell, Emily. Medicine as a
         Profession for Women. Printed for the Trustees of
         the New York Infirmary for Women, 1860.
         [Item not examined by editors.]

2966.   Bluestone, Naomi. "Marriage ... and Medicine." Journal
         of the American Medical Women's Association, 20:11
         (November 1965) 1048-1053.
         This article is primarily about how difficult a woman med-
         ical student or doctor who wants to marry a compatible
         man will find it. A woman desiring to become a doctor
         "will wonder if being doctor must mean giving up mar-
         riage.... Charges of masculinity, homosexuality and
         egg-headedness among female physicians will also be rapidly
         dismissed. The unwelcome and threatening fears are
         pushed aside; she wants to become a doctor, it is her
         privilege.... The heart-warming myth of the doctor wed
         only to her art and suffering humanity must bow to the
         more realistic position of most practitioners who go through
         life without a husband to enrich them. The unhappy truth
         is that if a woman fails in her task of maintaining a har-
         monious balance of all the great needs in her life, she may
         actually damage the image of the American woman in medi-
         cine by attitudes and emotional expressions which betray
         the truth."

2967.   Bodley, Rachel L. Valedictory Address to the Twenty-
         Second Graduating Class of the Woman's Medical Col-
         lege of Pennsylvania. Published by the class, Phila-
         delphia, Pennsylvania, 1874, 15 pp.
         Reminding the graduates that they are the last class to
         have been instructed by Professor Ann Preston (who died
         in April 1872), Dr. Bodley quotes from Dr. Preston's 1870
         valedictory address. Dr. Bodley further impresses upon
         the class the historical significance of the upcoming Amer-
         ican centennial. She gives examples of how the 19th cen-
         tury has proven to be the "Century of Woman," focusing
         upon advances in women's higher education and women's
         missionary work as a distinctive movement. Finally, the
         graduates are charged to "guide skillfully, guard-conscien-

tiously, mould wisely, and all this, in the interest of home,
of purity, and of Heaven!"

2968. [Bowling, W. K.] "Female Doctors." Nashville Journal of
       Medicine and Surgery, 2 (1852) 123-124. (Editorial.)
       While Dr. Bowling is "as gallant and fearless an advocate
       as any" of woman's progress, he feels that the practice
       of medicine is not "in the line of her progress." Medicine
       in practice is "too arduous, too exacting for her fragile
       mechanism." In addition, Dr. Bowling feels it is not true
       that women patients will turn to women physicians more
       readily than to men physicians, for "it is woman's nature
       to trust men in the hour of her affliction and calamity."
       "Shrewd women invariably choose their confidants from the
       opposite sex." Dr. Bowling concludes his article by label-
       ing women's efforts to enter the realm of medical practice
       as a "will-o'-the-wisp chase after an impossibility."

2969. Broome, Claire V. "Discrimination at Harvard." Harvard
       Medical Alumni Bulletin, 49:6 (July-August 1975) 42.
       port.
       Dr. Broome begins with a general discussion of the subtle-
       ties of discrimination against women physicians. She re-
       calls an anecdote which illustrates women's questioning
       their own perceptions of discrimination and men's often un-
       awareness of their own bias. Instances of discrimination
       have a cumulative effect and should be dealt with through
       "increased sensitivity and openness" in discussing them.

2970. Brown, William Symington. The Capability of Women to
       Practice the Healing Art. Ripley, Boston, Massa-
       chusetts, 1859.
       [Pamphlet not examined by editors.]

2971. Buchanan, J. Robert. "The Selection of Medical Students."
       Journal of the American Medical Women's Association,
       24:7 (July 1969) 555-560. (Presentation, the Josiah
       Macy, Jr. Foundation Conference on "The Future of
       Women in Medicine," Williamsburg, Virginia, 8-11
       December 1968.)
       If the subjective obstacles that women have to face when
       they have a professional career were to be eliminated,
       more female applicants would apply to medical school.
       "... the heart of the problem of the admission of women
       to medicine ... is that female graduates of medical school
       do not devote as much time to medical activities after
       graduation as do men...." He also says that there must
       be ways "of keeping the female physician as available for
       professional activities as her male counterpart while at the
       same time allowing for her role as a wife and mother."
       Until a solution is found, "admissions committees across
       the nation will be forced to continue their present practices
       with respect to female applicants." To fill the "pressing

medical and social needs of disadvantaged urban areas,"
this doctor suggests recruitment of black women. He notes
"the traditionally dominant role of the female in the black
community" would fit in with "the general preference of female physicians for careers in pediatrics, psychiatry and
internal medicine."

2972.   "The Bulletin's Line on Women, 1955-1975." Harvard Med-
            ical Alumni Bulletin, 50:1 (September/October 1975) 34-
            38.   cartoon.
        This section consists of excerpts from the last 20 years of
        the Harvard Medical Alumni Bulletin. Mildred F. Jefferson
        (class of 1951) wrote in October, 1955 of her struggles
        against prejudice since graduating from Harvard: "Were
        the situation less tragic, it would be downright comical."
        In 1972 the Bulletin announced a historic event: the first
        woman to be appointed to an associate deanship in the his-
        tory of Harvard Medical School--Mary C. Howell, M.D.,
        Ph.D.   In April, 1975, Dr. Howell resigned that post:
        "The job of 'woman administrator' would mean that a wo-
        man-identified woman would have some voice in the admin-
        istrative policies of the school, especially with regards to
        matters concerning students.... I have had little access or
        opportunity to affect policy...." Other alumnae who are ex-
        cerpted include Dr. Raquel Cohen and Dr. Doris Bennett.
        Dr. Leona Baumgartner wrote in 1972 to tell the story of
        why she went to Yale Medical School and not Harvard.

2973.   Byford, William Heath. "Doctorate Address." Chicago
            Medical Journal and Examiner, 48:6 (June 1884) 561-
            574.   (Original Communications.) (Commencement
            address, Woman's Medical College, Chicago, Illinois,
            22 April 1884.)
        Byford's address to the graduating class discusses prevalent
        arguments against the suitability of women for the practice
        of medicine and concludes, in each case, that the argument
        is erroneous. Labor-saving machinery frees women from
        full-time domestic duties; many women need an independent
        means of support; useful knowledge never degrades a per-
        son; women's physical strength is attested to by the labori-
        ous farm duties performed by so many; women can be
        trained to acquire nerve and courage; many women physi-
        cians and surgeons have proved their competence and skill.
        The address concludes with words of encouragement to the
        new graduates.

2974.   Caldwell, Ruth. "Women in Medicine: Chapter [V] The
            Present Status of Medical Women." Medical Woman's
            Journal, 37:9 (September 1930) 254-255.
        There are a variety of factors, this author proposes, that
        every woman in medicine should be aware of to alleviate
        further prejudice against women physicians. There is a
        reluctance of people to consult a first-rate woman doctor,

preferring instead to consult a mediocre man doctor under
the assumption that women would not have access to the
broadest experience and training possible. To overcome
this prejudice, the author suggests that "each woman in
medicine give the best kind of service available and ask for
no special privileges." Another reaction against women
doctors is that "women who take up medicine lose the
charm of a woman, becoming masculine in dress and man-
nerisms." As a solution to this objection the author proposes "each girl ... pay just a little more attention to her
appearance than she feels she has time to, remembering
that it is for the good of all medical women...." Another
objection to training women is that "they simply get married and never use it." In fact, 80.2 per cent of those
graduating between 1905 and 1910 and who are married were
in full-time practice, and 5.8 per cent were in limited
practice. Only 13.9 per cent did not practice. Of the
single women, 93.8 per cent were in full-time practice.
Because so many women patients are reluctant to see male
doctors, it is important to have women physicians.

2975. Carpenter, Elizabeth. "Address: Delivered at the Sixty-
seventh Annual Commencement of the Woman's Medical
College of Pennsylvania." Bulletin of the Woman's Medical College of Pennsylvania, (September 1919).
Elizabeth Carpenter congratulates the graduating class on
four points: becoming alumnae of the Woman's Medical
College of Pennsylvania; being women; graduating in 1919;
and having such diverse and unusual opportunities awaiting
them. While alumnae should be proud of Woman's Medical
College's unique position as the only U.S. medical school
for women and with a woman dean, it should be remembered
that the institution has been "aided and abetted by men."
Urging that more praise and credit be given to men who
help women, the speaker laments the "unreasoning and unnecessary antagonisms between the sexes." The "rare
privilege" of being a woman at this point in history carries
with it the obligation to find new solutions to world problems "and cultivate fields that men would never have cul-
tivated." As 1919 graduates, medical women follow the
glorious traditions of their counterparts who distinguished
themselves in the world war. Finally, the new work opportunities opening up to women physicians are discussed.

2976. Cartwright, Lillian Kaufman. "Conscious Factors Entering
into Decisions of Women to Study Medicine." Journal
of Social Issues, 28:2 (1972) 201-215.
"The data presented discuss the motivations and personality
of the female medical school student from the University of
California, San Francisco campus. Inductive analyses of
conscious reasons for entering medical school reveal the
importance of encouragement from others, long-standing interest, self-development motives, and altruism. In contrast

to studies reported on male subjects, economic and prestige factors as well as the unreachable aspect of other occupations are seldom mentioned by women." [Article abstract.]

2977.   Cartwright, Lillian K[aufman]. "The Personality and Fam-
           ily Background of a Sample of Women Medical Students
           at the University of California." Journal of the Amer-
           ican Medical Women's Association, 27:5 (May 1972)
           260-266. tables.
This article is a report of the empirical findings of a personality study of women medical students at the University
of California. Included are personality test data based on
the responses of 102 female medical school students from
the incoming classes of 1960-1967 and interview data collected on a sub-sample of 59 women drawn from the larger
group of 102. The California Psychological Inventory Test
was used. The women used in this study indicated an
overall effective social and intellectual functioning. They
were more self-accepting, dominant, independent, and active. Demographic group characteristics included high
paternal educational and occupational achievements, specific
sibling positions (only child, first, or second born), and
comparative stability in early family life.

2978.   "Challenge to Medical Women!" Bulletin of the Medical
           Women's National Association, 10 (October 1925) 23-
           24.
This article is a brief response to a speech given by Dr.
Hugh Cabot, dean of Ann Arbor Medical College, in which
he stated that "Women cannot stand the strain required in
the actual practice of medicine." At the same time he ad-
mires women who work in laboratories and in institutions
because "they work many more of the 365 days than men,
giving themselves less time and relaxation for football...."
Dr. Mabel Gardner's response included that this male physician would not know much about women physicians from
direct observations because none of the hospitals he attends
accepts women interns. In hospitals where women and men
act on services in rotation, women serve with at least as
much devotion and conscientiousness as men. Brawn is
irrelevant to the important criteria by which doctors should
be evaluated: ability to carry responsibility, endure loss
of sleep, make important decisions quickly. When women
physicians band together, then male physicians will value
them and cooperate with them.

2979.   Chappell, Amey. "The Time Is the Present." Journal of
           the American Medical Women's Association, 6:9 (Sep-
           tember 1951) 350-351. (Inaugural Address, American
           Medical Women's Association, Atlantic City, New Jer-
           sey, June 10, 1951.)
Equality of opportunity has not been achieved in the field of

medicine. This address constitutes a plea for women physicians to take an active role in the advancement of their
cause.

2980. Chesney, J. P. "Woman as a Physician." Richmond and
          Louisville Medical Journal, 11 (1871) 1-15.
       [Article not examined by editors.]

2981. Chiles, John A. "Patient Reactions to the Suicide of a
          Therapist." American Journal of Psychotherapy, 28:1
          (January 1974) 115-121.
       The rate of suicide among psychiatrists is high enough to
       consider suicide an occupational hazard. In this article the
       effects of a woman psychiatrist's suicide are examined in
       its relation to five male patients she served until the time
       of her death. One of her patients researched the possible
       causes of her death and found out from the psychiatrist's
       mother "that during the last six months of her life she had
       frequently asked, 'Why am I ugly when other people are
       beautiful?'" Another patient saw her as a "'Gertrude Stein-
       like figure,' masculine, low-voiced, chain-smoking--a veneer
       covering a lonely and depressed person, but a person with
       whom he could resonate because 'she was healthier than I
       but in the same kind of conflict.'"

2982. Clark, Margaret Vaupel. "Medical Women's Contribution to
          the Education of Mothers." Woman's Medical Journal,
          25:6 (June 1915) 126-128. (Presentation, Eighteenth
          Annual Meeting, Women's Medical Society of Iowa,
          Waterloo, Iowa, May 1915.)
       Women and children constitute four-fifths of the population
       and the larger part of the physician's patronage. Their
       needs are the first to be considered "as in them the future
       of the race is at stake." Women physicians are needed to
       care for these women, as many of them will only talk to
       another woman and submit to an examination only at the
       hands of another woman. Dr. Clark proceeds to discuss
       the education of young mothers by the woman physician.

2983. Clarke, Edward H. "Medical Education of Women." Bos-
          ton Medical and Surgical Journal, 4:24 (16 December
          1869) 345-346. (Original Communications.)
       Dr. Clarke presents excerpts from his address to the grad-
       uating medical class of Harvard College. His address con-
       cerns the subject of the medical education of women. Dr.
       Clarke feels that "whatever is right for [man] is right for
       [woman]. The real question is not of right, but of capa-
       bility or possibility." Here, Dr. Clarke considers the
       question one of "whether woman's organization will permit
       her to undertake the toil of the medical profession." A
       "complete experimental solution" to the question is suggested
       by Dr. Clarke: for if woman's organization is compatible
       with medical practice, she will succeed--if it is not com-

patible, she will fail.   Therefore, let her try--throw no
obstacles in her way.   Dr. Clarke feels they will master
the science of medicine, but to become practitioners they
must be strictly segregated from males, for it is not en-
nobling for men and women to aid "each other to display
with the scalpel the secrets of the reproductive system"; to
investigate "the constituents of the urine" together or to
"charmingly discuss together the labrynthine ways of syphilis."

2984.   Clarke, Miriam F.   "Stature and Body Build of Women
              Medical Students: A Study of Eight Classes at the Med-
              ical College of Pennsylvania."   Human Biology, 45:3
              (September 1973) 385-401.   figs., tables.
         "A sample of 401 women medical students aged 20 to 39
         years, the classes graduating 1960-67 at the Medical Col-
         lege of Pennsylvania," are measured in this study.   "The
         subjects of this study differed from other samples of women
         of the United States of America in: greater stature, lower
         weight for height in the fourth decade compared with the
         third, and lower percentage of overweight subjects."

2985.   Cleveland, E[meline] H.   Introductory Lecture on Behalf of
              the Faculty to the Class of the Female Medical College
              of Pennsylvania, for the Session of 1858-59.   Merri-
              hew & Thompson, Printers, Philadelphia, Pennsylvania,
              1858, 16 pp.
         Emeline Cleveland says that "though prejudice [against wo-
         men physicians] has not yet entirely worn away, we are
         most happy to know and to assure you that its strength has
         departed...."   Calling the medical profession "a truly wo-
         manly work," Dr. Cleveland reminds the new students that
         all rights carry with them responsibilities.   In addition to
         the duty to maintain a strong body as well as a strong in-
         tellectual and moral life, women medical students must re-
         member the worth of their cause and enter their studies
         with "'a spirit at once Roman in its sacrifice and Spartan
         in its simplicity.'"

2986.   Cleveland, Emeline H.   Valedictory Address to the Gradu-
              ating Class of the Woman's Medical College of Penn-
              sylvania, at the Sixteenth Annual Commencement,
              March 14, 1868.   Published by the Corporators, Phila-
              delphia, Pennsylvania, 1868, 12 pp.
         Emeline Cleveland's congratulations to the graduates in-
         cludes praise for choosing a life of "self-sacrifice and un-
         remitting labor," advice on obtaining success, and reflec-
         tions on the social and personal implications of being a wo-
         man in medicine.   She discusses the fear by some "who
         hold women in the highest reverence" that women's practice
         of medicine will "lessen their sense of delicacy and destroy
         that love of the pure and beautiful in nature and in life
         which constitutes one of the greatest charms of womanhood."

Such a fear is worthy of respect, but one should remember that the study of medicine strengthens "womanly feeling." Although prejudice against women physicians exists in some localities, such obstacles are "relics of a barbarous age," and friendly welcomes await most of the graduates. Dr. Cleveland goes on to outline the improving status of medical education for women in France and England. In conclusion, she warns the women to avoid "the unenviable distinction of being peculiar" by always being prudent in actions and by not abandoning the home.

2987.   Coates, Reynell. Introductory Lecture to the Class of the Female Medical College, of Pennsylvania. Delivered at the Opening of the Eleventh Annual Session, Oct. 17, 1860. Merrihew & Thompson, Printers, Philadelphia, Pennsylvania, 1861, 16 pp.
The College's professor of surgery, Dr. Coates, identifies and responds to the most prevalent arguments against women physicians. Florence Nightingale is held up as an example of one medical woman who was led into what many believed to be "improper exposures and associations destructive of feminine delicacy," yet she retained her refinement and received international acclaim. The moral objection to females studying anatomy and physiology, and to "feminine hands" being entrusted only to "feminine life," is discussed --then dismissed: "... the proper study, not only of mankind, but of womankind also, is man." To the accusation that women are weak, Dr. Coates answers that "weakness is not proof of inferiority," and goes on to list female characteristics that compensate for natural shortcomings. To those who say that "instances of superiority in woman are mere exceptions," Dr. Coates points out that those exceptions should not be condemned. Furthermore, even if the college never produces a great woman surgeon, its usefulness will not be doubted. The necessary attributes of a good woman surgeon are enumerated. Recalling the prejudices that have been evidenced in the past decade of the Female Medical College's existence, the speaker says that although each student will face similar prejudices, the rewards of a medical profession will be worth the struggle --"even if, in the battle of life, prosperity or woman's destiny remove you or entice you from the general practice of your profession...."

2988.   Cohen, Carol J. "Final Advice to Women MD's." New England Journal of Medicine, 285:23 (2 December 1971) 1329. (Letters to the Editor.)
This writer feels the "dialogue on the topic of female physicians has degenerated to the level of a nationally syndicated 'advice to the love-lorn' column." There should be no assumptions that the goal of most women is "to find a man ... whose masculinity tolerates domestic tasks." There should be no assumptions that everyone wants to live

in a nuclear family when in fact many people want to follow the lifestyle of their choice.

2989.   "A Condition, Not a Theory." Medical Woman's Journal,
            38:7 (July 1931) 178.
         An editorial in the Boston Transcript suggesting that pre-
         judice against medical women is still very strong, prompted
         a reply from Alice Stone Blackwell, Elizabeth Blackwell's
         niece. Recounting the early trials of women physicians
         (such as those described by Charles Reade in the novel, A
         Woman Hater), Alice Blackwell is confident that "all these
         prejudices will wear away in time."

2990.   "Co-operation Among Women Physicians." Woman's Med-
            ical Journal, 25:5 (May 1915) 104-105. (Editorial.)
         Women physicians must work "shoulder to shoulder" for the
         good of their profession as well as for the advancement of
         women everywhere.

2991.   Cornell, William M. "Woman the True Physician." Godey's
            Magazine and Lady's Book, 46 (January 1853) 82-83.
         "[Woman] can, from her very nature, more thoroughly un-
         derstand and more effectually assuage the diseases and suf-
         ferings of a sister than any man can."

2992.   Coste, Chris. "Women in Medicine; Progress and Preju-
            dice." The New Physician, 24:11 (November 1975) 25-
            33. charts, photos.
         The fact that the percentage of women in medical schools
         has doubled in the past four years does not necessarily in-
         dicate a disappearance of prejudice on the part of medical
         educators: federal laws have worked together to prohibit
         discrimination. "Faced with a cutoff of federal funds, med-
         ical schools are admitting more women--and in some cases
         actively recruiting them." Yet not a large percentage of
         women seem to be applying to medical schools. The author
         suggests the reasons for this phenomenon involve childhood
         conditioning, the hostile environment of the medical school,
         and a lack of role models for women medical students. In
         the future, however, medical schools may be forced to hire
         more women, when HEW begins enforcing the existing anti-
         discrimination laws. Women also have difficulties in inte-
         grating their woman/wife/mother roles with their profession-
         al roles. The ones who are most likely to "see beyond
         their own troubles and take action" are the other women.
         Flexible training programs are discussed, with special ref-
         erence to the undergraduate program at the University of
         Hawaii's medical school. The article concludes with an an-
         notated list of organizations willing to help women students
         form women's groups at their respective medical schools.

2993.   Craig, Alan G. and Pitts, Ferris N., Jr. "Suicide by
            Physicians." Diseases of the Nervous System, 29:11

(November 1968) 763-772.   tables.
"A systematic examination of the physicians records of
causes of death in physicians revealed 228 deaths by suicide in a two-year period.   The death rate by suicide for
male physicians was unchanged from that found 30 years
ago and did not differ from that of the age- and sex-matched
general population either of 30 years ago or the current
time.   Female physician suicides were four times as frequent as those in the female general population over age 25,
gave the highest reported rate for any group of females,
and indicate the desirability of examining a group of female
physicians for affective disorder.   Both female and male
physicians used drugs as a method of suicide significantly
more often than did the general population.   Within the medical specialties only board-certified otolaryngologists sui-
cided significantly more frequently and this difference is
probably a consequence of the fact that suicide rates increase with age and diplomates in otolaryngology are older
than diplomates of the other medical specialties."   [Article
summary.]

2994.   Cushman, Beulah.   "Married Women in the Medical Pro-
           fession."   Journal of the American Medical Women's
           Association, 18:7 (July 1963) 568.   (Editorial.)
This is a response to Dr. Mary Carter's "Notes on Married Women in the Medical Profession" [Journal of the Medical Women's Federation, 44:159-162, October 1962], in
which she says a woman who returns to medical practice
after marriage and children must begin a training course
in a junior position.   Dr. Carter "feels that although marriage enriches a professional woman's personality, it may
also be limiting, turning a woman in upon herself."   Beulah Cushman feels that a medical woman returning to her
practice is not "a late-motherhood recreation" and that
"returning" women physicians need not have to expect "dull,
non-dynamic type of employment."   Better yet, it should
not be necessary that a woman stop practicing during her
child rearing years.

2995.   Daniel, Annie Sturges.   "'A Cautious Experiment.'   The
           History of the New York Infirmary for Women and
           Children and the Women's Medical College of the New
           York Infirmary; Also Its Pioneer Founders: 1853-
           1899."   Medical Woman's Journal, 48:10 (October 1941)
           301-307.
This article in the series on the New York Infirmary reproduces excerpts from an address delivered at the commencement of the Women's Medical College of the New York
Infirmary, May 30, 1883, by Mary Putnam Jacobi.   Dr.
Jacobi admonishes the new graduates to remember that they
are first of all physicians, and secondarily women.   As
women, however, these graduates have a certain class of
interests, and while biological studies in health and disease

may be the most interesting of subjects, certainly the
"overthrow of social prejudices, tyrannies and monopolies"
is the second most interesting theme. "And of all monopolies, what has ever been more odious than that which has
restricted to one-half of the human race the advantages of
education and the facilities of increased life which that con-
fers, while the other half of humanity has been forcibly excluded from both?" The problem is to raise to an equality
the class [i.e., women] which has hitherto been kept at an
inferior status. The ways in which women physicians may
contribute to this effort are discussed.

2996. Davidson, Lynne R. Sex Roles, Affect, and the Woman
            Physician: A Comparative Study of the Impact of Later
            Social Identity Upon the Role of Women and Men Pro-
            fessionals. New York University, New York, New
            York, 1975, xvii, 609 pp. tables. (Ph.D. thesis.)
The purpose of this research report was to determine how
the sex of a woman influences her role as a physician. It
was hypothesized that women, because of their traditional
role in society, are less affectively neutral in their orienta
tion and performance as physicians than are men, and the
systematic comparison between men and women doctors-in-
training was an integral part of the study. The data are
qualitative as well as quantitative. A basic assumption was
that women doctors must deal with the two distinct statuses
of sex and profession, the dilemma being that affectivity
and emotional expressiveness have been expected from women in our society, but not from men or from physicians.
The research was conducted at a metropolitan hospital in
New York. Subjects were 48 women physicians and 48 male
physicians, matched on the three variables of ethnicity,
rank, and medical specialty. Methods included questionnaires, interviews, and self-reports. Findings indicated
that few doctors of either sex are as objective, detached,
or affectively neutral as traditional stereotype would indicate, but women measure higher on all items of affectivity
than men. Also, women more than men tend to regard as
desirable emotional involvement in fulfilling professional
objectives. And when physicians do control affect, persona
needs of the physician often govern this. Men and women
"use similar techniques to cope with affective feelings, and
manage the patient involved in similar ways ... both men
and women reported they gave better medical care ... [to]
patients with whom they felt sympathetic." It is recommended "that the medical system begin to accommodate women so that women can discontinue accommodating themselves, and thus compromising themselves, to the prevailing system." Further study is suggested. Tables accompany the text. Appendixes provide supplementary data and
samples of the questionnaire and code book. The report
contains a lengthy bibliography.

2997.   Davis, Paulina Wright. "Female Physicians." Boston
            Medical and Surgical Journal, 41 (1849) 520-522. (Let-
            ters to the Editor.)
         The author, while confessing no interest in practicing med-
         icine herself, speaks for women who do wish to enter the
         profession. In this letter to the editor, she recounts her
         difficulties in attempting to attend medical lectures. She
         emphasizes the need for women to administer to women and
         affirms that no power can prevent women from becoming
         physicians.

2998.   Denko, Joanne D. "Managing a Practice and a Home Simul-
            taneously: One Woman Physician's Solution." The Wo-
            man Physician, 25:1 (January 1970) 33-38.
         For a woman to be professional and to raise a family, this
         woman doctor says, "she must ... first decide what are
         the important aspects of each role, and she must then con-
         serve time and energy so as to implement both jobs without
         sacrificing anything essential in either." Determinants that
         will make her "two demanding careers" more compatible
         are the "help or hindrance from her husband," "the selec-
         tion of a specialty," and "the decision of how to practice."
         As a psychiatrist, she distinguishes between the types of
         patients she sees herself able to help, and those she can-
         not. For example, "Other patients with psychiatric prob-
         lems sound unsuited for interpretive therapy (too dull, low
         socioeconomic status)," and she sends those people to out-
         patient clinics at hospitals. She arranges her schedule so
         she can be with her son and at the same time has taught
         him "about the fact of compromise in life" so that she can
         be with her patients. There is a biographical inset on
         Joanne D. Denko.

2999.   Dolley, Sarah R. A. "Address." Woman's Medical Jour-
            nal, 18:4 (April 1908) 62-65. port. (Women's Medical
            Society of the State of New York, Rochester, New York,
            11 March 1908.)
         This address asks the question, Are women to be a power
         for good in the medical profession? Dr. Dolley thinks so,
         while at the same time she refuses to ignore the limitations
         women have. A portrait of Dr. Dolley precedes this arti-
         cle.

3000.   Dolley, Sarah R. A. Closing Lecture to the Class of
            1873-74, Delivered at the Woman's Medical College of
            Pennsylvania, March 5th, 1874. [Philadelphia, Penn-
            sylvania?, n.d.], 8 pp.
         In this address, Dr. Dolley reviews the obstacles which
         have been removed for women in medicine: "cultivated
         communities no longer regard the entrance of woman into
         the profession as an impertinence"; however, a medical
         woman must show a seriousness of moral purpose. Women
         have their limitations, and although they will not "revolu-

tionize medicine with startling discoveries or brilliant inventions" they may learn the science of medicine and become skillful in the practice of its art. A woman physician must be truthful, honest, tender, and sympathetic; she must achieve and succeed, and should she face great prejudice against women physicians, she must be patient until her actions are interpreted rightly.

3001.   Dublin, Louis I. and Spiegelman, Mortimer. "The Longevity and Mortality of American Physicians, 1938-1942: A Preliminary Report." Journal of the American Medical Association, 134:15 (9 August 1947) 1211-1215. tables. (Presentation, Ninety-Sixth Annual Session, American Medical Association, Atlantic City, New Jersey, 12 June 1947.)
This study, based on American Medical Association records of living physicians and physician deaths during 1938 through 1942, concentrates on males. Two statistical tables provide comparative data on men and women physicians, i.e., present ages, life expectation, and deaths according to sex and age. For the period studied, the average life expectancy for a 25-year-old man entering the medical profession is 43.5 years; for the 25-year-old woman, it is over 47 years.

3002.   Eckman, F. M. "Why Can't More Women Be Doctors?" Redbook, 137 (May 1971) 77, passim.
[Article not examined by editors.]

3003.   Ehrenreich, Barbara. "The Health Care Industry: A Theory of Industrial Medicine." Social Policy, 6:3 (November/December 1975) 4-11. photo.
The author attempts "to account for the subordination of women in the U.S. health industry by looking first for its origins in the preindustrial phase of medicine, then at some of the social factors which helped to perpetuate the original sexual division of labor and power, and finally by looking at the stabilizing role of sex stratification in the contemporary, industrialized health industry." Because of the pressure from the women's liberation movement, medical schools have been admitting more and more women. With these growing numbers of women in medicine and "with growing militancy among all women in health, sex differences will cease to be the automatic rationale for occupational stratification." Women health workers may find that "the greatest barrier to change is not so much sexism as it is the hierarchical divisions among women workers themselves."

3004.   Elliott, Susan J. "More Like a Woman ... More Like a Man." Inside Baylor Medicine, 6:6 (June-July 1975) 3. illus.
This article discusses a study of 640 Baylor College of

Medicine applicants undertaken by Dr. Robert L. Roessler, professor of psychiatry at Baylor [the study is entitled "Sex Similarities in Successful Medical School Applicants," and is published in the Journal of the American Medical Women's Association, 30:6 (June 1975) 254+].

3005.   Ellis, Ruth M. "Women Medical Dropouts." Journal of the American Medical Women's Association, 22:9 (September 1967) 666. (Open Forum.)
A response is given to the "President's Message" in the February 1967 issue of the Journal of the American Medical Women's Association, which advocated solving the attrition rate of women in medicine by arranging for childbirth leaves, baby sitters, maids, etc. Ruth Ellis responds, "Our best youngsters want to find challenge and best it; they'll not enter a field said to be so simple that one can master it, dropping babies along the way.... Perhaps a more effective way to attract young women would be to stress the unique imperative of excellence in medicine."

3006.   Ellison, Solon A.; Hollingsworth, Dorothy R.; Eilberg, Ralph G.; and Bunting, Joelle. "Open Forum." The Woman Physician, 26:8 (August 1971) 426-427. (Letters to the Editor.)
In response to Lewis T. Milic's letter in "Open Forum" [April, 1971, p. 217-218] commenting on being married to a woman physician, several people wrote various responses. Two other men with Ph.D.s who are married to women physicians disagree. Solon A. Ellison writes, "My wife did not depend upon our household help 'more than on any other person in the world.' They helped, but I rather think that she depended on me. And I was (and still am) flattered and delighted, and I hope good enough. At least, I enjoyed it, and it didn't inhibit my career." Ralph Eilberg writes, "I didn't marry a housekeeper. I am very happy to be married to a woman physician." Joelle Bunting, doctor and wife of Ralph Eilberg, observes that a woman physician is "not like [Mr. Milic's] watch-fob Phi Beta Kappa key; she is a dynamic, living human being on her own. She is not an ornament for him to show off at dinner." Another woman physician, Dorothy R. Hollingsworth, remarks, "It really is a tragedy when a gal gets stuck with a guy like Lewis T. Milic."

3007.   Ely, Allen. "What Do You Think of Women Doctors?" Medical Economics, (November 1948) 54-56. photo.
What do male physicians think of this country's "8,000-odd" medical women? A survey of "about a hundred chiefs of staff" showed that 1 per cent of male physicians rate the average woman physician as excellent, and 35 per cent of the respondents say women M.D.s are "good, or 'good as men.'" The remaining 64 per cent call women physicians "passable" or make such sweeping complaints as: they

"use more charm than brains," they "lose their heads in
emergencies," "they talk too much," and "they get pregnant."

3008.   Engleman, Edgar G.   "Attitudes Toward Women Physicians:
            A Study of 500 Clinic Patients."   Western Journal of
            Medicine, 120:2 (February 1974) 95-100.   tables.
         "A questionnaire was administered to 500 clinic patients [in
         New York City] and their replies about men and women phy-
         sicians were analyzed.   Ninety-six per cent stated that the
         typical doctor is a man, and 78 per cent expressed a pref-
         erence for a male doctor [although a higher percentage of
         women than men over all preferred a woman doctor.   "A
         significant percentage of the patients interviewed had never
         consulted a female physician yet did not hesitate to offer
         negative opinions..."].   A significant number of patients
         said they would be unwilling to discuss certain subjects with
         a woman doctor or to follow her advice.   Women physicians
         were considered less competent and less experienced than
         their male counterparts.   Attitudes toward women doctors
         were correlated with patients' sex, age, ethnicity, occupa-
         tion, and chief complaint.   Most impressive statistically
         were the negative attitudes of Spanish-speaking patients and
         the positive responses of obstetrics and gynecology patients
         and black women patients.   Patients who had previously con-
         sulted women physicians were more favorable toward them,
         suggesting that increased exposure may lead to reduced
         prejudice."   [Article abstract.]

3009.   "Equal Rights for Women Doctors."   Medical Woman's
            Journal, 29:10 (October 1922) 261.   (Editorial.)
         "Women doctors are not bestirring themselves to see that
         [their lives] are changed."   The four areas in which dis-
         crimination against women physicians is especially marked
         are training, hospital appointments, government service,
         and the military.   "It is time women physicians as a class
         recognized this situation, and worked for legislation to re-
         move the discriminations which restrict their activities in
         the field of medicine."

3010.   Feldman-Summers, Shirley and Kiesler, Sara B.   "Those
            Who Are Number Two Try Harder: The Effect of Sex
            on Attributions of Causality."   Journal of Personality
            and Social Psychology, 30:6 (1974) 846-855.   fig.
         "Two experiments were conducted [using students at the
         University of Kansas] in order to ascertain the causal at-
         tributions made by male and female subjects for identical
         performance (including success and failure) of males and
         females.   In both experiments, subjects made attributions
         along four dimensions: ability, motivation, task difficulty,
         and luck.   Whether evaluating undergraduates on an intel-
         lectual task (Experiment 1) or successful physicians (Experi-
         ment 2), subjects attributed greater motivation to females

than to males. In addition, males perceived the female
physician as being less able and having an easier task than
the male physician. However, female subjects perceived
the female physician as having a harder task than the male
physician. Implications for attribution theory and the perception of professional women in our society were discussed." [Article abstract.]

3011.   "Female Physicians." Boston Medical and Surgical Jour-
         nal, 48 (1853) 66.
         These musings on the novelty of admitting women to the
         medical profession were prompted by the conferring of the
         honorary M.D. degree on Harriot K. Hunt by the Female
         Medical College of Pennsylvania. "Female physicians seem
         to be on the increase among us ... in spite of the jeers,
         innuendoes and ridicule of us lords of creation.... It is
         not a matter to be laughed down, as readily as was first
         anticipated."

3012.   "Female Physicians." Boston Medical and Surgical Journal,
         54:9 (3 April 1856) 169-174. (Letters to the Editor.)
         The fact that females, by virtue of their "weak physical or-
         ganization," are unsuitable for the practice of medicine is
         so obvious that the writer confines his remarks to "the
         facts as regards midwifery alone." He first offers numer-
         ous examples to refute the claim that wild animals and
         primitive women birth their young with "immunity from pain
         and danger." As civilization advances, responsibilities at
         childbirth are appropriately transferred "from the midwife
         to the educated accoucheur," with a resultant decline (50
         per cent in half a century) in infant mortality. To the
         claim that midwifery is almost universal in France and
         Germany the writer declares that even after extensive gov-
         ernment training and regulation, these midwives have been
         found incapable of dealing with difficult cases. In Great
         Britain, midwives are sustained by the lower classes only.
         In one case a midwife, "after the patient had been delivered,
         dragged the womb itself out of the body," thinking it some-
         thing which ought to be removed. The support of midwifery
         is clearly a "retrograde step." Fortunately, the scheme to
         educate midwives "contains within itself the elements of
         failure; for ... 'the girls don't like to dissect.' They did
         not seem to like, either, to devote more than three months
         to a course of medical education."

3013.   "Female Practitioners of Medicine." Boston Medical and
         Surgical Journal, (2 May 1867) 272-274.
         Point by point, this article sets forth the reasons women
         are not adapted to the practice of medicine. They include:
         menstruation (an "abnormal" condition causing unreliable
         judgment); pregnancy; women's "uncurbed sympathy" (an ex-
         cess that interferes with efficiency); and the female intellect
         (prone to impulsive judgments). The author adds that wo-

men's "natural refinement" would be destroyed if women
were exposed to dissecting rooms, anatomy, and venereal
diseases.   "The pure-minded girl instinctively feels that
there are certain subjects which her maidenly dignity requires her to ignore."

3014.   "Females as Physicians."   Boston Medical and Surgical
               Journal, 53 (1 November 1855) 292-294.
           Women should have the right to practice medicine if they
           are able, but their ability is questionable.   "Those pursuits
           which require the exercise of the highest intellectual power
           ... are beyond her capacity."   Exceptions there are, "but
           what are they ... compared with the thousands of distin-
           guished medical men."   Obstetrics would seem an appropri-
           ate sphere for women, but "women in those hours ... feel
           the need of stronger support and assistance."   Woman's in-
           herent physical weakness is also a deterrent, as is the
           "social condition of females."   One woman physician, having
           been summoned in the middle of the night, then expected to
           be escorted home.   "It is obvious" that women must attend
           only women and children, so two doctors would then be re-
           quired for each family.   Nevertheless, if women can prac-
           tice medicine, they should.

3015.   Fischer-Pap, Lucia.   "My Mother, the Doctor: Another
               Solution to a Much-Discussed Problem."   Journal of
               the American Medical Women's Association, 21:6 (June
               1966) 509-511.   (Forum.)
           A woman physician tells how she re-entered medicine after
           a pregnancy and a year's absence.   Dr. Fischer-Pap lists
           the advantages and disadvantages of her decision to return
           to medicine.   Among the advantages are the finding of suit-
           able domestic help which "restore some style and a more
           dignified pace to our life"; the removal of worry over what
           would become of the family if her husband were to die.
           Third on the list of advantages, the author writes "I think
           I would have been a very frustrated person and a much
           more difficult woman to live with, had I not been able to
           continue my professional career."   A fourth advantage is
           that she can use her "title and license in many useful ways."
           As an example, Mrs. Fischer-Pap gives the fact that she
           could take her children to a girl's camp while she served
           as camp physician there.   Disadvantages include (heading
           the list) "my reminders ... my pace, and the multiplicity
           of duties that crowd my weekly schedule still make George
           [her husband] feel tense and nervous at times, especially
           when he is tired."   In addition, she does not have time for
           "fancy cooking."   Finally, she wonders if her children do
           not resent the diversity of her life.

3016.   Fishbein, Morris.   "Women in Medicine."   Postgraduate
               Medicine, 35:4 (April 1964) 448.   (Editorial.)
           Women score lower than men on the science portion of

medical college admission tests. And while women's enrollment in medical school is increasing, there are far
fewer women physicians in the United States than in many
other countries. Fishbein calls for sociological study as
the numbers of medical women increase. He adds that
while women are better suited for some specialties than
men, women seem less adapted for surgery. He recalls a
trip to Russia (where women make up 65 per cent of the
medical profession): a male professor of surgery told him
that women "make fine assistants but very poor chiefs."

3017.   Frye, Maud J. "The Health of the Physician a Neglected
            Factor of Success." Woman's Medical Journal, 26:6
            (June 1916) 145-146. (Presentation, Tenth Annual
            Meeting, Women's Medical Society of New York State.)
        Women physicians should be of sound health and mind and
        know themselves well enough to take vacations when they
        need rest and to exercise their bodies so that they feel joy
        lest their strength be dissipated.

3018.   Frye, Maud J. "Some Sensible Remarks." Woman's Med-
            ical Journal, 6:9 (September 1897) 283-285.
        Some thoughts on woman's place in medicine include the
        reflection that men and women are different physically,
        sexually, and mentally, but "there is equality with diversity."

3019.   Fullerton, Anna M. Woman in Medicine. Her Duties and
            Responsibilities. An Address to the Graduates of the
            Woman's Medical College of Pennsylvania, May 3, 1893.
            [Philadelphia, Pennsylvania?, n.d.], 16 pp.
        In this address, Dr. Fullerton presents the opportunities
        awaiting women physicians, the societal conditions which
        make the existence of women physicians a necessity, and
        the obligations of women physicians to live nobly, and act
        wisely. "The insight and attention to detail peculiar to the
        truly womanly nature" are an advantage in the healing art,
        especially as regards the care of women and children. By
        subtle persuasiveness and example the woman physician
        must "modify the artificial obligations of society-life," break
        the bonds of conventionalism which make of woman "an in-
        valid and a slave," and stretch out her hand to her fallen
        sister. She must, in addition, inspire respect by her skill.
        Both history and folklore record the universal appreciation
        of the fact that "intellect and influence may exist in indi-
        viduals regardless of sex." Dr. Fullerton presents ex-
        amples from both folklore and history to substantiate her
        statement. A view of 19th-century society and the woman
        physician's calling therein is presented, followed by Dr.
        Fullerton's assessment of woman's status in that society--
        "woman ... the mere toy or tool or slave of man." The
        history of medical education for women in the United States
        is reviewed, and Dr. Fullerton concludes with an overview
        of the Woman's Medical College of Pennsylvania and the Wo-
        man's Hospital of Philadelphia.

3020. Fussell, Edwin. Valedictory Address to the Graduating
       Class of the Female Medical College, of Pennsylvania,
       at the Tenth Annual Commencement, March 13th, 1861.
       J. B. Chandler, Printer, Philadelphia, Pennsylvania,
       1861, 16 pp.
       Edwin Fussell, professor of obstetrics at the Female Med-
       ical College, speaks of the rewards of a medical profession
       as well as its duties. Although the graduating students
       have turned away from the traditional activities of women,
       they still are fulfilling their "destiny," still following the
       "instincts of womanhood." Dr. Fussell expresses hope that
       as physicians, the graduating students "will be modest and
       unassuming; courteous, kind and patient ... cheerful and
       hope inspiring, as well as sympathetic and tender. You
       will be honorable, and true; devoted and self-sacrificing.
       In one word, you will be womanly." Although unenlightened
       male physicians and other opposers to women in medicine
       will persecute the new graduates, they should not permit
       such difficulties to overcome them, and let no temptations
       lure them from duty.

3021. Fussell, Edwin. Valedictory Address to the Graduating
       Class of the Female Medical College, of Pennsylvania,
       For the Session 1856-57. Published by the class,
       Philadelphia, Pennsylvania, 1857, 15 pp.
       Warning the women graduates that they must not expect a
       cordial reception from the medical profession at large, Dr.
       Fussell (professor of obstetrics) goes on to list the quali-
       ties of a good physician: "Whatever he does, he must do
       well!"

3022. Gardner, Mabel E.; [Rockhill, Margaret Hackedorn]; and
       Cabot, Hugh. "Resume of the Recent Correspondence
       with the Dean of the University of Michigan Regarding
       the Comparative Fitness of Women to Practice Medi-
       cine." Medical Woman's Journal, 33:4 (April 1926)
       112-113.
       Statements about the fitness of women to practice medicine
       made by Dr. Hugh Cabot, dean of the University of Michi-
       gan, prompt a letter from Mabel E. Gardner in which she
       charges that "Michigan is famous for its narrow-minded-
       ness with regard to women physicians.... [Since] no wo-
       man is allowed to give service in the hospital which he at-
       tends, or in nearby medical centers, he can have no first-
       hand observation to draw from." Two letters from Dr.
       Cabot state that he was misquoted, and that the University
       Hospital had no women interns prior to 1925 because "satis-
       factory accommodations could not be found." The Medical
       Woman's Journal's managing editor, Margaret H. Rockhill,
       defends Dr. Cabot, pointing out that he "comes from a
       Boston family in which there have been distinguished phy-
       sicians and surgeons all of whom have been helpful to med-
       ical women.... For one of that broad-minded family, and

the head of a coeducational medical school, to be unfriendly
to medical women would be almost unthinkable."

3023.   Gillmore, Emma Wheat. "A Call to Arms." Woman's
         Medical Journal, 27:8 (August 1917) 183-184. (Medical
         War Notes.)
         This article is a response to Dr. Isabella Vandervall's
         article, "Some Problems of the Colored Woman Physician,"
         which appeared in the July [1917] issue of the Woman's
         Medical Journal. Dr. Vandervall had attended the Woman's
         Medical College of Pennsylvania, had graduated but could
         not find a hospital in the State of Pennsylvania at which to
         serve an internship "on account of color prejudice," and
         therefore could not acquire a medical license in her resi-
         dent state. The author observes that "Dr. Vandervall suf-
         fers from no more pronounced injustice because she cannot
         obtain a license to practice in her native state than many
         a well qualified physician has experienced who has been
         forced to change his residence in middle age from one part
         of the country to another, and faces the necessity of passing
         a state examination which at his time of life is practically
         prohibitive." The author inquired of the Chicago Medical
         Society about this injustice. After the assistant secretary
         met with the general counsel of the society, a letter was
         written to the author suggesting that a writ of mandamus be
         issued "compelling the licensing board to issue a license
         non constat." The letter also suggests that another practical
         means of solving this problem is legislation limiting nurses
         and interns in hospitals to serving eight hours in each 24.
         This legislation would produce such a shortage that hospitals
         would then be glad to accept those who want to work, ir-
         respective of race or color. Dr. Gillmore herself suggests
         that Dr. Vandervall might consider hiring a lawyer so that
         she could "eventually save other colored medical graduates
         from the injustice with which she suffers. Meanwhile she
         must remember that Pennsylvania is not guilty of discrim-
         inating against a pigmented skin. For centuries, however,
         the general public have so discriminated, and with fearless
         veneration for the truth she should recognize that the pre-
         judice was originally founded upon a very real objection."
         As medical women applying to serve in the armed forces
         must prove their worth, so must colored women.

3024.   Glasgow, Maude. "Editorial." Medical Woman's Journal,
         56:9 (September 1949) 47, 52.
         In this editorial, Dr. Glasgow vigorously attacks the con-
         ditions that keep the number of women physicians "near
         the vanishing point." Medical schools purposely place low
         quotas on the admission of women. Of 400 hospitals, only
         about one-third accept women interns due to "lack of ac-
         commodation." The U.S. government provides medical edu-
         cation funds for male war veterans, while women desirous
         of entering medical school receive no encouragement or

financial aid. While discrimination in color, race, and religion is universally denounced, "the most extensive, devas-
tating and injurious" discrimination--that of sex--is ignored
because women "have not resorted to force or violence,
man's weapon." Dr. Glasgow urges women physicians to
withdraw support from public institutions that practice sex
discrimination and to actively recruit women for the medical profession.

3025.   "Glen R. Leymaster, M.D.: President and Dean, Woman's
               Medical College." Pennsylvania Medical Journal, 67:
               9 (September 1964) 19-23. port. (PMJ Interview.)
          In this interview Dr. Leymaster comments on women as
          medical students and physicians, pregnancy and marriage
          among women medical students, a possible shortage of phy-
          sicians, retraining women who have temporarily dropped
          out of the medical profession, and long-range plans for the
          Woman's Medical College. A photograph and biographical
          sketch of Dr. Leymaster are included.

3026.   Glenn, Georgiana. "Are Women as Capable of Becoming
               Physicians as Men?" Clinic (Cincinnati), 9 (1875) 243-
               245.
          [Article not examined by editors.]

3027.   Goldstein, Marion Zucker. "Preventive Mental Health Ef-
               forts for Women Medical Students." Journal of Med-
               ical Education, 50:3 (March 1975) 289-291. (Presenta-
               tion, 127th Meeting, American Psychiatric Association,
               Detroit, Michigan, May 1974.)
          In 1971 Dr. Goldstein began weekly group seminars for
          freshman women of the University of Pittsburgh School of
          Medicine. Her goal: "to help women medical students
          bridge the developmental lag of acquiring a comfortable
          professional identity in a male-dominated profession."
          Each year six students attended regularly; a total of 40
          women participated from the seminars' inception through
          1974. In 1974 the psychiatry department offered the sem-
          inar as an official elective. In this article, Dr. Goldstein
          offers a general description of the seminar format, the dis-
          cussion content, and the major problems that arose.

3028.   Graffis, Herb. "Her Turn to Treat." Esquire: The
               Magazine for Men, 25:3 (March 1946) 57-58. illus.
          This article on "lady docs" is interspersed with fictional
          dialogue on how "catty" women neighbors might feel about
          a woman treating a male patient. Women make good psy-
          chiatrists because a good expert psychiatrist in a criminal
          case can get a murderer off the hook with the right an-
          swers and "a bright woman always can come up with the
          right answer, especially if the jury is composed entirely
          of men." The reasons women are forcing their way into
          medical school are also discussed.

3029.   Graham, Davis W. "The Demand for Medically-Educated
        Women." Journal of the American Medical Association,
        6:18 (1 May 1886) 477-480. (Original Lectures.)
        (Commencement address, Woman's Medical College of
        Chicago, 6 April 1886.)
        Dr. Graham impresses upon the graduates the myriad duties
        and heavy responsibilities of a physician. Pointing out that
        while there is a demand for medical women in the United
        States, there are greater opportunities for American women
        physicians to work in Asia among "their oriental sisters."

3030.   Green, Marthalyn Johnson. "Marriage and the Woman Phy-
        sician." The Woman Physician, 25:7 (July 1970) 460-
        461.
        Can marriage and medicine be "happily mixed" in the United
        States? "An affirmative answer can only be made with res-
        ervation." The only marriages seen by the author that
        were "happy" were those in which the "physician-wife-moth-
        er" has a time-limited position (i.e., public health). "The
        woman who wishes to combine medicine with a family ...
        must be willing to sacrifice, without resentment, a part of
        the fulfillment of each role she plays for the combined sat-
        isfaction she receives from the two roles. This will be
        true until and unless the mores and the value systems of
        this country change or the health-care delivery system
        changes or maybe until children are born in test tubes and
        raised in nurseries without parents."

3031.   Gregory, George. Medical Morals, Illustrated with Plates
        and Extracts from Medical Works; Designed to Show the
        Pernicious Social and Moral Influence of the Present
        System of Medical Practice, and Its Importance of Es-
        tablishing Female Medical Colleges, and Education and
        Employing Female Physicians for Their Own Sex. Pub-
        lished by the author, New York, New York, 1853, 48
        pp. illus.
        The author wrote this book to "expose and correct" an evil
        in the medical profession, which he feels abounds with vi-
        cious and vulgar men who resort to deceit in discrediting
        women physicians. Examples are given of the lengths to
        which some male physicians have gone in order to discredit
        a female physician. Women physicians are very desirable,
        writes the author, brother to Samuel Gregory (moving force
        behind the founding of the New England Female Medical Col-
        lege), in order that women patients may be attended by wo-
        men physicians and thereby be spared the embarrassment
        and often extreme agitation caused by the indelicacies in-
        herent in examination by a male physician. The author
        quotes from medical texts, passages which instruct the phy-
        sician on how to examine an obstetrical patient. These
        methods are discussed by Gregory and used to highlight
        the imposition placed upon women by a male performing the
        examination. Several medical men are quoted on the subject

of "unnecessary" examinations of women by male physicians. Dr. Thomas Ewell of Virginia writes, "... there is a value in the belief that the husband's hands alone are to have access to his sacred wife." Male midwifery is "a crime against woman, and nature, and the sacredness of married life."

3032.   Gregory, Samuel. Doctor or Doctress? Published by the
         Trustees, Pratt Brothers Printers, Boston, Massachu-
         setts, 1868, 8 pp.
         Dr. Gregory makes a case for women physicians being re-
         ferred to as "Doctress" rather than doctor: "the distinc-
         tion of sex by a difference of termination in words is both
         elegant and convenient." "Doctor" is masculine, it sounds
         masculine, and carries the idea of a masculine occupation.
         Even if a woman were to call herself doctor or others were
         to call her so, "she would only be a Doctress still."
         Gregory quotes the opinions of other "authorities" on the
         matter, among whom are Professor Alpheus Crosby, Rev-
         erend William Jenks, Mrs. Sarah J. Hal, and Mrs. Almira
         Lincoln Phelps.

3033.   Gregory, Samuel. "Female Physicians." Living Age, 73
         (3 May 1862) 243-249.
         Dr. Gregory feels that women are particularly suited to
         medical practice and should have an education correspond-
         ing to their native abilities. Because three-fourths of the
         duties of the medical profession relate to the well-being
         of women and children, "there should be at least as many
         female as male physicians." Dr. Gregory cites a number
         of opinions on women in medicine, gives a history of their
         struggle, and discusses their current status.

3034.   Gregory, Samuel. Letter to Ladies, in Favor of Female
         Physicians For Their Own Sex, 3rd edition. New
         England Female Medical College, Boston, Massachusetts,
         1856, 48 pp.
         This booklet was first published in 1850 and was designed
         to elicit support from women for the education of women to
         become physicians. [The financial support was to under-
         write the costs of opening and operating the New England
         Female Medical College in Boston.] Dr. Gregory feels
         that women should attend women, and a school for their
         instruction should be established. In this pamphlet, he
         sets forth reasons that women should not be banned from
         practice as obstetricians, discusses the situation in other
         countries, and explicates biblical injunctions. Gregory
         speaks of the evil attending male physicians' care of wo-
         men patients.

3035.   Haar, Esther; Halitsky, Victor; and Stricker, George.
         "Factors Related to the Preference for a Female Gyne-
         cologist." Medical Care, 13:9 (September 1975) 782-

790. tables.

"This report investigates the characteristics of women who expressed a preference for a female gynecologist. It is part of a broader exploration of the attitudes and practices of women regarding gynecological examinations and gynecologists. Four hundred and nine female patients of both female and male physicians completed a self-administered questionnaire exploring their attitudes and practices regarding gynecologists and gynecological examinations. Responses to the question 'Would you prefer a woman gynecologist?' divided the sample into three groups: those responding 'yes' (33.9 per cent); those responding 'no' (19.3 per cent); and those responding 'no difference' (36.2 per cent). Results revealed that patients who preferred female gynecologists were most likely to find gynecological examinations difficult and to be critical of gynecologists' understanding of women's psychological and sexual problems. A subsample of patients in psychotherapy was especially apt to prefer female gynecologists. The 'no difference' group had the most positive attitudes towards gynecological examinations and gynecologists. Demographic differences were insignificant. The importance of judging a gynecologist's competence without sexual bias, of re-evaluating stereotypes of women physicians, and of increasing the proportion of women in gynecology is stressed." While a broad spectrum of socioeconomic levels was represented, most of the respondents tended to be well educated and in the higher income brackets. The authors indicate that their sample from the New York City area (Nassau County and Queens) might not be applicable to populations from other sections of the country. Because the authors only used one female gynecologist participant, they feel a comparative study is necessary to examine the responses of patients of female gynecologists with those of male gynecologists to determine if the patients seeing the female gynecologists would indeed feel more at ease.

3036. Hartshorne, Henry. Valedictory Address to the Twentieth Graduating Class of the Woman's Medical College of Pennsylvania. Jas. B. Rodgers Co., Printers, Philadelphia, Pennsylvania, 1872, 14 pp.

"Is the training and commissioning of women for intelligent, well-informed ministration to the sick, so as to use for their benefit the resources of science and the skill of art, right, or wrong?" asks Dr. Hartshorne. Can women reason? Is it proper for women to have charge of the sick? Should women be allowed to choose their own vocation? These are the questions presented and discussed by Dr. Hartshorne, who then proceeds to give the international picture of women in medicine. The Philadelphia Medical Society's attitudes towards women physicians must be seen as a response to conservatism. The address ends with a general exhortation to be good physicians and ways in which to

achieve this goal. "You, ladies," concludes Dr. Hartshorne, "now represent not only a profession, but a cause;
the noble and holy cause of woman's advancement."

3037.   Harvey, Ellwood. Valedictory Address to the Graduating
         Class of the Female Medical College of Pennsylvania,
         For the Session 1854-5. Published by the class, Phil-
         adelphia, Pennsylvania, 1854, 14 pp.
         Following a lengthy discussion of a physician's duties and
         importance, Ellwood Harvey (Professor of the Principles
         and Practice of Medicine at the Female Medical College)
         identifies the pitfalls peculiar to women physicians. Dr.
         Harvey warns the graduates of their "double danger."
         First, due to a huge demand for women physicians (the
         U.S. calls for "not less than" 5000 women doctors), newly
         degreed women do not have to endure the many years of
         perfecting skill and building a reputation that young male
         physicians face: "What I most fear is ... that your path
         to success will be too smooth...." The second danger is
         of acquiring premature popularity "so dangerous even to
         those who have been strengthened by long years of toil and
         effort." Dr. Harvey offers advice on handling male phy-
         sicians who have unfair opinions of women physicians. If
         such a man cannot be enlightened with facts, Dr. Harvey
         says, "you have just cause to pity [him]; but never, never
         quarrel about it. Never take advantage of his folly to in-
         jure him, but treat him tenderly and kindly and he may
         come to see the imprudence of his course...."

3038.   Henry, Frederick P. "Women in Medicine." Medical and
         Surgical Reporter, 76:21 (22 May 1897) 641-644. (Orig-
         inal Articles.) (Commencement address, Woman's
         Medical College of Pennsylvania, Philadelphia, Penn-
         sylvania, 19 May 1897.)
         Dr. Henry gives the graduates of the Woman's Medical Col-
         lege of Pennsylvania words of advice as they enter upon the
         practice of medicine: never betray anxiety to the patient,
         never argue with the laity on medical subjects, and never
         talk about yourself or your personal affairs in the sick-
         room. Specific to women physicians, Dr. Henry briefly
         catalogs the accomplishments of women and quotes from
         Bulwers's What Will He Do with It?: "'A good surgeon ...
         must have an eagle's eye, a lion's heart, and a lady's
         hand.'"

3039.   Hole, Judith and Levine, Ellen. Rebirth of Feminism.
         Quadrangle/the New York Times Book Company, New
         York, New York, 1971.
         Chapter II of this work is entitled "Feminist Analysis:
         Ideas and Issues." On pages 355-362 of this chapter med-
         icine is discussed. Facts and figures on women physicians
         are cited from various sources. Dr. Bernice Sandler,
         chairman of Women's Equity Action League (WEAL), states

that by 1971 some medical schools were increasing their
places for blacks, but only with a corresponding decrease
of places for women. Dr. Frances Norris feels the growth
of the women's movement "has elicited a backlash reaction
from the medical community rather than heightened sensitivity." The section concludes with a discussion of the
woman's health movement.

3040.   Holton, Susan Chapin. "The Woman Physician: A Study of
        Role Conflict." Journal of the American Medical Wo-
        men's Association, 24:8 (August 1969) 638-645. port.,
        tables.
        Role conflict and the woman physician is discussed using
        statistics from Lopate, and Panero, Wiesenfelder, and
        Parmelee. Some of the means whereby these difficulties
        might be resolved are "more adequate domestic help" and
        part-time internships and residencies. "While society pro-
        motes and reinforces role conflict for the educated woman
        by means of differential role expectations and socialization
        procedures, conceivably the social system could act to al-
        leviate or partially eliminate the dysfunctional effects."

3041.   Hosmer, William. Appeal to Husbands and Wives in Favor
        of Female Physicians. New York, New York, 1853.
        [Book not examined by editors.]

3042.   Hudson, Phoebe. "Women's Lib in Medicine? Thanks,
        But We've Got It Now." Medical Economics, (23 Octo-
        ber 1972) 118, passim.
        [Article not examined by editors.]

3043.   Hurd-Mead, Kate Campbell. "Amalgamation, Not Segrega-
        tion: Inaugural Address." Bulletin of the Medical
        Women's National Association, 4 (July 1923) 42-44.
        The author calls for cooperation of medical women world
        wide to solve the problems of public health and aid in the
        "peaceable work of reconstruction." "Pasteur has said that
        'science and peace will one day triumph over ignorance and
        war.' Men have been slow to prove this because, perhaps
        it is a work for women." "If women would only boost each
        other as men have boosted their sex, many a brilliant wo-
        men would have been discovered long before the days of
        the Great War." The author suggests that if women physi-
        cians had as much spare time as their male colleagues to
        sit around at smokers and medical meetings they too would
        be valued as indispensable consultants. Women physicians
        do not have wives at home to take care of the details of
        life. In consideration of these handicaps, the amount of
        work handled by medical women throughout the world is
        amazing. Women should unite to work together for the
        greatest value for the largest number of people.

3044.   Hurley, A. "I Am Not Happy to Be Married to a Woman

Doctor. I Would Not Do It Again." California's Health,
(December 1971) 4-5, 15.
[Article not examined by editors.]

3045.   Ingals, Ephraim Fletcher. "Lady Physicians." Chicago
Medical Journal and Examiner, 46 (April 1883) 390-392.
(Article VI.)
Speaking before an alumni banquet of the Women's Medical
College [Chicago], Professor Ingals affirms woman's right
to enter the medical profession. He goes on to say that
most women "cannot endure the hardships" of general practice and suggests that women physicians specialize in
pharmacy and dentistry.

3046.   Ingelfinger, Franz J. "Doctor Women." New England
Journal of Medicine, 291:6 (8 August 1974) 303-304.
(Editorial.)
Recalling the Harvard Medical School Alumni Day Program
of the Spring of 1974, the author pinpoints Dr. Penelope K.
Garrison's comments as she participated on a panel of four
women physicians who discussed "What It's Been Like":
women, she insisted, although certainly as capable and effective doctors as men, are different in their spiritual, attitudinal, and emotional make-up. From these comments,
the author extrapolates "the woman doctor is not only a
different, but, often as not, a better doctor."

3047.   Ingengo, A. P. "The Case Against the Female M.D."
Medical Economics, (4 December 1961).
[Article not examined by editors.]

3048.   "Is the Lady Doctor a Failure?" British Medical Journal,
1 (1 February 1902) 287.
Although "probably 6,000" lady doctors practice now in the
United States, there are indications in America that women
are failures as physicians. After a 30-years trial, the
trustees of Chicago's Northwestern University decided to
abolish the Women's Medical School. Explaining the impos-
sibility of making a doctor of a woman, one trustee said
that while medical coeducation at Northwestern was a failure,
the women's medical college "has been worse than a failure." This article further speculates that one reason for
women physicians' failure in America may be that supply
exceeds demand. Also, in America, there has been too
much engendering of "'artificial vocations.'" Women may
be able to pass the necessary medical examinations, but
without "physical vigour" they cannot be successful doctors.

3049.   Jacobi, A. ["Medical Studies for Women in America: Open
Letter to the Editors from Prof. A. Jacobi in New
York"]. Deutsche Medicinische Wochenschrift, 22:25
(18 June 1896) 401-403. (Ger)
Dr. Jacobi has practiced in New York for 42 years and has

become well acquainted with the women's rights movement.
The Americans are finding quite amusing the sentimental
publications in German journals advocating keeping women
out of medicine for their own good--they are physically
weaker, have less endurance, are more delicate, menstruate,
may have children, etc.--"as if men doctors were a combination of Apollo, Hercules and Methuselah." Even if the
world is becoming less ethical, a few thousand women doctors will not change its course; mass education of women
might even make the future more pleasant. American women met all the opposition Germans are now meeting, 30
to 40 years ago and responded by establishing their own
schools. Eventually they won their place in the medical
establishment; Dr. Jacobi himself sponsored the first woman member of the New York County Medical Society in
1872. Hospital positions are opening up to them, and at
least two states have laws requiring women staff physicians
to care for women inmates in mental hospitals. Most of
the women medical graduates are in general practice; few
have specialized, even in pediatrics and obstetrics and gynecology. The medical profession is becoming crowded, but
men no longer complain about being pushed aside by women.
They have been accepted by most of their colleagues, the
public, and the government.

3050. Jacobi, M[ary] Putnam. "An Address Delivered at the Com-
       mencement of the Woman's Medical College of the N.Y.
       Infirmary, May 30, 1883." Archives of Medicine, 10
       (1883) 59-71. (Editorial Department.)
The graduates are warned that because they will so often
be reminded that they are women physicians, they may forget they are first of all physicians. There is enough in
medicine to interest a woman, without diverting attention to
questions of social status. Nevertheless, medicine is still
a "class monopoly" characterized by brutal, densely organized, hypocritical opposition to women--especially in
England. Women physicians will continue to have "class
interests, which cannot, with either justice or safety, be
ignored." Dr. Jacobi presents examples of the monopoly
on clinical opportunities, and emphasizes the need for hospital appointments for women. She urges the graduates to
exert effort in extending educational opportunities for all
women. They should also remember that their own education must continue, for too often women, without the imposed discipline of medical school, "begin to drift like rud-
derless ships." Finally, Dr. Jacobi warns the women about
isolation.

3051. Jacobi, M[ary] Putnam. "Inaugural Address at the Opening
       of the Woman's Medical College of the New York In-
       firmary, October 1, 1880. Article I." Chicago Med-
       ical Journal and Examiner, 42:6 (June 1881) 561-585.
       (Original Lectures.)

Following a lengthy discourse on the difficulties involved in
the study and practice of medicine, Dr. Jacobi considers
the special difficulties encountered by women medical students. The entering class is urged "to look at yourselves
as a colony just landed in a new country, compelled to found
a state in spite of hardship and peril, and danger, and isolation, by means of the vigorous and intelligent co-operation
of each of its members."

3052.   Jacobi, Mary Putnam. "A Plea for Medical Women." Med
         ical Record, 37 (25 January 1890) 107. (Correspond-
         ence.)
         Dr. Jacobi comments on a recent Medical News editorial
         which "describes with horror" a case where men and med-
         ical students together watched a woman in labor. She re-
         iterates that "wherever there is a female patient there can
         be no impropriety in the presence of a female student or
         physician."

3053.   Jacobi, Mary Putnam. "Shall Women Practice Medicine?"
         North American Review, 134 (January 1882) 52-75.
         Dr. Jacobi attacks "the floating mass of vague ideas, pre-
         judices, preconceptions, and misconceptions concerning the
         study and practice of medicine by women." Examining the
         roots of society's opposition to medical women, she points
         to the "universal prejudice" towards all medical practition-
         ers, which is based in "the terror of sacrilege"; women
         who enter this "dirty, horrid, and irreverent" sphere not
         only "dehumanize" themselves as men do, but also "unsex"
         themselves. Dr. Jacobi discounts the "natural history" ar-
         gument, which believes women's mental and physical capa-
         cities to be lower than men's. Considering the problems
         of marriage and maternity in the practice of medicine, Dr.
         Jacobi calls for a re-arrangement of domestic work. In
         closing, Dr. Jacobi advocates women's pursuit of medicine
         "as a means of stimulating to better efficiency much exist-
         ing feminine occupation."

3054.   Joiner, Jane Herrod. "Women in Medicine: The Natural
         Thing." Rhode Island Medical Journal, 58:5 (May 1975)
         219-220.
         As long as women are expected to take the burden of re-
         sponsibility for maintenance of home and family, American
         medicine must make accommodations.

3055.   Jones, Jane Gaudette. Career Patterns of Women Physi-
         cians. Brandeis University, [Waltham, Massachusetts],
         May 1971, ix, 184 pp. figs., tables. (Ph.D. thesis.)
         This thesis is based on data collected from 265 women, 69
         per cent of whom were alumnae of the medical schools of
         Harvard, Tufts, or Boston University, and 31 per cent of
         whom were medical students at those schools. The intent
         was to examine the "decisions the woman made as she ad-

justed her progress through the institutionalized sequences
of medical training.   Also analyzed were those non-institu-
tionalized decisions such as marriage and childbearing."
The study examined background variables shared by the women, influences which directed their career choices, and
the problems they encountered in pursuing their career goals.
General findings included that the women tended "toward
being an elite group among American women"; they were
daughters of highly educated professional parents; their
career choice was congruent with their families' professional orientation; and their most frequent study interruptions
were related to marriage and childbearing.   This thesis
also contains comparative statistics on women in all U.S.
medical schools (taken from other sources).   The concluding chapter contains suggestions for recruiting women from
many strata of society and recommendations on how medical schools can help women students minimize role and
domestic conflicts.   An extensive bibliography concludes the
work.

3056.   Keyserling, Mary Dublin.   "Waste No Talent--Neglect No
         Skill."   Journal of the American Medical Women's
         Association, 24:2 (February 1969) 146-153.   (Presenta-
         tion, Annual Meeting, American Medical Women's Asso-
         ciation, Boston, 7 December 1968.)
Mary Keyserling, director of the Woman's Bureau of the
U.S. Department of Labor, addresses the problem of discrimination against women in the work force, and especially
in medicine, by recounting the proceedings of the 1967 Conference on Meeting Medical Manpower Needs--the Fuller
Utilization of the Woman Physician.   Introductory remarks
point out that the relative position of women in the labor
force has deteriorated rather than improved since 1940.
Statistics are cited to support this statement.   While "nearly half of all our women between the ages of 18 and 64 are
presently in the labor force ... [these] women remain very
highly concentrated in the least-skilled, lowest-paid jobs in
the economy."   Keyserling contends that the U.S. is failing
to utilize the talents, skills, and potential of its women:
"We educate and then waste that education in terms of professional activity.   Others educate a far smaller percentage
of their women but use their talents well."   In reviewing
the conference proceedings, three challenges to remedy the
physician shortage and encourage women to become physicians are cited: 1) to enlarge the medical schools; 2) to
eliminate the quota system; and 3) to explode the many attitudinal myths.   Another speaker whose comments were
reviewed pointed out that child rearing was a contribution
to society, and furthermore the years spent by physicians
in performing this task are not "wasted professionally" but
rather "increase human understanding."   Keyserling concludes with a discussion of the "forces at work" to remedy
the problem (e.g., federal equal-pay legislation of 1963,

Title VII of the Civil Rights Act of 1964, and State Commissions on the Status of Women).

3057.   Knopf, S. Adolphus. "The Woman Physician and Professor Cabot. A Reply to the Latter's Statement as to Her Unfitness for General Practice and Medical Research." Woman's Medical Journal, 25:7 (July 1915) 159-160.
In his address delivered before the graduating class of the Woman's Medical College of Pennsylvania, Professor Richard C. Cabot, of Harvard Medical School, is alleged to have said that women physicians "are not temperamentally and physically adapted for the more strenuous branches of the profession." Dr. Knopf refutes this assumption by listing the names and accomplishments of numerous women physicians.

3058.   Knopf, S. Adolphus. "Woman's Duty Toward the Health of the Nation." New York Medical Journal, 80 (1904) 865-867.
[Article not examined by editors.]

3059.   "The Lady Doctor: What Barriers Does She Meet?" Modern Medicine, 36:22 (21 October 1968) 54-56, 61, 64. photo., table. (Newsfeature.)
Opinions vary as to the nature and extent of barriers met by women physicians. An unnamed medical school dean prefers "a third-rate man to a first-rate woman," but questionnaires by Modern Medicine and the American Medical Women's Association reveal that some women physicians have met with few, if any, obstacles. Others suggested solutions: remove the stigma attached to all professional women, train counselors to encourage women to choose professional fields, make more scholarships available, get tax breaks because of the domestic help required, arrange flexible internships and residencies, make day-care available, offer refresher courses. Some 1966 statistics regarding women physicians are quoted.

3060.   Lake, Alice. "Drop Those Prejudices Against Women Doctors." Journal of the American Medical Women's Association, 22:6 (June 1967) 402-406.
In order to justify the statement that women physicians should not be discriminated against, Alice Lake writes that the stereotype of the female doctor is inaccurate: "hair in a tight bun, severe tweeds, shoes with thick rubber soles." Furthermore, women doctors "have more energy than most." They nurture husbands and a parcel of children. To earn the credibility of their patients, they perform wondrous feats: "In danger of being crushed [when a worker was pinned in a railroad accident, a woman doctor] inched her way on her stomach to give the man a shot of morphine...." Remarkable as women physicians might be, "most teenage

boys shun her, and some grown men blush at the thought
of allowing a female to check a hernia. Women can be
prejudiced too. Some secretly believe their own sex is inferior." Women "enjoy the half-flirtatious, half father-
daughter relationship that develops with a male obstetrician.
An occasional woman complains because a female doctor is
a spinster ('How can she understand a mother's problem?'),
another because she's married ('She's got half her mind on
her husband and children.').'' Other patients prefer seeing
a woman physician: children, teenage girls, and housewives who are more comfortable discussing "reproductive
complaints" and talking about their husbands or "a crush on
a friend's husband." Then too, some husbands "insist that
their wives see a female doctor whenever a pelvic examination is required." The "conflict between femininity and
medical success plays a greater role than academic failure
in the drop-out rate of girls from medical school." "My
philosophy is to be a good doctor, but never to look like
one," Dr. Mary Bazelon is quoted as saying. The author
adds: "For when a woman is feminine and a doctor to
boot, she tends to win over even the toughest opposition.
As a sixteen-year-old boy put it, when Dr. Maxine Schurter
was called in to repair his broken nose: 'Are you my doctor? Man, this is cool!'" [This article was reprinted
from Good Housekeeping, May 1967.]

3061.   Lanzoni, Phoebe Krey. "The Woman Doctor in the Medical
          Center." Boston University Medical Center Centerscope,
          (July/August 1971) 14-16.   port.   (Women in Medicine.)
     Through anecdotes of her children's reactions to their moth-
     er as a physician, Dr. Lanzoni illustrates the deeply in-
     grained traditions that place barriers before women seeking
     medical careers. She suggests ways in which medical train-
     ing could be altered in order to reduce the obstacles wo-
     men face.

3062.   Levine, Adeline. "Forging a Feminine Identity: Women in
          Four Professional Schools." American Journal of Psy-
          choanalysis, 35:1 (Spring 1975) 63-67.
     This article is based on a survey made in 1967 of 79 un-
     married women students in four professional programs at
     Yale, and on a follow-up questionnaire sent to these same
     women in 1973. The author identifies two groups: women's
     career field group, which includes nursing and teaching;
     and men's career field group, which includes law and medi-
     cine. The author concludes: "(1) choice of career field,
     as well as respondents' perceptions of familial attitudes to-
     ward proper adult roles for women, were each related to
     the level of the respondents' mothers' education. (2) Ex-
     periences in professional school were such that women in
     law and medical schools were learning to work with men,
     and many were having normal social experiences with men.
     The women in nursing and teaching were isolated from men

in their working life, as well as socially. (3) The plans
for future work differed considerably by career field.
Ninety-one per cent of [men's career field] and thirty-five
per cent of [women's career field] planned no withdrawal
from the labor force once children were born. (4) [Men's
career field] students had considered the problem of combining work and marital responsibilities in more detail than
had [women's career field] students and felt more able to
accommodate professional obligations to familial ones.
[Women's career field] planned to carry out professional
and familial activities at different periods in their future
lives. (5) A preliminary examination of a six-year follow-
up study shows [men's career field] members finding it a
bit more difficult than anticipated to work when children are
young, and [women's career field] members more concerned
about questions of equal pay and sharing of familial responsibilities than they had anticipated. Most are comfortable,
satisfied with careers, and have no regrets as they look
back.''

3063.   Levine, Adeline Gordon. Marital and Occupational Plans of
         Women in Professional Schools: Law, Medicine, Nurs-
         ing, Teaching. Yale University, [New Haven, Connecti-
         cut], 1968, 135, A10, 38 pp. tables. (Ph.D. thesis.)
The subjects of this study were all unmarried women students in four professional schools at Yale University. Two
of the professions (nursing and teaching) were characterized
as Women's Career Fields (WCF); the others (law and medicine), as Men's Career Fields (MCF). The two groups
were compared as to social class, background, future plans,
and current experiences. Findings included: the MCF group
came from a higher social class and had better educated
mothers than the WCF group; the MCF group did not plan
any withdrawal from the labor force, while the WCF group
planned withdrawal for child care; and, while work expectations were not related to social class in the MCF group,
work expectations were inversely related to social class in
the WCF group.

3064.   Liu, Felicia and Rothchild, Alice. "The Woman as Med-
         ical Student." Boston University Medical Center Center-
         scope, (July/August 1971) 6-8. ports.
The authors, students at the Boston University School of
Medicine, cite personal experiences of "daily oppressive
moments" in medical school. They call for changes in the
way men relate to women and for a restructuring of the
medical system. They note that they "feel closer ties to
the women who make up 80 per cent of the health care work
force than to the doctors who dominate it; for it is with
these women that we share the common experience of struggling with and defining ourselves within the health system."

3065.   Livezey, Abraham. Lecture, Introductory to the Course,

on the Practice of Medicine, to the Class of the N.E.
Female Medical College. Published by the class, Boston, Massachusetts, 1852, 14 pp. (Opening address,
New England Female Medical College, Boston, Massachusetts, 17 February 1852.)

Following generalized observations of medical study and
practice, Dr. Livezey (a professor at the Female Medical
College of Pennsylvania) discusses the suitability of women
for medical careers.

3066.   Lobdell, Mary. "Can Men and Women Doctors Be a Help
         to Each Other?" Woman's Medical Journal, 15:2
         (February 1905) 30-32. (Presentation, Kansas State
         Medical Society, Topeka, Kansas, May 1904.)

"A doctor's life is too short to spend any of it in petty
jealousies," says Dr. Lobdell, who makes suggestions on
how women physicians can unoffensively deal with antagonis-
tic male counterparts.

3067.   Longshore, Joseph S. A Valedictory Address Delivered Be-
         fore the Graduating Class at the First Annual Com-
         mencement of the Female Medical College, of Pennsyl-
         vania, Held at the Musical Fund Hall, December 30,
         1851. Published by the graduates, Philadelphia, Penn-
         sylvania, 1852, 14 pp.

Dr. Longshore admonishes the women of this graduating
class to remember the debt of deep gratitude they owe to
the State of Pennsylvania for "the high and noble stand she
has taken in behalf of woman's elevation and woman's interests." Dr. Longshore reiterates the historical importance of this event. He cautions that although the women
have proven themselves capable, have received a fine education, and may consider themselves particularly capable,
they must not let their anticipations rise too high, for there
will still be opposition (not the least of which will come
from other women). Dr. Longshore's advice to these women
physicians urges them to have self-confidence, to realize
their superiority but temper it with understanding, to take
on the mantle of authority and demand obedience: "Your
time, means, and energies have been directed towards a
higher and more responsible position than a performer of
the mere drudgery of the invalid's chamber.... But when
stern necessity requires of you a helping hand, be ever
ready, ever willing." Never allow interference, by anyone,
with your prescriptions, for "the responsibility of the case
rests with you alone." Do not use alcohol in medication;
be frank, candid, and truthful with patients; use no undue
influence to acquire patronage; never interfere with patients
of a neighboring practitioner; and "do not, because you are
women, regard yourselves inferior, or your judgment of
less value on that account ... yield only to conviction."

3068.   Lorber, Judith. "Women and Medical Sociology: Invisible

Professionals and Ubiquitous Patients." In: Another
Voice: Feminist Perspectives on Social Life and Social
Science. Edited by Marcia Millman and Rosabeth Moss
Kanter. Anchor Press/Doubleday, Garden City, New
York, 1975, 75-105.

"The studies of practicing women doctors and dentists, although done by medical sociologists, are static, lack cross-
national comparisons, and suffer from minimal conceptualiza-
tion or post hoc explanations." The author discusses such
concepts as "downward mobility," the "masculine mystique
in American medicine," and the woman as patient. The
chapter offers a review of major studies on women physicians.

3069.   Lueth, Carl Anthony. Selected Aspects in the Attainment
         and Use of the Doctor of Medicine, Doctor of Dental
         Surgery, and Bachelor of Laws Degrees by Women
         Graduates of Tulane University and Loyola University of
         the South. University of Mississippi, [University, Mis-
         sissippi], 1973, 204 pp. (Ph.D. thesis.)

Data was collected from 208 women who graduated in medicine, law, and dentistry from 1945 to 1972. The study's
purpose was to identify factors which impeded or facilitated
these women in their attainment and use of professional degrees, to describe the personal characteristics of women
who earn professional degrees, and to determine the women's
subsequent use of their training. Findings indicated that the
influence of others (especially parents) most facilitated the
attainment of professional degrees, while poor high school
and college counseling most impeded that progress. Most
of the women had upper-middle-class parents, married men
in professional fields, and bore two children. Only ten per
cent of the respondents were not professionally active. The
women experienced discrimination in entering the more
prestigious areas of their fields. A survey of available literature on the subject of women in professions was also
made, and conclusions drawn. Statistical tables throughout
the work segregate information by profession. One chapter
gives an overview of women in professions. The thesis contains an extensive bibliography. Appendixes include 28
pages of the respondents' personal comments, many of which
testify to discrimination.

3070.   Lyman, George H. "The Interests of the Public and the
         Medical Profession." Medical Communications (Massa-
         chusetts Medical Society), 2nd Series, 8 (1881) 1-44.
         (Presentation, Annual Meeting, Massachusetts Medical
         Society, 9 June 1875.)

Dr. Lyman discusses, among other interests of the public
in regard to the medical profession, the rights and suitability of women to medical education and hospital privileges,
and the question of coeducation in medical schools. A history is given of those times during which the society has

been called upon for its opinion on these matters. A discussion follows in which the fallacy of women's exclusive suitability for the practice of obstetrics is reviewed.

3071. McGrew, Elizabeth A. "To the Apteryx, an Anachronism."
        Journal of the American Medical Women's Association,
        22:5 (May 1967) 343. (AMWA President's Message.)
In response to another woman physician refusing to speak at a branch meeting of the American Medical Women's Association because, "women's professional organizations are anachronisms," Elizabeth McGrew points out the following areas of discrimination that continue to exist against women physicians: conflicting pressures in all stages of preparing for a medical career; women are not being recruited to fill medical "manpower" shortages nor to speak at governmental and educational conferences; the all-male committees of the American Medical Association do not represent the opinions and interests of women physicians; and women are being excluded from helping other countries develop medical care systems.

3072. McKusick, Marjorie J. K.; Anderson, Kathryn D.; and
        Garrison, Penelope. "A Panel Discussion: What It's
        Been Like." Harvard Medical Alumni Bulletin, 48:6
        (July-August 1974) 20-23. photos.
"What has Harvard meant to me, as a physician, as a member of my community and as a woman?" Three women graduates speak to this question. Dr. McKusick (a 1949 graduate) finds it difficult to relate her Harvard experience to being a woman. She was in the first class to admit women to Harvard, and after working through the we-made-it-in-a-man's-world-why-can't-they attitude, she realized that there is discrimination and it should be fought: "we should support the movement for women's liberation." Dr. Anderson (class of 1964) sees women in medicine as a three-stage phenomenon. Stage I was characterized by women entering medicine--a man's world--an extraordinary event. Stage II is that of women's liberation--calling attention to women's plight. Stage III will be that of assimilation of women into all branches of medicine. Dr. Anderson recalls experiences of prejudice against her as a woman physician. Dr. Garrison (class of 1969), following Dr. Anderson, notes that women have a way to go before they are completely assimilated, witnessed by the fact that they are last on the program. Dr. Garrison describes her experiences with child psychiatry and concludes with the hope that women will become "female individuals"--women are different from men, with different perspectives and different advantages.

3073. Mandelbaum, Dorothy Rosenthal. Factors Related to Per-
        sistence in Practice by Women Physicians. Bryn Mawr
        College, Bryn Mawr, Pennsylvania, 1974, xxiv, 389 pp.
        figs., tables. (Ph.D. thesis.)

This dissertation was based on the assumption that there are personality dispositions directly related to feminine self-definition that emerge in times of conflict and are decisive factors in the decisions of women physicians to persist or withdraw from practice. The major variables examined for differences between those who persisted with careers and those who withdrew (non-persisters) included: imbedding of the career goal; personality differences; marital and maternal status; women physicians as marginal persons; differences in role priorities; differences in work behaviors and attitude; and self-esteem. The study was conducted on 71 randomly selected women physicians in the Philadelphia area in 1973. Data were gathered by a mail questionnaire soliciting demographic information, an in-depth interview, and the Grough Adjective Check List. The 40 persisters were described as those who have always worked, those retired for reasons of age or disability but who had not worked for a cumulative period of less than one year, and those working at the time of the study who had not worked for a cumulative period of less than one year at some time. The 31 non-persisters included those not working for reasons other than age or disability and those working who had cumulative nonwork periods of one year or longer. The persisters and non-persisters were found significantly different on 45 variables. Although both groups followed similar patterns of professional socialization until at least their mid-twenties, the persister was found to have developed in an environment less favorable to her early imbedded unrealistic career wish. To achieve her goal it was necessary to channel her energies in one direction, at times denying her right to marriage and motherhood. The non-persister, however, was born a decade later than her colleague and matured in an environment with greater early support for her goal. Greater paternal closeness and more peer involvement contributed to increased feminine socialization. In situations of conflict between maternal and work demands, her priorities were more clearly in favor of maternity. In middle years, the persister enjoyed her work and its advantages while the non-persister was more conflicted and anxious for her appropriate identity.

3074. Marmor, Judd. "Women in Medicine: Importance of the Formative Years." Journal of the American Medical Women's Association, 23:7 (July 1968) 621-625. (Address, Conference on "Meeting Medical Manpower Needs The Fuller Utilization of the Woman Physician," January 12, 1968, sponsored by the U.S. Department of Labor, Women's Bureau, Washington, D.C.)

Only one-sixteenth of one per cent of the total feminine working force, or 15,500 women, are physicians. Therefore, the basic challenge "is no longer that of availability of vocational options, but rather that of making it possible

for more women to exercise those options that would enable them to realize their potentials fully." Regardless of
the fact that the practice of medicine would be "particularly
compatible with femininity" and because doctors as "private
practitioners, can elect to work as many or as few hours
as they like," as well as have "geographic mobility ...
[to] accompany her husband almost anywhere in the world,
and still be able to do remunerative work in her own field,"
culture patterns rather than basic biological differences between the sexes are the reasons why few women practice
medicine. "The challenge to society is to make it possible
for women, no less than men, to actualize themselves to
their fullest without feeling emotionally threatened in their
relationships with the opposite sex, or their basic sense of
femininity."

3075.   Marr, Judith. "Situation Improving, Say Michigan's Fe-
            male Physicians." Michigan Medicine, 74:2 (January
            1975) 15-17. illus., photo., ports.
         Four women physicians agree that there is still strong feel-
         ing against women in medicine but that the situation is im-
         proving. Ethelene Crockett, Detroit obstetrician, Jeanne
         McKune, Dearborn family practitioner, Marilyn Heins, as-
         sociate dean of Wayne State University Medical School, and
         Cecelia Hissong, Dearborn family physician, discuss their
         status and personal experiences as women physicians. The
         article quotes a survey reporting that 96 per cent of 500
         clinic patients felt the typical M.D. was male, and 78 per
         cent preferred a male doctor, but the women believe pref-
         erences will change when more women M.D.s graduate and
         begin practicing.

3076.   Marshall, Margaret. "Women and Medicine: or the Doc-
            tor's Dilemma." Case Western Reserve Medical Alum-
            ni Bulletin, 31:4 (Fourth Quarter, 1967) 4-7, 29. pho-
            tos., ports.
         Quotes from various studies and from interviews with women
         graduates of Case Western Reserve University School of
         Medicine identify the social, cultural, and economic road-
         blocks for medical women.

3077.   "Medical Education for Women Called Worthwhile." Science
            Digest, 44:5 (November 1958) 48. cartoon.
         Dr. Francis Hannett, a Chicago psychoanalyst, asserts that
         many women can be housewife-mothers and practice medi-
         cine at the same time, dropping out only temporarily for
         childbirth. It is not wasteful to train women as physicians:
         women "fill a vacuum" in the profession, taking jobs that
         male physicians do not want. Would women physicians urge
         their daughters to study medicine? An affirmative response
         came from 74 per cent of 1,040 women.

3078.   Menninger, Karl. "The Psychological Advantages of the

Woman Physician (1936)." Bulletin of the Menninger
Clinic, 37 (July 1973) 333-340. (Presentation, Meeting,
American Medical Women's Association, Kansas City,
Missouri, 13 May 1936.)
Dr. Menninger believes that women have "certain culturally
ingrained personality features" that especially suit them for
practicing medicine and psychiatry. Among those characteristics are "a better understanding of suffering and inferiority" and the related trait of intuition (defined as per-
ceptual sensitiveness to emotional reactions). In handling
patients, the woman physician's girlhood training is very use
ful. The techniques used by girls to attract love, which
can be carried over to the woman's professional work, include anticipating the needs of others, attracting attention
by listening to confidences, and disarming antagonists with
graciousness. Paraphrasing D. H. Lawrence's comment
that it is better to be "hen-sure" than "cock-sure," Dr.
Menninger affirms that "some of our most distinguished
psychiatrists are women...." He advises women physicians
not to imitate men, but to allow their "special gifts" as women to guide their work. This article also contains a description of psychiatric diagnosis and treatment.

3079.   Merritt, Doris H. "Discrimination and the Woman Execu-
             tive: Convention Blocks Use of a Resource." Business
             Horizons, 12:6 (December 1969) 15-22. illus.
         Dr. Merritt describes her experience in the medical pro-
         fession, "where women are better tolerated than in other
         fields," but where few achieve executive positions. The
         obstacle lies in society's social and economic attitudes.
         Women as women, however, have many advantages in at-
         tempting to gain management positions and in becoming suc-
         cessful as executives. Inherent female qualities--"patience,
         flexibility, tact, and attention to detail"--are desirable at-
         tributes for an executive. And the "fact we [married wo-
         men executives] do not have to work makes us better em-
         ployees" (e.g., job security does not affect decision mak-
         ing).

3080.   Middleton, William S. "Women in Medicine." Medical
             Woman's Journal, 43:11 (November 1936) 292-295.
             (Address, Twenty-sixth Biennial Convention, Alpha Ep-
             silon Iota, Madison, Wisconsin, 15 April 1936.)
         Dr. Middleton "sets forth many reasons for this conversion
         to and subsequent ardent support for the education of women
         in medicine, and at the same time points out the general
         principles which he considers responsible for the failure of
         medical women as a group to hold their own." [Journal
         summary.]

3081.   Milic, Louis T. "To the Editor." The Woman Physician,
             26:4 (April 1971) 217-218. (Open Forum.)
         In response to a previous article in this journal by Dr.

Mathilda Vaschak entitled "Household Help--The Woman Doctor's Gordian Knot," (June 1970), this male Ph.D. who is married to a woman physician points out that the major problems a woman physician has to solve go far beyond acquiring dependable household help. "The housekeeper does not want to bring up the doctor's children. She is forced to do so by economic necessity, usually the result of a lack of education or privilege." Besides the fact that medical school and training is essentially designed for young men without home responsibilities, and besides the fact that medicine is a business rather than an utility (which is not as it should be), "In the name of freedom from a woman's traditional duties, she has exchanged one form of servitude for another.... She chose to be always tired, often irritable, always in a hurry, the empty chair at the table."

3082.   Morantz, Regina Markell. "The Perils of Feminist History."
          Journal of Interdisciplinary History, IV:4 (Spring 1974)
          649-660.
      Morantz discusses in detail Ann Douglas Wood's work " 'The
      Fashionable Diseases': Women's Complaints and Their
      Treatment in Nineteenth-Century America" (Journal of Inter-
      disciplinary History, IV (1973), 25-52). Wood's article is
      at its weakest, suggests this author, in its discussion of
      19th-century medical therapeutics and the attitudes and self-
      images of pioneering women doctors. Morantz specifically
      takes issue with Wood's characterization of S. Weir Mitchell,
      a physician in the latter half of the 19th century. Morantz
      can find no substantiation for Wood's claim that Mitchell
      felt " 'women doctors would always be inferior to male phy-
      sicians.'" Wood also gives "special status to the 'sadism'
      of men and male doctors," a sadism which Morantz views as
      ill-defined and ill-supported. Wood's portrayal of the "atti-
      tudes and beliefs of the first-generation women doctors" is
      also reviewed, especially with emphasis on Harriot Hunt,
      an early physician and feminist. Wood presents Hunt as a
      man-hater--a portrayal which "lacks the richness which
      more attention to the historical background can provide."
      Morantz finds most interesting "the degree to which [women
      physicians'] own attitudes toward women mirrored those of
      their male colleagues. These professional women were not
      modern-day feminists charging the barricades of male privi-
      lege, but were very much Victorian women, prisoners of
      their own time and culture."

3083.   Morgan, Marcia Ruth. A Comparison of Selected Person-
          ality, Biographical and Motivational Traits Among Wo-
          men Athletes, Physicians, and Attorneys. Ohio State
          University, [Columbus, Ohio], 1973, vii, 147 pp. fig.,
          tables. (Ph.D. thesis.)
      This study's investigations indicate that many psychological,
      motivational, and biographical similarities exist among wo-
      men who are high achievers in male-dominated occupations

and that such women have personality patterns closer to the
general population of men than to the general population of
women.   Tables and explanatory text provide information on
women physicians in the following areas: birth order,
parental occupations and income, childhood play habits, attitudes towards medical practice, marital status, and religious affiliation.   The thesis includes copies of the questionnaires sent to the study's subjects (12 physicians were
included in the final sample of 34 women), and an extensive
bibliography.

3084.   Morrow, Laura E.   "Preliminary Report: Why Women Study
            Medicine."   Journal of the American Medical Women's
            Association,   30:3 (March 1975) 141.
         In 1974 the American Medical Women's Association (AMWA)
         sent questionnaires to 115 deans of U.S. medical schools
         asking them to identify the factors which they feel influence
         women to choose medical careers.   Fifteen influencing fac-
         tors were listed on the questionnaire.   The majority of the
         respondents (100) agreed that most women opt for medical
         careers due to society's changing attitudes which "encourage
         girls to aspire to a career as well as to marriage."   The
         least important influence on women's career choice, ac-
         cording to the deans: the "increasing demand for personal
         women physicians by members of women's organizations."

3085.   Morton, Mrs. Richard F.   "More Advice to Women MD's."
            New England Journal of Medicine, 285:15 (7 October
            1971) 862-863.   (Correspondence.)
         Mrs. Richard Morton, M.D., F.A.A.P. advises the woman
         medical student to select a husband "whose masculinity tol-
         erates domestic tasks," and whose "ego can survive spas-
         modic support."

3086.   Murphy, Claudia Q.   "Are Women a Failure?"   Woman's
            Medical Journal, 1:7 (July 1893) [144-145].
         The editor of the National Medical Review of Washington
         has stated that "women in medicine are a lamentable failure,
         unless they are able to quote someone else than Dr. Mary
         Putnam-Jacobi."   Dr. Murphy cites other examples of suc-
         cessful women physicians and states that women in medicine
         are a success and she will not try to convince this man,
         for "'the man convinced against his will, is of the same
         opinion still.'"   She suggests that what the male physician
         fears from women in the profession is what a male preacher
         she heard speak admitted: "... if they ordained woman,
         what would become of us men!"

3087.   Nadelson, Carol.   "'Increasing the Number of Women Phy-
            sicians: Problems and Directions.'"   Case Western Re-
            serve Medical Alumni Bulletin, 38:3 (1974) 4-6, 24.
            photo. (Presentation, Workshop on Women in Medicine,
            Case Western Reserve University School of Medicine,
            21 September 1974.)

3088.   Nadelson, Carol and Notman, Malkah T. "The Woman Phy-
         sician." Journal of Medical Education, 47:3 (March
         1972) 176-183.
         This article identifies some of the obstacles women physi-
         cians face in their careers. Passivity and compliancy, tra-
         ditionally seen as female attributes, preclude the considera-
         tion of a medical career for a great many women. Fe-
         male medical students feel hostility from peers and instruc-
         tors, have to deny their own personal identity needs and
         feelings, become the object of jokes, and feel the lack of
         women role models. Later difficulties include finding spe-
         cialty training, maintaining a social life, trying to maintain
         a traditional medical career and perform the activities of a
         traditional wife and mother, and finding support from other
         women who very well may be envious.

3089.   Norberg, Karen E. "A Critique of Pure Assimilation."
         Harvard Medical Alumni Bulletin, 50:1 (September/Oc-
         tober 1975) 33. ports. (The Harvard Medical Area
         Women Students Association.)
         Norberg, a member of the class of 1977, points out that
         when professionals speak of "women and medicine" they re-
         fer to problems of women professionals. In contrast, wo-
         men students feel sisterhood with other women workers and
         consumers in the health care system. While not entirely
         successful (few working class women attended), the 1975
         Conference on Women and Health was one attempt to exam-
         ine the problem of helping women claim control of their
         bodies and of their working situations.

3090.   Notman, Malkah T. and Nadelson, Carol C. "Medicine:
         A Career Conflict for Women." American Journal of
         Psychiatry, 130:10 (October 1973) 1123-1126. (Pre-
         sented at 125th Annual Meeting, American Psychiatric
         Association, Dallas, Texas, 1-5 May 1972.)
         The issues involved in a woman's choice of a medical ca-
         reer are explored by the authors: early patterns, paucity
         of acceptable role models for a variety of life and family
         patterns, and defining her identity as a woman in a "man's
         world." Women respond to these challenges in a variety of
         ways related to individual characterological and defensive
         styles. Specific recommendations for non-academically-
         related additions to medical school programs conclude the
         article.

3091.   "On the Opening of the Johns Hopkins Medical School to
         Women." Century Magazine, 19 (February 1891) 632-
         637. (Open Letters.)
         Cardinal Gibbons of Baltimore urges acceptance of women
         physicians: "The alleviation of suffering, for women of all
         classes, which would result from the presence among us of
         an adequate number of well-trained female physicians can-
         not but be evident to all." Mary Putnam Jacobi finds the

movement for women physicians to be solidly founded on a
democratic basis of support--popular demand from below,
rather than edict from government officials "above." Josephine Lowell states that only women can care for women
and cites various medical situations to substantiate this
view. William Osler feels that no obstacles should be
placed in the path of any woman who chooses to pursue
medicine as a career. Charles F. Folsom writes: "I am
quite sure there is no risk of lowering the intellectual
standard of medical education if women and men study together." In conclusion M. Carey Thomas points out that
"intellectual activity is the keenest of possible lifelong
pleasures and a safeguard against a multitude of evils,"
and women should certainly not be excluded from its pursuit.

3092.   Ortiz, Flora Ida. "Women and Medicine: The Process of
         Professional Incorporation." Journal of the American
         Medical Women's Association, 30:1 (January 1975) 18-
         19, 21-23, 27-30.
         "This study deals with the movement toward full incorpora-
         tion into a profession. The process is viewed in the con-
         text of the medical training of three female participants.
         The claim is made that a participant must undergo the 'rites
         of passage' (Van Gennep, 1960) in order to achieve complete
         professionalism. Acceptance into the profession is depend-
         ent on the bargain struck by the participant and the profes-
         sional organization. The participant identifies her role and
         the organization allocates an organizational 'space' congruent
         with the role identity." [Article abstract.]

3093.   "Our Joking Contemporaries." Woman's Medical Journal,
         5:8 (August 1896) 202-203. (Editorial.)
         "The Woman's Medical Journal believes in fun ... but be-
         cause we are doctors is no reason that we should cease to
         be ladies...." Obscene jokes have no place in medicine,
         and especially have no place among women physicians ("it
         is womanly to be clean").

3094.   "Panel Discussion--Women in Medicine Workshop." Case
         Western Reserve Alumni Bulletin, 38:3 (1974) 7-8, 24.
         ports. (Workshop on Women in Medicine, Case West-
         ern Reserve University School of Medicine, 21 Septem-
         ber 1974.)
         Panelists included Cathy Keating and Laurie Cappa (medical
         students), Drs. Ruth P. Owens, Doris A. Evans, Carol
         Nadelson, and Robert Weiss, and Dean Frederick C. Rob-
         bins. They touched upon such areas of concern as the
         origins of negative views towards women physicians, the
         pressures of minority status, discrimination and how to
         cope with it, and the sociological differences between the
         United States and the foreign countries that affect the per-
         centages of medical women.

3095.   Parker, E. "Why Not More Women in Medicine?" Med-
            ical Annals of the District of Columbia, 32 (November
            1963) 473-474.
        [Article not examined by editors.]

3096.   Parker, W. W. Woman's Place in the Christian World:
            Superior Morally, Inferior Mentally, to Man--Not Quali-
            fied for Medicine or Law--The Contrariety and Har-
            mony of the Sexes. J. W. Fergusson & Son, Printer,
            Richmond, Virginia, 1892, 26 pp.
        This treatise (which also appeared in Transactions of the
        Medical Society of Virginia in 1892, pp. 86-107) was writ-
        ten by an honorary fellow and ex-president of the Medical
        Society of Virginia. [Item not examined by editors.]

3097.   "Patients Found Mistrustful of Women MDs." Medical
            Tribune, (1 May 1974) 13.
        [Article not examined by editors.]

3098.   Patterson, Norma W. "Distaff Doctoral Candidates: A
            Sampling of Views & Goals." MCG Today [Medical
            College of Georgia], 2:2 (Fall 1971) 4-5, 30-33.   ports.
        This article is a result of interviews with students (ran-
        domly selected) from the Medical College of Georgia.
        Twenty-seven women are students at the College. Those
        interviewed were Libby Blanton, Becky Trowell, Katharyn
        Outzs, Lane Mathis, Gail Lamb, and Lou Frank. The wo-
        men discuss why they chose to enter medicine, whether
        they feel a medical career and family life are compatible,
        and whether or not they feel discriminated against.

3099.   Peterson, Frederick. "The Woman Physician--Her Future:
            Address to the Graduating Class of 1899, Woman's
            Medical College of the New York Infirmary." Woman's
            Medical Journal, 9[8]:10 (October 1899) 343-347.   (Orig-
            inal Articles.)
        "Women physicians have become so numerous now, and wo-
        men have so completely and perfectly assumed the role of
        merchant, tradesman, politician, lawyer, priest and doctor,
        that their presence no longer excites either comment or
        wonder." Women physicians are suited to the practice of
        medicine because of their "intuitive wit ... swift imagina-
        tion ... [and] deductive methods of philosophy."

3100.   Peterson, Robert A. "Vocational Interest Patterns of
            Male and Female Medical Students Over a Four-Year
            Period." Journal of Counseling Psychology, 19:1 (Jan-
            uary 1973) 21-25.   tables.
        "This study compared the vocational interests of matched
        samples of male and female medical students over a four-
        year period [1956-60]. Although several interest differences
        did occur between the samples, overall the samples ex-
        hibited more similar than dissimilar interest patterns.

Female students possessed slightly more 'nonpeople' interests [and scored significantly higher on the Academic
Achievement Scale] than did male students; both groups decreased in their preferences for science-related items over
the test-retest period." [Article abstract.]

3101.   Philbrick, Inez C. "Women, Let Us Be Loyal to Women!"
         Medical Woman's Journal, 36:2 (February 1929) 39-42.
         (Address, Nebraska Association of Medical Women, 19
         May 1928.)
         What is loyalty? "Are women not loyal to women? Is
         there that in women which deserves and demands the loyal-
         ty of other women? Has woman a part in the purposeful
         drama of a universe that she cannot play without the loyalty
         of women? As applying to medical women, are there not
         certain fields of medicine rightfully belonging to women
         physicians for reasons of propriety, racial experience, and
         aptness, which fields they cannot enter and cultivate and
         bring to fruition in best service without the loyalty of wo-
         men?" These questions are discussed in Dr. Philbrick's
         article.

3102.   Picot, L. J. "Shall Women Practice Medicine?" North
         Carolina Medical Journal, 16 (1885) 10-21.
         [Article not examined by editors.]

3103.   Pool, Judith G. and Bunker, John P. "Women in Medicine."
         Hospital Practice, 7:8 (August 1972) 109-116. photos.,
         table.
         The situation for women in medicine is improving. At
         Stanford University School of Medicine, for example, a
         conscious effort has increased women's representation on
         the faculty and raised to 25 per cent the proportion of fe-
         males in the 1972 entering class. But negative attitudes
         still exist towards women physicians. This article looks
         at the sources of those attitudes and their consequences,
         and offers suggestions on how opportunities for medical wo-
         men can be increased (e.g., part-time graduate training
         and retraining programs). "In the final analysis, more wo-
         men must themselves see medicine as a reasonable career
         goal and then articulate the special needs that must be met
         to enable them to pursue it and lead a full personal life as
         well."

3104.   Potter, Ellen C. "Woman As a Social Force." Journal of
         the American Medical Women's Association, 7:11 (No-
         vember 1952) 421-422.
         Dr. Potter believes women's feelings of inferiority are not
         justified by the facts. All but one medical school is open
         to them. They have had the vote for 30 years but why
         have women not taken more of a role in shaping public
         policy? "The facts are, and it is our own fault, that we
         have not prepared ourselves for public service in the polit-

ical field." Dr. Potter lists the various women who have
reached positions of power in different fields over the last
50 years and asks "Are we producing their like today? If
not, why not?"

3105.   Potter, Ellen C. "The Woman Physician and Public Wel-
        fare." Medical Woman's Journal, 37:7 (July 1930) 181-
        182. (Radio speech, Woman's Forum, Columbia Broad-
        casting Company, Conducted by the National Council of
        Women.)
During this broadcast, Dr. Potter, the returning president
of the Medical Women's National Association, speaks as a
representative of the 7,000 women physicians in the United
States. Women physicians are not a new product of the
feminist movement. They have been practicing for centuries
in some countries, and were exclusively in attendance to all
women in childbirth in America until the 18th century, when
men began to become involved in obstetrics. The time has
come when medical women need to be concerned with the
security and perpetuation of opportunity for future generations
of women. The door of opportunity is slowly closing for
women, and the Medical Women's National Association
"stands guard to keep the door of medical opportunity open."
Dr. Potter concludes the broadcast with a recounting of
some of the unique contributions made by medical women.

3106.   "Present Conditions." Woman's Medical Journal, 6:3
        (March 1897) 67-68. (Editorial.)

3107.   Preston, Ann. "Medical Classics: Introductory Lecture to
        the Class of the Female Medical College of Pennsylvania.
        Delivered at the Opening of the Tenth Session, October
        19, 1859." Medical Woman's Journal, 37:2 (February
        1930) 44-47. port.
Reviewing some of the changes in "occupations, modes of
living, habits of thought and general education of the people"
that have taken place over the preceding century, Ann Preston focuses attention on the movement, in the United States
and abroad, which put women into the labor force and expanded their range of employments. Correspondingly, women have realized and advanced in the standard of their edu-
cation--a standard which has carried them into the study and
practice of medicine. Those men who would regard such
education as "some abnormal social phenomenon" understand
neither the historical antecedents nor the present social
pressures. Neither do they understand the nature of woman. Ann Preston continues with an explication of the
state-of-the-art of medicine.

3108.   Preston, Ann. "Reply." Philadelphia Medical and Surgical
        Reporter, 4 May 1867. (Letter to the Editor.) In:
        Eighteenth Annual Announcement of the Woman's Medical
        College of Pennsylvania, North College Avenue and 22nd

Street, Philadelphia, For the Session of 1867-68. Jas.
B. Rodgers, Printer, Philadelphia, Pa., 1867, appended
pp. 2-4.
In this letter to the editor, Ann Preston "examine[s] the
arguments which support the resolution" adopted by the
Philadelphia County Medical Society to withhold encouragement to women who wish to become medical practitioners
and to decline to consult with such practitioners. Ann
Preston refutes each objection to women in medicine raised
by the Society: A woman's life is as long as a male's, and
"her power of surmounting its painful vicissitudes not inferior to his.... Women do practice medicine, [and] they
are able 'to bear up under the bodily and mental strain'
that this practice imposes." Nor does the practice of
medicine have a contrary effect on home influence and in
fact is often less exhausting than the ordinary home duties
of washing and serving. Her knowledge of preventive medicine will aid her in training her children about hygiene, and
the scope it will give to her intellectual cravings and powers
will only add to her enjoyment and satisfaction. The ethical
questions raised if a male and female physician were both
attending the same family is no different than if two males
were in attendance, as the matter of women physicians attending male patients is no different than the matter of
male physicians attending female patients. "We regard this
movement as belonging to the advancing civilization of the
age--as the inevitable result of that progressive spirit which
is unfolding human capabilities...."

3109.   Preston, Ann. Valedictory Address to the Graduating Class
of the Woman's Medical College of Pennsylvania, at the
Eighteenth Annual Commencement, March 12th, 1870.
Loag, Printer, Philadelphia, Pennsylvania, 1870, 15
pp.
Because of the prevalence of fashionable diseases among
women, women physicians have a duty to heal members of
their sex and teach them to "regard as pitiful and barbarous
the idea that uselessness is elegance, or that disease and
languor are womanly...." To be effective practitioners,
women physicians must maintain their own health, as well
as enjoy moderate recreation and social activity. Ann
Preston goes on to comment on the progress evidenced in
the medical education of women. She concludes with an
enumeration of womanly traits that will "enrich as well as
refine the profession...."

3110.   Preston, Ann. Valedictory Address to the Graduating Class
of the Female Medical College of Pennsylvania, at the
Twelfth Annual Commencement, March 16, 1864. Published by the Corporators, Philadelphia, Pennsylvania,
1864, 16 pp.
Although the graduates may encounter "embarrassments,
and the remnants of old prejudices," professional opposition

is decreasing and public demand for women physicians is unceasing. To retain society's confidence, women physicians must be firm, steadfast, truthful, knowledgeable, and sympathetic: the sentiment that "'the most perfect character of a woman is that she be characterless,'" would be fatal to a physician's success. The woman physician with these virtues will reap many rewards, one of which is gaining "the right, scarcely yet conceded to women, to grow old without reproach."

3111. Preston, Ann. <u>Valedictory Address to the Graduating Class of the Female Medical College of Pennsylvania, For the Session of 1857-58.</u> Published by the class, Philadelphia, Pennsylvania, 1858, 15 pp.
Because prejudice against women physicians is not based on reason, a woman physician should not "war with words," but demonstrate through deeds that her work is "natural and legitimate." Although many difficulties lie ahead, there will be many rewards too, one of which is having business relations principally with women.

3112. Preston, Ann. "Women as Physicians." <u>Medical and Surgical Reporter</u>, 16 (1867) 391-394.
[Article not examined by editors.]

3113. Ramey, Estelle. "An Interview With ... Dr. Estelle Ramey." <u>Georgetown Medical Bulletin</u>, 24:1 (August 1970) 4-11. photos., port.
This interview with Estelle Ramey, a woman Ph.D. physiologist who herself became one of the few women professors at the Georgetown Medical Center, identifies some of the obstacles women scientists and physicians face, demonstrated by the economic, political, and social stereotypes of women (all demonstrated by "statistics"). The flavor of the interview is best captured in Dr. Ramey's own words. In answer to the question of what are unique career problems of women doctors: "The unique problem for a woman is to be taken seriously." (She prefaces this answer with the assurance of her belief that men are "just as capable as women in medicine.") Does she think the attitudes toward women in medical sciences are changing rapidly: "No," and "It's enough to make a cat cry." Isn't it harder for a woman to be admitted to medical school in this country: "Curiously, our statistics do not bear this out.... The astonishingly small percentage of women doctors in this country reflects the psychological roadblocks thrown up for girls early in the game." And finally: "... it is not enough for a woman to be economically supported, cherished and long-lived if at the same time she is intellectually under-using herself."

3114. Reeves, Hila. "Woman's Sphere and Influence." <u>Syracuse Medical and Surgical Journal</u>, 6 (December 1854) 315-317.
[Article not examined by editors.]

3115. Richardson, George S. "My Daughter, the Doctor." Har-
           vard Medical Alumni Bulletin, 50:1 (September/October
           1975) 9. (Editorial.)
       The Bulletin editor introduces this issue, dedicated to wo-
       men at Harvard Medical School, by acknowledging the need
       for more women in medicine. He applauds Harvard's af-
       firmative action policies. Presenting an example of how
       established women in science do not always support their
       younger counterparts, the author wonders, "Does the bat-
       tered child become the battering parent?" He further hopes
       that women at Harvard "will be spared both the need to
       overuse aggressiveness and the paranoia that threaten the
       victim of many micro-inequities."

3116. Robens, Jane F. "Open Forum." Journal of the Ameri-
           can Medical Women's Association, 27:3 (March 1972)
           146. (Letters to the Editor.)
       A woman doctor of veterinary medicine writes that she "did
       not expect" to find an article like "Woman in Medicine:
       What Can International Comparison Tell Us," in The Woman
       Physician, "a magazine for and about professional women"
       without "editorial opinion." The male author of that article
       suggests that women enter the paramedical field and implies
       throughout that women will have "an infinitely more desir-
       able and ever present alternative of a presumably happy,
       economically easy and fulfilling role as a wife...." Dr.
       Robens observes that "women constitute 40 per cent of
       those granted baccalaureate degrees but little more than
       ten per cent of those entering medical schools, or for that
       matter schools of veterinary medicine, [her] own profes-
       sion."

3117. Robertiello, Richard C. "Rebuttal to 'Feminism, Psycho-
           therapy and Professionalism.'" Journal of Contempor-
           ary Psychotherapy, 4:2 (1973) 112-113.
       Responding to Dr. Tennov's paper, Dr. Robertiello calls
       the paper unscientific; "baldly a diatribe, and exhortation
       to the emotions." Now that there is an awareness of the
       prejudices practiced against women, psychotherapists have
       begun to see them also and alter their theories and tech-
       niques. Dr. Robertiello, who considers himself a "fem-
       ininist," feels that the abuses in therapy must be corrected,
       not all therapists dismissed.

3118. Roberts, Carol Lee. "Women in Medicine." New Physi-
           cian, 20:1 (January 1971) 9. (Editorial.)
       "If the freedom of choice were not taken from girls at a
       very early age, there would be no 'problems' of women in
       medicine or anywhere else ... we would be dealing with in-
       dividual human beings, not classes of more or less oppressed
       people."

3119. Robinson, Elizabeth. "Why Women Cannot Succeed." New

England Journal of Medicine, 285:5 (29 July 1971) 301.
(Correspondence.)

Part-time residencies, day care, and retraining opportunities will adequately aid medical women in making full use
of their training. "Only when the institution of wifehood in
its present form is either abolished or made available to
doctors of both sexes will women physicians be able to do
as much as their male colleagues."

3120. Rodgerson, Eleanor B. "And Female." Journal of the
American Medical Women's Association, 24:6 (June
1969) 510-512. (Open Forum.)

A woman doctor writes of her reaction to the remark that,
"I prefer a third-rate man to a first-rate woman doctor
any day!" She reminisces about some petty, irritating, and
irrational examples of discrimination during medical school.
"1. We women were excluded from the one senior year
lecture on contraceptives! 2. The urology course was
closed to us. That was all right with me then, but later,
specializing in obstetrics and gynecology, I needed that
knowledge of urology, and the exclusion has made me feel
inadequate in this field ever since. 3. One instructor in
gynecology refused to speak to women doctors. 4. One man
in obstetrics sweated and strained to turn a posterior in a
demonstration delivery and pointed out, with special emphasis, that this procedure obviously would be too much for
any woman doctor to perform. I wondered afterwards if
better judgment and more skill might not have been the real
remedy."

3121. Rodgerson, Eleanor B. "Out of Practice?" Journal of the
American Medical Women's Association, 19:7 (July
1964) 586-587.

A woman doctor who had four children describes the role
conflict she was made to feel by one of the children, her
mother, and another woman doctor, above and beyond the
conflict of time, housekeeping chores, and child rearing
responsibilities before she returned to practice part-time
as a gynecologist 15 years after she had "retired." "My
daughter who had been having a violent argument with a
neighbor's child ran to me crying, 'Mother, you're just a
mother aren't you? Just a mother?'" When the doctor
asked another woman doctor a question at a professional
conference about a paper she had presented, before answering the speaker asked, "Where are you practicing?" "When
I admitted I wasn't practicing she brushed me off and
bustled out."

3122. Roessler, Robert; Collins, Forrest; and Mefferd, Roy B.,
Jr. "Sex Similarities in Successful Medical School Ap-
plicants." Journal of the American Medical Women's
Association, 30:6 (June 1975) 254-257, 261, 265. tables.

This paper reports a study undertaken to examine sex dif-

ferences among medical school applicants, to test previously
reported results which frequently supported stereotypes of
women physicians and medical students, and to compare accepted applicants with rejected applicants on the variables
on which sex differences were defined. A comparison of
medical student applicants with college students for sex differences on cognitive and noncognitive characteristics was
also made. Participants were 523 of 640 applicants for
admission to the Baylor Medical School in 1974. Of these,
79 minority candidates were excluded for a separate study,
leaving 92 females and 352 males as subjects. Comparisons
were made on: 1) MCAT scores, 2) grade point averages
(GPAS), 3) number of medical schools applied to, 4) occupations of parents, 5) size of high school, 6) educational
level, 7) birth order and age. The principal noncognitive
test was the Edward's Personal Preference Schedule (EPPS).
Other tests used totally or partially included the Kaplan self-
degradation scale, the Barratt impulsivity scale, the MMPI,
and the California Psychological Inventory (CPI), the Eysenck
Personality Inventory, and the Birkman Vocational Interest
and Attitude Survey. A table displays the mean scores for
all applicants (accepted and rejected) by sex on the variables
on which they differ significantly. Items on this table are:
1) MCAT scores, 2) educational level, 3) Edwards Personal
Preference Schedule (EPPS) for succorance, dominance,
nurturance, change, and heterosexuality, 4) California Psychological Inventory (CPI) for capacity for status, tolerance, intellectual efficiency, and sociability, 5) Birkman attitudes
of individuality, depression, materialism, and 6) Birkman
Vocational Interests (persuasion, social science, mechanical,
artistic, literary, and musical). No differences were found
on the other tested factors. Another table displays mean
EPPS scores of college students (743 males and 1,077 females) with the Baylor applicants. A third table shows the
mean CPI scores of college students (1,133 males and
2,120 females) and the Baylor applicants. The results of
the study were compared with those found in a Toronto
study (Fruen, M. A., Rothman, A. I., and Steiner, J. W.,
"Comparison of characteristics of male and female medical
school applicants," Journal of Medical Education, 49:137,
1974). In general, accepted women scored lower than accepted men on the science subtest of the MCAT but did not
differ from accepted men on any other intellectual variables.
The women were like the men in measures of dominance,
nurturance, heterosexuality, and autonomy. The nonintel-
lectual differences between the accepted males and females
generally paralleled sex differences found in the college
sample.

3123.   Rosen, R. A. Hudson. "Occupational Role Innovators and
         Sex Role Attitudes." Journal of Medical Education, 49:
         6 (June 1974) 554-561. tables.

"This paper addresses itself to the attitudinal approach of role innovators to sex roles as found among women students and faculty members in medical schools. It was felt such attitudes were relevant to how they cope with discrimination and had implications for medical school policies. The data were gathered in late 1971 in 11 randomly sampled medical schools as part of a larger study. It was found that women in medical schools support the option of careers for women generally, although not necessarily at the expense of the maternal role. This pattern was stronger among students than faculty members. Also, more women in medical schools give careers priority than do women in nursing and social work schools. Men in medical schools have less clearly defined attitudes than do the women, but few state that women should be home centered." [Article abstract.]

3124. Rosow, Irving and Rose, K. Daniel. "Divorce Among Doctors." Journal of Marriage and the Family, 34:4 (November 1972) 587-598. tables.
An analysis of California divorce petitions of 1968 shows that physicians have a lower incidence of divorce than most professions. Both male and female physicians marry later (at age 30.3) than other divorcing professionals and file their initial divorce complaint at what is often the height of their careers (at age 43.1). Highest divorce rates in the profession appear among small-town doctors, blacks, and women. Reasons for women physicians having a higher annual "complaint rate" than men physicians (23.9 vs. 16.1) include the "chronic difficulties" of "legitimate professional claims on the wife's family obligations" and "the couple's equal work status as opposed to prevailing norms of their occupational inequality." Possibly in a "rational response to their higher prospect of divorce," women physicians marry less often than men (31 per cent are single, in contrast to 8 per cent of the men); 56 per cent of women doctors are married, compared with 90 per cent of the men [these figures are from the U.S. Bureau of the Census, 1964]. The authors point out, however, that these "deviant marital patterns ... are typical of female professionals in general." Speculating on the meaning of these patterns, the authors wonder if women who do not marry gravitate to the professions ("self-selection") or if professional schools favor non-marrying women and discourage others ("recruitment"), or if "family conflicts and divorce [are] the current price of women's serious professional commitment (sex roles)."

3125. Ross, Mathew. "Suicide Among Physicians: A Psychological Study." Diseases of the Nervous System, 34:3 (March 1973) 145-150. (Presentation, Annual Meeting, Southern Psychiatric Association, New Orleans, Louisiana, October, 1972.)
This study consists of a literature review. The study indicates that "(1) physician suicide varies from country to

country, (2) suicide among physicians is high, (3) suicide
among female physicians is very much higher than among
male physicians, (4) there is a high incidence of psychiatric
morbidity, alcoholism, and drug addiction among physician
suicides, (5) as in suicides among other age groups, there
are significant variable correlates of age, gender, type of
medical practice and specialty, the state of physical and
emotional health, the use of alcohol and drugs, professional
and psychosocial factors, (6) preventive action is both possible and desirable." The suicide rate among female physicians is four times that of the female general population of
U.S. women over age 25. This high rate of suicide in women physicians might be related to the personality constel-
lation of women who select male-oriented careers and to the
woman physician's knowledge of the lethality of readily available poisons.

3126.   Rossi, Alice S. "Women in Science: Why So Few?" Sci-
         ence, 148:3674 (28 May 1965) 1196-1202. tables.
         American society has been insensitive to those social hard-
         ships imposed because of sex. If we want more women
         scientists, both boys and girls must be educated for all
         their major adult roles, not merely gender roles. We
         must stop counseling girls to be "realistic" by lowering
         their occupational aspirations: the difficulties women might
         encounter as a result of trying to handle the triple roles of
         professional, wife, and mother, should be recognized as a
         social problem, not an individual problem. House-care
         firms should be considered as an alternative to the single
         domestic servant in handling the domestic responsibilities
         of working men and women. Men who have found marriage
         to a professional working woman a satisfying experience
         should be more articulate about themselves as males and
         about women.

3127.   Russell, Jane Anderson. "The Woman as Practicing Phy-
         sician." Boston University Medical Center Centerscope,
         (July/August 1971) 12-14. port. (Women in Medicine.)
         Men physicians, patients, and the public sometimes have
         difficulty "integrating the woman physician into their think-
         ing." To examine how these attitudes affect one's practice,
         Dr. Russell drew upon her own experiences and those of
         three others: Drs. Jean Arnold, Mary Donald, and Eliza-
         beth C. Spivack. All four women have private practices,
         and all are married. Discussed are each woman's experi-
         ence with referral patterns, colleague relationships, rela-
         tionships with nurses, and the difficulties of combining a
         practice with family responsibilities.

3128.   Ryder, Claire F. "President's Message." Journal of the
         American Medical Women's Association, 15:12 (Decem-
         ber 1960) 1178.
         A male doctor told Claire F. Ryder, president of the

American Medical Women's Association, that he was opposed to women entering medical school, and indeed dis-
suaded his daughter from becoming a medical student because he perceived that "each woman in medical school has
taken a man's rightful place, and that all too frequently
after graduation, marriage and family divert her from her
medical career. Thus, her 'spot' in that class has been
wasted and the final tally is one less practicing physician."
Dr. Ryder responds by saying that women do not waste
their medical education and furthermore that many women
physicians participate in community activities "which the
busy male practitioner cannot or does not take on ... the
responsibilities for these is a natural role for the woman
physician."

3129. Sadock, Virginia Alcott. "Where Are the Women Doctors
        Our Country Needs?" Parents Magazine, 47 (November
        1972) 66-67, 106, 108.
      [Article not examined by editors.]

3130. "St. Paul's Injunction to Women Still in Force." Medical
        Woman's Journal, 36:2 (February 1929) 44.
      On January 17, 1929, Vassar College dedicated the Minnie
      Cummnock Blodgett Hall of Euthenics. Despite the fact
      that women are so predominantly associated with Vassar,
      as students, alumnae, and faculty, they were poorly repre-
      sented on the program. The results of this and other such
      situations involving women are that women have inherited
      an inferiority complex while men have inherited a superior-
      ity complex. The home environment reinforces this psy-
      chology. The author suggests that a concerted effort be
      made to establish among medical women a superiority com-
      plex.

3131. Scarlett, Mary J. Valedictory Address of Prof. M. J.
        Scarlett, Before the Graduating Class of the Female
        Medical College, of Philadelphia, March 16, 1867.
        Spangler & Davis, Philadelphia, Pennsylvania, 1867,
        7 pp.
      A review of current public opinion regarding women in med-
      icine includes information on the State Medical Society of
      Pennsylvania's debate over possibly rescinding its 1859 reso-
      lution. That resolution made it an offense for members to
      consult with professors in a female medical college. Al-
      though opposition still exists, Mary Scarlett tells the grad-
      uating students, "You have cause to rejoice that you live in
      the nineteenth century ... an age when the right to labor in
      our own way is not denied us...." Dr. Scarlett further
      assures that marriage and domestic duties are compatible
      with a medical profession: "We would not advocate a posi-
      tion for women that would in the slightest degree remove
      her from the home throne." As for her professional role,
      despite popular belief that women physicians should administer

to "the degraded classes," Dr. Scarlett says that all
classes of society need women physicians. Finally, the
graduates are warned to be "true, modest, unpretending
women, and if you possess skill, as we believe you do,
there will be no need of pretentious display."

3132. Schwartz, Jane. "Medicine As a Vocational Choice Among
          Undergraduate Women." Journal of the National Asso-
          ciation of Women Deans and Counselors, 33:1 (Fall
          1969) 7-12.
During the past five years there has been a concern over
the small number of women entering medicine. More women than men shift their career interest from medicine between their freshman and senior years. Why do some females switch and others stay with medicine? Interviews
were held with 37 Barnard College seniors to find the answer and the results of those interviews are presented in
narrative form.

3133. Selections from Notices of the Press on the Valedictory Ad-
          dress to the Graduating Class of the Female Medical
          College of Pennsylvania. King & Baird, Printers,
          Philadelphia, Pennsylvania, 1863, 13 pp.
Editors of a variety of northeastern U.S. journals and newspapers respond favorably to Emeline Cleveland's valedictory
address, given March 14, 1863, which was an affirmation
of women's right to medical education.

3134. "Sermon." Woman's Medical Journal, 1:3 (March 1893) 47.
This article quotes from "Letters to a Young Physician,"
which was published in the National Medical Review. On
the question of whether women should study medicine, the
author stresses that "the motive and the object must be
first made clear; for ... questions enter into this problem
which are not present in the case of man."

3135. Shangold, Mona M. "Women Physicians." Journal of
          Medical Education, 50 (September 1975) 911. (Editor-
          ial.)
The author points out that the very need for support groups
for women in medical school highlights the gap in a culture
between reason (equality) and reality ("lingering tales of
tradition"). Development of such support programs should
be encouraged as long as they are needed, but, Dr. Shangold is quick to point out, "our goal should be to eliminate
their need and we are a long way from our goal." She
touches upon sample inequities and sexist practices in the
field of medicine which should no longer be tolerated: rest
rooms labeled "Nurses" and "Doctors"; the use of "nudie-
pictures" to stimulate interest at medical lectures; and the
practice of condescension toward patients, particularly female.

3136.   Shapiro, Edith T. "Women Who Want to be Women." Wo-
             man Physician, 26:8 (August 1971) 399-413.
         Dr. Shapiro studied married working women, predominantly
         from the upper-middle and middle class; overtly psychotic
         and overtly homosexual persons were excluded. The author
         sought to determine what conflicts there might be between
         working away from home and fulfilling the "feminine" role.
         Among other groups she examines in this study are mother-
         physicians, the only group that had an opportunity to live
         in a setting which acknowledged and attempted to integrate
         their double lives. The majority of the women in the study
         "wore attractive clothes, appropriate make-up and were
         much interested in personal appearance." Dr. Shapiro does
         not always distinguish between the physician-mother group
         and the other groups she studied. The areas of concern
         were marriage and divorce, motherhood, relationships with
         other women, domestic help, relationships with male col-
         leagues, choice of profession, and work schedule. The
         study indicated that most women found pleasure in feminine
         activities (e.g., sexual relations with men, breast feeding
         of infants, involvement in rearing a family). Men were
         very important in their lives and they were "eager to ac-
         commodate to the real needs of their husbands, if necessary,
         at the expense of their careers." The women wanted to
         have children and enjoyed domestic tasks. In short, "their
         real selves seemed to be composed of wishes to be fem-
         inine and maternal" while at the same time retaining a
         "drive for a career."

3137.   Shapley, Deborah. "Medical Education: Those Sexist Put-
             downs May Be Illegal." Science, 184:4135 (26 April
             1974) 449-451.
         A review of the report entitled Why Would a Girl Go into
         Medicine? Medical Education in the United States: A Guide
         for Women, gives also an overview of the various legal re-
         courses one might take in response to the "sexist putdowns"
         described in the report.

3138.   Sherbon, Florence Brown. "The Woman Physician in a
             Changing World." Medical Woman's Journal, 43:12
             (December 1936) 318-323. (Address, State Association
             of Iowa Medical Women, Des Moines, 16 April 1936.)
         Speculation about science's potential in reshaping the world
         precedes a discussion about the woman physician's role in
         man's social and scientific work. Women physicians should
         utilize their special female endowments--intuition, vicarious-
         ness, imagination, domestic predilection--and join with wo-
         men in nursing, elementary education, and children's social
         work, to concentrate on working with children. Women who
         try to demonstrate equality with men by competing "in his
         own specific fields" are making foolish gestures. Instead,
         women physicians, like all women, "must ever transform the
         elements of her body for the nutriment of the young of the
         species."

3139.   Sherbon, Florence Brown. "Women in Medicine." Medical
              Woman's Journal, 32:9 (September 1925) 240-243.
              (President's Address, Kansas Association of Medical
              Women, 7 May 1925.)
          After questioning a group of young college women, Dr.
          Sherbon compiled a list of reasons why these women were
          not considering becoming doctors, i.e., the length and in-
          tensiveness of training makes it especially difficult and ex-
          pensive for a woman who is self supporting; the medical
          course is so exacting and requires so much background in
          the abstract sciences that few women can do it; preparation
          and training is so demanding that few can withstand the
          strain on their health; and "many families violently oppose
          medicine as the daughter's vocation." Other deterrents are
          the anticipation of discrimination from medical men because
          of being female; not believing that financial security will be
          commensurate with the money and time invested; and "the
          difficulty the medical woman faces who wishes to realize
          the normal human experience of wifehood and motherhood."
          To examine some of these problems, Dr. Sherbon suggests
          the following: that a Medical Vocation Committee be formed
          "to discuss medical schools for women, costs, and condi-
          tions of training, the varied openings for medically trained
          women, etc..."; that these women be willing to give voca-
          tional talks for expenses only; and that the delegates to the
          National Medical Women's Association suggest the establish-
          ment of a national field secretary.

3140.   Southgate, M. Therese. "Remembrance of Things (Hope-
              fully) Past." Journal of the American Medical Associa-
              tion, 232:13 (30 June 1975) 1331-1332. (Commentary.)
          Besides the reasons commonly given for suicide among young
          professional women (role conflict, fear of success, and
          marginality), the author adds a fourth: singularity--isola-
          tion from a large number of other women with similar ideals
          and goals. Examples of the kinds of pressures faced by the
          woman medical student are discussed.

3141.   Spiro, Howard M. "Visceral Viewpoints: Myths and
              Mirths--Women in Medicine." New England Journal of
              Medicine, 292:7 (13 February 1975) 354-356.
          Dr. Spiro discusses the "women's lib" revolution in medi-
          cine. He finds it difficult to believe that overt discrimina-
          tion of the type described in the booklet, Why Would a Girl
          Want to Go into Medicine? by Margaret A. Campbell, repre-
          sents "outright hostility." Both men and women could well
          gain from adapting some of each other's traits. In discuss-
          ing those characteristics labeled "feminine" (e.g., nurtur-
          ance), Dr. Spiro states that medicine needs these psychic
          characteristics now: medicine has become too "scientific"
          in the hands of the male--"Even research has been seen as
          a contest with other researchers as much as with nature,
          and not a simple quest for truth. The syringe and the penis

may, after all, have much in common." In conclusion, the author credits "women's lib" as an "admirable movement although it is occasionally shriller than it need be."

3142.   "Staff of Women Physicians Appointed in Charge of Gyneco-
        logical Clinic." Woman's Medical Journal, 26:2 (Febru-
        ary 1916) 46.
Using the traditional male concept of chivalry, the author reinterprets the sense of the word to mean women support-ing women and respecting each other's skills, as those who struggle for professional, social, and economic recognition find fellowship and loyalty in each other's professional life work.

3143.   Standley, Kay and Soule, Bradley. "Women in Male-
        Dominated Professions: Contrast in their Personal and
        Vocational Histories." Journal of Vocational Behavior,
        4:2 (April 1974) 245-258. tables.
"Women in four high-status, male-dominated professions--architecture, law, medicine, and psychology--are described in terms of a variety of historical, social, and career vari-ables. The women share common antecedents of their voca-tional choices and similar perceptions of their work, but the occupational groups are dissimilar on a number of dimensions. Psychologists stand in particular contrast to the other three groups of professionals, describing experiences and career patterns less in conflict with stereotypic female roles. These contrasts may reflect differences in the sex-typed characterizations of the professions even though all are male-dominated." The authors also discuss discrimination faced by these women, and their emotional adjustments to their lives.

3144.   Standley, Kay and Soule, Bradley. "Women in Professions:
        Historic Antecedents and Current Lifestyles." In: Ca-
        reer Guidance for Young Women: Considerations in
        Planning Professional Careers. Edited by Richard E.
        Hardy and John G. Cull. Charles C. Thomas, Spring-
        field, Illinois, 1974, 3-16. tables.
A research project was carried out to "delineate certain aspects of the personal and career histories of some women physicians, lawyers and architects." It attempts to shed light on the questions, What are the roots of [these wo-men's] unusual choices? and What are the careers and per-sonal lives like for the women who have made such voca-tional commitments? The three professions are not differ-entiated in this article, but family background information, childhood experiences, self concepts, career expectations, and current lifestyles (especially of those married and with children) are discussed.

3145.   Steinmann, Anne and Fox, David J. "Male and Female Phy-
        sicians' Perceptions of Ideal Feminine Roles." Journal

of the American Medical Women's Association, 22:3 (March 1967) 184-188. tables.
The authors' "basic hypothesis was that despite the variables of socioeconomic class, ethnic or racial background, level of education, and occupational or professional status, women share a common set of life values." They used the Inventory of Feminine Values to test their hypothesis on samples of women differing on the variables mentioned in their hypothesis. The 44 female respondants were members of the American Medical Woman's Association of New York City and their answers were contrasted with 50 male physicians who practiced in New York. The data returned from female physicians "combine to delineate a group of female physicians who see their own role as slightly passive who have an ideal woman somewhat less passive or more self-assertive, but who think that men want women who are extremely passive and who place wifely and familial duties above their own development, and who seek satisfaction in these duties rather than in their own personal and professional development." The ideal woman for the male physicians responding "is slightly more passive than active ... and interestingly enough is almost identical to the woman physician's perception of her ideal woman." In contrast, the female physicians' perceptions of what the men would consider ideal was far more passive than the males' responses would indicate. The authors conclude that "there may be a serious failure in communication between men and women." In improved communication between the sexes, "a consensus could be reached where the ideal woman could be defined in terms of these shared opinions of both men and women."

3146.   Steinmann, Anne; Levi, Joseph; and Fox, David J. "Feminine Role Perceptions of Women Physicians: Self-Perception of Women Physicians as Compared to their Perception of Ideal Woman and Men's Ideal Women." Journal of the American Medical Women's Association, 19:9 (September 1964) 776-782. tables.
Based on 44 replies to a postal questionnaire sent to members of the Women's Medical Association of New York City, these authors make the following interpretation: "... there is a great discrepancy between the subjects' own concept of the feminine role and what these women think men want them to be. Actually, these women indicate that they accept a slightly passive, feminine role, but, at the same time, they are eager for fulfillment of their aims and ambitions and are desirous of self-realization. However, these professional women think that men's ideal woman is a very passive woman." Referring to an earlier study in which it was found "that men say that they do not desire as passive a woman as women think," the authors speculate that "there is a lack of understanding between men and women." Concerning conflict between role of professional woman, wife,

and mother, the authors found that "these professional women feel that husband and children come first, and further,
if necessary, that they, the women, should sacrifice their
achievements for the sake of the family.   On the other hand,
when their problems are not in opposition with their responsibilities toward the family, then these women are more
active and more self-assertive."   The self-perception scale
conflicted with the Men's Ideal Woman scale.   "Whereas
the [Men's Ideal] scale indicates that women think that men
make no compromises at all and wish the women to stay at
home, to have the home and family take precedence over
everything else in their lives.   The women think that men
want them completely to obliterate their own personalities
for the sake of the family.   The women feel that they should
have self-realization."

3147.   Steppacher, Robert and Mausner, Judith S.   "Suicide in
              Male and Female Physicians."   Journal of the American
              Medical Association, 228:3 (15 April 1974) 323-328.
              tables.
         "The frequency of suicide among physicians in the United
         States over the 5-1/2-year period March 1965 to August
         1970 was studied.   Suicides and possible suicides were
         identified through the obituary listings in JAMA.   Confirma-
         tion of suicide was attempted for equivocal cases where pos-
         sible.   Within this time period, 530 deaths by suicide were
         identified, 489 in men and 41 in women.   Analysis indi-
         cated that the rate in male physicians was approximately
         1.15 times that of the overall male population, whereas for
         female physicians the rate was fully three times that ex-
         pected on the basis of population values.   For physicians
         45 years of age and over, suicide rates were somewhat
         higher for men.   Below that age, there was a marked ex-
         cess among the women.   Twelve of the 41 women were in
         training.   The findings are consistent with reports of high
         rates of suicide among females in other professions."   [Ar-
         ticle abstract.]

3148.   Thelander, H[ulda] E.   "Aesculapius Beckoning: Some
              Thoughts on Medical Education for Women."   Journal
              of the American Medical Women's Association, 18:11
              (November 1963) 897-899.
         Because "the study and the practice of medicine are ex-
         ceedingly rewarding," women should consider medicine as
         a career.   "If the thought of being a physician is a passing
         fancy, or a selfish one, or if it is considered because it
         is a well-paying profession, or if a girl contemplates enter-
         ing it only to be different, or to invade a man's field, or to
         show that she can do it, the chances of a gratifying career
         are very remote."

3149.   Thelander, Hulda E.   "Is Medicine a Career for Girls?"
              National Association of Deans of Women Journal, 15:2

(January 1952) 74-77.
Dr. Thelander presents the results of a meeting held two
years ago in which women physicians discussed, with girl
medical students, the subject of marriage and medicine.
The meeting resulted in a study sponsored by the Women
Physician's Club of San Francisco, and directed by Dr.
Eschscholtzia Lucia. Questionnaires were filled out by 230
women in the Bay Area. General discussion given in this
article covers "The Need for Women Physicians," "Fitness,"
"Preparation," "Obstacles and Handicaps," and "Opportunities." Among the conclusions: candidates for school
should be "carefully selected for intelligence, adaptability,
sincerity and physical fitness." Although prejudice exists,
medical women find ample opportunity to live happy and
useful lives. Top leadership is available to women in many
branches of medicine. Marriage and a family, "coupled
with superior ability," are compatible with a successful
career.

3150.   Thelander, H[ulda] E. "Opportunities for Medical Women:
         On the Selection of Women for Medical Careers."
         Journal of the American Medical Women's Association,
         1:8 (November 1946) 284.
To alleviate the problems faced by women who want to become physicians, certain factors in training and acceptance
should be taken into consideration: women as professional
mothers have important direct and indirect influence on
their children and therefore "women should not be barred
from certain professions because of motherhood"; women
should have positions on medical admissions boards and on
certification boards to help "select women for the study of
medicine who have the mental, physical, and emotional
capacity and whatever else it takes to make use of the training obtained"; and "properly selected women should have a
right to study medicine, marry or not as they choose, and
have children or not as they choose."

3151.   Thelander, Hulda E. "Women for Internships." Medical
         Woman's Journal, 43:12 (December 1936) 324-326.
An article by a medical student [Virginia South] entitled
"Internships for Women" [Medical Woman's Journal, August
1936, p. 217] prompted this "analysis of the principles
underlying the success or failure" of medical women. Dr.
Thelander discusses, then dismisses, the questions of women's fitness for medicine that have to do with individual
characteristics, i.e., intelligence, dexterity judgment,
conscientiousness, and strength. The real problem for
most women physicians is the desire for children and motherhood. To solve the problem, each woman "should be
compelled to seriously consider the possibilities of her own
success in the field. If she is a woman of only average
college ability and has a strong attraction for the opposite
sex with a real urge for motherhood, it is a waste of time

and money to study medicine." "The easiest solution ...
is to remain single.... Celibacy is no problem to many
women, and it may be a boon." The author emphasizes
that grades alone should not determine who is admitted to
medical school, and recommends that "several interviews"
be conducted to "determine the fitness of a woman to enter
the field."

3152. Travell, Janet; Reid, Ada Chree; and Clapp, Mary P.
"Housework and the Physician-Mother: Report from the
U.S.A." Journal of the American Medical Women's
Association, 8:2 (February 1953) 63-64.
A written questionnaire was sent to a list of women doctors
with one or more children; about 80 per cent replied. The
first 300 replies formed the basis of this report on how professional women handle the problems of housework. After
reporting on the available appliances, kinds of heating systems, etc., the authors conclude that, "Half the women doctors felt that good domestic help was a highly important
factor in successfully combining home-making and medicine
as a career." Several women surveyed also felt that the
expense of domestic help should be an income tax deductible
expense.

3153. Vanderlip, Mrs. Frank A. [Narcissa Cox]. "Are Special
Provisions Necessary for Women Physicians Today?"
Women in Medicine, 69 (July 1940) 8-11. (Presentation, American Medical Women's Association, New York,
New York, 10 June 1940.)
In trying to raise money and gain support for the New York
Infirmary for Women and Children, Vanderlip points out why
provisions are desirable for women doctors. Her arguments
include the fact that few women are accepted at most medical schools and some medical schools "take no women students whatsoever." In most coeducational medical schools,
women are not allowed to take urology and surgery. Relatively few hospitals accept women as interns, and relatively
few women are able to get residencies and fellowships.
Because women only get appointments as directors of departments in hospitals and schools that are staffed by women, such women-run institutions need to continue to exist
so that women can have real experience that leads to real
competence in patient care. "It is only when leading, not
when following, that one becomes an authority. Frequently
it appears that as soon as a woman doctor has completed
her work in the lower posts and begins to show ability,
skill, or ambition other arrangements are made and she is
left in a subordinate position, this for no explicable reason
but her sex." Of the 450 to 500 women physicians in Manhattan and 248 in the other boroughs, 309 have no hospital
connections, 140 are on hospital staffs, 123 have only an
outpatient connection, 103 are connected with the New York
Infirmary; and of these only 16 have other hospital services.

[This article also appears in the Medical Woman's Journal, 47:9 (September 1940) 260-262, 277.]

3154.   Vandervall, Isabella.   "Some Problems of the Colored Wo-
             man Physician."   Woman's Medical Journal, 27:7 (July
             1917) 156-158.
         Dr. Vandervall blasts the new law of compulsory intern-
         ships as an almost insurmountable barrier to black women
         physicians.   She tells of her own struggles and humiliations
         in trying to obtain internships at various hospitals to illus-
         trate how compulsory internship seriously affects colored
         women who wish to be physicians and colored patients who
         have a right to have women physicians of their own race.
         Furthermore, the law "casts a serious reflection upon those
         white people--democratic and philanthropic Americans--
         who lavishly endow colleges and hospitals and allow colored
         girls to enter and finish their college course, and yet,
         when one steps forward to keep pace with her white sisters
         and to qualify before the state in order that she might do
         the same services for her colored sisters that the white wo
         man does for hers, those patriotic Americans figuratively
         wave the stars and stripes in her face and literally say to
         her: 'What do you want, you woman of the dark skin?
         Halt! You cannot advance any further! Retreat! You are
         colored! Retreat!'"

3155.   V[an] H[oosen], Bertha.   "Are English Women More Loyal
             to Sex Than American Women?" Medical Woman's
             Journal, 35:12 (December 1928) 353-354.
         In his book, Technique of Contraception, James F. Cooper,
         M.D., suggests that British women are more desirous of
         being cared for by women physicians than are American
         women patients.   Concluding that disloyalty springs from
         lack of confidence in women physicians--on the part of male
         and female patients and women physicians themselves--Dr.
         Van Hoosen believes publicity is one remedy.   She further
         offers: "The [Medical Woman's] Journal, without cost, will
         help you to ethically make yourself known."

3156.   [Van Hoosen, Bertha].   "Marriage--An Asset or a Handicap
             to the Medical Woman." Medical Woman's Journal, 36:
             9 (September 1929) 248.
         "The most normal life" for any woman is marriage and
         children.   The present trend, Dr. Van Hoosen points out,
         is that the medical woman "should eschew matrimony."
         Dr. Van Hoosen submits that motherhood would have a
         positive effect on one's practice of medicine.   "The argu-
         ment is not that a woman should have a right to marriage
         and a career, but more than that, she should have a right
         to become a part of everything in life that will enrich her
         mind and body, develop her character, and help to make her
         do her part in the world's work in as big a way as possible

3157.   Van Hoosen, Bertha. "Medical Women Defended." Medical
        Woman's Journal, 32:12 (December 1925) 322-324. (Ad-
        dress, Chicago Branch of the Michigan Alumnae.)
        As an alumna, Dr. Van Hoosen responds to a male dean
        of the College of Medicine at Michigan University who said
        that the reason fewer women were practicing medicine [in
        1924] than in 1872 was because despite women's boasts,
        women could not, in fact, stand the physical and nerve-
        testing strain it takes to practice medicine. After review-
        ing days and nights of continuous hard work in her own life,
        Dr. Van Hoosen makes the point that her mother, a farm-
        er's wife, worked ever harder and longer hours than "few
        men could or would elect to endure. But farmers' wives
        and mothers are common and are taken for granted." She
        then lists the records of accomplishments of women med-
        ical alumnae from Michigan University.

3158.   Van Hoosen, Bertha. "The Woman Physician--Quo Vadis?"
        Medical Woman's Journal, 36:1 (January 1929) 1-4.
        Inspired by action on the part of London medical schools
        to close the doors to women applicants, the Committee on
        Medical Opportunities of the Medical Women's National As-
        sociation communicated with the deans of all the medical
        schools in the United States "asking information in regard
        to the difficulty in securing internships for women students;
        if the reports from the hospitals where women were intern-
        ing were satisfactory; if the women students made good in
        their college work; if they caused the management any spe-
        cial trouble; and the attitude of the student body and the
        faculty toward the woman student." The responses are given
        in this article.

3159.   Van Hoosen, Bertha. "'Would It Were True.'" Medical
        Woman's Journal, 35:8 (August 1928) 232-233.
        The editor of Atlantic Medical Journal made several incor-
        rect statements regarding women physicians in a recent
        [1928] Atlantic editorial. Although he reports that 40 years
        ago "the last Medical Association capitulated" and admitted
        women members, many Southern medical societies and many
        gynecological and obstetrical organizations still refuse mem-
        bership to women. The editor also quoted Dr. [Eliza]
        Mosher as saying she never experienced discourtesy or an-
        tagonism as a woman physician. Dr. Van Hoosen explains:
        "Our senior editor is so courteous and kind herself that she
        does not recognize discourtesy or antagonism in any form."
        The Atlantic editor's belief that the type of woman entering
        medicine is changing and therefore they are treated with
        more respect, is also disputed by Dr. Van Hoosen.

3160.   Voorhis, Anna Harvey. "The Medical Woman of the Future."
        Medical Woman's Journal, 36:7 (July 1929) 174-176.
        (Address, Meeting of Woman's Medical Society of New
        York State, 3-4 June 1929.)

The most compelling reason for women (or men) to study
medicine seems to be "a combination of altruism and a desire for economic independence." Men take medicine more
seriously than women, who are "wedded to their medicine
until that co-respondent, marriage, appears." They then
often leave medicine permanently, and for this reason medical schools are reluctant to accept women. "This brings
us to the question," says Dr. Voorhis, "in the great plan
of the universe for what was a woman created?" She was
made for reproduction and "to be the cornerstone of the
home." Only leaders among women are adapted to the
study and practice of medicine: "This assuredly excludes
the vast majority" of women. Marriage and children handicap a woman physician in her profession and few women
doctors of reputation marry. Women physicians, as they
"advance and develop in medicine ... rise above the level
of sex themselves and realize, absolutely, there can be no
sex in medicine."

3161.   "What Has Happened to the Equal Rights Amendment?"
              Medical Woman's Journal, 49:10 (October 1942) 315-316
              (Editorial.)
          In July 1942 the Judiciary Committee of the House of Repre-
          sentatives voted the Equal Rights Amendment out of Com-
          mittee, but the House still has not received it. Because
          "... to no women does equality mean more than to women
          physicians" this amendment which says, "Men and women
          shall have equal rights throughout the United States and
          every place subject to its jurisdiction," is important. Every
          woman physician should write her congressman and repre-
          sentative so that the Equal Rights Amendment can become
          law.

3162.   Wheeler, Clementene Walker. "Barnard Women in White:
              Survey of 125 Alumnae Doctors Upsets Admissions
              Theories of Medical Schools." Barnard Alumnae Mag-
              azine, 44:5 (July 1955) 2-4. photos.
          A questionnaire was sent to 215 Barnard alumnae asking
          how they fared, whether they considered medicine worth the
          effort and sacrifice, and whether they were able to com-
          bine a medical career with a normal, happy life. A total
          of 125 questionnaires (57 per cent) were returned. The
          results are presented in narrative form. Over two-thirds
          of the women are married and nearly half have children.

3163.   White, Frances Emily. Valedictory Address to the Grad-
              uating Class of the Woman's Medical College of Penn-
              sylvania. Published by request, Philadelphia, Penn-
              sylvania, 1880, 16 pp.
          After lamenting that arguments against women of skilled
          labor and of professional work--particularly women physi-
          cians--"have been dragged to the front and paraded ad
          nauseam," Frances White lists and examines those argu-

ments.   The professor of physiology and hygiene concludes
that "the physiological law, that exercise increases muscu-
lar power, applies alike to men and women," and that in
intellectual ability, a similar law is true.

3164.   White, Martha S.   "Psychological and Social Barriers to
         Women in Science."   Science, 170:3956 (23 October
         1970) 413-416.   (Presentation, Symposium, Women in
         Science, Berkeley, California, 22 November 1969.)
The author submits that a major barrier to women in science, and especially those who wish to pursue the multiple
roles of scientist, mother, and wife, is the limited opportunities for colleague interaction.   For women with a dual
commitment to science and nonprofessional roles and identi-
fications, a new concept of professional "career" may be
necessary.   Suggestions are made as to what women can do
"to cope with these barriers and discriminatory practices
which intensify the effects of discontinuity in their lives."

3165.   Whitman, Howard.   "M.D. for Men Only?"   Woman's
         Home Companion, (November 1946) 32-33, 73, 76-77.
         photos.
The author discusses male prejudice against women physicians.   "How much longer must narrow prejudice bar women from their rightful opportunity in medicine...?"
The doors of admittance to medical school, which were
opened to women during the war, are being closed once
again.   Whitman reviews women's struggle to be recognized
as physicians, from Elizabeth Blackwell's difficulties in
finding a medical school which would accept her, through
their difficulties in serving with the armed services, to
their present dilemma of losing their jobs since the war
has ended: "Hospitals have pitched women off their staffs
as promptly as many shipyards told Rosie the Riveter to go
home and peel potatoes."   Whitman presents the many
problems women physicians encounter, supported with incidents from several women physicians' lives.

3166.   Williams, Josephine J.   "Patients and Prejudice: Lay At-
         titudes Toward Women Physicians."   American Journal
         of Sociology, 51 (January 1946) 283-287.   charts.
"A minority group within a profession is a group which, although technically qualified, deviates from an expected pattern of auxiliary characteristics, such as age, sex, and
religious or ethnic affiliation.   The situation in which a
layman selects a professional is distinguished from that in
which he exercises no choice but retains the right to protest.   The relative status of various minority group physicians in these two situations is reported on the basis of
data obtained from a sample of urban middle-class women.
Attitudes toward women physicians are compared with attitudes toward physicians of religious and ethnic minorities."
[Article abstract.]

3167.   Williams, Josephine J. "The Woman Physician's Dilemma."
          Journal of Social Issues, 6:3 (1950) 38-44.
          Women will, in the future, have a greater opportunity than
          ever before to study medicine and to specialize in the field
          of their choice. The author discusses the three major ex-
          planations for women's heretofore modest role in medicine:
          inherent sex differences, marriage-career conflict, and
          discrimination. [The following article in this issue of the
          Journal is a discussion by Margaret Mead of other articles
          including this one. The title of Dr. Mead's critique is
          "Towards Mutual Responsibility," and it begins on page 45.]

3168.   Williams, N. "A Dissertation on 'Female Physicians.'"
          Boston Medical and Surgical Journal, 43:4 (28 August
          1850) 69-75. (Presentation, Meeting, Clay, Lysander
          and Schroeppel Medical Association, [New York], 6
          June 1850.)
          Proposing "a calm, unbiased and rational view" of women's
          ability and right to enter the medical profession, Dr. Wil-
          liams reasons that women are unfit to become physicians.
          First of all, medicine is too laborious an occupation for wo-
          men: "It does not simply consist in riding about in an easy
          carriage, from patient to patient, whilst the weather is fair
          and pleasant, and all nature is rejoicing." Marriage and
          motherhood are incompatible with medicine: "... the though
          of married females engaging in the medical profession is
          too palpably absurd.... It carries along with it, a sense
          of shame, vulgarity and disgust." Referring to Elizabeth
          Blackwell's decision to remain unmarried, Dr. Williams re-
          minds his audience that celibacy is unnatural and morally
          wrong. As for woman's nervous and excitable temperament,
          education could "impose some improvements," but such al-
          terations would be unnatural. Bringing phrenology into the
          debate, Dr. Williams points to a female's mental constitu-
          tion and her innate love of the domestic duties. He warns
          that when a woman is not "content to labor in her sphere
          ... when she aspires to be the competitor of man, she
          must abandon all claim to the love, sympathy and affection
          which are so freely bestowed upon her."

3169.   Wistein, Rosina. "Answer to 'Women Physician--Quo
          Vadis?'" Medical Woman's Journal, 36:2 (February
          1929) 45-46.
          This article responds to Bertha Van Hoosen's article on
          women physicians which appeared in the January, 1929 is-
          sue of JAMWA (p. 1-4). "From a sociological and econom-
          ic standpoint women physicians will go 'just so far' as their
          knowledge, experience, judgment, business ability, patience,
          tact, energy, and courage will lead them, and no further."
          Men have no monopoly on qualifications, writes Dr. Wistein.
          They are not stenographers and lab assistants because they
          abhor detail. "There are any number of men in the prac-
          tice of medicine who are about as qualified theoretically,

practically, and morally as the dodo, and yet they practice
medicine, and some make money thereby." Dr. Wistein
also enumerates the reasons why medicine is not a particularly lucrative profession.

3170.   Wolman, Carol and Frank, Hal. "The Solo Woman in a
        Professional Peer Group." American Journal of Ortho-
        psychiatry, 45:1 (January 1975) 164-171. (Presentation,
        Annual Meeting, American Psychiatric Association,
        Honolulu, Hawaii, May 1973.)
The authors led or observed six peer groups (three work-
groups and three discussion groups) of graduate students
and psychiatric residents, each including a lone woman.
Findings, which are presented in the form of case studies,
show that all the women "became deviants, isolates, or low
status regular members of their groups." Among the suggestions the authors offer: if a woman finds herself in a
group where "the leader does not take responsibility for
... helping the men accept her," she should seek support
outside the group, "decrease her behavior in the group,
accept the role of deviant or isolate without becoming de-
pressed by it, and function as well as she can...."

3171.   "The Woman Doctor." Woman's Medical Journal, 25:1
        (January 1915) 13-14. (Editorial.)
Taking issue with an editorial entitled "The Business Problems of the Woman Doctor," recently published in the Medical Council (Philadelphia), this article asserts that discrimination against women physicians is generally a "thing
of the past."

3172.   "Woman's Place Is in the Home. Or Is It?" California's
        Health, (January 1970) 8-11.
Statistics regarding women physicians in the United States
show that women comprise a very low percentage of the
total "manpower" and that few women apply to medical
schools. [Article not examined by editors.]

3173.   "Women as Physicians." Philadelphia Medical and Surgical
        Reporter, 6 April 1867. In: Eighteenth Annual An-
        nouncement of the Woman's Medical College of Pennsyl-
        vania, North College Avenue and 22nd Street, Philadel-
        phia, For the Session of 1867-68. Jas. B. Rodgers,
        Printer, Philadelphia, Pa., 1867, appended pp. 1-2.
"In a recent discussion before the Philadelphia County Medical Society, upon the status of women practitioners of medicine, the following preamble and resolutions were adopted."
The preamble lists the reasons for the society's "grave objections" to women practicing medicine: their inability to
bear up under the bodily and mental strain to which they
would be subjected; the deleterious effects such practice
would have upon the household and children; the "embarrassments" which would be encountered on both sides, in

her visiting and prescribing for persons of the opposite sex;
and the chance for "breach of ethics, misunderstandings
and heartburnings" to ensue in the case where the services
of both a male and female physician are required in the
same household. "In no other country than our own, is a
body of women authorized to engage in the general practice
of medicine." In consideration of these points, it was resolved that "... this Society cannot offer any encouragement
to women becoming practitioners of medicine, nor, on these
grounds, can they consent to meet in consultation with such
practitioners."

3174.   "Women Doctors Speak on Women Doctors." Journal of
        the American Medical Women's Association, 14:5 (May
        1959) 434-435. ports.
        This article [reprinted from the Chicago Medical School
        Alumni News, November-December 1958] offers the opinions
        of six women physicians, alumnae, and faculty of Chicago
        Medical School, on the subject of whether it is worthwhile
        to train women for the medical profession, since they may
        quit to raise a family. Dr. Helen Button believes that the
        number of women who complete medical training is propor-
        tionately higher than that of men. Dr. Bella Hearst be-
        lieves it takes a lot of courage, but the woman doctor "cer-
        tainly is dedicated, or how else would it be possible for her
        to survive?" All would recommend medicine as a career
        for their daughters.

3175.   "Women Doctors Succeed Is the Conclusion after an Exhaus-
        tive Survey Made by One of Our Greatest American
        Newspapers." Woman's Medical Journal, 27:3 (March
        1917) 58.
        A Philadelphia newspaper ran a favorable article on women
        physicians which is reprinted in full. The conclusion of
        the article is that women have a field in which they can
        pioneer and be leaders. "With it all, they lose none of
        the charm of women nor in any way defeat the purposes of
        nature, but make themselves only more valuable to the
        world for their knowledge."

3176.   "Women in Medicine." Woman's Medical Journal, 16:2
        (February 1906) 23-24.
        This article consists of a letter from Dr. Maude Glasgow
        on the medical education of women. She refutes objections
        to women in medicine.

3177.   "Women MDs Join the Fight." Medical World News, (Octo-
        ber 23, 1970) 22-28.
        Discrimination against women trying to enter medicine and
        against physicians in institutional and administrative work
        is discussed, as well as discriminating practices by male
        physicians toward their female patients. Various physicians'
        opinions are presented.

3178. "Women M. D. s Need Home Aid." American Medical Asso-
       ciation News, (30 May 1966) 10.
       [Article not examined by editors.]

3179. "Women Physicians." Macmillan's Magazine, 18:107 (Sep-
       tember 1868) 369-380.
       This article is an apologia for the presence of women in
       the field of medicine. It begins with a history of the earli-
       est women physicians, from Laura Bassi (Bologna, 1732)
       to contemporaries, Elizabeth Blackwell in America and Miss
       Garrett in London. Two common substitute attitudes for
       full medical education for women are examined and refuted,
       i. e., that women could practice an abbreviated version of
       the doctor's art and that women could earn a special cer-
       tificate to be gained by far less effort. The standard
       should separate "not women from men, but the educated
       from the ignorant." If a woman spends at least ten years
       steady work in the profession, if a woman distinguishes
       herself like Dr. Jenner, it would be much to dissipate ex-
       isting prejudices. Intellectual capacity cannot be judged un-
       til women have the same educational opportunities as men.
       In regard to physical and nervous strength, it may be said
       that whenever these qualities have been called for in other
       areas, women have not been found wanting. Further, "a
       profession which brings ... lasting interest, and the dig-
       nity of a good social position, would remove the humiliation
       of celibacy, while it would not hinder the right kind of mar-
       riage." The article ends with a question: "Can it be that
       ... such a life would be less valuable to a woman than to
       a man... ?"

3180. "Women Physicians Get Widespread Publicity." Medical
       Woman's Journal, 54:5 (May 1947) 67.
       This brief article cites several favorable articles on women
       physicians which appeared around 1947 in nonmedical pub-
       lications.

3181. "Women Physicians; Professor Osler's Views." Woman's
       Medical Journal, 17:9 (September 1907) 356.
       Speaking at the London School of Medicine for Women, Pro-
       fessor Osler remarked that medicine is a satisfactory ca-
       reer for women "if they realize that it is not all roses and
       cream, and that they will not get a pecuniary return for
       everything they do." Listing the branches of medicine open
       to women, Osler commented that women are specially fitted
       for dealing with diseases of women, "but the chief trouble
       is that women--as a rule, men's women--do not believe
       much in women."

3182. "Women Students Say Med Schools Need Flexibility." BCM:
       Inside Baylor Medicine, 11:2 (February 1971) 1, 3.
       photo.
       "Most of Baylor's 17 women medical students are more

concerned with their commitment to their profession than
to their sex," yet they believe that more flexible scheduling
for both students and residents would make medicine more
open to women. The four married women medical students
interviewed for this article "agreed that being married has
made them more at ease in a predominantly male environment." Noting that "Baylor has a reputation for prejudice
against women," one woman recalls her surprise when,
during the admissions interview, she felt no antagonism towards her. "'The questions I was asked were legitimate
questions that should have been asked,'" she explains. The
article "supports" her statement with the following: "The
girls said their interviewers were concerned with their commitment to medicine, their desire to complete medical
school, how they planned to arrange their careers and family plans, and whether they will practice after graduation."

3183.   Wood, Ann Douglas. "'The Fashionable Diseases': Wo-
         men's Complaints and Their Treatment in Nineteenth-
         Century America." Journal of Interdisciplinary History,
         4:1 (Summer 1973) 25-52.
         American women of the middle class in the nineteenth cen-
         tury maximized their ill health to the point where they
         seemed to find their identity in the variety of nervous dis-
         eases they had--perhaps in order to escape the demands of
         the bedroom and kitchen. Male doctors of the time took
         advantage of these women by means of their (ignorant) pro-
         fessional superiority, masculine insensitivity, and compla-
         cency. Women's illnesses were one of the subjects to
         which pioneer women physicians first addressed themselves.
         They perceived women's diseases "as a result of submis-
         sion, and promoted independence from masculine domina-
         tion, whether professional or sexual, as their cure for
         feminine ailments." By specializing in hygiene and pre-
         ventive medicine, these early women doctors contributed
         much to the improved treatment of women's and children's
         diseases. To the feminists of the time, the appearance of
         women physicians provided hope that women's diseases
         would be treated differently for the benefit of all women and
         that women would no longer be victimized by male doctors.
         With women becoming healers, women could be self-reliant
         and not dependent upon men. By supporting and caring for
         their own sex, women physicians help women have self-
         esteem.

3184.   Wood-Comstock, Belle. "Attributes of a Woman Physician."
         Women in Medicine, 77 (July 1942) 25-26.
         If women physicians perform only the same tasks as male
         physicians, why bother having women physicians? A woman
         should realize she has a unique contribution to make in
         medicine--a contribution growing out of her femininity.
         Her gentleness and understanding render her uniquely quali-
         fied to practice medical gynecology (she need not practice

surgical gynecology in order to do medical gynecology). In
the treatment of women's diseases, the woman physician
"doesn't need to kill herself or overstrain her nervous
strength by doing a man's work, but is at her best in her
woman's sphere." Pediatrics and nutrition are two other
areas for which women physicians are well suited.

3185. Woodside, Nina B. "Women in Health Care Decision Mak-
       ing." Philadelphia Medicine, 71:10 (October 1975) 431,
       433, 435, 437, 439-441. (Presentation, International
       Conference on Women in Health, Washington, D.C., 17
       June 1975.)
Women are not only providers of health care but also are
active as consumers of health care services. Even though
more women are now in decision making positions since
federal regulations against discrimination by sex have been
in effect, there are still problems and disadvantages that
women (and men) have to face, i.e., reduced or otherwise
flexible schedules, the lack of child care alternatives, and
the lack of role models. Women hold a small percentage
of decision making jobs in health care but still do not have
equal access to exercise the rights and responsibilities that
would be equivalent to the role they exercise in the procurement of those services. Women do not have access (as do
men) for example, to informal channels of communications
(and connections) among their male peers; women still face
the real hardships of being the only token when they do hold
decision making positions; and women lack training in management skills and strategy. Women also have to face negative myths about what it means to be a woman by their
male colleagues as well as their male colleagues' general
insensitivity, and the pattern of behavior and negative self
perception among women themselves. Then too, once a
women achieves a position in the decision making sector,
she must face the criticism of her women colleagues that
she has identified with and become part of the male hierarchy to the exclusion of remaining aware of and able to
act upon women's issues--especially where she is the only
one and isolated from her primary identification group.
Women in health care need to support each other and encourage acceptance of leadership roles. Furthermore,
women need to remain in touch with people they have met
getting through the professional educational system at all
levels--students, faculty, and staff: men have always been
able to assume such networks for recruitment and placement. Women also need to know more about affirmative
action and legal routes to take to correct the inequities that
currently exist. Women must also support strategies to
change the socialization and traditional roles of women so
that women (as well as men) may enjoy a satisfying home
life and a more efficiently run household.

3186. Woolley, Alice Stone. "Rendevous [sic] with the Future." Medical Woman's Journal, 51:8 (August 1944) 17-20. (President's inaugural address, American Medical Women's Association, June 1944.)

In this speech, Dr. Woolley ponders the questions, "What are we [as a generation] to accomplish?" and "What should be the future pattern of the medical profession?" She hopes socialized medicine will not be one answer. Duties of women physicians include keeping medical schools and hospitals open to women, maintaining the strength found in women's medical organizations, and safeguarding national freedom.

3187.   Yarros, Rachelle. "Medical Women of Tomorrow." Woman's Medical Journal, 26:6 (June 1916) 146-149. (Annual Meeting, Medical Women's National Association, Detroit, Michigan, 13 June 1916.)

Because women physicians, per se, face difficulties, fewer women are studying medicine. Some of these difficulties are represented by the exclusion of women from holding hospital appointments at a large number of hospitals, and the exclusion of women from medical schools. If women physicians are to work collectively to put their demands and requests on a broader basis, many of these problems might be solved. Women need to gain confidence in themselves, learn how to face criticism, and make new opportunities for themselves.

3188.   Yarros, Rachelle S. "Women Physicians and the Problems of Women." Medical Woman's Journal, 50:1 (January 1943) 28-30.

"My work, my thought, and my time have been given in the fields that particularly concern women," writes the author. Because problems of obstetrics and gynecology more deeply concern women than men, women physicians are needed to research these problems. Dr. Yarros discusses various women physicians who have done outstanding work already in this field: Dr. Josephine Butler began in 1864 her famous attack on organized prostitution; Dr. Katharine Bement Davis was one of the first physicians to do research on the sex problems of women. Dr. Yarros, "still a feminist" after 50 years of professional experience and study, does not feel that men can or will solve the problems related to biological, psychological differences between women and men, and the problems relating specifically to women.

MEDICAL INSTITUTIONS, SOCIETIES,
AND THEIR JOURNALS

Included: general discussions and statistical
data primarily relevant to specific medical
schools; the experience of women in medical
societies or organizations; and, the history and
policies of medical journals. (For information
about medical education not focusing on specific
schools, see MEDICAL EDUCATION.)

AFRICA

3189.   Edwards, Phyllis M. "Women Doctors in University Col-
            lege Hospital: Ibadan, Nigeria--Conditions of Service."
            Journal of the Medical Women's Federation, 41:1 (Jan-
            uary 1959) 31-33.
        "The primary purpose of the hospital is the clinical train-
        ing of medical students of the College for the London M.B.,
        B.S. degree." This article discusses in part the steps
        that were taken to right a wrong that existed in respect to
        women members of the hospital medical staff, i.e., "Where-
        as women on the staff of the College, which pays the rate
        for the job irrespective of race, creed, sex or marital
        status, were in an acceptable position, women of house phy-
        sician/house surgeon grades and women registrars, if un-
        married, were offered contracts identical with those offered
        men, but automatically terminated on marriage."

ASIA

3190.   "Dr. Han So Jeai: Chief Girl Scout Executive." Medical
            Woman's Journal, 54:6 (June 1947) 32-33. port.
        Dr. Han is visiting the United States to "aid the girl scout
        movement in Korea." This article discusses conditions in
        Korea while that country was under Japanese government.
        Girl Scouting in Korea is also discussed.

3191.   Ferrer-Franco, Isabel. "Hospitals Run by Women Doctors:
            The Maternity and Children's Hospital." Journal of the
            American Medical Women's Association, 12:1 (January
            1957) 17-19. (Medical Practice Around the World.)
        A history of The Maternity and Children's Hospital of
        Manila is presented.

3192.   Griscom, Mary W. "Medical Women in China." Medical
            Woman's Journal, 33:8 (August 1926) 226-227.
        Dr. Griscom wrote this report of the Women's Union Med-
        ical College of Peking, China, because "the teaching of
        medicine and surgery to the Oriental women seems the only
        way to help countries like China, India, and Persia ever to
        rise and take their proper places in the world of work to-
        day."

3193.   Hall, Marian B. "East Gate Hospital, Seoul, Korea."
            Medical Woman's Journal, 33:10 (October 1926) 290-291.
        East Gate Hospital, the largest hospital for women in Korea
        was founded as the Baldwin Dispensary in 1892 by Dr.
        Rosetta Sherwood Hall. The first Western-trained Korean

physician was a woman, Dr. Esther Kim Pak, who graduated from Women's Medical College of Baltimore in 1900.
As of this article, there were 16 women doctors in Korea.
Although the Severance Medical College in Seoul is the logical place for women to study, women are refused admission, which is "not a reflection on all the [foreign] men
doctors in charge. Some of them are among the finest
Christian gentlemen I have met and not prejudiced against a
woman doctor...." In the meantime, "the girls are educated at much greater expense in non-Christian schools in
Japan."

3194.   Inouye, Tomo. "National Association of the Medical Women
        of Japan." Medical Woman's Journal, 30:8 (August
        1923) 238-240. photo., port.
        In order to give American women physicians an idea of the
        scope of subjects discussed at meetings of the Association,
        Dr. Inouye presents brief resumés of two meetings. She
        also states that the status of Japanese women physicians is
        very similar to that of American women physicians: while
        Japanese women are members of the medical associations,
        they serve in no official positions; while women practice in
        hospitals, they are not members of the staffs.

3195.   Isoda, Senzaburo. "Medical Education of Women in Japan."
        Journal of the American Medical Women's Association,
        15:10 (October 1960) 982-983.
        Dr. Yayoi [sic] Yoshioka founded, and in 1900 became the
        first president of, Tokyo Women's Medical College, Japan's
        oldest and longest surviving training medical institution for
        women. At the time she founded this school, Japanese
        society considered women subordinate to men. Dr. Yo-
        shioka believed that women should have economic independ-
        ence and that medicine was a suitable and an honorable
        career by which women might earn their living. As of
        1960, the situation for women studying medicine in Japan
        remained limited: 3,000 men pass the national board ex-
        aminations each year on the average, while only 250 wo-
        men do; medical schools that once were exclusively male
        admitted women but tended to admit only three or four each
        year. Therefore, the Tokyo Women's Medical College, with
        300 women students in 1960, remains an important institu-
        tion for the education of women physicians in Japan. In
        1960 the president of the college was Naotaro Kuji.

3196.   Lawney, Josephine C. "A Daughter Institution in the Ori-
        ent." In: 75th Anniversary Volume of the Woman's
        Medical College of Pennsylvania. Westbrook Publish-
        ing Company, Philadelphia, Pennsylvania, [1925?], 349-
        354.
        Elizabeth Reifsnyder, an 1881 graduate of Woman's Medical
        College of Pennsylvania, went to Shanghai, China where she
        founded the Margaret Williamson Hospital (in 1884) and the

Woman's Christian Medical College (in 1924). Dr. Lawney
(M.D., 1916), a faculty member of the College, reviews
the growth of the two Shanghai institutions.

3197.   Parish, Rebecca. "The Mary J. Johnston Memorial Hos-
         pital." Medical Woman's Journal, 36:9 (September
         1929) 231-232. (Special Article.)
         "Here is the story of what a hospital is doing for the peo-
         ple of the Philippine Islands." The Mary J. Johnston
         Memorial Hospital in Manila opened its doors in 1907.
         The hospital is affiliated with the Methodist Episcopal
         Church. Specific incidents in the history of this hospital
         are retold.

3198.   The Tokyo Women's Medical College: Introductory Bulletin,
         1937-1938. Ushigome, Tokyo, 1937, 21 pp. photos.,
         tables.
         An introduction to the school, its course of study and re-
         quirements, is followed by a history of the Tokyo Women's
         Medical College and a general history of Japanese medical
         women.

3199.   "The Tokyo Women's Medical College: Ushigome, Tokyo,
         Japan." Medical Woman's Journal, 43:3 (March 1936)
         75-77. photos., port.
         Given is a brief history of Japanese women in medicine,
         from the times when the terms "woman doctor" and "witch"
         were synonymous, to the present, when about 2000 women
         have graduated from the Tokyo Women's Medical College.
         A history of that institution constitutes the major portion
         of this article.

3200.   Whitmore, Clara B. "Letter from China: A Letter Writ-
         ten by Dr. Clara B. Whitmore, Elected President of
         the Society for 1916, But Unable to Serve Owing to Her
         Absence in China." Woman's Medical Journal, 26:8
         (August 1916) 198-199. (Presentation, Annual Banquet,
         State Society of Iowa Medical Women, Davenport, Iowa,
         9 May 1916.)
         Dr. Whitmore writes of her experiences and work at the
         Margaret Williamson Hospital in Shanghai, China.

3201.   "A Woman Physician in Charge of Dispensary for Indian
         Women and Children in Fiji." Medical Woman's Jour-
         nal, 28:12 (December 1921) 316.
         Dr. Mildred Staley was put in charge of the dispensary for
         women and children in Suva, Fiji. It is the first purely
         Indian dispensary for women and children.

3202.   "Women Physicians in Japan." Medical Woman's Journal,
         38:9 (September 1931) 236.
         The associations of Japanese women physicians are men-
         tioned, and impressions of the Japan Medical Woman's
         Journal are given.

3203.   Yoshioka, Y. "The Historical Outline of the Tokyo Women's
        Medical College." Medical Woman's Journal, 30:8 (Au-
        gust 1923) 240-242. port.
        Dr. Yoshioka relates events leading up to her founding of
        the College and her founding of hospitals for the purpose of
        giving women students practical experience. Included in this
        history is mention of the opposition to women's medical edu-
        cation in Japan.

AUSTRALIA & NEW ZEALAND

3204.   Cohen, Lysbeth. Rachel Forster Hospital: The First Fifty
        Years. Rachel Forster Hospital, Sydney, [New South
        Wales], 1972, 48 pp. photos., port.
        The Rachel Forster Hospital was founded in 1922 for the
        treatment of women and children by women, and for the
        training of medical women who were being excluded from
        positions in other hospitals. This history includes profiles
        of the six women physicians who established the institution:
        Drs. Lucy Bullett, Harriet Biffin, Constance D'Arcy,
        Margaret Harper, Susie O'Reilly, and Emma Buckley.
        Other women associated with the institution are mentioned
        as well. The current organizational and physical features
        of the hospital are contrasted with its modest beginnings.

3205.   MacKenzie, [Lady]. "The Flying Doctor Service." Med-
        ical Woman's Journal, 46:12 (December 1939) 376-377.
        (Editorial.)
        The Flying Doctor Service provides "aeroplane ambulances"
        for Australia's sparsely populated areas. One full-time
        "Flying Doctor" is Jean White, a British physician who
        graduated from Melbourne University.

3206.   Ravell, Marion. "Medical Women in Australia: Some Im-
        pressions." Medical Women's Federation Quarterly
        Review, (January 1935) 34-38.
        Dr. Ravell gives the history as well as the current status
        of the Queen Victoria Memorial Hospital in Melbourne,
        Australia. Several other hospitals are mentioned by Dr.
        Ravell, who visited Australia and New Zealand from Eng-
        land.

CANADA

3207.   "Canada's Medical Women Gain C. M. A. Affiliation." Cana-
        dian Doctor, (July 1963) 36-37.
        This article concerning women physicians' affiliation with
        the Canadian Medical Association, reports on the annual
        meeting of the Federation of Medical Women of Canada.
        [Article not examined by editors.]

3208.   Chase, Lillian A. "Women's College Hospital: Toronto,
         Canada." Medical Woman's Journal, 43:3 (March 1936)
         72-73.
         Forty women doctors constitute the staff of this new hos-
         pital. The building's physical features are described.

3209.   "Mid-Year Meeting of Canadian Medical Women." Medical
         Woman's Journal, 47:10 (October 1940) 310-311.
         This report includes new officers of the Federation of Med-
         ical Women of Canada.

3210.   "Report of Federation of Medical Women of Canada." Med-
         ical Woman's Journal, 48:3 (March 1941) 92-93.
         At the February 19, 1941, meeting of the Federation, Dr.
         Marion Hilliard delivered an address entitled "The Future
         of Women in Medicine." The essence of this address is
         given in the article.

3211.   Scriver, Jessie Boyd. "McGill's First Women Medical
         Students." McGill Medical Journal, (1947) 237-243.
         [Article not examined by editors.]

3212.   Stewart, Elizabeth L. A Brief History of the Women's Col-
         lege Hospital. Toronto, Canada, 1956.
         [Item not examined by editors.]

EUROPE, EASTERN

3213.   "Medical Education of Women in Russia." London Medical
         Record, 3 (27 January 1875) 60. (Miscellany.)
         Two hundred and forty women have been pursuing courses
         at the Academy of Medicine of St. Petersburg for three
         years. Most come from the provinces rather than from
         the capital and have their education paid for on the condi-
         tion they return to their province to practice.

3214.   Roubinovitch, Jacques. ["A Medical School for Women at
         St. Petersburg"]. Le Progrès Médical, Vol. 1 (3rd
         Series) (1 June 1895) 361. (Fre)
         On May 4 the Council of State at last voted favorably on
         the proposal to establish a medical school for women in St.
         Petersburg, since there are enough gifts and bequests avail-
         able to assure its financial future. It will be open to wo-
         men not less than 21 years of age, with written permission
         of the parents or husband; entrance requirements include
         Latin and Greek, as required for graduation from the boys'
         gymnasia. The curriculum will consist of exactly the same
         material taught in the Faculty of Medicine and will last five
         years. Women graduates will not be admitted as directors
         of general hospitals nor to the examinations of the recruit-
         ing board; some especially well qualified may be admitted
         as experts before the courts. The director of the school

will be appointed by the minister of public instruction and
will be responsible to a council of professors and to academic and administrative-economic commissions.

3215.   Sokoloff, D. A. ["New Clinic of Diseases of Children in
         the Woman's Medical School"]. Vrach. Gaz. (St.
         Petersburg), 11 (1904) 356. (Rus)
         [Article not examined by editors.]

3216.   Tkatchef, Alexandrine. ["Medical Curriculum for Women
         in St. Petersburg: Part 1"]. Gazette Hebdomadaire
         des Sciences Médicales de Montpellier, 9:26 (25 June
         1887) 301-305. (Fre)
         In this first of two installments, the author recalls the ear-
         ly history of this St. Petersburg institution. During the
         1860s a number of lyceums, normal schools, and other
         higher education facilities for women were established in
         Russia, all under private auspices. Courses for midwives
         were authorized by imperial decree in 1872, at the urging
         of the minister of war, M. Milioutine (Milutin), to be at-
         tached to the military medical school, which was the only
         medical school in St. Petersburg. Requirements for ad-
         mission included age over 20, a baccalaureate diploma in
         science, parental approval, a police certificate of good
         character, and an entrance examination. Classes were
         given separately from those of the military school, and the
         women lived under very strict rules of dress, conduct, etc.
         Officially, the courses were those suited to future midwives;
         actually the eminent professors taught the same material to
         the women as to the men. The women did so well in their
         studies that in a few years the curriculum was changed to
         five years and they became officially "medical courses for
         women." The men students accepted the women without
         resentment, helping them with their studies while the wo-
         men helped them out of scrapes with the police.

3217.   Tkatchef, Alexandrine. ["Medical Curriculum for Women
         in St. Petersburg: Part 2"]. Gazette Hebdomadaire
         des Sciences Médicales de Montpellier, 9:27 (2 July
         1887) 313-317. (Fre)
         The author describes student life at St. Petersburg. Many
         of the students had part-time jobs, and they usually shared
         apartments to save costs. The happy hours spent over tea
         and in heated discussion of the world and its problems com-
         pensated for hard work and frequent short rations. When
         the first five-year classes were completing their studies,
         the Turkish war broke out, and the women insisted on serv-
         ing in the army along with their male counterparts. Twenty-
         five of them were selected to serve with the ambulance
         corps, with the title of army surgeon. Their knowledge,
         surgical skills, patience, courage, and tireless care of the
         sick and wounded drew the admiration of foreign correspond-
         ents, military authorities, and even the emperor, who

awarded them a gold medal on the ribbon of the Order of
St. George. However, after the end of the war, these women still had to fight for the right to practice medicine.
Of the 450 graduates, a few became directors of hospital
clinics or laboratories; a few practiced in large cities.
Most, however, took civil service positions in the provinces,
where they quickly gained the trust and affection of the
peasant populations. They were especially in demand in the
Moslem provinces. The new minister of war soon decided
that the army could not support women's classes, although
government support during the ten years from 1872 to 1881
had totaled no more than 10,000 rubles. In 1882 gradual
closure of the courses was decreed and in the last year
(1886) they were closed completely.

3218.   Vestnik Oftalmologii, 22 (1905) 604-610. (Rus)
         Given are proceedings of a society [Moscow? Russia?] of
         ophthalmologists. The November meeting mentions the
         nomination of Evgenia Elizarovna Dikanskaya to full mem-
         bership; the December meeting reports that she was elected
         --one of two out of the half-dozen nominated.

EUROPE, WESTERN

3219.   "American Women Students at Zurich University." Woman's
             Medical Journal, 6:10 (October 1897) 303-304.
         American women studying for a doctorate at Zurich issued
         a circular offering advice and information to prospective
         students. A portion of the circular is given here, includ-
         ing information on such matters as fees, etiquette, course
         of study, and language requirement (German).

3220.   "'Before Women Were Human Beings.'" Medical Woman's
             Journal, 45:8 (August 1938) 246-247. (Editorial.)
         Ida H. Hyde was the first woman to obtain a Ph.D. at the
         University of Heidelberg (1894), and the first woman per-
         mitted to do research in that institution's medical school--
         thus establishing a precedent for women medical students.
         In an article entitled "Before Women Were Human Beings,"
         published in the June [1938] issue of the Journal of the
         American Association of University Women, Dr. Hyde re-
         calls her own struggles and depicts the changes in status
         of German women in medicine, and in other scientific fields,
         from 1893 to 1938.

3221.   Böhmert, Victor. [Women's Studies in the Experience of
             the University of Zurich]. Leipzig, Germany, 1874,
             12 pp. table. (Ger)
         Zurich was one of the first universities to offer complete
         equality of education to women (in 1854). This summary of
         the first ten years of education of women includes a table
         of yearly enrollment of women in political science, medicine,

and philosophy, the students' native countries, and the number leaving each year with and without taking the examinations in medicine or philosophy. The number matriculated in medicine ranged from one to eight in the first years, climbed to 88--comprised mostly of Russians--in 1872-3, then fell to 16 and 18 in 1873 and 1874 respectively, after the imperial decree ordering the Russian women to return home for political reasons. At about the same time the Swiss government ordered that foreigners as well as Swiss women would have to show evidence of suitable preparatory education to be admitted. The opening of the universities has demonstrated that women in general are capable of taking the medical course and of solving difficult scientific problems, but that they need better preliminary education to be the equals of men in academic life. The greatest attacks against women in professions have been against women in medical studies. The medical faculty, however, collectively and individually, have reported no problems resulting from mixed classes in theoretical and practical courses with no concessions made for women. The women also have said that they found little or no trouble adjusting to the situation, even though most of them had never studied with men before. Further evidence of the success of the program is that ten women have successfully taken the M.D. examination. Three Russians achieved the degree after only three years instead of the normal four and a half.

3222.   Carrier, Henriette. [Origins of La Maternité de Paris: The Chief Midwives and the Lying-In Department of the Old Hotel-Dieu (1378-1796)]. Georges Steinheil, Paris, France, 1888, xviii, 272 pp. illus. (Fre)
This history of the lying-in department of the Hotel-Dieu, the predecessor of the world-famous maternity hospital in Paris, was written by a graduate of the midwifery school of La Maternité and midwife of the Hôpital Lariboisiere. Part 1 (The Chief Midwives of the Hotel-Dieu, 1378-1775), includes names of midwives recorded as having practiced at the Hotel-Dieu from 1512 on. Part 2 (The Lying-In Department of the Hotel-Dieu) describes the physical and administrative arrangements; the personnel--chief midwife, apprentices, visiting medical-surgical staff and foreign visitors, and housekeeping and domestic staff--and the rules of the department at various times. Part 3 (The Directorship of Madame Dugès, Last Midwife of the Hotel-Dieu; Apprenticeship of Madame Lachappelle (1775-1797), describes a period of great change. Madame Dugès, born Marie Jornet, was "very capable at her craft, highly intelligent, zealous to a degree meriting high praise...." She took part in the reorganization after the fire which destroyed part of the Hotel-Dieu in 1772, and supervised the move to new quarters at the Oratory in 1795. Part 4 (The Hospice de la Maternité; Directorship of Madame Lachappelle 1797-1821) de-

scribes the maternity department and the school for midwives established in 1802. Madame Lachapelle, daughter
of Mme. Dugès, became her assistant in 1795, became
chief midwife or director in 1797, and was in sole charge
of the maternity department from 1797 to 1802. As chief
midwife, she was responsible for all deliveries, or for deciding when the attending obstetrician should be called.
She was also in charge of the school. This offered a six-
month course with lectures by the chief midwife, attending
obstetrician and pharmacist, and demonstrations in anatomy,
as well as practical instruction. Between 1802 and 1814
the school admitted nearly 1300 students and was considered
the best in France. Mme. Lachappelle died in 1821 at the
age of 52.

3223.   Chambers, Helen. "The Marie Curie Hospital." Medical
            Woman's Journal, 38:4 (April 1931) 79-82. photo.,
            port.
         Historical background is given and the facilities and pro-
         cedures are described for the Marie Curie Hospital, "the
         first research hospital to be started and staffed entirely by
         women for the primary object of the relief and cure of
         malignant disease."

3224.   Cohn, Hermann. ["On the Admission of Women to Lectures
            on Hygiene at Breslau (Germany) Medical Faculty"].
            Deutsche Medizinische Wochenschrift, 24 (1898) 530.
            (Ger)
         The author, a professor of ophthalmology at Breslau Uni-
         versity, comments on the exclusion of women from his lec-
         tures on eye care. He agrees to their exclusion from lec-
         tures on anatomy, physiology, and clinical medicine but
         feels that teachers and social workers should be allowed to
         attend his lectures as they might thereby be able to improve
         public health.

3225.   Dionesov, S. M. ["Russian Female Medical Students in
            Zurich in the Revolutionary Movement of the 70s in the
            19th Century"]. Sovetskoe Zdravookhranenie, 32 (1973)
            68-72. (Rus)
         After the new University charter in 1863 and the Order of
         the Minister of Defense in 1864, both prohibiting the study
         of sciences and medicine by Russian women, many of the
         women left for Zurich and entered the medical department
         of the University there. N. P. Suslova and M. A. Bokova
         were the first Russian women to graduate from the Univer-
         sity of Zurich as physicians and later defended doctoral
         theses. In 1869-70 there were nine Russian women stu-
         dents; in 1870-71, 13; in 1871-72, 17; and by summer 1873,
         76. They not only studied there, they also became inter-
         ested in the history and practice of the revolutionary move-
         ment in the West, the ideology of socialism, political econ-
         omy, and the history of the internationale. Under the pres-

sure of the Russian government, which was concerned about
its own security, they were forced to leave Zurich in 1874.
Some of the women stayed abroad. Many returned to Russia and joined the revolutionary movement; 63 of them became "outstanding revolutionary propagandists." The author
describes personalities, their activities in the '70s, their
participation in the revolutionary movement, and the fates
of many of them after they returned to Russia.

3226. "From Abroad--Lady Medical Students at Zurich--...."
        Medical Times and Gazette, 2 (7 September 1872) 261-
        262. (The Week.)
Following historical background on the admission of women
to medical courses in Zurich, the admissions of women over
the past decade are reviewed. During the past eight years,
89 women enrolled at the Zurich Medical School. Women
presently compose "about a fourth" of the total medical student population.

3227. Hurd-Mead, Kate Campbell. "The Bologna Medical School."
        Quarterly Bulletin of the Medical Women's National As-
        sociation, 18 (October 1927) 8.
Founded by Theodosius II in 425 A.D., the University of
Bologna practiced equality of the sexes in all of the faculties of the University. Dorothea Bocchi (1390-1436) was
professor of moral philosophy and practical medicine, and
Anne Morandi in 1760 became a famous professor of anatomy there. This article reviews women in medicine as portrayed in literature as well as women at the University of
Bologna.

3228. Jex-Blake, Sophia. "Female Physicians." The Spectator,
        41:2095 (22 August 1868) 991. (Letters to the Editor.)
Dr. Jex-Blake briefly expresses her satisfaction with the
Medical School of the University of Paris, which has final-
ly admitted women. A letter to her by the minister of
public instruction confirms the information; that letter [in
French] is also published herein.

3229. Lovejoy, Esther Pohl. The House of the Good Neighbor.
        The Macmillan Company, New York, New York, 1919,
        218 pp. photos.
During World War I, Dr. Lovejoy was associated with a
humanitarian venture in France called, unofficially, the
House of the Good Neighbor. Located in the factory district
of Levallois, the house was established and run as a community service by young French women of established social
position who "had had enough tea and macaroons to last
forever." Their goals were: "to help unfortunate people
help themselves; to afford them relief in emergencies ...
well-directed education ... [and] a spirit of self-respect and
responsibility...." Their efforts attracted official attention
and much war relief work was channeled to them.

3230.   Luhn, Antke. [The History of Women Students at the Med-
        ical Faculty of Göttingen University]. Göttingen, Ger-
        many, 1972, 168 pp. tables. (M.D. thesis.) (Ger)
        This extensively researched thesis on female medical stu-
        dents at Göttingen University (Germany) retraces the gen-
        eral history of women in medicine. The author then con-
        centrates on the controversy of women's admission in Gött-
        ingen starting in 1893 with the admission of the first fe-
        male auditors. She follows the evolution until present
        times, focusing on qualitative aspects of the problem.
        There are also chapters on women in residencies and as
        faculty members. The thesis contains extensive data on
        all aspects of women in medicine. A substantial bibliogra-
        phy is included.

3231.   Purnell, Caroline M. "Extracts from Report of Dr. Caro-
        line M. Purnell, Commissioner of the American Wo-
        men's Hospitals in France." Woman's Medical Journal,
        29[19]:2 (February 1919) 26-27.

3232.   Rohmer, Hanny. [The First 30 Years of Women in Medical
        Studies at the University of Zurich (1867-1897)]. Zuer-
        cher Medizingeschichtliche Abhandlungen, Neue Reihe
        #89, Juris Druck & Verlag, Zurich, 1972, 96 pp.
        table. (Ger)
        This issue in a series of monographs on the history of
        medicine deals with the particular problems and the indi-
        vidual destinies of the women who studied medicine during
        the first 30 years of their admission to the medical faculty
        of Zurich University. After a short summary of the most
        important steps in women's accession to medical studies,
        the author describes the situation of the groups and indi-
        viduals of different nationalities who came to Zurich to study
        medicine. She gives quite detailed bibliographies of the in-
        dividual students and captures the extreme determination and
        strength they showed in achieving their goals. The accounts
        quote from letters by the students and reports by their con-
        temporaries and professors. Three separate chapters de-
        scribe the attitudes of the faculty, the male students, and
        the general public to the controversial issue of women in
        medicine, using letters and quotes from contemporary arti-
        cles. An addendum lists the names, places of origin,
        topics of dissertation, and dates of graduation of the 61 wo-
        men of various nationalities who studied medicine in Zurich
        during the period under consideration. There is a list of
        the dates when other European universities admitted women
        to medical studies as regular students. The article ends
        with an extensive bibliography.

3233.   Rose, Edmund. "Zurich Female Students." Boston Med-
        ical and Surgical Journal, 101:13 (25 September 1879)
        460.
        Professor Rose has written a letter from Zurich in answer

to queries about the admission of women medical students
to the university there. "At first only very earnest and
industrious ladies entered, but later many coquettish and
hysterical ones, who have caused a strong prejudice against
the whole question." Once again the female students are
of the industrious type and "do not cause any great excite-
ment."

3234.   Sablik, Karl Von. ["The Admission of Women to the Med-
        ical Faculty of Vienna University"]. Wiener Medizin-
        ische Wochenschrift, 181:40 (5 October 1968) 817-819.
        table. (Ger)
        The author describes the medical training of women before
        their admission to the Vienna University faculty as regular
        students in 1900. The first women to obtain their medical
        degrees in Vienna had either not studied there or had
        changed from the faculty of philosophy (which then included
        most of the sciences) to the faculty of medicine after 1900.
        In 1901, however, two women came to medical school di-
        rectly from high school and became the first graduates of
        the Vienna University Faculty of Medicine to have followed
        a normal course similar to that of the male students. The
        women who came to medicine via philosophy successfully
        fought for the recognition of their previous science training.

3235.   "A Tribute to a Distinguished Medical Woman." Medical
        Woman's Journal, 44:2 (February 1937) 47-48. (Edi-
        torial.)
        A wing to the American Memorial Hospital at Reims,
        France was given as the gift of a number of American wo-
        men. This addition was a tribute to the services of Dr.
        Marie Louise Lefort, an American physician and director
        of the hospital.

3236.   "Women and the Berlin Medical Society." Woman's Medical
        Journal, 10:4 (April 1900) 164-165.
        A debate over the admission of women to the Berlin Medical
        Society took place at a January meeting. According to the
        Society's by-laws, women are ineligible as members be-
        cause German women physicians, all of whom obtained quali-
        fications abroad, are regarded as unqualified practitioners.
        During the debate, the galleries were crowded with specta-
        tors, including several women. The motion to admit wo-
        men members was rejected. This editorial further com-
        ments that German women must gain the right to study
        medicine in German schools.

GREAT BRITAIN

3237.   "Admission of Medical Women to the Obstetrical Society of
        London." The Obstetrical Journal of Great Britain and
        Ireland, 2 (April 1874) 23-25.

A resolution recently passed by the Obstetrical Society of
London banned women from membership. This editorial
agrees with the Society that the admission of women "would
be detrimental to the scientific objects and interests of the
Society." While female midwives are capable of handling
normal deliveries, women physicians would provide "frail
and imperfect help" in more serious obstetrical situations.

3238.   Aitken, Janet. "Elizabeth Garrett Anderson Hospital Cen-
             tenary." British Medical Journal, 2 (6 August 1966)
             354-355. sketch. (Medical History.)
         A history of the hospital is given in this article.

3239.   "The Annual General and Council Meetings of the Medical
             Women's Federation, May 2nd and 3rd, 1929." Medical
             Women's Federation News-Letter, (July 1929) 49-74.
         Among other activities and events reported, this article
         (which consists in a summary of the proceedings) presents
         principal items from the reports of the standing committees
         on public health, psychological medicine, venereal disease,
         National Health Insurance, and the working of the Midwives
         Acts.

3240.   "Annual General Meeting, June 17th, 1926." Medical Wo-
             men's Federation News-Letter, (July 1926) 20-39.
         Among other topics reported in this article (which consists
         in a summary of proceedings) are underpaid public health
         posts and the printing of leaflets on menstruation.

3241.   Balfour, Margaret I. "The Medical Women's Overseas
             Association News." Medical Women's Federation Quar-
             terly Review, (October 1945) 42-44.
         Brief notes are given on the progress of various overseas
         hospitals and the work of specific overseas physicians.

3242.   "The British Medical Women's Federation: Fifth Annual
             Meeting, London, England, May 6, 1922." Medical
             Woman's Journal, 29:7 (July 1922) 144-147.
         A list of the newly elected officers of the Federation is fol-
         lowed by a recounting of the resolutions discussed and car-
         ried. Reports of various standing committees are given.
         The Venereal Disease Committee discussed self-disinfection.
         The Committee for Cases of Unequal Treatment decided to
         support the claims to equal consideration of individual wo-
         men in government or local public bodies who are receiving
         salaries unequal to those of their male counterparts. On
         the dismissal of police women, the council "unanimously
         agreed that for social, moral and health reasons, it was
         most desirable" to retain the services of police women
         throughout the country. A letter describing the Federation's
         position and rationale was sent to the Prime Minister,
         Lloyd George, and is herein reproduced. Regarding a re-
         cent ad in the British Medical Journal for a job opening

which excluded married women physicians, the council
elected to write to the British Medical Association and point
out that such qualifications regarding the employment of
married women physicians are illegal.

3243.   Brittain, Vera. "Women and the Hospitals: The University
         Committee's Report." The Nation & Athenaeum, 44 (2
         February 1929) 609-610.
To complete a "memorable week for women" one thing was
required: the unequivocal acceptance of London medical
women on equal terms with men. However, when the report of the London University Committee on Medical Education of Women Students was issued, it was but a "tepid
document, conspicuous chiefly for its Laodicean ability to
blow neither hot nor cold." The author then discusses the
report and concludes, "The problem of the woman doctor,
like all questions affecting the position of women, can really be solved only in the nursery."

3244.   Brooks, Louie M. "Jubilee of the London (Royal Free
         Hospital) School of Medicine for Women." Medical
         Journal and Record, 121 (7 January 1925) 54-55. pho-
         tos.

3245.   Brown, John. "The Medical Women's Federation: How the
         Status of Medical Women Can Be Raised and How Med-
         ical Women Can Further the Reduction of Cancer and
         Other Diseases." Medical Times, (February 1925) 19-
         21.
No women physicians are represented on the General Council of Medical Education and Registration of the United Kingdom. Neither do the examining boards of the universities
and colleges have women examiners. The Medical Women's
Federation should seek to have women appointed to these
and other such organizations.

3246.   Carpenter, William Benjamin. "The University of London
         and Medical Women." Lancet, 2 (21 July 1877) 108-
         109. (Letters to the Editor.)
Dr. Carpenter seeks to correct a misapprehension regarding the Senate's intentions in modifying the regulations for
medical degrees. He states that "the existing regulations
in regard to medical degrees shall apply without distinction
of sex." He further elucidates the modifications that are
to take place as the listing of those foreign medical schools
from which degrees will be accepted.

3247.   Chadburn, M. M. "The Marie Curie Hospital." Medical
         Women's Federation News-Letter, (March 1929) 48-50.
         (Correspondence.)
The proposed Marie Curie Hospital will enlarge the scope
of work done by the Cancer Research Committee of the
London Association of the Medical Women's Federation.

The hospital will receive cancer cases from four hospitals
already carrying on the work of the committee. Dr. Elizabeth Hurden is director and research officer and sees the
work of all four hospitals, making her expertise available
to the rest of the staff. The letter ends with an appeal
for funds.

3248.   Chambers, Helen. "The Marie Curie Hospital." Medical
              Women's Federation News-Letter, (March 1930) 18-21.
              photo.
          Described are the evolution of and the treatments used at
          this institution, the first research hospital started and
          staffed entirely by women for the relief and cure of malig-
          nant disease.

3249.   Chisholm, Catherine. "A Retrospection and an Anticipation.
              Medical Women's Federation News-Letter, (November
              1928) 19-23. (Presidential Address, Council Meeting,
              Medical Women's Federation, Cheltenham, England, 25
              October 1928.)
          "By uniting women, by exercising pressure on women who
          have perhaps not quite realized the sin of under-cutting, by
          giving advice and encouragement to its members, and inci-
          dentally by exploding many myths as to the depths to which
          medical women were reduced," the Federation helps to
          maintain the spirit of pioneer women physicians, and safe-
          guard the interests of medical women. Dr. Chisholm re-
          flects upon the Federation's most valuable work: social
          services.

3250.   Crawford, Raymond. "Epsom College and Medical Women."
              Medical Women's Federation News-Letter, (July 1933)
              67-69. (Correspondence.)
          This letter encourages women to consider attending Epsom
          College, which has grown up around the nucleus of the
          Royal Medical Foundation.

3251.   "Demonstration of the Students of the University of Edin-
              burgh." Medical Times and Gazette, 1 (10 February
              1872) 180.
          This article describes the student demonstration at the Uni-
          versity of Edinburgh to protest the Lord Provost's actions
          regarding the education of lady medical students.

3252.   "The Edinburgh Female Medical Students." Medical Times
              and Gazette, 2 (16 November 1872) 547.
          The population of Edinburgh could be said to contain three
          sexes: "men, women, and avowedly female medical stu-
          dents." Renewing their efforts "to thrust themselves into
          medical schools founded for the education of male students,"
          these female agitators are out to damage a respected insti-
          tution and "bring a noble profession into disrepute."

3253.   "The Edinburgh Royal Infirmary." Medical Times and Ga-
              zette, 2 (14 December 1872) 656.
         Recently, a group of managers of the Edinburgh Royal In-
         firmary retired by rotation and were replaced by a group
         favorable to the matter of female clinical instruction.   This
         development may later seriously impair the Infirmary's
         prosperity.   The latest results of the "feminine vehemence"
         and efforts of "Miss Jex-Blake and her friends" would be
         "ludicrous" if the eminence of a great medical school and
         hospital were not threatened.   Not only is the hospital too
         small for female students, but hopefully "high-spirited and
         decent young men will never consent to study clinical medi-
         cine and surgery with persons of the opposite sex."

3254.   "Education of Women at Edinburgh. (From an old Corres-
              pondent)." Medical Times and Gazette, 1 (27 January
              1872) 106-107. (Provincial Correspondence: Scotland.)
         "The Senatus and Court have both found out that the med-
         ical education of women is both impracticable and illegal,"
         yet the battle still rages.   The women propose that if men
         and women cannot be taught together, then 30 or 40 beds
         in the infirmary should be set aside as a sort of hospital
         for the exclusive use of 16 "ladies."   The managers argue
         against this proposal on the technicality of the number of
         beds necessary to constitute a hospital (80 beds).   This
         agitation is inflicting much misery on the society of Edin-
         burgh.   The author of this correspondence wonders at the
         "curious" questions raised and asks, "Why has a portion
         of the press taken it up so generally on the women's side?"
         The writer suggests that the ladies "pressed their attention"
         upon these men and thereby gained their support.   Faculty
         politics at the University is also touched upon.

3255.   "Elizabeth Blackwell Memorial." Medical Woman's Journal,
              45:7 (July 1938) 212. (Editorial.)
         The Walker Dunbar Hospital, Bristol, England, plans to
         erect a new building as a memorial to Dr. Blackwell.

3256.   "Elsie Inglis Memorial Maternity Hospital." Medical Wo-
              man's Journal, [35]:1 (January 1928) 1-2.   port. (Fea-
              ture Article.)
         In an article requesting funds to endow an "Eliza M.
         Mosher Memorial Bed" to the one-year-old Elsie Inglis
         Memorial Maternity Hospital in Scotland--the only hospital
         in the world named after a woman physician--a brief pro-
         file of Dr. Inglis is given.   During World War I, although
         "treated with the same indifference and disdain by the
         [British] War Department as our own American medical
         women were treated by Washington," Dr. Inglis organized
         the Scottish Women's Hospitals.   Likening her courage dur-
         ing the war to a modern Joan of Arc, and recalling her
         tragic death, the article's author notes: "So many women
         have been burned at the stake of injustice, that it is not
         even unique."

3257.   "The English Medical Women's Federation and the Preven-
            tion of Venereal Disease." Medical Woman's Journal,
            47:11 (November 1940) 340. (Editorial.)
        Excerpted from The Lancet, this editorial applauds the work
        of the Medical Women's Federation in combating venereal
        disease through sex education.

3258.   "The Female Medical Students." Medical Times and Ga-
            zette, 1 (10 February 1872) 180.
        This brief paragraph notes in part the response of Edinburgh
        University Court to Sophia Jex-Blake in regards to the fe-
        male medical student question: that the Court will consider
        the fitness of Jex-Blake and the "other ladies" who have
        been matriculated students of the University, to practice
        medicine, but that "'It is ... to be distinctly understood
        that such arrangements are not to be founded on as imply-
        ing any right in women to obtain medical degrees....'"

3259.   Fowler, R. N. "The University of London and Medical
            Women." Lancet, 1 (30 June 1877) 953-954. (Cor-
            respondence.)
        The writer, a member of the [University of London] Senate,
        explains his voting decision on the issue of admitting wo-
        men to the University's medical program. Citing the "evil
        effects" of placing women on an equality with men as med-
        ical practitioners, Fowler fears that "the idea will grow up
        among ladies ... that there is something indelicate in con-
        sulting a gentleman.... It would be a most serious evil if,
        when a young lady is asked ... to consult some eminent
        physician, she takes it into her head that some lady doctor
        will do equally well."

3260.   "The Garrett Anderson Hospital." Medical Woman's Jour-
            nal, 37:2 (February 1930) 31-33. photo., ports. (Spe-
            cial Article.)
        Elizabeth Garrett Anderson was, in 1865, the second woman
        to enter medicine in England. A year after Drs. Elizabeth
        and Emily Blackwell and Marie Zakrzewska opened the New
        York Infirmary for Women and Children, Dr. Anderson
        founded the Garrett-Anderson Hospital in London to provide
        medical care and advice by competent women doctors to
        poor women and children, as well as medical opportunities
        for women doctors--the opportunity of getting bedside in-
        struction and holding resident and staff positions. A new
        wing, "the Queen Mary Wing," has enlarged the hospital's
        accommodations. The Garrett Anderson Hospital is "a
        special hospital only in the sense that it is one staffed en-
        tirely by women."

3261.   "General Correspondence: Scotland." Medical Times and
            Gazette, 1 (30 March 1872) 353. (Letters to the Ed-
            itor.)
        A Court of Session summons was "served on the Senatus

Academicus and Chancellor of Edinburgh University, with
the view of having it declared that the University is bound
to provide for and complete the Medical education (including
graduation) of lady students." The writer finds this "painful" and considers those responsible "a handful of wilful
women who will have their own way." He is now afraid
the argument will hinge on legal points, thus preventing the
legality of the case from being questioned in the first place.
This "may go far to turn the balance in favour of the
ladies," making it difficult to argue "the simple merits of
the case." He goes on: "It is almost self-evident that if
we admit the right of ladies to become matriculated students of the University, we must allow that they are entitled
to all the privileges of students of the University." But
perhaps the University authorities, "in allowing them to
matriculate at all ... have ... exceeded their powers."

3262.   "General Council Meeting." Medical Women's Federation
            News-Letter, (April 1933) 72-74.
         A letter sent to Federation members urges the support of
         candidature of Dr. Christine Murrell to the General Medical
         Council of the British Medical Association. The notice,
         published in its entirety, supplies reasons for female repre-
         sentation on the council. A separate memorandum, also
         published, lists Dr. Murrell's qualifications.

3263.   Gray, Sarah. "Women and the British Medical Association."
            Medical Women's Federation News-Letter, (November
            1926) 45-46.
         Dr. Gray writes an account of her recollections of the 1892
         meeting of the British Medical Association--at which time
         women were readmitted to the Association (Elizabeth Gar-
         rett Anderson being the first woman admitted, 23 years
         earlier, after which the rules were changed to debar wo-
         men).

3264.   "Great New Women's Hospital in London Dedicated: Med-
            ical and Surgical Staffs to be Composed of Women Phy-
            sicians and Surgeons." Woman's Medical Journal, 26:
            7 (July 1916) 181. (Editorial.)
         This article announces the opening of a new wing of the
         South London Hospital for Women, which should give women
         physicians full opportunity to serve women and children pa-
         tients. A male doctor hailed the opening as having a "bene-
         ficial effect upon the two evils [eugenists] most deplored--
         the falling birth rate and the mortality among children."

3265.   Hanson, H. B. "The Glut of Women Doctors." Lancet, 1
            (24 January 1925) 207-208. (Letters to the Editor.)
         Dr. Hanson comments on William Robinson's letter, which
         states that 78 women doctors applied for a junior post at
         Children's Hospital, Sunderland [Lancet, 17 January 1925].
         Mr. Robinson's report on the existence of a large number

of women physicians is gratifying, since medical women
are badly needed.

3266. Holland, Thomas. "The Medical Women's International
        Association Congress, Edinburgh, July, 1937. Inaug-
        ural Address." Medical Women's Federation Quarterly
        Review, (October 1937) 21-24.
        Sir Thomas Holland, principal and vice-chancellor of the
        University of Edinburgh, welcomes the Medical Women's
        International Association to Scotland. His address offers
        a historical overview of the struggle for medical education
        for women at Edinburgh. [This article was reprinted in
        Women in Medicine, 59 (January 1938) 15-16.]

3267. Inglis, Elsie M. "Medical Education of Women in Edin-
        burgh." Scottish Medical and Surgical Journal, 3
        (1898) 143-148.
        [Article not examined by editors.]

3268. "Jex Blake and Others v. the Senatus Academicus of the
        University of Edinburgh. The Lord Ordinary's Judg-
        ment." Medical Times and Gazette, 2 (3 August 1872)
        137-138.

3269. "The Lady-Students Again--Extra-Mural Courses--the
        'Potestas Docendi.'" Medical Times and Gazette, 2
        (26 October 1872) 471-472. (Provincial Correspondence:
        Scotland.)
        In a letter to the (Edinburgh) University Court, "Mr. Hog-
        gan, M.B., C.M." applied for recognition as an extra-
        mural anatomy lecturer. He wants to deliver courses to
        lady medical students. This article questions Hoggan's
        qualifications and further condemns the efforts of the lady
        medical students who continue to "amuse themselves with
        the exercise of feminine ingenuity."

3270. "The London Hospital and the Medical Women." Medical
        Times and Gazette, 2 (29 July 1876) 117-118.
        The Committee of the London Hospital decided to ban wo-
        men students from the wards of its new wing. Authorities
        of the Medical School for Women must provide themselves
        with a hospital: "such, we think, is the evil and the rem-
        edy."

3271. "The Lord Ordinary and the Edinburgh Lady-Students."
        Medical Times and Gazette, 2 (3 August 1872) 122-123.

3272. McLaren, Eva Shaw. A History of the Scottish Women's
        Hospitals. Hodder and Stoughton, London, England,
        1919, xv, 408 pp. facsims., map, photos., ports.,
        tables.
        The Scottish Women's Hospitals was founded in 1914 by
        Dr. Elsie Inglis through the Scottish Federation of Women's

Suffrage Societies. It was organized to offer medical care to soldiers and civilians in World War I, and was staffed by British women. Outstanding among the staff were Drs. Inglis, Alice Hutchinson, and Edith Stoney. A thoroughly documented history of the hospitals' work in Calais, Royaumont, Serbia, Troyes, Salonika, Corsica, Ostrovo, Vranja and Sallanches is illustrated with maps and photographs. Appended data include statistics on admissions, treatment, discharges, mortality, etc., for most of the units. Physicians photographed include Agnes Bennett, Isobel Emslie, Louise McLlroy and Eleanor Soltau.

3273. "Marie Curie Hospital." Medical Woman's Journal, 51:8 (August 1944) 36. (Editorial.)
The Marie Curie Hospital, which is staffed entirely by women physicians, recently suffered severe damage by enemy bombings. The extent of the destruction is described, and financial contributions for rebuilding are requested.

3274. "Married Medical Women." Medical Women's Federation News-Letter, (March 1925) 23-26.
Reprinted in full is the standing order of the London County Council, which requires resignation of medical women upon marriage. Following this is a letter of refutation drawn up by the Medical Women's Federation's standing committee for the defense of married medical women.

3275. "Medical Women and the University of London." Lancet, 1 (5 May 1877) 656-657. (Annotations.)

3276. "The Medical Women's Federation in War Time." Medical Women's Federation Quarterly Review, (October 1939) 45-46.
Because of the outbreak of war, meetings of the Federation may be irregular, but must be "carried on as far as possible." Publication of the Quarterly Review may also become irregular.

3277. "The Meeting of the Council: Birmingham, November 3rd and 4th, 1933." Medical Women's Federation News-Letter, (January 1934) 46-59.
Federation President Mabel Ramsay announced the death (on October 18) of Dr. Christine Murrell, who had actively participated in the Federation since its inception. The standing committee on the work of married medical women reported on its latest activities, as did the following other task groups: standing committee on psychological medicine, Scottish standing committee, committee on work in the colonies and dominions, menopause committee, sub-committee on dysmenorrhoea, committee for the promotion of a better health service for the women of India, British international standing committee, and the British Medical Association insurance acts committee.

3278.   "The Meeting of the Council Held in Leeds, October 21st
         to 23rd." Medical Women's Federation News-Letter,
         (November 1926) 47-61.
         This summary of events which took place at the Council
         meeting covers such topics as underpaid posts for women
         physicians, a report on the British Medical Association In-
         surance Acts Committee, and the appointment of a sub-
         committee "To make a report with the object of correcting
         any prevalent misconceptions about the inability suffered by
         women during the menopause, resulting in unnecessary loss
         of employment."

3279.   "The Meeting of the Council Held in London, May 11th and
         12th, 1928." Medical Women's Federation News-Letter,
         (July 1928) 40-61.
         The newly elected council for the year 1928-29 voted Dr.
         Catherine Chisholm (one of the Federation founders) as pres-
         ident. Other officers are listed. The problem of under-
         paid public health appointments of women was examined at
         length. Dr. Murrell reported on the action taken by the
         Federation on the decision of three London hospitals to ex-
         clude women students. In an effort to dispute statements
         regarding the high "wastage" rate among women physicians,
         the Federation gathered data from 1,000 British medical
         women; detailed results are published in this article.
         Further business by various committees is reviewed.

3280.   "The Meeting of the Council in Cheltenham, October 25th
         to 27th, 1928." Medical Women's Federation News-
         Letter, (November 1928) 28-51.
         The meeting included reports on the activities of the Med-
         ical Women's International Association, the Federation's
         position on nominating a woman for the General Medical
         Council, a report of the British Medical Association Insur-
         ance Acts Committee, as well as the election of officers
         and the Medical Women's Federation financial situation.
         The Committee on Psychological Medicine refers to a memo-
         randum to be published on the work of women in mental
         hospitals. The Public Health Committee's report deals
         with inequities in the payment of women public health phy-
         sicians, especially in Scotland, and in the Post Office. A
         letter was also sent from this committee to the Colonial
         Office, urging expansion of maternity and child welfare ser-
         vices in the Empire and opportunities for promotion for
         women in this work.

3281.   "The Meeting of the Council in Edinburgh, October 31st to
         November 2nd, 1929." Medical Women's Federation
         News-Letter, (November 1929) 27-44.
         Among the business discussed at this meeting: the appoint-
         ment of women physicians to venereal disease clinics and to
         mental hospitals, employment of married medical women,
         and salary inequalities between men and women medical

officers in the post office and in public health posts. Within her report on the Medical Women's International Association, Miss Martindale told of cooperation with Dr. Bertha
Van Hoosen to establish a library museum of medical women.

3282.   "The Meeting of the Council in Manchester, May 13th and
            14th, 1927." Medical Women's Federation News-Letter,
            (July 1927) 33-52.
         Comprehensive committee reports, reflecting the interests
         and activities of the 1,136-member Medical Women's Fed-
         eration, include the Council's stand on women's acceptance
         of public health posts paying below the salary scale fixed
         by the British Medical Association and the Society of Med-
         ical Officers of Health. In addition to sending protest let-
         ters to the public health bodies involved, a memorandum
         was distributed to women physicians. The communication
         warns that a woman who accepts "black-listed appointments"
         is contributing to the exploitation of women and the depre-
         ciation of women's work, and because of her betrayal, "can-
         not expect the support of her colleagues or of professional
         organizations at any time in her career." The report by
         the Standing Committee on Married Medical Women's Work
         includes its protest letter to the Durham County Council,
         which terminated the appointment of a married woman phy-
         sician and resolved to employ no wives of income-earning
         males. Also included in this article: results of a survey
         of medical women serving in mental hospitals; and a report,
         by a representative of the Medical Women's International
         Association, which details efforts to have women physicians
         appointed to the League of Nations' Health Committee.

3283.   "The Meeting of the Council: Liverpool, November 6th,
            1931." Medical Women's Federation News-Letter,
            (January 1932) 40-58.
         The council unanimously agreed that a concerted effort must
         be made to secure the nomination of a woman to the General
         Medical Council. Other business concerned the admission
         of women to postgraduate courses in London hospitals and
         the appointment of women physicians to venereal disease
         clinics. It was also announced that the Federation had re-
         ceived the gift of a letter autographed by Elizabeth Black-
         well.

3284.   "The Meeting of the Council. London, April 28th, 1939."
            Medical Women's Federation Quarterly Review, (July
            1939) 66-78.
         Proceedings of the meeting of the Council included the re-
         election of Elizabeth Bolton as president, a discussion of
         the disadvantages under which medical women were obliged
         to work during World War I and recent attempts to correct
         the situation (no definite action on the granting of commis-
         sions to women had been taken by the War Office), and re-

ports from the various committees (including public health, venereal diseases, psychological medicine, national health insurance, dysmenorrhoea, Scottish Standing Committee, coeducation watching, maternal mortality, etc.).

3285.   "The Meeting of the Council. London, November 4th and
            5th, 1932." Medical Women's Federation News-Letter,
            (January 1933) 42-55.
         Thirty-eight members attended the Council's meeting. One discussion concerned the choice of a woman candidate for the General Medical Council. The Standing Committee on Public Health reported discovering that women health officers serving in British colonies receive lower salaries than men. The Council discussed the general subject of appointing medical women to venereal disease clinics. It was resolved that the Scottish Union of Medical Women be dissolved, and that a Standing Scottish Committee of the Federation be formed. Other resolutions and topics discussed are summarized in this report.

3286.   "The Meeting of the Council, London, November 9th and
            10th, 1934." Medical Women's Federation Quarterly
            Review, (January 1935) 43-60.
         Reports of various committees of the Medical Women's Federation are given in summary. A few of the committees mentioned are those on public health, venereal disease, dysmenorrhea, and menopause, as well as committees on the Contraceptives Bill, co-education, and psychological medicine.

3287.   "The Meeting of the Council: London, October 31st and
            November 1st, 1930." Medical Women's Federation
            News-Letter, (November 1930) 49-63.
         Reports by the Federation's committees are summarized.

3288.   "Memorandum Regarding the Re-organization of Hospital
            Services in India: Committee of the Medical Women's
            Federation." Medical Women's Federation News-Letter,
            (January 1934) 41-46.

3289.   Moxon, W. "Men's Brains and Women's Brains, and the
            Convocation of the London University." Medical Times
            and Gazette, 1 (9 March 1878) 258-259.
         This article ridicules the decision of London University, which has decided to admit women to take the same degrees as men, but excluded them from the convocation of graduates, to which all men with degrees belong. "The thing is absurd, and suggests ridicule," says the author. "Perhaps it might be necessary to allow smoking, or to have a public gymnasium and bath in the chamber. Even this might, alas! fail to keep out horrid medical women." The author discusses the incompatibility of these two decisions and states that women are perfectly suited to the

impulsive decision-making of the convocation, because "cool reflection requires something that women are not born with." The author proposes this ability must be contained in the ten extra ounces of weight (on the average) of the male brain over the female brain. If the convocation had taken time to reflect, the author says, it would not have come to such a "preposterous" conclusion. "By all means let the ladies in."

3290.   Murrell, Christine. "British Medical Association Centenary Meeting." Medical Women's Federation News-Letter, (October 1932) 46-49.
Many medical women (including Dr. Maude Abbott of Montreal) took part in this meeting. Reported in full is the presentation, made by the Medical Women's Federation, of a portrait of Dr. Elizabeth Garrett-Anderson, the first woman member of the British Medical Association. Dr. Sarah Gray, the only living woman of the three who witnessed the Association's "historic decision of some forty years ago" to admit women members, recalls that occasion and Dr. Garrett-Anderson's speech.

3291.   "New Medical School for Women in London." Medical Woman's Journal, 45:2 (February 1938) 52.
Due to the inadequate number of undergraduate medical schools in London that accept women students, the West London Hospital's establishment of a full medical school "marks an advance in the movement for the medical education of women." "It is not proposed that the West London Hospital shall confine its school exclusively to women...."

3292.   "New School for Women." Medical Woman's Journal, 54:1 (January 1947) 45.
This article announces the recommendation of the Goodenough Committee in London that the West London Hospital be given over to an undergraduate training center. Many think the hospital might be used as the nucleus for a new women's medical school.

3293.   "Obstetrical Society of London." Lancet, 1 (7 March 1874) 352-353.
The Obstetrical Society of London met to consider the question of admitting medical women to its membership. Dr. Garrett-Anderson's petition for admission is the focus of the debate which constitutes this article. The meeting ended with the decision that "the by-laws of this society do not admit of the nomination of female practitioners to the Fellowship of the Society."

3294.   "Obstetrical Society of London. Meeting, March 4th, 1874. E. J. Tilt, M.D., President, in the Chair. Special Meeting to Consider the Interpretation of the Bye-laws Relative to the Admission of Medical Women." Obstet-

rical Journal of Great Britain and Ireland, 2:13 (April
1874) 28-38. (Abstracts of Societies' Proceedings.)
The question of admission of women to the Society comes
up as a result of Dr. Elizabeth Garrett-Anderson's applica
tion for admission.

3295.   "Opening of Helen Chambers Research Laboratories." Med
ical Woman's Journal, 44:4 (April 1937) 107-108. (Ed
itorial.)
In 1924 Dr. Helen Chambers urged the medical women of
Great Britain to carry out clinical research on radium trea
ment of the cervix. These research laboratories, named
in honor of Dr. Chambers, and part of the Marie Curie
Hospital, London, England, were opened on 19 March 1937.

3296.   "Opening of the Elsie Inglis Memorial Hospital, Edinburgh."
Medical Women's Federation News-Letter, (July 1930)
78-81. photo.
Although the Elsie Inglis Memorial Hospital has been open
since 1925, it became complete in February [1930] with the
formal opening of the nurses' home. Women comprise the
hospital's executive committee and staff. The ceremonies,
which many prominent women physicians attended, are reported.

3297.   Pickard, Ellen. "Ancient History." Medical Women's Fed
eration Quarterly Review, (April 1935) 42-46.
Dr. Pickard gives the history of the Association of Registered Medical Women of the United Kingdom from 1879-
1917. In 1917, when the Medical Women's Federation was
formed, the Association became the London Association of
the Medical Women's Federation.

3298.   "The Progress of Events in Edinburgh." Medical Times
and Gazette, 2 (21 December 1872) 681.
Describing the latest reports and meetings concerning the
question of female medical education at Edinburgh University, this article notes that the debate is working towards
settlement: "... we can only hope that the result will be
the removal from the Edinburgh School of a social fungus
[i.e., women medical students] which has already rendered
it unfavorably conspicuous...."

3299.   "Provincial Correspondence: Scotland." Medical Times
and Gazette, 1 (3 February 1872) 142-143.
The author of this correspondence submits that the present
election of managers for the Royal Infirmary at Edinburgh
who are favorably inclined to the admission of women students, was a circuitous move whose true intent was to
elect managers favorable to the relocation of the Infirmary
on a site other than the newly chosen one (to which many
people are opposed). The "lady-student" question is secondary to this main issue.

3300.   Ramsay, Mabel L. "The Annual General Meeting of the
          Medical Women's Federation. Newcastle-On-Tyne,
          May 8th and 9th, 1930." Medical Women's Federation
          News-Letter, (July 1930) 50-53.
          The article is comprised of the minutes of the thirteenth
          annual general meeting of the Medical Women's Federation
          and a description of the social functions provided for the
          gathering.

3301.   Ramsay, Mabel L. "The Glut of Women Doctors." Lan-
          cet, 1 (24 January 1925) 207. (Letters to the Ed-
          itor.)
          Dr. Ramsay refers to a letter by William Robinson [Lancet,
          17 January 1925], in which he reports that 78 women doctors
          applied for a junior post at Children's Hospital, Sunderland.
          Because most hospital posts are open only to males, it
          naturally follows that when one opens for medical women,
          a great number of women candidates apply. "Pure preju-
          dice on the part of the male colleague" is responsible for
          this situation, Dr. Ramsay writes. She adds that while Mr.
          Robinson's letter is meant as a deterrent to women seeking
          medical careers, "our movement has too strong a hold
          to be pushed back, much as the reactionary would like
          it."

3302.   Richards, Elizabeth. "The London School of Medicine for
          Women and the Royal Free Hospital: As I Knew Them
          --1933-1942." In: 100 Years of Medicine: 1849-1949.
          Modern Press Limited, Saskatoon, Saskatchewan, 1949,
          26-27.
          The London School of Medicine, associated with the Royal
          Free Hospital, was founded for the express purpose of
          teaching women medical students and was, for a time, the
          only place where women could learn medicine. This per-
          sonal memoir of the institution pays tribute to a num-
          ber of teachers associated with it during the years 1933-
          1942.

3303.   Ridler, M. E. "The South London Hospital for Women."
          Medical Women's Federation News-Letter, (July 1933)
          18-25. port.
          A brief history and description of the present organization
          of the Hospital, which was founded in 1911 and is staffed
          by women, credits its origin to Maud Mary Chadburn,
          M.D.

3304.   Robinson, William. "Glut of Women Doctors." Lancet,
          (17 January 1925) 157. (Letters to the Editor.)
          To illustrate the "glut of women doctors," this writer points
          to the fact that 78 women recently applied for the post of
          junior resident medical officer "(female)" at the Children's
          Hospital, Sunderland.

3305.   "Shall Women Be Admitted?" Woman's Medical Journal,
             18:10 (October 1908) 209.
         The debate over the admission of women to the Royal Col-
         lege of Surgeons is discussed.

3306.   [No entry.]

3307.   Stastny, Olga. "A Pioneer Among Pioneers." Medical
             Woman's Journal, 35:5 (May 1928) 121-122. photo.
             (Feature Article.)
         Dr. Stastny describes her visit to the Elsie Inglis Memorial
         Hospital and pays tribute to the memory of the woman phy-
         sician for whom it was named. She also salutes Dr. Fran
         Johnston, an American woman working for the hospital, and
         Dr. Eliza Mosher, in whose name a "Memorial Bed" was
         donated to the institution.

3308.   Sturge, Mary D. "The Aims and Work of the Medical Wo-
             men's Federation." Bulletin of the Medical Women's
             National Association, 2 (January 1923) 12-16.
         This article was written four and one-half years after the
         founding of the Federation, an organization which consists
         of ten distinct groups of associations of medical women.
         The author takes a critical look at the Federation and its
         effectiveness.

3309.   Sturge, Mary D. "The Aims and Work of the British Med-
             ical Women's Federation." Medical Woman's Journal,
             29:5 (May 1922) 77-81. (Address, Medical Women's
             Federation of Great Britain, Edinburgh, Scotland, No-
             vember 1921.)

3310.   Thorne, Isabel. Sketch of the Foundation and Development
             of the London School of Medicine for Women, Hunter
             Street, Brunswick Square, W.C., by Mrs. Isabel
             Thorne, Honorary Secretary. G. Sharrow, London,
             England, 1905, 45 pp.
         This book's author was one of the five women, including
         Sophia Jex-Blake, who matriculated at the University of
         Edinburgh in 1869 in hopes of receiving medical degrees.
         After four years of study, they were refused examinations.
         This refusal led to their cooperation with Elizabeth Garrett-
         Anderson in the establishment in 1874 of the London School
         of Medicine for Women. In 1877 an agreement was reached
         with the Royal Free Hospital for clinical instruction. Isa-
         bel Thorne, who had not completed her degree, was ap-
         pointed honorary secretary of the London school. This his-
         tory chronicles the growth and development of the school
         until 1904. It includes the names of numerous faculty, of-
         ficers, and students but lacks a name index. Administrativ
         and financial details are documented.

3311.   Thorne, May. "The Royal Free Hospital." Medical Woma

Journal, 31:4 (April 1924) 93-94.
The Royal Free Hospital in London is the first general
hospital in England which opened its wards for the clinical
instruction of women medical students (in 1877). A history
of the struggle of women in England to obtain medical training is recounted. A brief history of the hospital and a request for funds for the hospital conclude the article.

3312. "To Enter the Royal College." Woman's Medical Journal,
5:1 (January 1896) 7.
A petition to the Royal College of Physicians from the staff
of the School of Medicine for Women to admit its students
to examination is the subject of this brief article.

3313. Tod, Margaret C. "Christie Hospital and Holt Radium Institute." Medical Woman's Journal, 48:1 (January 1941)
28. (Correspondence.)
This letter to Dr. L'Esperance at the Strang Cancer Clinic
is to inform the medical women of the U.S. (through the
medium of the Journal) of the financial difficulties of the
Edinburgh Hospital for Women and Children, founded by Dr.
Sophia Jex-Blake, and the Elsie Inglis Memorial Hospital.
These two institutions were in imminent danger of being
closed and Margaret Tod, in this letter, appeals to women
physicians in the U.S. for help.

3314. The University Law Suit; a Brief Summary of the Action of
Declarator Brought by Ten Matriculated Lady Students
Against the Senatus of Edinburgh University. Edinburgh,
Scotland, [1872?].
[Article not examined by editors.]

3315. "University of London. Extraordinary Meeting of Convocation: Debate Upon the Action of the Senate." Lancet,
2 (4 August 1877) 164-168.
The article gives in detail the arguments of several persons
who attended the meeting of Convocation called to debate the
action of the Senate to admit women to medical degrees at
the University of London.

3316. "University of London. --Meeting of Convocation. Debate on
the Admission of Women to Degrees." Lancet, 1 (19
January 1878) 103-106.
At a meeting of Convocation to debate the draft charter proposed by the Senate to enable women to graduate in medicine
at the University of London, arguments for and against the
charter were presented. A majority of 110 voted in favor
of the charter.

3317. "University of London: Meeting of Convocation. The Admission of Women to Medical Degrees." Lancet, 1 (12
May 1877) 686-688.

3318.   Walker, Jane H. "Union--Was It Worth While?" Medical
              Women's Federation News-Letter, (March 1927) 19-21.
         Dr. Walker reviews the history of the Medical Women's
         Federation, formed when the medical women's associations
         of England, Scotland, Ireland, and Wales merged.

3319.   "The Women Medical Students." Medical Times and Ga-
              zette, 1 (13 January 1872) 45. (The Week.)
         This brief notice reports the University Court of Edinburgh'
         rejection of proposals to admit women to medical courses,
         on the grounds that decisions on the proposals were beyond
         the power of the Court. The Court, however, wishes to re
         move barriers to women, "provided that medical instruction
         to women be given to strictly separate classes."

3320.   "Women Physicians." Woman's Medical Journal, 12:5 (May
              1902) 111-112.
         Sir Thomas Smith's statements regarding the New Hospital
         for Women (London) are reported in this article, reprinted
         from the London Times.

3321.   "Women Physicians Finally Admitted." Woman's Medical
              Journal, 18:12 (December 1908) 258. (Editorial.)
         Finally, women have gained admission to the Royal College
         of Physicians and Surgeons.

3322.   "Women's Missionary Institute, London, England." Medical
              Missionary Record, 1:6 (October 1886) 153.
         The annual meeting of this mission included a report by
         Dr. Annie McCall, resident medical superintendent, which
         outlined the status of the women medical students.

3323.   "Work of Medical Women in Great Britain: Five General
              and Eight Special Hospitals." Medical Woman's Journal
              38:2 (February 1931) 45.
         Because it is becoming increasingly difficult for women to
         obtain staff appointments in male-administered hospitals, th
         "women-run" hospitals are of great importance to women
         physicians. In Great Britain there are five general and
         eight specialized hospitals staffed by women. Similar hos-
         pitals in India, Australia, and Yugoslavia are mentioned.

3324.   "The Work of the Council." Medical Women's Federation
              News-Letter, (July 1930) 53-78.
         Louisa Martindale was elected president of the Federation,
         and three vice-presidents were elected. Reports of the fol
         lowing committees were delivered: public health, psycholog
         ical medicine, National Health Insurance, venereal disease,
         the work of married medical women, the menopause, dys-
         menorrhoea, promotion of an improved health service for
         the women of India, insurance, maternal mortality and mor
         bidity, and international organization. There were also re-
         ports about the Medical Women's International Association,

several BMA committees, the London Association menstruation committee, women's training colleges, finance and sub-
scriptions, loan funds, and death of members.

3325.   "The Work of the Council." Medical Women's Federation
          News-Letter, (July 1931) 57-72.
        The reports of various committees of the Medical Women's
        Federation are summarized in this article, e.g., the com-
        mittees on public health, birth control, the work of married
        medical women, venereal diseases, and dysmenorrhea.

3326.   "The Work of the Council." Medical Women's Federation
          News-Letter, (July 1932) 44-60.
        The Federation's council, at its meeting on May 6, 1932,
        elected Mabel Ramsay president. Other officers were also
        named. The standing committee on venereal diseases re-
        ported that the public health and housing committee rejected
        a resolution to appoint women physicians as venereal dis-
        ease officers. The committee on public health noted that
        while appointments of medical women by the colonial office
        are satisfactory, post office women medical officers are
        still unequally paid. The standing committee on the work
        of married medical women stated that a debate in Decem-
        ber 1931 by the London County council showed 42 in favor
        of employment of married women and 73 against. The
        medico-political committee brought up the question of rep-
        resentation on a proposed national cinema enquiry commit-
        tee. The reports of the various other task groups are sum-
        marized.

3327.   "The Work of the Council." Medical Women's Federation
          News-Letter, (July 1933) 40-48.
        This article consists of a summary of the proceedings of
        the 1933 council meeting of the Medical Women's Federa-
        tion. Among many areas of interest to the council were
        the following items: work of medical women in the crown
        colonies and dominions, National Health Insurance, maternal
        mortality, and the work of married medical women.

3328.   "The Work of the Council." Medical Women's Federation
          News-Letter, (November 1927) 39-53.
        The council of the Medical Women's Federation met on
        November 4 in London. Reports of the committees are
        herein summarized.

INDIA

3329.   Badley, Mrs. M. A. "The National Association for Sup-
          plying Female Medical Aid to the Women of India."
          Calcutta Review, 85:170 (October 1887) 229-246.
        This article is divided into six sections: "(I) A history of
        medical work done prior to the organization of the Associa-

tion; (II) The Primary Course of the Organization of the
Association; (III) The Organization of the National Association; (IV) The Recognized Need of the Association; (V) Resumé of the Work Accomplished by Several Branches; and
(VI) Methods Proposed for Securing Funds."

3330.   Bhatia, S.   "The Association of Medical Women in India."
        World Medical Journal, 11:1 (January 1964) 31-33.
        Pioneer medical women in India came as missionaries after
        1867.   The response to establish schools for the training of
        women physicians, or to admit women to existing medical
        schools, was slow in coming.   In 1872 Madras Medical Col-
        lege agreed to admit women to the short certificate course.
        In January, 1907, medical women in Bombay formed the
        Association of Medical Women in India, whose objectives
        are reviewed by the author.

3331.   Brown, E.   "Training Indian Women Doctors: Ludhiana
        Women's Christian Medical College."   Missionary Re-
        view of the World, 62 (September 1939) 405-408.   illus.
        [Article not examined by editors.]

3332.   Chauduri, S.   "All-India Women's Reserve Medical Unit."
        Journal of the Association of Medical Women In India,
        37:3 (November 1949) 53-54, 56.
        The Unit, organized in 1942 to handle possible air raid
        casualties, has ministered to India's refugees and is com-
        posed of graduates of the Lady Hardinge Medical College.
        A need expressed is for the Unit to become a permanent or-
        ganization through which women physicians can volunteer
        for man-made as well as natural disasters.

3333.   Dufferin, (Countess of).   A Record of Three Years' Work
        of the National Association for Supplying Female Medical
        Aid to the Women of India.   Calcutta, India, 1888.
        [Item not examined by editors.]

3334.   "Female Medical Aid for the Women of India."   British
        Medical Journal, 2 (27 October 1888) 948-949.
        The organization and the achievements of the Countess of
        Dufferin's Fund--money for the training and supplying of
        medical women to attend to Indian women--is detailed.

3335.   "Female Students in the Madras Medical College."   Indian
        Medical Gazette (Calcutta), 12 (1877) 106.
        [Article not examined by editors.]

3336.   French, Francesca.   Miss Brown's Hospital: The Story of
        the Ludhiana Medical College and Dame Edith Brown,
        D.B.E., Its Founder.   Hodder and Stoughton, London,
        England, 1954, 120 pp.   illus.
        Following her medical studies at Edinburgh and receipt of
        her M.D. degree from Brussels, Edith Brown went (in

1891) to India. She was sponsored by the Baptist Zenana
Mission. In 1894 she opened the Women's Christian Medical College in Ludhiana, East Punjab, and served as its
principal until 1942. In 1915 this College incorporated the
Punjab Medical School for Women and accepted the transfer
of women students from the Government College in Lahore.
In 1948 the medical school was upgraded to offer the M.B.,
B.S. A hospital grew along with the school. Originally
known as the Charlotte Hospital, it was superseded by
Memorial Hospital in 1898. In 1952 the government of India offered to cosupport a new 500-bed hospital if the College could raise the remaining funds. (This booklet appears
to have been written as part of a fund raising effort for Ludhiana in commemoration of Dame Edith's 90th birthday in 1954.)

3337. Hunter, William Wilson. "A Female Medical Profession
         for India." The Contemporary Review, 56 (August
         1889) 207-215.
       Lady Dufferin's philanthropic effort to bring medical aid
       within the reach of the women of India involved recruit-
       ing English medical women--one solution to the problem
       of "how to freely throw open the British medical pro-
       fession to the female sex." In 1885 Lady Dufferin and
       her advisers founded the National Association for Sup-
       plying Aid to the Women of India after it was established
       that there was a large scale demand for such aid in India
       and that because of religious restraints, only women could
       bring the needed medical aid to Indian women. The asso-
       ciation had three objectives: (1) to import English medical
       women and train Indian women as nurses and doctors, (2) to
       establish hospitals and bring medical relief, and (3) to train
       midwives and nurses "for attendance at patients' houses."
       The association's "practical organization consists of a
       strong Central Committee and a number of Provincial
       Branches." No opposition was raised by missionaries
       despite the purely secular nature of the association. The
       Indian universities cooperated in every way, and the number
       of female medical students began to increase. The demand
       for qualified female practitioners increased, and it was es-
       timated that "a hundred thousand women and children will
       receive treatment or medicine during the present year from
       the agents and institutions under the control of the Associa-
       tion." India has done its part, but "for many years to
       come the supply of the directing staff of lady doctors must
       be obtained from England." The report boasts that "English
       liberality" has achieved "large and permanent results in the
       alleviation of human suffering."

3338. Kugler, Anna S. Guntur Mission Hospital: Guntur, India.
         The Women's Missionary Society, The United Lutheran
         Church in America, 1928, 135 pp. photos., ports.,
         tables.
       Anna S. Kugler joined the Guntur (India) Mission of the

American Lutheran Church in 1883. In this book, which
deals primarily with the years 1898-1923, she documents
the development of the medical mission and the work of the
women physicians and nurses associated with it during that
period. Included are members of the Guntur hospital staff
such as Mary Baer, Elsie Reed Mitchell, Eleanor B. Wolf,
Mary Fleming, the author, Lydia Woerner, and Betty Nilsson. The booklet includes the history and development of
the Guntur Hospital, its staff and patients, its cost and sup
port, the training school for nurses, and the extension of
medical work in Telugu, including the Chirala and Rajahmundry hospitals. Tabular appendixes include a statistical
summary of the medical mission such as numbers of patients classified by caste, expenditures and incomes, alumnae of the nursing program (1901-16), and lists of American physicians and nurses. The text is illustrated with
photographs of buildings, patients, and many staff and students.

3339.   "Lady Dufferin Fund." Woman's Medical Journal, 5:6 (June
        1896) 157. (News and Progress.)

3340.   "Lady Dufferin's Association." Medical Missionary Record,
        2:3 (July 1887) 71-72.
        Ladies working with the Dufferin Association in India are
        prohibited on pain of dismissal, from teaching Christianity
        to their patients. Women doctors in the Association have
        accomplished much. But the work of healing must never
        be severed from preaching God's Word, for Christianity
        gave man scientific and rational medical knowledge. Be-
        cause the Christian Church has failed in India to send med-
        ical aid as a companion of the Gospel, it is failing in its
        scriptural objective to "go in and possess the land."

3341.   McKibbin-Harper, Mary. "Lady Hardinge Medical College
        for Women." Medical Woman's Journal, 33:11 (Novem-
        ber 1926) 323-325. photos.
        Historical background and a description is given of the Lady
        Hardinge Medical College for Women-- "... the finest hos-
        pital in the world that is entirely staffed by women." Dr.
        Harper perceived the Delhi, India institution "for Indians
        and financed by them, a real Indian institution...." [emphasis
        hers]. At the head of the institution is Dr. Grace Camp-
        bell of Glasgow, England.

3342.   Maxwell, J. L. "Lady Dufferin's Scheme; Its Bearing on
        Christian Freedom." Medical Missionary Record, 2:9
        (January 1888) 230-231.
        Dr. Maxwell lists the objectives of the Dufferin Association
        --sometimes called the National Association for Supplying
        Female Medical Aid to the Women of India--and then attacks
        its rule that no Association employee may "'proselytise or
        interfere in any way with the religious beliefs of any section

of the people.'" While noting "the compliment which the
Association unintentionally pays to Christianity as a living,
aggressive system," Dr. Maxwell stresses that no Christian
sister has the right to work within the confines of such an
"utterly offensive" rule.

3343.   "Medical Aid to the Women of India." Medical Missionary
            Record, 1:2 (June 1886) 42-43.
         This article quotes from an article appearing in the June
         [1886] issue of Woman's Work for Woman, which discusses
         the importance of the Lady Dufferin Association's efforts to
         supply women physicians to the women of India.

3344.   "Medical Women in India." Medical Woman's Journal, 49:9
            (September 1942) 287.
         This article announces that the Second Triennial Conference
         of the Association of Medical Women in India was held in
         December, 1941. Primary concerns were childbirth, the
         availability of medical care during childhood, and the health
         of mothers during pregnancy.

3345.   "The Missionary Medical School for Women in India." Med-
            ical Woman's Journal, 47:11 (November 1940) 341.
         The school in Vellore, South India, founded by Dr. Ida
         Scudder in 1918, faces a financial crisis discussed in this
         article.

3346.   "News of the Association: Minutes of a Meeting of Council
            Held in Delhi at the Residence of Dr. Ruth Young on
            January 28th, 1936, at 10:30 A.M." Journal of the
            Association of Medical Women in India, 24:2 (May 1936)
            41, 45-48, 50-62. tables.
         The minutes of this meeting of the council of the Associa-
         tion of Medical Women in India reports on such topics as the
         means of increasing membership, the standards of medical
         education, a list of officers and representatives of the As-
         sociation, a financial report, and an extensive membership
         list complete with educational background and address for
         each member listed.

3347.   "What Indian Women Are Doing for Their Sisters." Med-
            ical Missionary Record, 2:1 (May 1887) 6.
         This report concerns activities of the Dufferin Fund Asso-
         ciation, which supports women physicians, hospitals, and
         medical schools in India.

INTERNATIONAL

3348.   "Banquet of the Medical Women's International Association:
            Geneva, Switzerland, September 7, 1922." Medical
            Woman's Journal, 29:10 (October 1922) 236-238. photo.
         The names of women called upon to say a few words at this
         banquet are given, as well as portions of their comments.

3349.   Barrett, (Lady). "President's Foreword." Medical Wo-
              men's International Journal, 1:2 (November 1925) 3-5.
         In her introduction to this issue of the Journal, Lady Bar-
         rett reviews the purpose of the Medical Women's Interna-
         tional Association, and the importance of separate organiza-
         tions for women physicians.

3350.   Brodie, Jessie Laird. "Our Part in the World Medical
              Program." Journal of the American Medical Women's
              Association, 17:8 (August 1962) 656-657. (Address,
              Eighth Congress, Pan American Medical Women's As-
              sociation, Columbia, 21 February 1962.)
         Jessie Laird Brodie, executive director of the American
         Medical Women's Association and past president of the Pan
         American Medical Women's Alliance, reminisces about the
         changes in these organizations over the years. "The fight
         for equal privileges is of little concern now. AMWA has
         gradually changed into a service organization...." The
         American Women's Hospital Service (AWHS), founded in
         1917, is AMWA's foreign service committee. The Medical
         Women's International Association was founded by the na-
         tional associations of women physicians.

3351.   Chapa, Esther. "Readjustment of Female Delinquents to
              Society." Medical Woman's Journal, 55:7 (June 1948)
              19-20. (Presentation, First Congress, Pan American
              Medical Women's Alliance, November 1947.)
         Dr. Chapa proposes that the Alliance study the problems of
         female delinquency in each Pan American country and lobby
         for the erection of female prisons that provide social read-
         justment programs.

3352.   "Convention of Medical Women's International Association:
              Association Internationale de Femmes Médecins." Med-
              ical Woman's Journal, 29:10 (October 1922) 234-235.
         This article gives an overview of the convention held in
         Geneva, Switzerland on September 4-7, 1922. A list of
         officers and members of the advisory board precede the dis-
         cussion. The women in attendance (c. 80 medical women
         from 19 countries) discovered the same prejudice against
         women in medicine existed in every country, with the ex-
         ception of Denmark and Italy.

3353.   "Geneva Meeting." Medical Woman's Journal, 29:7 (July
              1922) 148.
         Some of the topics to be discussed at this forthcoming meet-
         ing of the International Association of Medical Women are
         prevention of white slave traffic, drug traffic, and venereal
         disease; sex hygiene problems; women in obstetrics and
         gynecology; and the prevention of prostitution.

3354.   "The International Medical Woman's Association for the
              Promotion of Post-Graduate Study." Medical Woman's

Journal, 37:4 (April 1930) 104-105.
This article presents the address of Dr. Cora M. Ballard, chairman of the International Medical Woman's Association for the Promotion of Post-Graduate Study. Dr. Ballard presents the background of the New York Post-Graduate Medical School's opening of its doors to women. A second meeting was held at the residence of Mrs. Elizabeth Custer ("widow of General Custer of frontier fame") at which Dr. Nicholas Alter spoke of the purpose of the organization with an emphasis on its international scope.

3355. Lovejoy, Esther Pohl. "Historical Sketch of the Medical Women's International Association." Journal of the American Medical Women's Association, 1:8 (November 1946) 245-251. photo., ports.
The organization of the MWIA is traced from its inception in 1919 through its nine meetings held over the 27 years, to the date of this article. This sketch includes photographs of members of the "Committee of Twelve" elected to organize the Association in 1919.

3356. Lovejoy, Esther P[ohl]. "Letter Announcing Second Meeting of International Association." Medical Woman's Journal, 29:5 (May 1922) 94.

3357. Lovejoy, Esther P[ohl]. "The Possibilities of the Medical Women's International Association." Medical Woman's Journal, 30:1 (January 1923) 14-18. (Presentation, Convention, Medical Women's International Association, Geneva, Switzerland, 4-7 September 1922.)

3358. Lovejoy, Esther Pohl. Women Physicians and Surgeons: National and International Organizations. The Livingston Press, Livingston, New York, [1939], xvi, 246 pp. photos., ports.
This two-part work covers the history of the American Medical Women's Association (AMWA) and the Medical Women's International Association (MWIA) in the first "book," and the history of the American Women's Hospitals (AWH) in the second section. The author was president of the Medical Women's International Association (1919-1924) and president of AMWA in 1932-1933. Dr. Lovejoy was also general director of the American Women's Hospitals for 20 years. The section on the American Women's Hospitals gives each country in which a hospital was located and devotes three chapters to the AWH operation in the Appalachian region of the United States. Appendixes outline the number of hospitals and length of service in each country and give the names of AWH physicians. Although profusely illustrated with photographs of officers of the AMWA and the MWIA as well as the AWH staff, the book offers no name index. Many of the pictures depict hospitals and patients in the various areas of service. Dr. Kate Campbell Hurd-Mead wrote the introduction.

3359.   Lovejoy, Esther Pohl and Reid, Ada Chree. "The Medical
        Women's International Association: An Historical
        Sketch, 1919-1950." Journal of the American Medical
        Women's Association, 6:1 (January 1951) 29-38. ports.
        The founding of the Medical Women's International Associa-
        tion dates to a dinner given on October 21, 1919 by the
        American Women's Hospitals Committee of the American
        Medical Women's Association. The portrait of Esther P.
        Lovejoy who served as the first president is included as
        well as portraits of other presidents: Lady Barrett, second
        president; Alma Sundquist, fourth president; Louisa Martin-
        dale, fifth president; A. Charlotte Ruys, sixth president;
        Ada Chree Reid, seventh president. Of historical note, the
        council meeting held at Bologna in 1928 included among
        others, the Queen of Italy, Mussolini, and several other dig-
        nitaries of the Fascist Party as well as the Cardinal-Arch-
        bishop of Bologna. "At the end of the conference, the vis-
        itors were entertained by the Women's Section of the Fascist
        Party, and the Fascist hymn was the dominant musical and
        political note."

3360.   Lovejoy, Esther Pohl and Reid, Ada Chree. "The Medical
        Women's International Association: An Historical Sketch,
        1919-1950." Journal of the Association of Medical Wo-
        men in India, 39:3 (August 1951) 67-71, 73-75.
        The Association's history is traced from its founding in New
        York in 1919. Reports are given of the following meetings:
        Geneva, 1922; London, 1924; Prague, 1926; Bologna, 1928;
        Paris, 1929; Vienna, 1931; Stockholm, 1934; Edinburgh,
        1937; London, 1946; Amsterdam, 1947; Hameenlinna (Fin-
        land), 1949; and Philadelphia, 1950.

3361.   Martindale, Louisa. "The Bologna Meeting of the Medical
        Women's International Association, April 11th-14th,
        1928." Medical Women's Federation News-Letter,
        (November 1930) 19-29.
        About 100 women from 14 of the 24 countries affiliated with
        the Association attended this meeting, "a political event of
        importance in the history of medical women...."

3362.   "Medical Women's International Association." Medical and
        Professional Woman's Journal, 41:1 (January 1934) 32.
        A special meeting of the Women's International Association
        held in Paris on July 8, 1933 addressed the question of
        whether a permanent location for the international head-
        quarters would be better than the current arrangement,
        under which the office location changes every five years
        with the election of a new president. The "unfortunate
        position" of Jewish women physicians in Germany was also
        discussed. Although everyone "desired very earnestly to
        help their colleagues, none could hold out much hope ... as
        in the present economic crisis every country is cutting down
        its medical work...."

3363.   "The Medical Women's International Congress Meeting,
         Vienna, September 15-20." Medical Woman's Journal,
         38:11 (November 1931) 284-285.
         This Medical Women's International Congress addressed two
         main subjects: the work of medical women in "exotic coun-
         tries," and the legal protection of women workers. The
         delegates, who came from 47 different countries, adopted
         several resolutions, including one that labor of women be
         supervised by specially trained physicians, and another that
         equal pay for equal work for men and women be promoted.

3364.   Medical Women's International Association. Fourteenth
         Congress. Rio De Janeiro, Brazil, October 13-18,
         1974. Report. Number 26. Secretariat of the MWIA,
         Vienna, Austria, March 1975, 119 pp. chart. port.
         This publication consists of the Report on the XIVth Con-
         gress of the Medical Women's International Association
         (MWIA). A section entitled "Reports of National Cor-
         responding Secretaries" gives information on the status of
         women physicians for each of the 37 affiliated Associations
         in 37 different countries. Also given are reports of vari-
         ous committees and biographical information for outstanding
         members honored at the Congress. [For status-of-women-
         physicians-in-other-countries reports during preceding Con-
         gress years, see earlier Congress reports: 1926, 1929,
         1934, 1937, 1947, 1950, 1954, 1958, 1963, 1966, 1968,
         1970, and 1972. These reports are not cited in this bibli-
         ography.]

3365.   Montreuil-Straus, C. "The Fifth Congress of the Medical
         Women's International Association: Amsterdam, June
         24-30, 1947." Medical Woman's Journal, 55:1 (Janu-
         ary 1948) 54, 56, 58.
         About 350 women physicians representing 16 countries at-
         tended this organization's first postwar congress. Adminis-
         trative meetings, scientific sessions, and social activities
         are summarized.

3366.   Morani, Alma Dea. "A Short History of the Medical Wo-
         men's International Association." Transactions and
         Studies of the College of Physicians of Philadelphia,
         42:4 (April 1975) 422-432. fig., photos., ports.
         This is a chronological summary of the founding and his-
         tory of the Medical Women's International Association
         (MWIA). The Association began in 1919 in New York when
         Esther P. Lovejoy, then vice president of the American
         Medical Women's Association and chairman of the American
         Women's Hospital Service Committee, proposed its organ-
         ization to delegates honoring distinguished medical women
         who had just returned from war service in France. (Pho-
         tographs of the twelve organizers appear in the text.) The
         article's author, president of MWIA 1972-74, traces the
         history of the organization through its congresses, member-

ship growth, presidents, and professional accomplishments.
The sixth MWIA congress met in Philadelphia at the Woman's Medical College of Pennsylvania, which was then
celebrating its 100th anniversary (1950). In 1966 Marion
Fay, dean of the Woman's Medical College, summarized
the proceedings of the tenth congress, whose topic was
"The Optimal Utilization of Medical Woman Power." Permanent headquarters for the MWIA were established in Vienna, Austria in 1968.

3367.   "Pan American Medical Women's Alliance." Medical Wo-
          man's Journal, 53:4 (April 1946) 35-36. (Editorial.)
          The Alliance's objectives are listed, and its incorporators
          named.

3368.   "Pan-American Union of Women." Woman's Medical Jour-
          nal, 26:2 (February 1916) 39-40.
          A need for the organization of medical women from North,
          Latin, and South America was seen at meetings of the Wo-
          men's Auxiliary Conference of the Second Pan-American
          Scientific Congress. They perceived a need for the organ-
          ization of a permanent Pan-American Union of Women. A
          committee was established and assigned the duties of "the
          intelligent distribution of the proceedings of the conference
          in the countries represented; and, second, keeping alive the
          objects of this conference by correspondence, or otherwise,
          so that if in the future a more permanent women's organ-
          ization can be arranged, there will be a group of women
          ready to act as a nucleus of activity."

3369.   Reid, Ada Chree. "Medical Women and International Under-
          standing." Journal of the American Medical Women's
          Association, 6:1 (January 1951) 27-28. (Inaugural Ad-
          dress, Medical Women's International Association, Phil-
          adelphia, Pennsylvania, 15 September 1950.)
          There is a great need for international and personal under-
          standing among women physicians around the world. While
          the United Nations has not fulfilled its original promise,
          whenever possible "we must emphasize [its] positive ac-
          complishments...." The World Health Organization (WHO)
          is a model of international cooperation for the improvement
          of personal and public health and should receive increased
          financial and material support from all governments. Wo-
          men physicians should urge legislators to support the WHO.

3370.   "Report of Secretary Presented at Council Meeting, Medical
          Women's International Association, Held in Paris, April
          10, 1929." Medical Woman's Journal, 36:5 (May 1929)
          116-117.
          This report discusses membership, Journal distribution,
          and the organization of medical women into groups.

3371.   [Rockhill, Margaret Hackedorn]. "Power Attained Through

International Relationship." <u>Medical Woman's Journal,</u>
31:7 (July 1924) 214-215.
This article is an introduction to the paper of Dr. Louisa
Martindale of London, which appears in this issue of the
<u>Journal.</u> English medical women found that organizing "in-
creased their power and diminished the opposition." "American medical women have only recently been brought to an
appreciation of these truths."

3372.   Ruys, A. Charlotte. "The Medical Women's International
Association: Its Work and Aims." <u>Journal of the
American Medical Women's Association,</u> 6:1 (January
1951) 25-26. (Address, Sixth Congress, Medical Women's International Association, 11 September 1950,
Philadelphia, Pennsylvania.)
Among the Medical Women's International Association's immediate and long term functions are: to establish boards of
communication and cooperation so strong that they will hold
even if governments disagree; and to help medical women in
other countries fight for their rights.

3373.   Solis, Margarita Delgado de. "Greetings to the Women
Delegates to the Pan American Congress of Women Doctors." <u>Medical Woman's Journal,</u> 55:1 (January 1948)
39-40.
Dr. Delgado de Solis's speech (published in both Spanish
and English) refers to the "bonds of love" and the "intense
collaboration" that exist among the medical women of the
Americas.

3374.   Tayler-Jones, Louise. "The Medical Women's International
Association." <u>Medical Review of Reviews,</u> 37:3 (March
1931) 147-148.
A history of the Medical Women's International Association
is herein presented, dating from its inception in October
1919. Activities at this first meeting, held in New York
City under the sponsorship of the YWCA, are recounted;
names of officers elected and their respective countries are
given. The Association was created to foster international
friendships and provide for a "community of thought" on medical questions of international interest (e.g., human welfare
and international hygiene).

3375.   Thelander, H. E. "Is There Need for a Medical Women's
Association?" <u>Journal of the American Medical Women's Association,</u> 2:9 (September 1947) 410. (Editorial.)
From a recent trip to Europe the author reports the attitudes regarding a separate organization for women physicians. British women: minority groups everywhere and always needed to organize to present their own wishes and
needs. Male colleagues: "women [have] a contribution which
was desirable to add to medicine--their point of view [can]

best be formulated and expressed by women meeting in separate conference.''

3376.   Van Hoosen, Bertha. "Describes Trip to International
         Council Meeting." Bulletin of American Medical Wo-
         men's Association, 37:12 (September 1949) 4-7.

3377.   [Van Hoosen, Bertha]. "The Medical Women's Internation-
         al Association." Medical Woman's Journal, 36:5 (May
         1929) 135-136.
         Dr. Van Hoosen urges women physicians to join the Med-
         ical Women's National Association. The United States
         "placed" third, behind Great Britain and Germany, in at-
         tendance at the recent MWIA meeting in Paris (April 10-15,
         1929).

3378.   Van Hoosen, Bertha. "The Pan-American Medical Con-
         gress As Seen by a Woman Physician." Medical Wo-
         man's Journal, 37:8 (August 1930) 213-215.
         Dr. Bertha Van Hoosen reports that she was the only wo-
         man member of the Pan-American Medical Congress when it
         was held at Panama in January, 1930. "I was fully aware
         at the Pan-American Congress that I was representing,
         though it might be poorly, and surely without their knowl-
         edge and consent, all the medical women in North, South,
         and Central America." Because she perceived herself both
         as a doctor and as a woman, Dr. Van Hoosen attended the
         program for entertaining the visiting wives and daughters
         of the Congress as well as presented a paper on corrective
         obstetrics before the male doctors.

SOUTH, CENTRAL, LATIN AMERICA
AND MEXICO

3379.   Brodie, Jessie Laird. "If You Would Know Your Brother,
         Walk Three Miles in His Moccasins." Journal of the
         American Medical Women's Association, 22:12 (Decem-
         ber 1967) 959-960.
         A reminiscence of her work with the Pan American Med-
         ical Women's Alliance, past-president Jessie Laird Brodie
         reflects on its contributions to women and medicine: "...
         the prestige of the profession of medicine has made it an
         acceptable career for the young Latin American woman of
         the privileged class." Some of PAMWA's contributions in-
         volve: acceptance of Latin American women for internships
         and residencies in the United States when they could not ob-
         tain this necessary training in their own country; acquainting
         American women physicians with tropical diseases; women
         physicians sharing knowledge, encouragement, and training
         in parliamentary procedure, delivering scientific papers,
         achieving leadership positions; sharing translations of work;
         sharing necessary supplies, like vaccine when there was a
         polio epidemic in Bolivia.

3380.   Brodie, Jessie Laird. "Pan American Medical Women's
           Alliance, 1947-1967." Journal of the American Wo-
           men's Association, 22:9 (September 1967) 625-627.
         To facilitate the exchange of scientific information "to dis-
         cuss medical social problems of special significance to
         women and children, and to forge links of friendship, mu-
         tual help and understanding between the women physicians
         of the Americas," the Pan American Medical Women's Al-
         liance was founded in 1946 and held its first congress in
         Mexico in November of 1947. This article is a brief his-
         tory of all the places where this international body of med-
         ical women has held its meetings through the tenth con-
         gress, which was held in Lima, Peru.

3381.   Mason-Hohl, Elizabeth. "Report on the Third Congress of
           the Pan American Medical Women's Alliance." Med-
           ical Woman's Journal, 59:2 (February 1952) 19-22.
           photos.
         The names of women comprising the Commission of Honor
         and the names of those on the executive committee for the
         Congress are given. Events of the conference are re-
         counted.

3382.   Rosekrans, Sarah D. "Progress of the Pan American Med-
           ical Women's Alliance." Journal of the American Med-
           ical Women's Association, 15:11 (November 1960) 1082-
           1085. (Presented at the VII Congress, Pan American
           Medical Women's Alliance, San Juan, Puerto Rico, 4
           June 1960.)
         A brief history of those installed as presidents of the Pan
         American Medical Women's Alliance at the past congresses
         is included, as well as appreciation of many of the people
         and organizations who helped to make this one possible.
         One project of note, for example, that the cooperation of
         medical women in the western hemisphere made possible
         was the immunization program of 200 children in Bolivia
         against poliomyelitis with the assistance of CARE and of
         Eli Lilly's international corporation.

UNITED STATES

3383.   A. C. K. "Women at Johns Hopkins." Nation, 52:1334 (22
           January 1891) 71. (Correspondence.)
         A resolution adopted by the trustees of Johns Hopkins in
         October [1890] stated that the medical school be open to
         women "whose previous training has been equivalent to the
         preliminary medical course prescribed for men...." The
         resolution, however, further declared that "such preliminary
         training in all its parts shall be obtained in some other in-
         stitution of learning devoted in whole or in part to the edu-
         cation of women, or by private tuition." The letter-writer
         points out that no woman in Baltimore had access to the

proper preparation, since women were still barred from
undergraduate education at Johns Hopkins.

3384.   "The A. M. A. Meeting in St. Louis: Many Women Members
         Attended and an Unusually Large Number of Women
         Physicians Were on the Program." Medical Woman's
         Journal, 29:6 (June 1922) 120-121.
         Eight women among 500 men participated in the program--
         "quite a fair proportion." The large representation of wo-
         men is attributed to the fact that the meeting was held in
         the Middle West, where there are probably more women
         physicians than in the East.

3385.   "AMWA Presents ... the Only Woman Delegate to the AMA
         House of Delegates." Journal of the American Medical
         Women's Association, 19:2 (February 1964) 149-150.
         port.
         The only woman delegate to the American Medical Associa-
         tion House of Delegates, M. Louise C. Gloeckner, says,
         "every member of the American Medical Women's Associa-
         tion should be an active member of the American Medical
         Association." At the same time she admits, "I cannot at
         present think of any occasion on which problems of women
         physicians have been brought as such to the attention of the
         House."

3386.   "The Admission of Women to the Harvard Medical School."
         Lancet, (4 July 1878) 30-31. (Letters to the Editor.)
         This anonymous letter-writer objects to coeducational med-
         ical schools because, although most physicians can "meet
         each other on a basis of high ethics and science and forget
         sex ... students are not physicians." A one-year coeduca-
         tional experiment at Chicago Medical College, for example,
         resulted in great annoyance and embarrassment. While in-
         sisting that it "is no disparagement to women students" to
         say that they should be educated separately, the writer con-
         cludes, "The woman's movement, essentially just and cor-
         rect as it is, cannot afford to molest Harvard."

3387.   "The Admission of Women to the Massachusetts Medical
         Society." Boston Medical and Surgical Journal, 102:
         21 (20 May 1880) 501. (Miscellany.)
         This Fellow of the Society feels there is no reason to ad-
         mit women to the Society: "there is no evidence that more
         than a very few of the best reach the average male practi-
         tioners.... That a great society should modify its policy
         for the feelings of an utterly insignificant group is contrary
         to common sense."

3388.   "The Aim of This Journal." Woman's Medical Journal, 20:
         2 (February 1910) 34. (Editorial.)
         The Journal is "unalterably opposed to the segregation of
         women physicians or of their work," yet "how can women

work harmoniously and loyally with men unless they are
loyally in harmony with each other?" The purpose of the
Journal is to bring the work of women physicians to light
and to foster mutual support among them.

3389.   Alsop, Gulielma Fell. History of The Woman's Medical
College: Philadelphia, Pennsylvania, 1850-1950. J. B.
Lippincott Company, Philadelphia, Pennsylvania, 1950,
xi, 249 pp. photos.
Dr. Alsop's history of the College is told largely in terms
of personalities--the people involved in founding the College
and participating in its modern development. The "women
who came to study medicine and became its deans, surgeons,
clinicians, and professors" are especially highlighted--
Rachel Bodley (dean, 1874-88), Clara Marshall (dean, 1888-
1917), Martha Tracy (dean, 1917-40), Margaret Craighill
(dean, 1941-46), and Marion Fay (dean, 1946-). The author traces the development of the College from its beginnings in "two dark, rented lecture rooms, whose equipment
was a museum of papier-mâché models and one manikin" to
its present "modern, scientifically equipped unit, consisting
of a college and a hospital, under one roof and under one
management." There are references at the end of each
chapter, and there is an index.

3390.   "Amalgamation, Not Segregation." Woman's Medical Journal, 26:5 (May 1916) 132. (Editorial.)
Women physicians are hindered from obtaining the same
kind of professional opportunities as men: in Chicago, a
city of 100 hospitals, women may serve as internes at only
two; no gynecological or obstetrical society allows women
to be members. "The remedy for segregation is organization. Organization is the guiding star of the Twentieth
Century, and leads on to Liberty, Equality and Fraternity."

3391.   "American College of Surgeons: A Brief Summary of its
Origin and Function." Medical Woman's Journal, 39:3
(March 1932) 64-65. photo.
On October 18, 1931, the American College of Surgeons allowed three women--Emma K. Willits, Louisa Paine Ting-
ley, and Florence Duckering--to join their organization.
Emma K. Willits, gynecologist and surgeon of the San Francisco Hospital for Children, is quoted as saying, "If a woman is devoted to surgery, is willing to sacrifice the feminine side of life, and is a born surgeon, she will make her
mark in the field. She will not even know she is making a
sacrifice, so absorbed will she become.... Women are
fully capable of meeting emergencies, and the instant decisions and actions that a surgeon must handle are in line
with feminine temperament as a whole...."

3392.   "American Medical Women Needed in the Russian Caucasus."
Medical Woman's Journal, 28:11 (November 1921) 285-
286.

The American Women's Hospitals requires funding if it is
to provide medical service in Russia.

3393.   "American Medical Women's Association." Medical Wo-
         man's Journal, 44:7 (July 1937) 208. (News of the
         Month.)
         This article announces the official name change of the Med-
         ical Women's National Association to the American Medical
         Women's Association. The names of newly-elected officers
         are given. In addition, announcement is made of Dr. Alice
         Parker Ellsworth's gift to the Association of her home in
         Long Beach, California. This residence is given to be
         used by members "who are in poor health or suffering from
         economic difficulties."

3394.   "American Medical Women's Association Convention Group."
         Medical Woman's Journal, 49:7 (July 1942) 204, 228.
         photo.
         This article outlines the program of the Association's twenty-
         seventh annual convention.

3395.   "American Medical Women's Association Meeting." Medical
         Woman's Journal, 50:7 (July 1943) 185, 187.
         Dr. Emily Dunning Barringer and New York City attorney
         Dorothy Kenyon were the honored guests at the meeting of
         the AMWA Board of Directors. The meeting banquet was a
         "celebration" because of the recent passage of the Spark-
         man-Johnson Bill which permitted the commissioning of wo-
         men physicians in the Medical Reserve Corps of the U.S.
         Army and Navy. A listing of the new officers of the Board
         for 1943-1944 concludes the article.

3396.   "American Women's Hospitals." Medical Woman's Journal,
         33:12 (December 1926) 348-350. photos.
         Upon the death of Dr. Sue Radcliff, a treasurer of the
         American Women's Hospitals, "it seemed to her many
         friends that there was no way to more fittingly commemorate
         her life than to endow a bed in her memory." The article
         goes on to report on the activities of the American Women's
         Hospitals in Macedonia, Greece, and Albania.

3397.   "American Women's Hospitals." Medical Woman's Journal,
         34:9 (September 1927) 279-280. photo.
         The American Women's Hospitals' services in Japan, and
         Dr. Ruth Parmelee's activities within the organization are
         the topics of this report.

3398.   "American Women's Hospitals." Medical Woman's Journal,
         35:4 (April 1928) 109-110. photos.
         Completing ten years' work overseas, the American Women's
         Hospitals now includes 72 hospitals, 327 clinics, maternity
         services, nurses training, camps for pestilential diseases,
         and depots for food and clothing distribution.

3399.   "American Women's Hospitals." Medical Woman's Journal,
            49:11 (November 1942) 348. (Editorial.)
         Catharine Macfarlane, representing the executive board of
         the American Women's Hospitals, War and Medical Service
         Committee of the American Medical Women's Association,
         makes a request for funds so that this organization can
         continue its aid to Europe, China, and southern United
         States civilian populations--especially for the benefit of wo-
         men and children.

3400.   "The American Women's Hospitals." Medical Women's
            Federation Quarterly Review, (April 1941) 38-41.
         A brief history is given of the American Women's Hospitals,
         first organized in June, 1917.

3401.   "American Women's Hospitals: Medical Service Committee
            of Medical Women's National Association." Medical
            Woman's Journal, 32:12 (December 1925) 325-327.
            photos.
         The American Women's Hospitals, a medical service com-
         mittee of the Medical Women's National Association con-
         ducted 36 hospitals with clinics, dispensaries, and out-pa-
         tient service in Greek territory at different times and places
         in the early 1920s.

3402.   "American Women's Hospitals: Organized by War Service
            Committee of the Medical Women's National Associa-
            tion. Report of Meeting of the American Women's
            Hospitals." Woman's Medical Journal, 29[19]:1 (Janu-
            ary 1919) 6-10. port.
         This article includes a report of the work done by Dr. Bar-
         bara Hunt in France and extracts from the report of Dr.
         Caroline M. Purnell, also in France. A letter from Dr.
         Charlotte Fairbank, the surgeon of American Women's Hos-
         pital No. 1 (Luzancy, France), is also reprinted.

3403.   "American Women's Hospitals. Reconstruction Committee
            of the Medical Women's National Association, Head-
            quarters, 637 Madison Ave., New York: Splendid Work
            Done By Women Doctors of the A.W.H. in Serbia Dur-
            ing Disaster at Monastir." Medical Woman's Journal,
            29:5 (May 1922) 91. (Hospitals & Colleges.)
         An Associated Press news release is reprinted, which re-
         calls the explosion of 400 car loads of ammunition and ex-
         plosives in Monastir, Serbia. It describes the work done
         by the physicians of the A.W.H. Service during the dis-
         aster.

3404.   "American Women's Hospital Reserve Corps." Medical
            Woman's Journal, 49:12 (December 1942) 389.
         This article, reprinted from the New York Sun, October
         27, 1942, comments on the American Women's Hospital Re-
         serve Corps, founded in 1940 by Dr. Luvia Willard, who had

served in World War I. In 1942 the Manhattan unit was organized; this organization is looking for volunteers, to train under the direction of doctors and nurses, for home nursing hospitals, and clinic services. They are also seeking women for motor mechanic, nutrition, emergency canteen, and other defense work.

3405.   Baker, P. de L. "The Annual Oration. Shall Women Be Admitted into the Medical Profession?" Transactions of the Medical Association of Alabama, 33 (1880) 191-206. [Article not examined by editors.]

3406.   Banas, Felicia A. "The History of the New England Hospital." Journal of the American Medical Women's Association, 10:6 (June 1955) 199.
As chairman of the medical staff and senior surgeon at New England Hospital in Boston, Dr. Banas discusses the inception of her institution and lists its many "firsts": "First in New England to be staffed by women physicians; First in New England to admit women as interns; First to originate a school for training and graduating nurses; First to admit a colored woman for training as a graduate nurse; First to originate the idea of visiting nurses; First to originate social service; and First to qualify a woman surgeon as a Fellow of the American College of Surgeons."

3407.   "Banquet for Women Doctors of the A.M.A.; Blackwell Medical Women's Society. Detroit, Mich." Medical Woman's Journal, 37:8 (August 1930) 219-228.
This article prints the speeches presented at the banquet (sponsored by the Blackwell Medical Women's Society) for women doctors attending the American Medical Association convention in Detroit. Bertha Van Hoosen passed out a quiz which demonstrated with facts and figures the difficultie women have in obtaining medical education. Leda J. Stacy of the gynecology department of the Mayo Clinic assured the audience that women are accepted on the staff of the Mayo Clinic, although the surgical service area takes women "in only exceptional instances." Jeanne Solis, who was on the medical faculty of the University of Michigan, said women receive the same instruction as men and are accepted equally. She would like to see "the emphasis on women in medicine left behind." Alice Barlow Brown spoke of her medical missionary work in China and the health care needs there. Rachelle Yarros spoke of the equality of women physicians in the Soviet Union. Olga Stastny spoke of the pleasures in working with the American Women's Hospitals in serving the health needs of people in foreign countries. Vida A. Latham talked about the potential benefits of having the sciences coordinated; she used as a primary example how botany can be coordinated with related fields to alleviate medical problems. P. S. Bordeau-Sisco spoke of the benefits women physicians derive when they create organizations

to support each other. Lucy Nash Eames read an original poem entitled "The Strength of Organization."

3408. Bass, Elizabeth. "Scholarship Loan Fund of the Medical Women's National Association." Medical Review of Reviews, 37:3 (March 1931) 162-164.
The benefits and the administration of the fund, which was established by Dr. Grace N. Kimball, are described.

3409. Bates, Mary E. "A Friend in Need: A Personal Tribute by the Editor." Woman's Medical Journal, [8]:4 (April 1899) 131-132.
This obituary of Dr. James H. Etheridge focuses upon his role in the advancement of women in medicine. He was among the first men of Rush Medical College, Chicago, to admit women students to his medical lectures.

3410. Bauer, Franz K. "Dean's Message." USC Medicine, 24:1 (1974) 2. photos.
Because of the "recent clamor" about women's rights, this issue is dedicated to women faculty members. Long before "women's liberation," the University of Southern California (USC) School of Medicine recognized professional women. Says Dean Bauer, "there has never been any question about different standards of promotion or appointment, or working conditions."

3411. Beamis-Hood, Louise. "President's Address." Medical Woman's Journal, 38:6 (June 1931) 154-155. (Address, Twenty-fifth Annual Meeting, Women's Medical Society of New York State, Syracuse, New York, 1 June 1931.)
Women physicians can combat the effects of politics and "evil forces" that are undermining the medical profession by continuing to render "altruistic service" as well as by being "united in our loyalty to each other," says outgoing president Louise Beamis-Hood.

3412. Bennett, Alice. "Letter. A Word for Organization." Woman's Medical Journal, 26:11 (November 1916) 271. (Letters to the Editor.)
The organization of medical women is necessary for educating the public as well as other women physicians as to what women are doing in medicine. Dr. Bennett concludes her letter with this admonition: "... let us read the signs of the times and support our organization. Be forceful and strong, and advance by force of strength; demand instead of supplicate, command instead of obeying...."

3413. Blackwell, Elizabeth. "Address Delivered at the Opening of the Women's Medical College of the New York Infirmary, 126, Second Avenue. November 2, 1868." In: Essays in Medical Sociology, Vol. 11. Ernest Bell, London, England, 1902, 199-210.

Since its founding 15 years previously, the College has
struggled with financial problems. The second obstacle--
"want of professional support"--has been surmounted.
Blackwell contrasts this encouragement ("like breathing a
new and delightful atmosphere, which is, nevertheless,
strange and dream-like") to the rejection and hatred experienced by the College's founders. She discusses the new
plans of instruction at the school, and generally identifies
the importance of women physicians.

3414.   Blewett, Evelyn. "Women Pioneers in Medicine." Journal
         of the American Medical Women's Association, 1:1
         (April 1946) 20-21. photos.
Some facts are presented about the New York Infirmary for
Women and Children, established in 1857 by Elizabeth Blackwell. The event which occasioned this article was the announcement of a campaign to raise $5 million to build a
new hospital. Financial and statistical figures for the Infirmary are given as well as specific achievements of women who trained and practiced there. Some "firsts" which
occurred at the Infirmary are mentioned: the first training
of women as nurses in America; the first chair of hygiene
in a medical college; the first training of a Negro woman
physician; the first medical social service; and the first
visiting nurse service--before it was so called. Plans
for the proposed new hospital are discussed.

3415.   Blount, Anna E. "The Medical Women's National Associa-
         tion." Medical Review of Reviews, 37:3 (March 1931)
         143-146.
The Medical Women's National Association was founded in
Chicago in 1915 during an American Medical Association
convention. Bertha Van Hoosen served as the organization's
first president. This brief history touches upon the early
opposition to a separate women's organization, describes
the functions and accomplishments of various Association
committees, names the presidents, and discusses the official Bulletin.

3416.   Blount, Anna E. "President's Address." Medical Woman's
         Journal, 33:5 (May 1926) 134-136. (Address, Twelfth
         Annual Convention, Medical Women's National Associa-
         tion, Dallas, Texas, 18-20 April 1926.)
Outgoing president Anna E. Blount tackles the often-asked
question of why women in medicine need to organize along
sex lines. Recounting the struggles of pioneer women physicians, Dr. Blount writes that present-day women still do
not have equal opportunities with men. Less women were
enrolled in medical schools in 1925 than in 1924. Women
are financially handicapped, since parents are less willing
to give money to girls than to boys, and chances for girls
to earn it are fewer. Because many hospitals do not accept women on their staffs, women are forced to practice

in small towns and are "greeted with closed doors." Trying to study and work "in an atmosphere of chill solitude
and unappreciation," getting discouragement from "the
jealous male colleague, from the sneering lips of the con-
temptuous (and contemptible) 'parasitic' woman," the medical woman becomes defensive and "hard-boiled." Fellowship is the medical woman's greatest need: "We do not
mind even hanging if we hang together." A national woman's organization can offer comradeship and financial aid
and work to enlarge its numbers. "About three-fourths of
the medical profession should be women, enough to take
care of the bulk of the women and children and an occasional man."

3417.   Blount, Anna E. "Report of the Eleventh Annual Conven-
            tion of the Medical Women's National Association Held
            at Atlantic City, May 24-25-26, 1925." Medical Wo-
            man's Journal, 32:5 (May 1925) 169-171.
        Among other presentations on the agenda of the Convention
        of the Medical Women's National Association were two pro-
        posals for constitutional amendments concerning membership
        qualification eligibility for the American Medical Associa-
        tion, and the creation of junior memberships for senior
        medical students, internes, and first year graduates. The
        observation was made that women physicians are more ac-
        cepted in the west than in the south or east.

3418.   Borden, Isabelle F. "Minutes of the Thirty-Sixth Mid-
            Year Meeting of the Women's Medical Society of New
            York State, January 24, 1942." Medical Woman's
            Journal, 49:3 (March 1942) 69-70.

3419.   Borden, Isabella F. "Women's Medical Society of New York
            State: A Brief History." Journal of the American
            Medical Women's Association, 10:2 (February 1955) 59,
            62.
        This article includes a cataloging of some of the more il-
        lustrious members of the Society.

3420.   Boston University/School of Medicine: Centennial 1873/
            1973. "The Bright 100 Years." [Boston, Massachu-
            setts? 1973?], 32 pp. facsims., photos., ports.
        This historical account of the founding in 1873 and the
        growth of Boston University School of Medicine commences
        with the takeover by Boston University of the 25-year-old
        New England Female Medical College. Dr. Israel Tisdale
        Talbot, instrumental in the merger, was named the school's
        first dean.

3421.   Bourdeau-Sisco, P. S. "Woman's Medical Society of Mary-
            land: The History of Branch Three." Journal of the
            American Medical Women's Association, 7:11 (Novem-
            ber 1952) 417-418. ports.

Flora Pollack, the first president, and P. S. Bourdeau-
Sisco, a later president, helped to found the Woman's Medical Society of Maryland. "The objective of the society is
the closer association of women physicians, the reading of
medical papers, the presentation of cases, discussions and
general interchange of ideas." Portraits of Drs. Bourdeau-
Sisco, Abercrombie, Towles, and Shamer are included.

3422.   Bowditch, Henry I. "The Medical Education of Women.
         The Present Hostile Position of Harvard University and
         of the Massachusetts Medical Society. What Remedies
         Therefor can be Suggested?" Boston Medical and Sur-
         gical Journal, 105:13 (22 September 1881) 289-293.
Despite the fact that in this country at this time every adult
"has a right to such an amount and species of instruction,
that is offered to the public," both Harvard University Medical School and the Massachusetts Medical Society have seen
fit to bar women. Women are forced to go to Europe for
training, or to inferior schools, or they are driven into the
ranks of quackery. The author had presented a resolution
to the Massachusetts Medical Society, directing that women
be examined for admission into the Society, but to no avail.
The Society cannot "check the irresistible onward course of
human progress in giving all learning for woman as well as
man." He recommends that Harvard commence a separate
medical school for women. The Society should examine women who apply for license, grant diplomas to all who pass
the requisite examination, and invite these women to attend
their meetings.

3423.   "Branch Societies of the W.M.N.A. [sic]." Medical Wo-
         man's Journal, 37:10 (October 1930) 287.
In order to strengthen the Medical Women's National Association and to concentrate its influence, it was decided to
replace group memberships by branch societies with individual membership, each 25 members of same to have one
representative. It was anticipated that such reorganization
would increase membership, promote the good of individual
members, and in various ways secure tangible benefits for
women physicians.

3424.   "Brief History of the Women's Medical Society of Mary-
         land." Medical Woman's Journal, 36:11 (November
         1929) 302-303.
In addition to the history of the Society, this article lists
the names of some of the Society's members who occupy
public positions.

3425.   Brodie, Jessie Laird. "President's Message." Journal of
         the American Medical Women's Association, 15:3 (March
         1960) 278.
The American Medical Women's Association cannot " 'bother' "
the American Medical Association with those problems

unique to women in medicine. In the context of this thinking, the value of the AMWA is reviewed. "We believe that
AMWA members have an opportunity of being even better
members of AMA."

3426.   Brodie, Jessie Laird. "Service Unlimited-AMWA." Journal of the American Medical Women's Association, 14:
7 (July 1959) 605-612. (Inaugural Address, Annual
Meeting, American Medical Women's Association, Atlantic City, New Jersey, 6 June 1959.)
The American Medical Women's Association had a long history of enabling women who were led to be physicians to do
service (such as during World War I and in the foreign
mission field) through its medical service committee, the
American Women's Hospitals, during periods when other
countries were experiencing natural and man-made disasters.
"As individuals and as a prestige group, we can make ourselves felt as authorities in this field, developing public
opinion toward the support of private enterprise in medicine
and encouraging the dignity and independence of the individual
to provide his own security while keeping that laudable sympathy for the less fortunate that is so typical of our American Culture."

3427.   Bunker, John P. and Pool, Judith G. "The Case for More
Women in Medicine: The Stanford Program." New
England Journal of Medicine, 285:1 (1 July 1971) 53.
Inspired by an announcement of the faculty senate at Stanford University School of Medicine of its goal to increase
the proportion of women in its student body, this article
looks at the case for more women in medicine. In response to the "manpower" crisis in health, women represent a large and almost untapped potential pool. Their application to medical school should now be encouraged. One
of the major obstacles to the recruitment of women has been
the inflexibility of the curriculum. Stanford's curriculum is
now entirely elective, with no fixed timetable for completion
of the M.D. degree: students may arrange to take leave
without penalty. The author urges other members of the
medical profession to consider similar action and work
closely with parent groups, teachers, and vocational counselors to encourage young women to enter medicine.

3428.   "Capital of Medical Education for Women." National Business Woman, 46:7 (July 1967) 4-8. photos.
The Woman's Medical College of Pennsylvania (WMCP) has
made significant contributions for the training of women physicians. It gave women a chance to attend medical school
when male doctors resisted their acceptance in other medical
schools and resisted giving them an opportunity for clinical
training. WMCP was a pioneer in allowing flexible time
schedules which could be adjusted to the needs of their students, i.e., older women with families and women who had
medical training but who had taken time off to raise families.

3429.   Carew, Evangeline. "Serbia a Real Country." Medical
          Woman's Journal, 29:3 (March 1922) 61-62. (Hospitals
          & Colleges.)
        Dr. Carew describes through anecdotes the work of the
        American Women's Hospitals in Serbia.

3430.   "Catholic Medical Mission Sisters: Homecoming--Departure.
          Medical Woman's Journal, 55:2 (February 1948) 49-50.
          photo.
        This article reports the outcome of the Medical Mission Sis-
        ters' general election in August [1947] and describes the
        current activities of several of the medical missionaries.

3431.   Chadwick, James R. "The Admission of Women to the
          Massachusetts Medical Society." Boston Medical and
          Surgical Journal, 106:23 (8 June 1882) 547-549.
          (Miscellany.)
        This article is a recapitulation of the past action of the
        society in regards to an amendment to the bylaws which
        would permit the admission of women. The alteration of
        the bylaws is reprinted. In 1880 the author sent a ques-
        tionnaire to the secretary of every state medical society in
        the U.S., seeking information on women members. The
        results show that none of the societies shuts its doors to
        women.

3432.   "A Challenge: The Women's [sic] Medical College of Penn-
          sylvania." Pennsylvania Clubwoman, 42:3 (February-
          March 1955) 14-15, 17. illus. (Your State Project.)
        In 1954 the Pennsylvania Federation of Women's Clubs re-
        solved to help with the expansion of the Woman's Medical
        College of Pennsylvania. This article outlines how the
        Federation plans to carry out that pledge.

3433.   Cleaves, Margaret A. "Suggestions as to the Future Policy
          of the Journal." Woman's Medical Journal, 19:1 (Janu-
          ary 1909) 10-11. (Editorial.)

3434.   "The Conditions of Miss Garrett's Gift to the Medical School
          of Johns Hopkins University." Boston Medical and
          Surgical Journal, 128:3 (19 January 1893) 71-72.
        The letter of Miss Garrett of Baltimore in which she offers
        the $306,977 to complete the endowment of $500,000 to
        the Medical School, is reprinted. This endowment is given
        in order that the school might be opened to both sexes.
        The conditions of the gift are outlined in the letter.

3435.   Conrad, Agnes. "Women of the Staff of St. Elizabeth's
          Hospital." Medical Woman's Journal, 35:8 (August
          1928) 219-221. photos. (Feature Article.)
        In 1905, Mary O'Malley became the first woman physician
        appointed to the staff of Washington, D.C.'s St. Elizabeth's
        Hospital, which treats mentally ill women. Since Dr.

O'Malley's appointment, 34 women joined the staff; they are listed in this article.

3436.   Copple, Peggy. "How the AMWA Can Help Me in the Pursuit of My Career." Journal of the American Medical Women's Association, 12:1 (January 1957) 25.
A recent medical school graduate suggests the American Medical Women's Association can provide a source of unity and support for women medical students and women physicians.

3437.   "A Correction and Apology." Medical Woman's Journal, 36:5 (May 1929) 137.
Correcting the announcement in the April 1929 issue of the Medical Woman's Journal, this article explains that the New York Infirmary for Women and Children has not been merged with the Columbia-Presbyterian Hospital Medical Center.

3438.   Corson, Hiram. A Brief History of Proceedings in the Medical Society of Pennsylvania in the years 1859, '60, '66, '67, '68, '70 and '71 to Procure the Recognition of Women Physicians by the Medical Profession of the State to Which is Added an Account of the Measures Adopted by the Society at Its Annual Meetings in 1877, '78, '79 to Procure a Law to Authorize Trustees of Hospitals for the Insane Poor, Under Control of the State, to Appoint Women Physicians to have Entire Medical Control of the Insane of Their Sex. Herald Printing, Norristown, Pennsylvania, 1894, 53 pp.
The medical profession took no combined action against the women graduates of the Woman's Medical College of Pennsylvania until eight classes had graduated and many women established practice. On November 10, 1858, "the Board of Censors of the Philadelphia County Medical Society reported to the society their disapproval of any member who held professional intercourse with the professors or alumni of the Woman's Medical College. The history of the contest which followed the announcement of that report, and its adoption by the county society, is recorded in this pamphlet."

3439.   Crane, J. H. "Protest Against Receiving Females as Members of the State Medical Society." Pacific Medical and Surgical Journal, 19 (1876-1877) 22-25.
[Article not examined by editors.]

3440.   Crawford, Mary Merritt. "Report of Chairman: American Women's Hospitals for the Year 1918-1919." Woman's Medical Journal, 29 [19]:8 (August 1919) 164-168.
Dr. Crawford's report reviews the organization's policies, domestic and foreign activities, and lists the women who hold executive positions.

3441.   Cruikshank, Marion. "American Women's Hospitals: Med-

ical Service Committee of Medical Women's National Association." Medical Woman's Journal, 32:2 (February 1925) 47-53. photos.
A surgical nurse recounts her experiences working with American Women's Hospitals in Serbia, Turkey, Greece, and Armenia. She observes that "American women have gone into a land where women counted as nothing, have taken charge, have been looked up to, from the highest government official down to the lowest bedraggled refugee, and that their words have been taken as Gospel.... We have demonstrated in Greece that women are capable of doing what has always been considered 'a man's job.' And not only the men in that country realize it, but the women with whom we have come in contact have begun to sit up and imbibe some of the American notions."

3442.   Curtis, Arthur C. "The Woman as a Student of Medicine." Association of American Medical Colleges Bulletin, 2 (April 1927) 140-148. graphs, tables.
This article reports on the activities of women medical students at the University of Michigan, the first medical school to become coeducational. The report reveals that women compose approximately 6.2 per cent of the graduating classe of the University. Of the women, 84.8 per cent had bachelor degrees for entrance as compared to 44.1 per cent of the men. Of students entering the medical school, practically the same proportion of women and men graduate. Female students do better than male students during the first two years and equal them during the last two years. The average woman medical student meets numerically about a ten per cent higher standard than the average male.

3443.   Daniel, Annie Sturges. "'A Cautious Experiment.' The History of the New York Infirmary for Women and Children and the Women's Medical College of the New York Infirmary; Also Its Pioneer Founders: 1853-1899." Medical Woman's Journal, 46:6 (June 1939) 168-174, 183. facsims., port.
A reproduction of the original "Incorporation Certificate of intention to incorporate the New York Infirmary for Indigent Women and Children" makes up the major portion of this second installment in the series about the Infirmary. One of the men who obtained the Infirmary's charter was Theodore Sedgwick; a biography and portrait of him is given.

3444.   Daniel, Annie Sturges. "'A Cautious Experiment.' The History of the New York Infirmary for Women and Children and the Women's Medical College of the New York Infirmary; Also Its Pioneer Founders: 1853-1899." Medical Woman's Journal, 46:7 (July 1939) 196-202.
This article in the series presents excerpts from Elizabeth Blackwell's Pioneer Work, Agnes Vietor's A Woman's Quest: The Life of Marie E. Zakrzewska, the first annual report

of the New York Dispensary for Women and Children (February 8, 1855), and newspaper accounts of the Dispensary.
A biography is given of Mary L. Booth, a journalist whose newspaper articles about the dispensary made her an invaluable "early friend of the Infirmary."

3445.   Daniel, Annie Sturges.   "'A Cautious Experiment.' The History of the New York Infirmary for Women and Children and the Women's Medical College of the New York Infirmary; Also Its Pioneer Founders: 1853-1899." Medical Woman's Journal, 46:8 (August 1939) 229-238. port.

This installment in the series about the Infirmary's history reviews newspaper accounts of the hospital's opening (May 1857).   Biographies are given of speakers "who were willing to publicly endorse" the Infirmary at the opening ceremony: Henry Ward Beecher (preacher), William Elder (physician and author), Dudley Atkins Tyng (clergyman), and Stacy Budd Collins (publisher).

3446.   Daniel, Annie Sturges.   "'A Cautious Experiment.' The History of the New York Infirmary for Women and Children and the Women's Medical College of the New York Infirmary; Also Its Pioneer Founders: 1853-1899." Medical Woman's Journal, 46:9 (September 1939) 269-277, 280.

This article in the series about the New York Infirmary gives biographies of Charles A. Dana (an Infirmary trustee), Elizabeth and Emily Blackwell, and Marie Zakrzewska.
Also included: a history of Manhattan Island, and of 64 Bleecker Street (the building which initially housed the Infirmary); excerpts of Infirmary reports from 1855 to 1858; and quotes from Blackwell's Pioneer Work.   Marie Zakrzewska's recollections of daily work routines at the Infirmary is an account of struggle made bearable due to "youthful enthusiasm."   She also describes two occasions in which angry mobs, convinced that the women doctors were killing patients, threatened the Infirmary.

3447.   Daniel, Annie Sturges.   "'A Cautious Experiment.' The History of the New York Infirmary for Women and Children and the Women's Medical College of the New York Infirmary; Also Its Pioneer Founders: 1853-1899." Medical Woman's Journal, 46:10 (October 1939) 295-299, 309.

Drs. Blackwell's and Zakrzewska's comments on the first 20 months of practice at the Infirmary (ending December 1857) begin this article.   Excerpts of the executive committee minutes for 1858 include information on finances, advertising, and staff changes.   The first medical students to train at the Infirmary are mentioned, as is the nursing staff situation.   This article concludes with a discussion of the introduction of "gas and baths" in the building.

3448.   Daniel, Annie Sturges. "'A Cautious Experiment.' The
         History of the New York Infirmary for Women and Chil-
         dren and the Women's Medical College of the New York
         Infirmary; Also Its Pioneer Founders: 1853-1899."
         Medical Woman's Journal, 46:11 (November 1939) 335-
         339.
         "Biographical sketches" given in this article in the series
         about the Infirmary include the following men who served
         the Infirmary as consulting physicians: Valentine Mott,
         John Watson, and Willard Parker. Also profiled: Edith
         Parker Stimson, an Infirmary trustee.

3449.   Daniel, Annie Sturges. "'A Cautious Experiment.' The
         History of the New York Infirmary for Women and Chil-
         dren and the Women's Medical College of the New York
         Infirmary; Also Its Pioneer Founders: 1853-1899."
         Medical Woman's Journal, 46:12 (December 1939) 357-
         360.
         Biographical sketches of Drs. Richard Sharpe Kissam,
         Isaac E. Taylor, and George Phillip Camman--all of whom
         served the Infirmary in its formative years--are given in
         this installment.

3450.   Daniel, Annie Sturges. "'A Cautious Experiment.' The
         History of the New York Infirmary for Women and Chil-
         dren and the Women's Medical College of the New York
         Infirmary; Also Its Pioneer Founders: 1853-1899."
         Medical Woman's Journal, 47:1 (January 1940) 10-12.
         This article in the series about the New York Infirmary
         opens with excerpts of letters by distinguished European
         physicians who offered testimonials to and support of Emily
         Blackwell.   The occasion was her assignment as supervisor
         of the Infirmary, when Elizabeth Blackwell went to England
         for a vacation and Marie Zakrzewska departed for work in
         Boston.   Also presented are extracts from the Infirmary's
         executive committee reports for 1859 and 1860.

3451.   Daniel, Annie Sturges. "'A Cautious Experiment.' The
         History of the New York Infirmary for Women and Chil-
         dren and the Women's Medical College of the New York
         Infirmary; Also Its Pioneer Founders: 1853-1899."
         Medical Woman's Journal, 47:2 (February 1940) 40-45,
         62.
         Subtitled "Medical Education," this installment opens with
         statements of the institution's goals to assist women in
         practical medical study by offering opportunities within the
         Infirmary itself and by opening other institutions to its stu-
         dents.   Intentions regarding nurses' training are also men-
         tioned.   Excerpts from Infirmary reports and from Eliza-
         beth Blackwell's Pioneer Work tell of the Infirmary's ef-
         forts in response to the Civil War.   Nurses were trained
         for military hospitals, and Dr. Blackwell helped form the
         Women's Central Relief Association of New York.

3452. Daniel, Annie Sturges. "'A Cautious Experiment.' The
         History of the New York Infirmary for Women and Chil-
         dren and the Women's Medical College of the New York
         Infirmary; Also Its Pioneer Founders: 1853-1899."
         Medical Woman's Journal, 47:3 (March 1940) 67-69.
This installment offers biographies of two supporters of the
institution: Horace Greeley, who served as a trustee from
1853-1858; and Henry Jarvis Raymond, a trustee from 1853-
1868. Greeley, best known for establishing the New York
Tribune, supported women's rights but "opposed the suffrage
because all women did not want it." He also supported the
medical education of women but did not perceive any obstacles to women obtaining that education. Raymond, at
one time a Tribune journalist, had a daughter--Aimee Ray-
mond--who graduated from the Women's Medical College of
the New York Infirmary in 1889.

3453. Daniel, Annie Sturges. "'A Cautious Experiment.' The
         History of the New York Infirmary for Women and Chil-
         dren and the Women's Medical College of the New York
         Infirmary; Also Its Pioneer Founders: 1853-1899."
         Medical Woman's Journal, 47:4 (April 1940) 98-101.
The major portion of this installment quotes from the Infirmary's annual reports of 1862 and 1863. Also presented
is historical background on the Society of Friends; the role
of Quaker support of the Infirmary is emphasized.

3454. Daniel, Annie Sturges. "'A Cautious Experiment.' The
         History of the New York Infirmary for Women and Chil-
         dren and the Women's Medical College of the New York
         Infirmary; Also Its Pioneer Founders: 1853-1899."
         Medical Woman's Journal, 47:5 (May 1940) 135-139, xi.
This installment is subtitled "The Evolution of the College:
Address on the Medical Education of Women, prepared by
Drs. Elizabeth and Emily Blackwell and read before a meeting held at the New York Infirmary, December 19, 1863."
The speech, presented in direct quotes and paraphrases,
opens with emphasis on the necessity for educating good
nurses and the woman physician's role in that training. An
examination of the status of women's medical education includes discussions of women's many disadvantages, e.g.,
inferior training as girls, poverty, domestic slavery, and
general nonsupport from the (male) profession. Elizabeth
Blackwell draws upon her own experiences to illustrate these
obstacles. Detailed are four points in which a women's
medical college should differ from other institutions now established: (1) changes must be imposed on the examinations
for conferring the M.D.; (2) emphasis must be placed on individual discipline and practical medicine; (3) attitudes assumed by the profession towards medical women must be
changed; (4) and a woman's college must receive an endowment. The last part of the speech proposes ways in which
the Infirmary can fulfill these four points in its founding of
the Women's Medical College of the New York Infirmary.

3455.   Daniel, Annie Sturges. "'A Cautious Experiment.' The
          History of the New York Infirmary for Women and Chil
          dren and the Women's Medical College of the New York
          Infirmary; Also Its Pioneer Founders: 1853-1899."
          Medical Woman's Journal, 47:6 (June 1940) 167-171.
In this installment, subtitled "The Evolution of the College,"
biographies are given of the following: Samuel Willets, who
served the Infirmary as a trustee and as its president;
Robert Haydock, a treasurer, secretary, and president of
the Infirmary; Hannah Wharton Haydock, a chairman of the
executive committee; and Merritt Trimble, who served as
a trustee and secretary. Excerpts from the Infirmary reports of 1864 and 1865 conclude this article.

3456.   Daniel, Annie Sturges. "'A Cautious Experiment.' The
          History of the New York Infirmary for Women and Chil-
          dren and the Women's Medical College of the New York
          Infirmary; Also Its Pioneer Founders: 1853-1899."
          Medical Woman's Journal, 47:7 (July 1940) 199-204,
          228.
Subtitled "The Evolution of the College," this article in the
series opens with a biography of Richard H. Bowne, a
trustee and a member of the finance committee. Following that is a collage of primarily financial information extracted from executive committee minutes from 1862-1868.

3457.   Daniel, Annie Sturges. "'A Cautious Experiment.' The
          History of the New York Infirmary for Women and Chil-
          dren and the Women's Medical College of the New York
          Infirmary; Also Its Pioneer Founders: 1853-1899."
          Medical Woman's Journal, 47:8 (August 1940) 234-239.
Subheaded "The Evolution of the College," this installment
opens with the incorporation announcement for the College
and a summary of a lecture by Elizabeth Blackwell concerning the procurement of funds for the College. Press
notices about the institution are reproduced.

3458.   Daniel, Annie Sturges. "'A Cautious Experiment.' The
          History of the New York Infirmary for Women and Chil-
          dren and the Women's Medical College of the New York
          Infirmary; Also Its Pioneer Founders: 1853-1899."
          Medical Woman's Journal, 47:9 (September 1940) 263-
          268, 282. illus.
This article in the series is subtitled "An Era Begins:
November 2, 1868, at 126 Second Avenue (Address Delivered at the Opening of the Women's Medical College of
the New York Infirmary by Dr. Elizabeth Blackwell)." Following the text of this speech are excerpts from Infirmary
reports of 1869-1870.

3459.   Daniel, Annie Sturges. "'A Cautious Experiment.' The
          History of the New York Infirmary for Women and Chil-
          dren and the Women's Medical College of the New York

Infirmary; Also Its Pioneer Founders: 1853-1899."
Medical Woman's Journal, 47:10 (October 1940) 296-300.
Subheaded "An Era Begins November 2, 1868, at 126 Second Avenue," this installment discusses the activities of the
College and presents excerpts from executive committee reports (1869-1870) and faculty minutes (November 1868-May
1870). A "postscript" tells of Elizabeth Blackwell's intention to visit England to renew her strength and assist in
pioneer work in London. She did not return to America.

3460. Daniel, Annie Sturges. "'A Cautious Experiment.' The
History of the New York Infirmary for Women and Children and the Women's Medical College of the New York
Infirmary; Also Its Pioneer Founders: 1853-1899."
Medical Woman's Journal, 47:11 (November 1940) 323-
329, 345.
Reproduced in this installment is the content of the College's
first annual catalogue and announcement. The 1869 class
consisted of 17 women, five of whom graduated in 1870.
The remainder of the article reprints comments made by
the medical and consumer press about the College's opening.

3461. Daniel, Annie Sturges. "'A Cautious Experiment.' The
History of the New York Infirmary for Women and Children and the Women's Medical College of the New York
Infirmary; Also Its Pioneer Founders: 1853-1899."
Medical Woman's Journal, 47:12 (December 1940) 357-
362, 370.
Biographies are given in this installment of Simson Draper,
a trustee from 1853 to 1866, and of Dennis Harris, trustee
from 1853-1854. Reprints of articles by the press tell of
the first College commencement (April 1870). Of those
first five graduates, one married the chemistry professor,
one went to India as a missionary, and another later adopted
homeopathy. An extensive biography is presented of Sophia
Jex-Blake, the first woman to matriculate at the College
(in October 1868). Highlighted are excerpts from her diary
which tell of her father's opposition to her career ambitions.

3462. Daniel, Annie Sturges. "'A Cautious Experiment.' The
History of the New York Infirmary for Women and Chil-
dren and the Women's Medical College of the New York
Infirmary; Also Its Pioneer Founders: 1853-1899."
Medical Woman's Journal, 48:1 (January 1941) 10-13.
Excerpts of faculty minutes (1871-1882), discuss examina-
tions, lectures, grades, and other matters pertaining to the
administration of the College.

3463. Daniel, Annie Sturges. "'A Cautious Experiment.' The
History of the New York Infirmary for Women and Chil-
dren and the Women's Medical College of the New York
Infirmary; Also Its Pioneer Founders: 1853-1899."

Medical Woman's Journal, 48:2 (February 1941) 33-39.
This article in the series presents excerpts from faculty
minutes (1871-1882). Such items are discussed as the hour
and room locations of lectures, whether or not to permit
students to retake final exams if they did not pass them,
the financial situation at the College, Dr. Blackwell's succeeding to the presidency of the faculty, and the discontent
of the student body with the poor showing of professors for
lectures.

3464.   Daniel, Annie Sturges. "'A Cautious Experiment.' The
             History of the New York Infirmary for Women and Chil-
             dren and the Women's Medical College of the New York
             Infirmary; Also Its Pioneer Founders: 1853-1899."
             Medical Woman's Journal, 48:3 (March 1941) 74-79, 91.
Excerpts from faculty minutes (1871-1882) comprise this installment about the Infirmary's history.

3465.   Daniel, Annie Sturges. "'A Cautious Experiment.' The
             History of the New York Infirmary for Women and Chil-
             dren and the Women's Medical College of the New York
             Infirmary; Also Its Pioneer Founders: 1853-1899."
             Medical Woman's Journal, 48:4 (April 1941) 102-104.
Press notices of college commencements, recording prizes
awarded, commencement speakers, and excerpts from commencement addresses, make up this installment.

3466.   Daniel, Annie Sturges. "'A Cautious Experiment.' The
             History of the New York Infirmary for Women and Chil-
             dren and the Women's Medical College of the New York
             Infirmary; Also Its Pioneer Founders: 1853-1899."
             Medical Woman's Journal, 48:5 (May 1941) 134-138.
Excerpts from Infirmary reports (1871-1881) make up this
installment.

3467.   Daniel, Annie Sturges. "'A Cautious Experiment.' The
             History of the New York Infirmary for Women and Chil-
             dren and the Women's Medical College of the New York
             Infirmary; Also Its Pioneer Founders: 1853-1899."
             Medical Woman's Journal, 48:6 (June 1941) 167-173.
This article in the series on the New York Infirmary presents excerpts from Infirmary reports (1871-1881). Treasurer's and trustees' reports offer a glimpse of the full range
of Infirmary operations.

3468.   Daniel, Annie Sturges. "'A Cautious Experiment.' The
             History of the New York Infirmary for Women and Chil-
             dren and the Women's Medical College of the New York
             Infirmary; Also Its Pioneer Founders: 1853-1899."
             Medical Woman's Journal, 48:8 (August 1941) 233-240.
Excerpts from the college faculty minutes of October 10,
1882, the first meeting of the college year, to September
27, 1889, comprise this installment.

3469. Daniel, Annie Sturges. "'A Cautious Experiment.' The
       History of the New York Infirmary for Women and Chil-
       dren and the Women's Medical College of the New York
       Infirmary; Also Its Pioneer Founders: 1853-1899."
       Medical Woman's Journal, 48:9 (September 1941) 272-
       278, 288.
       This article in the series on the New York Infirmary pre-
       sents excerpts from the college faculty minutes of October
       10, 1882, the first meeting of the college year, to September
       27, 1889, the end of the college year. Correspondence
       is read from students, faculty, and deans of other medical
       schools, desiring information about the college. The re-
       sults of students' examinations are read and discussed.

3470. Daniel, Annie Sturges. "'A Cautious Experiment.' The
       History of the New York Infirmary for Women and Chil-
       dren and the Women's Medical College of the New York
       Infirmary; Also Its Pioneer Founders: 1853-1899."
       Medical Woman's Journal, 48:11 (November 1941) 331-
       338, 346.
       Excerpts from executive committee minutes, 1871-1874,
       make up this installment.

3471. Daniel, Annie Sturges. "'A Cautious Experiment.' The
       History of the New York Infirmary for Women and Chil-
       dren and the Women's Medical College of the New York
       Infirmary; Also Its Pioneer Founders: 1853-1899."
       Medical Woman's Journal, 48:12 (December 1941) 364-
       371.
       This article in the series on the New York Infirmary con-
       sists of excerpts from college catalogues, 1883-1889 in-
       clusive. Number and composition of faculty, length of col-
       lege year, student course load, and examination schedules
       are given, as well as the order of lectures and clinics,
       division of studies, method of instruction, and course con-
       tent.

3472. Daniel, Annie Sturges. "'A Cautious Experiment.' The
       History of the New York Infirmary for Women and Chil-
       dren and the Women's Medical College of the New York
       Infirmary; Also Its Pioneer Founders: 1853-1899."
       Medical Woman's Journal, 49:1 (January 1942) 12-15,
       26.
       Excerpts of annual catalogues and announcements from the
       years 1885 to 1889 comprise this installment.

3473. Daniel, Annie Sturges. "'A Cautious Experiment.' The
       History of the New York Infirmary for Women and Chil-
       dren and the Women's Medical College of the New York
       Infirmary; Also Its Pioneer Founders: 1853-1899."
       Medical Woman's Journal, 49:2 (February 1942) 37-40,
       59.
       This installment reproduces the Infirmary's twenty-ninth
       annual report for the year 1882.

3474.   Daniel, Annie Sturges. "'A Cautious Experiment.' The
          History of the New York Infirmary for Women and Chil-
          dren and the Women's Medical College of the New York
          Infirmary; Also Its Pioneer Founders: 1853-1899."
          Medical Woman's Journal, 49:3 (March 1942) 71-74.
        This installment in the series about the Infirmary repro-
        duces the Infirmary's report for the year 1883.

3475.   Daniel, Annie Sturges. "'A Cautious Experiment.' The
          History of the New York Infirmary for Women and Chil-
          dren and the Women's Medical College of the New York
          Infirmary; Also Its Pioneer Founders: 1853-1899."
          Medical Woman's Journal, 49:4 (April 1942) 105-109.
        The institution's thirty-first annual report (1884) is repro-
        duced in this installment.

3476.   Daniel, Annie Sturges. "'A Cautious Experiment.' The
          History of the New York Infirmary for Women and Chil-
          dren and the Women's Medical College of the New York
          Infirmary; Also Its Pioneer Founders: 1853-1899."
          Medical Woman's Journal, 49:5 (May 1942) 137-138.
        This article in the series about the Infirmary reproduces
        the Infirmary's thirty-second annual report (1885).

3477.   Daniel, Annie Sturges. "'A Cautious Experiment.' The
          History of the New York Infirmary for Women and Chil-
          dren and the Women's Medical College of the New York
          Infirmary; Also Its Pioneer Founders: 1853-1899."
          Medical Woman's Journal, 49:6 (June 1942) 165-166,
          189.
        "Women's Medical College of the New York Infirmary:
        Thirty-second Annual Report of the New York Infirmary for
        Women and Children for the Year 1885" is the subtitle for
        this installment.

3478.   Daniel, Annie Sturges. "'A Cautious Experiment.' The
          History of the New York Infirmary for Women and Chil-
          dren and the Women's Medical College of the New York
          Infirmary; Also Its Pioneer Founders: 1853-1899."
          Medical Woman's Journal, 49:7 (July 1942) 208-212,
          228.
        This installment reproduces the thirty-second annual report
        of the New York Infirmary for Women and Children for
        the year 1886.   Included are the reports from the executive
        committee; reports of patients, of the Infirmary, and of the
        dispensary; and the treasurer's report including donations
        received.

3479.   Daniel, Annie Sturges. "'A Cautious Experiment.' The
          History of the New York Infirmary for Women and Chil-
          dren and the Women's Medical College of the New York
          Infirmary; Also Its Pioneer Founders: 1853-1899."
          Medical Woman's Journal, 49:8 (August 1942) 241-243.

Reproduced in this installment: the thirty-fourth annual report for the year 1887. Included are the reports of the
executive committee, the dispensary, and the children's department, and listings of the patients and the diseases
treated during the year.

3480.   Daniel, Annie Sturges.   "'A Cautious Experiment.'   The
        History of the New York Infirmary for Women and Chil-
        dren and the Women's Medical College of the New York
        Infirmary; Also Its Pioneer Founders: 1853-1899."
        Medical Woman's Journal, 49:9 (September 1942) 274-
        275.
This installment reproduces a portion of the thirty-fourth
annual report for the year 1887: patient data, the treasurer's report, and a record of donations are included.

3481.   Daniel, Annie Sturges.   "'A Cautious Experiment.'   The
        History of the New York Infirmary for Women and Chil-
        dren and the Women's Medical College of the New York
        Infirmary; Also Its Pioneer Founders: 1853-1899."
        Medical Woman's Journal, 49:10 (October 1942) 306-309,
        319.
This article reproduces the thirty-fifth annual report for
the year 1888.

3482.   Daniel, Annie Sturges.   "'A Cautious Experiment.'   The
        History of the New York Infirmary for Women and Chil-
        dren and the Women's Medical College of the New York
        Infirmary; Also Its Pioneer Founders: 1853-1899."
        Medical Woman's Journal, 49:11 (November 1942) 342-
        344.
This installment reproduces the thirty-sixth annual report
(1889) which includes a description of the physical conditions, student training facilities, and a memorial to the
late teacher, Lydia Wadleigh; the record of dispensary
cases; the record of medical practice away from the hospital; the druggist's report; and other patient care and oper-
ational information.

3483.   Daniel, Annie Sturges.   "'A Cautious Experiment.'   The
        History of the New York Infirmary for Women and Chil-
        dren and the Women's Medical College of the New York
        Infirmary; Also Its Pioneer Founders: 1853-1899."
        Medical Woman's Journal, 49:12 (December 1942) 373-
        375, 392.
This installment reproduces the thirty-sixth annual report of
the New York Infirmary for the year 1888-1889. Statistics
included in this report represent the respective department
dispensaries and the number and variety of cases identified
and treated, the causes of death, and the treasurer's report noting gifts to the Infirmary and gifts, in turn, to tene-
ment house patients.

3484.   Daniel, Annie Sturges. "A Cautious Experiment. Thesis:
         Great Events Affect All Peoples." Medical Woman's
         Journal, 43:10 (October 1936) 268-271.
         Given is historical background on the opening of the Women's
         Medical College of the New York Infirmary and the estab-
         lishment of the New York Infirmary for Women and Chil-
         dren. [This article appears to be the first in Dr. Daniel's
         series of articles on the New York Infirmary.]

3485.   Daniel, Annie S[turges]. "The Mary Putnam-Jacobi Fellow-
         ship: A Worthy Memorial to 'A Pathfinder in Medicine.'
         Medical Woman's Journal, 43:4 (April 1936) 94-95.
         port. (Presentation, Mid-Year Meeting, Women's Med-
         ical Association of New York City, January 1936.)
         Contributors to and recipients of the Fund are mentioned,
         along with a few observations about Dr. Jacobi's life.

3486.   Daniel, Annie S[turges]. "Report of the Legislative Com-
         mittee of the Woman's Medical Society of the State of
         New York." Woman's Medical Journal, 29:8 (August
         1919) 174.

3487.   "Daughters for Harvard." Time, (9 October 1944) 90.
         port.
         In 1945 Harvard will break with its 163-year tradition and
         admit women medical students. Nevertheless, U.S. preju-
         dice against women in medicine is still evidenced by the low
         percentage of women's enrollment in U.S. medical schools
         compared with medical schools in other countries, and the
         fact that the U.S. government will not subsidize women
         students in the same way they subsidize men. For those
         who still agree with the medical men of 1850 Boston who
         resolved to oppose the medical education of females, there
         are still four "all-male medical strongholds" in the U.S.:
         Georgetown, St. Louis, Dartmouth, and Jefferson.

3488.   Dean-Throckmorton, Jeanette. "History of the State Society
         of Iowa Medical Women: Part I. From 1898 to 1905."
         Journal of Iowa State Medical Society, 25:12 (December
         1935) 694-697. (History of Medicine in Iowa.) (Pre-
         sentation, Thirty-eighth Annual Session, State Society
         of Iowa Medical Women, Davenport, Iowa, 8 May 1935.)
         A historical summary of the first eight years work of the
         State Society of Iowa Medical Women is expected to inspire
         future meetings to include scientific programs of equal
         value.

3489.   "The Discussion on the Female Physician Question in the
         American Medical Association: [Part I]." Medical and
         Surgical Journal, 84 (25 May 1871) 350-355.
         This article consists of an abstract of the debate over the
         female physicians question [i.e., whether or not to admit
         representatives from female medical colleges as AMA dele-

gates] which occurred at the San Francisco American Medical Association (AMA) convention.   Dr. Hartshorne of
Philadelphia, Pennsylvania proposed an amendment to the
constitution which would permit women to be received into
the AMA.   Several men give their opinions on the issue:
Professor N. S. Davis of Illinois, in asking that the question be carefully considered, says "the female in her proper
sphere is just as far superior to man as man in his proper
sphere is superior to women. [Applause.] You, sir, and
I can no more do properly the work that God designed for
woman than she can do the work designed for you and me
to do. [Applause.]" Dr. James King of Pittsburgh, Pennsylvania feels that "this war against the women is beneath
the dignity of a learned society of scientific men."   Professor Johnson of Missouri feels that women should be permitted
to have as many medical associations as they wish, and "let
them attend to their own business and we will attend to ours
....   This body will stultify itself by the admission of women, or the reception of any representatives of women from
any college or other institution."   The next day the resolution was defeated by a vote of 45 to 41.   In conclusion, Dr.
Davis suggested they take their planned excursion to Oakland, California for the day and finish this business "tomorrow....   It is a question only of Tweedle-dum and Tweedle-
dee."

3490.   "The Discussion on the Female Physician Question in the
          American Medical Association: [Part II]." Medical
          and Surgical Journal, 84 (1 June 1871) 371-374.
     The American Medical Association discussion regarding the
     right of members to meet in consultation with women phy-
     sicians continues.   Dr. Storer argues that women, although
     they make the best nurses, do not inspire confidence as
     doctors since their judgment varies from month to month.
     Dr. Gibbons counters with the observation that male judg-
     ment fluctuates depending on the amount of alcohol con-
     sumed.   Dr. Atlee insists on his right to consult whom he
     pleases, and Dr. Stillé reminds members that the presti-
     gious College of Physicians in Philadelphia "left everybody
     to do as seemed good in his conscience."   The resolution
     to restrict consultation with women physicians was indefinite-
     ly postponed.

3491.   "The Dispensary for Women and Children--The New York
          Infirmary for Women and Children--The Woman's Med-
          ical College--The Olivia Sage Training School of Prac-
          tical Nursing." Medical Woman's Journal, 30:3 (March
          1923) 80-87. port.
     Within this section, which tells how a one-room dispensary
     grew to the present hospital, Eliza M. Mosher writes about
     the Infirmary and Elizabeth M. Cushier presents a history
     of the Infirmary's college.

3492.   "Distaff Doctors." Saturday Evening Post, (9 May 1959)
             28-29. photo.
         A large color photograph shows a group of women physicians
         at the Woman's Medical College of Pennsylvania working
         over a hand injury on a child. The writeup accompanying
         the picture focuses on the 2550 well-trained women the
         College has graduated in its 109-year history and shows the
         international flavor of its student body.

3493.   "Dr. Stella Quinby Root Memorial Nursery." Medical Wo-
             man's Journal, 50:6 (June 1943) 143-144, 160. photo.
         A description of Stamford Hospital is included in this article
         along with biographical data on Dr. Root, who practiced in
         Stamford, Connecticut and devoted much of her time to the
         hospital there. The nursery was named in her honor after
         her death (in 1941).

3494.   Duff, Jane. "Stanford's Young Women in Medicine." Stan-
             ford M.D., 7:2 (Spring-Summer 1968) 10-15. ports.
         In 1968 women made up 12 per cent of Stanford's first-year
         medical school class--the highest percentage in the school's
         history. Upon completion of that year, seven of those wo-
         men give their opinions "on becoming a doctor," "on Stan-
         ford," and "on becoming doctor, wife, and mother."

3495.   Dufner, Mary Elizabeth. "National Fraternities for Women
             in the United States." Medical Woman's Journal, 56:
             11 (November 1949) 24-27. table.
         This article gives facts and figures for medical fraternities
         for women in the United States: Alpha Epsilon Iota, Nu Sig-
         ma Phi, and Zeta Phi.

3496.   Earle, Charles Warrington. The Demand for a Woman's
             Medical College in the West: An Address, Delivered
             at the Commencement of the Seventh Annual Course of
             Lectures and Dedication of the Woman's Medical College,
             Chicago, Illinois. Printed at the Gazette office, Wau-
             kegan, Illinois, 1879, 13 pp.
         [Item not examined by editors.]

3497.   Earle, Charles Warrington. "The Woman's Medical College
             of Chicago. Twenty-One Years of Success [Part I]."
             North American Practitioner, 3 (August 1891) 381-389.
             (Commencement address, Woman's Medical College of
             Chicago, Chicago, Illinois, 1891.)
         Dr. Earle contrasts historical opposition to higher education
         for women with the success evidenced by the approximately
         300 women who have graduated from Woman's Medical Col-
         lege of Chicago. Responses to questionnaires reveal that
         alumnae have met with little prejudice and that few women
         have been refused membership in medical societies (those
         societies refusing to admit women should not be criticized,
         says Dr. Earle, since ladies have clubs which exclude men).

Alumnae also report good health and incomes equal to male
physicians.

3498.   Earle, Charles Warrington. "The Woman's Medical College
             of Chicago. Twenty-One Years of Success [Part II]."
             North American Practitioner, 3 (September 1891) 429-
             436. (Commencement address, Woman's Medical Col-
             lege of Chicago, Chicago, Illinois, 1891.)
         Continuing his reports on the activity and status of the Col-
         lege's alumnae, Dr. Earle focuses upon the work of med-
         ical missionaries and women on the staffs of insane asylums.
         He then generalizes about the rewards and the tribulations
         that await the graduating class and assures them, "The
         world is open to you today. You are not invited into a cold
         unfurnished home. The graduate of twenty-one years ago
         was. For you the light is burning, there is a fire on the
         grate...."

3499.   "Eclectic Department. 'Carpere et Colligere.' Art. I--
             Female Doctors--Amendments Proposed to the Consti-
             tution of the American Medical Association--Views of
             the Advocates for and Against the Movement--Spirited
             Discussions." The Richmond and Louisville Medical
             Journal, 12:1 (July 1871) 16-55.
         In response to an amendment which would admit representa-
         tives from female medical colleges as delegates to the Amer-
         ican Medical Association, individual arguments for and
         against the subject were presented at the annual session.
         Dr. Harding: "I can see no good reason ... why they
         should not be regarded as legally and in fact members of
         the medical profession." Professor N. S. Davis: "We will
         destroy that which God has imprinted upon our race as the
         distinction between male and female in the operations of
         this world." Dr. James King: "Is there anything [in the
         practice of medicine] that does not call forth all there is
         in the heart of a ... woman?" Professor Henry Gibbons:
         "The promiscuous intermingling of [the sexes] in our schools
         and hospitals I utterly repudiate." Professor Johnson: "I
         say let her stay at home and put on an apron, and attend
         to her children, and not come to a Medical Association."
         Dr. Atlee: "Many women earn their livelihood over the
         wash-tub, and many others by the needle, and why should
         they not as well by the profession of medicine? ... Quali-
         fication, and not sex, ought to be the discriminating point
         between members of the medical profession." The proposi-
         tion to amend the constitution was indefinitely postponed.
         Following this discussion, a resolution was offered acknowl-
         edging the right of members to consult with graduates and
         teachers of women's medical colleges. Although arguments
         were offered to suggest the inferiority of women physicians
         on the basis of "uncertain equilibrium," inferiority of judg-
         ment and intellectual ability, etc., the general opinion was
         that the code of ethics was not violated by consulting with

female practitioners and the resolution was indefinitely post-
poned.

3500.   "Editorial." Medical Woman's Journal, 29:12 (December
             1922) 335-336.
         "Possibilities" and "probabilities" for the Medical Woman's
         Journal in the future are discussed. It is hoped the Jour-
         nal will become the "mouthpiece" for medical women.

3501.   "Editorial." Medical Woman's Journal, 50:7 (July 1943) 181
         A medical woman's journal is necessary to aid in maintain-
         ing a united front on issues vital to medical women. Wo-
         men physicians are such a minority that it is necessary to
         publicize their existence in order to encourage other women
         to study and practice medicine.

3502.   Elliott, Mabel. "American Women's Hospitals...." Med-
             ical Woman's Journal, 30:2 (February 1923) 54-55.
         Published is a letter written by Dr. Elliott to the Ameri-
         can Women's Hospitals headquarters. She vividly describes
         the wretched conditions in Greece, which due to an influx
         of war refugees and an outbreak of typhus and smallpox, has
         become "a pest hole." Dr. Elliott tells of her efforts in
         establishing a quarantine station on the island of Macronissi.

3503.   Ellis, Ruth M. "How the AMWA Can Help Me in the Pur-
             suit of My Career." Journal of the American Medical
             Women's Association, 11:6 (June 1956) 213-214.
         "How the AMWA Could Have Helped Me and Didn't, But
         Might Yet," is the alternative title Ruth M. Ellis would
         have preferred for this first-prize winning essay "sponsored
         by AMWA for medical students, interns or residents." The
         American Medical Women's Association could be doing con-
         siderably more than it does to advertise its existence and to
         formulate programs that actually would help women medical
         students, interns, and residents. Suggestions for a more
         effective American Medical Women's Association include:
         ask AMWA members to contact women medical students and
         offer to be available for questions about problems, help stu-
         dents find loans if necessary, establish a small monetary
         award at medical school graduation for the outstanding wo-
         man student (to give itself publicity), offer a form of em-
         ployment clearinghouse information, really urge and then
         welcome women interns and residents to attend meetings,
         send every woman medical student a pamphlet about the his-
         tory of women in medicine. There is a brief biographical
         inset on Ruth M. Ellis.

3504.   "Equal Rights for Men and Women." Medical Woman's
             Journal, 38:5 (May 1931) 126. (Editorial.)
         Advance program announcements of medical association con-
         ventions for May and June, 1931 have one thing in common:
         women doctors are represented on the programs of only one

convention (California). The omission of women from these
programs indicates that men prefer to keep medical experiences within their own group, and that they "are determined
to circumscribe [the woman physician's] opportunities and
minimize her importance." The omission also indicates that
women "are a bit too ready to accept the valuation put on
their ability and importance by men physicians."

3505. "Eureka! Women to Be Admitted to the Medical Department
of Columbia University." Woman's Medical Journal, 26:
3 (March 1916) 70.

3506. "Extension Campaign for the Woman's Medical College:
Medical Women Should Rally to the Support of the Only
Woman's Medical College in the United States." Wo-
man's Medical Journal, 29[19]:10 (October 1919) 215.
(Editorial.)

3507. Fall Announcement of the Penn Medical College of Philadelphia. Female Session. G. S. Harris, Printer,
Philadelphia, Pennsylvania, 1853, 16 pp.
This pamphlet describes the philosophy, course of instruction, and expenses for the female session of Penn Medical
College. Costs for two sessions, which include matricula-
tion, instruction, practical anatomy, and board, add up to
$210. The reader is assured that "the useless employment
of the bleeding lancet, the scarificator, and the loathsome
leech, will find no countenance among the teachings of our
school."

3508. "Fame Has a Feminine Gender." Philadelphia Magazine,
(December 1950) 28. ports.
The Woman's Medical College of Pennsylvania celebrated
its centennial by conferring honorary degrees on nine distinguished Americans, four of them women physicians:
Florence Barbara Seibert, whose techniques made intraven-
ous injections safe; Elise Strang L'Esperance, who set up
the first cancer preventive clinic in the U.S.; Florence R.
Sabin, public health worker in Colorado; and Alice Hamilton,
assistant professor in industrial medicine at Harvard Medical School.

3509. Fay, Marion. "The First Woman's Medical College: 1850-
1975." Philadelphia Medicine, 71:10 (October 1975)
413-421.
Background on the establishment of the Female Medical College of Pennsylvania is given, beginning with Sara Josepha
Hale's enthusiastic support and Dr. Joseph Longshore's and
William Mullen's securing on March 11, 1850, a charter
for the College. A history of the various locations of the
school and the several name changes are included by the
author, a former president and dean of the College. Outstanding women who played a major role in the development
of the College are discussed.

3510.   Fay, Marion. "To the New Century." Journal of the
        American Medical Women's Association, 5:9 (Septem-
        ber 1950) 367.   illus.
        "The first century [of the Woman's Medical College of Penn-
        sylvania] has demonstrated that a medical school for women
        can successfully train students for practice, for training,
        and for research--the three important functions of any med-
        ical school."

3511.   Fay, Marion. "The Woman's Medical College of Pennsyl-
        vania: 1850-1950." The Scalpel, 11:1 (November 1950)
        6, 7-10, 31.   illus., photo., port.
        This brief history of the Woman's Medical College of Phila-
        delphia covers its founding in 1850, the early graduates
        whose accomplishments helped insure the school's success
        (Ann Preston, Emeline Cleveland, Elizabeth Shattuck, and
        Clara Swain), barriers of prejudice encountered in the ef-
        fort to educate women as physicians, and the development
        of the College into a modern medical school and hospital.

3512.   "Female Medical Colleges." Boston Medical and Surgical
        Journal, 45 (1851) 106-107.
        This article presents a review of these institutions. [Arti-
        cle not examined by editors.]

3513.   Female Medical Education Society (Boston). Report from
        November, 1848, to December, 1850; Containing the
        Charter, Constitution, By-laws, Names of Officers and
        Members, Together with Information Respecting the
        Boston Female Medical School and the Proposed Clinical
        Hospital, Which Is to Form a Part of the Institution,
        etc.   Boston, Massachusetts, 1851.
        [Item not examined by editors.]

3514.   Finkler, Rita S. "A Committee for the Relief of Distressed
        Women Physicians." Medical Woman's Journal, 49:5
        (May 1942) 135-136.
        The Committee, formed by the American Medical Women's
        Association in 1938, gives advice, financial aid, and em-
        ployment guidance to refugee women physicians who came to
        the U.S. from Austria and Germany.

3515.   "The First Annual Meeting of the Medical Women's National
        Association." Woman's Medical Journal, 26:5 (May
        1916) 133.   port.
        This article announces the first annual meeting of the Med-
        ical Women's National Association which was to be held on
        June 13, 1916.   The intended goals of this organization in-
        clude: helping to increase the number of women studying
        medicine as well as upholding the standards of women stu-
        dents, making it possible for women to be represented on
        staffs of hospitals and on the faculty at universities, and
        helping medical women serving in foreign countries keep in-
        formed about the progress in medicine and surgery.

3516.   "First Woman Delegate to the A.M.A." Medical Woman's
        Journal, 35:4 (April 1928) 108.
        As a delegate from the Illinois State Medical Society, Sarah
        Hackett Stevenson became the first woman physician to be
        elected a member of the American Medical Association.
        She is listed on the minutes of an AMA meeting held in
        Philadelphia, June 6-9, 1876. Confirmation of these facts
        was obtained by Bertha Van Hoosen in a letter she re-
        ceived from the Association.

3517.   Fleming, Ruth. "Equal Rights." Journal of the American
        Medical Women's Association, 28:6 (June 1973) 321.
        (AMWA President's Message.)
        American Medical Women's Association members should
        support Equal Rights Amendment legislation.

3518.   Forbes, Shirley J. "Future Aspects of the American Med-
        ical Women's Association." Journal of the American
        Medical Women's Association, 29:11 (November 1974)
        494-495.

3519.   Fraade, Estelle and Reid, Ada Chree. "The American Wo-
        men's Hospitals: A Half-Century of Service." Journal
        of the American Medical Women's Association, 22:8
        (August 1967) 548-571. photos., ports.
        A review is given of the history of American Women's Hos-
        pitals (AWH) upon the occasion of their 50th Anniversary.
        First conceived by the American Medical Women's Association's
        War Service Committee in 1917, the AWH was formed to
        "offer medical aid wherever needed" during World War I.
        The services of AWH did not terminate after the war. The
        article is organized into five decades. The various geo-
        graphical areas of service covered by AWH are discussed
        under each decade.

3520.   Frankfeldt, Gwen. "Doing Women's Work." Harvard Med-
        ical Alumni Bulletin, 50:1 (September/October 1975) 29-
        32. ports. (The Joint Committee on the Status of
        Women.)
        The Joint Committee on the Status of Women, formed in
        1973, reviews and recommends improvements in the status
        of women at the Harvard Schools of Medicine, Dental Medi-
        cine, and Public Health. The 26-member committee draws
        from faculty, employees, students, and hospital house offi-
        cers. This article is an interview with committee repre-
        sentatives.

3521.   Frazer, Mary Margaret. "Elizabeth Blackwell Centennial:
        1949." Medical Woman's Journal, 56:4 (April 1949)
        40-41.
        Detroit medical women honored Dr. Blackwell in 1944 by
        naming their branch of the American Medical Women's Asso-
        ciation after her.

3522.   Frost, Lorraine. "Student News." Medical Woman's Jour-
         nal, 53:5 (May 1946) 64, 62. photo.
         In a special meeting, students of the Woman's Medical Col-
         lege of Pennsylvania voted to oppose merger plans between
         the College and Jefferson Medical College. A brief biogra-
         phy of Dr. Martha Tracy is presented.

3523.   Frost, Lorraine. "Student News: Woman's Medical Col-
         lege." Medical Woman's Journal, 53:3 (March 1946)
         56. photo.
         The 36 graduates of the Woman's Medical College of Penn-
         sylvania's class of 1946 are listed.

3524.   Frost, Lorraine and Frank, Mary. "Student News." Med-
         ical Woman's Journal, 53:2 (February 1946) 56, 58.
         photos.
         Described is the ninety-fourth annual commencement of the
         Woman's Medical College of Pennsylvania, during which 36
         women received degrees.

3525.   [Gaillard, E. S.] "Tweedle Dum and Tweedle Dee; or The
         Proceedings of the American Medical Association."
         The Richmond and Louisville Medical Journal, 12:1
         (July 1871) 114-117. (Editorial.)
         The proceedings of the 1871 meeting of the American Med-
         ical Association "amounted to about the difference between
         tweedle dum and tweedle dee," because the spirited discus-
         sion of the "woman question" was the chief work of this
         meeting and no consensus was reached. "Nothing of a sci-
         entific character [was] done by the Association." In the
         future it is hoped the Association "will confine itself to
         strictly scientific labors, and resign the functions of a ju-
         dicial regulator to a new and now necessary organization."

3526.   Gassett, Helen M. Categorical Account of the Female Med-
         ical College, to The People of the New England States.
         Printed for the author, Boston, Massachusetts, 1855,
         138 pp.
         The author has written this book in an attempt to seek re-
         dress for having been placed in an unfavorable position be-
         fore the public in regard to events at the Female Medical
         College of Boston. In 1845, Helen Gassett agreed to be-
         come an agent for the distribution of circulars and other
         material of the American Medical Education Society in order
         to solicit support and funds for the Female Medical Col-
         lege of Boston. She attempted to persuade wealthy and in-
         fluential ladies of the worth of the proposed Female Medical
         College and to persuade women to attend the school when it
         opened. The book deals with the author's efforts to influ-
         ence people, the towns she visited, and the tactics she used,
         in addition to events leading up to her public discrediting by
         Samuel Gregory who on 16 June 1852 had printed a "Caution
         to the Public" which stated that "Hellen Maria Rice, alias

Hellen Maria Gassett ... [is] still continuing to collect
[funds]" even though she had been dismissed by the directors of the Society because she was "found unworthy of confidence." Gassett refutes these claims and offers a summary of the libel suit she brought against the directors.
The author claims the directors turned against her because
she refused to be a party to their motives which were not
to "advance the cause of true medical science, so much as
to promote private pecuniary gain."

3527. Gibbons, Marion N. "A Note on Women in Medicine Among
Graduates of Western Reserve University." Medical
Woman's Journal, 52:10 (October 1945) 45-46, 57.
In 1944 a questionnaire was sent to the 61 living women
medical graduates of the Medical School of Western Reserve
University. This questionnaire was inspired by a desire to
know "whether the investment the Medical School has made
in educating women students has paid dividends worthy of
its continuance." Fifty-six women responded to the questionnaire. A breakdown of the responses is given.

3528. Gillett, Josephine D. "The Woman's Hospital of Cleveland,
Ohio." Medical and Professional Woman's Journal,
40:10 (October 1933) 300-301. photo., port.
This article traces the history of the Woman's Hospital of
Cleveland, Ohio from its founding in 1878, as the Women's
and Children's Free Medical and Surgical Dispensary.

3529. "Girls' Medical School: Woman's Medical College of Pennsylvania, Now 95 Years Old, Is the Only One in the
U.S." Life, (10 December 1945) 91-94.
Several pages of photographs illustrate the training which
future women doctors receive at the Woman's Medical College of Pennsylvania.

3530. "The Gotham Hospital." Medical Woman's Journal, 36:4
(April 1929) 87-89.
The Gotham Hospital plan is herein discussed. The Hospital will "assist in the advancement of women physicians
and surgeons by breaking down a spurious and unwarrantable
distinction in medical work. The chiefs-of-staff are to be
women.... The establishment of the Gotham Hospital will
mark a transitional stage from the time when women physicians were obliged to use separate colleges and hospitals
to the time when there will be physicians in institutions
with no discrimination as between the sexes." This hospital (as well as this article) is the result of a need felt
by the women physicians of New York City upon the merger
of the New York Infirmary for Women and Children with the
Columbia-Presbyterian Hospital Medical Center [a "Correction and Apology" for this inaccurate information appeared
in the May, 1929 issue of this journal, p. 137].

3531.   "Greetings: First in the Field--a Journal Devoted to the
            Interests of Women Medical Practitioners." Medical
            Woman's Journal, 50:1 (January 1943) 20.
         This article [reprinted from the Toledo Daily Commercial,
         January 1893] welcomes the Woman's Medical Journal as a
         new publication in Toledo, Ohio.

3532.   "Greetings to the AMWA." Medical Woman's Journal, 48:
            5 (May 1941) 155-156. (Editorial.)
         A Welcome-to-the-Ohio-Convention greeting to AMWA mem-
         bers briefly discusses the value of the Journal.

3533.   Greisheimer, Esther M. "Woman's Medical College of
            Pennsylvania: Department of Physiology." Women in
            Medicine, 75 (January 1942) 17-18. photo.
         This, the first in a series of articles about different depart-
         ments of the College, describes the organization and func-
         tions of the Department of Physiology.

3534.   Grigg, Tony. "Medical Magazine Fifty Years Old." Med-
            ical Woman's Journal, 50:9 (September 1943) 242.
         This is a very brief overview of the history of the Medical
         Woman's Journal, whose offices are in Cincinnati, Ohio.
         [This note was apparently reprinted from the Cincinnati
         Times-Star on 12 July 1943.]

3535.   Grigg, Tony. "Medical Woman's Society of New York
            State." Medical Woman's Journal, 51:12 (December
            1944) 24.
         Postwar medical education was the topic of discussion at
         the Society's meeting, held in November [1944]. Several
         speakers are quoted.

3536.   Griscom, Mary W. "History of Woman's Hospital of Phila-
            delphia. On Adventure Bound: 1861-1934." Medical
            Woman's Journal, 41:11 (November 1934) 291-295. pho-
            tos.
         The first article in a two-part account of the formative
         years of the Woman's Hospital of Philadelphia extracts de-
         tails from minutes of the early meetings of the institution's
         founders.

3537.   Griscom, Mary W. "History of Woman's Hospital of Phila-
            delphia. On Adventure Bound: 1861-1934." Medical
            Woman's Journal, 41:12 (December 1934) 318-325.
            photos.
         The second and final article about the early years of the
         Woman's Hospital of Philadelphia traces events up to the
         present (1934).

3538.   Griswold, Bernice. "The New York Infirmary for Women
            and Children." Medical Woman's Journal, 36:11 (No-
            vember 1929) 289-290. sketch.

This article discusses new-building plans for the New York Infirmary for Women and Children. A sketch of the proposed new building is included.

3539. "Hahnemann Medical College." Medical Woman's Journal, 48:8 (August 1941) 253.
This article, reproduced from the Philadelphia Inquirer of 23 May 1941, was written upon the announcement that the College would admit women students the next year for the first time in its 93-year history. Beginning in the fall, 10 per cent of approximately 150 students admitted each term were to be women. "'With more women in practice,'" Dr. Von Rapp is quoted as saying, "'it naturally will release more men for government service.'"

3540. Hale, Sarah J. "An Appeal to American Christians on Behalf of the Ladies' Medical Missionary Society." Godey's Lady's Book, 64:18 (March 1852) 185-188.
The preamble from the "Rules of the Ladies' Medical Missionary Society" is quoted to explain the purpose of the Society. The author then proceeds to discuss the propriety of admitting women to the study of medicine. The Female Medical Education Society in Boston and its consequent New England Female Medical College are covered.

3541. Hamilton, Edith Hulbert. "New York Medical College and Hospital for Women." Woman's Medical Journal, 26:3 (March 1916) 64-67. photo., port. ("The Field for Women of Today in Medicine: College, Hospital, Laboratory and Practice." Mary Sutton Macy, editor.)
Founded by Dr. Clemence Sophie Lozier in 1863, the New York Medical College and Hospital for Women was an institution where women who wanted medical training and practical experience could obtain it. This article includes a brief history of this school.

3542. Harvard University Medical Alumni Association. The First Decade of Women in the Harvard Medical School, 1949-1959. Harvard University, Cambridge, Massachusetts, 1959.
[Item not examined by editors.]

3543. Harvard University Medical School. [Majority and Minority Report Upon the Offer of Miss Marian Hovey, Made March 21, 1878, Proposing to Give the Sum of Ten Thousand Dollars to the Harvard Medical School, if its Advantages Can be Offered to Women on Equal Terms with Men. May 3, 1879]. [Boston, Massachusetts, 1879].
[Item not examined by editors.]

3544. "Health Legislation Promoted by Women Physicians." Medical Woman's Journal, 45:11 (November 1938) 342. (Editorial.)

The New York State legislature passed several laws that were advocated and worked out by the Women's Medical Society of New York State. Among those laws were ones requiring premarital couples and pregnant women to have Wassermann tests, and one which stated that "all birth control measures and advice be in the hands of physicians only."

3545. Heinz, Margaret S. "How the AMWA Can Help Me in the Pursuit of My Career." Journal of the American Medical Women's Association, 11:9 (September 1956) 322. This essay won second prize in the AMWA-sponsored contest for medical students, interns, and residents. AMWA can best help this recent medical graduate to secure her goals "by offering the woman physician intellectual stimulation, concrete aid, and sympathetic colleagues."

3546. "Help Finish This Job." Medical Woman's Journal, 28:3 (March 1921) 72-74. photos., ports. (Hospitals & Colleges.) The work of Dr. Etta Gray and her associates in Serbia, and other activities of the American Women's Hospitals organization, are mentioned.

3547. Hewitt, Dorothy. "History of Branch Thirty-Eight." Journal of the American Medical Women's Association, 10: 12 (December 1955) 431. This article is a short history of the Long Beach, California branch of the American Medical Women's Association. This branch was organized in 1950.

3548. Hillman, Sara Frazer. The Founding of Scholarships in the Medical School of the University of Pittsburgh By the Congress of Women's Clubs of Western Pennsylvania and a Sketch of the Woman Doctor of Yesterday and Today. [Pittsburgh, Pennsylvania], 1916, 39 pp. ports. This book, which is in recognition of the establishment in 1912 of scholarships for women in the University of Pittsburgh Medical School, includes sketches of the work of some women physicians in the early 20th century. There are photographs of several women, including Luba Robin Goldsmith, president of the Women's Medical Society of Pittsburgh (1913-14), and Evangeline Young, founder of the School of Eugenics, Boston.

3549. Hocker, Elizabeth Van Cortlandt. "The Laura Memorial Woman's Medical College." Medical Woman's Journal, 53:9 (September 1946) 46-49. sketch. (History of Women in Medicine, Bertha Selmon, ed.) "The history of this college is a short, short story, but full of action." In 1887 the Cincinnati College of Medicine and Surgery established a department known as the Woman's

Medical College of Cincinnati. In 1890 the College became an independent institution, but closed five years later. Its students were transferred to the newly-established Laura Memorial Woman's Medical College of Cincinnati which, in turn, lasted eight years. In 1903 the Miami Medical College absorbed it, and in 1910 the University of Cincinnati absorbed the Miami Medical College.

3550.   Houghton, Dorothy D. "Woman's Opportunity for Service: A Mid-Century Look." Journal of the American Medical Women's Association, 10:5 (May 1955) 161-165. (Address, Woman's Medical College of Pennsylvania, Philadelphia, 9 June 1954.)
The past struggles are viewed as creating a present in which equality of opportunity for women physicians has arrived--"the dream materialized"; the future is seen as a medical challenge. Women physicians' work with the Foreign Operations Administration is highlighted.

3551.   [Hurd-] Mead, Kate Campbell. "The American Medical Women's National Association, Inc." Medical Women's Federation News-Letter, (April 1933) 48-52.
The work of some of the Association's 16 committees is explained: the American Women's Hospitals; the committee of medical opportunities for women; the committees on public health and race betterment; the history of women in medicine committee; and the legislative committee. In conclusion, Dr. Mead informs her British readers that "America is over-supplied with doctors and surgeons, and ... women as a rule do better, financially, than men...."

3552.   Hurd-Mead, Kate Campbell. "Forty Years of Medical Progress: Reminiscences and Comparisons." In: 75th Anniversary Volume of the Woman's Medical College of Pennsylvania. Westbrook Publishing Company, Philadelphia, Pennsylvania, [1925?], 171-183. photo., ports.
In a backward glance through the years since she graduated in 1888, Dr. Hurd-Mead finds "much to praise and very little to criticize" in Woman's Medical College of Pennsylvania. Dr. Hurd-Mead's reminiscences include descriptions of many faculty members.

3553.   Hurrell, M. Louise. "Most Interesting Report from Dr. Louise Hurrell, Director of A.W.H. at Luzancy." Woman's Medical Journal, 29[19]:3 (March 1919) 49. port., photo.

3554.   Hurrell, [M.] Louise. "Thrilling Story of American Women's Hospitals in France." Woman's Medical Journal, 29[19]:11 (November 1919) 227-228. photo., port.

3555.   "In Command of an American Woman Doctor." Medical Woman's Journal, 27:1 (January 1920) 20.

Dr. Virginia Murray's American Red Cross unit in Eastern
Poland is discussed, as well as the work of Dr. Emily A.
Pratt.

3556.   "An Interesting and Pertinent Retrospect." Medical Wo-
         man's Journal, 42:3 (March 1935) 78-79. (Editorial.)
         This article gives a historical overview of the Medical
         Women's National Association and the Medical Woman's
         Journal.

3557.   J. Mc. "The State Society of Iowa Medical Women." Wo-
         man's Medical Journal, 12:7 (July 1902) 170-171.
         The oldest if not the only state medical society composed
         entirely of women, the State Society of Iowa Medical Women
         disclaims all "idea of antagonism" to male physicians.
         The purpose of a separate society was to bind women to-
         gether in "fraternal helpfulness."

3558.   Jacobi, Mary Putnam. "Progress in Medical Education--
         The Women Taking the Lead." Medical Record, 38
         (21 November 1885) 584.
         Dr. Putnam-Jacobi writes this letter to the editor to in-
         form readers of the separation of the study of therapeutics
         and materia medica at the Woman's Medical College of
         Pennsylvania.

3559.   Johnston, Pauline. "College's Archives Preserve History
         of Women in Medicine." Alumnae News [Medical Col-
         lege of Pennsylvania], 26:1 (February 1975) 8-9. ports.
         The author, an archives assistant at the Medical College
         of Pennsylvania's Florence A. Moore Library of Medicine,
         describes the institution's historical collection. Books, per-
         sonal correspondence, and artifacts tell the history of the
         College and the life stories of many of the women graduates.
         A sidebar to the article lists many of the more distinguished
         graduates of the College.

3560.   "The Journal." Medical Woman's Journal, 52:6 (June 1945)
         49. (Editorial.)
         A brief history of the Woman's Medical Journal is herein
         given.

3561.   "The Journal and Directory of Alpha Epsilon Iota Fraternity."
         Woman's Medical Journal, 26:10 (October 1916) 246.
         The Alpha Epsilon Iota Fraternity, founded at the University
         of Michigan in 1890, has branches at other medical schools
         in the United States. This article announces that there is
         now a Journal and Directory of the Alpha Epsilon Iota Fra-
         ternity which will publish news of the programs and meetings
         of the various chapters of this medical women's society, as
         well as scientific articles.

3562.   "The Journal's Platform for Women Doctors." Medical

Woman's Journal, 52:11 (November 1945) 33.   (Editorial.)

The 11 "planks" which constitute this platform are listed. Among them are "encouragement of college women to enroll in medical schools," "establishment of a requirement that all institutions housing women patients or inmates have women physicians in attendance," and various demands for equal opportunities.

3563.   Kandravy, Anna M. and Ahlum, Carol.   "Programs of the Center for Women in Medicine."   Alumnae News [The Medical College of Pennsylvania], 26:1 (February 1975) 10-11.

The Medical College of Pennsylvania's 1974 Summer Premedical Program, in which ten women pre-med students spent eight weeks attending seminars and observing routine at the College's hospital, is explained.   Another project of the Center is a three-year contract to study physician inactivity.   Funded by the Office of Health Resources Opportunity, U.S. Department of Health, Education and Welfare, the study also includes a retraining program.

3564.   Kanof, Naomi M.   "Memo from the Editor."   Journal of the American Medical Women's Association, 30:11 (November 1975) 436.

In the 1930s Bertha Van Hoosen suggested that the American Medical Women's Association create a doll collection depicting distinguished women physicians.   In 1975 the dolls (some of which are portrayed on the cover of this month's Journal) were presented to the Smithsonian Institution.   Included in this "memo" is a brief profile of Dr. Anna Dengel, the only living person represented in the doll collection.

3565.   Kazmierczak, Mary J.   "Mid-Year Meeting of the Women's Medical Society of the State of New York: Women Physicians go on Record as Opposed to State Medicine. Official Report."   Medical Woman's Journal, 38:4 (April 1931) 97.   (Meeting, Women's Medical Society of New York State, Buffalo, New York, 28 February 1931.)

Dr. Louise W. Beamis, president of the Women's Medical Society of the State of New York, urges women physicians to "present a solid front against the insidious attempts, made under the cloak of charity, to destroy our medical ethics and permit the State in its impersonal way to supplant the family physician."   She speculates that with state medicine, "Our professional pride will slump to political expediency."

3566.   Keene, Mrs. Charles M.   "Women and Children's Hospital of Chicago."   Medical Woman's Journal, 34:2 (February 1927) 49.   illus.

The publicity chairman for the Women and Children's Hospital outlines the history of the hospital.

3567.   Kittredge, Elizabeth. "Woman's Medical Society of District
        of Columbia: The History of Branch One of the
        A.M.W.A." Journal of the American Medical Women's
        Association, 6:11 (November 1951) 443-445.

3568.   Kleinert, Margaret Noyes. "Medical Women in New Eng-
        land: History of the New England Women's Medical
        Society." Journal of the American Medical Women's
        Association, 11:2 (February 1956) 63-64, 67.
        A history of branch thirty-nine of the American Medical
        Women's Association is presented.

3569.   Lakeman, Mary R. "Annual Meeting of Association Women
        in Public Health: [Official Report]." Medical Woman's
        Journal, 42:11 (November 1935) 311-312.
        A history of the Association is given, following its growth
        from its inception in 1920 in New York, through its succes-
        sive annual meetings, to its accomplishments. The purpose
        of the organization, according to its sponsors, should be
        "to afford women who make public health their profession
        an opportunity of studying together the problems and inter-
        relationships of public health activities and to keep in touch
        with national and international developments in public health."

3570.   Lakeman, Mary R. "Association of Women in Public
        Health." Medical Woman's Journal, 31:7 (July 1924)
        212-213.
        One-hundred and twenty-six women physicians belong to the
        Association of Women in Public Health, a composite organ-
        ization that includes ten health professions: medicine, nurs-
        ing, social work, teaching, laboratory technique, publicity,
        vital statistics, nutrition, oral hygiene, secretarial science.
        Women in these health fields and other fields which were
        beginning to open to women felt "that there was a growing
        demand for freer interchange of thought and experience
        among public health women than has been found possible with-
        in any existing organization ... more important than any
        material accomplishment the Association can point to in its
        four years of life may be counted its service in fostering
        the acquaintanceship of women workers in the field of public
        health endeavor--its own members--and in making them feel
        themselves a part of the great world-wide movement for a
        stronger and a healthier race."

3571.   Lakeman, Mary R. "The Women's Field Army." Medical
        Woman's Journal, 45:2 (February 1938) 51-52.
        Dr. Lakeman, regional director of the Women's Field Army
        of the American Association for the Control of Cancer, ex-
        plains the organizational structure of the Army. Because
        many women will more readily submit to examination by an-
        other woman, the woman physician has special responsibility
        in the control of breast and cervical cancer. Medical wo-
        men should lend their fullest support to the endeavors of the
        Women's Field Army.

3572.   Leaman, William G. "Woman's Medical College of Penn-
          sylvania: Historical Sketch." Journal of the Ameri-
          can Medical Women's Association, 2:10 (October 1947)
          460-462. facsims.
          This article traces the history of the Woman's Medical Col-
          lege of Pennsylvania from its charter, granted on March
          11, 1850, to the article's present. Faculty, fees, enroll-
          ment, and geographical moves of the College are touched
          upon.

3573.   "Legitimate Force." Medical Woman's Journal, 45:5 (May
          1938) 140. (Editorial.)
          Women's medical societies must unite and exert pressure
          to increase the educational and service opportunities avail-
          able to medical women, and to direct legislation that af-
          fects women and children.

3574.   L'Esperance, Elise S. "The Advantages of Women's Med-
          ical Societies." Medical Woman's Journal, 43:6 (June
          1936) 150-151. (Presentation, 30th Annual Meeting,
          Women's Medical Society of New York State, New York
          City, 27 April 1936.)
          "Segregation is not the purpose of a women's medical asso-
          ciation." The purposes of such organizations include: unit-
          ing to influence legislation that is beneficial to women phy-
          sicians; raising and distributing educational funds; and bring-
          ing to the attention of medical women the achievements of
          their counterparts.

3575.   L'Esperance, Elise S. "The Future of the Woman's Med-
          ical Association of New York City." Medical Woman's
          Journal, 31:4 (April 1924) 87-89. (Read before the
          Woman's Medical Association of New York City, May
          1923.)
          The Woman's Medical Association of New York City has
          been in existence for 53 years. This Association was
          founded for two primary reasons: to assist and further the
          efforts of Drs. Elizabeth and Emily Blackwell with the
          struggling Women's Medical College of the New York In-
          firmary, and to give the alumnae of that school an oppor-
          tunity to keep in touch with their alma mater. In 1885
          three women decided to expand their intent "to promote the
          knowledge of science and medicine; to advance the mutual
          interest of its members, as well as those of the College
          and the Infirmary, and to secure regular, accurate and
          permanent records of the Alumnae." In 1900 the Associa-
          tion expanded membership to all women physicians. In
          answer to criticisms that women do not need to maintain a
          separate medical society, Dr. L'Esperance responds, "Un-
          doubtedly we have far greater medical advantages than the
          brave, early pioneers, but I hasten to add--we are still a
          long way from attaining the opportunities granted our more
          fortunate brother medical men."

3576.   L'Esperance, Elise S. "Influence of the New York Infir-
         mary on Women in Medicine." Journal of the Ameri-
         can Medical Women's Association, 4:6 (June 1949) 255-
         261. photos., ports. (Inaugural Address, American
         Medical Women's Association, Chicago, Illinois, 19
         June 1948.)
         The Infirmary was founded as part of the pioneer movement
         described in an 1855 address by Elizabeth Blackwell as "a
         revival in advanced form of work in which women had al-
         ways been engaged, but in a form suited to the enlarged
         capabilities of women." A history of the establishment of
         the Infirmary is given, and distinguished alumnae are men-
         tioned.

3577.   L'Esperance, Elise S. "Suggestions for the Development of
         the Woman's State Medical Association." Medical Wo-
         man's Journal, 44:6 (June 1937) 175-176.
         Dr. L'Esperance offers suggestions to increase the useful-
         ness of the Women's Medical Society of New York State,
         the second organization for medical women in the United
         States.

3578.   Lichtenstein, Julia V. "Address by President of Women's
         Medical Association of New York City (Branch Four-
         teen)." Journal of the American Medical Women's
         Association, 15:8 (August 1960) 778-779. (Presentation,
         Annual Spring Meeting, Women's Medical Association of
         New York City, 28 April 1960.)
         During Dr. Lichtenstein's tenure as president of the Wo-
         men's Medical Association of New York City, all the min-
         utes and other written materials of the Association since
         its 1892 beginning were collected. The New York Academy
         of Medicine is storing these records. Dr. Romaine be-
         came the first woman to be elected to the Comita Minora
         of the New York County Medical Society. The Women's
         Medical Association of New York City should consider more
         active participation and show greater concern in working
         with the New York County Medical Society on legislative is-
         sues.

3579.   Lichtenstein, Julia V. "Introductory Remarks at Fiftieth
         Anniversary of Women's Medical Association of New
         York City (Branch Fourteen)." Journal of the American
         Medical Women's Association, 15:8 (August 1960) 780.

3580.   Longshore, Joseph S. Introductory Lecture Delivered in
         the Female Department of the Penn Medical University
         of Philadelphia, October 1, 1860, Being a Review of
         the Action of the Pennsylvania State Medical Society,
         in Relation to Female Physicians and Female Medical
         Colleges. Published by the class, Philadelphia, Penn-
         sylvania, 1861, 18 pp.
         Dr. Longshore begins his lecture with a tribute to Mary

Elizabeth Frost, a medical student at the university who
had recently died. Following a discussion of the courses
to be pursued and the various existing branches of medicine, Dr. Longshore reviews in general the struggle of women to obtain medical training, the objectives of Penn
Medical University in particular. Finally, Dr. Longshore
reviews the attitude toward women physicians held by the
Pennsylvania State Medical Society, and answers their remarks with his own.

3581.   Loomis, Metta. "Medical Societies: Chicago Council of
         Medical Women." Medical Woman's Journal, 39:2
         (February 1932) 44-45.
         The Quine Library, College of Medicine, University of
         Illinois, sponsored a library display on the activities of
         women in medicine when the Chicago Council of Medical
         Women met there on January 8, 1932.

3582.   Lovejoy, Esther Pohl. "American Women Physicians in
         Serbia." Medical Woman's Journal, 27:2 (February
         1920) 44-57. photos., ports. (Newsletter.)
         This report of the work of the American Women's Hospitals
         in Serbia, Turkey, Armenia, and France during 1919 in-
         cludes portraits of and information on several women phy-
         sicians.

3583.   Lovejoy, Esther Pohl. "The American Women's Hospitals."
         Medical Review of Reviews, 37:3 (March 1931) 149-156.
         Given is a history of the American Women's Hospitals,
         which was founded by the Medical Women's National Asso-
         ciation during the world war. Past and current work in
         foreign countries and proposed activity within the U.S. are
         described. Also mentioned: the rewards American women
         reap while serving the organization, e.g., discovering that
         European and other peoples are similar to Americans.

3584.   Lovejoy, Esther Pohl. "American Women's Hospitals."
         Medical Review of Reviews, 39:5 (May 1933) 204-214.
         This article discusses the work of the Rural and Mountain
         Medical Service of the American Women's Hospitals (AWH).
         The article is divided into several sections, each written
         by a different woman physician. Dr. Rosa L. Gantt de-
         scribes services of the AWH in North Carolina; Dr. Hilla
         Sheriff writes of AWH work in South Carolina; and Dr.
         Lillian South covers the Kentucky sector.

3585.   Lovejoy, Esther Pohl. "American Women's Hospitals:
         Reconstruction Committee of the Medical Women's Na-
         tional Association. Headquarters, 637 Madison Ave.,
         New York: Summary of Work of Year." Medical Wo-
         man's Journal, 27:4 (April 1920) 100-106. photos.
         (Hospitals and Colleges.)

3586.   Lovejoy, Esther P[ohl]. "American Women's Hospitals:
        637 Madison Ave., New York." Medical Woman's Jour-
        nal, 29:8 (August 1922) 199-201. photos., port. (Hos-
        pitals & Colleges.)
        A brief narrative and pictorial account of the American
        Women's Hospitals discusses in part the work of Dr. Etta
        Gray in Serbia.

3587.   Lovejoy, Esther P[ohl]. "Annual Report of the American
        Women's Hospitals to the Medical Women's National
        Association." Medical Woman's Journal, 32:8 (August
        1925) 215-218.
        Dr. Lovejoy prints the communications received from the
        American Women's Hospitals representatives for 1924-1925,
        describing general medical service, the operation of hos-
        pitals and clinics, distribution of food and clothing for
        Greece, Turkey, Serbia, Russia, France, Japan, and Ar-
        menia. She also reports that during her chairmanship,
        despite the arduous and trying work of the American Wo-
        men's Hospitals Committee, "no member of the Committee
        has resigned, but the spirit of devotion and loyalty to this
        service and to each other has grown stronger with the pass-
        ing years."

3588.   Lovejoy, Esther Pohl. "Annual Report of American Wo-
        men's Hospitals to the Medical Women's National Asso-
        ciation." Medical Woman's Journal, 36:8 (August 1929)
        211-215.
        In Dr. Lovejoy's annual report, the spread of tuberculosis
        is discussed. The work of American Women's Hospitals in
        various parts of the world is reviewed.

3589.   Lovejoy, Esther Pohl. Certain Samaritans. The Macmil-
        lan Company, New York, New York, 1927, 302 pp.
        photos.
        In this book on the American Women's Hospitals (AWH),
        Dr. Esther Lovejoy, former chairman of the AWH execu-
        tive board, tells of her efforts in establishing the first
        American Women's Hospital in France in 1917 as an out-
        growth of the desire of American medical women to con-
        tribute to the war effort. (The U.S. government would not
        commission women physicians in the medical reserve corps
        of the armed services.) More than 1000 American women
        physicians volunteered to serve the noncombatant popula-
        tion in France, Italy, Poland, and the Balkans. Several
        chapters deal with these hospitals in France and Serbia,
        but the bulk of the book describes the American Women's
        Hospitals founded after World War I in the Balkans, where
        epidemics followed hundreds of thousands of Christian refu-
        gees fleeing from Turkish-ruled Armenia and Anatolia.
        The author describes conditions as physicians and nurses
        from the hospitals moved with the refugees from island to
        island. Many women physicians are mentioned in the book,

and portraits are liberally scattered throughout.   There is,
however, no index to the book.

3590.   Lovejoy, Esther [Pohl].   "Commendation of Work of Amer-
              ican Medical Women in Turkey by a Rear Admiral of
              the United States.   Also Letter from the Ministry of
              Serbia."   Medical Woman's Journal, 28:12 (December
              1921) 308-309.   (Hospitals & Colleges.)

3591.   Lovejoy, Esther Pohl.   "Looking Backward."   Journal of
              the American Medical Women's Association, 11:4 (April
              1956) 137-139.   ports.   (Tenth Anniversary Section.)
         When the Medical Women's National Association was or-
         ganized in 1915, the Medical Woman's Journal served as
         the official organ for its first seven years.   Elmina M.
         Roys-Gavitt had founded this journal in 1893 to serve as a
         vehicle of communications between women doctors around the
         country and to further their progress.   Many distinguished
         women doctors published in this journal, and it constitutes
         an historical record of a certain group of women in medi-
         cine through its publication history.   In 1922, when Grace
         N. Kimball became president of the Medical Women's Na-
         tional Association, that organization severed ties with the
         privately owned journal and established its own official pub-
         lication, the Quarterly Bulletin of the Medical Women's Na-
         tional Association.   Grace N. Kimball served as manager
         and editor until 1926, when she became associate editor, in
         which capacity she served for 12 years.   In 1934 this pub-
         lication changed its name to Women in Medicine, and in
         1946, when it became a monthly, it was changed to Journal
         of the American Medical Women's Association.   When the
         Pan American Medical Women's Alliance was organized,
         the Medical Woman's Journal became its official organ.

3592.   Lovejoy, Esther Pohl.   "President's Address."   Bulletin of
              the Medical Women's National Association, 37 (July
              1932) 8-9.
         This article advocates that women physicians support each
         other professionally and personally by forming local organ-
         izations.   Such organizations, namely branches of the Med-
         ical Women's National Association, would facilitate the pre-
         sentation of scientific papers which in turn would be polished
         for presentation at the American Medical Association--"prac-
         tice on one another, as it were, and thus prepare excellent
         papers...."   When women physicians from various branches
         and forms of medicine meet, there is more to be gained
         "... educationally, socially, and from the standpoint of
         travel, recreation, and personal relations."

3593.   Lovejoy, Esther Pohl.   "Report of American Women's Hos-
              pitals Reconstruction Committee M.W.N.A."   Medical
              Woman's Journal, 27:5 (May 1920) 142-147.   (Annual
              Reports: Committees of Medical Women's National

Association.)
Activities of American women physicians in Serbia, Turkey,
Armenia, and France during 1919 are described.

3594.   Lovejoy, Esther [Pohl]. "The Report of Medical Service
            Committee of Medical Women's National Association."
            Medical Woman's Journal, 28:12 (December 1921) 313.
         Work of the American Women's Hospitals in France, Serbia,
         Asia-Minor, and Russia is very briefly touched upon in this
         article, which consists of a letter from Elizabeth Bass.

3595.   Lovejoy, Esther P[ohl]. "Report of the American Women's
            Hospitals." Medical Woman's Journal, 31:7 (July 1924)
            202-208. (Presentation, Annual Meeting, Medical Wo-
            men's National Association, Chicago, Illinois, 9-10
            June 1924.)
         In this, her review of the work of American Women's Hos-
         pitals for the fiscal year 1923-24, Dr. Lovejoy, chairman
         of the executive board of the American Women's Hospitals,
         highlights the contributions of this organization's members
         whose working conditions in foreign countries include inade-
         quate supplies, funding, space, supportive medical person-
         nel, and, of course, personal comfort. Included is a brief
         eulogy for Sue Radcliffe, who had been commissioner for
         the American Women's Hospitals to Europe in 1922. Dr.
         Radcliffe contributed much of her time and paid her own
         expenses in order to be an effective behind-the-scenes work-
         horse for this organization. Places serviced by American
         Women's Hospitals include Greece, Serbia, France, Japan,
         Constantinople, and Russia. Specific contributions of this
         organization include such activities as initiating antimalarial
         work, giving employment to large numbers of well-qualified
         physicians--men and women--in war-wrecked countries who
         might otherwise have been in the bread line themselves,
         contributing to the establishment of children's hospitals,
         and supplying medical care in obscure places that otherwise
         would have none. American Women's Hospitals works
         closely with the American Red Cross.

3596.   Lovejoy, Esther [Pohl]. "Report of the Armenian Service
            of the American Women's Hospitals." Medical Woman's
            Journal, 28:4 (April 1921) 91-94. photos., port.
         The work done by the American Women's Hospitals in Ar-
         menia is recounted, especially that of Dr. Mabel Elliott,
         director of the cooperative work in Ismid. A large portion
         of this article consists of a letter from Dr. Elliott relating
         conditions.

3597.   Lovejoy, Esther P[ohl]. "Report of the Chairman of the
            American Women's Hospitals." Medical Woman's Jour-
            nal, 34:6 (June 1927) 175-178. port. (Report, Thir-
            teenth Annual Convention, Medical Woman's National
            Association, Washington, D.C., 15-17 May 1927.)

Work performed by the American Women's Hospitals, founded in 1917 by the Medical Women's National Association, "constitutes the greatest achievement of any group of women in the world organized during this decade." Dr. Lovejoy summarizes the organization's activities within the U.S. and in foreign countries.

3598.   Lovejoy, Esther P[ohl]. "Report of the Twelfth Annual Convention of the Medical Women's National Association: Report of the Chairman of the American Women's Hospitals." Medical Woman's Journal, 33:6 (June 1926) 161-163.
Activities of the American Women's Hospitals during 1925 and 1926 are detailed.

3599.   Lovejoy, Esther [Pohl]. "A Report to the Executive Board of the A.W.H." Medical Woman's Journal, 28:10 (October 1921) 246-252. photos., port. (Hospitals & Colleges.)
Following an investigative visit to Europe, Dr. Lovejoy presents an overview of the work of the American Women's Hospitals, highlighting activities in Turkey and France.

3600.   Lovejoy, Esther P[ohl]; Stewart, Clara; Campbell, Janet M.; and Barringer, Emily Dunning. "American Women's Hospitals." Medical Woman's Journal, 48:7 (July 1941) 215. (Correspondence.)
This correspondence from the Medical Women's Federation of Great Britain thanks the American Women's Hospitals Service for its generosity in providing financial assistance in the form of contributions. A list is included which shows the distribution of the funds.

3601.   "Luvia Willard, M.D., F.A.C.P., F.A.A.P., Organizer and Founder." Medical Woman's Journal, 51:6 (June 1944) 22. photo., port.
In 1940 Dr. Willard suggested to American Women's Hospitals that lay women be trained as a medical assistance group to serve in times of disaster. She organized that group, the Reserve Corps of the American Women's Hospitals, which has grown to more than 10,000 members.

3602.   Lyman, T., et al. "The Medical Education of Women at Harvard: Report on a Committee." Medical News (Philadelphia), 40 (1882) 476.
[Article not examined by editors.]

3603.   M. "Northwestern University Woman's Medical School." Chicago Clinical Review, 3 (October 1893) 57-62. photos.
This article consists of a historical overview of the University.

3604.   McCrea, Eppie S. "History of the State Society of Iowa
            Medical Women: Part II. From 1906 to 1935." Jour-
            nal of Iowa State Medical Society, 26:1 (January 1936)
            60-61. (History of Medicine in Iowa.) (Presentation,
            Thirty-eight Annual Session, State Society of Iowa Med-
            ical Women, Davenport, Iowa, 8 May 1935.)

3605.   Macfarlane, Catharine. "The Department of Gynecology of
            the Woman's Medical College of Pennsylvania." Women
            in Medicine, 78 (October 1942) 9-11.
         For the 80 years the Woman's Medical College of Pennsyl-
         vania's Department of Gynecology has existed, it has always
         been "controlled by women physicians," and the head of the
         department has always been an alumna of this school.
         From 1862 until 1879, Emeline Horton Cleveland was pro-
         fessor of obstetrics and diseases of women and children.
         In 1879 Anna E. Broomall became professor of obstetrics
         and gynecology. Diseases of children was assigned to some
         one else. In 1880 Dr. Broomall remained professor of
         obstetrics and Hannah T. Croasdale was appointed professor
         of diseases of women and children. Ella B. Everitt suc-
         ceeded Dr. Croasdale in 1902. Catharine Macfarlane suc-
         ceeded her in 1922. Women doctors who assisted her in-
         cluded Margaret Castex-Sturgis, Faith Skinner-Fetterman,
         and Dorothy Laing Ashton. The article also gives a descrip
         tion of the way in which gynecology is taught to third-year
         students. At the time this article was written, Dr. Sturgis,
         Dr. Fetterman, and Dr. Macfarlane were trying to deter-
         mine the value of periodic pelvic examinations in the control
         of cancer of the uterus.

3606.   [Macfarlane, Catharine]. "Presidential Address--Catherine
            [sic] Macfarlane, M.D., F.A.C.S.: Annual Meeting--
            June 7, 1937." Women in Medicine, 57 (July 1937) 19-
            20. port.
         In this, Catharine Macfarlane's outgoing presidential address
         to the Medical Women's National Association, she sum-
         marizes her concerns about the direction she hopes this
         group takes: continuing membership drives; continuing to
         create an atmosphere where professional and personal friend
         ships can be made; realizing the need for a salaried full-
         time secretary for publicity and recruitment of women to
         the field of medicine and to this organization; founding fel-
         lowships for demonstrated professional ability along clinical
         or research lines.

3607.   Macfarlane, Catharine. "A Temple of Learning." Journal
            of the American Medical Women's Association, 2:10
            (October 1947) 423-424. photos. (Editorial.)
         Founded in Philadelphia, Woman's Medical College of Penn-
         sylvania was the first medical college for women and the
         only one that has survived. One out of six women physi-
         cians practicing in the United States is a graduate of this

school. Sixty per cent of the teaching staff are women.
While there can be no doubt that women physicians have
made invaluable contributions to medicine, perhaps women
do best when they themselves control the institutions where
they work, do research, and attend school.

3608.   Macfarlane, Catharine. "The Woman's Medical College
             Faces the Future." Journal of the American Medical
             Women's Association, 11:4 (April 1956) 134-135.   photo.
         A brief history of the College is given, and the need for a
         larger endowment is discussed: "Funds for endowment are
         more needed than funds for scholarships."

3609.   Macfarlane, Catharine. "The Woman's College of Pennsyl-
             vania: The First Hundred Years." Journal of the
             American Medical Women's Association, 5:5 (May 1950)
             194-195.
         This article observes the occasion of the 100th anniversary
         of the Woman's Medical College of Pennsylvania, the only
         women's medical college still extant.   The author explores
         the questions, "What made it possible for this particular
         college to weather the various crises that beset educational
         institutions?" and "What made it possible for this college
         to meet the demands of the regulating bodies that control
         medical education?"   A number of distinguished alumnae are
         mentioned and discussed briefly.

3610.   McGrew, Elizabeth A.   "The Junior Membership Program."
             Journal of the American Medical Women's Association,
             21:1 (January 1966) 39.   (Editorial.)
         Elizabeth Kahler of Washington first directed the junior
         membership program of the American Medical Women's
         Association in 1950.   The primary aim of this organization
         is to compete with the squandering of almost 50 per cent
         of the United States' intellectual talent on housewifery and
         to recruit women for medicine.

3611.   McGrew, Elizabeth A.   "The Woman's Medical College of
             Pennsylvania." Journal of the American Medical Wo-
             men's Association, 22:9 (September 1967) 659-660.
             (AMWA President's Message.)
         Elizabeth McGrew, president of the American Medical Wo-
         men's Association, was appointed to ex officio membership
         of the board of corporators of the Woman's Medical College
         of Pennsylvania.

3612.   McGuinness, Madge C. L.   "The President's Address."
             Medical Woman's Journal, 45:6 (June 1938) 178-181.
             (Address, 32nd Annual Meeting, Women's Medical So-
             ciety of New York State, New York City, 9 May 1938.)
         Incoming president Madge McGuinness reviews presentations
         made before the Society's annual meeting, including the
         scientific program and reports by the legislation committee,

the committee on medical education, and the committee on
public health. Noting that the membership committee admitted little progress, Dr. McGuinness laments that the
younger women physicians are too satisfied with their personal careers to help their medical sisters by supporting
women's medical organizations. United bodies of women
physicians can widen medical opportunities for women and
can be instrumental in preserving the family and protecting
the public.

3613. McGuinness, Madge C. L. "President's Address: Annual
        Meeting of the Women's Medical Society of New York
        State at Syracuse, April 23-24, 1939." Medical Wo-
        man's Journal, 46:10 (October 1939) 300-305.
This speech stresses the importance of medical women helping each other, attending organizational meetings, preparing
papers and exhibits, urging women to patronize women physicians, and occupying leadership positions. The article
concludes with a review of the activities of the Society's
various committees.

3614. McKibbin-Harper, Mary. "Editorial." Bulletin of the Med-
        ical Women's National Association, 14 (October 1926) 8.
Men in medicine get appointed to the significant chairs in
colleges and executive positions, while women in medicine
do work without such honors. Women physicians need to
develop an esprit de corps which will create many benefits
by association on a national level and enable women to share
in some of the honors and privileges of being in the field
of medicine.

3615. McKibbin-Harper, Mary. "The New Women and Children's
        Hospital of Chicago." Medical Review of Reviews, 37:
        3 (March 1931) 165-166. (Editorial.)
Following a review of the history of the Women and Children's Hospital (formerly the Mary Thompson Hospital, in
honor of its founder), this editorial describes the institution's new five-story building.

3616. McKibbin-Harper, Mary. "The New York Infirmary for
        Women and Children." Medical Review of Reviews, 37:
        3 (March 1931) 167-168. (Editorial.)
Along with a review of the history of the Infirmary and its
founders, this editorial mentions the plans for erecting a
modern 21-story hospital on the present institution's site.

3617. Macnutt, Sarah J. "Medical Woman, Yesterday and To-
        day." Woman's Medical Journal, 28:8 (August 1918)
        173-177. (Presentation, meeting, Women's New York
        State Medical Society, Albany, New York, 20 May
        1918.)
This article was written in response to requests for "information regarding the woman doctor's preparation and ex-

periences." Dr. Macnutt draws from her experience at the
New York Infirmary for Women and Children.

3618.   Macy, Mary Sutton. "The Field for Women of Today in
            Medicine: College, Hospital, Laboratory and Practice."
            Woman's Medical Journal, 26:2 (February 1916) 41-42.
            photo.
         Dr. Macy proposes in this introduction to the series she
         will edit, "The Field for Women of Today," that it will
         cover the general practice of medicine by women. Included
         in this article are extracts from "The Endowment Fund
         Campaign of the Woman's Medical College of Pennsylvania."

3619.   Magier, Nina G. "Careers in the Veterans Administration."
            The Woman Physician, 26:6 (June 1971) 314-316.
         Veterans Administration hospitals welcome women physicians.
         As of October 31, 1967, the VA employed full-time 4,804
         male physicians and 385 female physicians; as of January
         31, 1968, 1023 male physicians and 62 females were em-
         ployed part-time; 3,245 residents were male and 183 resi-
         dents female. Marriage, years of study, and cost of edu-
         cation need not discourage women from entering medicine.
         A woman physician can marry "satisfactorily with careful
         planning, flexibility, good health, proper motivation, average
         intelligence, work endurance, emotional stability, plus some
         outside help when the children come along. An understand-
         ing husband is a blessing!" A woman working for the VA
         system receives various benefits: "continuous educational
         opportunity, comfortable salary, set hours, 30 days annual
         vacation, and 15 days sick leave annually, group insurance,
         and a retirement plan." She considers another benefit the
         fact that, "should your health or fancy require a change of
         climate, or should your husband relocate," there is prob-
         ably a Veterans Administration facility at which to work
         nearby. Included is a biographical inset on Nina G. Magier.

3620.   Malisoff, Vera. "Reflections on Our Past, Present and Fu-
            ture." Alumnae News [Medical College of Pennsylvania],
            26:1 (February 1975) 1. port.
         The president of the Medical College of Pennsylvania's
         alumnae association, Dr. Malisoff points out that although
         the College has gone coeducational, its historical importance
         in women's education and its commitment to women contin-
         ue. She warns that women must not be naive about having
         achieved unshakable equality with medical men. Alluding to
         the country's economic difficulties, Dr. Malisoff reminds
         her readers that when society suffers, minority groups suf-
         fer most.

3621.   Manning-Spoerl, Jacolyn Van Vliet. "Excerpts from an
            Argument Accompanying a Request that Women Be Re-
            Admitted to the Medical Department of Northwestern
            University." Woman's Medical Journal, 25:6 (June

1915) 130-131.

The author presents her retorts to the "arguments" that
medical women are not desired by the faculty or the male
students; that women physicians are not agreeable to man
physicians or the public; that women are insufficiently prepared for medical study, and unable to practice medicine;
and that medical study "unsexes" women and makes them
unfit for the duties of wife and mother.

3622.   Mara, Joy R. "Jefferson Alumnae: Making It." Jeffer-
          son Medical College Alumni Bulletin, 24:1 (Fall 1974)
          10-13.

The history of women at Jefferson Medical College began
with Elizabeth Blackwell's application for admission in 1846.
One professor suggested that admission might be arranged--
if she disguised herself as a man. Not until 1961 did Jefferson begin admitting women. To date it has graduated
over 100 women. The new freshman class contains 39 women (17 per cent of a 223-member class), and there are
90 other female students in the school. About 65 women
(one a full professor) are on the Jefferson Medical College
faculty of over 1200. Most of the information contained in
this article is based on questionnaire responses and personal
interviews with Jefferson women graduates. All respondents
practiced medicine after graduation, salary levels were for
the most part equal to those of male alumni, and specialty
selections conformed with nation-wide trends for women.
Most of the women defer to their husbands' career plans,
and report the use of household help as one means of managing marriage and career. Women students at Jefferson
note instances of subtle discrimination, but no "substantive"
opposition. A women's group on campus, the 1961 Society,
"is not a raving, demanding enclave of medical Betty Frie-
dans"; men regularly attend its programs, and through sharing experiences with other women, Society members receive peer support.

3623.   Marble, Ella M. S. "The Real Facts." Woman's Medical
          Journal, 1:7 (July 1893) 149-150.

One year ago--after admitting women medical students for
ten years--Columbian College in Washington, D.C. closed
its doors to women. The faculty vote to exclude women was
not unanimous, and there seems no substantial reason for
this backward step. Women wanting to study medicine at
the capital, however, can look to the National Medical and
Dental University, which welcomes women to share all
privileges with male students. Professors there feel no
resentment or embarrassment in the presence of women.
One even told Ella Marble that "there are only two stupid
students in the College and neither of those are women."

3624.   Marion, John Francis. "The Medical College of Pennsyl-
          vania: 3300 Henry Avenue." In: Philadelphia Medica:

Being a Guide to the City's Historical Places of Health
Interest. Smithkline Corporation, 1975, 131-135. photo.
The author traces the history of the Medical College of
Pennsylvania from its inception as an idea of William J.
Mullen, to the present. The women who were trained in
those early years after the College's 1850 opening are noted
and their achievements set in the context of the College's
history.

3625.   Marshall, Clara. The Woman's Medical College of Pennsylvania: An Historical Outline. P. Blakiston, Son &
Co., Philadelphia, Pennsylvania, 1897, 142 pp. port.
Clara Marshall, while dean of the Woman's Medical College
of Pennsylvania, produced this overview of the history and
development of the institution, "the first college in the world
regularly organized for the education of women for the medical profession" (incorporated March 11, 1850). William J.
Mullen was the first president of the College, and Mary E.
Mumford was the first woman president 44 years later.
"The idea of establishing a college for the medical education
of women originated with Dr. Bartholomew Fussell, a member of the Society of Friends," and from humble beginnings
("the days of small things") arose an enterprise of unanti-
cipated magnitude. The first faculty consisted of six men,
and 40 students matriculated for the first session. "With
the exception of a few annual donations from interested
friends, there was not a dollar in the treasury for compensation of professors or illustration of lectures." In order
to secure a manikin for the college, Dr. Elwood Harvey devised a daring plan leading to the collection of a reward of
$300. Two rewards had been offered for the return of a
particular slave girl, one by her master and one by a New
York friend of the antislavery cause. Dr. Harvey arranged
for the girl to be taken to Philadelphia and then, via the
Underground Railroad, to Canada and freedom. The duly
earned reward for this perilous service made possible the
purchase of the needed manikin. The work of Ann Preston
and Emmeline H. Cleveland on behalf of the hospital and
medical school is outlined, with liberal quotes from professional correspondence. The fight against various impediments to the study of medicine by women is chronicled,
often via correspondence. Included is a list of institutions
where graduates of the College have received appointments
and a list of medical papers written by alumnae prior to
1897.

3626.   "Martha Tracy Memorial Fund." Medical Woman's Journal,
49:10 (October 1942) 319.
The June convention of the American Medical Women's As-
sociation voted to collect a fund to memorialize Martha
Tracy, formerly dean of the Woman's Medical College of
Pennsylvania and assistant health officer of Philadelphia.
The fund will be used to provide a health service for women
medical students.

3627.   Marting, Esther C. "The Whys and Wherefores of the
           AMWA." Journal of the American Medical Women's
           Association, 15:2 (February 1960) 147-148. (Editorial.)

3628.   Mason-Hohl, Elizabeth. "Address of Retiring President
           Elizabeth Mason-Hohl: Annual Meeting, June 2, 1941."
           Women in Medicine, 73 (July 1941) 23-27.
       Some issues of general interest to medical women that re-
       tiring president of the American Medical Women's Associa-
       tion, Elizabeth Mason-Hohl, identified in this address were:
       scholarship funds have to increase to be able to help all the
       medical women students who apply; funds must be appro-
       priated for the AMWA Committee on Relief to Distressed
       Women Doctors in Europe and Asia as well as native United
       States women doctors; recognition in terms of equal rank,
       pay and veteran rights must be sought for women doctors who
       want to serve in the armed forces; scientific exhibits at
       American Medical Association conventions should be en-
       couraged; recommendation should be made to the postmaster
       general that Elizabeth Blackwell be put on a postage stamp;
       relatives of Kate Mead should be aided in the publication of
       her uncompleted books; and AMWA should publish a monthly
       rather than a quarterly magazine.

3629.   Mason-Hohl, Elizabeth. "Annie Sturges Daniel and the
           Cautious Experiment: Dr. Blackwell's Dream Come
           True." Medical Woman's Journal, 49:12 (December
           1942) 372, 392.
       Annie Sturges Daniel's "A Cautious Experiment" records
       the struggles and accomplishments of Elizabeth and Emily
       Blackwell, Harriot Hunt, and Marie Zakrzewska in founding
       the New York Infirmary for Women and Children and the
       Women's Medical College of the New York Infirmary. Dr.
       Daniel bases her work on her memories as a colleague and
       friend of these women, as well as on the minutes of the
       board of trustees, on hospital records, and on medical,
       surgical, and outpatient yearly reports. Included in this
       article is a brief review of the Infirmary's 79th annual re-
       port (1941).

3630.   [Mason-Hohl, Elizabeth]. "Loan Fund." Medical Woman's
           Journal, 54:5 (May 1947) 35-36. (Editorial.)
       This article responds to comment received on the proposed
       loan fund for women as students and postgraduates. "The
       Journal's Platform for Medical Women of the Americas," in
       list form, precedes this article.

3631.   [Mason-Hohl, Elizabeth]. "Our Platform--Plank Number
           Three." Medical Woman's Journal, 54:4 (April 1947)
           35-36. (Editorial.)
       The third plank in the Journal's platform concerns "ac-
       quaintance of women doctors with the medical work and aims
       of the Office of Inter-American Affairs."

3632.   [Mason-Hohl, Elizabeth]. "Semi-Centennial." Medical Wo-
          man's Journal, 50:1 (January 1943) 13-20. illus.,
          ports. (Editorial.)
        Fifty years of continuous publication of the Medical Woman's
        Journal is herein celebrated with a biography of the Journal's
        first editor-in-chief, Dr. Elmina Roys Ganitt. Portraits of
        various other editors are also included: Dr. Elise Strang
        L'Esperance, Dr. Eliza Root, Dr. Eliza Mosher, Dr.
        Elizabeth Mason-Hohl, and Margaret H. Rockhill.

3633.   Mason-Hohl, Elizabeth. "To the Women Physicians of
          America." Medical Woman's Journal, 49:2 (February
          1942) 52. (Editorial.)
        This editorial laments the loss to the Journal of two editors,
        Margaret H. Rockhill and Elise S. L'Esperance (through
        death and resignation, respectively).

3634.   Mason-Hohl, Elizabeth. "Woman's Medical College of Balti-
          more." Medical Woman's Journal, 53:12 (December
          1946) 58-63. port. (History of Women in Medicine,
          Bertha Selmon, ed.)
        This article traces the history of the College, from its
        incorporation in 1882 to its closing in 1910. Commenting
        on the brevity of the school's career, one of its graduates,
        Johanna T. Zelwis Baltrusaitis, said, "the great mistake
        made in the founding of the college was to have men, man
        and steer the craft on which women expected to reach
        shore." The article concludes with biographies of many of
        the College's 129 graduates.

3635.   Matthews, Margie R. "The Training and Practice of Women
          Physicians: A Case Study." Journal of Medical Edu-
          cation, 45:12 (December 1970) 1016-1024. tables.
        Duke University Medical Center, complex institution that it
        is, has not been responsive to the needs of women who
        might have become physicians, or to those who might have
        required more flexible schedules. A study done at Duke
        during the academic year 1967-68, on the training of women
        physicians from the pre-medical through the post doctoral
        years and the situations women physicians face in Duke's
        immediate community, presented the following statistics:
        23 per cent of freshman women at Duke in 1967 indicated
        some interest in medicine as a career. In the 1968 gradu-
        ating class, 38.9 per cent of the women were science ma-
        jors in what were traditionally held to be appropriate pre-
        medical programs, yet only 5.1 per cent applied to medical
        schools. In the fall of 1968, about the same percentage of
        total applicants (8.9 per cent) and of total acceptances (8.3
        per cent) were women. In 1968, almost the same percent-
        age of women applicants and of men applicants (11.6 per
        cent to 12.7 per cent) were accepted at Duke for entrance
        in 1968. In 1965-66 nationally, 47.7 per cent of women ap-
        plicants and 48.2 per cent of men applicants were accepted.

In 1967-68, 8.8 per cent of the students enrolled in the
Duke School of Medicine were women. This compares with
7.7 per cent women enrolled in 1966-67, which then ranked
Duke University School of Medicine forty-third among the
nation's 89 medical schools. Attrition in the sense of total
dropouts has been almost nonexistent at Duke. In 1967-68,
42.8 per cent of the enrolled women were in the upper
thirds of their classes, with 28.6 per cent each in the middle and lower thirds. In 1967-68 the women medical students at Duke ranged in age from 21 to 35: 24 per cent
were married; only one had a child. At least 83 per cent
planned residencies, and all juniors and seniors had chosen
specialty fields. At least 59 per cent of the total expressed
goals of full-time practice. During 1967-68 women in full-
time training accounted for four per cent of the house staff
at Duke. Their greatest perceived need as a group was for
financial aid, followed equally by part-time schedules and
child care. Those with family commitments saw child care
centers as the greatest single need. When the chairmen of
clinical departments in the medical school were questioned
about their attitudes toward women in the profession, five
of the nine were positive, two were neutral, and two were
negative toward the possibility of increasing the flow of women into medicine. In 1968 there were 70 women physicians of pre-retirement age in Durham and Orange Counties,
North Carolina. Of these women, 95.7 per cent were active professionally. At least 60 per cent were known to be
in full-time activity. These included the women house staff
members at the two university medical centers. Very few
of the total group were in high-level posts. The United
States with its 6.7 per cent of women physicians in 1967
does not compare well with the other major nations of the
world. Reasons for the small number of women in medicine appear to be rooted both in the circumstances unique
to the medical profession as it has been traditionally organized in this country, and in the conflicts American women have felt in adopting multiple roles. In recent years,
women seem more willing to adopt more than marital roles
and continue with education and careers. The situation at
Duke appears to be a microcosm of the national picture.

3636.   "Medical Education of Women at Harvard." Medical News,
              40 (29 April 1882) 476. (News Items.)
           At an April 12 meeting of the Board of Overseers of Har-
           vard University, the committee on medical education of
           women presented the opinion of the medical faculty. While
           not opposing the medical education of women in general, the
           faculty strongly opposes it in the Harvard Medical School.
           Because the school was founded and endowed for men, the
           school's purpose would "be seriously perverted" if women
           were admitted. In addition, accommodations for women
           would probably result in a lowering of the school's standards.
           Only two out of 20 faculty members dissented in the report.

3637.   Medical Woman's Journal, 30:1 (January 1923) 27-28.
         This editorial reminds readers of the services the Journal
         has provided and gives a preview of services the Journal
         editors plan to offer.

3638.   Medical Woman's Journal, 56:2 (February 1949) 55.   (News
             Notes.)
         This untitled news item discusses the American Medical
         Women's Association's book collection and its drive--co-
         ordinated by Bertha Van Hoosen--to raise funds for a li-
         brary.   The Woman's Medical College of Pennsylvania
         guarantees the site and care of the library if AMWA pro-
         vides the building.   A dollar from each sale of Dr. Van
         Hoosen's book, Petticoat Surgeon, goes to the fund.

3639.   "Medical Women on the A.M.A. Program at Atlantic City."
             Medical Woman's Journal, 42:6 (June 1935) 166.   (Ed-
             itorial.)
         This editorial was inspired by the "unusually large number
         of medical women [who] appear on the program" of the
         American Medical Association meeting.   "The fact that so
         many women will take part in the Atlantic City sessions is
         indicative of the increasing interest in public affairs among
         women physicians."

3640.   "Medical Women's Library Memorial Building."   Medical
             Woman's Journal, 54:3 (March 1947) 41.
         This article discusses the American Medical Women's Asso-
         ciation's plans to raise funds for a medical women's library
         to house the literature and memorabilia of women physi-
         cians' collections.   The Woman's Medical College of Penn-
         sylvania has donated a site on its campus for the library.
         Names of women physicians working on the campaign are
         given.

3641.   "The Medical Women's Press."   Medical Woman's Journal,
             39:6 (June 1932) 158.   (Editorial.)
         Founded in 1902, the Medical Woman's Journal in this ed-
         itorial congratulates itself for being "the first [journal] in
         the field in this or any other country, and still retains the
         distinction of being the only scientific medical journal for
         medical women."

3642.   "Medical Women's Society of New York State: Twenty-
             Seventh Annual Meeting."   Medical Woman's Journal,
             40:4 (April 1933) 90-91.
         An official program of the meeting is included in this article
         along with "an important resolution pertaining to Amendment
         365 introduced in the Senate of New York State."   This
         amendment applies to Section 306 of the Civil Practice Act
         which reads "and if the party to be examined in action to
         recover damages for personal injuries shall be a female,
         she shall be entitled to have examination before a physician

of her own sex." The Society opposes striking this Section.
A history of cases and debates appertaining to Section 306
is also included.

3643.   "Membership List of Women's New National Association
        Growing Rapidly." Woman's Medical Journal, 26:3
        (March 1916) 69.
        The Medical Women's National Association is growing rapid-
        ly and should serve as a means of promoting efficiency and
        harmony as women physicians work together toward their
        common goal of serving mankind.

3644.   "Memorial to Dr. Anna Howard Shaw: National American
        Woman Suffrage Association Helps Woman's Medical
        College of Pennsylvania." Medical Woman's Journal,
        27:3 (March 1920) 80-81. port.
        A pledge of $30,000 from the League of Women Voters and
        the National American Woman Suffrage Association will help
        establish a memorial for Dr. Shaw in the College's new De-
        partment of Preventive Medicine.

3645.   Miller, Deborah W. "Sex Is the Issue." Harvard Medical
        Alumni Bulletin, 50:1 (September/October 1975) 9.
        (Editorial.)
        Surveying "the precarious nature of women's liberation" at
        Harvard, the author notes the proportion of women students
        and faculty and the reasons for "a nascent optimism."

3646.   Morse, Marion S. "President's Address." Medical Wo-
        man's Journal, 39:6 (June 1932) 155-156. (Address,
        Annual Meeting, Medical Women's Society of New York
        State, Buffalo, New York, 23 May 1932.)
        The Women's Medical Society of New York State was founded
        in 1907 as a joint meeting for four women's medical organ-
        izations: The Physicians' League of Buffalo, the Women's
        Medical Association of New York City, the Blackwell Med-
        ical Society of Buffalo, and the Dr. Cordelia A. Greene
        Society of Castile. Medical meetings such as this one,
        where women physicians share health prevention insights as
        well as identify problems of health care, where women may
        give support to each other's professional ambitions, are im-
        portant. Just as important is the consideration of how iso-
        lated many women physicians are from others and their
        meetings give them a chance to have "the companionship of
        women of their own profession."

3647.   Mosher, Eliza M. "New England Hospital for Women and
        Children." Medical Woman's Journal, 30:6 (June 1923)
        178-183. photos.
        Dr. Mosher traces the history of the Hospital, from its
        opening in 1862 to the present. The contributions of the
        women physicians associated with the institution are empha-
        sized.

3648.   Mosher, Eliza M. "Report of the Annual Meeting of the
         Medical Women's Association of New York State."
         Medical Woman's Journal, 30:6 (June 1923) 173-174.
         This report of the meeting held in May 1923 lists officers
         elected and names of a few of the 119 attendees who parti-
         cipated in the program. Among the scientific papers pre-
         sented was one by Dr. Alberta Green concerning prison in-
         mates; commenting upon the paper, Dr. Mosher states that
         from a eugenic standpoint, "the great army of defective
         girls and women loose in our cities should be legally segre-
         gated as promptly as possible." A member of the Ameri-
         can Medical Association's Woman's Auxiliary (composed of
         wives of AMA members) asked that women physicians co-
         operate in the social activities of the AMA's meetings.

3649.   Mosher, Eliza M. "The Smyrna Disaster and the Part
         Taken by the A.W.H. in the Relief of Appalling Con-
         ditions." Medical Woman's Journal, 30:1 (January 1923)
         22-25. port. (Hospitals & Colleges.)
         Under the direction of Dr. Mabel Elliott, the American Wo-
         men's Hospitals will install and manage a facility in Greece
         to handle 10,000 refugees. The medical station on the is-
         land of Macronisi will be the largest of its kind in the
         world. Extracts of a report by Dr. Elliott are included in
         this article.

3650.   Mosher, Eliza M. "The Value of Organization--What It
         Has Done for Women." Woman's Medical Journal, 26:
         6 (June 1916) 141. (Original articles.) (Address, An-
         nual Meeting, Medical Women's National Association,
         Detroit, Michigan, 13 June 1916.)
         Women, unlike men, have tended not to organize and band
         together. Now that preparedness is needed, it is important
         that medical women organize so that the organized unit will
         be able to exert a power that no individual standing alone
         can match. Such an organization not only will enlarge the
         power and opportunities of its individual members, but also
         will give intellectual companionship and common bonds of
         spirituality.

3651.   Moyer, Elizabeth. "Women in the Female Medical College."
         Boston University Medical Center Centerscope, (July/
         August 1971) 5-6. port. (Women in Medicine.)
         A brief history of the New England Female Medical College
         relates how the institution "fell apart" when Dr. Samuel
         Gregory died in 1872.

3652.   "National Association of Medical Women." Woman's Med-
         ical Journal, 26:1 (January 1916) 14-15.
         The history of women in medicine was marked by the forma-
         tion of the Medical Women's National Association in Chicago
         on November 18, 1915, during the semi-centennial celebra-
         tion of the founding of the Mary Thompson Hospital. The

officers included Eliza H. Mosher as honorary president,
Bertha Van Hoosen as president-elect, Marion Craig Potter [first vice-president], Mary McLean as second vice-
president, Mary H. Bates as third vice-president, Martha
Welpton as recording secretary and treasurer, and [Mar-
garet Hackedorn Rockhill] as corresponding secretary. The
Woman's Medical Journal was chosen as the official organ
of the Association.

3653.   Natural Guardians of the Race. Woman's Medical College
            of Pennsylvania, Philadelphia, Pennsylvania, 1926,
            27 pp. photos., ports.
         This booklet gives a history of the College and presents
         the plans for the new college and hospital on Henry Avenue
         in north Philadelphia.

3654.   Nemir, Rosa Lee. "AMWA--Six Decades of Progress (in
            the Service of Women in Medicine)." Journal of the
            American Medical Women's Association, 29:11 (Novem-
            ber 1974) 486-490. figs., tables.
         Dr. Nemir considers a "few significant highlights" in the
         history of the American Medical Women's Association
         (AMWA). Tables show the geographic distribution and spe-
         cialties of AMWA presidents. A graph illustrates the num-
         ber and amount of scholarships distributed to women stu-
         dents.

3655.   Nemir, Rosa Lee. "Women Doctors Educating Others:
            50th Anniversary of the American Medical Women's
            Association Scholarship Loan Fund." Journal of the
            American Medical Women's Association, 28:9 (Septem-
            ber 1973) 475-477. port.
         A history of the AMWA Scholarship Loan Fund includes ex-
         cerpted letters from various recipients as well as a photo-
         graph of the author.

3656.   Nemir, Rosa Lee; Crawford, Mary M.; Guion, Connie M.;
            and Sharp, Dorothy J. "History of the Women's Med-
            ical Association of New York City (Branch Fourteen):
            1909-1959." Journal of the American Medical Women's
            Association, 15:8 (August 1960) 781-783. ports.
         The history of this Association is traced from its evolution
         out of the alumnae association of the Women's Medical
         College of the New York Infirmary for Women and Children.

3657.   "New Cancer Prevention Clinic." Medical Woman's Journal,
            49:5 (May 1942) 151. (Editorial.)
         Elise Strang L'Esperance--who with her sister founded, in
         1937, the Kate Depew Strang Tumor Clinic at the New York
         Infirmary for Women and Children--is directing a new can-
         cer prevention clinic at New York City's Memorial Hospital.

3658.   "New Name Approved." Woman's Medical College: Today,

1:6 (March 1970) 1.
Following the decision to admit male students, the Board of
Corporators of the Woman's Medical College of Pennsylvania
unanimously voted to change the College's name to the "Medical College of Pennsylvania." The committee reasoned
that the new name "comes closest to maintaining the traditional name of the institution and removes only the word
'Woman's' from the title...."

3659. "The New Women and Children's Hospital of Chicago."
        Medical Woman's Journal, 36:2 (February 1929) 31-33.
        illus.
        A history of the Women and Children's Hospital of Chicago
        is given on the occasion of the opening of the new hospital.

3660. Newman, Meta R. Pennock. "Twenty-First Annual Meeting
        of the Association of Women in Public Health." Med-
        ical Woman's Journal, 50:1 (January 1943) 8, 12.
        (Public Health Section.)
        Proceedings of the meeting are briefly outlined in this arti-
        cle.

3661. "News Items from the Woman's Medical College of Penn-
        sylvania." Medical Woman's Journal, 47:12 (Decem-
        ber 1940) 375.
        The "items" focus upon recent professional activities (ap-
        pointments, papers presented, grants received) of faculty
        members.

3662. "Nineteenth Annual Banquet of Women's Medical Society of
        New York State in Honor Dr. Eliza M. Mosher's Fifty
        Years in Medicine; Monday Evening, May 11, 1925."
        Medical Woman's Journal, 32:8 (August 1925) 220-223.
        At this banquet held in honor of Eliza M. Mosher's 50
        years in medicine, Dr. Mosher reminisced about the great
        women physician teachers she had known whom she felt
        had helped her career: Elizabeth Blackwell, Emily Black-
        well, Marie Zakrzewska, Lucy E. Sewall, Helen Morton,
        and Susan Dimock. She urged the women members of this
        society to speak at their meetings of those women physi-
        cians who have helped them become successful physicians.
        Susan Moody also spoke about women's health care in Persia
        where women physicians were especially needed because of
        the cultural practice specifying that women may only be seen
        by the men of their own families.

3663. "92nd Annual Commencement of Woman's Medical College of
        Pennsylvania." Medical Woman's Journal, 51:6 (June
        1944) 36. (News Notes.)
        Information is given on the 21 graduates and on the com-
        mencement exercise itself.

3664. "No Medical Women in House of Delegates of A.M.A."

Medical Woman's Journal, 28:6 (June 1921) 163.
The author of this brief reminder urges the matter to be
taken up by the "Councillor and Executive Committee of
our Association," and expresses the hope that next year a
goodly number of women will be in the American Medical
Association (AMA) House of Delegates.

3665.   "No Woman Physician Desired in A. M. A. House of Dele-
         gates." Medical Woman's Journal, 46:7 (July 1939)
         216. (Editorial.)
The Women's Medical Association of New York City requested the House of Delegates of the New York State Medical Society to recommend that the American Medical Association grant a seat in its House of Delegates to a woman.
The resolution stated that the seat would be permanent and
filled each year by a woman delegate. Although the New
York State Medical Society favorably received the resolution,
the AMA's House of Delegates voted it down, "and there
will be no woman physician in that body this year."

3666.   Noble, Mary Riggs. "The Women Doctors of the Children's
         Bureau." Medical Woman's Journal, 40:1 (January
         1933) 5-10.
Upon the occasion of the 20th anniversary of the Children's
Bureau of the United States Department of Labor, this article was written to commemorate the achievements of the
Bureau and the medical women who had a share in its pioneering work. A history of the Bureau, its departments
and organization, is given. The history is presented in
terms of the women physicians who made it possible.

3667.   Norris, Frances S. "Medical Womanpower." New England
         Journal of Medicine, 281:16 (16 October 1969) 910-911.
         (Letters to the Editor.)
In a criticism of medical school admission policies, Dr.
Norris attacks recent events at the Woman's Medical College in Philadelphia, where, for the first time since 1850,
men students will be admitted. "With virtually untapped
national womanpower available to them, the male leadership at the College wish to restrict admission of women so
that male applicants rejected elsewhere can be admitted."
Dr. Norris adds that not only is the College promoting discriminatory policies now toward women applicants, but women faculty are being "programmed into extinction." She
believes the government should withhold federal funds from
the College because it is "so bent on mediocrity."

3668.   "Northwestern University Woman's Medical School." Chi-
         cago Clinical Review, 3 (October 1893) 59-62. illus.
         [Article not examined by editors.]

3669.   "The Northwestern University Woman's Medical School."
         Woman's Medical Journal, 12:3 (March 1902) 56-57.
This article discusses the discontinuance of the school.

3670.   "A Notable Record Service: Woman's Medical College."
         Medical Woman's Journal, 55:5 (May 1948) 45-46.
         (Notes from the Woman's Medical College of Pennsyl-
         vania.)
         Professors and department heads for 1947-1948 are listed
         in this article, which presents a general history of the Col-
         lege. Also described is a dinner held in honor of Dr.
         [Catharine] Macfarlane, upon her completion of 50 years of
         medical achievement. "Dr. Macfarlane, being a woman,
         had the last word, and was charming and witty in her
         reminiscences of her early practice."

3671.   "Notes from the Woman's Medical College of Pennsylvania."
         Medical Woman's Journal, 54:6 (June 1947) 50.   table.
         A table lists the names of foreign countries and the number
         of medical students from each country to attend the College
         between the years 1850-1945. Dr. Marian Shaffner Morse
         is also mentioned in this news column.

3672.   "Notes from the Woman's Medical College of Pennsylvania."
         Medical Woman's Journal, 55:4 (April 1948) 49.   photo.
         Dr. Isabella H. Perry, a 1921 graduate of Woman's Med-
         ical College of Pennsylvania, will direct a new cancer
         teaching program at the College. A biography of her ac-
         companies a description of that program. Also described
         in this article are the College's Founders Day ceremonies,
         during which a bust of S. Josephine Baker was presented.

3673.   "Notes from the Woman's Medical College of Pennsylvania."
         Medical Woman's Journal, 55:9 (September 1948) 64.
         The College's 1948 commencement, during which 35 women
         received degrees, is briefly described. Also mentioned in
         this article is Gerty T. Cori, M.D., who won the Nobel
         Prize in 1947.

3674.   "Notes from the Woman's Medical College of Pennsylvania."
         Medical Woman's Journal, 55:11 (November 1948) 57.
         Two women physicians named the Woman's Medical College
         of Pennsylvania as beneficiary to their wills: Margaret
         Delmore (class of 1899), in the amount of $47,000; and
         Grace Sherwood (M.D., 1904)--$17,000. Honorary degrees
         conferred, and other awards received are also included.

3675.   "Notes from the Woman's Medical College of Pennsylvania."
         Medical Woman's Journal, 56:1 (January 1949) 55.
         A new laboratory in Middletown, Connecticut's Middlesex
         Hospital has been named after Jessie Weston Fisher, an
         1893 graduate of Woman's Medical College and a distinguished
         bacteriologist and pathologist. Awards, new appointments,
         and activities of several other College alumnae are men-
         tioned in this column.

3676.   "Notes from the Woman's Medical College of Pennsylvania."

Medical Woman's Journal, 56:3 (March 1949) 56, 58.
Founders' Day ceremonies are described and new faculty
appointments are announced in this article.

3677.   "Notes from the Woman's Medical College of Pennsylvania."
Medical Woman's Journal, 56:8 (August 1949) 45-46.
Among other College events mentioned in this article is a
description of the [1949] commencement ceremony, during
which 30 women received degrees.

3678.   "Notes on the National Woman's Party Convention." Medical Woman's Journal, 49:12 (December 1942) 385.
(Editorial.)
Dr. Catharine Macfarlane introduced a resolution at the
eleventh biennial convention of the National Woman's Party
which "urge[s] that the women physicians of this country
be not discriminated against but that they be admitted to
full membership in the Medical Reserve Corps of the United
States Army and Navy."

3679.   O'Connor, Katheryn and Forbes, Lorna. "Student News."
Medical Woman's Journal, 52:9 (September 1945) 54-
55. photo., ports.
A cameo of the entering freshman class at the Woman's
Medical College of Pennsylvania is given, including names
of undergraduate schools attended, number of women married, family backgrounds, and former occupations of the
students.

3680.   O'Connor, Katheryn and Forbes, Lorna. "Student News."
Medical Woman's Journal, 52:12 (December 1945) 59,
64.
This article discusses the structural changes in course and
clinical work at the Woman's Medical College of Pennsylvania. Lectures by various women physicians at the College are alluded to.

3681.   "Our Journal." Woman's Medical Journal, 1:5 (May 1893)
97-98.
Men as well as women are invited to subscribe to the Journal. The Journal provides a place where women physicians
may write and be heard and thereby "bring their names before the public through meritorious articles," as male physicians have done to attain eminence.

3682.   "Outline of Activities the American Women's Hospitals: Organized 1917." Medical Woman's Journal, 29:4 (April
1922) 78-80. (Hospitals & Colleges.)
This article briefly outlines the work of the American Women's Hospitals (AWH) in France, Serbia, Armenia, and
Russia. Letters from Drs. Mabel E. Elliott and Lucy Mac-
Millan Elliott as well as "letters from grateful patients" are
reproduced.

3683.   Pearce, Louise. "A Century of Medical Education for
         Women." Independent Woman, 29:4 (April 1950) 104-
         106, 122. photos.
         The president of Woman's Medical College of Pennsylvania
         (now celebrating its 100th anniversary), emphasizes the ac-
         complishments of Clara Swain and other medical mission-
         aries in this article about the College's early graduates.
         The life of Anandibai Joshee is highlighted as well.

3684.   Peck, Phoebe. "Women Physicians and Their State Med-
         ical Societies." Journal of the American Medical Wo-
         men's Association, 20:4 (April 1965) 351-353.
         Early admissions of female practitioners to state medical
         societies was rarely accomplished without controversy. In
         1872 Kansas, North Carolina, Michigan, and Rhode Island
         took the actual step of accepting women. Nine states fol-
         lowed suit in the subsequent three years. Circumstances
         surrounding these admissions are briefly summarized.

3685.   "The Personnel and Scope of the Medical Women's National
         Ass'n." Woman's Medical Journal, 26:10 (October
         1916) 245. (Editorial.)
         The first slate of officers of the Medical Women's National
         Association is given.

3686.   Pincock, Carolyn S. "New Horizons for the American
         Medical Women's Association." Journal of the Amer-
         ican Medical Women's Association, 30:1 (January 1975)
         9-11.
         The American Medical Women's Association should adopt a
         unified program to provide change in discriminatory be-
         havior towards women in medical schools.

3687.   "Pioneer Medical Women of Cleveland and the Story of the
         Women's and Children's Free Medical and Surgical Dis-
         pensary." Journal of the American Medical Women's
         Association, 6:5 (May 1951) 186-189. photos., ports.
         A history is presented (in narrative and excerpts of reports)
         of the Women's and Children's Free Medical and Surgical
         Dispensary of Cleveland, Ohio, founded by Dr. Myra K.
         Merrick in 1878.

3688.   "Plastic Surgery Clinic: Director, Alma Dea Morani, M.D.,
         F.A.C.S., F.I.C.S." Medical Woman's Journal, 55:1
         (January 1948) 53.
         Described is Philadelphia's first plastic surgery clinic, the
         Plastic Surgery and Hand Clinic of Woman's Medical Col-
         lege Hospital. Its director, Dr. Alma Dea Morani--one of
         the first women surgeons to specialize in plastic surgery--
         describes the work at the clinic.

3689.   "Progress--Not Segregation." Medical Woman's Journal,
         30:6 (June 1923) 190. (Editorial.)

The importance of medical women's organizations is emphasized.

3690.   Purnell, Caroline M. "American Women's Hospitals: Or-
         ganized by War Service Committee of the Medical Wo-
         men's National Association." Woman's Medical Journal,
         29[19]:2 (February 1919) 26-27.

3691.   Putnam, James Jackson. "Women at Zurich." Boston Med-
         ical and Surgical Journal, 101:16 (16 October 1879) 567-
         568.
         This letter to the editor supports medical education for wo-
         men at Harvard, as proposed by Dr. Bowditch and Profes-
         sor Rose. The medical coeducation experiment at Zurich
         has been a great success, contrary to what has been im-
         plied in the Journal. The author also objects to the Journal's
         protest that a female medical college at Harvard would
         oblige smaller colleges to close their doors. Harvard has
         never been influenced by such a consideration before. It is
         important to make first-rate practitioners of women, and
         not relegate them to inferior schools. An editorial note in-
         sists that the objection has been to medical coeducation
         alone.

3692.   Qua, Julia Kimball. "President's Address." Medical Wo-
         man's Journal, 32:7 (July 1925) 195-197. (Address,
         Annual Meeting, Women's Medical Society of New York
         State, Syracuse, New York.)
         In this address, the retiring president of the Women's Med-
         ical Society of New York State, Dr. Qua, reviews the rea-
         sons why a separate medical organization for women needs
         to exist and identifies some of the problems of medical
         practice to solve in the future. Women need their own med-
         ical organization because "in this smaller body the members
         would have more opportunity for presenting papers and be
         less timid in their discussions, a better chance of acquaint-
         ance with each other's aims and ideals, and by this inter-
         change of thought be strengthened in our work."

3693.   "A Record of the Work of Medical Women." Medical Wo-
         man's Journal, 29:10 (October 1922) 260. (Editorial.)
         The Medical Woman's Journal "faithfully [records] the
         achievements of women physicians" and contains the only
         extensive history of this group. This article expresses
         hope for the support of medical women in the continuation
         of the Journal.

3694.   Reid, Ada Chree. "Those Were the Days!" Journal of the
         American Medical Women's Association, 11:4 (April
         1956) 140-141.
         An editor of the Journal describes the difficulties of the wo-
         men who worked on the Journal for its first ten years: ob-
         taining material, learning printing, editing information, meet-
         ing deadlines, etc.

3695.   "Report of the Fourth Annual Meeting of the Medical Wo-
          men's National Association Held in Atlantic City, June
          9-10, 1919." Woman's Medical Journal, 29[19]:7 (July
          1919) 137-149.
          Dr. Angenette Parry, president, presided at this meeting.
          New officers elected included Etta Gray, president.   Dr.
          Gray's speech, giving recommendations for Association work
          of the coming year, is printed.   Also published in full are
          reports by Maude Glasgow (committee on opportunities for
          medical women), Kristine Mann (committee on industrial
          diseases of women and children), Emma Wheat Gilmore
          (committee, women physicians, general medical board,
          Council National Defense), Isabelle Thompson Smart (intern-
          ship committee), and Willa F. Davis (committee on publi-
          cations).

3696.   "Report of the Semi-Annual Meeting Women's Medical So-
          ciety of New York State." Medical Woman's Journal,
          46:2 (February 1939) 55-57.
          Among the debates of this thirty-third semiannual meeting
          was the question of general affiliation of state societies with
          the national medical women's organization.   Resolutions
          adopted include the dissolution of the affiliation between the
          Women's Medical Society of New York State and the Med-
          ical Woman's Journal.

3697.   "Report of World Fair Committee Women's Medical Asso-
          ciation of New York City." Medical Woman's Journal,
          46:3 (March 1939) 90-91.
          The American Women's Association and the Women's Med-
          ical Association of New York City in cooperation will pro-
          vide entertainment for women visiting the World's Fair.
          Among the arrangements are "Career Tours" of several city
          hospitals.

3698.   "Representation for Medical Women." Medical Woman's
          Journal, 46:5 (May 1939) 148.   (Editorial.)
          At its April [1939] meeting, the New York State Medical
          Society unanimously adopted a resolution to urge the AMA
          to grant a permanent seat in its house of delegates to a
          woman delegate.

3699.   "Resolutions Adopted at the Annual Convention." Medical
          Woman's Journal, 37:7 (July 1930) 196-197.   (Meeting,
          Medical Women's National Association, Detroit, Michi-
          gan, 22-24 June 1930.)
          Among the resolutions adopted at this convention were those
          in the following areas: women medical students must not
          be discriminated against because of their sex, and the MWNA
          "condemns the resolution against the participation of women
          in Olympic Games...."   In addition, it was resolved that
          contraception counseling is a "wholly proper medical func-
          tion."   MWNA also endorses "the movement looking to the
          abolition of child labor."

3700.   Ridlon, John. "Dr. Marie J. Mergler, Dean." Woman's
             Medical Journal, 9:4 (April 1899) 117-118.
         The announcement of Dr. Mergler's appointment as dean of
         Northwestern University Woman's Medical School is incor-
         porated into information on other changes in the School.

3701.   Robinson, Alice. "American Woman's Association Club-
             house." Medical Woman's Journal, 38:6 (June 1931)
             147-150. photo.
         The 4500-member American Woman's Association (AWA)
         boasts a multi-facility clubhouse in New York City that at-
         tracts many prominent women physicians including Florence
         R. Sabin, and Mary M. Crawford. Explaining why the
         Association has special interest for women physicians, Dr.
         Crawford, a founder and vice-president of AWA, says "Here
         [at the AWA Club] we see people who are doing things so
         differently from us and we can listen and enjoy them with-
         out the slightest responsibility." The author adds that wo-
         men physicians often prefer "when pleasure-bound to mingle
         with women not especially interested in medicine."

3702.   Robinson, Daisy M. O. "President's Address." Medical
             Woman's Journal, 37:6 (June 1930) 166-168. (Address,
             Annual Meeting, Women's Medical Society of New York
             State, Inc., Rochester, New York, 2 June 1930.)
         Women physicians have to band together to promote the
         interchange of ideas and to support the contribution and ad-
         vancement of women in medicine. The early women pio-
         neers of medicine give us models of character and service,
         and prove that women in medicine can make important con-
         tributions.

3703.   Rochford, Grace E. "The New England Hospital for Women
             and Children." Journal of the American Medical Wo-
             men's Association, 5:12 (December 1950) 497-499.
             photo., port.
         From the premise that the history of the New England Hos-
         pital for Women and Children closely parallels the history
         of the progress of education of women in medicine in the
         United States, the author traces that hospital's history,
         from its stated purpose in 1863 through the approach of
         its centenary.

3704.   Rockhill, Margaret H. "Report of the Sixteenth Annual
             Meeting of the Medical Women's National Association
             Held in Detroit, Mich., June 22-24, 1930." Medical
             Woman's Journal, 37:7 (July 1930) 191-195.
         Besides highlighting the social events and the program of
         this annual meeting, this article also points out the diffi-
         culty in raising scholarship funds for women medical stu-
         dents: that "medical women themselves, some of those
         formerly interested have withdrawn their support." As a
         result, the Medical Women's National Association should

look to more stable support from foundations to fund scholarships for women medical students.

3705.   Rudd, Helga M. "The Women's Medical College of Chicago:
        Later Called the Northwestern University Woman's Med-
        ical College. 1870-1902." Medical Woman's Journal,
        53:6 (June 1946) 41-46, 64. (History of Women in
        Medicine, Bertha Selmon, ed.)
The first of three articles about the College, this article
traces the events leading up to the founding of the Women's
Medical College. Dr. Mary Harris Thompson's role in establishing the school is described; other women who figured
prominently in the school's history are also mentioned.   In
1891 the College united with Northwestern University and
assumed the name, Northwestern University Woman's Medical College. In 1902 the University declared the woman's
school extinct.

3706.   Rudnick, Sarah. "A Story of the Work Being Done in Ser-
        bia Under the Supervision of Dr. Etta Gray." Medical
        Woman's Journal, 28:11 (November 1921) 281. port.
The institution with which Dr. Gray is associated is part of
the American Women's Hospitals organization.

3707.   Sanford, Mary B. "Letters to the Editor." Medical Wo-
        man's Journal, 50:4 (April 1943) 110.
This letter was written in response to a request from the
editor of the Journal for information about the Salvation
Army. Dr. Sanford gives her personal feelings about the
"army" and tells of one experience she had with the Salvation Army offering medical aid to storm victims in Ohio.

3708.   Scarlett-Dixon, Mary J. Valedictory Address to the Twenty-
        Third Graduating Class of the Woman's Medical College
        of Pennsylvania. Published by request, Philadelphia,
        Pennsylvania, 1875, 16 pp.
Alluding to the religious and governmental evolution that
gave rise to women's medical education, Mary Scarlett-
Dixon reviews the history of the Woman's Medical College
as well as its present organization. Also discussed are the
special duties of women physicians, most of which have to
do with exerting "purifying and refining" influences upon society. Following the text of this speech is an appendix
which details the October 1874 ceremony commemorating
the erection of the new building of the Woman's Medical
College.

3709.   Scharnagel, Isabel M. "Minutes of the Thirty-Fifth Annual
        Meeting of the Women's Medical Society of New York
        State." Medical Woman's Journal, 48:6 (June 1941)
        164-166.
These minutes cover such topics as the resolution regarding
the eligibility of women physicians in the U.S. Army and

Navy Medical Reserve Corps. A second resolution was passed which dealt with an expression of gratitude to Western Reserve University (WRU), Cleveland, Ohio (where the AMWA Convention was to meet in June of this year) for granting women physicians the privilege of graduating from WRU in 1854.

3710. Scharnagel, Isabel M. "Minutes of the Thirty-Fourth Annual Meeting of Women's Medical Society of New York State: New York--May 6, 1940." Medical Woman's Journal, 47:6 (June 1940) 185-187.
A resolution concerning efforts to have Emily Dunning Barringer appointed a delegate to the 1940 American Medical Association convention was passed at this meeting. Other business included: reports by the legislative committee and the committee on medical education; a debate of the question of amalgamation with the national women's society; and a discussion of the status of women physicians during wartime.

3711. Scharnagel, Isabel M. "Official Report Mid-Year Meeting: Women's Medical Society of New York State." Medical Woman's Journal, 47:2 (February 1940) 59-61.
During this meeting, it was agreed that the Medical Woman's Journal be made the official organ of the Women's Medical Society of New York State. Dr. Emily Barringer reported on the question of affiliation with the national women's society.

3712. Schlachter, Jo. "The American Women's Hospitals Reserve Corps." Medical Woman's Journal, 51:6 (June 1944) 18-21. photos.
The organizational structure, activities, and reward system of the corps (a semimilitary "lay" committee that aids the work of the American Women's Hospitals) is outlined.

3713. Schwartz, Neena B. "Why Women Form Their Own Professional Organizations." Journal of the American Medical Women's Association, 28:1 (January 1973) 12-15.
"Four functions are subserved when women form their own professional organizations. The first of these functions is an attempt to achieve equal opportunity and rights with regard to their professional aspirations. The second function subserved by women's professional organizations is to promote, recognize and act on women's own perspectives in their professional field. These perspectives do not always coincide with those of the men. The third function is to train women in the administrative and political aspects of their professions so that they are better able to move back into the parent professional organizations and achieve influence and power. Finally, women's professional organizations serve a 'consciousness arousal' function for women by means of sharing the common problems women have in achieving career goals." [Article abstract.]

3714.   "Second Annual Meeting of Association of Southern Medical
             Women." Woman's Medical Journal, 25:1 (January
             1915) 15-16.
         The report includes biographical sketches of the Associa-
         tion's newly elected president Dr. Mary E. Lapham, vice-
         president Dr. Mary A. Parsons, and secretary-treasurer
         Dr. Rosa H. Gantt.

3715.   "Second Century of Building Progress for the Woman's Med-
             ical College of Pennsylvania." Journal of the Ameri-
             can Medical Women's Association, 14:3 (March 1959)
             240-241.
         On December 9, 1958 construction began at the Medical Col-
         lege of Pennsylvania on a $2 million research wing whose
         projected completion date was to have been 1961.   This ad-
         dition would provide teaching space to enable 20 per cent
         more students to enroll, as well as more room for labora-
         tories.   Renovations in the main building will provide addi-
         tional space for diagnosis and treatment of patients.   This
         additional wing is the third major expansion since 1950.   In
         1952 a nursing wing was completed, and in 1954 a preven-
         tive medicine wing was completed.

3716.   Selmon, Bertha L.   "The Homeopathic Medical College for
             Women: Cleveland--1868-1870." Medical Woman's
             Journal, 53:5 (May 1946) 29-32.   facsim., ports.   (His-
             tory of Women in Medicine.)
         Biographies are given of Cleora Augusta Seaman, M.D.,
         principal founder of the Cleveland Homeopathic Medical Col-
         lege for Women, and of Myra K. Merrick, M.D., president
         of the College.   The institution merged, after three years'
         operation, with the Western Homeopathic Medical College.

3717.   Selmon, Bertha L.   "The New York Medical College and
             Hospital for Women (Homeopathic): 1863-1918." Med-
             ical Woman's Journal, 53:4 (April 1946) 43-46.   port.
             (History of Women in Medicine.)
         This article opens with a description of the differences of
         opinion between women in homeopathy--represented by
         Clemence Sophia Lozier--and the women who remained
         "strictly allopath"--represented by Elizabeth and Emily Black-
         well.   The professional antagonism between the "regular
         and irregular schools" contributed to the "icy gulf" between
         Lozier and the Blackwells.   A history of the New York
         Medical College and Hospital for Women, founded by Dr.
         Lozier in 1863, was written by Cornelia Chase Brant and
         mentions the women who ran the institution.   A biography
         is given of Dr. Lozier, written by her granddaughter, Jes-
         sica Lozier Payne.

3718.   Selmon, Bertha L.   "The Woman's Medical College of
             Pennsylvania." Medical Woman's Journal, 52:7 (July
             1945) 46-50, 55.   illus., ports.   (History of Women in

Medicine.)
This serialized history [continued in the October, November, and December 1945 issues of the Journal] begins with background information on the College and its early outstanding women physicians (e.g., Clara Marshall, Ann Preston, Hannah E. Longshore, and Emeline H. Cleveland, among others).

3719.   Selmon, Bertha L. "Woman's Medical College of Pennsylvania: 1888-1900." Medical Woman's Journal, 52:12 (December 1945) 45-48. (History of Women in Medicine.)
The growth and success story of the College concludes this four-part series. [The first three installments appear in the July, October, and November issues of the Journal.] Dean Clara Marshall's letter, an excerpt of which appears in this article, relates the story of the acceptance of a woman into the Philadelphia County Medical Society. Statistics on the College and a discussion of various departments are also included.

3720.   "The Semi-Annual Meeting of the Woman's Society of New York State." Medical Woman's Journal, 48:2 (February 1941) 55, 57.
An outline of the proceedings of this meeting lists the presentations as "Women's Place in the Defense Program," by Judge Dorothy Kenyon, and "The Role of Physicians in these Historical Times," by Colonel Samuel Kopetsky of the U.S. Army Medical Corps.

3721.   "Semi-Centennial Celebration of Mary Thompson Hospital of Chicago for Women and Children--1865-1915." Woman's Medical Journal, 25:12 (December 1915) 280-283. port.

3722.   "Semi-Centennial of the Medical Woman's Journal." Medical Woman's Journal, 50:5 (May 1943) 128.

3723.   "Seventy-Fourth Annual Commencement of the Woman's Medical College." Medical Woman's Journal, 33:7 (July 1926) 208.
Out of the 29 women graduating from the Woman's Medical College of Pennsylvania in 1926, ten expect to serve as medical missionaries; 17 will intern in Pennsylvania hospitals--four in Philadelphia. Since the first class in 1852, 1,600 have graduated from the college, which is the only U.S. school exclusively for the training of women doctors.

3724.   "Shall the Identity of the New York Infirmary for Women and Children Established by Doctors Elizabeth and Emily Blackwell in 1857 Be Lost? Now Entirely Staffed by Women Physicians. Under Reorganization, But 5 Percent of Women Eligible as Members of Staff." Medical Woman's Journal, 33:4 (April 1926) 111. (Editorial.)

The proposed merger of the New York Infirmary for Women
and Children--the only hospital in the city controlled by
women--with Columbia University-Presbyterian Hospital, is
firmly opposed in this editorial stand.

3725.   Sinkoff-Goldstein, Jean. "Some Background on the Blackwell
            Chapter, AMWA." Michigan Medicine, 74:2 (January
            1975) 19.   port.
        In addition to outlining the history and the current organiza-
        tional structure of the 200-member Blackwell [Michigan]
        chapter, Dr. Sinkoff-Goldstein (the chapter's president)
        identifies the organization's goals and major concerns.
        Among the severe problems these Michigan women physicians
        are preoccupied with: the high cost of medical education and
        the difficulty of obtaining part-time residencies and proper
        household childcare workers.

3726.   "Sixteenth Annual Meeting of Women's Medical Society of
            New York State Was Held at the Hotel Ten Eyck, Al-
            bany, on Monday, April 17, 1922." Medical Woman's
            Journal, 29:5 (May 1922) 95-96.
        Proceedings of this meeting are herein recorded.   Names
        of newly elected officers are given as well as titles of papers
        read by various women physicians.

3727.   "Sixty-Sixth Annual Meeting of A.M.A.--Banquet of Medical
            Women--A Great Success." Woman's Medical Journal,
            25:7 (July 1915) 158-159.

3728.   Slater, Robert J. "Memorandum from the President on the
            125th Anniversary of the College." Alumnae News, 26:
            1 (February 1975) 2-3.   port.
        As the number of women physicians increases, the impact of
        the woman's point of view on medical care will mean "ac-
        commodation and adjustment for men as well as women."
        Reflecting upon the College's move to coeducational status
        and its subsequent name change [from Woman's Medical Col-
        lege of Pennsylvania to the Medical College of Pennsylvania],
        Dr. Slater asserts that the school's historical importance to
        women has not diminished.   He further points out that co-
        education "provides all of our students with experience more
        reflective of the situations they will be meeting in later
        life."

3729.   "Some of the Women Physicians Expected to Attend the Med-
            ical Women's National Association." Bulletin Medical
            Women's Club of Chicago, 12:9 (May 1924) 6.
        Dr. Martha Tracy, Dr. Elizabeth Thelberg, Dr. Rosalie
        Slaughter Morton, Dr. Mabel Elliott, and Dr. Maude E.
        Abbott are among those women expected to attend the Asso-
        ciation meeting.

3730.   "Something About Ourselves." Medical Woman's Journal,

44:6 (June 1937) 170.   (Editorial.)
A rationale for the existence of the Medical Woman's Journal is presented.

3731.   "The Southern Medical Women's Association."   Woman's Medical Journal, 24:5 (May 1914) 103-104.

3732.   Spencer, Everett R.   "The Ten-Year Debate."   Massachusetts Physician, (July 1972) 36-37, 42.
Basing his remarks on Walter L. Burrage's book, History of the Massachusetts Medical Society 1781-1922, this executive secretary of the Massachusetts Medical Society reiterates the debate and methodology of getting women accepted into the Society.   He traces events from the application of the first woman, Susan Dimock, in 1872, until the acceptance of the first woman, Emma Louisa Call, in 1884.

3733.   Spurlock, Jeanne.   "New Recognition for Women in APA."   American Journal of Psychiatry, 132:6 (June 1975) 647-648.   (Editorial.)
Dr. Spurlock announced that the Committee on Women in Psychiatry--"a new member of the family of APA organizational components"--has become a part of the American Psychiatric Association's structure.   This editorial further provides background information on women's membership in the APA.

3734.   Starr, Sarah Logan Wister.   "What the Woman's Medical College of Pennsylvania Stands For."   Medical Woman's Journal, 31:11 (November 1924) 317-319.   photo., port.
A history of the College is given, and of Ann Preston, a member of the first graduating class and subsequent dean of the faculty.

3735.   Stephens-Walker, Hasseltine.   "Report of the President of the Medical Staff of the Mary Thompson Hospital of Chicago."   Woman's Medical Journal, 25:12 (December 1915) 283-286.   (Presentation, Meeting, Chicago Woman's Club, 16 November 1915.)

3736.   Storer, H. B.   "The Gynaecological Society of Boston and Women Physicians: A Reply to Mr. Wm. Lloyd Garrison."   Journal of the Gynaecological Society of Boston, 2 (1870) 28-38.
[Article not examined by editors.]

3737.   "Student News."   Medical Woman's Journal, 53:8 (August 1946) 60.   photo., port.
Included in the "News" is the information that of the 77 U.S. medical schools, four do not admit women students.

3738.   "Student News."   Medical Woman's Journal, 53:11 (November 1946) 60.

This mention of the opening exercises of the ninety-seventh session of Woman's Medical College of Pennsylvania includes data on the new students.

3739.   "Student Women in White." Newsweek, (16 June 1947) 23-
         26.   photos.   (Picture Review.)
         This review consists of photographs of women physicians
         and students performing various tasks at the Woman's Med-
         ical College of Pennsylvania.

3740.   Taylor-Jones, Louise.   "President's Address."   Medical
         Woman's Journal, 35:7 (July 1928) 189-190.   port.
         (Address, Annual Meeting, Medical Women's National
         Association, Minneapolis, 10-12 June 1928.)
         Incoming Medical Women's National Association president
         Louise Taylor-Jones reviews the advances the organization
         has made over the preceding five years.

3741.   Tenney, Rachel.   "New Medical Opportunities."   Woman's
         Medical Journal, 1:8 (August 1893) 167.
         Dr. Tenney writes of the value of coeducation in medical
         schools.   She also announces the faculty appointments of
         women physicians at the Hering Homeopathic Medical College
         of Chicago.

3742.   Thelander, H. E.   "Children's Hospital of San Francisco."
         Medical Woman's Journal, 41:7 (July 1934) 184-186,
         198.   chart, photos. , port.
         A biography is presented of Charlotte Blake Brown, a
         principal founder of the Pacific Dispensary for Women and
         Children (now known as Children's Hospital).   A history of
         that San Francisco-based institution is given along with a
         description of its current organization.   "The physicians
         who have figured prominently in the history of the hospital's
         growth ... have been women of vision and ideals."

3743.   Thelberg, Elizabeth B.   "Report of Medical Women's Na-
         tional Association of the National Council of Women."
         Medical Woman's Journal, 28:12 (December 1921) 312.
         A brief history of the Medical Women's National Association
         is herein given.

3744.   "The Thirty-Third Annual Meeting of the Women's Medical
         Society of New York State."   Medical Woman's Journal,
         46:5 (May 1939) 149-151.
         Among the business of the meeting held in Syracuse, April
         23 and 24 [1939], the following resolution was passed: "Re-
         solved, that the Women's Medical Association of New York
         City in Executive Session, respectfully request and urge the
         House of Delegates of the Medical Society of the State of
         New York to recommend to the House of Delegates of the
         American Medical Association that they grant a seat to a
         woman delegate in the House of Delegates."

3745.   "This Journal." Medical Woman's Journal, 45:1 (January
             1938) 18. (Editorial.)
         The Journal's importance is emphasized in this article.

3746.   "This Journal the Official Organ of the Organization of Iowa
             Medical Women." Woman's Medical Journal, 12:7
             (July 1902) 171.

3747.   "The Title in the Library and Memorial Building." Med-
             ical Woman's Journal, 54:6 (June 1947) 35-36.
         This article on the proposed library and memorial building
         to be built by the American Medical Women's Association
         on a site donated by the Woman's Medical College of Penn-
         sylvania, contains a letter from George A. Hay, comptrol-
         ler of the College. In his letter, Mr. Hay answers ques-
         tions relevant to the title and use of the library.

3748.   Tracy, Martha. "Address of Incoming President of Med-
             ical Women's National Association, New Orleans, April
             28, 1920." Medical Woman's Journal, 27:5 (May 1920)
             133-135. port.
         "We exist, not for segregation from medical men in scien-
         tific work, but as machinery to accomplish certain things
         in the interest of women to which men have given scant at-
         tention, and which must be done by women if done at all."

3749.   Tracy, Martha. "The Medical Student of Today." Women
             in Medicine, 55 (January 1937) 14-15.
         Woman's Medical College of Pennsylvania accepted 32 stu-
         dents from 100 applicants in the entering class of 1936.
         The qualities looked for in applicants were: capacity for
         amassing factual knowledge, potential of earning the respect
         of their teachers and the confidence of their patients, fam-
         ily background, native intelligence, college record, "reputa-
         tion as to integrity of character, of poise and steadfastness
         of purpose," score on the Aptitude Test for Medical Stu-
         dents, health status, personality, and neatness in person
         and dress.

3750.   Tracy, Martha. "Report of Chairman on Medical Opportun-
             ities for Women." Medical Woman's Journal, 33:5
             (May 1926) 136-138.
         Speaking before the twelfth annual convention of the Medical
         Women's National Association, Martha Tracy lists the cre-
         dentials of recipients of the Association's scholarship fund.
         "In regard to the continuance and the increase of opportun-
         ities for women physicians ... I continue to believe there is
         no need or advisability for special drive. I am more em-
         barrassed by the fact that I do not find women trained and
         ready to accept the opportunities now available.... There
         are more higher places for women physicians today than
         there are qualified candidates to fill them. The will to
         work and to qualify is our greatest need."

3751.   Tracy, Martha. "A Retrospect." In: The 75th Anniver-
         sary Volume of the Woman's Medical College of Penn-
         sylvania. Philadelphia, Pennsylvania, 1926, 1-6. (Re-
         print.)
         Dr. Tracy outlines the history of the College by describing
         the efforts of the personalities involved in its founding
         (Joseph S. Longshore, Bartholomew Fussell, and William
         J. Mullen) and the alumnae who returned to teach (Ann
         Preston, Mary Putnam Jacobi, Anna E. Broomall, Hannah
         T. Croasdale, Frances Emily White, and Clara Marshall).

3752.   Tracy, Martha. "Woman's Medical College of Pennsylvania."
         Bulletin of the Medical Women's National Association,
         38 (October 1932) 17-18.
         The establishment of a medical school for women in 1850
         was the natural outcome of the "social, economic, and edu-
         cational revolution which has been part of the so-called
         'woman movement' of the past 125 years." A history of
         the College and common attitudes towards women in medicine
         at the time are given. A discussion of Drs. Ann Preston
         and Hannah Longshore is also included with mention of oth-
         er eminent faculty members.

3753.   Tracy, Martha. "The Woman's Medical College of Penn-
         sylvania: A Glimpse at History and a Personal Retro-
         spect." Bryn Mawr Alumnae Bulletin, (May 1935).
         Dr. Tracy's account of the Medical College of Pennsylvania's
         history recalls the struggles and achievements of the first
         25 years of the College: the hard fight to obtain funds for
         equipment and support, the fight for recognition in the county
         medical society, the part played by alumnae in medical mis-
         sions, and the standardization of courses before schools like
         Harvard and the University of Pennsylvania had done so.
         Dr. Tracy concludes this article with comments upon her
         own years as faculty (appointed in 1907) and later as dean
         (appointed in 1918) of the College.

3754.   Tracy, Martha and Potter, Ellen C. "The Woman's Med-
         ical College of Pennsylvania; Its Relation to All Women
         in Medicine." Woman's Medical Journal, 29[19]:10
         (October 1919) 202-208.
         An examination of the social climate of the times and the
         struggle of women elsewhere to obtain medical education and
         establish women's schools provides context for this history
         of the Woman's Medical College of Pennsylvania. Ann Pres-
         ton, Emeline Cleveland, and Hannah Longshore are pro-
         filed as representative of some of the "refined, cultured,
         beautiful" women of the college's early years who were "in-
         sulted in the streets [and] spat upon...." The article con-
         cludes with a listing of the College's contributions that more
         than justify its perpetuation as an exclusively female medical
         school.

3755.   "Transactions of Annual Meeting of Medical Women's Na-
            tional Association, Tuesday June 13, 1916--4 p.m.,
            Hotel Statler, Detroit, Mich., Dr. Eliza Mosher, Pre-
            siding." Woman's Medical Journal, 26:6 (June 1916)
            163-164.
        At this meeting, Mary Thompson, the founder of the hos-
        pital named after her in Chicago, was honored for having
        established a place where women and children could receive
        medical care and where medical women could work and
        train.

3756.   "Twenty Women Enrolled for Study of Medicine at New York
            University." Medical Woman's Journal, 27:1 (January
            1920) 22. (Notes and Comments.)

3757.   "The Value of Organization to Medical Women." Medical
            Woman's Journal, 29:5 (May 1922) 92-93.

3758.   [Van Hoosen, Bertha]. "Address of President at Second
            Annual Meeting of the Medical Women's National Asso-
            ciation. Held in New York, June 5 and 6, 1917." Wo-
            man's Medical Journal, 27:6 (June 1917) 129.
        This speech stresses the necessity for women's organizations
        and the necessity for cooperation among all medical organiza
        tions.

3759.   Van Hoosen, Bertha. "The Children's Mercy Hospital."
            Medical Woman's Journal, 35:6 (June 1928) 172-173.
            port.
        Biographies are given of two sisters, Dr. Alice Berry
        Graham and Dr. Katherine Berry Richardson, who together
        founded the Children's Mercy Hospital in Kansas City, Mis-
        souri.

3760.   Van Hoosen, Bertha. "The Clinical Congress of the Amer-
            ican College of Surgeons From the Viewpoint of a Wo-
            man Surgeon." Medical Woman's Journal, 29:12 (De-
            cember 1922) 305-308.
        Women have always been freely admitted to membership in
        the American College of Surgeons whenever they could meet
        the requirements. In 1922 there were 30 women members.
        Dr. Van Hoosen lists the names of the new members at the
        Boston convocation in October 1922 and gives a description
        of the Congress itself. One of the "clinical attractions" was
        the program offered by the New England Hospital for Women
        and Children. Dr. Van Hoosen's description of this program
        is complete with case histories.

3761.   [Van Hoosen, Bertha]. "Do Women Doctors Need Their Own
            Medical Journal?" Medical Woman's Journal, 36:1 (Jan-
            uary 1929) 16.
        In 1926 the Journal printed five-eighths of all the articles
        that had been produced by medical women in America. The

Journal stimulates medical women to unite, and reflects each month the growing history of women in medicine.

3762. Van Hoosen, Bertha. "Looking Backward." Journal of the American Medical Women's Association, 5:10 (October 1950) 406-408.
Dr. Van Hoosen offers a brief accounting of women physicians' efforts to organize within the American Medical Association and a reminiscence of the incipient American Medical Women's Association's War Service Committee struggles.

3763. Van Hoosen, Bertha. "Medical Women's National Association--Reasons for Its Existence--Its Scope and Its Work." Woman's Medical Journal, 26:4 (April 1916) 97-98. (Editorial.)
Medical women as a class have problems that cannot be solved in the already existing medical societies. Functions which a medical woman's society could serve include: fostering a better communicative spirit; setting up a reference service so that women physicians may refer patients to other women, hear about job openings, and exchange professional information; obtaining and publishing information about where women can get training in the specialty of their choice; establishing support systems so that women will be more active in the various medical societies and associations; establishing a fund to take care of women physicians and medical students in need; and working to increase the opportunities and choices of women in medicine.

3764. Van Hoosen, Bertha. "Opportunities for Medical Women Internes." Medical Woman's Journal, 34:1 (January 1927) 4-7. illus.
A description of the growth of the Women and Children's Hospital of Chicago includes a salute to its founder, Dr. Mary Thompson. The author also calls for contributions for the institution's current fund drive.

3765. Van Hoosen, Bertha. "Opportunities for Medical Women Interns." Medical Woman's Journal, 34:2 (February 1927) 36-39. photo.
Established by the "Jean [sic] d'Arc of Temperance," Dr. Mary Weeks Burnett, the Frances E. Willard National Temperance Hospital in Chicago forbids the use of alcoholic medications. Managed by women, the hospital has accepted 11 women interns over the past seven years, although it has "been unfortunate in its selection in many instances." One woman interne was a drug addict; another left after serving a month in order to marry; two others were foreign-educated and unable to adapt themselves to American life; still another left after three months' service to take a salaried position. In spite of these discouragements the medical staff (all men with one exception) still give to women

internes every advantage and treat them absolutely without
prejudice." The article concludes with a plea for women
physicians to wrestle with and drive the "curse alcohol"
from its "final stronghold": the medicine chest of the physician.

3766.   Van Hoosen, Bertha. "Outline of Work for Year. Instruc-
          tions to Committee." Woman's Medical Journal, 26:6
          (June 1916) 159-160. port. (Address, Annual Meeting,
          Medical Women's National Association, Detroit, Michi-
          gan, 13 June 1916.)
The priorities of the committees of the Medical Women's
National Association are identified. The committee on women's hospitals is to report on the activities of the various
women's hospitals and on the opportunities for postgraduate
work. The committee on internships, by publishing a list
of hospitals that accept women as interns, provides a broader base from which to choose a place that offers good training. The committee on scholarships could organize scholarships and loan funds from funds contributed by wealthy women physicians and appreciative wealthy patients. The committee on state society transactions and on city and district
committees will share news, reports, and abstracts of the
activities of medical women. The committee on postgraduate work will publish the names and addresses of women
in medical centers where postgraduate work may be done,
in order that women physicians may know where to seek
help and advice from other women physicians. The committee on publications will use the Woman's Medical Journal
as its official organ.

3767.   Van Hooseen [sic], Bertha. "Shall Medical Women Hold
          Official Positions in the A.M.A.?" Medical Woman's
          Journal, 34:10 (October 1927) 287-288. (Feature Arti-
          cle.)
Inspired by the debate over whether the American Hospital
Association should elect a woman president, Dr. Van Hoosen
advocates that women become officers within the American
Medical Association.

3768.   Van Hoosen, Bertha. "Why Not Women Speakers?" Med-
          ical Woman's Journal, 35:7 (July 1928) 205.
At a National League of Woman Voters convention, a "score
of men [speakers] had such a wonderful opportunity to talk
down to the women and receive their adoration," despite the
fact that "woman speakers are more enthusiastic, briefer,
more entertaining, and can hold an audience much better."
Dr. Van Hoosen hopes that the Medical Women's National
organization will continue to have meetings for and by women.

3769.   Van Hoosen, Bertha. "Woman's Hospital of Detroit." Med-
          ical Woman's Journal, 35:12 (December 1928) 352-353.

Detroit's Woman's Hospital began 40 years ago as "a small affair ... in a disagreeable part of the city," with one woman physician playing multiple roles: no task was too menial. "The Board of Women Managers were indefatigable in their attention and interest to the institution." Although at present this hospital affords women physicians a better representation than most other institutions, "it is deeply to be regretted that [it] is not entirely staffed by women...."

3770.   [Van Hoosen, Bertha]. "Women Doctors as Members of Medical Societies." Medical Woman's Journal, 36:10 (October 1929) 276-277.
This article was written upon the sixteenth anniversary of the American College of Surgeons. Dr. Van Hoosen reminisces about her experience with this association, of which she was a member.

3771.   "WMC Becomes Co-Educational." Woman's Medical College: Today, 1 (October 1969) 1.   photo.
Mrs. Paul Kaiser, chairman of the Board of Corporators at Woman's Medical College of Pennsylvania, announces the College's plan to begin admitting male students. Benefits of coeducation include increased financial support and the ability to attract "high caliber" faculty, interns, and residents. A photograph introducing the first male students, and captioned "Girls Meet the Boys," accompanies this article.

3772.   Waite, Frederick C.   History of the New England Female Medical College: 1848-1874.   Boston University School of Medicine, Boston, Massachusetts, 1950, 132 pp. facsim.
This short history of the New England Female Medical College attempts to trace the history of the school as related to the general history of medicine in the U.S. The school was founded in 1848 by Samuel Gregory for instruction in midwifery. The first session in which a full course was offered was 1852, and the first M.D. degrees were awarded in 1854. The school awarded degrees to 98 women until it merged with the Boston University, then a homeopathic institution, in 1874. Appendixes to this work list all trustees, directors, teaching staff, graduates, and some non-graduated students during the life of the school. The history is based on manuscript records, reports, catalogues, legislative records, and articles in medical journals and newspapers.

3773.   Waite, Frederick C.   "Medical Education of Women at Penn Medical University." Medical Review of Reviews, 39 (1933) 255-260.
[Article not examined by editors.]

3774.   Waite, Frederick C.   "The Pioneer Medical College for

Women." The Pharos, 12:1 (May 1949) 7-8. (Presentation, Installation Beta Chapter, Boston University School of Medicine, Boston, Massachusetts, 12 November 1948.)

Highlights of the history of the New England Female Medical College are given, from its inception to its consolidation into Boston University.

3775.   Waitzkin, Evelyn D.   "Sex at Harvard."   Harvard Medical Alumni Bulletin, 49:6 (July-August 1975) 21-22.   photo., port.

Dr. Waitzkin, a general psychiatrist, presents in capsule form statistics on the number of women who have attended Harvard Medical School. In 1949, the first year women were admitted, 13 of 112 students were women. The 1975 class admitted 54 women in a total of 165 students. Dr. Waitzkin sees the problem of "femininity and medicine" as one involving both males and females. "All of the ways in which men and women relate to each other are subjected to scrutiny," and the sexual relationship is a major area of concern. As people often go to physicians for sex information, and as physicians do not necessarily know more about sex than any other college graduate, Harvard Medical School, in response to requests from students, began a course in human sexuality (in 1971). Dr. Waitzkin discusses this course and its dynamics.

3776.   Wakefield, Alice E.   "New York Infirmary for Women and Children: A Sketch of its Past and Plans for its Future."   Woman's Medical Journal, 29[19]:9 (September 1919) 186-190.   photos., plans.

3777.   Walker, Gertrude A.   "Many Happy Returns!"   In: 75th Anniversary Volume of the Woman's Medical College of Pennsylvania. Westbrook Publishing Company, Philadelphia, Pennsylvania, [1925?], 162-170.

Following a history of the College and the women associated with it, Dr. Walker (class of 1892) urges alumnae to think of their alma mater "as a spiritual entity of vastly greater importance than any one person or group of persons...."

3778.   Walker, Gertrude A.   "The Woman's Medical College of Pennsylvania."   Woman's Medical Journal, 26:2 (February 1916) 42-44.   photo., ports.

Written in the sixty-sixth year of the Woman's Medical College of Pennsylvania, this article reviews a portion of the College's history and gives a description of its physical facilities. In several instances this college has led others in the advance of medical education. In 1888 an obstetrics outpatient department was established and later, ward cases were received which enabled students at this college to have clinical experience. Besides enabling women to hold faculty

positions, the College has also contributed up to one-fourth
of all medical missionaries sent out each year by the United
States.   As a woman's college, this school has been active
in securing the rights of women.

3779.   Walker, Stella Ford. "A Library of the Writings of Med-
            ical Women." Medical Woman's Journal, 37:6 (June
            1930) 149.
        In order to collect a comprehensive library of materials by
        women physicians that could be used not only as a practical
        working library but also as "a source of inspiration to wo-
        men thinking of entering the medical field," Bertha Van
        Hoosen helped to direct the establishment of a collection at
        the Library of the American College of Surgeons.

3780.   Wallace, Ellen A. "The New Hampshire Memorial Hospital
            for Women and Children." Medical Woman's Journal,
            35:10 (October 1928) 275-276.   photo.
        The growth of the New Hampshire Memorial Hospital for
        Women and Children, founded by Julia Eastman Wallace-
        Russell in 1876, is traced to the present.

3781.   Waugh, Elizabeth S. "History of the Library Trust Fund."
            Journal of the American Medical Women's Association,
            28:11 (November 1973) 590-594.   port.
        Dr. Waugh traces the history of the American Medical
        Women's Association Library Trust Fund from Dr. Julia
        Donahue's initial $75 contribution to the building of the
        Florence A. Moore Library of Medicine at the Medical Col-
        lege of Pennsylvania.

3782.   Waugh, Elizabeth S. "The Pioneer Spirit." Journal of the
            American Medical Women's Association, 5:10 (October
            1950) 409. (Inaugural Address, American Medical Wo-
            men's Association, Pebble Beach, California, 21 June
            1950.)
        This article is a very brief tribute to Dr. Bertha Van
        Hoosen, the first president of the American Medical Wo-
        men's Association.

3783.   Wells, Mrs. S. E. F. "Women in Medicine and Their Col-
            leges." Medical-Literary Journal (San Francisco), 4:3
            (1881-1882) 9-14.
        [Article not examined by editors.]

3784.   "What Price--The M.W.N.A.?" Medical Woman's Journal,
            36:6 (June 1929) 152.
        The benefits derived from having formed a separate associa-
        tion for women physicians are discussed.   This article ap-
        pears fifteen years after the organization of the Medical
        Women's National Association.

3785.   "A Wise Decision." Woman's Medical Journal, [8]:7 (July

1899) 247-248.
The formal announcement of the "wise decision" to close
the Women's Medical College of the New York Infirmary
for Women and Children is reprinted along with excerpts
of remarks by Dr. Emily Blackwell. The College, which
has been in existence for 40 years, "fulfilled its purpose"
and women can now obtain medical education with men on
an equal basis.

3786.   "Woman's Medical College." Medical Woman's Journal,
         33:10 (October 1926) 299.
The Woman's Medical College of Pennsylvania began its
seventy-seventh year with exercises at which Dr. Ellen C.
Potter, the Pennsylvania State Secretary of Welfare, warned
the 30 entering students against isolation from cultural interests. In 1926 Dr. Ai Hee Kim became the first Korean
woman to study at the College.

3787.   "The Woman's Medical College of Penn." Woman's Med-
         ical Journal, 5:11 (November 1896) 297-298.
Quotes from the student handbook of the Woman's Medical
College of Pennsylvania provide historical background and
reasons for the importance of the institution.

3788.   "The Woman's Medical College of Pennsylvania." Club Wo-
         man's Journal, 6:3 (February 1940) 7.
On the occasion of its 90th year, the history of the Woman's
Medical College is reviewed.

3789.   "The Woman's Medical College of Pennsylvania." Journal
         of the American Medical Women's Association, 1:1
         (April 1946) 22.   photo.
After the Woman's Medical College of Pennsylvania was
founded in March 1850, Ann Preston was in the first graduating class and was the first woman given a faculty appointment: the chair of physiology and hygiene. In 1867 she
became dean of the faculty. Since Emeline H. Cleveland
was appointed to the chair of obstetrics in 1862, women have
held that position. Nineteen hundred women have been graduated from this college in its 95-year history. Faith S.
Fetterman is medical director of the hospital affiliated with
the College. Margaret D. Craighill, the dean of the College, was the first woman ever to be commissioned as an
officer in the U.S. Army. After serving as chief of the
Women's Health and Welfare Unit of the Office of the Surgeon General, she received the Legion of Merit and rose to
the rank of lieutenant-general. She was appointed consultant
for the medical care of women veterans.

3790.   "The Woman's Medical College of Pennsylvania." Journal
         of the American Medical Women's Association, 14:3
         (March 1959) 240.
The Woman's Medical College of Pennsylvania, founded in

1850, has given women a chance to study medicine when other medical schools would not accept them. Currently, only 50 students per entering class are admitted, which makes classes small enough for individual teaching and large enough for stimulating and lively discussion. Students get clinical experience not only at the College hospital but also at other Philadelphia hospitals. Students came from all over the United States and from many foreign countries, as well as from Pennsylvania, to attend Woman's Medical College.

3791. "The Woman's Medical College of Pennsylvania." Medical Woman's Journal, 37:4 (April 1930) 85-86. photo.
After first meeting in rented rooms when it was founded in 1850, the Woman's Medical College of Pennsylvania in 1875 erected the first building in the world to be used exclusively for the education of women in medicine. The College, which is about to celebrate its eightieth anniversary, has outgrown its former building and is about to complete its latest structure which is to accommodate students, nurses, doctors, patients, modern equipment and "numerous memorials to the women who were pioneers in the profession of medicine and surgery."

3792. "Woman's Medical College of Pennsylvania." Medical Woman's Journal, 47:10 (October 1940) 311.
At the opening of the College's ninety-first annual session, Dr. Catharine Macfarlane announced minor faculty changes and reported an enrollment of 115 students, including 41 in the first-year class.

3793. "Woman's Medical College of Pennsylvania." Medical Woman's Journal, 48:1 (January 1941) 27.
Announcement is made of faculty activities at the Woman's Medical College.

3794. "Woman's Medical College of Pennsylvania." Medical Woman's Journal, 48:4 (April 1941) 119. (News of the Month.)
News of the College is given which includes mention of a lecture course during 1941 in applied medico-genetics.
This was believed to be the first symposium on this subject sponsored by a medical school in the United States.

3795. "Woman's Medical College of Pennsylvania." Medical Woman's Journal, 48:5 (May 1941) 150.
This brief announcement concerns the appointment of Dr. Ellen C. Potter as acting president of the Woman's Medical College of Pennsylvania, and Dr. Margaret D. Craighill as dean of the College.

3796. "Woman's Medical College of Pennsylvania." Medical Woman's Journal, 48:10 (October 1941) 324. (News of the

Month.)
A list of new appointments to the Woman's Medical College
of Pennsylvania is given. At the time of this article, 115
students were enrolled in the College.

3797.   "Woman's Medical College of Pennsylvania." Medical Wo-
             man's Journal, 53:3 (March 1946) 34.
         The 36 women who received degrees at the College's ninety-
         fourth annual commencement are listed. Information is also
         provided on Margaret D. Craighill, who returns from mili-
         tary duty as dean of the institution.

3798.   "Woman's Medical College of Pensylvania [sic]." Medical
             Woman's Journal, 53:8 (August 1946) 22-23.
         This report includes details of a merger proposed by Mar-
         garet D. Craighill, dean of Woman's Medical College, with
         Jefferson Medical College. All assets of Woman's Medical
         College and its hospital (valued at over $3 million) were to
         be turned over to Jefferson. In return, women would be
         admitted to Jefferson on a 20 per cent quota basis; no pro-
         visions were made for staff members. Dr. Craighill's
         proposal was rejected at an April 10, 1946 meeting of the
         board of corporators. On April 24, 1946, Dean Craighill's
         resignation was presented and accepted.

3799.   "The Woman's Medical College of Pennsylvania: Founded
             1850." Medical Woman's Journal, 55:6 (June 1948) 59-
             60. (Notes from the Woman's Medical College of Penn-
             sylvania.)
         The College's importance to women is the subject of this
         article, which also reports on a testimonial dinner in honor
         of Catharine Macfarlane, grants received by the College,
         and the inauguration of a chapter of the Association of In-
         ternes and Medical Students.

3800.   "Woman's Medical College of Pennsylvania: News of Activi-
             ties." Medical Woman's Journal, 45:4 (April 1938) 115-
             116.
         The "news" consists of recent lectures, ceremonies, and
         other activities held at the college.

3801.   "The Woman's Hospital of Philadelphia." Medical Woman's
             Journal, 39:11 (November 1932) 285-286.
         The Woman's Hospital of Philadelphia which merged with
         the West Philadelphia Hospital for Women in 1929 continues
         both institutions' tradition of having women interns. The
         Woman's Hospital of Philadelphia, founded in 1861, is prob-
         ably the oldest hospital to employ women interns.

3802.   "Woman's [sic] Medical College of the New York Infirmary."
             Medical Record, 7 (1925) 215. (Medical Items and
             News.)
         Eight ladies received degrees during the recent commence-

ment exercises. This report of that ceremony includes summaries of the main address, delivered by Professor Mary C. Putnam, M.D., as well as a speech by Joseph H. Choate, Esq.

3803.   "Women at Mayo: a Steady Climb up a Steep Staircase." Mayovox (August 1974) 1-4. photo., ports.
Female residents comprise five per cent of Mayo physicians-in-training. Citing some reasons why women are not found in large numbers in the medical profession, the author admits that "unconscious chauvinists attitudes on the part of some male physicians" is a factor. Women have also "been held back by their own preconceived notions of what their role in business should be." The article then discusses three successful women at Mayo: Margaret Thompson, a political activist and Mayo Medical School's first registrar (in 1971); Diane Casper, administrator in research services; and Dr. Ann Schutt, a Mayo Clinic consultant.

3804.   "Women Hold Positions of Responsibility." Medical and Professional Woman's Journal, 40:9 (September 1933) 275.
A large number of women hold positions of responsibility at the Medical Center of the New York Hospital, Cornell Medical College Association. Thirty-three are associated with the faculty and 42 women hold "responsible" positions in the hospital departments. The number of women in each department is given as well as the names of many of the women at the organization. Mentioned are Dr. Connie M. Guion, Dr. Evelyn Holt, Dr. Phyllis Greenacre, Dr. Mary G. Wilson, and Dr. Lucy Crawford.

3805.   "Women in Medicine at the University of Michigan Medical School." Journal of the American Medical Women's Association, 18:7 (July 1963) 566-568.
Historical notes and faculty reaction to women as medical students are included in this article about the University of Michigan Medical School. The article concludes with a roster of distinguished medical alumnae.

3806.   "Women in Medicine at UNM: A Better Place in Transition." University of New Mexico School of Medicine Alumni News, 1:3 (December 1974) 4. photo., port.
Women number 63 of 265 medical students at the University of New Mexico School of Medicine. On the 292-member faculty, 40 (or 13 per cent) are women; in administration, there is one woman dean, one associate dean, four assistant deans, and no women department chairpersons. Men receive proportionately more financial aid than women students, because more men have non-working spouses and have greater financial need. While special women's service, such as daycare and gynecological health care, are not specifically provided, very few other medical schools offer such

services. Some women students report encountering subtle
discrimination, such as "female pin-up slides used to 'en-
liven'" lectures, and female patients sometimes prefer male
doctors: one woman patient said "she'd feel 'absolutely
queer' if she were treated by a woman." Most UNMSOM
women students feel, however, that medical school is a good
place for a woman.

3807.   "Women in Medicine: Philadelphia Has Solely Female Med-
         ical School." See, (July 1949) 33-35. photos.
         A brief introduction to the history and outstanding graduates
         of the Woman's Medical College of Pennsylvania precedes
         a photo essay of the College's students and facilities. The
         College, to date, has graduated 2,142 women, including 212
         from 30 foreign countries.

3808.   "Women in Science." Medical Woman's Journal, 44:1 (Janu-
         ary 1937) 19-20. (Editorial.)
         Of the 45 medical officers on the staff of the National Insti-
         tutes of Health (NIH), one third are women. The work of
         several women scientists at NIH is cited, including the re-
         search in bacteria by Drs. Alice Evans and Alda Bengtson.

3809.   "Women Man the White Coats." Case Western Reserve
         University INSIGHT, 3:1 (Fall 1974) 27-28. port.
         This article is primarily about women attending the medical
         school of Western Reserve College (WRC) in Cleveland,
         Ohio. Dr. Nancy Clark was the first woman student at
         the College (M.D. 1852) and the "second woman doctor in
         the world." Five other women physicians who attended
         WRC are discussed: Emily Blackwell, Sarah Chadwick,
         Cordelia A. Green, Marie Elizabeth Zakrzewska, and Eliza-
         beth Griselle. "These six women medical graduates con-
         stitute the 'Golden Age' of coeducational medical training."

3810.   "Women of Pennsylvania." The 1970-71 Pennsylvania Man-
         ual, 100 (1972) 847-857.
         Under the "Women and Medicine" section of this manual
         (pages 850 and 851) a brief history is given which focuses
         upon the Woman's Medical College of Pennsylvania.

3811.   "Women Praised as Physicians: Baruch Speaks at Opening
         of Infirmary Drive." Medical Woman's Journal, 53:6
         (June 1946) 53. (News Notes.)
         At a fund-raising dinner for the New York Infirmary for
         Women and Children, Bernard Baruch (United Nations
         Atomic Energy Commission representative) asserted that
         woman is "a natural" physician because she "knows about
         the beginning of life, about bringing up children." Norman
         T. Kirk (army surgeon-general) discussed how women phy-
         sicians have proved their worth in the army.

3812.   "Women's [sic] Medical College of Pennsylvania Celebrates

Its Ninetieth Anniversary." <u>Medical Woman's Journal</u>, 47:4 (April 1940) 101.

Since its founding to the present, the Woman's Medical College of Pennsylvania graduated more than 2,000 physicians, more than 150 of whom became medical missionaries. The institution's anniversary program included a series of lectures on genetics.

3813.   "Women's Medical Society of New York State." <u>Medical Woman's Journal</u>, 48:11 (November 1941) 351.

This article consists of a fund-raising letter sent out by the Medical Education Committee of the Women's Medical Society of New York State. The letter is sent to each of the 1500 women physicians in the state of New York. The amounts received annually in the past 15 years of this drive would not support one medical student in the United States, "but it will help a few in Korea...."

3814.   "Women's Medical Society of New York State: Annual Meeting May 19, 1941, Buffalo." <u>Medical Woman's Journal</u>, 47:12 (December 1940) 375.

This article, consisting of a scholarship fund-raising announcement, states that although the Society is supporting the medical education of three women in Korea, it has not received enough money to support any students in this country.

3815.   "Women's Medical Society of New York State: 31st Annual Meeting, Rochester, N.Y., May 24, 1937 (Official Report)." <u>Medical Woman's Journal</u>, 44:6 (June 1937) 173-174.

3816.   "Women's Rightful Place in Medicine: Board Certifications won by CME-LLU Alumnae." <u>Alumni Journal</u> [Loma Linda University, School of Medicine], 44:3 (May 1973) 16-17.

The names and locations of 58 alumnae of the College of Medical Evangelists, Loma Linda University, who have been granted certification by an American board, are listed according to specialty. Notes on various "firsts" are given, and it is noted that 20 women are in residency training, preparing for certification.

3817.   Woodside, Nina B. "What is CWIM?" <u>Journal of the American Medical Women's Association</u>, 29:5 (May 1974) 222-226.

The organization as well as the objectives of the Center for Women in Medicine at the Medical College of Pennsylvania are discussed, i.e., research and information, recruitment, training, elimination of discrimination, and placement. In addition, current and proposed activities, such as workshops, premedical student summer applications, and a program for high school students are reviewed.

3818.   Woolley, Alice Stone. "'United Front': Address by Dr.
              Alice Stone Woolley, President of the Women's Medical
              Society of New York State, in a Joint Banquet Meeting
              with the New York State Medical Society." Medical
              Woman's Journal, 47:6 (June 1940) 188, 171.
         Following a justification for women physicians maintaining
         separate medical societies, Dr. Woolley calls for men and
         women physicians to unite "to help break down a disabling
         apathy" that currently characterizes the American youth.

3819.   "Work of American Women's Hospitals in Serbia and the
              Near East: President of National Association Goes to
              Serbia to Organize this Field." Woman's Medical Jour-
              nal, 29 [19] 8: (August 1919) 162. photo.

3820.   "World Institution, The Woman's Medical College: A Cen-
              tury of Service." American Soroptimist, 24:8 (April
              1951) 5-7. photos., ports.
         The history and services of the Woman's Medical College
         [of Pennsylvania], 100 years old in 1950, are given in this
         article.

3821.   Wright, Elizabeth S. "Federation's Gifts to Woman's Med-
              ical College: Salute to Women in Medicine." Ameri-
              can Soroptimist, 28:9 (June 1955) 5-6. photo. (Ser-
              vice Objectives--Phase VI.)

3822.   Wright, Katharine W. "President's Message." Journal of
              American Medical Women's Association, 14:3 (March
              1959) 242.
         The Woman's Medical College of Pennsylvania is a place
         for women medical students and teachers to work together,
         learn together, and cooperate together. It serves as a
         model for women physicians to pool their interests, time,
         and abilities in working for the American Medical Women's
         Association.

3823.   Wynekoop, Alice Lois Lindsay. "The Relation of the Wo-
              man Physician to Social Service." Woman's Medical
              Journal, 25:12 (December 1915) 272-274. (Presenta-
              tion, Semi-Centennial Celebration, Mary Thompson Hos-
              pital of Chicago, Chicago, Illinois, 18 November 1915.)
         In addition to discussing the responsibilities of medical wo-
         men in social services, Dr. Lindsay-Wynekoop reminisces
         about the women who were associated with the Mary Thomp-
         son Hospital.

3824.   X. "The Admission of Women to the Philadelphia County
              Medical Society." The Polyclinic, 1 (15 October 1883)
              62-63. (Correspondence.)
         This article ridicules the results of secret balloting in
         which the Philadelphia County Medical Society voted 95-70
         to continue excluding women physicians. Because state and

national associations will not admit practitioners unless they belong to county organizations, the author hopes to change minds by presenting arguments in favor of women. To the argument that women would interfere with discussion, the author replies, "what cannot be properly said in the presence of women had better not be said in the presence of men," and calls for freedom of speech in medical societies.

3825.   Young Women's Christian Associations. International Conference of Women Physicians and Convention of Delegates from National Women's Organizations: By Invitation of Social Morality Committee, War Work Council, National Board of the Young Women's Christian Associations. Conference: September 15-October 25. Convention: October 17-24. [n. p.], [1919?], 32 pp. ports.

"This conference is called that it may bring women physicians together from all nations to consider ways in which the physical condition of women may be improved and their ignorance and immaturity of attitude toward sex and emotional health eliminated." Portraits and thumbnail sketches are given for several women physicians who were speakers at the conference.

GENERAL

The literature cited here mentions multiple
aspects of women in medicine, and gives
overviews of the situation for women physicians.

AFRICA

3826.   Klempman, Sarah. "Women Doctors." <u>South African Med-</u>
            <u>ical Journal</u>, 44:15 (11 April 1970) 460. (Letters to the
            Editor.)
         If women doctors take a leave of absence, it is temporary.
         When male doctors emigrate, as they do in great numbers,
         their absence is permanent. The Medical Council and Med-
         ical Association of South Africa should open up enough med-
         ical schools so that every one who fulfills the requirements,
         regardless of sex or color, may acquire medical training.

ASIA

3827.   Balfour, Margaret I. "Medical Women in India." <u>Hospital</u>
            <u>Social Service</u>, 11 (1925) 239-243.
         Dr. Balfour explains why India needs medical women, the
         organizations which supply India with medical women, the
         conditions under which one must practice in India, and the
         medical education available there.

3828.   Barrett, (Lady). "Impressions of India." <u>Medical Wo-</u>
            <u>men's Federation News-Letter</u>, (July 1929) 26-29.
         In this article [reprinted from the <u>Journal of the Associa-</u>
         <u>tion of Medical Women in India</u>, February 1929], Dr. Bar-
         rett describes poverty in India, the people's subsequent
         health problems, and the country's great need for women
         physicians.

3829.   Beals, Rose F. "The Woman Doctor in India." <u>Medical</u>
            <u>Woman's Journal</u>, 33:7 (July 1926) 204-207.
         Although there is a tremendous satisfaction and "profession-
         al thrills enough" for the woman doctor practicing in India,
         there are "drawbacks to life in these Eastern countries."
         "Learning the language and understanding the people are
         equally difficult and also exceedingly necessary. Next, one
         must be willing to live in a rather primitive way ... But
         one can have as many books and magazines as in America.
         One can have one's own piano and typewriter and sewing
         machine." Dr. Beals gives anecdotes about the patients
         she administers to at the hospital in Wai, India.

3830.   Cambel, Perihan. "The Status of Women Physicians in
            Turkey." <u>Journal of the American Medical Women's</u>
            <u>Association</u>, 4:1 (January 1949) 25-28. ports.
         Perihan recounts her first meeting with Müfide Kâzim (one
         of the first women in Turkey to study medicine) at a tea
         party where Müfide Kâzim (later Müfide Küley), at that time

a medical student, and her friend Süreyya Agaoglu, a lawyer, arrived in tailor-made black suits, and advocating
dress reform. Women's struggle for admittance to medical
school and residencies is briefly discussed as well as the
lives of Dr. Rasim Kizi Suat, one of the first women physicians in Turkey, and Dr. Suat Giz, who practices surgery
in a private hospital. Pediatrics, internal medicine, and
gynecology and obstetrics head the list of specialties for
Turkey's 277 women physicians, which indicates that "Turkish women prefer certain branches where they are relatively more assured of individual freedom and success." Memberships of Turkish women physicians in professional organizations and government posts is reviewed, and the author states that "there never has been any discrimination
against women by medical societies" in Turkey. Certain
points of the Turkish woman's "historical evolution" are high
lighted.

3831.   "Chinese Women Good Doctors. Commission Finds Remark-
         able Ability--Three Medical Colleges for Women in
         China." Bulletin Medical Women's Club of Chicago, 4:1
         (September 1915) 5.
         The three medical colleges for women in China are listed:
         Hackett Medical College, North China Union Medical College,
         and the Women's Medical College at Soochow.

3832.   "Education for Medical Women in India." British Medical
         Journal, 1 (20 January 1923) 128.
         This very brief news item concerns a proposed medical
         school for women in Madras, India. It is noted that in
         1920 there were only 135 qualified women medical practi-
         tioners for India's female population of more than 21 million.

3833.   Fischer, Golda. "Medical Women in Israel: Historical
         Background." Journal of the American Medical Wo-
         men's Association, 7:4 (April 1952) 137-138.
         Part I in a series of three articles gives a historical back-
         ground of Israel itself as well as information on women
         physicians in Israel, and the formation of the Israeli Wo-
         men's Medical Association in 1936 in the home of Dr. Anna
         Jacob[-Peller]. Currently, 20 per cent of the total number
         of physicians in the country are women. [Part II of this
         series deals with biographical data, and Part III considers
         professional activity.]

3834.   "Four Hundred Million Women in Asia Appeal for Relief
         from Physical Suffering." Medical Woman's Journal,
         30:[4] (April 1923) 117-121. photos., port.
         A review of the work of Dr. Ida Scudder initiates this arti-
         cle, which discusses, in addition, the native Indian woman
         physician. Various women's colleges in the Orient are
         described.

3835. Gomez, Trinidad. "Demand for Philippine Medical Woman-
          power." Journal of the American Medical Women's
          Association, 22:7 (July 1967) 478-480.
       This paper, presented at the tenth Congress of the Medical
       Women's International Association, discusses the great de-
       mand for medical power in the Philippines, a demand which
       women physicians can help meet.   The problems of the
       country are reviewed, e.g., malnutrition and public health.
       Women constitute 25 per cent of the Philippines medical
       population.   The author concludes with a list of Filipino
       women physicians who have achieved national and interna-
       tional fame.

3836. "Japanese Medical Women." Medical and Professional Wo-
          man's Journal, 41:1 (January 1934) 31.
       The three women's medical colleges in Japan annually gradu-
       ate approximately 150 doctors each.   Other general observa-
       tions about Japanese professional women are given.

3837. Kawai, Yaeko. "Medical Women in Japan." Journal of
          the American Medical Women's Association, 6:9 (Sep-
          tember 1951) 352-353.   photo., port.   (Status of Wo-
          men Physicians.)
       The efforts of Dr. Yaoi Yoshioka, a pioneer medical woman
       in Japan, are presented.   Dr. Yoshioka (although not the
       first woman licensed to practice medicine in the country--
       Dr. Ginko in 1890 was the first) concerned herself with,
       and contributed greatly to, the education of medical women
       in Japan.   Japanese women are socially considered inferior
       to men, and this status affects women in Japan in a way
       United States women cannot fully appreciate.   Dr. Yoshioka
       established, in 1899, the Tokyo Women's Medical College,
       the buildings of which were twice destroyed in 20 years--
       by the earthquake of 1924 and by air raids in 1943.   At the
       time of this article, the Tokyo Medical Society for Women
       boasts 5000 members (out of 10,000 women doctors).   There
       are five medical colleges for women.   Specialties chosen
       most frequently are internal medicine, pediatrics, and gyne-
       cology and obstetrics.   "All Japanese medical women ad-
       mire and envy the social position ... of our colleagues in
       the United States."

3838. Lloyd-Green, Lorna. "Supply." Journal of the American
          Medical Women's Association, 22:5 (May 1967) 337-338.
       This article consists of a report to the Medical Women's
       International Association on the countries of the Western
       Pacific and Southeast Asia.   The author had difficulty col-
       lecting the data because the directories of the various coun-
       tries did not list physicians by sex.   No charts are included;
       the report is a brief narrative highlighting conditions for
       women physicians in various countries.

3839. Lovejoy, Esther P. "Philippine Medical Women." Journal

of the American Medical Women's Association, 7:8
(August 1952) 304-306.   ports.

There are over a thousand women doctors registered for
practice in the Philippine Islands.   Because women students were not admitted to Santo Tomas University until
1930, many of these women received their degrees from the
College of Medicine of the University of the Philippines established in 1908.   Manila Central University allowed women to enroll for M.D. degrees in 1931.   By the late
1940s, these three schools were graduating about 70 women
yearly.   Included are portraits of Dr. Honoria Acosta-
Sison and Dr. Olivia Salamanca, both of whom attended
Woman's Medical College of Pennsylvania and graduated in
1909 and 1910; the former is considered the first Philippine
woman physician, and became professor of obstetrics and
gynecology at the College of Medicine, University of the
Philippines and head of its Department of Obstetrics; Dr.
Fe del Mundo, president of the Philippine Medical Women's
Association and editor of its official organ, The Philippine
Medical World; Dr. Marie Paz Mendoza-Gauzon, in 1912,
was the first woman to receive an M.D. degree in the
Philippines and was the first dean of women at the University of the Philippines and the first president of the Philippine Association of University Women.   Her field was path-
ology.

3840.   McKibbin-Harper, Mary.   "Medical Women in India."   Med-
         ical Woman's Journal, 33:10 (October 1926) 287-289.
         Dr. McKibbin-Harper complements a sketchy account of the
         work of women physicians in India with her impressions of
         that country's religious and social customs.   Dr. Turner-
         Watts heads the Cama and Albless Hospitals "with only na-
         tive assistants," who include surgical assistants Miss
         Jhirad, M.D., and Miss Dadabohg, M.D., M.R.C.P.
         Margaret Balfour, an English physician, does research in
         maternal morbidity and infant mortality.   The Countess of
         Dufferin's Association funded the training of Indian women
         as nurses and sub-surgeons.   The Servants of India Society
         and the Poona Seva Sadan Society have trained 150 women
         doctors: "Thus it will be seen that the Indians are doing
         something for themselves."   The greatest obstacle for med-
         ical women to overcome is "the dense ignorance of the mass
         of Indian humanity, built up through many generations of
         superstition and religious fanaticism."

3841.   "Medical Women of Japan."   Medical Woman's Journal, 40:
         3 (March 1933) 67.
         In 1900 there were four women doctors in Japan; in 1933
         there were 1,247 practicing [women] doctors in Japan,
         China, Korea, Formosa, and "other neighboring countries."
         This increase is credited to the Tokyo Women's Medical Col-
         lege.   The Japanese Medical Women's Society is described,
         also.

3842.   Morrow, Laura E. "Women Physicians of Israel." Jour-
         nal of the American Medical Women's Association, 18:
         4 (April 1963) 312-313. photos.
         This article is a review of data on women physicians in
         Israel. The data are gathered from a meeting of the au-
         thor with six leading women physicians of Tel Aviv and
         from an informative letter prepared by one of these six
         women, Dr. Krieger, "a grandmother." The aims of the
         Medical Women's Association in Israel are discussed.

3843.   Morton, Rosalie Slaughter. "Report of Work of Women
         Physicians in the Near East." Medical Woman's Jour-
         nal, 43:8 (August 1936) 203-214. (Presentation, 30th
         Annual Meeting, Women's Medical Society of New York
         State, New York City, 27 April 1936.)
         The professional activities, status, and difficulties faced by
         women physicians in the Middle East are discussed, and the
         work of specific women is mentioned.

3844.   Ohara, Kazue. "Women Doctors in Japan: Past and Pres-
         ent." Journal of the American Medical Women's Asso-
         ciation, 12:6 (June 1957) 175-180. tables.
         Before World War II, there were three women's colleges
         in Japan and about 15 per cent of the medical students in
         Japan were women. Since the war, every medical school
         of a university has at least one woman student and the total
         percentage of women students in all medical schools in 1956
         was 8.4 per cent. While women are found in every area
         of medical specialty, their salaries are lower than men's.
         There was a medical school for women in Japan more than
         1200 years ago.

3845.   "Opportunities for Women Physicians in Far East." Medical
         and Professional Woman's Journal, 40:11 (November
         1933) 338. (Editorial.)
         The fact that women physicians in the Orient seem to be
         gaining equality more rapidly than women in the United
         States is attributed, in part, to the tradition which pro-
         hibits women there from consulting men physicians. "Even
         in China ... the position of women physicians has become
         more secure."

3846.   "Opportunities in Korea." Medical Woman's Journal, 42:4
         (April 1935) 107. (Editorial.)
         Esther Kim Pak was the first Korean woman physician.
         This and a few other facts relating to medical women in
         Korea are given in this editorial.

3847.   Pak, Rhoda Kim. "Medical Women in Korea." Journal of
         the American Medical Women's Association, 5:3 (March
         1950) 116-117. port. (Status of Women Physicians.)
         Esther Kim Pak, in 1900, was the first Korean physician
         (man or woman) to practice Western medicine in Korea.

In 1914 two women succeeded in obtaining admission into
the Government Medical College in Seoul, and in 1918
three other women graduated from the College which,
shortly thereafter, closed its doors to women.   In 1928 Dr.
Rosetta Hall founded the Women's Medical Institute in Seoul.
At the time of this writing, there are four coeducational
medical colleges in Korea and 476 women physicians (compared to 2,934 men physicians).   While theoretically men
and women have equal opportunity now to obtain a medical
education and practice, "there are in Korea certain old
customs which tend to limit, somewhat, the practice of
medicine by women."

3848.   Pennell, Alice M. Sorabji. "A Medical Woman in India."
          Medical Women's International Journal, 1:2 (November
          1925) 52-56.
          The author talks in general terms about opportunities for
          women physicians in India.   A major portion of this article,
          however, relates anecdotes about a particular woman doc-
          tor's experiences in India, a woman referred to only as
          "Doctor Miss-Sahiba."

3849.   Platt, Kate. "The Annual Reports for 1925 of Four Indian
          Medical Activities." Medical Women's Federation News-
          Letter, (March 1927) 33-35.
          This report includes some statistics on women in Indian
          medical schools as well as a general discussion of women's
          work in hospitals.

3850.   Richey, Margaret C. "Medical Opportunities for Women in
          China." Medical Woman's Journal, 45:5 (May 1938)
          124-125.
          Following a generalized discussion of the educational oppor-
          tunities for Chinese medical women, the author (director
          of the Church Hospital, Changshu, Kiang Province, China)
          addresses the need for additional woman physicians to be-
          come "fellow-workers with our Chinese friends."

3851.   Scott, Agnes C. "Medical Work for Women in India." Med-
          ical Women's Federation News-Letter, (March 1927) 29-
          32.
          Based upon her personal observations, Dr. Scott reports on
          the education and the professional activity of Indian women
          physicians.   In addition, she offers advice to the British
          woman physician who wishes to work in India.

3852.   "A Survey of Medical Women's Work in India: Government
          Medical Work for Women." Medical Woman's Journal,
          36:12 (December 1929) 326-327.
          In India, two colleges and one medical school (The Lady
          Hardinge Medical School in Delhi) are maintained exclusively
          for the training of women.   The Countess of Dufferin Fund
          devotes its funds chiefly to the training of Indian women as

doctors and gives grants to hospitals for women in India.
Indian medical women's service under the government and
in the medical college is discussed.   Other funds and organizations, which in some way support the training and
work of women physicians in India, are also mentioned.

3853.   Tao, S. M. "Medical Education of Chinese Women." Med-
         ical and Professional Woman's Journal, 41:3 (March
         1934) 73-76.
         "Information on the medical education of women in China is
         very meagre," and although general histories of modern
         medical education in China are available, the most recent
         report--by Faber to the League of Nations (1931)--contains
         no reference whatsoever to women in any of its discussions
         or recommendations.   There are, however, over 550 quali-
         fied women physicians in China.   The Chinese Medical Asso-
         ciation estimates that the proportion of women to men doc-
         tors is about one to ten.   Out of China's 23 coeducational
         and two women's medical colleges, women make up 16.9
         per cent (619) of the total student registration (3,655).
         "Medicine is the only profession in this country in which
         women have thoroughly established themselves."   Stressing
         the need for China to make more educational opportunities
         available to women, the article discusses the history of
         Chinese medical women, and the social traditions which have
         affected them.   (This article was reprinted from the Chinese
         Medical Journal, xlvii (1933) 1010-1028.)

3854.   "A Terrible Memorial. Fifty-Five Lady-Doctors, Mission-
         ary and Otherwise, Petition the Indian Government on
         the Subject of Child-Marriage." Medical Missionary
         Record, 6:12 (December 1891) 271-272. (Woman's
         Needs and Woman's Work.)
         These women presented a petition which catalogues 24 cases
         of bodily injury done to female children by adult Indian
         males who have had sexual intercourse with them (as their
         prerogative in marriage).

3855.   "The Woman Doctor in India." Medical Woman's Journal,
         51:11 (November 1944) 24, 30.
         This generalized discussion of Indian women physicians
         touches upon social conditions, i.e., the purdah system,
         medical education opportunities for women, and the status
         of women MDs in the military.

3856.   "Women Doctors in Japan." Literary Digest, 101:48 (20
         April 1929).
         Following a review of the history of Japanese medical wo-
         men, Dr. Yayoi Yoshioka is quoted on the founding and the
         present activity of the Tokyo Women's Medical College.

3857.   Wynen, Elise. "Women Surgeons in India." Journal of the
         American Medical Women's Association, 8:7 (July 1953)

248-249.
There is a tremendous doctor shortage in India, and due to
the traditional modesty and strict seclusion of women, women physicians are much in demand. Missionary hospitals
in India and the medical specialties that are needed are
discussed.

3858.   Yamazaki, R. ["Current Status of Women Physicians in
         Japan"]. Journal of the Japan Medical Association, 56:
         5 (1 September 1966) 527-528. (Jap)

3859.   Yamazaki, Rinko. "The Demand for Medical Women."
         Journal of the American Medical Women's Association,
         22:7 (July 1967) 485-487.
         Comparative data on men and women physicians in Japan
         is cited, where women at the time of this article repre-
         sented 9.3 per cent of the total physician population. The
         author also looks at "what types of specialties are best
         suited for women physicians" in relation to the socioeco-
         nomic conditions of a given country. In discussion of apti-
         tudes, Dr. Yamazaki submits that "Japanese women physicians,
         because of their natural aptitudes, are best suited for work
         as general practitioners, pediatricians, gynecologists or
         obstetricians."

3860.   Yoshioka, Yayoi. "The Story of Medical Education for Wo-
         men in Japan." Medical Woman's Journal, 36:3 (March
         1929) 69-71.
         Ginko Ogino became, in 1885, the first woman doctor in
         Japan. The author received her M.D. degree in 1892 from
         the Saisei Gakusha (Saisei Medical School). Some facts
         about the Tokyo Women's Medical College are also given.

AUSTRALIA & NEW ZEALAND

3861.   Dawson, Elizabeth. "Medical Women of Australia." Med-
         ical Woman's Journal, 56:1 (January 1949) 43-47. pho-
         tos.
         Although Australian universities did not admit women med-
         ical students until the 1890s, Australian women physicians
         now have distinguished themselves in most branches of the
         profession, and they have no difficulty obtaining appoint-
         ments in any hospital. The "firsts" of Australian medical
         women are reviewed, and several notable physicians are
         profiled. Hospitals staffed and conducted by women for
         women are also described in this article.

CANADA

3862.   Abbott, Maude E. "Women in Medicine." University Maga-
         zine [Toronto], (April 1911).
         [Article not examined by editors.]

3863.   Corbet, G. G. "The Profession of Medicine for Women."
             Maritime Medical News (Halifax), 16 (1904) 54-57.
         [Article not examined by editors.]

3864.   Gray, Jessie. "Women's Place in Medicine." University
             of Toronto Medical Journal, 18 (November 1940) 46-49.
         [Article not examined by editors.]

3865.   "Women and Medicine." Canadian Association of Medical
             Students and Internes Journal, (February 1964) 8-10.
         [Article not examined by editors.]

EUROPE, EASTERN

3866.   Child, Richard Washburn. "Professional Women in Russia."
             Woman's Medical Journal, 26:7 (July 1916) 183.
             (From the August Century.)
         Because Russian medical schools were closed to women, a
         Russian woman had to attend medical school in Zurich to
         receive her medical degree (in 1867). By 1876 there were
         enough women surgeons to distinguish themselves in mili-
         tary service at the front in the Serbian-Turkish War, the
         Russo-Japanese War, and World War I. "Today women
         physicians are as prominent as men, and in some cities
         there are more female than male dentists."

3867.   Conta, (Mme.). ["The Medical Woman in Romania"].
             Cong. Intérnat. d. Oeuvres et Inst. Fêm. 1900 (Paris),
             4 (1902) 167. (Fre)
         [Article not examined by editors.]

3868.   ["Female Doctors in Bosnia"]. Wiener Medizinische Wochen-
             schrift, 30 (1896) 1349-1351. (Ger)
         Female doctors work in Bosnia and the Herzegovina, hired
         by the state government to treat Muslim women. For a
         fixed salary they provide free medical care for the poor and
         collect information on the sanitary conditions among female
         Muslims. The article lists the number of patients and the
         diseases treated in different cities. Under the influence of
         these women physicians the general health of Muslim women
         and their attitude towards modern hygiene markedly im-
         proved, underlining the advantage of having female doctors
         in Bosnia and the Herzegovina, as Muslim women could not
         be treated by male physicians.

3869.   Freminville, Bernard de. ["Medicine and the Modern
             World: Medical Students in the USSR"]. Concours
             Medical, 87:5 (30 January 1965) 755-762. charts, pho-
             tos. (Fre)
         The author was one of a group of French exchange students
         who recently visited the USSR, spending eight days in the
         provincial city of Ryazan, southeast of Moscow, and eight

days in Moscow. In the USSR, 80 per cent of physicians
are women, as compared to about 40 per cent in 1926.
Women make up more than half the medical chiefs and directors of various institutions and more than 80 per cent
of the dentists. The majority of the medical candidates
are or have been nurses, who continue to work and take
evening courses for the first two years and then follow the
same course as the other students. All students receive
a stipend, although medical students receive less than chemistry or physics students--35 rubles a month plus supple-
ments for extra or especially good work. Many of the students live in communal lodgings which they manage themselves. The French students visited the Institute of Medicine in Ryazan and the Sechenov Institute in Moscow, and
de Freminville compares the two schools with French teaching institutions. He also discusses the health care system
in the USSR, with some statistics on hospital beds and numbers of patients. No further details are given on women
specifically.

3870.   ["More on the Question of Female Doctors in Russia"].
              Med. Vestnik (St. Petersburg), 3 (1863) 261-263.   (Rus)
         [Article not examined by editors.]

3871.   Murav'eva, E. F.   ["Women-Physicians in Russia and So-
              viet Graphic and Fine Arts (On the Occasion of the In-
              ternational Woman's Year)"].   Sovetskaia Meditsina
              (Moscow), 12 (December 1975) 112-118.   (Rus)
         [Article not examined by editors.]

3872.   "One Way to Meet the Doctor Shortage."   Independent Wo-
              man, 26 (February 1947) 44-46, passim.
         [Article not examined by editors.]

3873.   Waite, Lucy.   "A General Resumé of the Moscow Meeting:
              The Women Delegates."   Woman's Medical Journal, 6:
              10 (October 1897) 309-310.
         Dr. Waite reports that the most interesting feature of an
         international medical congress held in Moscow was a banquet
         given by the Russian women physicians to all the female
         delegates. The Russian women were jubilant because the
         University of Russia is being reopened to women. Dr. Waite
         calls the Russians a "fine appearing body of women ... in
         every sense the 'new woman,' as the champaign and ciga-
         rettes conclusively proved [that] evening...." There are
         50 women physicians in Moscow and about 100 in St. Peters-
         burg.

EUROPE, WESTERN

3874.   Berwig, Elsie.   "Berlin Letter."   Woman's Medical Journal,
              14:8 (August 1904) 174-176.

The third quinquennial of the International Council of Women, held in Berlin, Germany, in 1904, included a session on women in medicine. Dr. Agnes Bluhm of Berlin reviewed the history of German women's entrance into the profession. Dr. Ellen Sadelin of Stockholm lectured on the status of Swedish women physicians. Dr. Tiburtins [sic] of Germany spoke on German women's medical education and present status. Other speakers and topics are also reported.

3875. Bono, Silvia Maria. [The Swiss Woman Physician]. Medizin-Historisches Institut der Universitaet Zurich, Zurich, Switzerland, 1958, 60 pp. tables. (M.D. thesis.) (Ger)
The author was born in Zurich, completed her secondary education in Basel, and studied medicine in Basel and Zurich, taking the state examination in the spring of 1956. Her dissertation contains a historical review of medical activities of women from antiquity to the present, with emphasis on the role of Swiss schools and of Zurich in particular. Chapter 2 describes the prerequisites for medical study and the curriculum in Switzerland. Chapter 3 covers the postmedical school options and the course followed by most women graduating from Swiss schools. Of 7665 registered physicians in the country in February 1958, 942 were women; of these, 173 were in general practice, 215 in specialty practice, 13 in salaried positions, 138 were not in practice, and 403 were hospital assistants. Tables in the text include numbers of females taking the state examination in certain years, practitioners by the various cantons, and practitioners by specialty.

3876. Bonsignorio, (Mlle.). ["The Real Situation of the Women Doctor in Medicine: What Has Been Done, What Is Left to Do."] Cong. Intérnat. d. Oeuvres et. Inst. Fém. 1900 (Paris), 4 (1902) 135-144. (Fre)
[Article not examined by editors.]

3877. Carpuppino-Ferrari, (Dr.). "The Work of Women Physicians in Italy." Medical Woman's Journal, 29:12 (December 1922) 323-325. (Presentation, Convention, Medical Women's International Association, Geneva, Switzerland, 6 September 1922.)
During the last 25 years in Italy, women have been permitted to study medicine without restriction. The author discusses current attitudes which create the favorable situation; she suggests also that women physicians locate themselves where they can be contacted easily in case of emergencies, and not simply cling to large city practices. Dr. Carpuppino-Ferrari very briefly reviews the history of women in medicine in Italy and the founding and activities of the National Italian Association of Women Physicians.

3878. D'Ancona, Silvia. "Women in Medicine: Italy." British

Medical Journal, 4 (17 November 1973) 404-405.
In Italy today, most women doctors work in large towns,
and many specialize in pediatrics. No obstacles are imposed on the employment of either married or single women, but "it is still relatively difficult for women to get
university jobs." In some medical schools, 40 per cent of
the student enrollment are women.

3879.   Darcanne-Mouroux. "French Medical Women Have Done
          Such Excellent Work as to Change Public Opinion.
          Many Young French Women Are Now Studying Medicine."
          Medical Woman's Journal, 29:5 (May 1922) 85.
This letter to the editor was written in response to a request for information on the work of women physicians in
France. A history of French medical women is given. In
1900 it was not the "fashion" for a French girl to study
medicine, as it is in 1922. Since the war, the public opinion has been entirely won over to the cause of the woman
physician. In 1901 there were 95 women physicians practicing throughout France. In 1922 there were 150 in Paris
alone.

3880.   Darcanne-Mouroux. ["Women Doctors"]. Le Siècle Médi-
          cal, 3:44 (1 March 1929) 1-4. (Fre)
[Article not examined by editors.]

3881.   Dorveaux, P. ["Women Physicians: Notes by Mademoiselle
          Biheron"]. Journal de Méd. de Paris, 13 (1901) 322.
          (Fre)
This article also appears in Med. Anecdot., (1901) 1965-
1971. [Article not examined by editors.]

3882.   Esch, Margaret, comp. [The Academic Professions: The
          Woman Doctor]. Academic Information Office in Berlin,
          in cooperation with the Office for Vocational Education
          and Management in the German Labor Front, Berlin,
          Germany, 1939, 16 pp. (Ger)
This small booklet is part of a series titled Academic Professions for Women, compiled by Dr. Margaret Esch of the
Academic Information Office. The publication contains an
introductory section on the problems and demands of the
medical profession for women ("of all the academic professions, that of physician is the most womanly and motherly").
A brief statement on the prerequisites, courses, examinations, probationary year, licensing, doctoral examination,
and costs of education and examinations follows. Sections
on the professional paths open, the economics of medical
practice, and professional prospects are included next. The
information on courses required is current as of 1939.

3883.   Esch, Margaret, comp. [The Academic Professions: The
          Woman Doctor]. Academic Information Office in Berlin,
          in cooperation with the Office for Vocational Education

and Management in the German Labor Front, Berlin,
Germany, 1940, 20 pp. (Ger)
This publication is a revised edition of a booklet by the
same title published in 1939. The material is unchanged
from the first edition, except for Section 2: "Course of
Education and Examinations" has been updated and expanded
to cover additional requirements for wartime service. Women are required to put in six months of nursing service
with the Red Cross or in a hospital before starting medical
school, and several periods of prescribed service in clinics,
with a practitioner, or on a rural post between semesters
and before qualifying for practice.

3884.   "Facts and Figures About Dutch Women in Medicine." Jour-
            nal of the American Medical Women's Association, 13:
            6 (June 1958) 251-253. table. (Special Article.)
Twenty per cent of the physicians in the Netherlands are
women at the time of this article: most are married and
are in general practice. Data is given on Dr. Aletta
Jacobs, the first woman physician in the Netherlands (1879),
as well as on Dr. J. W. van den Blink-Rolder, the first
woman elected president of the Royal Netherlands Company
for the Promotion of Medical Science. Midwifery in the
Netherlands is also discussed.

3885.   Forkl, Martha and Koffmahn, Elisabeth. [Women's Studies
            and Academic Work of Women in Austria]. Wilhelm
            Braumüller, Vienna, Austria, 1968, 128 pp. charts,
            tables. (Ger)
This book contains statistical data and a historical survey
of women in academe and in professions. For each profession, the author first deals with the evolution of women's
education, then discusses the situation of women in actual
professional work. Two short chapters deal specifically
with Austrian women in medicine. Following a survey of
the main steps in women's admission to medical school, the
situation of practicing physicians is illustrated.

3886.   Fragan, Till. ["The Question of Women as Service Physi-
            cians"]. Allm. Sven. Läkartidn., 3 (1906) 769-775.
            (Swe)
[Article not examined by editors.]

3887.   Freitas Pereira, Maria Joana de. "Medical Women of
            Portugal." Medical Woman's Journal, 57:1 (January
            1950) 45-46, 54.
Of the approximately 5,000 doctors in Portugal, 390 to 400
are women, according to Dra. Maria Joana de Freitas
Pereira, herself a radiologist and one of Portugal's pioneers
in this field.

3888.   Gundersen, Herdis. "The Status of Women Physicians:
            Medical Women in Norway." Journal of the American

Medical Women's Association, 6:7 (July 1951) 281-282. port.

In 1882 women were first admitted to the University of Norway, and in 1893 Norway's first woman physician, Marie Spaangberg Holth, obtained her medical degree from the University. In 1951 women comprised approximately 9 per cent of the medical profession in Norway. Of this 9 per cent, only 19 per cent specialized as compared with 30 per cent of the men. Sixty per cent of the women physicians were married and had one or more children. "Medical women in Norway have better working conditions than those in many other countries."

3889.   Hellstedt, Leone McGregor. "Interrelationships." _Journal of the American Medical Women's Association_, 22:6 (June 1967) 413-414.

"Women physicians as a group have little influence on Scandinavian culture." The women physicians in Sweden face such favorable environment that they do not feel the need to organize for female colleague support (25 per cent of the medical students are "girls"). Yet there are only eleven women in top clinical or research posts in Sweden, and only 45 women in second to top posts. A major socio-cultural factor affecting the life of women physicians in Sweden is the paucity of domestic and child help. "Concrete factors" preventing the recruitment of women physicians do not seem to exist, yet the author feels that psychological factors do exist--factors related to role stereotypes and the need to postpone marriage for a woman who enters medical training. Finally, the author explores the questions "What are our goals in life for our little daughters?" and "How ... as women doctors can we help and encourage more young girls ... to choose medicine as a life profession?"

3890.   Hurd-Mead, Kate Campbell. "Medical Women in Spain." _Bulletin of the Medical Women's National Association_, 16 (April 1927) 19-20.

"Ideas and points" on medicine in Spain and Portugal are presented in this article. In these countries "men and women study together under exactly the same conditions, except that the number of women students is always very small." The leading medical woman in Madrid is Dr. Elise Soriano whose article "Why do not more women in Spain study medicine?" provides the source for this author's facts. Martina Castello was the first woman in Spain to receive a degree in medicine (1883). In the next 35 years, only 12 other women had taken degrees in medicine, while in Madrid alone, 1700 men had been made MDs. Dr. Soriano feels that "the young women and their parents fear the dissecting room work; fear that a girl's morals would be tainted and that she would not have as good chances of marriage, the goal of every Spanish girl; fear that as doctors their working hours would be too long, and meal times too often interrupted; fear that they would see unpleasant cases of skin disease or even syphilis; fear that they would lose social prestige if they were known to be able to examine urine; fear that seven years of study would unfit them for domestic work at the family altars." The women who do go into medicine are "individualistic." Dr. Soriano says that "although they belong to the Federation of University Women they do not consult with one another but with men who usually take all the 'plums' and leave the 'stones' for the women who have to be satisfied with anything."

3891.   Kühn, Wilhelm. ["Female Physicians in Foreign Countries"].
          Muenchener Medizinische Wochenschrift, 52:34 (22 Au-
          gust 1905) 1644. (Ger)
          Woman doctors were not uncommon in France in the Middle
          Ages, being officially permitted to practice surgery in
          Paris in the 14th century. In the 19th century, noblewomen
          who studied medicine included the anatomists Marquise
          Voyer d'Argenson, Countess Colgny, Mme. Staal de Launay,
          and Mlle. Thecle-Felicite du Fay. A Mlle. Biheron made
          artificial anatomical preparations so natural that "all they
          lacked was the smell." A Mme. d'Arconville published a
          number of articles in surgery, physiology, and other fields.
          Among the midwives, Boivin and Lachapelle were well known.
          At present, however, only a few women doctors practice in
          France; of the 77 in Paris, less than half are Frenchwomen.
          Austria only recently opened medical practice to women and
          so far only 29 have received degrees there. Spain has no
          women physicians, but midwives and practitioners give
          basic care in areas without doctors. (The information in
          this article is taken from a review published in the British
          Medical Journal.)

3892.   Lollini, Clelia. "The Italian Medical Women's Association:
          Held the First Congress of Italian Medical Women."
          Medical Woman's Journal, 29:5 (May 1922) 82-84. pho-
          tos.
          A short history of women in academia in Italy is followed
          by a discussion of, and statistics on, Italian women physi-
          cians, of which there were about 300 in 1922. The work
          of specific Italian medical women is reviewed.

3893.   McKibbin-Harper, Mary. "Medical and Other Women of
          Norway." Medical Woman's Journal, 33:3 (March 1926)
          74-77.
          Dr. Harper's study of medical women in northern Europe
          includes the following observation: In Norway, Sweden, and
          Denmark, medical women occupy positions on an equality
          with men.

3894.   McKibbin-Harper, Mary. "Medical Women in France."
          Medical Woman's Journal, 33:4 (April 1926) 105-107.
          Dr. Harper discovered that French medical women "work

very quietly, for I had to hunt them out, seek and pursue them, so I conclude that they are modest...." Men and women enter medical school "and work on equality and together." In 1926, 4,158 men and 803 women were enrolled in France's medical schools. Currently less than 1000 women practice medicine in France. No woman does general surgery. No woman has yet been appointed to a chair or professorship "though there is no ruling to prevent them from competing" in the examinations. Dr. Harper observed that French newspapers bewail the fact that English and American women have a bad influence upon young French women, "teaching them independence." Several notable women physicians are mentioned.

3895.   McKibbin-Harper, Mary. "Medical Women in Sweden."
          Medical Woman's Journal, 33:2 (February 1926) 47-49.
          photo.
          From Stockholm University, the only medical school in
          Sweden, approximately 50 or 60 graduate each year, and
          two or three of these are women. In 1888 Karoline Wider-
          strom became the first woman to graduate in medicine.
          Alma Sundquist--one of the leading physicians in Stockholm
          --was connected with the Polyclinic Hospital's Department
          of Venereal Diseases for 16 years. In Sweden, "there is
          no organization of medical women, and none needed or de-
          sired, for women are members of all medical organizations
          and have the same standing and opportunities as men."

3896.   McKibbin-Harper, Mary. "Medical Women of Denmark."
          Medical Woman's Journal, 32:11 (November 1925) 302-
          305.
          The first woman to earn her medical degree in Denmark
          was Mathilde Nielson who graduated in 1885. Fifty women
          who are practicing medicine in Denmark do not have a sep-
          arate medical society for women. "It is generally con-
          sidered that the opportunities for men and women are equal.
          The women of Denmark have never had to make any fight
          for recognition, and they account for this by co-education,
          and doubtless it is a strong factor."

3897.   "Medical Women in Spain." Medical Woman's Journal, 39:
          10 (October 1932) 259.
          When Spain's first woman physician, Martina Castaneda,
          was graduated in Madrid in 1882, all the schools were
          closed and the students had parades. Today about 100 wo-
          men are registered as physicians in Spain. Drs. Elise
          Soriano and Garcia de Cosa hold positions in the Spanish
          civil navy.

3898.   Nilsson, Hjordis. "Status of Medical Women in Sweden."
          Journal of the American Medical Women's Association,
          4:8 (August 1949) 345-346. port. (The Status of Wo-
          men Physicians, IV.)

Women have been allowed to practice medicine in Sweden
since 1870. Karolina Widerstrom, Sweden's first woman
physician, did not begin her medical studies until 1879 and
did not open her practice in Stockholm until 1889. Women
physicians were not employed in public service until 1907
and then were only appointed to inferior posts. A portrait
of Nanna Svartz, Sweden's first woman professor with a
doctor of medicine, is included. The present generation of
medical women is concentrated in children's diseases and
psychiatry.

3899.   Odier-Dollfus. "Status of Medical Women in France."
         Journal of the American Medical Women's Association,
         3:10 (October 1948) 413-414.
         While women had begun to practice medicine in France in
         the second half of the nineteenth century and attend the
         same medical schools as men, receive the same diplomas,
         and practice under the same conditions, "custom" has in
         fact excluded most women from hospital appointments and
         the practice of surgery; no woman has yet been elected to
         the French Academy of Medicine. Women who do practice
         tend to take jobs that fix hours, such as in dispensaries,
         in schools, or in industrial plants. Some work in govern-
         ment service. The highest proportion of women are con-
         centrated in pediatrics and gynecology.

3900.   "Official Report of Dr. Esther Clayton Lovejoy." Woman's
         Medical Journal, 28:5 (May 1918).
         This report of Dr. Lovejoy is made to the members of the
         Woman's Committee, Council of National Defense. The re-
         port deals with the conditions of women and children before,
         during, and after childbirth. Dr. Lovejoy writes particular-
         ly about the sage-femmes (learned women) of France and
         the "valuable literary contributions" relating to obstetrics
         made by women such as Marie Bourgeois.

3901.   Pereira-d'Oliveira, E. [Women Feminists Who Practiced
         Medicine: About Women Physicians in the Netherlands].
         Wetenschappelijke Uitgeverij, Amsterdam, The Nether-
         lands, 1973. 123 pp. photos., ports. (Dut)
         This book was published in commemoration of the 40th an-
         niversary of the founding of the Society of Women Physicians
         of the Netherlands in November 1933. The author, a prac-
         ticing family doctor, is also a writer of medical books for
         the general public. She traces the emergence of women as
         physicians in the Netherlands, starting with the first eight
         who began their studies before 1900, through the "second
         generation" (1900-1910), the pre-World War II period, the
         occupation and postwar recovery. Included are tables of
         entering medical students in the years 1900-1970. The
         founding of the Society of Women Physicians is described,
         along with its cooperation with the International Association
         of Medical Women. The problems of combining medicine

with marriage and a family are discussed briefly. The author's introduction mentions early problems of discrimination; a later chapter is titled "A Doctor is Still Always
'He'." A number of chapters are devoted to statistics or
discussion of individuals: practicing outside the country,
family doctors, women specialists, other fields of practice
in the Netherlands, and Dutch women with professorial or
other high status at home and abroad. One chapter includes
a list of papers published by women in the Nederlands
Tijdschrift voor Geneeskunde from 1907 to 1931. There is
no bibliography and there are no indexes. Illustrations are
used, including 16 portraits.

3902. Petersen, Julius. ["Women Physicians in Past and Pres-
        ent"]. Ugeskrift for Laeger, 36 (1905). (Dan)
      [Article not examined by editors.]

3903. Poli, U. ["The Italian Woman in Medicine"]. Ann. di
        Ippocrate (Milano), 3 (1908-1909) 590. (Ita)
      [Article not examined by editors.]

3904. "Present Position of Medical Women in Germany." Medical
        and Professional Woman's Journal, 40:12 (December
        1933) 367. (Editorial.)
      Women physicians in Germany deeply resent the Nazi-uni-
      fication-inspired segregation of men and women, and their
      consequent relegation to the classification of trade and
      office workers if they wish "a place in the front." Since
      their hard-won equality with men physicians was wiped out
      by the Hitler government, an attempt was being made to
      organize a woman's medical group in Germany.

3905. Schindler-Baumann, Jida. "Interrelationships." Journal
        of the American Medical Women's Association, 22:6
        (June 1967) 419-421.
      The first female medical student at the University of Zurich
      was a Russian named Nadya Suslova. The first Swiss wo-
      man to study medicine was Marie Vogtlin. Switzerland pre-
      sents a paradoxical situation in that although the "canton of
      Zurich distinguished itself [100 years prior] by an outstand-
      ingly progressive attitude [toward educating women] ... to-
      day, on the question of female suffrage, it has to be con-
      sidered as shamefully reactionary."

3906. Selvini, Mara Palazzoli. "Medical Women in Italy." Jour-
        nal of the American Medical Women's Association, 5:11
        (November 1950) 460-461. ports. (Status of Women
        Physicians.)
      As early as the eleventh century women were allowed to
      teach as well as to practice medicine in Italy. Anna
      Morandi Manzolini held the chair of Ordinary Professor of
      Anatomy at Bologna in the eighteenth century. Until the
      turn of the century, only women "of exceptional character

and ability" were allowed to enter medicine.   From 1942
to 1947 approximately 15 per cent were enrolled at the
Faculty of Medicine at Milan University and of these, ten
per cent took their degrees.   More women enter medicine
from northern and central Italy than from the south.   Fewer women enter obstetrics and gynecology in Italy than in
other countries.   Until the present era women were excluded from holding posts of director and vice-director in
hospitals.   Only one woman holds the position of Ordinary
University Professor: Angela Borrino, Professor of Pediatrics at the University of Perugia.

3907.   Seppanen, Anni. "Medical Women in Finland." Journal of
        American Medical Women's Association, 5:7 (July 1950)
        291-293.   ports.   (The Status of Women Physicians.)
Rosina Heikel became the first woman physician in Scandinavia in 1875.   Not for another 20 years did any other women try to become doctors.   Women physicians are still
having difficulty obtaining positions as assistant physicians
in special clinics.   At the beginning of 1949, there were
361 women physicians.   Prominent Finnish women physicians include Laimi Leidenius, Gota Tingvald-Hannikainen,
and Rakel Jalas.   Dr. Leidenius was appointed professor of
obstetrics and gynecology in 1930 and was active in the
planning and building of the Women's Clinic in Helsinki.
Dr. Tingvald-Hannikainen started regular tuberculosis examinations of Helsinki State University students in 1932
which was later extended to include all schoolchildren, and
helped organize Student Health Welfare in 1946-48.   Dr.
Jalas, a psychiatrist, was the first woman doctor elected
to the Finnish Parliament.   An important law she helped to
prepare was one concerning state-supported maternal allowances for all women who want to apply for it.   She is a
Finnish delegate to the World Health Organization.

3908.   Tiburtius, Franziska. "The Development of the Study of
        Medicine for Women in Germany, and Present Status."
        Canadian Practitioner and Review, 34 (August 1909)
        492-500.   (Presentation, Meeting, International Council
        of Women, Toronto, Canada, 30 June 1909.)
Dr. Tiburtius, who began her medical studies in 1870 in
Switzerland and started practice in 1876 in Berlin, draws
upon personal experience to discuss the social and economic
conditions responsible for the "relatively late" appearance
of German women physicians.   The resistance of German
universities to admitting women medical students, partially
attributed to the German "tendency to conservatism and respect for everything of historical growth," came to a legal
end in 1904.   The idea of women's medical colleges was
fought by women physicians who feared that graduates of
such institutions would be considered second-class.   "Now
it is as easy for women to enter on the study of medicine
in Germany as it is in [Canada]," says Dr. Tiburtius, who

goes on to outline the current position of German women physicians. The work of women as school physicians is especially detailed.

3909.   Vallinkoski, Jorma V. "Some Features of the Medical Science in Finland in Former Times and Now." Medical Woman's Journal, 54:8 (August 1947) 17-21. chart, ports.
This history of medicine in Finland is followed by a brief history of women in medicine in Finland. Dr. Karolina Sidonia Eskelin was the first degreed woman physician. Dr. Laimi Leidenius was the first woman physician to receive the title of university professor.

3910.   "Women and the Medical Profession in Germany." Woman's Medical Journal, 1:4 (April 1893) 76.
Although four German women who obtained medical degrees abroad are practicing in Berlin, the German medical profession still refuses women the right to take the state examination. Essentially, women are refused admission to the medical profession.

GREAT BRITAIN

3911.   Aldrich-Blake, L. B. "London (Royal Free Hospital) School of Medicine for Women." Woman's Medical Journal, 11:3 (March 1901) 88-91.
In addressing a class of students just beginning their work at the London School of Medicine, Dr. Aldrich-Blake chose to speak in general terms on the subject: "Our Common Work, the Preparation for the Practice of the Profession of Medicine." Her advice for becoming a good doctor was to be the best person you possibly can be--in terms of kindness, thoroughness, courage, intellect, energy, and self-reliance.

3912.   "Bits of News." Woman's Medical Journal, 6:2 (February 1897) 48-50.
News of the activities of 11 women physicians is briefly stated. Included is a quote from a review of Elizabeth Blackwell's book, Pioneer Work in Opening the Medical Profession to Women, and an appeal for funds by Elizabeth Garrett-Anderson to support the New Hospital for Women and the London School of Medicine for Women.

3913.   Breakell, Mary L. "Women in the Medical Profession: By An Outsider." Nineteenth Century, 54 (November 1903) 819-825.
After describing the work of Agnodice, a woman physician of ancient Greece, the author discusses medical women in England in historic perspective. She also covers the prevailing attitudes of the public to men and women physicians.

3914.   Crosse, V. Mary. "Interrelationships." Journal of the
           American Medical Women's Association, 22:6 (June
           1967) 410-412.
        The author shares the knowledge about recruitment, training,
        and the practice of medicine of women physicians in the
        United Kingdom which was gained through two nationwide
        surveys and from an advisory service run by the Medical
        Women's Federation.

3915.   "General Memoranda." Medical Women's Federation News-
           Letter, (November 1926) 79-91.
        A variety of appointments, accomplishments, and issues
        concerning medical women in England are covered. In 1924
        the Cancer Research Committee of the London Association
        of the Medical Women's Federation was formed. Reprinted
        is a paragraph from The Vote for September 3, 1926, which
        deals with discrimination against women physicians in hos-
        pitals.

3916.   "General Memoranda." Medical Women's Federation News-
           Letter, (November 1927) 72-76.
        Notes on several women physicians describe their various
        appointments and awards. The article briefly mentions the
        resolution by the British Medical Association (BMA) affirm-
        ing the right of medical women to marry and to share equal
        status and salary with medical men. Dr. Laura Fowler is
        mentioned as one of the earliest women members of the
        South Australia branch of the BMA. A list of recent papers
        and publications by medical women is given. A final note
        describes a meeting on maternal mortality which was at-
        tended by political and social reform workers and led by
        Lady Barrett, M.D.

3917.   "General Memoranda." Medical Women's Federation Quar-
           terly Review, (April 1942) 71-75.
        The award of the MBE (Civil Division) was given to Dr.
        Adaline Nancy Miller, ship surgeon aboard the Britannia,
        for her courage in battle. This and other general news
        items constitute this article.

3918.   "Interesting London Letter [From Our Own Correspondent]:
           Medical Women in Great Britain." Medical Woman's
           Journal, 28:5 (May 1921) 126-128.
        A discussion of the situation of medical women in Great
        Britain is followed by a notice that Serbian medical students
        are being offered scholarships to the London School of Med-
        icine for Women.

3918a. Ivans, Frances. "An Address to Junior Members." Med-
           ical Women's Federation News-Letter, (March 1925) 13-
           18. (Presentation, Meeting, Junior Branch, Liverpool
           and District Association of the Medical Women's Fed-
           eration, 18 March 1925.)

The author advises women entering the medical profession
on how to obtain the best training and how to best make use
of that training. She recommends postgraduate courses
abroad after a "good general education" and training at a
medical school chosen with discrimination. Public health
appointments are scarce, but "there is ample scope for
women in general practice." Good gynecological training is
expected of women physicians. She warns of the difficulty
in obtaining capital to start a practice and the necessity of
accepting the standard remuneration fixed by the British
Medical Association and Society of Medical Officers of Health.
She mentions the alternative of medical missions as an opportunity for women.

3919.   Jex-Blake, Sophia. "The Practice of Medicine by Women."
            Fortnightly Review, 23 (1 March 1875) 392-407.
         No monopolies can be tolerated in the British Empire, yet
         many occupations are restricted to one sector of the com-
         munity as completely as if there were a law. The author
         gives several examples of such restriction and then discus-
         ses the one instance in England where the law supports "a
         stupendous monopoly," i.e., "the forcible exclusion of wo-
         men from the legalized practice of medicine." This exclu-
         sion is effected by abuse of the Medical Act of 1858 which
         limits the legal practice of medicine to those whose names
         appear on the government medical register. The purpose
         of the act and the flaws in its construction are discussed by
         the author, who feels that in spite of its flaws, it was not
         intended by Parliament to produce a monopoly of any special
         body of practitioners. She relates how the act has been
         abused and women excluded from medical practice. Jex-
         Blake then covers the history of the admittance of women
         to the medical courses at the University of Edinburgh. The
         Cowper-Temple bill, which would make it legal for any
         Scottish university to instruct and graduate women, is re-
         viewed. Jex-Blake closes her discussion with a quote from
         "Mrs. Mill": "The proper sphere for all human beings is
         the largest and highest which they are able to attain to."

3920.   Kelynack, Violet. "Women in the Medical Profession: A
            Retrospect for the Year 1929." Medical Women's Fed-
            eration News-Letter, (March 1930) 55-58.
         This article [reprinted from Woman's Leader, 3 (January
         1930)] generalizes about the position of women physicians
         within Britain and its Commonwealths. Issues discussed in-
         clude different treatment of women medical officers, dis-
         crimination against married women physicians, and the ef-
         fects of the "great rush of women, many wholly unsuitable,
         into the medical profession" after the war.

3921.   Keyes, Muriel. "The Value of Insurance to Medical Wo-
            men." Medical Women's Federation News-Letter, (Oc-
            tober 1932) 56-58. (Correspondence.)

3922.   Laurie, Jean. "More About Women in Medicine--In Eng-
              land." Journal of the American Medical Women's As-
              sociation, 18:5 (May 1963) 402-403. (Letters to the
              Editor.)
         Despite different economic systems, the difficulties women
         physicians face are similar in the United States and Eng-
         land. Proceedings of the Council at Bournemouth are re-
         ported.

3923.   Martindale, L. The Woman Doctor and Her Future. Mills
              & Boon, Limited, London, England, 1922, 196 pp.
              illus., photos.
         This book, written when Dr. Martindale was an honorary
         surgeon at the New Sussex Hospital for Women and Children
         in Brighton, reviews the history of medical women, espe-
         cially in Great Britain, to the time of this writing. Eliza-
         beth Blackwell's life is presented as characteristic of wo-
         men's struggle for education and licensing. Appended
         is a list of women registered in Great Britain from
         1858 to 1885. An overview of the work of women army
         surgeons during the world war includes details of the work
         of the Scottish Women's Hospitals in Royaumont, France.
         Also discussed: the current position of women in private
         practice, government service, and hospital work (comple-
         mented, in the appendix, by lists of woman-staffed hos-
         pitals); and the activities of women physicians in govern-
         ment, research, as teachers and lecturers, in India and se-
         lected foreign countries. Recommendations for education
         and training programs and speculation about the woman phy-
         sician's future conclude the book. An undated bibliography
         is included, as is an index.

3924.   Richelot. ["Women Physicians in England"]. L'Union Médi-
              cale, (1875) 219-220. (Fre)
         A news note reports that the General Medical Council in
         London has received and approved a report from a commis-
         sion appointed to consider the questions, posed by the gov-
         ernment, of admitting women to practice and of accepting
         diplomas earned in foreign schools by women. The com-
         mission concluded that women should give up the idea of
         becoming doctors, which requires qualities of strength, per-
         severance, and lack of feeling, foreign to their nature; but
         if they persist in their determination to have a medical ca-
         reer, they should not be excluded. If one of the 19 au-
         thorized bodies admits women to its examination, the Coun-
         cil will register their diplomas; if not, special examinations
         might be established for women. At present the only wo-
         man legally qualified to practice medicine in England is
         Elizabeth Garret [sic] Anderson, a diplomate of the Society
         of Pharmacy; no other women have been admitted to the ex-
         aminations because they are not from "recognized" schools.

3925.   Scharlieb, Mary. "The Medical Woman: Her Training, Her

Difficulties, and Her Sphere of Usefulness." Nineteenth Century, 78 (November 1915) 1174-1185.
The struggles of Dr. Sophia Jex-Blake and the "ladies of
Edinburgh" are recalled, after which Dr. Scharlieb reviews
the history of the Royal Free Hospital in London and its
admitting of medical women. The author then proceeds to
describe medical women's struggle for an education, for
hospital staff positions, and for public acceptance; she also
describes the work of women physicians in various areas
during World War I.

3926.   Wilson, Robert. "Aesculapia Victrix." Fortnightly Review
             (London), 45 (January 1886) 18-33.
The author gives examples of contributions made by Elizabeth Garrett-Anderson and her counterparts in England,
America, and other countries. He presents a thorough
history of the London School of Medicine for Women and a
review of the success of the Countess of Dufferin's Association in India. Wilson concludes with an affirmation of woman's right to study and practice medicine.

INTERNATIONAL

3927.   Balfour, Margaret I. "The Medical Women's Overseas
             Association News." Medical Women's Federation
             Quarterly Review, (April 1942) 62-63.
The government of India will recruit European women medical officers to serve in the India medical services.

3928.   Baumgartner, Leona. "Optimal Utilization of Medical Wo-
             manpower." Journal of the American Medical Women's
             Association, 21:10 (October 1966) 832-837.
Addressing the Xth Congress of the Medical Women's International Association, Dr. Baumgartner suggests that doctors
are "illiterate" about social and economic factors, the understanding of which is basic "to any real understanding of
the problems of utilization of human resources." The author
identifies these factors and discusses them, after which she
asks: since women are human resource that can be tapped
to meet the world's health care demands, "what ... stands
in the way?" The customs and conditions in various countries are discussed and a plea for appropriate guidance
counseling, greater flexibility, and better utilization of all
physicians is made.

3929.   Bowers, John Z. "Wife, Mother and Physician." Journal
             of the American Medical Women's Association, 22:10
             (October 1967) 760-764. (Commencement Address,
             Woman's Medical College of Pennsylvania, 6 June 1967.)
A cursory overview of women physicians in other countries
is followed by a generalized discussion of the socioeconomic
factors governing the situation in the United States.

3930.   Bowers, John Z. "Women in Medicine: An International
              Study." New England Journal of Medicine, 275:7 (18
              August 1966) 362-365.
         The medical schools and teaching hospitals should "face up
         to the question, should there be a higher percentage of wo-
         men entering medicine." If the answer is affirmative,
         measures should be taken to attract larger numbers of wo-
         men and make it possible for them to complete their train-
         ing. Having gathered data on women physicians in other
         countries during overseas visits and from colleagues, Bow-
         ers discusses the factors which contribute to the percentage
         of women entering medicine in Europe, Australia, Asia,
         Africa (south of the Sahara), Latin America, and the United
         States.

3931.   "Demand for Women Physicians Is Increasing in All Parts
              of the World." Medical Woman's Journal, 42:4 (April
              1935) 106. (Editorial.)
         The Journal is continually receiving communications from
         all countries regarding the need for women doctors. "The
         evidence would seem to indicate that medical women are
         coming into their own."

3932.   Ernest, Elvenor. "The Present Status of Women in Medi-
              cine." Bulletin of the Medical Women's National Asso-
              ciation, 31 (January 1931) 11-14. (Read before the
              Annual Meeting, Kansas Medical Society, Topeka, Kan-
              sas, May 7, 8, and 9, 1930.)
         After reviewing the international achievements of women in
         medicine since Elizabeth Blackwell became the first woman
         doctor in modern times, this author feels that the argu-
         ments against women being in medicine are best answered
         by looking at the accomplishments of outstanding women in
         surgery, scientific research, the specialties, literature, at
         the lecture platform, and as heads of colleges and hospitals,
         AMA sections, government offices, etc. In 1929, 4.43 per
         cent women were admitted as medical students, but the
         average admittance of women for the last ten years has not
         been above four per cent. Included is a summary of Kan-
         sas medical women's practice patterns.

3933.   Fontanges, Haryett. [Women Doctors in Medicine Through-
              out the World: Historical, Statistical, Documentary,
              and Anecdotal Studies of Medicine as Exercised by Wo-
              men]. Alliance Cooperative du Livre, Paris, France,
              1901, 275 pp. illus., photo., ports. (Fre)
         The first half of this study of women in medicine reviews
         women physicians in France. Along with anecdotes of their
         careers, lists of publications and prize-winning theses at
         the Medical Faculty in Paris are given. A list of French
         medical faculties which accept women also includes statis-
         tics on the number of students now studying at these facul-
         ties. There are also chronological lists of theses presented

by women for the doctorate, beginning with "Mlle. Garret"
in 1870, the addresses of women physicians in Paris, and
a brief description of prizes available. The second half of
the book gives a very brief resumé (including lists of
names) of women physicians in America, Russia, the British Isles, India, the Near East, Europe, Africa, South
America, and the Orient. The book finishes with a brief
look at women physicians active in Paris in 1292, and others in Germany, Poland, England, and Constantinople. The
book includes several illustrations of French doctors and
their hospitals. There is no index.

3934.   MacMurchy, Helen. "Medicus et Medica [Part II]." Amer-
        ican Medicine, 7 (13 February 1904) 270-272. (Special
        Articles.)
        Information is provided on the historical background and cur-
        rent activity, including enrollment figures of the following
        medical schools: London School of Medicine for Women,
        Edinburgh School of Medicine for Women (which operated
        only from 1887-1898), Medical College for Women (Edin-
        burgh), and the Queen Margaret College of the University
        of Glasgow. The article goes on to survey the situation of
        medical women in Canada, India, Germany, Russia, and
        other countries.

3935.   Nemir, Rosa Lee. "Interrelationships: Rapporteur."
        Journal of the American Medical Women's Association,
        21:10 (October 1966) 839-841.
        Reported are the proceedings of a session on the interre-
        lationship of the woman physician and her environment, as
        presented at the Tenth Congress of the Medical Women's
        International Association. The author reviews salient points
        of the session which touched upon socioeconomic, cultural,
        religious, and political factors "that affect the supply of
        women medical students, and the practice of medicine by
        women in various countries."

3936.   "Personal." Woman's Medical Journal, 6:5 (May 1897) 132-
        134.
        Contained in this column are many news items concerning
        women's medical education and the work of specific women.
        Among items reported: Baroness Possaner von Ehrenthal
        recently became Austria's first woman physician; Emma
        Wakefield became the first woman of her race to receive
        a medical license in the South; trustees of Des Moines'
        Drake University reversed the medical faculty order ex-
        cluding women students; and the Woman's Medical College
        of the New York Infirmary suffered a devastating fire.

3937.   "Personal." Woman's Medical Journal, 6:10 (October
        1897) 315-319.
        Mention is made of Dr. M. Isabella French, a medical
        missionary to China; the death of Dr. Amelia Lange; and

the work of Dr. Maria Keith, house physician and superintendent of the Phyllis Wheatley Sanitarium and Training School for Nurses. The exclusion of women medical students in New Orleans receives criticism, and the advances of the North India School of Medicine for Christian Women (Ludhiana) is discussed, along with several other short news items.

3938.   "The Record of Advance." Woman's Medical Journal, 5:4
         (April 1896) 101-102.
         General news items include information on the status of women's admittance to German medical schools, as well as the latest appointments granted Dr. Eliza Maria Mosher (literary department dean at the University of Michigan) and several other physicians.

3939.   Sanderson, Susanne. "Women in Medicine." Journal of
         the Michigan State Medical Society, 30 (May 1931) 339-
         344.
         Reviewing the history of medical women of Europe and the United States, Dr. Sanderson identifies the years during which medical coeducation was initiated in various countries. The work of several notable personalities is mentioned. The second half of the article summarizes the history and current activities of Michigan women physicians.

3940.   Schultze, Caroline. [Female Physicians in the 19th Cen-
         tury]. Peter Hobbing, Leipzig, Germany, 1889, 65 pp.
         port. (Ger)
         This article describes the situation of women in medicine in Europe and elsewhere at the end of the nineteenth century. The author reports the difficulties encountered by Madeleine Bres in Paris where she fought for recognition as a physician, and by Tkatcheff and Ribard in Montpellier where female students were still a problem. Concerning the situation in Russia, the author describes the political and social problems leading to the foundation of an academy for female studies which was closed after a short time. This closing led to massive emigration of Russian medical students to other European countries. In Great Britain, the main problem was resistance of professors and male fellow students to women in clinical training, creating considerable hardship for Miss Jex-Blake and her fellow women students. In the U.S., Elizabeth Blackwell found more support from faculty and peers. Germany had very few women doctors, most of whom, like Franziska Tiburtius, had studied abroad. [A French edition of this work was also published in Paris, France, 1888, 76 pp.]

3941.   "Women-Doctors in Switzerland and Melbourne." Medical
         Times and Gazette, 2 (1872) 111, 261.
         [Article not examined by editors.]

SOUTH, CENTRAL, LATIN AMERICA
AND MEXICO

3942.   Delgado de Solis Quiroga, Margarita. "Mexico and the
             Women in Medicine." Journal of the American Med-
             ical Women's Association, 11:10 (October 1956) 355-
             356.
         Summarized is a paper presented during a symposium on
         "Women as Medical Students and Physicians in the Countries
         of the Americas." There is still much prejudice to be
         overcome for educated women in the work force, especially
         among the wealthy classes. "We should strive for woman
         to get an adequate preparation for life; and develop a vigor-
         ous personality, a sense of responsibility, and a conscious-
         ness of her rights. Thus there will be no incompatibility
         with home, love, and motherhood." In 1887, Matilde Mon-
         toya "opened the breach" in Mexico and received her title
         of medical surgeon.

3943.   Finkler, Rita S. "The South America Women Doctors I
             Met." Medical Woman's Journal, 54:7 (July 1947) 23-
             29, 56.
         There are about 300 women doctors in Chile: 130 of them
         are in Santiago. Many government jobs (which pay very
         little) are open to women physicians. In Chile, the law re-
         quires a certified midwife to attend every obstetrical case
         and therefore the physician spends comparatively little time
         with obstetrical cases (only if complications arise). Fees
         charged by physicians range from three dollars to five dol-
         lars per visit. Dr. Finkler's visits to various other cities
         in South America are detailed.

3944.   "Medical Women of Uruguay: They Are Only Eight in Num-
             ber, but Full of Enthusiasm and Zeal. Letter from a
             Medical Woman of Montevideo." Medical Woman's
             Journal, 29:5 (May 1922) 86.
         This letter to the editor was written in response to a re-
         quest for information on women physicians in Uruguay.
         There are eight women physicians in Uruguay, and a re-
         ception was given recently for the two newest graduates.
         At this reception, there were several males in attendance,
         which "goes to prove that men no longer consider profes-
         sional women in the light of rivals, but rather as co-work-
         ers and companions." The names of these eight physicians
         are given, as well as the specialty of each.

3945.   Morton, Rosalie Slaughter. "Work of Medical Women in
             Mexico." Medical Woman's Journal, 36:11 (November
             1929) 293-295.
         Dr. Morton gives an account of women physicians in Mexico,
         the status and activities of whom she learned through her
         visit as "Ambassador of Good Will" of the Women's Medical
         Society of New York State.

3946. Shepherd, Gwendolyn. "Medical Women in Argentina."
Journal of the American Medical Women's Association,
9:1 (January 1954) 20.
There are four medical schools in Argentina; all are national (not private). Women constitute 15 to 20 per cent of the medical school population. While women have no difficulty entering medical school, they do have a problem securing internships. "Senorita Paso" in 1879 was the first woman to be admitted to a medical school in Argentina. Dr. Cecilia Grierson was the first woman to graduate as a "medica" in Argentina (1889).

3947. Tichauer, Ruth W. "Problems of the Woman Physician in Bolivia." Journal of the American Medical Women's Association, 11:10 (October 1956) 359-361.
Versatility is necessary for the woman physician working in Bolivia. Characteristics of the fewer than 50 women physicians practicing in Bolivia indicate that most come from local families, marry, and practice in cities (mainly gynecology and pediatrics). Feelings about women physicians are never indifferent, but are either approving or disapproving. Patient-physician relationship is discussed as well as Bolivian customs. Two professional duties which are almost exclusively relegated to women physicians in Bolivia are those of childbirth and mental hygiene.

3948. Vargas, Tegualda Ponce de. "Women Doctors of Chile."
Journal of the American Medical Women's Association,
7:10 (October 1952) 389.
There are 225 women doctors in Chile. Women have been allowed to enter medicine since 1877 when a government decree declared women should be able to obtain degrees, provided they fill all the requirements that men are expected to fill. Eloiza Diaz Inzunza received her medical degree in 1887 and in doing so became the first woman physician in Latin America. Ernestina Perez Barahona graduated shortly after her. Agrupacion Medica Femenina was founded in 1938 by government decree to be the organization of women doctors in Chile. It serves two functions: scientific education of its members and the promotion of maternal and child welfare. In 1950 it opened a cancer detection clinic for women in downtown Santiago.

3949. "Women Physicians in Ecuador." Journal of the American Medical Association, 78:5 (4 February 1922) 365.
(Foreign Letters.)
Matilda Hidalgo of Ecuador just obtained a medical degree from Quito University. Three women have so far practiced medicine in Ecuador.

3950. Wright, Katharine M. "Supply--The Americas." Journal of the American Medical Women's Association, 22:5 (May 1967) 340-342.

This article gives statistics for women physicians in Argentina, Brazil, Columbia, and Peru; also given are comparative data on the United States and Canada. The report is sketchy and brief.

UNITED STATES

3951. Ahlem, Judith. "Fruits of the Spirit." Journal of the American Medical Women's Association, 8:9 (September 1953) 305-307. (Inaugural Address, American Medical Women's Association, New York, 31 May 1953.)
A review of past inaugural addresses and a recounting of the "spiritual rewards" of being a woman in medicine are given.

3952. American Medical Women's Association; The President's Study Group on Careers for Women; and U.S. Department of Labor, Women's Bureau. Conference on Meeting Medical Needs: The Fuller Utilization of the Woman Physician. Washington, D.C., January 12-13, 1968. Report. U.S. Department of Labor, Women's Bureau, Washington, D.C., [1968], viii, 104 pp. photos., ports.
Various speakers' thoughts and recommendations on women in medicine are herein given. Speakers refer to statistics contained in a previously distributed booklet, not included with this publication. [The booklet is entitled U.S. Department of Labor, Women's Bureau, Wage and Labor Standards Administration. Facts on Prospective and Practicing Women in Medicine, and appears elsewhere in this bibliography.]

3953. "Armistice Day Reflections." Medical Woman's Journal, 36:11 (November 1929) 298. (Editorial.)
Where are the women physicians eleven years after the Armistice was signed? "... only in isolated instances are individual women doctors being accorded such recognition as [their splendid war service] record deserves." Women doctors should utilize their organized "power of concerted action" to achieve the professional success to which they are entitled.

3954. Ashby, T. A. "Abstract of an Address on the Medical Education of Women, Delivered at the Opening of the First Course of Lectures of the Woman's Medical College of Baltimore." Maryland Medical Journal, 9 (15 October 1882) 267-275.
The reasoning behind the founding of the Woman's Medical College of Baltimore (Maryland) is given, followed by a history of woman's place in medicine over the centuries. Dr. Ashby gives arguments against the admission of women to the medical profession and refutes these arguments. A history of woman's struggle to obtain a medical education fol-

lows.   Statistics on the number of women studying medicine
in various countries are given.   In conclusion, Dr. Ashby
cites statistics and responds to questions considered by Dr.
Rachel L. Bodley in her valedictory address to the 29th
graduating class of the Woman's Medical College of Pennsylvania [1881].

3955.   Atkinson, Dorothy W.   "'Give Us the Courage-'" Journal
            of the American Medical Women's Association, 4:9
            (September 1949) 374-377.   (Inaugural Address, Annual
            Meeting, American Medical Women's Association, Atlan-
            tic City, New Jersey, 5 June 1949.)
        "... to demand of our women physicians, and from them,
        more adequate training freed from a sense of group frustra-
        tion; for a tenacious and unyielding belief in the dignity of
        our profession in its stand against all the marshalled forces
        of bureaucracy...."

3956.   Baker, S. Josephine.   "Address of the Eighty-Eighth Annual
            Commencement of the Medical College of Pennsylvania."
            Medical Woman's Journal, 48:4 (April 1941) 95-100.
        This address, delivered in the 1940's turn-of-the-decade
        tension, reflects medical concerns of the time, i.e., pre-
        ventive medicine, general practice, and uncertainties of
        choosing a specialty.

3957.   Barringer, Emily Dunning.   "Address Delivered at the
            Eighty-Seventh Opening of W. M. C. of PA."   Women in
            Medicine, 55 (January 1937) 15-17.
        Women physicians have occupied a "mentally isolated, truly
        colonial position" in the medical field of the United States.
        "... now that prohibition has gone the cocktail has lost its
        lure, but Lady Nicotine is getting in much deadly work."
        Dr. Barringer also warns the students about the occupa-
        tional hazard of narcotic addiction.

3958.   Beshiri, Patricia H.   The Woman Doctor: Her Career in
            Modern Medicine.   Cowles Book Company, Inc., New
            York, New York, 1969, xiv, 240 pp.
        Statistical answers have been sought to statistical problems
        of the number of women physicians in the United States.
        This book attempts to present the "personalized informa-
        tion" on women physicians which has been lacking for so
        long.   The author addresses the questions: "what are the
        personal requirements for a medical career as they specif-
        ically apply to women?   What are the personal experiences
        of such a career?   What are the personal rewards for such
        effort?"   The book is indexed.

3959.   Blackman, Julia Cole.   "Address to the Graduating Class
            of the Northwestern University Woman's Medical School."
            Woman's Medical Journal, 10:7 (July 1900) 289-291.
            (Address, Alumnae Association, Northwestern University

Woman's Medical School, 20th Annual Meeting, 14
June 1900.)
Dr. Blackman offers words of advice and encouragement to
the graduating class. She urges patience in diagnosis and
restraint in the use of medications. A physician must learn
to "think in her profession" the way one learning a foreign
language must learn to think in that language. She must
be discrete, and if she feels a "stronger call in another
direction--even a matrimonial one," she should not feel
"abashed or abased," for whatever one decides to do, the
years of study have not been wasted.

3960.   Branson, Laura H. "The Woman Physician." Woman's
               Medical Journal, 15:4 (April 1905) 74-75. (First An-
               nual Mid-Winter Banquet, Johnson County Iowa Medical
               Association, Johnson County, Iowa, 8 February 1905.)
          In this host of general comments concerning the status of
          women in medicine, Dr. Branson mentions the work of Dr.
          Margaret Cleaves, Dr. Margaret Sharp, and Dr. Anita New-
          comb McGee. She also describes the unveiling in Chicago
          of the first statue ever erected to the memory of a woman
          physician in the United States: Dr. Mary H. Thompson.

3961.   Brodie, Jessie Laird. "The Woman Physician in the United
               States Today." World Medical Journal, 11:1 (January
               1964) 25-28. tables.
          What can be done to encourage women to enter medicine?
          What can be done to keep women in the profession once
          they begin their studies or obtain their degrees? The au-
          thor speaks to these questions by discussing on a general
          level such areas as recruitment, motivation and counseling,
          scholarship loans, graduate training opportunities, part-time
          residencies and medical work, and income tax relief. Sta-
          tistical data from other sources on women physicians in the
          United States is reported.

3962.   Brown, Edith Petrie; McGrew, Elizabeth; Christine, Bar-
               bara; Kerr, Charlotte; Mermod, Camille; Gilmore,
               Marguerite; Nemir, Rosa Lee; and Helfand, Toby.
               "Medical Womanpower--Can It Be Used More Efficiently?"
               Journal of the American Medical Women's Association,
               17:12 (December 1962) 973-985. ports.
          This article is based on a panel discussion for women phy-
          sicians held at the American Medical Association annual
          meeting, June 24, 1962, in response to Dr. A. P. Inge-
          gno's article, "The Case Against the Female M.D.," pub-
          lished in Medical Economics, December 1961. Seven wo-
          men physicians discuss the problems women face going
          through medical training and entering practice. Women face
          heavy competition getting into medical school because such
          a low percentage of women are accepted. There is a lack
          of part-time hospital jobs. One panel member suggests that
          when any physician stops practicing for more than 12 months,

she should be reexamined for medical licensure. Women physicians "risk the success of marriage and motherhood," and feel the conflict of "selfishly curing humanity" while depriving their children of their presence. Another problem for women physicians is finding the right man to marry (one who is proud to have his wife in medicine and glad she has something all-consuming to occupy her time and energy so he might be spared the excessive attention of "henpecking"). Another difficulty is finding reliable household help. As one women physician on the panel points out, "There are many domestic workers who like to work for a professional woman. They feel that they are fulfilling themselves, in part through their employer's fine work. It is also extremely important to select domestic help that will give one a feeling of approval and not a feeling of guilt."

3963.   Burnet, Anne. "The Status of Medical Women in Iowa." Woman's Medical Journal, 14:7 (July 1904) 148-149.
In 1903 there were 28 women members of the Iowa State Medical Society. Women physicians have a better standing in Iowa than in any other state, and the opposition of male physicians "is a delusion in the majority of, if not in all, cases." In this address to the seventh annual session of the State Society Iowa Medical Women, Burnet enumerates the contribution of a number of contemporary women physicians in Iowa.

3964.   Bryn Mawr College. Bryn Mawr Alumnae Bulletin: An Issue on Medicine. Bryn Mawr College, Bryn Mawr, Pennsylvania, 1974, 48 pp. ports.
In this issue, several women physician graduates of Bryn Mawr College contribute original articles on women in medicine. Topics covered include "The Applicant Explosion"; "Affirmative Action"; "The Doctors' Dilemma," a discussion of the criteria of death; and a historical view of women (especially Bryn Mawr women) in medical schools.

3965.   Campbell, Elizabeth. "Medical Reforms (Valedictory Address)." Woman's Medical Journal, 6:5 (May 1897) 140+.
Dr. Campbell was the first woman physician in Cincinnati, Ohio chosen to deliver the valedictory address at the commencement exercises of Laura Medical College. Her remarks make liberal use of allegory to illustrate the search for truth, which is the lifelong occupation of the dedicated physician.

3966.   Center for Women in Medicine, comp. Resource Booklet Prepared by the Center for Women in Medicine, the Medical College of Pennsylvania for Use of Participants at Its First Workshop Women in Medicine: Action Planning for the 1970s. March 14 and 15, 1974. Medical College of Pennsylvania, Philadelphia, Pennsylvania,

[1974], 156 pp. charts, tables.
This booklet contains four types of information. The first
is a compilation of statistical data covering undergraduate
and graduate medical education of women, women physicians
in the U.S., foreign medical graduates, and studies of students at the Medical College of Pennsylvania. This section
of more than 60 pages pulls together and reproduces data
and tables from published studies and articles in professional journals. Among the findings highlighted: (1) accepted
women students increased from 10.1 per cent of the total
students in 1967-68 to 13.7 per cent in 1971-72; (2) in 1973-
74 first year women students filled almost 20 per cent of
the U.S. medical school places; (3) in 1973-74 women comprised 15.4 per cent of all medical students; (4) in 1973
women represented eight per cent of the total U.S. physician
population; (5) women represented 21.3 per cent of all pediatricians in the U.S. and 18.8 per cent of all physicians in
public health in 1971; (6) the percentage of active women
physicians in western European countries ranged from 7.3
per cent in Spain to 36 per cent in Austria; and (7) in 1970,
15.3 per cent of the foreign medical graduates in the U.S.
were women. The booklet's second section summarizes
recent relevant literature on medical women in their various professional, personal, and social roles. A third section is devoted to highlights of conferences: the 1968 workshop on the utilization of the woman physician sponsored by
the AMWA, the President's Study Group on Careers for Women, and the Woman's Bureau of the U.S. Department of
Labor; the 1968 study on the woman physician in training
and practice conducted at Duke University; and the 1973
Carnegie Commission on Higher Education findings. The
booklet closes with a bibliography, taken from MEDLINE
searches.

3967.   Center for Women in Medicine. The Medical College of
        Pennsylvania. Women in Medicine: Action Planning
        for the 1970s: Report of a Workshop, Philadelphia,
        March 14 and 15, 1974. Center for Women in Medi-
        cine, Philadelphia, Pennsylvania, [1974?], 84 pp.
Reports and recommendations from each of five groups at
the workshop are summarized. Each group focused on a
different major issue: (1) recruitment, education, and retraining, (2) specialization, practice, and career, (3) family
and professional responsibilities, (4) communications and
coordination, and (5) interaction with other agencies and organizations. Group leaders were Mary Howell, June Kling-
hoffer, Jeannette Haase, Doris Bartuska, Nancy Roeske,
Doris Howell, Mary Hartman, Amber Jones, Maggie Matthews, and Gerald Escovitz.

3968.   Chappell, Amey. "The Obligations of a Medical Woman."
        Journal of the American Medical Women's Association,
        5:3 (March 1950) 107-108. (Editorial.)

Obligations to one's profession, patients, and continuing education, as well as to one's family and community, are discussed.

3969. Chenoweth, Alice Drew. "Exploring Medical Talent." Journal of the American Medical Women's Association, 23:1 (January 1968) 22-26. (Inaugural Address, Annual Meeting, American Medical Women's Association, Atlanta, Georgia, 2 December 1967.)
A review of both the statistics on women in medicine and possible etiology for the relatively few numbers of women physicians is given.

3970. Cornell, William M. An Introductory Lecture Delivered to the Class of the Female Medical College of Pennsylvania, September 13th, 1852. Published by the class, Philadelphia, Pennsylvania, 1852, 16 pp.
Beginning with comments upon female education in general, Dr. Cornell states that he is not an advocate of "Ultraism" (i.e., woman's rights) although he is not opposed to them having their rights. He proceeds to catalogue the qualities women possess which make the practice of medicine a natural sphere for them: they are gentle, persevering, less easily disheartened than men, and more understanding of children. The medical curriculum is next reviewed; and finally Dr. Cornell refutes the various oppositions to women in medicine. In conclusion, Dr. Cornell talks briefly of the opportunities open to women physicians.

3971. Craighill, Margaret D. "An Analysis of Women in Medicine Today." Women in Medicine, 71 (January 1941) 7-8.
This article reviews the statistics of women in medicine from 1905 to 1940. The summary includes the facts that the number of women studying medicine is not increasing rapidly; men's and women's applications are being accepted in almost equal proportion; a slightly smaller percentage of women than of men is graduated; there are adequate opportunities for women to study medicine in the United States; relatively fewer women than men are being qualified as specialists.

3972. Dodge, Eva F. "Women Physicians of Arkansas." Journal of the American Medical Women's Association, 19:10 (October 1964) 865. (Editorial.)
While the University of Arkansas School of Medicine was organized in 1879, the first woman did not graduate until 1901 and then, of the 90 women who have attended this school, 80 have received their degrees since 1935. This article is a report of a survey taken of the women who could be found from this group. Some of the highlighted careers include one woman from the class of 1938 who served in the navy during World War II as a psychiatrist

and who remained to make her career there. Her promotion to captain in 1957 made her the second woman physician to achieve that rank. A member of the class of 1934 became the first woman doctor in Panama.

3973.   Fay, Marion. "The Woman Doctor." In: Listen to Leaders in Medicine. Edited by Albert Love and James Saxon Childers. Holt, Rinehart, and Winston, New York, New York, 1963, 299-320.
Dr. Fay reviews the progress of women in medicine in the U.S. since the mid-19th century and emphasizes the opportunities for medical study and practice currently available. She discusses the problems unique to women selecting medical careers (e.g., combining a career and family), and suggests ways to handle these problems, frequently citing examples of practicing women physicians. Attributes, such as integrity and stamina, of a good physician are reviewed; examples of how these characteristics are demonstrated by both students and practitioners are given. Dr. Fay makes suggestions for evaluating one's interest and ability to cope with medical study and a career and indicates how admissions committees and advisers assess students. Financial planning suggestions are included. The chapter concludes with a bibliography of books, mostly biographies, that would familiarize an interested student with the history and contributions of women in medicine.

3974.   Fay, Marion; Travell, Janet; Powell, Virginia; Means, James H.; and Ryder, Claire F. "Women in Medicine --Letters from Other Desks." Journal of the American Medical Women's Association, 16:5 (May 1961) 394-396.
A selection of letters reprinted from other sources constitutes this article. By appointing Janet Travell as his personal doctor, President Kennedy helped to give a positive role model to younger women who might now consider medicine as a career. A child of a woman physician writes, "Mom takes vacations from her work, not from us." A male M.D. is "worried about whether the married ones [women physicians] really do enough for medicine as the great cost of their education really demands of them.... The spinsters ... do excellent and complete professional jobs." Dr. Claire Ryder responds that fewer women drop out of medical school than men so that part-time service by a woman physician means more service than that provided by a male dropout. Women physicians do invaluable volunteer service that male physicians cannot afford to do because males perceive themselves as carrying full family support responsibilities.

3975.   Fishbein, Morris. "Women in Medicine: Breaking the Sex Barrier." Medical World News, 15:31 (23 August 1974) 56. (Editorial.)

Dr. Fishbein looks at the increasing number of women entering medical school and contemplates the changes one can
expect to see in medicine as a result (e.g., the availability
of doctors for deprived areas and rural districts).   Fewer
women than men are among the foreign physicians coming
to the U.S.   Dr. Fishbein states that "if ... society is to
benefit from the services of highly trained women in any
field, it must recognize woman's role as a mother and keep-
er of the household."   Certain specialties are, however, by
their nature, not constituted to be practiced by women, e.g.,
orthopedic surgery.

3976.   Florence, Loree.   "Women in Medicine."   Journal of the
        Medical Association of Georgia, 31 (1942) 1-14.
        [Article not examined by editors.]

3977.   Gloeckner, M. Louise C.   "The Challenge of Medicine for
        Women Today."   Journal of the American Medical Wo-
        men's Association, 15:3 (March 1960) 271-274.   (Open-
        ing address, Woman's Medical College of Pennsylvania,
        Philadelphia.)
        From history we know women were comforters, healers,
        and midwives.   Women lost the position of being the pri-
        mary healers.   Now the Woman's Medical College of Penn-
        sylvania has given young women physicians models of good
        woman-physician health care.   General practitioners are
        needed.   Women physicians should consider becoming active
        in professional organizations.   Physicians should be prepared
        to serve their communities: in civil defense, in natural dis-
        asters, in responding to cultists, in educating about serums,
        in learning more to solve the problems of diseases whose
        cures are not known today.   The physician should take as
        careful care of herself as she does of her patients.

3978.   Gordon, Burgess.   "Women in Medicine."   Minnesota Medi-
        cine, 36 (July 1953) 724-725, 735.
        A serious shortage of doctors makes it desirable to fully
        integrate women into the field of medicine.

3979.   Gordon, Burgess.   "The Privileges of Medicine."   Journal
        of the American Medical Women's Association, 6:12
        (December 1951) 472-473.   (Address, opening exer-
        cises, Woman's Medical College of Pennsylvania, Phila-
        delphia, 12 September 1951.)
        In his first opening exercises as new president, Dr. Gordon
        discusses the achievements of Woman's Medical College
        graduates and also mentions the contributions of women
        educators and researchers in the basic sciences.

3980.   "Governor to Proclaim Women in Medicine Week: Mrs.
        Paul R. Kaiser to Accept Governor Shafer's Proclama-
        tion at Commonwealth Committee Luncheon in Harris-
        burg on March 4."   Viewpoint: The Woman's Medical
        College of Pennsylvania, 22:1 (Winter 1967) 1.   photo.

3981.   "Great Day in Harrisburg Launches 'Women in Medicine
         Week.'" Viewpoint: The Woman's Medical College of
         Pennsylvania, 22:2 (Spring 1967) 3. facsim., photos.

3982.   Hall, Wesley W. "Ms. and M.D." Journal of the Ameri-
         can Medical Women's Association, 27:4 (April 1972)
         179-180, 196. (Address, Annual Meeting, American
         Medical Women's Association, New Orleans, Louisiana,
         December 1971.)
         A general discussion, by the president of the American
         Medical Association, is given on the health-care system.

3983.   Haycock, Christine E. and Weiss-Schwartz, Sandra. "New
         Jersey Women Physicians--Their Opinions on Today's
         World." Journal of the American Medical Women's
         Association, 28:6 (June 1973) 296-312. ports.
         Results of a survey sent to 184 active members of the New
         Jersey Medical Women's Association on a number of social
         and medical questions. A 33 per cent response was re-
         ceived. "The attitudes appear to be relatively conserva-
         tive." Questionnaires and number of total responses are
         included as well as narrative summaries.

3984.   Hill, Lister. "The Challenge to Women in Medicine."
         Philadelphia Medicine, 51:50 (13 July 1956) 1619-1621.
         (Commencement Address, Woman's Medical College of
         Pennsylvania, Philadelphia, Pennsylvania, 7 June 1956.)
         Senator Hill (Alabama) opens his lecture by discussing the
         role of government in health care. He speaks of the cen-
         tral position health care has in society today and the doctor
         as the central figure in the battle for better health care.
         The challenges this situation presents to women in medicine
         involve maintaining intellectual integrity and high standards,
         the challenge of understanding the importance of close and
         continuing contact between the scientist and the doctor. A
         third challenge is to preserve "the wonderful missionary
         spirit" characterized by graduates of the Woman's Medical
         College of Pennsylvania. Senator Hill, in conclusion, ex-
         presses surprise that out of 28,000 medical students in the
         U.S. in 1955, only 1,500 of them were women. He calls
         for more women to enter medicine.

3985.   Hintze, Anne Augusta. "Women in Medicine." Clifton
         Medical Bulletin, 11:1 (March 1925) 12-25.
         [Article not examined by editors.]

3986.   Hurd-Mead, Kate Campbell. "Women Doctors: Today and
         Yesterday." Independent Woman, (May 1939) 138-140,
         150-151. ports.
         Many contemporary women physicians are given mention in
         this general article on women in the medical profession.
         The article focuses on contemporary situations for women in
         medical schools, in hospitals, and in practice.

3987.   [Hurd-]Mead, Kate C[ampbell].   "No Other Vocation for
         Women as Useful." Woman's Medical Journal, 29[19]:
         1 (January 1919) 12.
         [Article not examined by the editors.]

3988.   Hurd-Mead, Kate Campbell. "Women Have Arrived: And
         They Intend to Hold Their Place in Medicine." Med-
         ical Economics, (January 1936) 23-26. ports.
         An overview of women's struggle to gain a place in the
         medical profession is followed by a report of the current
         status of women in the profession. In the United States in
         1936 there were over 7,000 licensed women doctors. In
         1932, eight per cent of the medical women had incomes of
         $10,000. The names of leading women in medicine in the
         United States are given and their work discussed: Dr.
         Florence R. Sabin, Dr. Anna W. Williams, Dr. Bertha
         Van Hoosen, Dr. Yung Ting, and Dr. Alice Hamilton,
         among others.

3989.   H[uth], E[dward] J. "Women in and out of Medicine."
         Annals of Internal Medicine, 66:5 (May 1967) 1022-
         1023. (Editorial.)
         This editorial introduces the Rosenlund and Oskii study on
         women physicians which appears in this issue of the Annals.
         The editor also makes a few general comments upon the
         numbers and percentages of women "in and out" of medi-
         cine.

3990.   James, Selwyn. "What's the Matter with Women Doctors?"
         Redbook, (June 1949) 36-37, 89+. photo.
         The reasons that so few women practice medicine in the
         United States (less than 8,000) can be found in the "myth
         of male superiority"--a mixture of "professional jealousy
         and lay superstition." Women first face medical school
         quota systems. Then, "guardians of male supremacy will
         do their best to embarrass the girls." Even after earning
         medical degrees, women discover that the men have only
         just begun to fight. Training opportunities and hospital
         staff positions for women are limited. Organizations of
         medical specialists often bar women members. Finally,
         there are the arguments that women do not remain in active
         practice, and that a medical career and marriage do not
         mix. The author of this article affirms women's contribu-
         tion to medicine, concluding that "good medicine knows no
         barrier of sex."

3991.   Jones, Harriet B. "The Woman Physician." Transactions
         of the Medical Society of West Virginia, (1896) 1329-
         1336.
         [Article not examined by editors.]

3992.   Kaplan, Harold. "Challenge to AMWA." Journal of the
         American Medical Women's Association, 19:7 (July

1964) 577. (Editorial.)
Women physicians are urged to "inform their male peers
how they feel" about the need for special programs to
facilitate women entering medicine and utilizing their medical educations. "Women physicians should not feel reluctant, ashamed, or guilty to ask for special treatment because they are women and mothers ... they should be proud
of their multiple roles and their unique ability to assume
them as well as they do."

3993.   Larsson, Elisabeth. "Women's Rightful Place in Medicine:
              The Role of Women in Medicine." Alumni Journal
              [Loma Linda University, School of Medicine], 44:3 (May
              1973) 10-15. illus., photo.
Dr. Larsson, professor emeritus at Loma Linda University,
has divided her remarks into three parts: past, present,
and future. Past: She discusses the medical contributions
of two Hebrew midwives mentioned in Exodus 1:15-21, of
Agnodice of Athens, of Trotula of Salerno, of Elizabeth
Blackwell, and of Mary Putnam Jacobi. Present: Armed
with statistics, especially regarding Seventh-day Adventist
medical schools, she asks why there are so few women
doctors, concluding that the prospects for women doctors
in America are improving. Future: Quoting several authorities, Dr. Larsson predicts that women, "who have
one-half of the nation's most valuable resource--human
talent," will soon make up half of America's medical profession. Special flexible training programs for women doctors with small children will help to make this possible.

3994.   Longshore, J. S. An Introductory Lecture, Delivered Be-
              fore the Class, At the Opening of the Female Medical
              College of Pennsylvania: October 12th, 1850. James
              Young, Printer, Philadelphia, Pennsylvania, 1850, 28
              pp.
Dr. Longshore opens his lecture with a discussion of the
laws of progress in chemistry, electricity, and medicine.
Concerning this latter field, Dr. Longshore reviews the various practices prevalent: homeopathy, mesmerism, hydrop-
athy, and allopathy, the latter of which is the school em-
braced by the Female Medical College of Pennsylvania. A
discussion of the fields of medicine which might interest
women and be appropriate to their study follows (e.g., obstetrics and pediatrics). A justification of women in medical
practice is followed by comments on the propriety and safety of the practice. Concluding his introductory remarks,
Dr. Longshore impresses upon the students the uniqueness
of this institution and their unique position as students there:
"Do the women of Pennsylvania, of America, duly appreciate
the relation in which they stand to this magnificent enter-
prize? Can they realize the vastness of the project? Have
they yet become impressed with the great truth--that in this
Institution is the germ of their emancipation from mental

bondage and physical suffering?" An appendix to the lecture expresses Dr. Longshore's experiences after the lecture was delivered and those in the medical profession learned of his views. He discovered there is much more evil in the medical profession than he had even anticipated--evil he hopes women physicians can rectify. Extracts "from legitimate sources" follow, which express the favorable opinion and high hopes of others as well as himself, regarding the entrance of women into medical practice.

3995. Lopate, Carol. Women in Medicine. Johns Hopkins Press, Baltimore, Maryland, 1968, xvii, 204 pp. tables.
The Macy Conference on Women for Medicine held in 1966 provided the impetus for this book, and the author's intention: "to communicate what it is like to be a woman in medicine in the United States." Data from statistical studies (taken from other sources) illustrate women's experience in medical education and practice. The book also incorporates personal interviews with women physicians and Lopate's critical examination of the social systems that influence medical women. Lopate's inquiry into the nature of women physicians' lives begins with a historical overview of the struggles faced by the modern medical woman's professional ancestors. While early prejudice found its basis on assumptions concerning women's biology and intelligence, Lopate notes that more recent objections to recruiting medical women take more subtle forms ("often indistinguishable from 'official planning'"), i.e., women's lower practice rates. The forms of that resistance and its effects are discussed in relation to: influences that motivate women to become doctors ("and why many do not"); the role of high school and premed counseling; problems of coeducational and sex-segregated medical schools; stresses of graduate education and specialty selection. A separate chapter is devoted to marriage and medicine, in which Lopate suggests how the medical profession and the government can be more responsive to the woman's "double burden." Many suggestions are offered throughout the work for the improvement of women's position: increased scholarship aids, more flexible scheduling during the training years, and child-care tax deductions. In her conclusion, however, Lopate points out the futility of demanding, for example, that medical schools increase their admission of women: "What seems necessary is that the national climate of opinion concerning sexual roles be changed so that many more high-caliber women will, of their own choice, decide to become doctors and will squeeze their way into the medical world." Lopate admits the difficulty of accomplishing such a task in the United States, "a country meek about taking committed action to resolve its social problems." Sweeping reform within the medical profession itself may also be necessary to make the field more inviting to women. This book contains a foreword by John Z. Bowers and a preface by Mary

Bunting. Appendixes (containing statistical tables) and an
index conclude the work.

3996.   McGrew, Elizabeth A. "The 'Fair Sex.'" Journal of the
         American Medical Women's Association, 22:1 (January
         1967) 32-34. (Inaugural Address of AMWA President,
         Annual Meeting, Washington, D.C., 2-5 November
         1966.)
    After Elizabeth McGrew defines the Fair Sex as "not really
    more 'pleasing to the eye'--at least, the eyes of most of
    us are more likely to be pleased by men," she goes on to
    say that women physicians, "unencumbered by power and
    undazzled by glory, can play a crucial role" in helping med-
    icine serve "those citizens least able to pay." She then
    goes on to say that to make it easier for women to practice
    medicine, "high priority" ought to be given to "obtaining
    tax relief for women who can practice only if they can hire
    suitable people to care for their families, and modifying
    medical training programs so that women with family re-
    sponsibilities can become qualified specialists."

3997.   McGrew, Elizabeth A. "The History of Women in Medi-
         cine; A Symposium: The Present." Bulletin of the
         Medical Library Association, 44:1 (January 1956) 23-24.
    In the days when medicine was "a highly strategic and
    stoutly defended ... citadel of male supremacy," women
    had to be fighters, scientists, as well as humanitarians to
    become physicians. Now, any serious girl can obtain an
    M.D. degree (only two medical schools--Jefferson and Dart-
    mouth--do not admit women). Today, women physicians'
    identity as women is lost in the exciting activity of modern
    medicine.

3998.   McKibbin-Harper, Mary. "Contemporary Women in Medi-
         cine." Medical Review of Reviews, 41:8 (August 1935)
         381-388. (Foreword.)
    In this "foreword" to this journal's "Woman's Number--
    III," Dr. McKibbin-Harper mentions journals, collections,
    and books devoted to the subject of women in medicine.
    Contributions of specific women physicians are recounted,
    along with the activities of the Medical Women's National
    Association and women physicians in California. Affirming
    that women are not "invaders in medicine," the author rea-
    sons that women's difficulties in entering the profession
    have been due to generalized competition rather than sex-
    based prejudice. Women have been excluded from medical
    schools because schools are crowded, and medical schools
    have difficulty securing internships for women graduates
    since some hospitals refuse women on the ground of not
    having suitable accommodations. "I do not believe that men
    have ever been less generous with women than they have
    been with each other," Dr. McKibbin-Harper writes. She
    points out that "men have not kept women from posts of

honor or emolument except as they have needed them for
themselves."

3999.   "Mary Putnam Jacobi Fellowship Fund."   Women in Medi-
             cine, 71 (January 1941) 18-19.   port.
         This article includes a description of how to apply for a
         fellowship which is named in honor of Mary Putnam Jacobi,
         and is made available by the Women's Association of New
         York City.   The fellowship is for medical research and is
         open to any woman doctor, either American or foreign.
         An appreciation by Clara Raven of Mary Putnam Jacobi's
         life as a pioneering international medical woman, as well
         as of her understanding of the fruitlessness of nationalist
         wars of aggression for material gain, is included.

4000.   "The Mary Putnam Jacobi Fellowship of the Women's Med-
             ical Association of New York City."   Journal of the
             American Medical Women's Association, 15:8 (August
             1960) 784-785.
         In honor of Mary Putnam Jacobi, the Women's Medical
         Association of New York City established a fellowship to en-
         able graduate women physicians from America to study
         abroad and foreign women physicians to study in America.
         One award is given each year.

4001.   Mason-Hogle, Kate A.   "Annual Address."   Woman's Med-
             ical Journal, 18:7 (July 1908) 137-139.   (Original Arti-
             cles.)   (Presentation, 11th Annual Meeting, State Soci-
             ety of Iowa Medical Women, Des Moines, Iowa, 19 May
             1908.)
         Dr. Hogle reviews the struggle of women for the right to
         practice medicine and expresses the opinion that women
         physicians should be sought because of their worth, and not
         because of their sex.

4002.   Mott, Lucretia.   A Sermon to the Medical Students, De-
             livered by Lucretia Mott at Cherry Street Meeting
             House, Philadelphia, on First-Day Evening, Second
             Month 11th, 1849.   W. B. Zeiber, Philadelphia, Penn-
             sylvania, 1849, 21 pp.
         [Item not examined by editors.]

4003.   Nemir, Rosa Lee.   "The American Woman Physician:
             Doorway to the Second Century."   Journal of the Amer-
             ican Medical Women's Association, 19:1 (January 1964)
             45-50.   (Inaugural Address, Annual Meeting, American
             Medical Women's Association, San Antonio, Texas, 15
             November 1963.)
         Dr. Nemir reviews major developments in the "community"
         served by women physicians: developments in infectious
         disease, health care, and the use of paramedical personnel.
         She reviews the status of women in medicine and asks why
         there are so few women entering medical schools when

"there seems to be no appreciable discrimination against
women who apply for admission." An overview of women
pioneers in medicine follows. A discussion of recruitment
yields four possible deterrents for women entering medicine:
finances, length of medical studies, role conflict, and lack
of reliable information about a medical career.

4004.   "News Notes." Medical Woman's Journal, 56:8 (August
          1949) 43.
        Among the medical women mentioned in this article are the
        first four women to obtain medical degrees from Harvard
        and Dr. Sushila Nayar, who was once physician to Ma-
        hatma Ghandi.

4005.   "Notes and Comments." Medical Woman's Journal, 30:6
          (June 1923) 192-193.
        The topics reported in this column include: the resignation
        of Dr. S. Josephine Baker as director of the Bureau of
        Child Hygiene, New York City Department of Health; the
        building of a women's medical school in Madras, India; the
        merging of the North China Union Medical College for Wo-
        men with the Shantung Christian University; and the appoint-
        ment of Dr. Blache N. Epler as contract physician to Coast
        Guard stations.

4006.   "Notes and Comments." Medical Woman's Journal, 30:10
          (October 1923) 311-312.
        Among the announcements appearing in this news column:
        the founding of a $5,000 scholarship for women of Italian
        descent to study at the Woman's Medical College of Penn-
        sylvania and the appointment of Canadian physician Winifred
        Blampin to the faculty at that college.

4007.   "Number of Women Physicians Increasing." Medical Wo-
          man's Journal, 36:4 (April 1929) 100.
        According to Dr. Martha Tracy, dean of the Woman's Med-
        ical College of Pennsylvania, there are 7,000 women physi-
        cians in the United States. That number is ever increas-
        ing. Dr. Tracy's comments on women in the medical pro-
        fession are given.

4008.   "The Number of Women Physicians Increasing." Medical
          Woman's Journal, 38:9 (September 1931) 233.
        According to the American Medical Association, 990 women
        registered in medical schools during the 1930-1931 session
        --an increase of 35 from the previous year, and the larg-
        est number since 1904. In 1931, 217 women received their
        M.D.s (4 per cent of the total number of graduates).
        "While the number of hospitals which still have no women
        on their staff, and are still refusing to admit women for
        one reason or another, is large, the foregoing facts would
        indicate the discrimination ... is being replaced by a policy
        of equal rights...."

4009.   O'Conner, Katheryn and Forbes, Lorna. "Student News."
            Medical Woman's Journal, 52:3 (March 1945) 52.   photo.
        A list of residency appointments for the graduating students
        at the Woman's Medical College of Pennsylvania is given.
        A brief biography of Dr. Mary Easby is also presented upon
        the occasion of her election as president of the Philadelphia
        Heart Association.

4010.   "Opportunities for Medical Women Sixty-Five Years Ago--
            And Now." Medical Woman's Journal, 28:3 (March
            1921) 79. (Editorial.)
        This editorial draws generalized comparisons between condi-
        tions of Dr. Cleora Seaman's day and the opportunities of
        the present.

4011.   "PMJ Interview with Marion Spencer Fay, Ph.D.: Former
            President and Dean, Woman's Medical College." Penn-
            sylvania Medical Journal, (February 1964) 25-26.
            port.
        Dr. Fay, dean of the Woman's Medical College of Pennsyl-
        vania, responds to questions on discrimination against wo-
        men in medicine ("There is some discrimination"), marriage
        and medicine ("... medicine lends itself very nicely to the
        combination"), the future of women doctors in the U.S.
        ("I'd like to see more women going into medicine"), medical
        students and medical schools, and fund raising, among oth-
        er topics.

4012.   Phelps, Charles E. "Women in American Medicine." Jour-
            nal of Medical Education, 43:8 (August 1968) 916-924.
            tables.
        Because the emergence of women in medicine is having a
        poorly understood effect on the "medical community," this
        report is presented to supply information on that topic: the
        type of women who become physicians, the specialties they
        enter, the amount of time they practice medicine, and the
        barriers they encounter. Calling the anti-women-physicians
        viewpoint unenlightened, the author quotes Dr. Glen Ley-
        master, dean of the Woman's Medical College of Pennsyl-
        vania, who opined, "'Discrimination against women in medi-
        cine is largely a thing of the past.... A few male physi-
        cians hold reservations toward females as a class. But
        even these minority voices evaluate individual doctors on
        their qualifications without regard to sex. That's all any-
        one can ask.'" And, while the acceptance of women in
        medicine is far from complete, the percentage of women as
        medical students, although still very low (7.7 per cent),
        represents a "rather remarkable change considering that
        there were no women in medicine only a hundred years
        ago." Two major factors contributing to the "grudging ad-
        mission" of women to medical schools are the obvious lag-
        ging of the United States compared to other countries in the
        percentage of women physicians, and the "realization that a

vast source of talent was remaining untapped." A large
section of this article reiterates the finding of the 1957
Dykman and Stalnaker study ["Survey of Women Physicians
Graduating from Medical School: 1925-1940," Journal of
Medical Education, 32 (March, Part 2) 1957]. This author
makes additions to that study and a few others, and points
out factors overlooked in these surveys, i.e., the influence
in patient acceptance of women physicians. He feels that
whether or not women return to practice after marriage
and childbirth is a "moot point" since no study verifies this
contention. The author reviews the difficulties women face
when practicing medicine and the methods for alleviating
these problems (e.g., retraining programs, part-time employment). He concludes that "women are more marginally
valuable to the medical complex at this time because of
their propensity to enter specialties in which there is presently the greatest shortage of physicians."

4013. Platz, Carol; O'Conner, Katheryn; Piccone, Louisa; Zolliker, Margaret; Imperi, Lillian; Brekke, Viola; Raven,
Clara; and McLean, Brita. "Women in Medicine: Opportunities and Problems." Journal of the American
Medical Women's Association, 18:11 (November 1963)
885-890. (Panel Presentation, Executive Board Meeting, American Medical Association, Detroit, Michigan,
20 June 1963.)

Excerpts from this panel comprise the article. Dr. O'Conner, a 1946 graduate of the Woman's Medical College of
Pennsylvania, has "not experienced any problems from being
a woman in [medicine]." She gives the "3 H's" necessary
to a successful medical woman as "Health, adequate household Help, and an understanding Husband." Dr. Piccone, a
1944 graduate of Wayne State University, says "medicine is
a woman's field and has been through the ages." She feels
medicine has become less interesting to men "lately" because of the social and economic problems involved. She
feels this waning of interest on the part of the men accounts
for less prejudice against women in medicine (with the exception of women in surgery). Dr. Piccone feels the government should give more consideration to child care services for women physicians. Dr. Margaret Zolliker, a
1946 graduate of Wayne State, feels that "pediatrics is a
natural for women." A married woman in any field "must
realize that she is going to have to make some compromises.... With the domestic chores that she must carry
out, a woman cannot give her all to a career unless she is
very unusual. Part of her time must be spent being a woman." Dr. Imperi, a psychiatrist and 1955 graduate of the
University of Michigan, discusses psychiatry as a career
and says "a woman psychiatrist's horizon may be further
widened by volunteer service in foreign areas." Discussing
her experience with medicine in the armed services, Dr.
Clara Raven, a 1936 graduate of Northwestern University

and a colonel with 20 years service in the Army Medical
Reserve Corps, states that prejudice against women physicians in the service is unusual, and where there are difficulties, "it is usually with a man who is a poorly adjusted
or alcoholic individual." Dr. Olson adds in conclusion, "I
think we are inclined to forget the times we are discriminated against."

4014.   Preston, Ann. <u>Introductory Lecture, to the Course of In-
         struction in the Female Medical College of Pennsylvania,
         For the Session 1855-6.</u> Published by the audience,
         Philadelphia, Pennsylvania, 1855, 14 pp.
In this lecture [printed by Anna E. McDowell, Woman's
Advocate Office, Philadelphia] Dr. Ann Preston notes the
occasions in civilization when truths which ran counter to
convention were scorned, and conservatism shrank from innovation. She moves on to discuss the history of women in
the healing art and the opposition to women in medical studies. While this opposition exists, Dr. Preston continues,
women physicians will not realize the advantages "in some
directions" which their medical brothers enjoy (e.g., the
privilege to practice in hospitals). The second half of the
lecture is devoted to a discussion of the actual course of
medical study the student will pursue at the Female Medical College of Pennsylvania. The woman physician must
be prudent, above-board in her actions, self-disciplined,
and reliable. In conclusion, Ann Preston extends to these
women medical students "the warm hand of sisterly sympathy. I know the heart of a woman, and especially that
of one entering upon a new and untried course, like that
before you." [A letter to Ann Preston requesting a copy
of her lecture for publication is signed by, among others,
William S. Peirce and Lucretia Mott.]

4015.   Pullum, Carla A. "Women, Medicine and Misconceptions."
         <u>Journal of the American Medical Women's Association,</u>
         <u>18</u>:7 (July 1963) 563-565. tables.
Women who do not consider applying to medical school are
"victims of misinformation." To determine more recent
trends than those of the Dykman and Stalnaker study about
women physicians, the author interviewed 40 of the 58 women physicians who attended classes at Wayne State University College of Medicine. She proposes that since 25 per
cent of the women interviewed had degrees in medically related fields, they may not have considered medical school
itself as an initial career choice [because they had no confidence of getting in]. Another 25 per cent of women interviewed had at least one physician in their immediate
family. This survey about women physicians included a
section on marriage and family. Since being a doctor means
prestige, title, and higher salary, husbands of women physicians may feel social insecurity. A woman physician may
decide to choose a specialty that she can anticipate will be

compatible with marriage and family life. Of the women
surveyed in this study who married, over 50 per cent married physicians, 25 per cent married other professionals,
and the remainder married men with business careers.

4016.   Rabinowitsch, Lydia. ["American Women and Their Achieve-
            ments"]. Die Frauenbewegung, 3:15 (1897) 1-4. (Ger)
        A lecture given before the women's welfare society of Ber-
        lin on 25 May 1897 summarizes the author's impressions
        gained during two years of teaching and travel in America.
        She speaks of the freedom of young women, of family life,
        the women's rights movement, higher education, social life,
        women's clubs, the voluntary welfare system, etc. She
        notes that in 1892 there were 4555 women physicians and
        surgeons in the U.S. Included is a description of a visit
        to a settlement house in an unnamed city, a house apparently
        run by an organization of college graduates. The staff in-
        cludes a woman doctor and two nurses who are on call at
        all times, free to the people in the area.

4017.   Rayne, Mrs. M. L. What Can a Woman Do; or, Her Posi-
            tion in the Business and Literary World. Eagle Pub-
            lishing Co., Petersburgh, New York, 1893, 552 pp.
            illus.
        This discussion of occupations open to women in 1893 in-
        cludes chapters on literature, journalism, law, medicine,
        telegraphy, beekeeping, and homemaking, among others.
        Several poems by women authors are interspersed. The
        chapter on medicine (pp. 65-80) lists medical colleges open
        to women and gives a chronological account of women's ad-
        mittance to medical schools in various countries. Many
        women physicians are mentioned, and incidents from their
        life stories are given. The chapter includes a paper by
        Dr. Emily Pope, showing the extent of the practice of medi-
        cine by women and how this practice has affected their
        health. Dr. Pope's report reveals that 390 women physi-
        cians (of the 470 who received questionnaires on the subject)
        were in active practice. Seventy-five per cent were single
        when they began the study of medicine (which they did at
        an average age of 27 years). A majority of the women
        (269) were in general practice. The average annual income
        of a woman physician was $1,000. The chapter concludes
        with a brief paragraph by Dr. Alice Stockham entitled
        "Requisites for a Physician."

4018.   "Report of Convention: Medical Women's National Associa-
            tion. Atlantic City, New Jersey." Medical Woman's
            Journal, 42:7 (July 1935) 189-192.

4019.   Romaine, Adelaide. "Future of Women in Medicine."
            Journal of the American Medical Women's Association,
            4:5 (May 1949) 197-198. (Editorial.)
        To retain exclusively "feminine" medical colleges and hos-

pital staffs, and to build good public relations between the American Medical Women's Association and other medical associations, such is the future of women in medicine.

4020. Root, Eliza H. "The Distribution of Medical Women in the State of Illinois." Woman's Medical Journal, 14:5 (May 1904) 100-101.

4021. Rutherford, Frances A. "New Force in Medicine and Surgery." Woman's Medical Journal, 1:9 (September 1893) 181-184. (Presentation, Michigan State Medical Society, May 1893.)
Vice president of the Michigan Medical Society, Dr. Rutherford scans the record of the first 20 years of the American medical women's movement. She contrasts the early struggles with the current situation, speaking in general terms of women's work in hospitals and missions. Finally, she congratulates the Society for being the first state medical organization to admit women members; she urges the gentlemen to continue using their influence for placing women in positions commensurate with their abilities.

4022. Sherbon, Florence Brown. "Our Novitiates." Medical Woman's Journal, 33:7 (July 1926) 191-193.
As the retiring president of the Kansas State Medical Women's Association, Dr. Sherbon addresses women graduating from the Kansas University Medical School. The true philosophy of feminism is embodied in a quote by H. G. Wells: "You'll never run parallel with men, you free women. You've got to work out a way that is different." Women physicians must have the courage "to express our real interests and our real personalities, our feminism ..." rather than remain "content to do and think only as men do and think." Rather than "resist our destiny" for "emotional expression and human service," women physicians should concentrate on public health work and obstetrical research. Dr. Sherbon also urges women to join or start medical women's organizations--"not for producing a demarcation from the regular medical group, but for one purpose of working out together the specific contributions women have to make...."

4023. Spencer, Steven M. "Do Women Make Good Doctors?" Saturday Evening Post, (13 November 1948) 15-17, 134, 137-138, 141. photos.
This is a review of the status of women physicians in the U.S. during the postwar period. In 1948, 2,159 women were enrolled in 27 U.S. medical colleges and comprised 9.5 per cent of the medical student body. At the same time, professional groups such as the New York Obstetrical Society and the Boston Obstetrical Society refused to admit women. Of 807 hospitals in the U.S. offering internships in 1948, 437 said they would accept women; 318 of 1,102

hospitals providing residency training would admit women.
A popular male educator's prejudice was that medical
schools have to admit two or three women to get one who
will practice. However, a poll of 1,240 women graduating
from seven large medical schools between 1920 and 1940,
showed 91.5 per cent actively engaged in full-time practice,
research, teaching, or institutional work. The article reviews the education of women in medicine, citing in particular the Woman's Medical College of Pennsylvania [now the
Medical College of Pennsylvania]. The admission of women
to the leading medical schools in the U.S. is chronicled
along with enrollment statistics for 1947-1948. The decline of the enrollment of women that accompanied the
return of World War II [male] veterans to school is also
noted. Examples of women in medical practice who are
cited in the article are Margaret Castex Sturgis, F. Marian
Williams, Catharine Macfarlane, May Baker, Mary Larney
Hansen, Elise Strang L'Esperance, and Ida S. Scudder.

4024. Sullivan, Margaret P. "A New Era: Challenges for the
         Woman Physician: (Hey, No Fair! There are Hardly
         any Lady Doctors!)." Journal of the American Medical
         Women's Association, 29:1 (January 1974) 9-11. tables.
This article reviews the data [taken from other sources] on
characteristics of women medical school applicants, women
medical students, women physicians, and women medical
faculty.

4025. Tayler-Jones [sic], Louise. "Medicine as a Field for Wo-
         men.... An Age-Old Profession for Women: Some
         Notes on Requirements Today." Journal of the Ameri-
         can Association of University Women, 31 (April 1938)
         152-155.
Statistics on the number of women physicians and medical
students are discussed in historical retrospect, after which
the situation of the medical woman in 1938 is reviewed.
Despite the injustices, the sacrifices, and the struggle,
there is no more rewarding career than medicine.

4026. "Three Generations Look at Their Profession." Texas
         Medicine, 71:1 (January 1975) 91-100. photos.
Drs. May Owens (M.D. 1921), Margaret P. Sullivan (contemporary practitioner), and Peggy Hostetter (medical student), discuss their feelings about medicine, advertising depicting women physicians, problems of women medical students, medical school admissions policies, and role models.

4027. Todd, Malcolm C. "Address to Annual Meeting of the
         American Medical Women's Association." Journal of
         the American Medical Women's Association, 29:4 (April
         1974) 161-163. (Palm Beach, Florida, 10 November
         1973.)
"You're like the cigarette ad, 'you've come a long way,

baby!'" A recounting by this president elect of the American Medical Association of the point to which women in medicine have come, precedes a discussion of the contemporary medical issues.

4028. Tracy, Martha. "The Profession of Medicine and Women's Opportunity in This Field." Journal of the American Association of University Women, 21:1 (October 1927) 5-10.
Dr. Tracy discusses the increasing demand for medical women's services which she has witnessed during her nearly 20 years on the faculty of the Woman's Medical College of Pennsylvania. The woman physician need no longer limit her services to general practice, yet the woman medical student is often given no guidance nor encouragement at her university regarding opportunities for her in the medical profession. Dr. Tracy gives concrete advice on how women should approach medical education, its costs, securing a license, doing postgraduate work, and deciding upon a practice.

4029. Tyson, J. R. Address at the First Annual Commencement of the Pennsylvania Female College, at Harrisburg. Harrisburg, Pennsylvania, 1854, 24 pp.
The speaker devoted a portion of his talk to women in medicine. [Item not examined by editors.]

4030 U.S. Department of Labor, Women's Bureau, Wage and Labor Standards Administration. Facts on Prospective and Practicing Women in Medicine. Washington, D.C., Government Printing Office, 1968, 78 pp. tables.
This booklet was prepared for the Conference on Meeting Medical Manpower Needs: The Fuller Utilization of the Woman Physician (Washington, D.C., January 12-13, 1968) and sent to registrants for that Conference. The booklet contains statistical data on women in medicine. General "source" information as well as a brief narrative is given for each table and chart. [The reports given at the Conference itself, and their reference to this statistical data may be found in the publication: American Medical Women's Association; The President's Study Group on Careers for Women; U.S. Department of Labor, Women's Bureau. Conference on Meeting Medical Manpower Needs: The Fuller Utilization of the Woman Physician. Washington, D.C., January 12-13, 1968. Report, which appears elsewhere in this bibliography.]

4031. Van Hoosen, Bertha. "Annual Report of Committee on Medical Opportunities for Women." Medical Woman's Journal, 36:8 (August 1929) 216-217.
In 1928 and 1929, the work of this committee was directed towards "ascertaining opportunities for women physicians in the State Insane Institutions." Two questionnaires were sent

out: one to women physicians and one to the superintendents of various state institutions. Based on responses to
these questionnaires, the committee recommended that "a
concerted effort be made through our Legislative Committee
to pass a law providing for insane female patients the care
of a woman physician." St. Elizabeth's Hospital in Washington, D.C. may be used as a model. The response of its
superintendent, Dr. Arthur P. Noyes, is given in this article. The committee also "felt greatly the need of a directory of women physicians of the United States."

4032.   Van Hoosen, Bertha. "Opportunities for Medical Women."
          Medical Review of Reviews, 37:3 (March 1931) 139-142.
          Dr. Van Hoosen begins her article by discussion of the op-
          portunities not available to women physicians, i.e., engaging
          in hospital work, attending medical societies, and teaching
          in medical schools. Women, in order to have hospitals in
          which to practice, had to build those hospitals; and from
          them sprang women's medical colleges. Women physicians
          were denied membership in medical societies until 1876
          when Dr. S. H. Stevenson (Sarah Hackett) was accepted as
          a delegate to the AMA convention in Philadelphia, becoming
          the first woman member of the AMA as well as the first
          woman delegate. Dr. Van Hoosen next discusses the emer-
          gence of women's medical colleges (14 in the U.S. by the
          beginning of the 20th century) and the increasing numbers of
          women physicians seeking faculty positions. At the begin-
          ning of the 20th century there were as many as 1100 women
          medical students in the U.S. This figure steadily decreased
          as the women's medical schools folded, until the beginning
          of World War I. Wars have been for the woman physician
          "an avenue for broader entrance into her profession," and
          by the end of World War I, the number of women medical
          students had again risen to more than 1,000. Many hos-
          pitals in need of more physicians also opened their doors
          to women interns during the war. The U.S. government,
          however, failed to recognize women physicians in the armed
          services, and once again women had to create their own op-
          portunities--the American Women's Hospitals. In conclusion,
          Dr. Van Hoosen calls for the abolishment of sex barriers
          to women physicians in hospitals, medical schools, and on
          teaching faculties.

4033.   V[an] H[oosen], B[ertha]. "What's in a Name?" Medical
          Woman's Journal, 37:9 (September 1930) 260-261.
          In trying to contact women physicians by means of first
          names in the American Medical Association directory, the
          Journal received a variety of responses from men whose
          first names could be mistaken for women's. A sample re-
          sponse reads: "Please take my feminine name off your list,
          because I am anything but a woman, and to prove it, just
          look up my world war record, and you will see I was a
          major in M.C. and I still retain the same sex features and

build--six feet four and weigh two hundred fifty-five pounds,
and I thank you. He-man."

4034.   Wager, Mary A. E. "Women as Physicians." The Galaxy,
        6 (December 1868) 774-789.
        Biographies of Elizabeth Blackwell, Sarah R. Adamson Dol-
        ley, Emily Blackwell, and Marie E. Zakrzewska include
        descriptions of their latest activities and their physical ap-
        pearances. Information on the founding of women's medical
        schools and hospitals staffed by women in the U.S. is pro-
        vided. The U.S. now boasts over 300 women physicians,
        some of whom have incomes of $10,000 a year. Among
        their number there are "some bold, bad women" who "try
        to be as much like men as possible," but the majority of
        medical women are "gentle, modest, and womanly." The
        article concludes with "a hurried glance" at women's med-
        ical education and practice in Europe.

4035.   Walters, Josephine. "Address: President of the Women's
        Medical Association, New York City ... Delivered May
        6, 1909." Medical Woman's Journal, 27:6 (June 1920)
        161-165.
        Following a tribute to Mary Putnam Jacobi, Dr. Walters
        presents an overview of the present opportunities for wo-
        men in medicine and affirms woman's right to practice
        medicine.

4035a. Warwick, Margaret. "Women in Medicine." Medical Wo-
        man's Journal, 48:12 (December 1941) 372-375.
        The history of women physicians in the United States began
        in 1847 when Elizabeth Blackwell applied to medical school
        and was accepted by the Medical Institute of Geneva. Male-
        run medical schools have discriminated against women both
        as students and as interns, as well as against their study-
        ing certain specialties. When this article was written, wo-
        men were admitted to only 71 of the 77 approved medical
        schools in the United States, and only 5.4 medical students
        were women. In 1934 only one-third of approved hospitals
        would accept women as interns. Women who are already
        physicians should make a concerted effort to fight for equal
        opportunities for women: educate laity and male physicians;
        financially support medical training facilities, housing, and
        scholarships for women; use influence to get women ac-
        cepted as interns; and seek support from women's organiza-
        tions in the community. Women should in turn fulfill their
        contracts and not let personal desires interfere with the
        good of the hospital, for males who will be physicians may
        assume their right to that training and position, while women
        who train to be physicians, and the women who follow, may
        not yet feel so assured of their right to training and title.
        Some comparative figures on women physicians in other coun-
        tries include: England has 5,971 women physicians; Japan,
        1,247; and the American Medical Association lists 7,470

women physicians in the U.S.   And for the first time in
400 years, in 1934, a woman, Dr. Helen Mackay, was
elected a Fellow of the Royal College of Physicians in London.   Women have practiced medicine and made important
contributions: as writers of medical books, as teachers,
as researchers, as specialists and as healers in a variety
of ways.

4036.   Weiss, Robert.   "'Changing Patterns of Health Care: Ef-
            fects on and of Women Physicians.'"   Case Western
            Reserve Medical Alumni Bulletin, 38:3 (1974) 4-6.
            photo.   (Presentation, Workshop on Women in Medicine,
            Case Western Reserve University School of Medicine,
            21 September 1974.)
Dr. Weiss calls for greater flexibility in time arrangements
and commitments of physicians, as well as a shift in the
medical value system.

4037.   White, Frances Emily.   "The American Medical Woman."
            Medical News, 67 (3 August 1895) 123-128.   (Original
            Address.)   (Address, Woman's Medical College, Phila-
            delphia, Pennsylvania, May 1895.)
Dr. White, after a cursory review of women in medicine
throughout the ages, discusses the American medical woman
from the colonial period in New England--where much of
the medical practice was in the hands of women--through
the increasingly scientific years and their concomitant restrictions in the practice of medicine.   Midwifery developed
into the formal training of the medical woman, commencing
with the granting of a medical degree to Elizabeth Blackwell in 1849.   Dr. White traces the history of the New
England Female Medical College and the Woman's Medical
College of Pennsylvania, after which she discusses the field
of medicine and woman's participation in it.   In order for
a professional field to be occupied successfully by women,
it must offer the following conditions: (1) the work must
fall within the scope of woman's physical and mental abilities, (2) it must afford an opportunity for exercise of the
"'peculiarly feminine'" qualities, (3) it must develop to a
satisfactory degree the physical and mental energies of women, and (4) it must pay well enough to enable women to
devote their best efforts to the work.   Medicine fulfills
these requisites and in fact engages more women (from between 3,000 to 5,000 in the United States) in its practice
than do all other professions put together.

4038.   Wilbur, Ray Lyman.   "Address of Dr. Ray Lyman Wilbur
            (President Elect of the A.M.A.)."   Bulletin of the
            Medical Women's National Association, 4 (July 1923)
            13-14.
The author gives an overview of the structure and function
of human society, using a bee-hive analogy.   Lyman then
brings the doctor into the picture and briefly discusses his

role. Women physicians have a unique opportunity to serve humanity, especially the child and the family, through public health. They are a minority "and they are going to be a minority for a long long time." As a minority, the way they can have the greatest influence inside the profession is to "scatter throughout the majority," not to separate themselves.

4039.   Williams, Phoebe A. "Women in Medicine: Some Themes and Variations." Journal of Medical Education, 46 (July 1971) 584-591. tables.
The author, a research associate at Radcliffe Institute, Cambridge, Massachusetts, reports on part of a study of Radcliffe College alumnae in medicine. The study probes the basic question: What is it like for women who choose to become doctors? In 1967, 253 Radcliffe alumnae who had enrolled in medical school over the last 60 years were sent questionnaires which dealt with personal characteristics, attitudes, and experiences at various career stages. A total of 212 (84 per cent) replies were received. Of these replies, 203 had received their M.D. or were currently in medical school, and nine had dropped out. Several themes thread their way across generations for these Radcliffe women who enter medicine: an interest in the subject matter, a desire to be of service, the need for independence, and encouragement from an adult. Concerns reflected were for the cost of a medical education and combining marriage and a medical career. The study does not presume that Radcliffe alumnae are representative of women college graduates in general.

4040.   "The Woman Physician: A Symbolic Study." Survey, 36 (22 July 1916) 435.
Dr. Rosalie Slaughter Morton presented a bas-relief (a photograph of which appears on the cover of this issue of Survey) to the Woman's Medical College of Pennsylvania. "An interpretation of Dr. Morton's conception of the maternal spirit which especially animates women to lessen suffering and heal the sick," the work was sculpted by a woman artist, Clara Hill. The bas-relief is described in detail.

4041.   "Women as Physicians." Medical Missionary Record, 8:12 (December 1893) 279.
Although it is not yet 50 years since Elizabeth Blackwell's graduation in medicine, women physicians numbering in the hundreds are now welcome everywhere--especially in the field of medical missionary work.

4042.   "Women in Medicine." Journal of the American Medical Women's Association, 1:3 (June 1946) 93-95. tables.
The New York Infirmary conducted a survey of employment opportunities for women among hospitals and medical col-

leges throughout the country to obtain certain facts about
the status of women at these institutions. Of the questionnaires sent to 967 hospitals, replies were received from
491 (50.7 per cent); 64 (82 per cent) of the medical colleges
responded of the 78 addressed. The questions are reproduced with the tabulated answers.

4043.   "Women in Medicine." Medical Woman's Journal, 54:1
              (January 1947) 45.
         This article, reprinted from the Medical Pocket Quarterly,
         September 1946, cites the "unfortunately" low number of
         women in medicine and the difficulties they have in securing
         hospital residencies.

4044.   "Women in Medicine." New Physician, 7:2 (February 1958)
              42-46, 82-83. photos. (Wyeth Roundtable.)
         Panelists, all women physicians and medical students, dis-
         cuss women physicians, their problems, abilities, and op-
         portunities. Participating in this roundtable discussion are
         Dr. Alma Morani, Dr. Elinor Glauser, Dr. Louise Gloeck-
         ner, Dr. Katharine Boucot, Dr. Betty Gorman, Dr. Marion
         Fay, and Hazel Broberg and Rita Welton (medical students
         at the Woman's Medical College of Pennsylvania).

4045.   "Women in Medicine in the United States." Medical Wo-
              man's Journal, 43:10 (October 1936) 279. (Editorial.)
         During 1936 in the United States, 1,133 women were study-
         ing medicine, 246 women graduated from medical school
         (33 from Woman's Medical College of Pennsylvania; 213 from
         coeducational institutions), and "more than 7,000" women
         physicians were practicing. A few figures concerning Cana-
         dian medical women are also given.

4046.   "Women Physicians." Outlook for Women in Occupations in
              the Medical Services. U.S. Department of Labor, Wo-
              men's Bureau, Bulletin 203:7 (1945) 1-28.
         The bulletin presents statistics and summaries on the pre-
         war situation of women physicians, changes occurring con-
         comitant with World War II, and the postwar outlook for
         women in medicine.

4047.   "Women Physicians in Texas." Woman's Medical Journal,
              18:9 (September 1908) 192-193. (Editorial.)
         "The woman physician in the South has had much more to
         overcome in the practice of medicine than her northern
         sister." The status of Texas medical women is reviewed.

4048.   "Women Physicians to Have Important Postwar Role." Med-
              ical Woman's Journal, 52:9 (September 1945) 45.
         The Women's Bureau of the U.S. Department of Labor re-
         ports that women physicians will have a larger part in fill-
         ing postwar medical needs [than they had in filling prewar
         medical needs]. "Only four out of 77 approved U.S. med-

ical schools refuse admission to women." It is expected that after the war, women physicians will expand their areas of practice into medical research and teaching.

4049. Yarrell, Zuleika. "Women in Medicine." Journal of Educational Sociology, 17:8 (April 1944) 492-497.
Dr. Yarrell (senior psychiatrist at Bellevue Hospital, New York City) makes a case for her belief that the position of women physicians in the postwar world will be secure and that the role need be no different from that of her male colleague. Specialties that will open up include psychiatry, rehabilitation, and public health.

4050. Young, R. "Your Daughter's Career if She Wants to be a Doctor." Good Housekeeping, 61 (August 1915) 168-174.
[Article not examined by editors.]

FICTION

References appear for literature which deals
with non-historical figures.

4051. Alsop, Gulielma F. <u>My Chinese Days</u>. Little, Brown,
and Company, Boston, Massachusetts, 1918, ix, 271
pp. photos.
Dr. Gulielma Alsop has woven a romantic novel around her
own experiences as a missionary doctor in Shanghai after
1911. The plight of Chinese women of this period is again
and again cause for reflection for Dr. Wilhelmina, the
novel's main character, who is herself in the throes of a
love affair. Her first medical case in Shanghai was a suicide who died with the help of her lover so she would not
have to go back to her hated Mandarin husband. "Love is
the great adventure," says the lover as the girl dies. And
more than 200 pages later, Edward slips a ring on Wilhelmina's finger as she recalls the same words, "Love is the
great adventure." In between there has been much reflection over whether Edward's feeling for her differs significantly from Chinese relationships she has observed: "When
a river man takes a river woman to wife, the only change
in the life of the woman is to step across from the boat of
her father to the boat of her husband." In a specific case,
she had found a mother and baby drowned after a dragon of
a mother-in-law had made it clear that the baby should
have been a boy: "Take the little dog out of my sight,"
she would say. Wilhelmina wonders about the relationship
between these extremes of prejudice and Edward's remark
that "a man must have his work ... a woman has love ...
and home and babies." She herself admits: "Work and independence, how passionately I had wanted them! And now
I was ready to cast them away for the touch of a man's
fingers." There is no resolution or speculation about the
effect of her romance and intended marriage on the future
course of her career.

4052.   Baudouin, Marcel.   ["Women Doctors in Drama and Novels"].
        Gazette Médicale de Paris, Series 12, 1:38 (21 Septem-
        ber 1901) 297-299. (Medicine and Literature.) (Fre)
        The article identifies highlights in the history of women doc-
        tors and healers in literature from their first appearance
        in Shakespeare's All's Well That Ends Well. The emphasis
        is on French literature beginning with the 1731 play, Woman
        Doctor or Theology on the Distaff Side, and proceeding
        through Besnard and Pompigny's Woman Doctor or the Se-
        cret Door (1806) to Koenig's Reversed World. Fourteen
        plays are cited, all equally as well known as those previ-
        ously mentioned. Florian Pharaon's Madame Maurel, Doc-
        tor, published in 1885, was the first French novel whose
        heroine was a woman doctor. Other novels discussed are
        Roger Dombre's Woman Doctor (1891), Philippe Louvet's
        Doctor Jeanne Lemoine (1891), and J. M. Rosny's The In-
        domitable (1895). Not all of these works present a positive
        picture of women physicians: Jeanne Lemoine murders the
        illegitimate child of her sailor lover before beginning her
        medical studies. Pierre Boyer's "Memoires of a Woman
        Doctor," which appeared in serial form in Temps, is the
        only work credited with literary merit. The author sug-
        gests that similar reviews of other national literatures
        would prove interesting.

4053.   [Gardner, Mabel] E. "Medicine on the Stage and the
        Films." Medical and Professional Woman's Journal,
        41:1 (January 1934) 31.
        In the theater and on the movie screen, women physicians
        are being presented "with a sympathetic touch." Also, the
        woman physician's "sex does not interfere with the execu-
        tion of her professional career, but is taken for granted
        with no apologies. While it is necessary, in order to make
        an appealing picture, to bring romance into the plot, the
        fine character of the woman who bears the part of the phy-
        sician is made paramount...."

4054.   Hall, Marjory. Quite Contrary: Dr. Mary Edwards Walker.
        Funk and Wagnalls, New York, New York, 1970.
        This book, designed for "grades seven to eleven," is a fic-
        tionalized story of the life of Dr. Mary Edwards Walker,
        Civil War physician who eventually received the Congression-
        al Medal of Honor for her work during the war: the Medal
        was revoked when the United States government changed its
        award criteria.

4055.   Hiestand-Moore, Eleanor M.; Moore, Rebecca; Grice, Julia;
        Fullerton, Anna M.; Slaughter, B. Rosalie; Walker,
        Gertrude A.; Hurd-Mead, Kate C.; Hatton, Julia Eliza-
        beth; Hewlings, Hester A.; and Seabrook, Alice M.
        Daughters of Aesculapius; Stories Written by Alumnae
        and Students of the Woman's Medical College of Pennsyl-
        vania. George W. Jacobs & Co., Philadelphia, Penn-

sylvania, 1897, 155 pp. photos.
The authors believe this collection to be "the first book of
stories by medical women." Rebecca Moore, class of 1883,
wrote on "The Domestic and Professional Life of Ann Preston." Kate (Hurd) Mead, class of 1888, recalls her travels
and foreign studies in an essay titled "Reminiscences of
Medical Study in Europe (1889-1890)." The remaining articles are presented as fiction, most of which have women
physicians or medical students as the central characters.
One story, by B. Rosalie Slaughter (class of 1897), is a
romance in which the female character chooses a medical
career over marriage. Other stories--like "The Home
Side" by Alice Seabrook, class of 1895--describe the affection and mutual respect which existed among women medical
students.

4056.   Howells, William D. Dr. Breen's Practice: A Novel.
                Houghton, Mifflin and Company, Boston, Massachusetts,
                1881, 272 pp.
            This 19th-century American novel is set in a New England
            summer resort where the heroine, Dr. Grace Breen, is
            vacationing before entering medical practice. She is intro-
            duced to the reader as having entered the medical profes-
            sion after an unfortunate love affair, as her counterpart
            in another time and place would have entered the convent.
            While caring for a woman friend undergoing marital prob-
            lems, she meets a wealthy young man whom she eventually
            marries. (She turns down a proposal from the local physi-
            cian in the course of the courtship.) The author leaves the
            reader and heroine alike with the dilemma of selecting an
            appropriate practice. Dr. Breen cares for the children of
            her husband's employees in the manner in which many ladies
            of her position devote themselves to charity. In the eyes
            of those who espouse the cause of women, she has sacri-
            ficed herself for marriage. In the words of Howells, "...
            the conditions under which she now exercises her skill cer-
            tainly amount to begging the whole question of woman's fit-
            ness for the career she had chosen."

4057.   Jex-Blake, Sophia. "Medical Women in Fiction." Nine-
                teenth Century, 33 (1893).
            [Article not examined by editors.]

4058.   Kenton, Edna. "The Pap We Have Been Fed On: VIII--
                'Lady Doctresses' of Nineteenth Century Fiction."
                Century Magazine, 44:3 (November 1916) 280-287.
            The author examines the mid-Victorian novel by Charles
            Reade entitled A Woman Hater, which has as its heroine the
            first woman doctress in English fiction. Next, Kenton turns
            her attention to Ruth Bolton, created by Mark Twain and
            Charles Dudley in The Gilded Age; Dr. Zay, an Elizabeth
            Stuart Phelps creation; and Dr. Breen by W. D. Howells.
            A discussion of Helen Brent, M.D., an anonymous work of

1892, and <u>Dr. Janet of Harley Street</u>, Arabella Kenea[?]y's 1890s work, concludes the article.

4059.   Lees, Hannah. <u>Women Will Be Doctors</u>.   Triangle Books,
          New York, New York, 1940, 271 pp.
        The protagonist of this novel becomes embroiled in roman-
        tic intrigue while working as an intern in a large city hos-
        pital.   Love affairs with two male doctors provide Dr.
        Amanda Paull with the conflict of finding fulfillment as a
        woman and as a physician.

4060.   Lin, Hazel.   <u>The Physicians: A Novel</u>.   The John Day
          Company, New York, New York, 1951, 250 pp.
        Wang Kung, a wealthy Peking physician, doted on his young
        daughter-in-law and wished for a grandson.   But his daughter-
        in-law died in childbirth, and in his grief, he was outraged
        to learn that the child was a female.   Naming her Hsiao-
        Chen, which means a particle of dust, he shunned her for
        five years before finally accepting her into the Wang family.
        Later, against much opposition, Hsiao-chen studied medicine
        in China and in the United States.   She distinguished herself
        in kidney research and credits the success of her program
        to a combination of her own skills in "Western" medicine
        and of her grandfather's teachings in Chinese medicine.

4061.   McElfresh, Adeline.   <u>Calling Doctor Jane</u>. Avalon Books,
          New York, New York, 1957, 224 pp.
        This novel opens with Dr. Jane Langford's decision to prac-
        tice medicine in Indiana instead of following her lover--the
        Reverend Bill Latham--to his missionary work in Africa.
        Doctor Jane's subsequent adventures as a rural practitioner
        include implication in a murder and a malpractice suit.   At
        the close of the novel, Doctor Jane joins her lover in Afri-
        ca, realizing that she "almost was an awful fool."

4062.   Phelps, Elizabeth Stuart.   <u>Doctor Zay</u>.   Houghton, Mifflin
          and Company, Boston, Massachusetts, 1882, 258 pp.
        This novel is written from the point of view of a young
        male, Waldo Yorke, who, on a visit to Maine, sustains in-
        juries in a buggy accident and finds himself in the care of
        a woman homeopathist, "Dr. Zay."   While initially shocked
        and apprehensive about possibly receiving inferior care,
        Yorke learns to trust Dr. Zay's "firm and fearless touch."
        As Yorke begins to fall in love with Dr. Zay, he is faced
        with a conflict about this "useful woman, who has not time
        to be admired, and perhaps less heart ... how was a man
        going to approach this new and confusing type of women?
        The old codes were all astray.   Were the old impulses
        ruled out too?"   When he accuses Dr. Zay of being cold
        and unnatural, she replies, "I do not doubt I have seemed
        unwomanlike to you in many other respects.   Your ideal
        and my fact are a world's width apart."   She adds: "I have
        had different things to do from thinking what would be pleas-

ing to men. My life is not like other women's...." "A
Vassar girl," Dr. Zay tells Yorke about studying medicine
at New York, Zurich, and Vienna, and how the need for
women to attend women in country towns led her to practice
in Maine's wilderness. Throughout the book, this character
is portrayed as courageous, pragmatic, honest, and skilled
in her profession. At the conclusion of the novel, she suc-
cumbs to Waldo Yorke's romantic ambitions for her.

4063.   Reade, Charles. A Woman Hater. The Aldine Publishing
             Company, Boston, Massachusetts, 1910, 533 pp. illus.
         Most of the women in this Victorian novel of manners and
         romance are frivolous creatures, overly involved with music
         and the "three Cs--croquet, crochet, and coquetry." An
         exception is Doctress Rhoda Gale, who loves "science as
         other women love men." She would be allowed to practice
         legally in France, but practices illegally in England. When
         financial difficulties arise, friends advise her to "give up
         medicine, and fall into some occupation in which there are
         many ladies already to keep you in countenance." But Doc-
         tress Gale asks them to "suppose you had loved a man you
         were proud of ... and then they came to you and said,
         'There are difficulties in the way ... you must give him
         up.'" At the close of the narrative, the author offers sev-
         eral pages in defense of greater opportunities for women,
         especially in the field of medicine, where women's "less
         theoretical, but cautious, teachable, observant kind of in-
         tellect" can be put to good use.

4064.   Rogers, (Major) E. A Modern Sphinx. John and Robert
             Maxwell, Publishers, London, [England], 1895, 314 pp.
             illus., photos., ports.
         Colonel Rogers bases this novel on the life, and events sur-
         rounding the life of Dr. James Barry, inspector general
         of hospitals for the British army. Dr. FitzJames, a char-
         acter in this novel, portrays James Barry, the British offi-
         cer who, upon death, was discovered to be a woman. In
         his introduction, the author discusses the discovery of Dr.
         Barry's true sex and quotes from correspondence regarding
         the matter, which appeared in the British medical journal
         Lancet in 1895. [This novel was originally published in
         three volumes in 1881--the present edition being a republica-
         tion in one volume by the author.]

4065.   Seifert, Elizabeth. Girl Intern. Triangle Books, New York,
             New York, 1944, 242 pp.
         The central character of this novel is Dr. Chris Metcalf,
         "girl intern" in a small town hospital. She was hired on
         the assumption that she was a male. The chief of staff is
         a handsome male of "virile charm" who was reputed to be
         both prejudiced against women and fearful of them. The in-
         tern moves through a succession of situations which test her
         ability as a physician and as a woman. She ultimately wins

the love of the chief of staff, who realizes his feelings for
her when he is emotionally incapable of performing an ap-
pendectomy on her. "'I don't care about being a doctor,'"
she tells him at the book's conclusion, "'I'm most glad
about being a girl--and that you're a man....'"

4066.   Truax, Rhoda. This Dynasty of Doctors. The Bobbs-Mer-
              rill Company, Indianapolis, Indiana, 1940, 397 pp.
         This book presents a fictional story of Marie Chestwick,
         her desire to become a doctor, her dream realized, and
         the experiences she had.

4067.   Wells, Helen. Doctor Betty. Messner, New York, New
              York, 1969, 190 pp. (Career-Romance Series.)
         This Career-Romance was written for grades six through
         nine. [Book not examined by editors.]

4068.   Whitten, Kathryn M. The Horses of the Sun. Meador Pub-
              lishing Company, Boston, Massachusetts, 1942, 314 pp.
         To a little girl being reared in a hard-working, Calvinistic
         farm family, the goal of becoming a successful surgeon can
         seem remote indeed. Although everyone Ellin Grayson
         knew seemed to believe that "deformed people, sick people,
         people who dropped dead had defied an angry God," Ellin's
         determination and common sense led her eventually to a
         medical career. Her sister Anne had encouraged her to
         persevere, insisting that with "great and unremitting effort"
         she would be able to break out of the family pattern of fe-
         male drudgery and low expectations. She proved to be
         right. [Although this book is a novel, Dr. Whitten was
         quoted in a book review as saying that "all incidents of the
         story fell within my own experience and observation."]

4069.   Woody, Regina J. The Young Medics. Julian Messner,
              New York, New York, 1968, 187 pp.
         Amanda Davis is a student nurse at an eastern U.S. hos-
         pital, but she yearns to take part in the thrill and excite-
         ment of differential diagnosis and decision making. The
         solution: she applied to medical school. The fictional
         metamorphosis of one young woman from nurse to pedia-
         trician is intended to inspire others to surmount all ob-
         stacles if they are serious about pursuing a career in medi-
         cine. Dedicated to "the girl who wants to be a doctor," the
         book quotes Marion Fay, president and dean of Woman's
         Medical College of Pennsylvania: "If you are serious about
         a medical ambition, you can succeed. You can open doors,
         you can find funds, you can study medicine--and practice
         it--for all your active life." One in a series of Career
         Romances for Young Moderns, the novel ends on a romantic
         note: "The next time she saw Seattle [where she planned
         to intern] she'd be a bride as well as Amanda David,
         M.D."

NONMEDICAL ACTIVITY

4070.   Cole, Carol Skinner. "Where Are You Going for Your
         Vacation?" Medical Woman's Journal, 38:7 (July 1931)
         174-177. photos.
         "Men doctors seem to be more proficient in the art of com-
         plete relaxation than women, because men do not accept
         responsibilities with a woman's fanatical zeal." Therefore,
         women physicians need relaxing vacations, and should bud-
         get time, money, and family demands in order to get away
         from the devitalizing routine of home, hospital, and office.
         In addition to recommending specific places at which to va-
         cation, the author suggests, "no woman doctor should carry
         her profession and title along on a vacation; it is excess
         baggage, and half the fun is 'getting out of character.'"

4071.   Eberly, Marion Stevens. "Rx for Financial Security."
         Journal of the American Medical Women's Association,
         5:1 (January 1950) 32-34.
         This article speaks to the question, "Can you advise me
         regarding retirement plans for women physicians?" Ways
         to build a reserve against the three hazards of interrupted
         income, premature death, and cessation of income are dis-
         cussed.

4072.   "English Medical Women up in Arms." Medical Woman's
         Journal, 34:3 (March 1927) 84-85.
         The Factories Bill before the House of Commons provides
         "protective" measures for women workers. Among the
         feminists who vocally oppose the bill are two women phy-
         sicians: Jane Walker and Christine Murrell.

4073.   "Financial Planning for the Woman Physician: Part I."
         The Woman Physician, 25:4 (April 1970) 244-249.
         This is the first in a series of three articles developed un-
         der the direction of Betty S. Martin, Director of the Wo-
         men's Division, Institute of Life Insurance, New York.

This series is a repeat of its initial appearance in the January, February, and March 1964 issues of Journal of the American Medical Women's Association. A few of the financial figures have been updated for this 1970 rerun. Part I offers a suggested approach to taking stock of one's financial situation and planning for the future which involves determining available assets; creating a "money plan" which will provide for emergencies, cover day-to-day spending, accumulate funds for some special project, and provide for building upon income for later years; seeking advice; and choosing the right plan. Two case examples of young physicians are used as illustration.

4074.   "Financial Planning for the Woman Physician: Part II. The Young Physician." The Woman Physician, 25:6 (June 1970) 386-389.
This second part of a three-part series on financial planning deals with the woman physician just entering her profession. Two case histories are offered as examples, one of a single intern, the second of a married woman in part-time group practice.

4075.   ["Financial Planning for the Woman Physician:] Retirement and Estate Planning." The Woman Physician, 25:7 (July 1970) 454-458.
This third and final part of a three-part series on financial planning for the woman physician is addressed to the established woman physician who is not married. A case illustration is given in which assets and financial planning are discussed.

4076.   Gardner, Mabel E. "Women Physicians Should Enter This Field." Medical Woman's Journal, 35:7 (July 1928) 204-205.
The "regular practitioner" should follow the example of osteopaths who are active in business and professional women's clubs. By associating with those who may be in "a sister field of endeavor," women physicians can "prevent ... industrious independent women from becoming one-sided in their ideas of medical treatment."

4077.   McGrew, Elizabeth A. "Tax Deductions." Journal of the American Medical Women's Association, 22:8 (August 1967) 585. (AMWA President's Message.)
Congress, heads of university departments, and husbands are insensitive to the energy and time-consuming household and homemaking tasks that are the responsibilities of all 18,000 women physicians and other career women. For these women, the lack of reliable and competent domestic help is the biggest problem. A cartoon on page 580 of the Journal is referred to which shows a woman doctor on her knees scrubbing a floor, a nurse saying, "Your first patient is here, Doctor," and captioned with the remark, "Anyone

care to start a college for domestic engineers whose graduates would be available exclusively to professional women?"

4078.   McGrew, Elizabeth A. "Taxes Which Punish Professional-
          ism." Journal of the American Medical Women's Asso-
          ciation, 22:7 (July 1967) 493. (AMWA President's
          Message.)
          Women physicians pay punitive taxes. Women physicians
          are proposing, through the Medical Women's International
          Congress and the American Medical Women's Association,
          that professional women ought to be able to deduct the ex-
          pense of household help and child care from their income
          taxes. Because of these expenses, it hardly pays the wo-
          man physician to work.

4079.   "'March Hares.'" Medical Woman's Journal, 49:3 (March
          1942) 93. (News Notes.)
          Not once in the 44 years since their graduation from the
          Woman's Medical College of Pennsylvania have Alla Grim,
          Florence Richards, Jeanette Sherman, and Mary Buchanan
          missed their annual get-together, where they celebrate their
          March birthdays. "Neither time nor disaster has changed
          the loyalty and devotion of the four of us for each other,"
          explains Dr. Sherman.

4080.   "Medical Women in Suffrage Parade at Washington." Wo-
          man's Medical Journal, 23:3 (March 1913) 63-65.
          Over 5000 women marched in a pageant procession on March
          3 in Washington. The parade's medical section, comprised
          of women physicians, dentists, and pharmacists was headed
          by a float on which stood a woman and a man--illustrating
          that men and women stand side by side in the medical pro-
          fession. Over 70 delegates from 14 states, many of them
          carrying banners, marched in this section. Dr. A. Frances
          Foye, who led the group, was mounted on a horse; she
          "rode most gracefully and made an admirable leader." Spe-
          cial banners honored pioneer medical women. Dr. Mary
          Getty headed a large delegation of alumni from the Woman's
          Medical College of Pennsylvania. The only other U.S. med-
          ical college for women, the New York Medical College and
          Hospital for Women, was represented by eight delegates.
          All the marchers and their affiliations are named.

4081.   "News Notes." Medical Woman's Journal, 51:7 (July 1944)
          36. photo.
          Dr. Rosalie Slaughter Morton presented to her birthplace--
          Lynchburg, Virginia--a ten-foot high statue. The group of
          three heroic white limestone female figures represent Vi-
          sion, Fortitude, and Kindliness. A photograph of Dr. Mor-
          ton's gift is included in this brief news item.

4082.   "Noted Sculptor Early Day Medical Student." Medical Wo-
          man's Journal, 51:7 (July 1944) 45.

The first woman to matriculate in a St. Louis medical school, Harriett Hosmer entered McDowell's Medical School in 1850. Her studies and interest in anatomy led her to sculpting, however, and she became a famous artist.

4083. "Resolution of Medical Women." Medical Woman's Journal, 48:3 (March 1941) 73.
Whereas the United States Constitution fails to grant to women the same protection against discrimination as it grants to men; whereas the Equal Rights Amendment to the Constitution is pending before the judiciary committee of the Senate and the House; and whereas two congressmen from Illinois are on that committee, it was resolved that the Medical Women's Club of Chicago, Inc. and the Chicago Council of Medical Women endorse the amendment and call upon the congressmen to expedite its passage.

4084. "San Francisco Woman Doctor Wins Short Story Prize." Medical Woman's Journal, 37:1 (January 1930) 15.
Chief of the psychiatric clinic of the University of California, Eva Charlotte Reid won a short story contest for writing the best social work short story, "Fighting Through," a tale of an orphan who is committed to an institution for the feeble-minded by officials of the orphanage who tired of her mischievousness.

4085. Saunders, A. M. "A National Home for Aged Women Physicians." Medical Woman's Journal, 33:6 (June 1926) 172-173.
An article published in the November, 1925 issue of the Illinois Medical Journal announces an endowment campaign to construct a national home for aged and incapacitated physicians who are left without financial resources. Following an abstract of that article, Dr. Saunders suggests that such an institution would be of particular interest to women physicians who "give a large proportion of their time, skill and knowledge without receiving any or adequate compensation." She asks that financial contributions be made, and invites suggestions.

4086. "Where Are Our Medical Women Leaders?" Medical Woman's Journal, 40:5 (May 1933) 114. (Editorial.)
Will the women of America meet the challenge of leadership expected of them since they have been elevated by the nineteenth amendment to the Constitution, from their pre-1919 political ranking on par with "children, idiots and criminals"? This editorial urges women to become active in public affairs.

4087. X. Y. Z. "B. M. A. Pension and Insurance Scheme." Medical Women's Federation News-Letter, (January 1934) 66-67. (Correspondence.)
X. Y. Z. writes that she is dissatisfied with the terms for

women practitioners in the British Medical Association's
(BMA) pension scheme. She points out the inequities and
relates a personal experience with an insurance company.

APPENDIX I

DIRECTORIES

A-1.   American Medical Association. Directory of Women Physi-
            cians in the U.S. 1973. American Medical Association,
            Chicago, Illinois, xl, 432 pp.
        This first edition is published as a supplement to the 1973
        American Medical Directory. It is a joint effort of the
        American Medical Association and the American Medical
        Women's Association. An introductory section of the Di-
        rectory comments statistically upon the increasing number
        of women physicians in the United States: as of 31 Decem-
        ber 1973, there were 30,568 women physicians in the U.S.
        and possessions (or 8.3 per cent of all physicians in this
        part of the world). A geographical section follows the al-
        phabetic name index and lists the women physicians by state
        and city. The following information appears for each phy-
        sician: address, year of birth, medical education informa-
        tion, year of license, primary specialty, secondary special-
        ty, type of practice, and American Board Specialty.

A-2.   "Directory of Women Physicians of California, Alabama,
            Arizona, Florida, Idaho, Georgia, Arkansas and Colo-
            rado." Woman's Medical Journal, 20:3 (March 1910)
            65-69.
        Names and addresses are given for the women physicians
        in these states. In addition, an indication is made of med-
        ical affiliations (i.e., regular, homeopathic, eclectic), state
        medical society membership, and American Medical Asso-
        ciation membership.

A-3.   "Directory of Women Physicians of California, Alabama,
            Arizona, Florida, Idaho, Georgia, Arkansas, and Colo-
            rado." Woman's Medical Journal, 20:6 (June 1910) 132-
            138.
        Names, addresses, state medical society and American
        Medical Association memberships and medical affiliations
        (i.e., regular, homeopathic, eclectic) are given for women
        physicians in these states.

A-4.   "Directory of Women Physicians of New England, Massa-
            chusetts, Connecticut, Maine, New Hampshire, Vermont

963

and Rhode Island." Woman's Medical Journal, 20:1
(January 1910) 20-23.
Names, addresses, state medical society and American
Medical Association memberships, and medical affiliations
(i.e., regular, homeopathic, eclectic) are given for women
physicians in these states.

A-5.   "Directory of Women Physicians of States of Iowa and New
York." Woman's Medical Journal, 19:9 (September
1909) 191-196.
Names, addresses, state medical society and American
Medical Association memberships, and medical affiliations
(i.e., regular, homeopathic, eclectic) are given for women
physicians in Iowa and New York.

A-6.   "Directory of Women Physicians of States of Pennsylvania,
New Jersey, Delaware and Iowa." Woman's Medical
Journal, 19:10 (October 1909) 215-220.
Names, addresses, state medical society and American
Medical Association memberships, and medical affiliations
(i.e., regular, homeopathic, eclectic) are given for women
physicians in these states.

A-7.   Fraternity of Alpha-Epsilon-Iota: Founded at University of
Michigan, 1890. McElroy Publishing Company, Chicago,
Illinois, [191?], 32 pp.
A list of members, addresses, and social notes comprise
this directory. [The organization is a "fraternity" of medical women. Directories were published periodically by the
Grand Chapter at the University of Michigan. Each directory includes also a list of the different chapters located at
various medical schools throughout the United States. Other
issues of this fraternity's directory have not been cited in
this bibliography.]

A-8.   Grigg, Bessie, comp. Directory of Medical Women: 1949.
Elizabeth Press, Newport, Kentucky, 1949, 303 pp.
The names of several thousand women physicians appear on
248 pages of this second Directory of Medical Women produced by the Medical Woman's Journal. The directory is
arranged alphabetically by states and cities in the United
States, with a section for territories, countries of South
and Latin America, and Canada. Each entry gives the woman's name, her medical school, date M.D. was received,
medical specialty, professional memberships, and address.
In addition to these 248 pages, there is a 52-page name
index.

A-9.   Grigg, Bessie, comp. Medical Woman's Directory: 1945.
The Elizabeth Press, Cincinnati, Ohio, 1944, 236 pp.
This first Directory of Medical Women of the United States
prepared by the Medical Woman's Journal contains the names
of several thousand women physicians in the United States.

The names are listed alphabetically by state and city. In
addition to the name, each physician's medical specialty,
professional membership, and address are given. An index
of names concludes the directory.

A-10.   U.S. Council of National Defense, General Medical Board,
         Committee of Medical Women, comps. Census of Wo-
         men Physicians: November 11, 1918. American Wo-
         men's Hospitals, New York, New York, [1918], 125 pp.
The initial pages of this census describe the American Women's Hospitals (AWH), giving the names on the executive
board of the War Service Committee as well as the names
of those women on the executive board of the AWH units of
the American Red Cross. A letter from Dr. Martha Tracy
entitled "A Campaign of Propaganda for Recruits to Medical
Colleges" also appears here. The census is arranged alphabetically by state. The women physicians' name, status
(retired or out-of-practice indications), medical school, date
of graduation, and present address are given. In addition
there are symbols to indicate membership in county medical
societies, the American Medical Association, American Institute of Homeopathy, Medical Women's National Association [which later became the American Medical Women's
Association], and an incomplete indication of whether or not
the woman is registered with the Council of National Defense or the AWH. The names of several thousand women
physicians are listed.

APPENDIX II

COLLECTIONS

Selected Collections Holding Materials Relating to
Medical Women's Organizations and Women Physicians

THE SOPHIA SMITH COLLECTION.   Women's History Archives.
Smith College, Northampton, Massachusetts.
Material on the New England Hospital (ca. 1820-1955), established in 1862 in Boston, and the first hospital in New
England both to train women physicians, and to provide
medical care for women by women: hospital records, annual reports, meeting minutes, correspondence, and biographical information on women associated with the hospital;
includes correspondence from well-known contemporaries in
the medical, literary, and political worlds.   Collection also
contains personal papers of several individual women physicians, most notably Dorothy M. Reed Mendenhall (1874-
1964), and Florence Rena Sabin (1871-1953).

DEPARTMENT OF MANUSCRIPTS AND UNIVERSITY ARCHIVES.
Cornell University Libraries, Ithaca, New York.
American Medical Women's Association material (1895-
1970).   The Association, founded in 1915, has as members
women physicians and women medical students: annual reports, minutes, correspondence, printed matter, and miscellaneous records are included.   Also, the Women's Medical Society of New York State records (1907-1966).

ARTHUR AND ELIZABETH SCHLESINGER LIBRARY ON THE HIS-
TORY OF WOMEN IN AMERICA.   Radcliffe College, Cambridge,
Massachusetts.
Located in this collection are papers of several women doc-
tors including Elizabeth Blackwell (1821-1910), Martha May
Eliot (b. 1891), Mary Putnam Jacobi (1842-1906), Ida
Sophia Scudder (1870-1960), and Alice Hamilton (1869-1970).
Collection also contains numerous books about women phy-
sicians.

ELIZABETH BASS COLLECTION.   Rudolph Matas Medical Library.
Tulane University, New Orleans, Louisiana.

Personal collection of Elizabeth Bass, M.D. (1876-1956). 1200 items. Articles, letters, photographs, memoranda, memorabilia.

WOMEN IN MEDICINE COLLECTION. Florence A. Moore Library of Medicine. Medical College of Pennsylvania, Philadelphia, Pennsylvania.

Comprehensive repository for published and unpublished material about women physicians (ca. 1850-). Includes the Kate Hurd Mead and American Medical Women's Association Collections. 300 monographs. 3500 photographs. Papers of several medical women's associations. Numerous personal collections of women physicians, including Martha Tracy (1876-1942), Ellen Culver Potter (1871-1958), Emiline Horton Cleveland (1829-1878), and Catharine Macfarlane (1877-1969). 19th century M.D. theses. Archives of the College (formerly Woman's Medical College of Pennsylvania).

At this writing a comprehensive directory of collections pertaining to women is being prepared by the Social Welfare and History Archives Center of the Universities Libraries, University of Minnesota. Tentatively titled Women's History Sources: A Guide to Archives and Manuscript Collections in the U.S. and scheduled for publication in 1978, this work will report dozens of collections of individual women physicians, and should provide a useful resource for accessing the lesser-known collections such as the Dr. and Mrs. Edwin Elliott Calverley collection in the Archives of the Hartford Seminary Foundation, Connecticut, which contains papers of Eleanor Jane (Taylor) Calverley, M.D.; and the Dr. Mary Walker collection in the George Arents Research Library for Special Collections at Syracuse University, New York.

AUTHOR INDEX

AAMC see Association of
American Medical Colleges
Abbott, Maude E. 8, 307,
353a, 3862
Abramowitz, Christine V.
2949
Abramowitz, Stephen I. 2949
Ackerman, Emma M. 127
Acres, E. Louis 493
Adam, H. B. 2880
Adamson, Rhoda H. B. 260,
494, 2694
Aggebo, Anker 415
Aguirre de Gonzales, Amelia
1944
Ahlem, Judith 3951
Aigner, Reinhold 416
"Aiken Heart, M.D." 2950
Aird, L. A. 1915
Aitken, Janet K. 128, 495,
2688, 2911, 3238
Albert, Edouard 2881
Aldrich-Blake, L. B. 3911
Alexander, Ida M. 749
Alexander, Leslie L. 750
Alexander, W. S. 2128
Alexeyev, Y. A. 2267
Allee, Ann Silver 753
Allen, Belle Jane 2510
Allen, Maud 2594
Alpert, H. 2951
Alpha Kappa Alpha Sorority,
Inc. 756
Alsing, I. 2176
Alsop, Gulielma Fell 757,
758, 3389, 4051
Alvarez, Pola Pelaez de 1945
Alvarez Ricart, Maria Del
Carmen 18, 2858
Amat, Ana 2948
American Medical Women's
Association 1852, 2722,

3952
Amira, Stephen 2949
Anderson, Elizabeth Garrett
see Garrett-Anderson, Eliza-
beth
Anderson, Kathryn D. 3072
Anderson, Louisa Garrett 496
Anderson, M. Camilla 760
Anderson, Olive M. 497
Andreae, Horst 418
Andreen, Andrea 419, 420
Andrews, Mabel L. V. 498
Andriole, Vincent T. 761
Angela, Sister M. 2511
Angwin, Maria L. 129
Anneler, H. 1912
Anthony, Catherine W. 2416,
2954
Antipenko, E. S. 2266
Apgar, Virginia 2417
Appelbaum, Ann Halsell 2955
Apter, Julia T. 2418
Arak, Gladys 2441
Arie, Tom 2047
Arnold, Anna W. 2956
Arnold, Charles B. 2490
Arnold, Jeannie Oliver 772
Arons, Elissa 2460
Arthurs, Ann Catherine 773
Ashby, T. A. 3954
Association of American Med-
ical Colleges 1946
Atkinson, Dorothy Wells 1739,
3955
Austin, Grace Baliunas 2958
Austin, Margaret 130

Back, Marjorie 261
Bacon, (Dr.) 1774
Bader, Christine 2380
Badley, Mrs. M. A. 3329

Bain, Katherine 2496
Bainbridge, Lucy Seaman 775
Baker, A. H. 500
Baker, P. De L. 3405
Baker, Rachel 777, 778
Baker, Sara Josephine 776, 779, 2090, 2728, 3956
Baker-Hyde, Harriet 988
Baker-McLaglan, Eleanor Southey 288
Baksh, Ilahi 2596
Balfour, Andrew 2389
Balfour, Frances 501
Balfour, Margaret I. 309, 2116, 2253, 3241, 3827, 3927
Ball, Elizabeth B. 780
Ballintine, Eveline P. 2280
Balsam, Alan 2420
Balsam, Rosemary Marshall 2420
Banas, Felicia A. 3406
Bancroft, Jessie Hubbell 781
Bancroft, Mabel H. F. 2682
Barbosa y Sabater, Antonio 2859
Barclay, E. R. 503
Barclay, William R. 2959
Barker-Ellsworth, Alice 784
Barkman, E. 722
Barlow-Brown, Alice 2682
Barrett, (Lady) Florence E. Willey 504, 621, 3349, 3828
Barrie, Susan 289
Barringer, Emily Dunning 210, 211, 785, 2281, 2728-2737, 2785, 3600, 3957
Barsness, Nellie N. 786, 787
Bartholow, Roberts 788
Bartley, Eileen 421, 505
Barton, Ethel M. 612
Basden, Margaret M. 597
Bass, Elizabeth 131, 692-694, 789-804, 2717, 2961, 3408, 3594
Bastman, A. E. 2154
Bates, Mary Elizabeth 805, 3409
Batt, Roberta 2962
Battersby, Cameron 2129
Battino, Barbara 806
Baudouin, Marcel 19-22, 132, 4052
Baudouin de Courtenay, Romualda 1887
Bauer, Franz K. 3410
Bauknecht, Ruth 2178
Baum, O. Eugene 2421
Baumann, Frieda 807-809
Baumer, Gertrud 1904
Baumgartner, Leona 3928, 3952
Bayon, H. P. 23
Bazanov, V. A. 197, 376
Beals, Rose F. 3829
Beamis-Hood, Louise 3411
Bean, E. S. 9
Beaton-Mamak, Mary 10
Beattie, Lillian M. 309
Beatty, Geneva 811
Beatty, J. 812
Beatty, William K. 167
Beaugrand, A. 133-135
Beauperthuy de Benedetti, Rosario 195
Beck, Sr. M. Bonaventure 2658
Becker, Jane 1991
Becker, W. 79
Becker-Manheimer, Olga 2381
Beckh, H. 24
Beiswenger, Immanuel 80
Bejnarowicz, Janusz 1889
Belicza, Biserka 13
Belitskaia, E. La. 198, 199
Bell, Ellen Cary 3964
Bell, Enid Hester Chataway Moberly 109
Bell, (Sir) Gordon 297
Benedek, Elissa P. 2422, 2423
Benedict, Sister M. 2512, 2513
Benetar, Judith 814
Bennett, A. H. 2193
Bennett, Alice G. 2963, 3412
Bennett, Granville A. 1366
Bennett, Jane E. 815
Bennett, Laura B. 2964
Bennett, Ruth Blount 816
Benson, Annette M. 506
Beregoff-Gillow, Pauline 310, 704, 705
Berger, E. 81
Berman, Ellen 2424, 2425

Bermudez, Laura Contreras de
2948
Bernard, Marcelle T.   507,
706, 817-834
Berry, F. May Dickinson   504,
508, 2194
Berwig, Elsie   3874
Beshiri, Patricia H.   3958
Beske, Fritz   2179
Best, Katharine   838
Bett, W. R.   311
Beveridge, W. H.   1916
Bewley, Beulah R.   2195
Bewley, Thomas H.   2195
Beyer, M. Virginia   1948, 2080
Bhatia, S.   3330
Bickel, Beatrix A.   2945
Bieder, Martha   1912
Biermer, Leopold   477
Billig, Anton Hermann   82
Binder, Sidonie   2882
Birch, Carol L.   2282
Birdsall, Helen Brant   902
Bishoff, Theodor L. W. von
2883
Bisiarina, V. P.   723
Bittner, Christina   841
Black, Dora   2196
Blackledge, Joan   509
Blackman, Julia Cole   3959
Blackwell, Alice Stone   842,
1263
Blackwell, Anna   843
Blackwell, Elizabeth   844,
1949, 2912, 2965, 3413
Blackwell, Emily   1949, 2965
Blain, Daniel   2426
Blain, M.   845
Blair, Mary A.   510, 597
Blake, John B.   212, 846
Bland, Bessie Farinholt   847
Blechmann, Jane   2382
Blewett, Evelyn   3414
Bliss, Barbara E.   2427
Bloch, Harry   213
Block, Jean Libman   848, 849
Blodgett, F. M.   1794
Blount, Anna Ellsworth   3415-
3417
Bluemel, Elinor   850
Bluestone, Naomi   2428, 2966
Bluhm, Agnes   1894, 2884
Blumenthal, Annemarie   83

Blythe, Legette   1705
Bochalli, R.   136
Bodley, Rachel L.   851, 2284,
2967
Boedeker, Elisabeth   478
Boerner, F.   2885
Böhmert, Victor   1895, 3221
Bolton, Elizabeth   511, 512
Bolton, H. Carrington   137
Bone, Honor   607
Bono, Silvia Maria   3875
Bonsignorio, (Mlle.)   3876
Booth, Alice   852
Borden, Isabella F.   3418,
3419
Borrino, Angiola   2156, 2383
Bothma, J. H.   513
Boucot, Katharine R.   1950
Bourdeau, Patience see Bour-
deau-Sisco, Patience S.
Bourdeau-Sisco, Patience S.
853, 3421
Bourke, Geoffrey J.   2168
Bouzarth, William F.   2429
Bowditch, Henry Ingersoll
1896, 3422
Bowen, Earl A.   1951
Bowers, John Z.   1952, 3929,
3930, 3952
Bowling, W. K.   2968
Brackett, Elizabeth R.   854
Braid, Frances   576
Branson, Helen Kitchen   855,
856
Branson, Laura H.   3960
Brant, Cornelia Chase   3717
Breakell, Mary L.   3913
Breeze, Gabrielle   2505
Brekke, Viola   4013
Brindley, Clare Evalyn   2430
Brittain, Vera   3243
Brodie, Jessie Laird   707-709,
858-860, 1866, 2118, 3350,
3379, 3380, 3425, 3426,
3961
Brody, Irwin A.   861
Brohl, Ilse   84
Brooks, Benjy F.   862
Brooks, Louie M.   3244
Broome, Claire V.   2969
Brown, Adelaide   863
Brown, Caree Rozen   2431
Brown, E.   3331

Brown, Edith M.   2597, 2598, 2844
Brown, Edith Petrie   3962
Brown, Elizabeth B.   864
Brown, Gwendolen   591
Brown, Harrison J.   865
Brown, John   3245
Brown, Mary   2540
Brown, Sara W.   866
Brown, William Symington   2970
Brunner, Lois   867
Brunton, Lauder   138
Brupbacher, Fritz   2886
Brussel, James A.   868
Bryant, Ruby F.   869
Bryant, W. S.   870
Bryn Mawr College   3964
Bryson, Louise Fiske   871
Bucar, F.   377
Buchanan, J. Robert   2971
Buchheim, Liselotte   85, 2887
Buck, Carol   2144
Buck, Ruth Matheson   312, 313
Buckley, Olive B.   2514
Bui-dang-ha-doan, J.   2157
Bundy, Elizabeth R.   1953
Bunker, John P.   3103, 3427
Bunting, Joelle   3006
Burger, Elisabeth   86
Burgess, Alan   514
Burkett, Gary L.   2057
Burnet, Anne   3963
Burns, Margaret V.   1267
Burr, Elizabeth see Thel-
  berg, Elizabeth Burr
Burstyn, Joan N.   110
Burt, Charles   2913
Burt, O. W.   872
Burton, Katherine   515
Bushnell, Katharine C.   873
Butavand, Arlette   2646
Butler, A. S. G.   874
Butler, Miriam   875
Butlin, Henry T.   2390
Buxton, R. St. J.   1917
Buzek, Joanna   2050
Byers   2391
Byford, William Heath   2973

Cabot, Hugh   3022
Cabot, Richard C.   2432

Calderone, Mary S.   877
Caldwell, Ruth   25-27, 139, 2974
Call, Emma L.   244
Calverley, Eleanor T.   878
Cambel, Perihan   3830
Campbell, Elizabeth   3965
Campbell, Grace   1787
Campbell, Janet M.   516, 517, 2392, 2690, 2691, 2708, 3600
Campbell, Margaret A. [aka Mary Howell]   1955
Campbell-Mackie, Mary   518, 519
Campion, Nardi Reeder   879, 880
Canals, Dolores   422
Carew, Evangeline   3429
Carling, Esther   512
Carpenter, Elizabeth   2975
Carpenter, William Benjamin   3246
Carpuppino-Ferrari, (Dr.)   3877
Carr, J. Walter   2515, 2599
Carrier, Henriette   3222
Carroll, Barbara Anne   3494
Carter, Charlene A.   2433
Carter, Mary   2197
Carter, R. Adelaide   521
Cartwright, Lillian Kaufman   2976, 2977
Cary, Helen A.   885
Caspari-Rosen, Beate   1636
Cass, Victoria   886
Casson, Elizabeth   522
Center for Women in Medicine (Medical College of Pennsyl-
  vania)   3966, 3967
Chadburn, Maud M.   524, 3247
Chadwick, James R.   140, 3431
Chambers, Helen   3223, 3248
Chambers, Peggy   888
Chapa, Esther   3351
Chapman, John E.   1956
Chapman, Rose Woodallen   889
Chappell, Amey   2979, 3968
Charlton, Ethel   890
Chase, Lillian A.   315, 3208
Chaudhuri, S.   3332, 3862
Chenoweth, Alice Drew   3969

Chêreau, A. 28
Chesney, J. P. 2980
Chesser, Elizabeth Sloan 525
Chikin, S. Y. 2267
Child, Richard Washburn 3866
Chiles, John A. 2981
Chisholm, Catherine 512, 526, 3249
Chizea, Dora Obi 3964
Chojna, J. W. 14
Chow, Rosalie see Han, Suyin
Christian Medical Service in India, Burma and Ceylon 2517
Christie, A. F. Mary 527
Christine, Barbara 3962
Clapp, Mary P. 3152
Clark, Ida Clyde 528
Clark, Margaret Vaupel 2982
Clarke, Ann D. 2141
Clarke, Edward H. 2983
Clarke, G. G. 1880
Clarke, Miriam F. 2984
Cleaves, Margaret A. 895, 3433
Cleveland, Emeline Horton 2985, 2986
Clower, Virginia Lawson 2434
Cloyes, S. A. 897
Coates, Reynell 2987
Cobb, Sidney 1910
Cobb, W. Montague 898, 899
Cockram, E. Joyce 111
Coghill, Violet A. P. 529
Cohen, Carol J. 2988
Cohen, Frances 2785
Cohen, Lysbeth 290, 3204
Cohn, Hermann 3224
Coker, Robert E. 2452
Cole, Carol Skinner 4070
Cole, Helen Grady 2435
Collins, A. Dorothy 2198
Collins, Forrest 3122
Colver, Alice Ross 902
Comandini, Adele 903
Committee of Medical Women of the General Medical Board of the U.S. Council of National Defense see U.S. Council of National Defense
Comstock, Elizabeth 905, 906
Condict, Alice B. 2600

Conrad, Agnes 3435
Constable, Judith A. 2130
Conta, (Mme.) 3867
Contreras de Bermudez, Laura see Bermudez, Laura Contreras de
Copple, Peggy J. 2436, 3436
Corbet, G. G. 3863
Corcoran, Paul J. 2437
Cordell, Eugene F. 141
Corea, Gena 913
Cormier, Hyacinthe M. 530
Cornell, William M. 2991, 3970
Corson, Hiram 3438
Coryllos, Elizabeth 2438
Coste, Chris 2992
Cote, Marie M. 914, 2518
Coues, William Pearce 29
Coulter, Molly P. 2052
Council of National Defense see U.S. Council of National Defense
Coury, C. 30
Coutard, Vera L. 915
Coveny, Mary A. 2439
Cox, Alfred 598
Cox, Narcissa see Vanderlip, Mrs. Frank A.
Cox, Pearl Bliss 916-920
Craig, Alan G. 2993
Craighill, Margaret D. 3971
Crane, J. H. 3439
Crawford, Margaret D. 2393
Crawford, Mary Merritt 921, 2785, 3440, 3656
Crawford, Raymond 3250
Crawford, Susan A. 1959
Creutz, Rudolf 31, 87
Crocker, Geraldine H. 922
Crosse, V. Mary 3914
Crovitz, Elaine 1978
Crowley, Anne E. 1959, 1960
Cruishank, Marion 3441
Cullis, Winifred C. 597
Cullum, Iris M. 2406
Cummings, Emma J. 2601, 2602
Cunningham, Gladys Story 2541
Curcio, Mary R. 923
Curran, A. P. 2199

Currie, Muriel G.   317, 318
Curtis, Annie N.   924
Curtis, Arthur C.   3442
Cushier, Elizabeth M.   925,
   926, 3491
Cushman, Beulah   2994
Cushman, Mary Floyd   2506
Cuthbert, Sister M.   142, 2507
Cybulski, Napoleon   2850
Czajecka, Boguslawa   378

Dale, James G.   928
Daley, Dorothy E.   319
Dall, Caroline Healey   265,
   929
Dally, Ann   533
Daly, Flora M.   2394
Damour, Felix   32
D'Ancona, Silvia   3878
Danforth, I. A.   930
Dangotte, C.   423
Daniel, Annie Sturges   214,
   931-935, 2995, 3443-3486
Daniels, Robert S.   2268
Darcanne-Mouroux   33, 3879,
   3880
Davidson, Gisela K.   938
Davidson, Lynne R.   2996
Davis, Loda Mae   939
Davis, Paul J.   940
Davis, Paulina Wright   2997
Davis, Willa F.   3695
Dawson, Elizabeth   3861
Dawson, Kathleen A.   536
Day, Emerson   2071
Deal, Louise B.   2782
Dean, Jennie A.   2682
Dean-Throckmorton, Jeannette
   3488
de Azevedo, Nair   424
De Bermudez, Laura Contreras
   see Bermudez, Laura Con-
   treras de
de Blainville   2686
De Garis, Mary C.   291
Delgado de Solís Quiroga,
   Margarita   3942
Dempsey, Lillian E.   945
Dengel, Anna   2604, 2605,
   2647, 2648, 2659, 2660
Denko, Joanne D.   2998
Department of Health for Scot-

land, Ministry of Health,
   Inter-Departmental Commit-
   tee on Medical Schools see
   Ministry of Health, Depart-
   ment of Health for Scotland,
   Inter-Departmental Commit-
   tee on Medical Schools (Good-
   enough Report)
De Procel, Matilda Hidalgo
   see Hidalgo de Procel,
   Matilda
Deschamps, (Mlle.)   2860
De Solís, Margarita Delgado
   see Delgado de Solís Quiroga
   Margarita
Dethan, G.   2861
Dettelbacher, Werner   379, 479
DeVore, Louise   2743
Dickerman, Marion   946
Diggs, Marguerita C.   3964
Dionesov, S. M.   200, 380,
   724, 3225
Dissosway, Carolyn F.-R.   948
Dixon, C. W.   2131
Dixon, Dorothy   509
Dixon, Mary J. see Scarlett-
   Dixon, Mary J.
Dobbie, Mina L.   538
Dobrski, Konrad   381
Dobrzycki, Henryk   2851
Dodds, Gideon S.   2354h
Dodge, Eva F.   3972
Doherty, Winifred J.   555
Dohrn, R.   2384
Dole, Mary Phylinda   1068
Dollar, Jean M.   556
Dominik, M.   384
Dolley, Sarah Read Adamson
   2999, 3000
Donahue, Julia   1069
Donegan, Jane Bauer   216
Dopson, Laurence   112
Dorpat, Klarese   1073
Dorveaux, P.   3881
Douglas, G. W.   287
Douglass, M. Ellen   325
Dowkonitt, Mrs. George D.
   2522
Downes, Helen R.   2285, 2316
Doyle, Helen MacKnight   1074
Drew, Nellie L.   1075
Drinkwater, H.   143
Drooz, Irma Gross   1076

Drouillard, Louisa C.   217
Drysdale, C. R.   1918, 2915
Dubé, Waltraut F.   1962, 1963,
    1964, 1965, 1966, 1967,
    1968, 1969, 1970, 1971,
    2023, 2024
Dubin, Nathan I.   326
Dublin, Louis I.   3001
Ducker, Dalia Golan   2440
Duff, Jane   3494
Dufferin, (Countess of)   3333
Dufner, Mary Elizabeth   3495
Dunn, Fannie see Quain,
    Fannie Dunn
Dunnahoo, Terry   1077
Dunnett, Agnes   557
Dunning, Emily see Bar-
    ringer, Emily Dunning
Durie, Ethel   303
Dutton, William S.   1078
Dyer, Florence M.   1336
Dyer, Helen M.   1079
Dykman, Roscoe A.   1972,
    2286

Earle, Charles Warrington
    3496, 3497, 3498
East, Marion Reed   1080
Eberly, Marion Stevens   4071
Eckman, F. M.   3002
Eddy, Mary Pierson   1082,
    2523, 2524
Edmunds, J.   2202
Edward, Mary Lee   1083
Edwards, Linden F.   1084,
    1085
Edwards, Muriel   1086
Edwards, Phyllis M.   3189
Edwards, Sally   2203
Egan, Lenora Horton   1087
Egan, Richard L.   1959
Ehlers, Kathryn H.   3964
Ehrenreich, Barbara   144,
    3003
Eilberg, Ralph G.   3006
Eisenberg, Leon   2287
Elia, Joseph J.   1091
Eliot, Martha M.   1836
Elkin, Edward M.   2288
Elliot, H. B.   1105
Elliott, Mabel Evelyn   1106,
    3502

Elliott, Patricia M.   2216,
    2220
Elliott, Susan J.   3004
Ellis, Ruth M.   3005, 3503
Ellison, Solon A.   3006
Ellsworth, Adelaide   2718
Elmes, Margaret   2916
Ely, Allen   3007
Emanuel, Vera   262
Engbring, Gertrude M.   89
Engleman, Edgar G.   3008
English, Deirdre   144
Ernest, Elvenor   3932
Ernst, Alice L.   2525
Esch, Margaret   3882, 3883
Eskin, Frada   2048, 2205
Essex, Nina   2203, 2206
Essex-Lopresti, Michael   2207
Esterly, Nancy B.   2441
Eulenburg, Albert   1897
Evans, Barbara   565
Everitt, Ella B.   2290

Fabricant, Noah D.   1121
Fahimi, Miriam   270
Fairbanks, Virgil F.   1122
Fairfield, Letitia   582, 598,
    2395, 2693, 2694
Fancourt, Mary St. J.   566
Farkhadi, R. R.   726
Farrer, Ellen M.   567
Fawcett, Millicent Garrett   2917
Fay, Marion   568, 1853, 1854,
    2071, 2649, 3509, 3510, 3511,
    3952, 3973, 3974
Fearn, Anne Walter   1124
Fehling, Hermann   2180
Feilchenfeld, Wilhelm   2888
Feldman, Judith   2460
Feldman-Summers, Shirley
    3010
Felker, Gertrude   988
Female Medical Education So-
    ciety (Boston)   3513
Fenninger, Leonard D.   2054,
    3952
Fenten, D. X.   1855
Fenwick, Dorothy   2695
Fenwick, E. D.   2686
Fernandez-Fox, Eva   2055
Ferrer-Franco, Isabel   3191
Ferrier, (Miss)   2650

Fett, M. Ione 2132, 2133, 2134
Fichna, Margarete 34
Fickert, Auguste K. 1898, 1899
Field, G. W. 90
Field, Mark G. 2269
Fielde, Adele M. 2543
Fiessinger, C. 2862
Figueredo, Anita V. 1127
Filar, Zbigniew 385
Finkler, Rita S. 3514, 3943
Fischer, Golda 273, 2119, 3833
Fischer, J. 35
Fischer-Hofmann, Hedwig 2385
Fischer-Pap, Lucia 3015
Fish, D. G. 1880, 1884, 1886
Fishbein, Morris 2292, 3016, 3975
Fisher-DeFoy, Werner 91
Fisk, Dorothy 569
Fitter, Clara 570
Flatow, E. 36
Fleming, Alice 1134
Fleming, Ruth 3517
Flemming, Roberta M. 274
Fletcher, Grace Nies 1135
Fletcher, Walter 2919
Flexner, Abraham 1976
Florence, Loree 3976
Floyd, Olive 1139
Flynn, Ann C. 2211
Fog, E. 2686
Fohlmeister, Gisela 3494
Folsom, Charles F. 3091
Fontanges, Haryett 3933
Forbes, Lorna 1540-1544, 3679, 3680, 4009
Forbes, Shirley J. 3518
Forkl, Martha 3885
Forrer-Gutknecht, E. 1912
Forster, Emily L. B. 1921
Foulks, Sara E. 1141
Fowler, R. N. 3259
Fox, Christie 1142
Fox, David J. 3145, 3146
Fox, Ida E. 2212
Fraade, Estelle 3519
Frågan, Till 3886
Francis, Sister M. 2609
Frank, Hal 3170

Frank, Julia Bess 92
Frank, Mary 3524
Franke, Meta E. 2265
Frankfeldt, Gwen 3520
Franklin, C. L. 1977
Franz, Nellie Alden 113
Fraser, Margaret E. V. 2684
Frazer, Mary Margaret 3521
Frederic, Sister M. 2610, 2611
Freedman, Alfred M. 2063, 2064
Freitas Pereira, Maria Joana de 3887
Freminville, Bernard de 3869
French, Francesca 3336
French, John R. P., Jr. 1910
Fried, Frederick E. 2056
Friedenwald, H. 37
Frolund, A. 2176
Frost, Lorraine 3522, 3523, 3524
Fruen, Mary A. 1881
Frye, Maud J. 1144, 3017, 3018
Fullerton, Anna Martha 3019, 4055
Furey, Nancy 2441
Furman, Bess 218
Furtos, Norma C. 2749
Fussell, Edwin 3020, 3021

Gabrielson, Ira W. 2057
Gael, A. 2864
Gaffikin, Prudence E. 572
Gaffin, Ben 2294
Gage, Asa Franklin 1145
Gage, Simon Henry 1145
Gaillard, E. S. 3525
Galbraith, Maurice J. 2282
Gambrell, W. Elizabeth 1146
Gantt, L. Rosa 3584
Garcia Arroyo, Maria Luisa 2948
Gardiner, Mary S. 3964
Gardiner, Mildred White 2090
Gardner, Emily 1147, 1148
Gardner, Frances 2211
Gardner, Mabel E. 1149, 1150, 1460, 1550, 2058, 2090, 2295, 2296, 2413, 2442, 2920, 3022, 4053, 4076
Gardner, Penney 1151

Garis, Mary De see De
    Garis, Mary C.
Garrett-Anderson, Elizabeth
    114
Garrison, Penelope 3072
Gassett, Helen Maria 3526
Gates, Irene 1152
Gautsch, H. 2908
Gauvain, Suzette 1924
Gavrilovic, Vera S. 388, 388a,
    389
Gay, Claudine Moss 1153
Geib, M. Eugenia 1154
General Council of Medical
    Education and Registration
    (Great Britain) 1922
General Medical Board of the
    U.S. Council of National De-
    fense see U.S. Council of
    National Defense
Georgi, Audrey Adele 716
German, William J. 1155
Gerrish, Frederic H. 1336
Gevorkov, A. A. 726
Ghrist, Jennie 145
Gibbons, James 3091
Gibbons, Marion N. 3527
Gibson, Julia R. 1157
Gill, P. F. 2041
Gillett, Josephine D. 3528
Gillett, Richenda 574
Gillette, Harriet E. 2443
Gillie, Annis 583, 1158,
    2213
Gillie, K. Annis 575
Gillmore, Emma Wheat 2750-
    2754, 3023, 3695
Gilmore, Hugh R. 329
Gilmore, Marguerite 3962
Gingras, Rosaire 2163
Ginsberg, Michele 2441
Ginzberg, Eli 3952
Giraud-Teulon 2865
Glasgow, Maude 146, 147,
    1159, 1160, 2671, 2696,
    3024, 3695
Glenn, Georgiana 3026
Glick, Ruth 2297
Glinsky, B. B. 2379
Gloeckner, M. Louise C.
    3977
Gnauck-Kühne, Elisabeth 2889
Godden, J. O. 2044

Godfrey, C. M. 11
Goldowsky, Seebert J. 1161
Goldstein, Marion Zucker 3027
Gomes, Beverly 2949
Gomez, Trinidad 3835
Goodbody, Norah C. 576
Goodcell, Roscoe 1162
Goodell, William 38
Goodenough Report see Min-
    istry of Health, Department
    of Health for Scotland, Inter-
    Departmental Committee on
    Medical Schools (Goodenough
    Report)
Goodwin, Occa Elaine 1163
Gordon, Burgess 3978, 3979
Gordon, Charles Alexander 39
Gordon, Doris Jolly 295, 296
Gordon, Elizabeth Putnam 1164
Gordon, J. Elise 40
Gorinevskaya, Valentina 2672
Gosswiller, Richard 1165
Gough, Harrison G. 2444
Gourfein-Welt, L. 1912
Goz, R. 2445
Grace, Sister M. 2526
Gracey, Mrs. J. T. 2254,
    2527
Grad, Marjorie A. 1168
Graetz-Menzel, Charlotte 2890
Graffis, Herb 3028
Graham, Davis W. 3029
Grainger, R. M. 1882
Grangée, F. M. 41
Gray, Etta 3695
Gray, Jessie 330, 3864
Gray, Sarah 3263
Great Britain. General Council
    of Medical Education and
    Registration see General
    Council of Medical Education
    and Registration (Great
    Britain)
Green, Marthalyn Johnson 3030
Green, Pearl 577
Greenbie, Marjorie Barstow
    2755
Greenslade, N. F. 2135
Gregory, George 3031
Gregory, Samuel 3032, 3033,
    3034
Gregory Society of Boston 2059
Greisheimer, Esther M. 3533

Grice, Julia 4055
Gridley, Marion 1170
Griffith, G. de Gorrequer
2651
Griffiths, Sheila M. 2931
Grigg, Tony 3534, 3535
Grigoréva, N. N. 2673
Griscom, Mary W. 1171, 1172,
3192, 3536, 3537
Griswold, Bernice 3538
Groff, Margaret T. 2298
Gross, Wendy 1978
Grove, Jessica 650
Grundy, Betty L. 1856
Guardia, J. M. 42
Guest, Edna M. 331, 353a,
2669
Guion, Connie M. 219, 3656
Gulesen, Ozdemir 1924
Gundersen, Herdis 3888
Guthrie, Sylvia K. 578

Haar, Esther 3035
Hacker, Carlotta 12, 333
Haffner, V. B. 1174
Haines, Frances E. 2756
Hale, Sarah J. 3540
Halitsky, Victor 3035
Hall, Alice K. 1175
Hall, Marian B. 3193
Hall, Marjory 4054
Hall, Rosetta Sherwood 2528,
2529
Hall, Wesley W. 3982
Hall, Winifred S. 2396
Hamilton, A. 1176
Hamilton, Alice 1177
Hamilton, Edith Hulbert 3541
Hamilton, George L. 43
Han, Suyin (aka Rosalie Chow)
363-365
Hanaford, Phebe A. 1178
Handley-Read, Eva 580
Hannak, Emanuel 2891
Hannett, Frances 1979
Hano, Helene 1180
Hansen, O. S. 1181
Hanson, Helen B. 2674,
2675, 2697, 3265
Harding, B. 2686
Harding, Frances Keller 148,
2299

Harlem, O. K. 434
Harper, Anita Wilson 1182
Harper, Mary McKibbin see
McKibbin-Harper, Mary
Harrell, George T. 3952
Harris, Harry 390
Hartshorne, Henry 3036
Hartt, Rollin Lynde 220
Harvard University Medical
Alumni Association 3542
Harvard University Medical
School 3543
Harvey, Ellwood 3037
Harvey, Ruth A. Johnstone
334, 335
Haskins, Grace 2698
Hatton, Julia Elizabeth 4055
Hawkins, Lucy Rodgers 1186
Haycock, Christine E. 2446,
3983
Hay-Cooper, L. 1187
Hayes, A. J. 435
Hays, Elinor Rice 1188
Hazzard, Florance Woolsey
1189-1191
Hedvall, Gunnel 44
Heggie, Barbara 1192
Heimrath, Susan L. 2490
Heinz, Margaret S. 3545
Heischkel, Edith 93
Heise, Agnete 45, 436
Helfand, Toby 3962
Hellinger, Marilyn Levitt 2431
Hellstedt, Leone McGregor
3889
Helz, Mary K. 1980, 1981
Hemenway, Ruth V. 1194,
1641, 2544-2579
Henderson-Smathers, Irma 221,
1195-1220
Hendricks, Anne M. 1221
Hendrickson, Robert M. 2300
Henius, Dr. von 2892
Henry, Frederick P. 3038
Henry, Lydia M. 2397
Hercus, [Sir] Charles 297
Herring, Christina 2421
Herzenstein, G. M. 1888
Herzfeld, Gertrude 517, 581
Heslop, Barbara F. 2136
Heusler-Edenhvizen, Hermine
480
Hewitt, Dorothy 3547

Hewlings, Hester A. 4055
Hick, Ford K. 1366
Hidalgo de Procel, Matilda 2948
Hiestand-Moore, Eleanor M. 4055
Hilberman, Elaine 1982
Hill, Emma Linton 1225
Hill, Lister 3984
Hillis, William C. 1959
Hillman, Sara Frazer 3548
Hillyer, Katharine 838
Hinche, Charles L. 1800
Hind, E. Cora 338
Hintze, Anne Augusta 3985
Hirsch, Max 2893
Hjort, G. 1900
Hobson, Sarah M. 1226
Hocker, Elizabeth Van Cortlandt 2758, 3549
Höfstatter, Robert 1901
Hogarth, Margaret 582
Hoggan, Frances Elizabeth 2120
Hole, Judith 3039
Holland, R. 2137
Holland, Thomas 3266
Hollingshead, Frances 1227
Hollingsworth, Dorothy R. 3006
Holloway, Lisabeth M. 223
Holmberg, Anton 2165, 2166
Holmes, Merrilee Illsley 3964
Holmes-Siedle, Monica 2214
Holmstrom, Marta 2167
Holsti 2866
Holt, Mary C. 2206
Holton, Susan Chapin 3040
Hood, Louise Beamis see Beamis-Hood, Louise
Hoover, Nancy 1234
Horan, Margaret B. 298
Horwitz, L. 94
Hoskins, Mrs. Robert 1235
Hosmer, William 3041
Houghton, Dorothy D. 3550
Houston-Patterson, Anne 1237
Hovorka, Ostar 46
Howard, Meta 2530
Howell, Mary C. 1983, 1984
Howell, Sarah E. 2441
Howells, William D. 4056

Howes, Joyce 1884, 1885
Howqua, June L. 2042
Hubert, Marjorie B. 583
Hübsch, M. 438
Hudson, Phoebe 3042
Hughes, Muriel Joy 149
Hume, Edward H. 2652
Hume, Ruth Fox 697
Humpal-Zeman, Josephine 439
Humphrey, Tryphena 1690
Hunt, Harriot Kezia 1238
Hunt, Sharon 3494
Hunter, Gertrude T. 1239
Hunter, Rosemary 1982
Hunter, William Wilson 3337
Huppert, M. P. 15
Hurd, Annah 1240
Hurd-Mead, Kate Campbell 47-49, 150-154, 224, 440-442, 512, 584, 727, 2531, 3043, 3227, 3551, 3552, 3890, 3986-3988, 4055
Hurdon, Elizabeth 2215
Hurley, A. 3044
Hurrell, M. Louise 3553, 3554
Hutchins, Edwin B. 1985, 1987
Hutchison, Robert 2921
Huth, Edward J. 3989
Hutton, Isabel Emslie 585, 686, 1241, 2694
Hutton, Jack G. 2023, 2024

Imperi, Lillian 4013
Ingals, Ephraim Fletcher 3045
Ingelfinger, Franz J. 3046
Ingengo, A. P. 3047
Ingersoll, Louise M. 1267
Inglis, Elsie M. 3267
Innes, Elizabeth 686
Inouye, Tomo 3194
Inter-Departmental Committee on Medical Schools, Department of Health for Scotland, Ministry of Health see Ministry of Health, Department of Health for Scotland, Inter-Departmental Committee on Medical Schools (Goodenough Report)
Irwin, Inez Haynes 225, 226
Isambert, Emilie 2867
Isoda, Senzaburo 3195

Ivens-Knowles, Mary H.
    Frances 587, 2699, 2922,
    3918a

Jack, Bridget 2203
Jacobi, A. 3049
Jacobi, Abraham 1263
Jacobi, Mary Putnam 227,
    1270, 1271, 2304, 2995,
    3050-3053, 3091, 3558
Jacobs, Aletta Henrietta 445
Jacobson, Beverly 228
Jacobson, Wendy 228
Jadassohn, Werner 446
Jäderholm, Axel 1940
Jakoby, Ruth Kerr 2447
James, Selwyn 3990
Jameson, Florence I. 1550
Jancovicova, J. 2852
Janisch, Ruth N. 589, 590
Janosik, J. 2853
Jantsch, Marlene 51
Jarecky, Roy K. 1986
Jasicka, Janina 378
Jasinska, W. 391
Jaworski, Józef 392, 393
Jeffery, Mary Pauline 1275-
    1278
Jefferys, Margot 1924, 2216
Jeffries, L. M. Blackett 591
Jelliffe, S. E. 447
Jenison, Nancy 2785
Jennings, Dana C. 1280
Jerger, B. 1281
Jervis, J. Johnstone 592
Jex-Blake, Sophia 115-117,
    678, 1925, 3228, 3919,
    4057
Jhirad, J. 3, 2121
Johnson, Davis G. 1968-1970,
    1986-1988
Johnson, Edith E. 1283
Johnson, Evelyn 1284
Johnson, Lyndon B. 3952
Johnson, Sophie E. 2613,
    2614
Johnston, Helen 1285
Johnston, Malcolm Sanders
    1286
Johnston, Pauline 3559
Johnstone, Rutherford T.
    1287

Joiner, Jane Herrod 3054
Jolly, Doris see Gordon,
    Doris Jolly
Jolly, H. Paul 2305
Jones, D. E. 1288
Jones, Grace G. 1289
Jones, Harriet B. 3991
Jones, Jane Gaudette 3055
Jones, Louise Taylor see
    Taylor-Jones, Louise
Jones, Mrs. Edward see
    Taylor-Jones, Louise
Jones, R. O. 340
Jones, Sarah Van Hoosen 1550
Jones, Vera Heinly 2448
Jordan, Elizabeth 1694
Josephi, Marion G. 2761, 2762,
    2763, 2764
Jougla, G. 52
Journal of the American Med-
    ical Association, "Education
    Number" see Crowley,
    Anne E.
Joyce, Margaret 587, 593
Joyce, Nessa M. 2168, 2170
Judson, Eliza E. 1291
Jussim, Judith 2306

Kahan, J. 2217
Kahler, Elizabeth S. 2307
Kaiser 95
Kalopothakes, Mary 448
Kaltreider, Nancy B. 1294
Kalyan, Valentina see Gorinev-
    skaya, Valentina
Kandravy, Anna M. 3563
Kanof, Naomi M. 2449, 3564
Kaplan, Harold I. 1989, 1990,
    2062-2064, 3992
Kaplan, Helen Singer 2063-
    2065
Karnaukhova, E. I. 201
Kashade, R. 481
Kass, Joan S. 2014
Katona, Ibolya 395
Katscher, Leopold 367
Katzeff, Miriam 1301
Kaufman, Martin 229
Kavinoky, Nadine R. 2450
Kawai, Yaeko 3837
Kazmierczak, Mary J. 3565
Kearney, Elizabeth F. 2451

Keefer, Dorothy Campbell   230
Keegan, B.   231
Keenan, Margaret   3494
Keene, Mrs. Charles M.   3566
Kehrer, Barbara H.   2308,
  2309
Kelly, Gertrude B.   1263
Kelly, Howard Atwood   1302
Kelynack, Violet   3920
Kempe, G.   929
Kempler, K.   16
Kennedy, Agnes   495
Kennedy, Melanie   2310
Kenton, Edna   4058
Kenyon, Dorothy   2765, 2766
Kerr, Charlotte Herman   1857,
  3962
Kerr, Laura   1303
Kettle, M. H.   2218
Keyes, Joseph A.   1991
Keyes, Muriel   3921
Keyes, Regina Flood   2682
Keyserling, Mary Dublin   3056
Kidd, Mary   595
Kiesler, Sara B.   3010
Kilham, Eleanor B.   2683
Killain, Maud   2580
Kimball, Grace N.   1304
King, Caroline R.   1305
King, Gordon   276
King, John W.   1305
King-Salmon, Frances W.
  1306
Kinney, Dita H.   1307
Kirby, Percival R.   596
Kirchhoff, Arthur   2868
Kirkpatrick, Martha J.   2311
Kirschner, Barbara S.   2441
Kitchin, Kathleen F.   53
Kittredge, Elizabeth   988,
  1308-1311, 2581, 3567
Kleiner, Charlotte A.   1312
Kleinert, Margaret Noyes
  3568
Klempman, Sarah   2112, 3826
Klenerman, Pauline   263,
  2113
Klinefelter, Lee M.   1858
Klodzinaki, S.   396
Knabe, Lotte   96
Knapp, Sally Elizabeth   699,
  1313
Knauber, Connie   1314

Knauf, John   1315
Kneen, B. D.   1316
Knight, Charlotte   1317
Knill-Jones, R. P.   2398, 2414
Knopf, S. Adolphus   3057, 3058
Knowles, Frances Ivens   2694
Kobayashi, Aya   277
Koelsch, F.   1318
Koeneke, Irene A.   2080
Koenig-Warthausen, G. von   97
Koffmahn, Elisabeth   3885
Köhnecke, Ingeborg   482
Konanc, Judy   1982
Korchilava, D. S. H.   728
Korman, Belle   1320
Korobkin, Rowena Lichtenstein
  3964
Kosa, John   2452
Koscialkowska, Wila   397
Kraetke-Rumpf, Emmy   98
Kral, J. J.   2312
Krasne, B.   1321
Kress, Daniel Hartman   1322
Kress, Lauretta Eby   1322
Kritskii, E. I.   2270, 2271
Kronfeld, M.   2869
Kroslakova, E.   2854
Krug, Else see Weyman, Else
  Krug
Krüger, Gisela   483
Kubankova, V.   2152
Kubie, Lawrence S.   1323
Kugler, Anna S.   2615, 2616,
  3338
Kühn, Wilhelm   3891
Kuhnke, Laverne   1
Kull-Schaffner, R.   54
Kunn, Carl   1902
Kusta, Charlotte E.   1324

Ladova, Rosalia M.   203, 204
Laird, Jessie see Brodie,
  Jessie Laird
Lake, Alice   3060
Lakeman, Mary R.   2313,
  3569-3571
Lambson, Roger O.   1992
Lamont, Margaret   2617
Lamotte, S.   2686
Landau, Richard   155
Landry, L. Thuillier   449
Lange, Helene   484, 1903, 1904

Lansdown, Frances S. 2029
Lanzoni, Phoebe Krey 3061
Lara, Maria Julia de 717
La Roe, Else K. 485
Larsell, O. 1325
Larson, Thomas A. 2305
Larsson, Elisabeth 3993
Lassar, O. 2894
Last, John M. 2240
Latham, Vida A. 156, 1326, 2663
Lathrop, Julia 398
Lathrop, Ruth Webster 2314
Lathrop, Virginia T. 1327
Lattin, Cora Billings 2182
Lauer, Hans H. 486
Laurie, Jean 3922
Lawney, Josephine C. 3196
Lawrie, Jean Eileen 2219, 2220, 2399, 2911
Lax, Ruth F. 2454
Lazar, Szini C. 399
Lazarewitch, Radmilla 17
Leaman, William G. 3572
Ledgerwood, Hilary 598
Lees, Hannah 4059
LeMarquis, Antoinette 1328
Lenden, E. 157
Leney, Lydia 599
Lentz, J. 1329
Lerner, Raymond C. 2490
Lesky, Erna 55
Lesnikova, R. V. 2676
L'Esperance, Elise S. 1333, 2071, 3574-3577
Levi, Joseph 3146
Levine, Adeline Gordon 3062, 3063
Levine, Ellen 3039
Lewin, Octavia 600
Lewis, Faye Cashatt 1335
Lewis, Harriet M. 1336
Lewis, Margaret C. 2315
Lewis, Nancy R. 601
Lewis, Robert E. 368
Leymaster, Glen R. 1959, 1993, 1994, 3952
Lichtenstein, Julia V. 3578, 3579
Lide, Frances 450
Ligertwood, Laura M. 2923
Lightbody, Georgia Meaus 1338
Lin, Chiao-chih 369
Lin, Hazel 4060
Linde, Harry W. 1995
Lindemann, Lillian C. 1339
Lindsay-Wynekoop, Alice Lois see Wynekoop, Alice Lois Lindsay
Link, Eugene P. 1340, 1341
Lion-Meitner, Gisela 1905
Lipinska, Melanie 56, 57, 158, 1342
Lister, John 2221-2223
Little, Ernest Gordon Graham 1926
Little, Marjory 300
Liu, Felicia 3064
Livezey, Abraham 3065
Lloyd, Hilda 118
Lloyd-Green, Lorna 3838
Lobdeli, Effie L. 2768
Lobdell, Mary 3066
Lobo, F. B. 718
Logie, Iona Robertson 1344
Lollini, Clelia 3892
LoMonaco, Carmine J. 2958
Longshore, Joseph S. 3067, 3580, 3994
Loomis, Metta M. 160, 3581
Lopresti, Michael Essex see Essex-Lopresti, Michael
Lorber, Judith 3068
Lopate, Carol 3995
Love, Minnie C. 232
Lovejoy, Esther Pohl 161, 988, 1346-1348, 1460, 2677, 2700, 2719, 3229, 3355-3360, 3582-3600, 3839
Lowell, Josephine 3091
Lowenstein, Leah M. 2068, 2069
Lowther, Florance deL. 2285, 2316
Loyola, Sister M. 162
Lucas, Chris 1349, 1350
Lueth, Carl Anthony 3069
Luhn, Antke 3230
Lull, George F. 2769
Lunn, John E. 2224
Lutzker, Edythe 119, 602-606
Lyman, George H. 3070
Lyman, T. 3602

Lynch, Frank W. 1352
Lynn, Ethel 1353
Lyons, Dorothy J. 1354

McCall, Eva 2933
McCloskey, Bertram P. 287
McCombs, A. Parks 2455
MacCorquodale, Donald W.
  2122
McCrea, Eppie S. 3604
McDade, Dorothy 2376
MacDermot, H. E. 342
MacDonald, Carolyn Nicholas
  1358
MacDonald, Eva Mader 2146
MacDonald, J. Ramsay 607
McElfresh, Adeline 4061
McEwan, Lena E. 2138
Macfarlane, Catharine 1359-
  1363, 1996, 3605, 3609
Macfaul, M. 2217
McFerran, Ann 1364
McGeachy, Jessie A. 343
McGee, Anita Newcombe 2770
M'George, Mary 2620
McGill, M. Isabel 2400
McGraw, Harriet G. 1365
McGrew, Elizabeth A. 1366,
  1997, 1998, 3071, 3610,
  3611, 3962, 3996, 3997,
  4077, 4078
McGuinness, Madge C. L.
  1367, 3612, 3613
McIlroy, A. Louise 608, 621,
  2685
McIntyre, A. D. 2225
MacKay, Jean Sinclair 344
Mackenzie, Joan 2226
MacKenzie, K. A. 345
Mackenzie, Marion E. 2401
MacKenzie, [Lady] Muir 57,
  3205
MacKenzie, Ridley 609
McKibbin-Harper, Mary 120,
  163, 233, 451, 701, 988,
  1368-1373, 3341, 3614-
  3616, 3840, 3893-3895,
  3998
McKusick, Marjorie J. K.
  3072
McLaren, Alice J. 610
McLaren, Barbara 611

McLaren, Eva Shaw 612, 3272
MacLaren, Gertrude D. 613
McLaughlin, Kathleen 2771
McLean, Brita 4013
McLean, Mary H. 370, 2653
Macleod, J. W. 1883-1885
Macleod, Jessie McGeachy see
  McGeachy, Jessie A.
MacMurchy, Helen 164, 347,
  353a, 614, 2255, 3934
McNamara, Mary 2050
Macnicol, Mary 615
MacNutt, Sarah J. 234, 1374,
  3617
MacRobert, Rachel N. 2678
Macy, John W., Jr. 3952
Macy, Mary Sutton 165, 166,
  1375, 2045, 2256, 2317,
  2318, 2772, 3541, 3618
Madarasz, Erzsebet 400
Maffett, Minnie L. 2071
Magier, Nina G. 3619
Magilnitskii, S. G. 729
Maher, Irene E. 1999, 2773
Maher, Margaret M. 2958
Maisel, Albert Q. 1377
Malampus 1451
Malisoff, Vera 3620
Malleson, Hope 616
Mandelbaum, Dorothy Rosenthal
  3073
Manley, D. C. E. 2131
Mann, Helen 1380
Mann, Kristine 2072, 3695
Manning-Spoerl, Jacolyn Van
  Vliet 3621
Manroe, Barbara 3494
Manson, Cecil 301
Manson, Celia 301
Manton, Ann P. D. 1381
Manton, Jo 617
Mara, Joy R. 3622
Marble, Ella M. S. 1382,
  2320, 3623
Marion, John Francis 3624
Markó, Miklós 401
Marks, Geoffrey 167
Marmor, Judd 3074, 3952
Marr, Judith 3075
Marshall, Clara 235, 1398,
  3625
Marshall, Margaret 3076
Marshall, R. R. 1399

Martin, Elisabeth 1401, 1402
Martin, Pete 262
Martindale, Louisa 512, 597,
    619-621, 1403, 2257, 2702,
    3361, 3923
Marting, Esther C. 1404,
    3627
Martland, E. Marjorie 622
Mason, Henry R. 1959
Mason-Hogle, Kate A. 4001
Mason-Hohl, Elizabeth 58,
    236, 237, 1420-1425, 2321,
    2775-2777, 3381, 3628-
    3634
Matlin, Margaret W. 2322
Matthews, Margie R. 3635
Mattson, Dale E. 1986
Mausner, Judith S. 2346,
    3147
Maxwell, J. L. 3342
Maynard, Edith L. 2402
Mead, Kate Campbell Hurd
    see Hurd-Mead, Kate Camp-
    bell
Mead, Margaret 3167
Means, James H. 3974
Mears, Mary 623
Medical College of Pennsyl-
    vania 1860
Medical Women's International
    Association 1449, 2686,
    3364
Mefford, Roy B., Jr. 3122
Melampus 1451
Melville, Mildred McClellan
    1452
Memant, (Mlle.) 279
Menendian, Rose V. 1459,
    1460
Menninger, Karl 3078
Mermod, Camille 1461, 1462,
    2326, 3962
Merritt, Doris H. 3079
Merritt, Emma L. 1463
Mesnard, Elise Marie 1464
Meyer, Blanche M. 2456
Meyer-Plath, Maria 478
Michel, Auguste Marie 454
Middleton, William S. 3080
Miles, May S. 1465
Milic, Louis T. 3081
Miller, Deborah W. 1466,
    3645

Miller, Florence Fenwick 624
Miller, George 2071
Miller, Helen Markley 1467
Miller, Janet 1468
Miller, Janet Goucher 1469
Miller, Marilyn 2441
Miller, Neal 1470
Millican, Edith F. 2532
Ministry of Health, Department
    of Health for Scotland, Inter-
    Departmental Committee on
    Medical Schools (Goodenough
    Report) 1933
Minney, Doris 1471
Minor, T. C. 171
Miracle, Marian 625
Mirek, Roman 2855
Miskowiec, O. L. 1473
Mitchell, Elsie Reed 2782
Moenckeberg, A. 487
Moffatt, Agnes K. 2147
Moir, D. D. 2398
Mole, Joyce B. 626
Moll, Albert 2186
Molloy, Robyn J. 2136
Monk, Mary A. 2359
Montanier, Henri 2871
Montreuil-Straus, G. 455,
    2169, 3365
Moon, George R. 2282
Moore, Rebecca 4055
Morani, Alma Dea 1474-1476,
    3366
Morantz, Regina Markell 239,
    3082
More, V. 240
Moreno, Ldo. Bonifacio Ramir-
    ez 2872
Morgan, Beverly C. 2006
Morgan, Elma Sandford 5
Morgan, Marcia Ruth 3083
Morris, James Polk 1482
Morrison, Ann 1483
Morrow, Laura E. 3084,
    3842
Morse, Marion S. 3646
Morton, Barbara G. 627
Morton, Jane 1935
Morton, Rosalie Slaughter
    1484, 1485, 2457, 2458,
    2783-2785, 3843, 3945,
    4055
Morton, Mrs. Richard F. 3085

Mosher, Clelia Duel 1486,
  1487
Mosher, Eliza M. 241, 1488-
  1502, 2786-2788, 3491,
  3647-3650
Moss, Margaret Steel 1503
Mott, Lucretia 4002
Moulten, Barbara 3952
Mouroux see Darcanne-
  Mouroux
Moxon, W. 3289
Moyer, Elizabeth 3651
Mugan, Monica 2670
Mühl, Anita M. 1505
Muller, Charlotte 2306
Müller, P. 2895
Munson, Arley 2622
Münster, Ladislao 59, 60
Murav'eva, E. F. 3871
Murdoch, Virginia C. 2584
Murphy, Claudia Q. 3086
Murphy, Thomas 2170
Murray, Flora 2231, 2705
Murray, Florence Jessie 351
Murrell, Christine M. 2927,
  3290

Nadelson, Carol C. 2007,
  2459, 2460, 3087, 3088,
  3090
Nagatoya, Yoji 280
Naish, A. E. 2933
Nanson, E. M. 1879
Nauck, E. th. 99
Naudé, Anneke te Water 2112,
  2114
Nekrasova, E. 202
Nelson, Bonnie C. 1970, 1971,
  2008
Nelson, Selwyn 2043
Nelson-Jones, Richard 1886
Nemeth, Magdalene C. 2461
Nemir, Rosa Lee 1510, 1865,
  1866, 3654-3656, 3935,
  3962, 4003
Nesterenko, A. I. 730
Neumann, Isidor 2873
Newhouse, Muriel L. 2219,
  2220
Newman, Barbara J. 2414
Newman, Meta R. Pennock
  3660

Nichols, Mary Sargent Neal
  Gove 1531
Nichols, R. Bond 352
Nicholson, J. Fraser 2148
Niles, Mary W. 2585, 2586
Nilsson, Ada 456
Nilsson, Carl-Axel 2171, 2172
Nilsson, Hjordis 3898
Noall, Claire 1533
Noble, Iris 1535
Noble, Mary Riggs 3666
Noble, Nellie S. 1534, 2790
Norberg, Karen E. 3089
Norris, Frances S. 3667
Norris, W. 2404
Notman, Malkah T. 2007,
  2460, 3088, 3090
Nuysink-Steinbuch, D. C. 2261

Oblensky, Florence E. 1539
O'Conner, Katheryn 1540-1544,
  3679, 3680, 4009, 4013
Odier-Dollfus 3899
Offenbach, Bertha 1545
Office of Student Records,
  AAMC see Association of
  American Medical Col-
  leges
Ohara, Kazue 3844
O'Hara, Margaret 2623
Okunkova-Goldinger, Z. 203,
  204
Oliphant, Beverly A. 1549
Olson, Avis M. 1550
O'Neill, Frederick William
  Scott 637
Orchard, Ethel 638
Oreman, Jennie G. 2331
Orr, Ellen B. 512
Ortiz, Flora Ida 3092
Osborn, Stellanova 1554
Oski, Frank A. 2342
Osler, William 3091
Ostler, Fred J. 1555
Ostrowska, Antonina 1889
Owens, Joan Llewelyn 1851
Owens-Adair, Bethenia Angelina
  1561, 1562

Packard, Francis R. 242
Pailthorpe, Mary E. 2624

Pak, Rhoda Kim 3847
Palmieri, Vincenzo Mario 2874
Paluszny, Maria 2462
Pam, Millicent 639
Pantin, Amy 640
Paolone, Clementina J. 1563
Papara, Dora 62
Parbrook, G. D. 2404
Parish, Rebecca 3197
Parke, Davis & Company 2332
Parker, E. 3095
Parker, W. W. 3096
Parkhurst, Genevieve 1564
Parks, John 3952
Parmelee, Ruth A. 1565,
    2728, 2737
Parmelle, Rexford D. 2336
Parrish, John B. 2272
Parrish, Rebecca 1566
Parry, K. M. 2225
Parsons, Florence M. 641
Parsons, John L. 1567
Paterson, Susanne J. 2077
Patterson, Norma W. 3098
Pattison, Jean H. 2684
Paulin, L. Estelle 2233
Pavluchkova, A. V. 197
Payne, Jessica Lozier 3717
Payne, Sylvia M. 642
Pearce, Louise 3683
Peck, Phoebe 3684
Pecker, A. 30
Pelaez de Alvarez, Pola see
    Alvarez, Pola Pelaez de
Pelzel, Jane Barksdale 1571
Pennell, Alice M. Sorabji
    3848
Pennell, Maryland Y. 2333,
    2334, 2338
Penzoldt, Franz 2896, 2897
Peo, Evalene E. 172
Péraud, J. M. 2115
Percival, Eleanor 173
Pereira-d'Oliveira, E. 3901
Perera, George A. 3952
Perez-Reyes, Maria 1982
Perrin, Edwin N. 1573
Petersen, Edward S. 1959
Petersen, Julius 3902
Peterson, Frederick 3099
Peterson, Robert A. 3100
Petrén, Gustaf 63
Petrov, B. D. 2273, 2274

Petteys, Anna C. 1575
Phelan, Mary Kay 1576
Phelps, Charles E. 4012
Phelps, Elizabeth Stuart 4062
Phifer, Mary H. 1577
Philbrick, Inez C. 3101
Phillips, Bessie 1578
Phillips, Dennis H. 1579
Phillips, Josephine Dirion 1580
Piccone, Louisa 4013
Pickard, Ellen 643, 3297
Pickett, Elizabeth P. 1584
Picot, L. J. 3102
Pierce, Clara M. 2080
Piercy, Harry D. 1585
Pierrel, Rosemary 1867
Pincock, Carolyn S. 1586,
    1587, 2347, 3686
Pirami, Edmea 65, 457, 2173
Pitts, Ferris N., Jr. 2993
Platt, Kate 3849
Platt, Lois Irene 1594, 2335
Platz, Carol 4013
Platzer, Elisabeth 488
Plechl, Pia Maria 1595
Plum, Gunnar 2175
Pocock, Dorothy 644
Podgórska, Klawe Zofia 404
Poglubko, K. A. 405
Pohl, Esther see Lovejoy,
    Esther Pohl
Polcino, Sister M. Regis 2665
Poli, U. 3903
Polk-Peters, Ethel 1596
Pondrom, Cyrena N. 2009
Ponetaeva, N. E. 207
Pool, Judith G. 3103, 3427
Pope, C. Augusta 244
Pope, Emily F. 244
Popova, A. P. 732
Porter, Sarah K. 281
Porth, Edna 1597
Potter, Ada 66
Potter, Ellen C. 1598, 1868,
    3104, 3105, 3754
Potter, Marion Craig 174, 1800
Pouzin, Yvonne 2174
Powell, Janet Travell 1599
Powell, Virginia 3974
Power, Eileen 175
Powers, Lee 2336, 3952
Poynter, Lida 1600
Poznanski, Elva 2462

President's Study Group on
   Careers for Women 3952
Preston, Ann 3107-3112,
   4014
Preston, Frances I. 304
Price, Mary C. 458
Pringle, Julia 660
Prior, Mary A. 1606
Procel, Matilda Hidalgo de
   see Hidalgo de Procel,
   Matilda
Pruett, Patricia Onderdonk
   3964
Pryor, Helen B. 1608
Przerwa, Tetmajer A. 407
Puckett, Pearl 1610
Pulido, (Dr.) 2875, 2876
Pullum, Carla A. 4015
Purdy, Ann 1611
Purnell, Caroline M. 3231,
   3690
Putnam, James Jackson 3691
Putnam, Ruth 1612

Qua, Julia Kimball 3672
Quain, Fannie Dunn 1613
Quentin, E. 100
Quiroga, Margarita Delgado de
   Solís see Delgado de Solís
   Quiroga, Margarita

Rabinowitsch, Lydia 4016
Racster, Olga 650
Radcliff, Sue 2785
Radford, Muriel 651
Rae, Isobel 652
Rall, Jutta 101
Ramey, Estelle 3113
Ramirez, Ldo. Bonifacio see
   Moreno, Ldo. Bonifacio
   Ramirez
Ramsay, Mabel L. 467, 2694,
   2922, 3300, 3301
Rankin, Hattie Love 2587
Rath, F. 2187, 2188
Ratterman, Helena T. 1363
Ratzan, R. Judith 2029
Ratzer, Maria A. 2241
Raulin, Louis 67
Ravell, Marion 3206
Raven, Clara 1550, 2794, 4013

Rayne, Mrs. M. L. 4017
Rea, Marion Hague 1614
Reade, Charles 4063
Reardon, Rosalie M. 2078,
   2079, 2625
Redaksie, Van Die 2843
Reddy, D. V. S. 176
Redman, Helen C. 1615
Reed, Marjorie E. 1616
Rees, Florence M. 1617
Reeve, Arthur B. 177
Reeve, J. C. 246
Reeves, Hila 3114
Regnault, Paule 460
Reid, Ada Chree 247, 1618,
   1619, 2797, 3152, 3359,
   3360, 3369, 3519, 3694
Reimerdes, Ernst Edgar 102
Rennie, Joan 2112
Renshaw, Josephine E. 2012,
   2333, 2334, 2338, 2463
Reti, Ende 408
Rew, Mabel 654
Ricart, Maria Del Carmen Al-
   varez see Alvarez Ricart,
   Maria Del Carmen
Rice, Helen Maria see Gas-
   sett, Helen Maria
Richards, Elizabeth 3302
Richardson, George S. 3115
Richelot, G. 3924
Richey, Margaret C. 3850
Riddell, (Lord) 655
Ridler, M. E. 3303
Ridlon, John 3700
Rifkind, Arleen Brenner 3964
Ritter, Mary Bennett 1621
Robb-Smith, A. H. T. 2236
Robens, Jane F. 3116
Robertiello, Richard C. 3117
Roberts, Carol Lee 3118
Roberts, E. Louise 2406
Roberts, Sheila M. H. 2340
Robertson, D. E. 353a
Robertson, Elizabeth E. 2706
Robinson, Alice 3701
Robinson, Daisy M. O. 2090,
   3702
Robinson, Elizabeth 3119
Robinson, Marion O. 354
Robinson, Victor 1622, 1623
Robinson, William 3304
Rochford, Grace E. 3703

Rockhill, Margaret Hackedorn
   1226, 1624, 3022, 3371,
   3704
Rockstro, Enid 1625
Rodgerson, Eleanor B. 2341,
   3120, 3121
Rodrigues, L. V. 2398
Roeske, Nancy A. 2464
Roessler, Robert 3122
Rogers, Fred B. 1626
Rogers, (Major) E. 4064
Rohmer, Hanny 3232
Rolant-Thomas, Catherine M.
   656
Rolleston, (Sir) Humphry 2929
Romaine, Adelaide 4019
Romieu, Claude 657
Romm, May E. 2465
Rooney, James F. 2031
Root, Eliza H. 1627-1631,
   2466, 4020
Root, Pauline 2654
Rosdahl, Nils 2175
Rose, Blanche E. 1632
Rose, Edmund 3233
Rose, Joan K. 659, 660
Rose, K. Daniel 3124
Rose, Katherine S. 1633
Rosekrans, Sarah D. 3382
Rosen, George 1636
Rosen, R. A. Hudson 3123
Rosenfeld, Siegfried 1943,
   2898-2901
Rosenlund, Mary Loretta 2342
Rosow, Irving 3124
Rosqvist, Ina 2866
Ross, Isabella Younger see
   Younger Ross, Isabella
Ross, Ishbel 1637
Ross, Mathew 3125
Ross, Nancy Wilson 1638
Rossi, Alice S. 3126
Roth, Nathan 702
Rothchild, Alice 3064
Rothman, Arthur I. 1881
Roubinovitch, Jacques 3214
Roughton, E. W. 2930
Roussy, Gustave 460a
Roy, J. H. 1639
Rozova, K. A. 205
Ruben, R. J. 178
Rudd, Helga M. 1640, 3705
Rudnick, Sarah 3706

Rue, Rosemary 2049, 2237
Ruland, Dora 2467
Runge, Hans 103
Runge, Max 2902
Russell, Jane Anderson 3127
Russell, M. P. 661
Russell, Violet 2407
Rutherford, Frances A. 4021
Rutherford, N. J. C. 662
Ruud, Helen 1642
Ruys, A. Charlotte 461, 3372
Ryan, T. M. 2275
Ryder, Claire F. 1643, 1644,
   1869, 2343, 2468, 3128,
   3974
Rydygier, Ludwig Ritter v.
   Ruediger 2903

Sabater, Antonio see Barbosa
   y Sabater, Antonio
Sabin, Francene 1646
Sablik, Karl von 3234
Sachs, Bernice C. 2013
Sadock, Virginia Alcott 3129
Safford, Pearl 1647
Sahli, Nancy Ann 1648
St. John, Christopher 663
Salmond, G. C. 2140
Salzi, Francesco 68
Samilowitz, Hazel 2469
Sandelin, Ellen 179, 1909
Sanders, Shirley 1982
Sanderson, Susanne 3939
Sandes, Gladys M. 122
Sanes, Samuel 1650
Sanford, Mary B. 3707
Sargent, Eva R. 1651
Satran, Richard 462
Saul, Ezra V. 2014
Saunders, A. M. 4085
Saunders, Ida B. 2141
Savage, Anne 2238, 2931
Sawyers, Martha 373
Scagnelli, Joan 1982
Scanlan, Theresa 2080
Scarlett, Mary J. see Scar-
   lett-Dixon, Mary J.
Scarlett-Dixon, Mary J. 3131,
   3708
Schaefer, Jane 1653
Schaefer, Romanus Johannes
   489

Scharlieb, Mary Ann Dacomb
    Bird 664-666, 2015, 2116,
    2533, 3925
Scharnagel, Isabel M. 3709-
    3711
Schelenz, Hermann 69
Scher, Maryonda 2470
Schidler, K. 2848
Schindler-Baumann, Jida 3905
Schlachter, Jo 3712
Schmidt, Otto 1774
Schmidt-Schütt, Margarete 490
Schnabel, Ilse 463
Schneider, Margaret Jane 2344
Schoch, Agnes Selin 1654
Schoenfeld, W. 2386
Schondel, A. 2176
Schönfeld, Walther 180, 491
Schrack, Helen F. 2728, 2737
Schrattenbach, Vilma 2667
Schreiter, Anneliese 2904
Schuck, R. F. 1870
Schultze, Caroline 3940
Schurter, Maxine 2471
Schw., W. 667
Schwalbe, Julius 2905
Schwartz, Adolf W. 181
Schwartz, Barry J. 2016
Schwartz, Jane 3132
Schwartz, Joseph M. 2949
Schwartz, Neena B. 3713
Schwendener, Hattie 1655
Schwerin, Ludwig 2906
Scoffield, Mary 2144
Scott, Agnes C. 3851
Scoutetten, Henri 182
Scriver, Jessie Boyd 3211
Scudder, Dorothy Jealous 2626
Seabrook, Alice M. 4055
Seaman, Barbara 2472
Sebesta, Vilma 409
Sechenov, I. M. 734
Sedlacek, William E. 1988,
    2017
Segre, Marcello 70
Seifert, Elizabeth 4065
Selmon, Bertha L. 183, 248-
    252, 1662-1689, 2534-2537,
    2589, 2655, 2656, 3716-
    3719
Selvini, Mara Palazzoli 464-
    466, 3906
Semenoff, A. M. 2856

Sensenig, E. Carl 1690
Seppanen, Anni 3907
Severinghaus, A. E. 2071
Severinghaus, E. L. 1691
Seward, S. C. 2627
Shainess, Natalie 2473
Shamer, Bertha Tapman 1692
Shanahan, Kathleen 1693
Shane, Jessie F. 2345
Shangold, Mona M. 3135
Shapiro, Carol S. 2346
Shapiro, Edith T. 3136
Shapley, Deborah 3137
Sharp, Dorothy J. 3656
Sharp, Helen Carmeleta 2538
Shaver, Phillip 1910
Shaw, Anna Howard 1694
Shaw, Lillian E. 1739
Shea, Petrena Abbe 2347
Sheehan, Donal 2018
Sheets, Emily T. 374
Shepherd, Gwendolyn 3946
Sheppard, Amy 467
Sherbon, Florence Brown 1697,
    3138, 3139, 4022
Sheriff, Hilla 1698, 3584
Shibokov, Anatotii Aleksovich
    206
Shmigelsky, Irene 1699
Shore, E. 2239
Shrubshall, Nancy K. 2916
Shryock, Richard Harrison 253
Siebel, Johanna 468
Silva, Alberto 721
Silver, George A. 2348
Silver, P. H. S. 1915
Simecek, Angeline Frances 1701
Simon, William E. 2474
Singer, Charles 104
Singer, Joy Daniels 1702
Sinkoff-Goldstein, Jean 3725
Skachilov, V. A. 735
Skirving, R. Scot 305
Slater, Robert J. 3728
Sloop, Mary T. Martin 254,
    1705
Smart, Isabelle Thompson 2081-
    2085, 3695
Smith, Alice M. 1706
Smith, B. 1937
Smith, E. D. Chalmers 610
Smith, Frederick C. 2720
Smith, Isabel 2203

Smith, Joseph T.   1707
Smith, Katharine   1708
Smith, Margaret H. D.   2496
Smith, Mary Sloan   668
Smith, Myrtle Lee   2475
Smith, Olive W.   2476
Smith, Stephen   1263, 1709
Snelgrove, Erle E.   1710
Snell, Elsie K.   1711
Snow, Laurence H.   2016
Snyder, Charles McCool   1712
Snyder, Ruth E.   2477
Sokoloff, D. A.   3215
Solis, Margarita Delgado de
     3373
Solomon, Barbara Miller   1714
Solomon, Rebecca Z.   2478
Soltau, B. Eleanor   669
Soriano, Victor   1715
Sorrel-Dejerine, Y.   469
Soule, Bradley   3143, 3144
South, Lillian H.   3584
South, Virginia   2086
Southgate, M. Therese   3140
Spaeth, Joseph   2877
Spalding, Warren F.   1716
Speer, Alma Jane   2728, 2737
Spence, A. A.   2398, 2414
Spencer, Everett R.   3732
Spencer, R. B.   2805
Spencer, Steven M.   4023
Spiegelman, Mortimer   3001
Spiller, Violet   2406
Spillman, Ramsay   1717
Spiro, Howard M.   3141
Spurlock, Jeanne   3733
Stack, N.   1718
Stalnaker, John M.   1972,
     2020, 2286
Standley, Kay   3143, 3144
Stanley, Gillian R.   2240
Stanton, Rosamond Wilfley   880
Starbird, Adele C.   2806
Starr, Sarah Logan Wister
     3734
Stastny, Olga Frances   1719,
     1720, 2349, 3307
Steinberger, S.   184
Steinbuch, D. C. see Nuy-
     sink-Steinbuch, D. C.
Steiner, Jan W.   1881
Steinmann, Anne   3145, 3146
Stelzner, Helene Friderike

2189, 2190
Stenhouse, Evangeline E.   185,
     2352
Stephen, James A.   686
Stephens, Nannie A.   2
Stephens, Nora   3494
Stephenson, Kathryn L.   460
Stephens-Walker, Hasseltine
     3735
Steppacher, Robert   3147
Steppanen, Anni   470
Stern, Madeleine B.   1721
Stetler, Pearl M.   1722
Steudel, Johannes   72, 73
Stevens, Audrey D.   1723
Stevens, Marion C.   2682
Stevenson, Sarah Hackett   2021
Stewart, Clara   670, 671, 2707,
     2708, 3600
Stewart, Eleanor Wolf   2629
Stewart, Elizabeth L.   3212
Stewart, George Walter   1724
Stewart, Margaret R.   1725
Stewart, Marguerite   643
Stewart, Marian   306
Stewart, W. Brenton   355
Stibler, Barbara-Jean   2346
Stieda, Ludwig   1911
Stimson, Barbara B.   2709
Stinson, Mary H.   2125
Stochik, A. M.   207
Stokvis-Cohen Stuart, N.   1850
Stoll   2907
Stone, Berenice   1727
Storer, H. B.   3736
Storkan, Margaret Ann   1728
Storrie, V. Marie   2022
Stötzer, F.   2908
Straight, William M.   1729
Strashun, I. D.   736
Strassmann, P.   74
Strawn, Julia C.   2807
Strecker, Gabriele   105
Stricker, George   3035
Stricker, W.   106
Stritter, Frank T.   1971, 2023,
     2024
Strong, R. M.   1550
Strott, George G.   2808
Stuard, Susan Mosher   75
Stuart, Madeleine   672
Stuart, N. see Stokvis-Cohen
     Stuart, N.

Stuart, N. G. 1730
Sturge, Mary D. 3308, 3309
Sturgis, Katharine R. 1733
Sturgis, Margaret Castex 1734
Sugden, Louisa Grace 2590
Sullivan, Margaret P. 4024
Summerfield, G. P. 2932
Sutherland, Joan K. 673, 2408
Svartz, Nanna 471
Svejcar, J. 410
Svendsen, H. J. 2387
Swain, Clara A. 2631
Swanson, A. Maud 674
Swartz, Philip Allen 1739
Swayne, Walter C. 2933
Swiss Association of University
   Women 1912
Sydenstricker, (Mrs.) 2591
Sylk, Ellen 675
Szenajch, Wladyslaw 411
Szkop-Frankiel, Susana 2126

Tackabury, Patty 3494
Tait, L. 1938
Tao, S. M. 3853
Tattersall, Joan 2409
Taylor, L. Dorothea 676
Taylor, Ruth E. 1740
Taylor, William 2509
Taylor-Jones, Louise 988,
   3374, 3740, 4025
Tayson, Juyne M. 2479
Teffeau, Cleora 1741
Tenbrinck, Margaret S. 1742
Tenney, Rachel 3741
Terry, Robert J. 1743
Thelander, Hulda Evelyn 1744,
   1745, 2353, 2354, 2809,
   2810, 3148-3151, 3375,
   3742
Thelberg, Elizabeth Burr 926,
   988, 2480, 3743
Thomas, Belle 2785
Thomas, Caroline Bedell
   2359
Thomas, Laurel 2847
Thomas, M. Carey 3091
Thomas, Mary A. 1871,
   2089
Thomas, Mary F. 2025
Thompson, Theodis 2354a
Thomson, Bertha M. 2127

Thomson, Constance M. 686
Thomson, St. Clair 512
Thorburn-Johnstone, Mabel
   677
Thorne, Isabel 3310
Thorne, May 123, 124, 678,
   3311
Tiburtius, Franziska 492, 3908
Tichauer, Ruth W. 2415, 3947
Tikotin, M. A. 208
Timbury, G. C. 2934
Timbury, Morag C. 2241, 2934
Tissue, Florence 1748
Tkatchef, Alexandrine 3216,
   3217
Todd, Malcolm C. 4027
Todd, Margaret C. 679, 3313
Toland, Gertrude M. B. 2710
Tolstoi, K. 1891
Toropoff, D. I. 2277
Touff, Roselyn 1750
Tower, Elizabeth 1751
Tracy, Martha 1872, 2354b,
   3748-3754, 4028
Tracy, Rose H. 2054
Travell, Janet 1752, 3152,
   3974
Trenholme, Marilyn 2377,
   2378
Tripp, Wendell 1755
Truax, Rhoda 1756, 4066
True, Mabelle 1757
Tucker, B. Fain 1366
Tyson, J. R. 4029
Tyson, Judith Weigand 3964

Ulrich, Mabel S[imus] 1759
Ulyatt, Kenneth W. 2935-
   2937
Ulyatt, Frances Margaret 2935-
   2937
United States Congressional
   House Committee on Mili-
   tary Affairs 2814
U.S. Council of National De-
   fense 718
U.S. Department of Labor
   (The Outlook for Women in
   Occupations in the Medical
   Services...) see Zapoleon,
   Marguerite Wykoff
U.S. Department of Labor,

Women's Bureau 3952, 4030
Upjohn, William 287
Uzemack, Edward A. 1959
Uzman, Betty Geren 2481

Vallinkoski, Jorma V. 3909
Van Cortlandt, Elizabeth see Hocker, Elizabeth Van Cortlandt
Vanderlip, Mrs. Frank A. [Narcissa Cox] 3153
Vandervall, Isabella 3154
Van Der Velden, Friedrich 107
Van der Vlugt, Martha 1761
Van Erp, Ymkje M. 1762
Van Gasken, Frances C. 2816
van Heerden, Petronella 264
Van Hoosen, Bertha 186, 988, 1763-1774, 2027, 2028, 2040, 2090-2101, 2354c, 2354d, 2354e, 2354f, 2354g, 2482-2484, 2592, 2817, 2946, 3155-3159, 3376-3378, 3758-3770, 4031-4033
Van Leeuwen, Kato 2485
Van Liere, Edward J. 2354h
Vargas, Tegualda Ponce de 3948
Vaschak, Mathilda R. 1775, 2355, 2356, 2486, 2487
Vasilievskaya, O. 722
Vaughan, E. 1776
Vautin, Joy M. 2141
Velin, Connie 1380
Vida, Trivadar 412
Vietor, Agnes C. 1778, 2488
Vilar, Lola 472
Villard, Mrs. Henry 1263
Vilmon, Gyulane 408
Vines, Charlotte S. 2635
Vladimirova, G. A. 376
Vlasenko, V. I. 2278
von Sholly, Anna I. 2489
Voorhis, Anna Harvey 3160
Vysohlid, J. 2152

Waal-Manning, Hendrika J. 2136
Wade, Phyllis 682

Wager, Mary A. E. 4034
Wagner, Marianne 2878
Wagner, Wyonia 1779
Wainer, Robert A. 2029
Waite, Frederick C. 255, 256, 1780-1784, 3772-3774
Waite, Lucy 257, 3873
Waitzkin, Evelyn D. 3775
Wakefield, Alice E. 2281, 3776
Walker, Emma E. 2358
Walker, Gertrude A. 3777, 3778, 4055
Walker, Jane H. 187, 683-685, 2711, 3318
Walker, Stella Ford 3779
Wallace, Ellen A. 3780
Wallace, Joyce 2102
Wallin, Mathilda K. 1785
Walsh, James Joseph 76, 188, 2712
Walsh, Ngaire M. 2136
Walters, Josephine 4035
Walton, H. J. 2938
Ward, Vera Chance 1786
Warren, Elsie 2599
Warren, Fidelia 2030
Warwick, Margaret 4035a
Warwick, O. H. 2144
Wassertheil-Smoller, Sylvia 2490
Watkins, Rachel A. 1787
Watson, Anne Mercer 686
Watson, Jeanne M. 1550
Wattie, Nora I. 2410
Wauchope, Gladys Mary 687
Waugh, Elizabeth S. 1788-1790, 3781, 3782
Webb, Elizabeth M. 2146
Webb-Johnson, Alfred 125
Weber, Mathilde 2909
Webster, Augusta 1791
Weinberg, Ethel 2031, 2103, 2104
Weinstein, Morton R. 2491
Weiss, Robert 4036
Weiss-Schwartz, Sandra 3983
Weitz, Lawrence J. 2949
Welch, William H. 1263
Wells, Dorothy see Atkinson, Dorothy Wells
Wells, Helen 4067
Wells, Mrs. S. E. F. 3783

Welsh, Lilian 258, 1792
Wensel, Louise Oftedal 1599
Wessel, M. A. 1794
West, Charles 2939
Westling-Wikstrand, Helena
    2359
Weyman, Else Krug 2492
Weyrauch, Helen B. 2354
Wharton, May Cravath 1796
Wheaton, Walter F. 1798
Wheeler, Clementene Walker
    3162
Wheeler, Emily C. 1799
Whipple, Dorothy V. 3952
White, Agnes H. T. 357
White, Frances Emily 3163,
    4037
White, Marguerite 2713
White, Maria 2637-2642
White, Martha S. 3164
White, Paul D. 358
White-Thomas, Cornelia
    1800
Whitfield, A. G. W. 2243-
    2245
Whitlock-Rose, Elise 1873
Whitman, Howard 3165
Whitmore, Clara B. 3200
Whitten, Kathryn M. 189,
    2737, 4068
Whittier, Isabel 1801
Wickner, Hali 1802
Widerström, Karolina 473,
    474
Wigginton, R. M. 1803
Wijnen, M. Elise 2846
Wilberforce, Octavia M. 688
Wilbur, Ray Lyman 4038
Wild, Ella 1912
Wilder, Dora Lee 259
Wilks, Samuel 2940, 2941
Willard, L. 2105
Willey, Florence E. 2824
Williams, Anna W. 2494
Williams, Ethel M. N. 689,
    690, 2411
Williams, Josephine J. 3166,
    3167
Williams, Marjorie J. 2363,
    2495
Williams, Mary Edith 1804
Williams, N. 3168
Williams, Phoebe A. 4039

Williams, Stanley 287
Wilson, Dorothy Clarke 285,
    1805, 1806, 2643
Wilson, Isabel G. H. 522
Wilson, Jno. Stainback 2032
Wilson, Marjorie Price 1991,
    2364, 3964
Wilson, Mary Lena 1807
Wilson, Robert 3926
Wilson-Davis, Keith 2168
Winckel, Franz von 77
Winkelvoss, E. 929
Winner, Albertine 2246, 2714
Wisenfelder, Harry 2336
Wissler, Robert W. 1808
Wistein, Rosina 3169
Withington, Alfreda 1809-
    1812
Witthoff, Evelyn 1813
Wittke, Carl F. 1814
Wlodarska, H. 2153
Wojcik, Ladislas D. 2496
Wolfe, Claire V. 2497
Wolfe, Mary M. 2365
Wollstein, Martha 191
Wolman, Carol 3170
Women's Bureau see U.S.
    Department of Labor, Wo-
    men's Bureau
Women's Bureau, U.S. Depart-
    ment of Labor (The Outlook
    for Women in Occupations in
    the Medical Services...)
    see Zapoleon, Marguerite
    Wykoff
Wong, Helena 375
Wong, K. Chimin 4
Wood, Ann Douglas 3183
Woodbridge, Helen McFarland
    1833
Wood-Comstock, Belle 3184
Woodroffe, Helen 2684
Woodruff, Frieda Wagoner
    3964
Woodruff, Kay H. 2503, 2504
Woodside, Nina B. 2264, 3185,
    3817
Woodward, Helen Beal 1834
Woody, Regina J. 4069
Woolley, Alice Stone 1835-
    1837, 2080, 3186, 3818
Woolsey, Florance see Haz-
    zard, Florance Woolsey

Worcester, Blandina   1838
Wright, Elizabeth S.   3821
Wright, Katharine W.   1842,
   3822, 3950
Wu, Lien-Teh   4
Wulsin, John H.   1875
Wylie, A. M. McElroy   2644
Wylie, I. A. R.   1836
Wyne, Sister M. Elise   2645
Wynekoop, Alice Lois Lindsay
   3823
Wynen, Elise   3857

Yakovlev, Paul I.   1843
Yamazaki, Rinko   3858, 3859
Yarrell, Zuleika   4049
Yarros, Rachelle Slobodinsky
   1844, 1845, 2090, 3187,
   3188
Yoshioka, Yayoi   286, 3203,
   3860
Young, R.   4050
Young, Ruth   2116
Young, T. K.   2593
Young Women's Christian
   Association   3825
Younger Ross, Isabella   7

Zabludovskaia, Elena Davy-
   dovna   738
Zakrzewska, Marie A.   929,
   1846
Zapoleon, Marguerite Wykoff
   2375
Zaunick, Rudolph   108
Zehender, Wilhelm von   2910
Zelkovic, Audrey A.   2346
Zenil, Sara   2947
Zhbankoff, D. N.   1892
Zikeev, P. D.   209, 739
Zink, Pearl L.   1848
Zolliker, Margaret   4013
Zurbrugg, Jo   2441

Abolitionists 1340, 1398
Abortion
    Attitudes towards 2331, 2472, 2490, 3983
    Spontaneous in physicians 2398, 2414
Academy of General Practice of San Antonio (Texas) 1848
Academy of Medicine of St. Petersburg (USSR) see St. Peters-
        burg Academy of Medicine (USSR)
Academy of Science (Paris, France)
    Lallemand prize 466
Acupuncture, Attitudes towards 3983
Adamless Eden 1085
Addams, Jane 1177, 1567, 1774
Administrative positions for women physicians 2348, 2428, 2451,
        3079, 3177, 3185
        See also Hospitals--Administration, Women in
Admissions see under Medical schools
Adolescent girls, Work with 771, 2448
        See also Pediatrics
Advertisements depicting women physicians 4026
Affectivity see Characteristics of women physicians--Sympathy;
        and Patients--Emotional involvement with
Affirmative action 2009, 3185, 3964
Afghanistan
    British physicians (specific) 547, 664
Africa (See also specific countries)
    Employment opportunities (1920s) 2389
    Foreign physicians (non missionary) 454, 1272, 1379
    Missionary activity 608, 1042, 1201, 1468, 2646, 2648, 2652,
        2665
    Need for women to attend women 2253
African Research Foundation 1272
Age distribution of physicians 2230, 2267, 2270, 2271, 2375, 3001,
        4030
        See also Longevity
Age of consent law (U.S.) 787
Agra, Women's Medical School of (India) 1876
Agriculture, United States Department of 1192
Ahmedabad, India see India, Ahmedabad
Air Force (Great Britain) see Armed services (Great Britain)
Air Force (U.S.) see Armed services (U.S.)
Ajmer, India see India, Ajmer
Ajmer Women's Hospital see under India, Ajmer

Alabama
    Medical Association of Alabama   3405
    Physicians   2475
Alaska
    Physicians   1261, 1751
Albert, Professor E.
    Comments on his essay on women in medical study   2869, 2891
Alcoholism control, Physicians' work in   586, 3765
Algeria
    French physicians   440, 455
All-India Women's Reserve Medical Unit   see   India Women's Re-
                serve Medical Unit
Allahabad, India   see   India, Allahabad
Allergy and immunology (See also Pediatric allergy, Women in)
    American College of Allergy, Board of Regents   1216
    Women in (specific)   761, 1216, 1847
Alpha Epsilon Iota Fraternity   2106, 3495, 3561
Ambulance service   785, 1077, 1535, 2095
American Academy of Obstetrics and Gynecology   811
American Academy of Pediatrics   806
American Association of Anatomists   795
American Association of Obstetricians, Gynaecologists and Abdom-
                inal Surgeons   2323
American Association of University Women   417
American College of Allergy   1216
American College of Surgeons   756, 1532, 2100, 3391, 3406, 3760,
                3770, 3779
American Diabetes Association   1532
American Heart Association   1008
American Indian medical students, statistics   see   Medical students--
                Minority statistics
American Indian physicians and healers   233, 693, 824, 1131, 1288,
                1592
American Medical Association
    Attitudes towards women physicians   1764, 2729
    Delegates   1497, 3516, 3664, 3665, 3710, 4032
    Meetings   3384, 3407, 3639, 3727
    Officers   1439, 3767
    Question of admitting women   235, 3489, 3490, 3499, 3525
    Role of women physicians   2483, 3385, 3425
American Medical Women's Association (See also branches in spe-
                cific cities; and American Women's Hospitals Service.
                For resolutions see under specific topics)
    Activities (pre-1930)   3401, 3685, 3748, 3766
    Activities (post-1930s)   2722, 3105, 3395, 3551, 3686
    Awards   1345, 1366, 1549, 1587
    Branches   3423
    Campaign for women physicians in the armed services   1108,
                2781, 2819
    Committee for the relief of distressed women physicians   3514,
                3628
    Committees on medical opportunities   1857, 2028, 2354d, 3022,
                3158

Committees on war service opportunities   2761, 2785, 2787,
        2788, 2820, 3762
Cooperation with American Medical Association   3385, 3425
Criticism of   3071, 3503
Doll collection   3564
History   3315, 3358, 3393, 3415, 3426, 3556, 3652, 3743
Journal   3591, 3694, 3761
Library fund   3638, 3781
Medical College of Pennsylvania liaison   3611, 3822
Meetings (pre-1920s)   2780, 3695, 3755
Meetings (1920s-1940s)   3394, 3417, 3699, 3729, 4018
Membership programs   3610
Necessity for   3412, 3643, 3763
Preceptorship programs   1980, 1981
Presidents   1149, 3654, 3782
Purpose   1865, 3416, 3436, 3518, 3545, 3592, 3606, 3614,
        3627, 3740, 3784
Scholarship and memorial funds   3408, 3626, 3654, 3655, 3704,
        3750
American Memorial Hospital   see under   France, Reims
American Mother of the Year   1705
American Pediatric Society   1250
American Posture League, Founders   781
American Psychiatric Association   2464, 3733
American Public Health Association   795, 939, 1230, 1400
American Red Cross work   see   Red Cross work
American Social Hygiene Association   1066
American Society for the Control of Cancer   1513
American Society of Clinical Pathologists   1747
American Telephone and Telegraph Company physicians   1524
American Trauma Society   882
American University of Beirut, School of Public Health   see   Beirut,
        American University of, School of Public Health (Lebanon)
American Women's Hospitals Service (See also under specific coun-
        tries)
Activities (pre-1920)   1485, 2723, 2788, 2790, 3440, 3585,
        3593
Activities (1920s)   1106, 3396-3398, 3401, 3441, 3546, 3586,
        3588, 3590, 3595, 3597, 3598, 3682
Activities (World War II)   2700, 3600
Affiliation with Red Cross   2795
Benefits to physicians who serve   3583
Fund raising   2786, 3399
History   161, 988, 1475, 1742, 1785, 3358, 3400, 3519, 3583,
        3589, 3690
Reserve corps   3404, 3601, 3712
Rural and mountain medical service   3584
Amritsar Medical School (India)   1876
Anatomy
American Association of Anatomists   795
History of women in   53, 3891
Specific women in   795, 992
Anesthesiology

Hazards for women in 2398, 2414
Women in 335, 508, 1381, 2404, 2417, 2756
Anglican Mission Dispensary see under New Guinea, Dewade
Angola
American missionaries 2506
Ani, India see India, Ani
Anita Newcomb McGee Award recipients (Daughters of the American
Revolution) 769
Ann Arbor, Michigan see Michigan, Ann Arbor
Ann Arbor Private Hospital for the Mentally Disturbed see under
Michigan, Ann Arbor
Anthony, Susan B. 1094, 1694
Physician to 698
Anxiety in medical students see Medical students--Anxiety
Apgar score 1064
Apothecaries' Hall (London, England) 1932
Appalachia (U.S.)
Physicians 828, 1705
Apprenticeships for medical students see Preceptorship programs
Arabic physicians 152
See also under specific countries
Archbishop Attipetty Jubilee Memorial Hospital see under India,
Thuruthipuram
Architects compared with physicians 3144
Argentina
Physicians (specific) 703, 706, 721
Physicians (status) 3364, 3946
Arizona
Physicians 1723
Arkansas
Physicians 3972
Arkansas, University of, Medical School (Fayetteville) 744, 756,
2729, 3972
Armed Forces Institute of Pathology, Medical Museum of (U.S.)
218
Armed services (Canada)
Commissions for women 2669
Physicians (specific) 2670
Armed services (Great Britain)
American physicians (specific) 699, 2701, 2709
Commissions for women 2690, 2693, 2703, 2704, 2708, 3284
History of physicians in 2714, 2717
Inspector-general of army hospitals 650, 652, 661, 667
Physicians (status) 2686, 2692, 2695, 2702, 2706, 2707, 2720,
2815
Armed services (USSR)
Physicians 204, 2671-2673, 3217
Armed services (U.S.) (See also Hospitals--Military)
Association of military surgeons 1539
Commissions for women 768, 981, 2728, 2732, 2739, 2773,
2797, 2809, 2818
American Legion activities 2721
American Medical Association activities 2729, 2730, 2781,

2798, 2825
First physicians commissioned 1129, 2748
History of struggle 2757, 2794, 2838
Women's organizations activities 1108, 2781, 2782, 2800,
      2819
Contract surgeons defined 2770
Exemption and financial aid for medical students 1948, 2026,
      2801, 2815
History of physicians in 2717, 2794
Legislation 2724, 2746, 2765, 2766, 2770, 2778, 2813
   Celler Bill (U.S. Bill H.R. 824) 2731, 2734, 2735, 2792,
      2814
   Sparkman-Johnson Bill (U.S. Bill H.R. 1857) 2721, 2733,
      2738, 2757, 2777, 2792, 2814
Physicians (specific) 2741, 2742, 4013
   Army 900, 909, 911, 1128, 1378, 1573, 1656, 1657, 1824,
      2745, 2758, 2799, 2826
   Navy 1142, 1317, 1337, 1659-1661, 2749
Physicians (status) 2722, 2727, 2736, 2737, 2751, 2762, 2763,
      2793, 2810, 2834, 2839
Recruitment 2725, 2775, 2789, 2820, 2827, 2841
Requirements for serving 2808, 2837
Uniforms 2812
Volunteer medical service corps 2750, 2753, 2754, 2802
Women's auxiliary services 2776
Armed services (Yugoslavia)
   Physicians 388
Armenia (See also Iran; and Turkey; and USSR)
   American physicians 1004, 1106
   American Women's Hospitals 3596
   Native physicians 406
Armour, South Dakota see South Dakota, Armour
Army (Great Britain) see Armed services (Great Britain)
Army (USSR) see Armed services (USSR)
Army (U.S.) see Armed services (U.S.)
Army (Yugoslavia) see Armed services (Yugoslavia)
Army Nurse Corps (U.S.) 869, 1539, 2747
Art depicting women physicians 92, 185, 218, 353a, 453, 1136,
      1530, 1819, 3672, 3871, 3960, 4040
            See also Portraits of women physicians
Arthur S. Gillow Foundation for Scientific Research and Preventive
      Medicine (Columbia) 704, 705
Asbury Hospital see under Minnesota, Minneapolis
Asheville, North Carolina see North Carolina, Asheville
Assertiveness training for physicians 3185
Association of Internes and Medical Students 1947
Association of Medical Women in India see India Association of
      Medical Women
Association of Military Surgeons 1539
Association of Southern Medical Women see Southern Medical
      Women's Association (U.S.)
Association of Women in Public Health 3569, 3570, 3660
Athens, University of, Medical School (Greece) 448

Atlanta, Georgia see Georgia, Atlanta
Atomic radiation training programs   2429
Attitudes of women medical students see Medical students--Atti-
        tudes of
Attitudes of women physicians 1668, 2935, 2937, 3145, 3146, 3947
        See also under specific topics
Attitudes towards women physicians
    Catholic church   162
    Compared with attitudes towards other minority physicians   3166
    Family 2473, 3055, 3974
    Hospital administration   2854
    Male physicians 220, 2032, 3007
    Medical community 212, 1867, 1978, 2018, 2166, 2180, 2905,
        3158
    Patients and general public 1867, 2007, 2465, 3008, 3035,
        3097, 3166, 3913
    Press 2817, 2858, 2875, 3175
    Prison council (Sweden) 2166
    Self-image 2962, 3082, 3083, 3130, 3155, 3183, 3184
    Sociocultural determinants of 3008, 3010
    Stereotypes 3010, 3060, 3113
Auckland, School of Medicine (New Zealand) 1879
Augusta, Georgia see Georgia, Augusta
Australia
    Hospitals run by women 2257
    Physicians (specific) 638, 694
    Physicians (status) 300, 1505, 1768, 3364, 3838, 3885
Austria
    Medical education 51, 72, 1893, 1901, 1905, 1913, 3885
    Physicians (specific) 34, 51, 55, 416, 427, 2385, 2667, 3936
    Physicians (status) 2173, 2312, 2869, 3364, 3891
    Practice patterns 55, 2158, 2177
Austria, Graz
    First woman physician 416
Austria, Hernels
    Institute for Officers' Daughters 475
Austria, Vienna
    Physicians 430, 431, 438
    Post-graduate medical education 2045
    Vienna Medical Women's Association 427
Austrian Institute for Urban Research Survey 2158
Automobile drivers, Comparisons with women physicians 2419
Aviation pathology training programs see under Pathology
Aylsbury, England see England, Aylesbury

B. J. Medical School (Ahmedabad, India) 1876
B. J. Medical School (Poona, India) 1876
Babies' Hospital see under New York City
Bacteriology, Women in 968, 1217, 1445
Baghdad, Iraq see Iraq, Baghdad
Bahia, University of (Brazil) 721
Bakwin, Harry 1510

Baltimore, Maryland see Maryland, Baltimore
Baltimore University Medical School (Maryland) 1674
Baltimore, Woman's Medical College of 141, 164, 1692, 3634,
        3954
Bangladesh (See also Pakistan)
     American missionaries 2513
Bangladesh, Mymensingh
     St. Michael's Hospital 2511, 2512
Banting Medal recipients (American Diabetes Association) 1532
Bapalta, India see India, Bapalta
Bareilly, India see India, Bareilly
Barnard College (New York City) 3162
Baroda, India see India, Baroda
Barry, Kitty 219
Baruch, Bernard 3811
Bass Collection on Women in Medicine (Tulane University) 240,
        1482
Battle Creek, Michigan see Michigan, Battle Creek
Baylor College of Medicine (Houston, Texas) 1117, 1140, 1874,
        3004, 3122, 3182
Beirut, American University of, School of Public Health (Lebanon)
        821
Belgian Congo see Congo
Belgium
     Physicians 417, 423, 450, 2155
Bellevue Hospital see under New York City
Benares, India see India, Benares
Berekum, Ghana see Ghana, Berekum
Berlin, Germany see Germany, Berlin
Berlin Medical Society see under Germany, Berlin
Bermondsey Medical Mission see under England, London
Bethany Dispensary see under Philippine Islands, Manila
Bethel Mission (Kiukiang) see under China, Kiukiang
Bethel Mission (Shanghai) see under China, Shanghai
Bible (Ecclesiastes) see Ecclesiastes, Book of
Billings, Frank 2100
Bingen, Germany see Germany, Bingen
Binghamton, New York see New York, Binghamton
Biochemistry, Women in 1433
Bird watching 1589
                (For other non medical activities see Non medical
                activities)
Birmingham, England see England, Birmingham
Birmingham General Hospital see under England, Birmingham
Birmingham, University of, Medical School (England) 2243-2245
Birth control
     Attitudes towards 2122, 2490, 3325, 3699, 3983
     Contraceptive bill (Lord Damson's) 3286
     Physicians' work in 445, 461, 744, 1066, 1647, 2399
     Planned Parenthood Federation of America 877
Bishop's College Medical School (Quebec Province) 8
Black American medical students, Statistics see Medical students
                --Minority statistics

Black American physicians
    Attitudes of 1777
    Attitudes towards 3023
    Employment and practice problems 855, 859, 2375, 3154
    Internship opportunities 2093
    Recruitment 2971, 3929
    Role conflict 1140
    Specific women 699, 756, 855, 856, 1173, 1180, 1201, 1239,
            1526, 1639
        Firsts 750, 866, 899, 1015, 1033, 1052, 1272, 1532, 1559
    Statistics 223, 2256, 2354a
Black Americans
    Missionary activity among 2648
Blackwell, Alice Stone 1637
Blackwell, Antoinette Brown 1094, 1188
Blackwell, Elizabeth
    Comments on her "Pioneer Work" 1302
Blackwell, Elizabeth, Award see Elizabeth Blackwell Award
Blackwell, Elizabeth, centennial see Elizabeth Blackwell centen-
            nial
Blackwell, Hannah 1483
Blackwell, Samuel 777, 1483
Board Certification statistics (1970s) 2300, 2309
Bolivia
    Physicians 708, 713, 3364, 3947
Bologna, University of, Medical School (Italy) 457, 3227
Bombay, India see India, Bombay
Bombay, University of, Medical School (India) 605
Bookstores run by physicians 1633
                    (For other non medical activities see Non medical
                    activities)
Booth, Mary L. 3444
Bosnia, Yugoslavia see Yugoslavia, Bosnia and Herzegovina
Boston Female Medical College see New England Female Medical
            College (Boston, Massachusetts)
Boston, Massachusetts see Massachusetts, Boston
Boston State Hospital see under Massachusetts, Boston
Boston University Medical School (Massachusetts) 230, 3055, 3064,
            3420, 3772
                    See also New England Female Medical College (Boston,
                    Massachusetts)
Bowne Memorial Hospital see under New York, Poughkeepsie
Bowne, Richard H. 3456
Bratislava, Czechoslovakia see Czechoslovakia, Bratislava
Brazil
    Medical education 721
    Physicians 196, 718, 721, 3364, 3943
Brazilian College of Surgeons 196
Breast feeding, Attitudes towards 2441
Breshkovsky, Catherine 1721
Breslau University Medical School (Germany) 3224
Bridgeton Hospital see under New Jersey, Bridgeton
Bridgeton, New Jersey see New Jersey, Bridgeton

Brighton, England see England, Brighton
Bristol, England see England, Bristol
Bristol, University of, Medical School (England) 1917, 2933
British Columbia
    British Columbia Medical Association 356
British Medical Association
    Cooperation with the Medical Women's Federation 1929
    General Medical Council 539, 1922, 3924
    Resolutions concerning women physicians 3916
    Women as members 496, 617, 2927, 3262, 3263, 3290
British Medical Register see Medical Register (Great Britain)
British Medical Women's Federation see Medical Women's Fed-
            eration (Great Britain)
British Paediatric Association 1051
Brooklyn, New York see New York, Brooklyn
Bryn Mawr College (Pennsylvania) 1825, 3964
Buffalo Medical Journal and Monthly Review
    First article by a woman physician published in the U.S. 1650
Buffalo, New York see New York, Buffalo
Bulgaria
    Physicians 405
Burma
    American physicians 914
    Missionaries 1104, 1504, 2517-2519
Burma, Moulmein
    Ellen Mitchell Memorial Hospital 2519
Bush Church Aid Society's Flying Medical Service (Australia) 294
Bussing, Attitudes towards see School bussing, Attitudes towards
Busts of women physicians see Art depicting women physicians
Butler, Charles 932
Butler Memorial Hospital see India, Baroda--Mrs. William Butler
            Memorial Hospital
Byron, Lady Noel 844

Calcutta Medical School (India) 1876
California
    California Academy of Medicine 1611
    Milk commission 1501
    Physicians (specific) 236, 863, 1074, 1343, 1425, 1432, 1463,
        1621, 1665, 1704
    Problems for black women physicians 855
    State and county medical societies 236, 993, 3439
California Academy of Medicine see under California
California, Catalina Island
    Physicians 1458
California, Compton
    Women's and Children's Hospital 1832
California, Long Beach
    American Medical Women's Association (Branch 38) 811, 3547
California, Los Angeles
    Los Angeles County Hospital 1370, 2078
    Urban poor clinics 856

California, Madera
    Public health officers   801
California, Nevada City
    Physicians   236
California, Palo Alto
    Physicians   806
California, Pasadena
    Lutheran Hospital   855
California, San Diego
    Guadalupe Clinic   881
    Physicians   1127
California, San Francisco
    Children's Hospital of San Francisco   978, 3742
    Langley Porter Neuropsychiatric Institute   2491
    Pacific Dispensary for Women and Children   236
    Physicians (specific)   892, 953, 1610
    Presbyterian Medical Center retraining program   2051
    San Francisco County Medical Society   863, 1463
    Women Physicians' Club of San Francisco   1022, 1745, 3149
California, Stanford
    Stanford University Hospital   1611, 1802
California, University of, Medical School (Berkeley)   2977
California, University of, Medical School (Davis)   774
California, University of, Medical School (Los Angeles)   1281
California, University of, Medical School (San Francisco)   2976
California, Vallejo
    Physicians   945
Camille Mermod Award recipient (American Medical Women's Asso-
            ciation)   1587
Campbell, Margaret A.
    Comments on her "Why Would A Girl Want To Go Into Medi-
            cine"   3137, 3141
Campbell Medical School (Calcutta, India)   1876
Canada
    Colombian physicians   704
    Interns and residents (statistics)   2054, 2087
    Medical education   1858, 1960
    Native physicians (status)   2256, 2258, 3364
Canada and United States
    Comparative statistics on physicians   3950
Canada Department of National Health, Division of Child Welfare
            see   Child Welfare Division, Department of National
            Health (Canada)
Canada, Federation of Medical Women of   3207, 3209, 3210
    Retraining program   2044
Canadian Medical Association   337, 2145
Cancer clinics   see   Cancer control--Clinics
Cancer control (See also specific clinics under their hospital names)
    American Society for the Control of Cancer   1513, 3571
    Cancer research committee of the Medical Women's Federation
            3915
    Clement Cleveland Cancer Award   896
    Clinics   881, 921, 2313

National Cancer Institute of Canada   356
Women in (specific)
    Great Britain   541, 620, 621, 647
    Sweden   474
    U.S.   741, 823, 1015, 1272, 1314, 1438, 1444, 1618, 1750,
      2283, 2298
Cancer research   see   Cancer control
Cape Province, South Africa   see   South Africa, Cape Province
Capital Hospital   see under   China, Peking
Capitalism, Attitudes towards   454
Cardiology
    American Heart Association   1008
    Philadelphia Heart Association (Pennsylvania)   4009
    Women in (specific)   309, 311, 331, 342, 348, 1008, 1653
Career counseling   see   Vocational guidance
Carl Gustav Carus Medical Academy (Dresden)   2908
Carnegie Commission on Higher Education   2287
Carnegie Foundation for the Advancement of Teaching
    Flexner report on medical education in the U.S.   1976
Carroll L. Birch Award (American Medical Women's Association)
    1366
Case Western Reserve University Medical School (Cleveland, Ohio)
    Alumnae (specific)   255, 256, 1585, 1783, 1814, 3809
    Alumnae (survey)   2297, 3076, 3527
    Workshop on women in medicine   3094
Castile, New York   see   New York, Castile
Catalina Island, California   see   California, Catalina Island
Catholic Maternity Institute   see under   New Mexico, Santa Fe
Catholic Medical Missionary Society   see   Society of Catholic Med-
      ical Missionaries
Catholic physicians   162, 1873, 2661, 2665
Celler bill   see under   Armed services (U.S.)--Legislation
Cellular research, Women in   1576
Center for Women in Medicine (U.S.)   3563, 3817, 3966, 3967
Central Medical College of Syracuse (New York)   212
Central University of Venezuela   195
Certification statistics   see   Board certification statistics
Ceylon   see   Sri Lanka
Chambers (Helen) Research Laboratories   3295
Characteristics of women medical students   see   Medical students--
      Characteristics
Characteristics of women physicians
    Compared with those of automobile drivers   2419
    Compared with those of men   2878, 2901, 2921, 3018
    Compared with those of women athletes and lawyers   3083
    Relation to practice patterns   2297, 3073
    Stereotype   1955
Characteristics of women physicians (specific)   1856, 2390, 2411,
      2987, 3046, 3078, 3141, 3947
      See also specific characteristics, e.g., Longevity; and
      Determinants of medical careers (specific)
Aggression   1978
Anxiety   2359

Avoidance of responsibility 2854
Dominance 1978
Endurance 1978, 3973
Humanism 2947, 3911, 3970
Independence 3612, 3613, 4039
Insecurity 3613
Intuition 4022
Maternalism 1978, 2382, 2912
Modesty 3894, 4034
Motor ability 2419
Sexlessness 2870, 2874, 2879, 2923, 2945, 3053, 3621
Sympathy 2996, 3184
Charing Cross Hospital Medical School (England) 1921
Charlatan physicians see Quack physicians
Chelmsford League see Lady Chelmsford League (India)
Chengtu, China see China, Chengtu
Chicago Council of Medical Women see under Illinois, Chicago
Chicago, Illinois see Illinois, Chicago
Chicago Medical School (Illinois) 3386
Chichester Hospital for Women and Children see England, Brighton
              --Lady Chichester Hospital for Women and Children
Child care centers (See also Domestic help; and Children of women
              physicians)
    Attitudes towards 2130, 2356, 3983, 4013
    Day nursery for children of working women (USSR) 727
Child psychiatry see Psychiatry, Child
Child Welfare Division, Department of National Health (Canada)
              322
Childbirth see Obstetrics and gynecology
Children
    Education of 418, 464
    Labor of 3699
    Legislation affecting 424
    Marriage of 3854
Children, Handicapped, Work with see Handicapped children, Work
              with
Children of women physicians (See also Marriage; and Child care
              centers)
    Alternative care needs 1571, 2932
    Career advice to daughters 2963, 3174
    Congenital abnormality 2398, 2414
    Effects on medical activity 2197, 2216, 2217, 2237, 2440, 2847,
              2911, 2916, 2937, 3015, 3121
    Statistics 2133, 2286, 2354, 2354h, 2890
Children, Retarded, Work with see Retarded children, Work with
Children's Bureau (U.S.) 1822, 3666
Children's Free Kindergarten see under Michigan, Jackson City
Children's Hospital of San Francisco see under California, San
              Francisco
Children's Hospital (Sunderland) see under England, Sunderland
Children's Hospital Luetic Clinic (Washington, D.C.) see under
              Washington, D.C.
Children's Mercy Hospital see under Missouri, Kansas City

Chile
    Physicians (specific) 709, 721
    Physicians (status) 1945, 3943, 3948
Chile Women Physicians' Society 3948
China
    American physicians' observations 1172, 1369, 1372, 1764,
            1769-1771, 1773
    Foreign physicians 4, 503, 1124, 1194, 1237, 1596, 3200
    History of women in medicine 3853
    Medical education 2541, 3192, 3831, 3853
    Missionaries (specific) 835, 950, 1030, 1040, 1298, 1306,
            1410, 1641, 2527, 2531, 2534-2536, 2649, 2656
    Missionary activity 4, 2539, 2646, 2648, 2652
    Native physicians (specific) 4, 368, 699
    Native physicians (status) 3831, 3845, 3853
    Need for women physicians 359, 3850, 3853
China, Canton
    American missionaries 2585, 2586
    Hackett Medical Center 2532
China, Chengtu
    Canadian missionaries 2580
China, Chungmou
    Friends Hospital 1180
China, Foochow
    Mintsing Hospital 2575
    Missionaries 2583
    Woolston Memorial Hospital 1194
China, Kiukiang
    Bethel Mission 371
    Elizabeth Skelton Danforth Memorial Hospital 374
China, Manchuria
    British physicians 637
China Medical Association 2587, 3853
China, Mintsing
    Nathan Sites Memorial Good Shepherd Hospital 1194
China, Nanchang
    Women's and Children's Hospital 4
China, Nanking
    Friends Hospital 370
    Physicians 359, 1744
China, Peking
    Capital Hospital (formerly Peking Union Medical College Hos-
            pital) 369
China, Shanghai
    Bethel Mission 4
    Fearn Sanitarium 969, 1124
    Margaret Williamson Hospital 1306, 1654, 2653, 3196,
            3200
China, Soochow
    American missionaries 1212
    Women's Hospital 969
            See also Soochow Woman's Medical School
China, Su-Tsierr-Ku

Missionaries 1207
China, Tzechow
    Hospital 2579
China, Wei Hien
    Missionaries 2540
China, Wuchang
    Church Mission Hospital 1519
China, Wuhu
    American missionaries 1242
Chirala Mission Hospital see under India, Chirala
Chiropractic education see Education, Chiropractic
Chorus girls, Physicians as 1200
Christ Hospital see under Ohio, Cincinnati
Christian Medical College see Vellore Medical School (India)
The Christian Register, Editor 1721
Christianity effects on physicians 162, 370
Chungmou, China see China, Chungmou
Church Mission Hospital see under China, Wuchang
Cincinnati College of Medicine and Surgery see Cincinnati, Uni-
                versity of, Medical School (Ohio)
Cincinnati, Ohio see Ohio, Cincinnati
Cincinnati, University of, Medical School (Ohio) 238
Cincinnati, Woman's Medical College of see Laura Memorial Wo-
                man's Medical College (Ohio)
Cinema see Theater and films, Portrayal of women physicians
City Hospital (Minneapolis) see under Minnesota, Minneapolis
City Hospital of New Orleans see under Louisiana, New Orleans
City University of New York see New York, City University of,
                Medical School (New York)
Civil War (U.S.)
    Congressional Medal of Honor recipients 1084
    Physicians (specific) 247, 788, 1009, 1084, 1196, 1578, 1712,
                2755, 2794, 3451
    Sanitary Aid Commission 1637, 2755
Clapham Maternity Hospital see under England, London
Clapp, Cornelia Mary 692
Clara Swain Hospital see under India, Bareilly
Clement Cleveland Cancer Award 896
Clergy, Physicians as 1694
Cleveland Academy of Medicine see under Ohio, Cleveland
Cleveland Homeopathic College 1498, 3716
Cleveland Medical College see Case Western Reserve University
                Medical School (Cleveland, Ohio)
Cleveland, Ohio see Ohio, Cleveland
Clinic of Notre-Dame des Malades see under Pennsylvania, Phila-
                delphia
Clinics see under specific topics
Coeducation in medicine see Medical schools--Coeducational ques-
                tion
College Equal Suffrage League see under Woman suffrage
College of Medical Evangelists see Loma Linda University (Cali-
                fornia)
College of Midwifery of the City of New York 2033

College of Physicians and Surgeons (Ontario) see under Ontario
College of Physicians of Philadelphia see under Pennsylvania,
          Philadelphia
Collingswood, New Jersey see New Jersey, Collingswood
Colombia
     Physicians 704, 705
Colorado
     History of women in medicine 232
     Physicians 838, 850, 1377, 1576
     Public health department 901
Colorado, Denver
     Physicians 700, 850, 1101, 1471
Colorado, Fraser
     Physicians 1738
Columbia College (Washington, D. C.) see George Washington Uni-
          versity Medical School (Washington, D. C.)
Columbia County Health Department see under New York State
Columbia Presbyterian Medical Center see under New York City
Columbia University College of Physicians and Surgeons (New York
          City) 2071, 3505
Columbian College (Washington, D. C.) see George Washington Uni-
          versity Medical School (Washington, D. C.)
Columbus, Ohio see Ohio, Columbus
Communes, Attitudes towards 3983
Communism, Effects on physicians 363, 2587
Compton, California see California, Compton
Concord, New Hampshire see New Hampshire, Concord
Conference on Meeting Medical Manpower Needs--The Fuller Utiliza-
          tion of the Woman Physician 3056, 3952, 4030
Congo
     Missionaries 514, 1351
Congress of Women's Clubs of Western Pennsylvania see under
          Pennsylvania
Congressional Medal of Honor recipients 1084
Connecticut
     Physicians 2317
Connecticut, Middletown
     Middlesex Hospital 3675
Connecticut, Stamford
     Stamford Hospital, Stella Quinby Root Memorial Nursery 3493
Consciousness raising 908, 2311, 3713
Conscription, Attitudes towards 3983
Consultants, Medical, Women as see Medical consultants, Women
          as
Continuing education 2058
Contraception see Birth control
Contraceptive bill (Lord Damson's) see under Birth control
Contract surgeons see Armed services (U. S.)--Contract surgeons
          defined
Cook County Hospital see under Illinois, Chicago
Cooper Medical College see Stanford University Medical School
          (California)
Copenhagen, Denmark see Denmark, Copenhagen

Copenhagen, University of (Denmark) 45
Coping mechanisms of women physicians and medical students 1955,
          2852, 2969, 3055, 3066, 3127, 3164, 3170
Cornell University Medical School (New York) 880, 921, 1021, 1077,
          1134, 1535, 3804
Coroners see Forensic medicine, Women in
Cosmetic surgery, Women in see Plastic surgery, Women in
Council Bluffs, Iowa see Iowa, Council Bluffs
Counseling see Vocational guidance
Countess of Dufferin's Association see Dufferin Association
County medical societies see specific societies under their states
Court testimony see Criminal law--Physicians as expert witnesses
          and jurors
Cowper-Tempel bill (Scotland) 3919
Crimean War, Physicians in 206
Criminal law (See also Forensic medicine)
     Court appointed women physicians for women 2361
     Physicians as expert witnesses and jurors 2291, 2395
Criminology, Physicians' work in 1506
Crittenden Home (Iowa) see Iowa, Sioux City--Florence Critten-
          den Home
Crittenton General Hospital see under Minnesota, Rochester
Croatia see Yugoslavia
Crossnore, North Carolina see North Carolina, Crossnore
Cuba
     Physicians 711, 717
Curriculum see under Medical schools
Cushing, Harvey 1155
Cystic fibrosis differentiated from coeliac disease 290
Czechoslovakia
     Physicians (specific) 390, 403, 410, 1548, 1701
     Physicians (status) 2152, 2852, 2854
Czechoslovakia, Bratislava
     Municipal Hospital and Polyclinic 2853
     Physicians 384a

Dacca Medical School (Bengal, India) 1876
Dalhousie University, Medical School (Nova Scotia) 2148
Damson's bill see Birth control--Contraceptive bill (Lord Dam-
          son's)
Darmstadt, Germany see Germany, Darmstadt
Daughters of the American Revolution 769, 1307, 1539
Day care centers see Child care centers
DeKalb, Illinois see Illinois, DeKalb
Delancey, Margaret Munro 1755
Delhi, India see India, Delhi
Del Lowther and Downs
     Comments on their survey 2352
Delphi survey 1991
Denmark
     Physicians (specific) 45, 71, 415, 417, 441
     Physicians (status) 2167, 2175, 2176, 2258, 3364, 3896, 3902

Denmark, Copenhagen
    Eli Moeller's Clinic   45
Dentistry, Physicians in   1441, 1448
Denstists compared with physicians   3069
Denver, Colorado   see   Colorado, Denver
Department of Labor, Children's Bureau (U.S.)   see   Children's
            Bureau (U.S.)
Dermatology
    Careers in   2449
    French Society of Dermatology and Syphilology   1437, 1824
    Women in (specific)   13, 446, 656, 1538
Deseret Hospital   see under   Utah, Salt Lake City
Des Moines, Iowa   see   Iowa, Des Moines
Determinants of medical careers
    Surveys   2452, 2976, 3055, 3069, 3073, 3083, 3084, 3132
Determinants of medical careers (specific)   253, 861, 1121, 1714,
            1889, 2032, 3144, 3148, 3995
            See also Characteristics of women physicians
    Adult encouragement   1239, 2007, 2934, 4039
    Concern about health care   258, 1889
    Financial need   2869, 2891
    Independence it offers   1764, 2930, 4039
    Need for women to attend women
        India   2120, 2844, 3337
        U.S.   2997, 3029, 3031, 3034, 3183
        Western Europe   2864, 2873, 2898, 2906, 2909, 2930
    Religious sentiment   1340, 1533, 2603
    Scientific curiosity   1889, 4039
Deterrents to medical careers
    Suggestions for resolving   3056, 3059, 3103
    Surveys   3069, 3132
Deterrents to medical careers (specific)   228, 1858, 2995, 3113,
            3139, 3144, 3995
            See also Role conflict
    Biological makeup   1901, 2883, 2892, 2902, 3168
    Class antagonism   144
    Conditioning   2900, 3243
    Domestic duties   2852, 2854
    Feminine nature   253, 2877, 3013, 3954
    Inadequate income of physicians   2196, 2219
    Inferior intellect   2876, 2877, 2901, 2910, 2929, 3013, 3096,
        3179
    Inferior physiology   110, 2877, 2880, 2883, 2903, 3048, 3179
    Inferior preparatory education   3454
    Influence of anti-feminist attitudes to psychoanalysis   2297
    Loss of innocence   2858, 3890
    Male attitudes   2957, 3165, 3168, 3990
    Medical school conditions   2027, 2960, 3182, 3217, 3998, 4003
    Over-crowded medical profession   2896, 2897, 2924
    Poverty   3416, 3454, 4003
    Racial prejudice   1559
    Satan   370
    Social inertia   253

Societal pressure 2966, 3167, 3177
Traditional roles 3088, 3118, 3126, 3164, 3847
    U.S. 3040, 3061, 3087
    Western Europe 59, 2867, 2903, 3890
Victorian prudery 248
Vocational guidance 1863, 1875, 1952, 2006, 2949, 3088, 3090,
    4003, 4015
Detroit, Michigan see Michigan, Detroit
Dewade, New Guinea see New Guinea, Dewade
Dhar, India see India, Dhar
Diabetes control
    American Diabetes Association 1532
    Women in 817, 1444, 1447
Dickens Society see under Illinois, Chicago
Dietetics, Women in see Nutrition, Women in
Diphtheria, Work in 786, 834, 1312, 1616
Disarmament Conference (1932) 710
Disaster medicine see Emergency medicine
Discoveries and descriptions (medical) by physicians 290, 462, 533,
    552, 1075, 1250, 1576
        See also Inventions and innovations by physicians
Distinguished Daughters of Pennsylvania Award (Pennsylvania Fed-
    eration of Women's Clubs) 1572, 3432
District of Columbia see Washington, D.C.
Divorce statistics 3124
        See also Marital status
Dix, Dorothea Lynde 804
Dixon, Illinois see Illinois, Dixon
Dr. Susan Smith McKinney Junior High School see under New York,
    Brooklyn
Doctress used instead of "Doctor" 3032
Domestic help 3962, 3996
        See also Child care centers; and Housework, Attitudes
            towards
    Attitudes towards 2858, 2937, 3081
    House-care firms 3126
    Necessity for 2952, 3178, 3889, 4077
    Surveys 2136, 2355, 2356, 3152
Dominion Women's Enfranchisement Association (Canada) 356
Dover Emergency Medical Service Hospital see under England,
    Dover
Dover, England see England, Dover
Downstate Medical Center (New York) 2952
Drama see Literature
Dress reform 419, 789, 1048, 1712, 3109, 3830
Dropouts see Medical schools--Attrition...
Drug addiction, Physicians' work with 1444
Drug control, Attitudes towards 3983
Drug industry careers 2430
Dryden Springs, New York see New York, Dryden Springs
Duchess of York Hospital for Babies see under England, Man-
    chester
Dufferin Association 2116, 3852, 3926

Activities (1885-1895) 3333, 3334, 3339, 3347
   Criticism of its secular objectives 3340, 3342
   History and goals 3329, 3337, 3343
Duke of Richmond and Gordon Bill (England) 1931
Duke University, Medical School (Durham, North Carolina) 1978,
      3635
Dunedin, New Zealand see New Zealand, Dunedin
Duties of women physicians 3019, 3050, 3058, 3968
   Cooperate with male physicians 3066
   Disseminate health information 2349
   Exercise authority 3067
   Exercise moral leadership 2884, 2912, 2967, 3020, 3708,
      3984
   Maintain personal health 2985, 3017, 3109
   Make value judgments 2299
   Participate in community activities 3128
   Practice religion 2913, 3340, 3342
   Provide health care for women 2296, 2321
   Publish medical literature 2362
   Refuse to perform abortions 2331
   Retain femininity 2923, 2974
   Work for equal rights 2979, 3009, 3161, 3186
   Work towards racial preservation and improvements 2884, 2890
   Work with the lower class 2860, 3131
Dykman and Stalnaker
   Comments on their study 1979, 2336, 4012

Earnings see Medical practice--Earnings
East Gate Hospital see under Korea, Seoul
East Germany see Germany
East Pakistan see Bangladesh
Ecclesiastes, Book of
   Written by a woman physician 187
Ecuador
   Physicians 2948, 3364, 3949
Edinburgh Hospital for Women and Children see under Scotland,
      Edinburgh
Edinburgh Royal Infirmary see under Scotland, Edinburgh
Edinburgh School of Medicine for Women (Scotland) 679, 3934
Edinburgh, Scotland see Scotland, Edinburgh
Edinburgh, University of (Scotland)
   Debate over medical education of women
      Action brought against senatus by women students 3268,
         3314
      Admission to courses 3258, 3261, 3269, 3319
      Attitudes of the press 3252, 3254, 3271, 3298
      History 119, 124, 3266, 3919
      Personal memories 117, 624
      Student demonstrations 3251
   First woman medical graduate 661
   Medical students
      Examination marks (1870) 1932

        Survey (1960s) 2938
Education, Childhood see Children--Education of
Education, Chiropractic 3983
Education, Graduate medical see Internships and residencies; and
        Continuing education; and Retraining programs
Education, Medical (See also Medical schools; and Medical students)
        Cost effectiveness of educating women 2114, 2306
        Effects of World War II 276, 2737
        Opinions and predictions 1991, 2018, 3826, 3983, 4011
Education, Paramedical 2272, 3983
Education, Undergraduate and premedical 2286
Egypt
        Foreign physicians 379, 628
        Medical education 1
        Missionary activity 1521, 2526, 2646
        Native physicians 3364
Egypt (ancient)
        Healers 2, 25
Eighteenth century healers and physicians 30, 36, 79, 96, 152, 227
Electrotherapy, Physicians' work in 1110
Eleventh century healers see under Middle Ages
Eli Moeller's Clinic see under Denmark, Copenhagen
Elizabeth Bass Collection see Bass Collection on Women in Medi-
        cine (Tulane University)
Elizabeth Blackwell Award 245, 887, 1710, 1775
Elizabeth Blackwell centennial 695, 1092, 1093
Elizabeth Garrett Anderson Hospital see under England, London
Elizabeth Skelton Danforth Memorial Hospital see under China,
        Kiukiang
Elizabeth Steel Magee Hospital see under Pennsylvania, Pittsburgh
Ellen Mitchell Memorial Hospital see under Burma, Moulmein
Elsie Inglis Memorial Hospital see under Scotland, Edinburgh
Emergency Hospital see under Poland, Warsaw
Emergency Medical Service (Great Britain) see under World War
        II
Emergency medicine
        American Trauma Society 882
        Women in 2429, 3332
Emigrant physicians 478, 2244
Emily Blackwell Memorial see under New York City--New York
        Infirmary for Women and Children
Emmaus Home for Girls see under Missouri, St. Louis
Emory University Medical School (Atlanta, Georgia) 1732
Emotional involvement with patients see Characteristics of women
        physicians--Sympathy; and Patients--Emotional involve-
        ment with
Employment opportunities and services for women physicians 1857,
        2330, 4028
Endell Street Military Hospital see England, London--Military
        Hospital, Endell Street
Endocrinology, Women in 687, 699, 706, 1448, 1620
        See also Gynecologic endocrinology, Women in
England

American physicians   1827
Native physicians   1092, 1806
Nottingham and Notts Chirurgical Society   569
Oxford Regional Hospital Board   2049
Post-graduate medical education   2045
England, Aylesbury
  Female Convict Prison and Borstal Institution for Girls   627
England, Birmingham
  Birmingham General Hospital   2228, 2928
England, Brighton
  Lady Chichester Hospital for Women and Children   2193
  New Sussex Hospital   620
England, Bristol
  Walker Dunbar Hospital   3255
England, Dover
  Dover Emergency Medical Service Hospital   2710
England, Essex
  Goodmayes Hospital   2047
England, Gillingham
  Gillingham Welfare Association for the Care of the Aged Sick
        639
England, Hastings
  Physicians   112
England, Hull
  Physicians   616, 620
England, Lincolnshire
  Retraining program survey   2205
England, London
  American physicians   1514
  Bermondsey Medical Mission   627
  Clapham Maternity Hospital   2193
  Elizabeth Garrett Anderson Hospital (formerly New Hospital for
        Women, and St. Mary's Dispensary)   496, 3236, 3260,
        3320
  London County Council   2208, 3274, 3326
  London Homeopathic Hospital   559
  London Hospital   2248, 3270
  Marie Curie Hospital for Cancer and Allied Diseases   561, 3223,
        3247, 3248, 3273, 3295, 3323
  Military Hospital, Endell Street   2705
  Royal College of Physicians   629, 653, 3312
  Royal College of Physicians and Surgeons   3321
  Royal College of Surgeons   125, 282, 3305
  Royal Free Hospital   655, 2924, 3302, 3311
        See also London School of Medicine for Women
  South London Hospital for Women   2193, 3264, 3303
  West London Hospital   3291, 3292
England, Macclesfield
  Macclesfield Infirmary   525, 2229
England, Manchester
  Duchess of York Hospital for Babies   507, 2193
  Police physicians   2412
England, Sheffield

Women doctors' retraining scheme   2048
England, Sunderland
    Children's Hospital   3265, 3301, 3304
Epidemiology, Careers in   2393
Epsom College (Great Britain)   3250
Equal rights (See also Women's rights movement)
    Deferred in time of war   2751, 2768
    League of Equal Rights for Women (Tel Aviv, Israel)
        273
    Legislation   2364, 3137, 3161, 3517, 4083
    Physicians' support of   339, 420, 635, 940, 1340, 1462,
        4072
    Price   2874
Eskimos
    Missionary activity among   2648
Esthetic surgery, Women in   see   Plastic surgery, Women in
Etheridge, James H.   3409
Eugen Kahn Award (Baylor College of Medicine)   1117
Eugenics, Work in   816, 2884
Executions of physicians   70
Expert testimony   see   Criminal law--Physicians as expert wit-
        nesses and jurors
Eye and Ear Infirmary   see under   Massachusetts, Boston

Factories bill, Opposition by physicians   4072
Factory health inspectors   see   Occupational medicine--Careers in
Faculte de Medecine de Toulouse   see   Toulouse, Medical School of
        (France)
Faculty   see under   Medical schools
Faculty of Medicine   see   Paris, Ecole de Medicine (France)
Families in medicine   796
Familistere of Guise   see under   France
Family life, Attitudes towards   2299, 2988, 3983
Family planning   see   Birth control
Family practice (See also General practice)
    Careers in   2415, 2492
    Retraining program (Australia)   2041
    Suitability of women for   1864, 2029, 2268, 2499
    Women in (statistics)   2377, 2378
Farmers, Physicians as   304
Fearn Sanitarium   see under   China, Shanghai
Federal Women's Award recipient (U.S.)   1053
Federated Farmers Movement, Women's Division (New Zealand)
        304
Federation of Children's Agencies   see under   New York City
Federation of Medical Women of Canada   see   Canada, Federation
        of Medical Women of
Federation of Women's Dental Societies   1448
Female Medical College (Boston)   see   New England Female Medical
        College (Boston, Massachusetts)
Female Medical College of Pennsylvania   see   Medical College of
        Pennsylvania (Philadelphia)

Female Medical Education Society see under Massachusetts, Boston
Femininity conflict 2459, 3062, 3136, 3145
          See also Deterrents to medical careers (specific)--Fem-
          inine nature
Ferdman Hospital see under Washington, D. C.
Fett, Ione
          Comments on her article on Australian medical graduates 2143,
          2264
Fiction, Physicians and healers in see Literature--Physicians and
          healers in
Fifteenth century healers see under Middle Ages
Figure skating 1646
          (For other non medical activities see under Non med-
          ical activities)
Fiji, Suva
     Dispensary 3201
Films see Theater and films, Portrayal of women physicians
Financial planning 57, 78-80, 530
Finland
     Physicians (specific) 441, 470
     Physicians (status) 2167, 2863, 3364, 3907, 3909
Finland, Helsinki
     Helsinki Women's Clinic 3907
First century (AD) healers 20
First century (BC) healers 20
Fischer-Stevens Report statistics 2351
Florence Crittenden Home see under Iowa, Sioux City
Florida
     Physicians 1530, 1546, 1729
Flying Doctor Service (Australia) 301, 3205
Foochow, China see China, Foochow
Ford Motor Company, First woman physician 951
Foreign medical graduates 2327, 3924, 4030
Foreign Operation Administration (U.S.) 3550
Forensic medicine, Women in 318, 1130, 2395
          See also Criminal law
Fourteenth century healers see under Middle Ages
France
     American physicians (specific) 696, 749, 1486, 1487
     American Women's Hospitals 2804, 3231, 3402, 3554, 3599
     Familistere of Guise 844
     Healers 19, 32, 38, 74
     Medical education 3933, 3940
     Native physicians (specific) 428, 429, 437, 447, 449, 454, 455,
          460, 462, 469, 2382, 2387
     Native physicians (status) 2161, 2173, 2233, 3364, 3879, 3880,
          3891, 3894, 38999, 3933
     Practice patterns 1092, 2157, 2163, 2174
     Scottish physicians 585, 657
     World War I
          American physicians 1041, 1232, 1478, 2681-2684, 2744,
          2784, 3229
          British physicians 2699

Red Cross work   1115, 3900
World War II
    Physicians' activities   2169
France, Luzancy
    American Women's Hospitals   3553
France, Paris
    House of the Good Neighbor   3229
    La Maternité   844, 1364, 3222
    Medical education   1906, 1914
    Physicians   30, 452, 460a, 462
France, Reims
    American Memorial Hospital   3235
France, Royaumont
    Royaumont Hospital   2699
    Scottish Women's Hospitals   3923
Frances E. Willard National Temperance Hospital   see under   Illi-
        nois, Chicago
Fraser, Colorado   see   Colorado, Fraser
Freiburg, University of (Germany)   99
French Neurological Society   452
French Society of Dermatology and Syphilology   1437, 1824
French Society of Sanitary and Moral Prophylactics   428
Friends Hospital (Chungmou)   see under   China, Chungmou
Friends Hospital (Nanking)   see under   China, Nanking
Frontier Nursing Service (U.S.)   811
Full-time medical practice   see   Practice patterns--Full time
Fuller, Margaret   212
Fussell, Bartholomew   220

Gael, Mme. A.
    Comments on her book   2871
Galen Hall   see under   New York City
Garfield Memorial Hospital   see under   Washington, D.C.
Garrett, Mary E.   3434
Garrison, William Lloyd   3736
Gassett, Helen   3526
Gastroenterology, Women in   13, 1447
General Medical Council (Great Britain)   see under   British Medical
        Association
General practice
    Academy of General Practice of San Antonio (Texas)   1848
    Suitability of women for   1951, 2376, 2411, 2921, 3045, 3057
    Women in (status)   2213, 2394, 2408, 2479
Geneva College   see   Hobart College (Geneva, New York)
Geneva Disarmament Conference representatives   770
Geneva, New York   see   New York, Geneva
Geographical distribution of physicians   2177, 2184, 2189, 2256,
            2267, 2333, 2334, 2338, 2375, 4030
            See also Practice patterns
George Washington University Medical School (Washington, D.C.)
            1515, 1644, 2320, 2335, 3623
Georgetown University (Washington, D.C.)   2335

Georgia
    Physicians   802, 803, 1269, 1597, 2317
Georgia, Atlanta
    Physicians   1146
Georgia, Augusta
    Lenwood Division of the Veteran's Administration Hospital   1034
Georgia, Medical College of (Augusta)   1746, 2360, 3098
Geriatrics, Work in   618, 2343
German Association of Medical Women   105
German Society of University Women   488
Germany (See also Nazism, Effects on women physicians)
    Attitudes towards women medical students and physicians   1899,
        1903
    Comparisons with United States   3049
    Medical education   72, 73, 1895, 1897, 1898, 1902, 2889, 3882,
        3938, 3940
    Physicians (specific)   1434, 2386, 4016
    Physicians (status)   2258, 3364, 3882, 3883, 3904, 3908, 3910
    Responsibilities of physicians in racial preservation and im-
        provement   2884
Germany, Berlin
    Berlin Medical Society   3236
    Clinics for women   491, 492
    Physicians (specific)   2884
    Practice patterns   2186
Germany, Bingen
    Ruppertsberg Abbey   100
Germany, Darmstadt
    Heidenreich-von Siebold Foundation (for indigent expectant moth-
        ers)   479, 481
Germany, Hamburg
    American physicians   810, 2945
Germany, Quedlinburg
    Physicians   98
Germany, Wiesbaden
    Medical meeting (1898)   1899
Ghana
    British physicians   533
Ghana, Berekum
    Holy Family Dispensary   893
Ghandi, Mahatma
    Personal physician to   4004
Giessen, University of (Germany)   479
Gillingham, England see England, Gillingham
Gillingham Welfare Association for the Care of the Aged Sick see
        under England, Gillingham
Gillow Foundation (Colombia) see Arthur S. Gillow Foundation for
        Scientific Research and Preventive Medicine (Colombia)
Gimbel Philadelphia Award recipients   976, 1435
Girl Scouts Organization   1384, 2315, 3190
Girton College (England)   617
Glasgow Award see Janet M. Glasgow Award (American Medical
        Women's Association)

Glasgow, University of, Medical School (Scotland) 2199, 2241, 2934
Goethe, Johann Wolfgang 2386
Gold Coast see Ghana
Golden Diploma Award (Graz, University of Austria) 416
Goodenough Report (Great Britain) 109, 113, 1933
            See also Medical schools--Coeducational question
Goodmayes Hospital see under England, Essex
Gotham Hospital see under New York City
Gothenburg, Sweden see Sweden, Gothenburg
Göttingen University Medical School (Germany) 3230
Goucher College 1792
Gouverneur Hospital see under New York City
Grace Hospital see under Michigan, Detroit
Grand Rapids, Michigan see Michigan, Grand Rapids
Grant Medical College (Bombay, India) 1876
Graz, Austria see Austria, Graz
Graz, University of, Medical School (Austria) 416, 1901, 2158
Great Britain
    History of women in medicine 224
    Hospitals run by women 2257
    Medical education 1961, 2018, 3940
Greece (See also American Women's Hospitals Service--Activities;
            and Scottish Women's Hospitals--World War I activities)
    American Women's Hospitals 1719, 3502, 3649
    Foreign physicians 677, 833, 1437, 1485, 1807
    Native physicians 62, 433, 448, 451
    Scottish Women's Hospitals 291, 2687
Greece (ancient)
    Healers 20, 21, 25, 68, 132, 133, 152
Greeley, Horace 3452
Greene Sanitarium see under New York, Castile
Gregory, Samuel 212, 223, 253, 3526, 3651, 3772
Groningen, University of (Netherlands) 445
Guadalupe Clinic see under California, San Diego
Guatemala
    Physicians 3364
Guidance counseling see Vocational guidance
Guntur, India see India, Guntur
Guntur Mission Hospital see under India, Guntur
Gynecologic endocrinology, Women in 1708
            See also Endocrinology, Women in
Gynecology see Obstetrics and gynecology

Hackett Medical Center see under China, Canton
Hackett Medical College for Women (Canton, China) 4, 3853
            See also China, Canton--Hackett Medical Center
Hadassah Hospital see under Israel, Haifa
Hahnemann Medical College (Philadelphia, Pennsylvania) 3539
Haifa, Israel see Israel, Haifa
Haiti
    German physicians 490
Halle, University of (Germany) 91

Halle-Wittenberg, University of (Germany) 1899
Hamburg, Germany see Germany, Hamburg
Handicapped children, Work with 800, 822
Handicapped physicians 285, 1442, 2375
Harvard University Medical School (Cambridge, Massachusetts)
    Alumnae 1466, 2972, 3046, 3055, 3072, 4004
    Coeducation controversy 249, 1238, 2476, 3386, 3422, 3543,
            3602, 3636, 3691
    Faculty 1091, 1567
    Joint committee on the status of women 3520
    Proposed absorption of New England Female Medical College
            248
    Students 2969, 3055, 3089, 3487, 3542, 3645, 3775
Harvey, Elwood 220
Hastings, England see England, Hastings
Havana, University of (Cuba) 717
Hawaii
    Physicians' impressions of 1766
Hawaii, University of, Medical School (Honolulu) 2992
Health care
    Maternal and child 353a, 582
        Sheppard-Towner Act 1815, 2354e, 4031
    Students 2409
Health care system
    Necessity for changes 3003, 4036
Health occupations, Vocational guidance see Vocational guidance
Health of women physicians 895, 2278, 2398, 2414, 2533, 4017
Health Protection Clinic see under Public health
Hebrew healers 150
            See also Jewish physicians
Heidelberg, University of, Medical School (Germany) 3220
Heidenreich-Von Siebold Foundation see under Germany, Darm-
            stadt
Helsingfors, University of (Finland) 727
Helsinki, Finland see Finland, Helsinki
Helsinki, University of (Finland) 3909
Helsinki Women's Clinic see under Finland, Helsinki
Hematology, Women in 761, 1138, 1699
Hering Homeopathic Medical College of Chicago (Illinois) 3741
Hermaphrodite physicians 596
Hernels, Austria see Austria, Hernels
"Hero of Labor" Award (USSR) 730
Herzegovina, Yugoslavia see Yugoslavia, Bosnia and Herzegovina
Higher education amendments (of 1972) 1983
            See also Medical schools--Admissions policies--Legisla-
            tion
Higher Women's Courses (Moscow, USSR) 207
Hindu physicians 265, 279
Historians see Medical historians
History of women in medicine (See also under specific institutions
            and organizations. See also Medical historians)
    Asia 3198, 3199, 3853, 3856
    Cuba 717

Debate over identity of first woman physician 190
International 3933
Medical and graduate medical education 452, 1057
Sources 3998
USSR 736, 3216
Western Europe 441, 448, 484, 678, 3875
Hitler, Adolf
Physicians' encounters with 1434
Hobart College (Geneva, New York) 844
Elizabeth Blackwell's association with 1286, 1364, 1650, 1755
Elizabeth Blackwell Citation 245, 887, 1710
Hoffman-La Roche plant physicians see under New Jersey, Nutley
Holland see Netherlands
Holy Family Dispensary see under Ghana, Berekum
Holy Family Hospital (Mandar) see under India, Mandar
Holy Family Hospital for Women and Children (Rawalpindi) see
under Pakistan, Rawalpindi
Home of the Friendless see under Michigan, Jackson City
Homeopathy, Women in 748, 1681
Hong Kong
Medical students 276
Paediatric Society 571
Physicians 271, 275, 278, 282, 284, 571, 3364
Hong Kong, University of, Medical School 276, 283, 571
Hospital of the Good Shepherd see under Illinois, Chicago
Hospitals see specific hospitals under their geographic locations.
See also Internships and residencies; and Psychiatric
hospitals
Administration, Women in 2467, 2649, 2922, 2942
Appointment of women physicians, Necessity for 1954
Debarment of women students 1920, 1927
Established and run by women 47, 161, 300, 3215, 3923
First woman appointed house physician to mixed-sex hospital
525, 531
Housing accommodations for women interns 2094
Military 611, 742, 1337, 1426, 2832
Missionary 2646, 3857
Nunneries as 26
Staff positions
Exclusion of black women 855, 2229
Flexibility for married physicians 2210
Goodenough Report recommendations 1933
Status of women in 224, 2160, 2174, 2255, 2711
Surveys 2054, 2088, 2154, 2172, 2212, 4042
Temperance 3765
Veteran's Administration 1034, 1725, 3619
Wartime acceptance of medical women 1939, 2711
Hospitals, Women's see specific hospitals under their geographic
locations.
See also American Women's Hospitals Service; and
Scottish Women's Hospitals
Eastern Europe 204, 2153
History 2193

Medical school affiliations 2096
Missionary established 2517
Run by women 2257, 2368, 3323
House of a Thousand Babies see China, Shanghai--Margaret Williamson Hospital
House of the Good Neighbor see under France, Paris
Household help see Domestic help
Housework, Attitudes towards 3136, 3152
            See also Domestic help
Housing reform, Physicians active in 616
Howard University Medical School (Washington, D.C.) 859, 1559, 2335
Howe Kai Po (Ida Kahn's mother) 2592
Howell, Mary C.
    Comments on her article on what medical schools teach about women 2037
Hull, England see England, Hull
Hull House see under Illinois, Chicago
Hungary
    Medical education 1890
    Physicians 16, 386, 387, 395, 400, 401, 408, 409, 412
Husbands see Marital partners
Hussey, Cornelia 844
Hyderabad Medical School (Sindi, India) 1876
Hygiene see Social hygiene
Hygiene movement 253
Hysterectomy techniques see under Obstetrics and gynecology

Ibadan, Nigeria see Nigeria, Ibadan
Iceland
    Mental Hygiene Conference 1727
    Physicians 1365
Illinois
    Hospital survey 2088
    Occupational Disease Commission 1177, 1567
    Physicians (specific) 1196-1198
    Physicians (statistics) 4020
    Shawmut Mining Company 1061
    Waukesha County Medical Society 905
Illinois, Chicago
    Chicago Council of Medical Women 1534, 3581
    Chicago Medical Society 1830
    Chicago Woman's Club 2100
    Chicago Woman's Shelter 1591
    Cook County Hospital 805, 1347, 1424, 1471, 1764, 2099
    Dickens Society 800
    Frances E. Willard National Temperance Hospital 3765
    Hospital of the Good Shepherd 1498
    Hull House 1177, 1567
    Lewis Maternity Hospital 1764
    Medical Women's Club of Chicago 1642, 2088, 2779, 4083
    Michael Reese Hospital 2092

Municipal Tuberculosis Sanatorium 1229
    Physicians 970, 1169, 1186, 1617, 1652
    Social Hygiene Council of Chicago 1845
    Women and Children's Hospital of Chicago (formerly known as
          Mary Thompson Hospital) 771, 1722, 3615, 3735
          History 1253, 1455, 3566, 3659, 3721, 3764, 3823
Illinois, DeKalb
    Physicians 1334
Illinois, Dixon
    Physicians 1184
Illinois, Quincy
    Physicians (specific) 780
Illinois, University of, Medical School (Urbana) 2005, 2282
Immunology see Allergy and immunology
Imperial Medical-Surgical Academy (USSR) 200, 207
Inactive physicians see Practice patterns--Inactive
Income see Medical practice--Earnings
India
    American missionaries 515, 1118, 1135, 1157, 1235, 1581,
          1805
    American physicians 812, 1369, 1373, 1799, 2116, 3829
    British physicians 502, 546, 549, 603, 666, 669, 2116, 2120,
          3336, 3851
    History of women in medicine 3, 2123
    Hospitals run by women 2257, 2517
    Medical education 1876, 1877, 2844, 3849, 3852
    Missionaries (specific) 315, 435, 2527, 2531, 2534-2536, 2656
    Missionary activity 2116, 2517, 2539, 2646, 2648, 2652, 2665
    Native physicians (specific) 265, 267, 269, 272, 285, 2123,
          3840
    Native physicians (status) 2116, 2121, 2126, 2127, 2846, 3364,
          3827, 3834, 3855
    Opportunities for physicians 2117, 2121, 2258, 2389, 2510,
          2596, 3828, 3848, 3851, 3857
    Recruitment 3927
    Social conditions 666, 3854
India, Ahmedabad
    Missionaries 2620
India, Ajmer
    Ajmer Women's Hospital 2608
    British missionaries 634
India, Allahabad
    Missionary activity 2612
India, Ani
    Missionaries 2618
India Association of Medical Women 2595, 3330, 3344, 3346
India, Bapalta
    American missionaries 2602
India, Bareilly
    Clara Swain Hospital 2643
India, Baroda
    Mrs. William Butler Memorial Hospital 1581
India, Benares

Missionaries   2624
India, Bombay
    Missionaries   2600
India, Chirala
    Chirala Mission Hospital   3338
India, Delhi
    St. Stephen's Hospital   435
India, Dhar
    Missionaries   2537, 2623
India, Guntur
    Guntur Mission Hospital   3338
    Missionaries   2616, 2629
India, Kashmir
    Missionaries   2632
India, Ludhiana
    Memorial Hospital   3336
India, Madras
    Royal Victoria Hospital for Caste and Gosha Women   666
India, Madura
    Women's Hospital   1799
India, Mandar
    Holy Family Hospital   2611
India, Medak
    American missionaries   2622
India, Nasik
    Pechey-Phipson Sanitarium   603
India, Neemuch
    Missionaries   2606
India, Palwal
    Rohmatpur Hospital   669
India, Patna
    American missionaries   2645
India, Punjab (See also Pakistan)
    Physicians' activity   2597, 2639
    Women's and Children's Hospital   2637
India, Rajahmundry
    Rajahmundry Mission Hospital   3338
India, Ramapatam
    Missionaries   2601
India, Rawalpindi   see   Pakistan, Rawalpindi
India, Sialkot
    American missionaries   2640, 2642
    Memorial Hospital   2636, 2638
India, Thuruthipuram
    Archbishop Attipetty Jubilee Memorial Hospital   2609
India, Vellore
    American missionaries   1277, 2630
    Mary Taber Schell Memorial Hospital   1277, 1805, 2634
India, Wai
    American physicians   3829
India Women's Reserve Medical Unit   3332
Indiana
    Medical education   2025

Medical societies   1784
Indies see Indonesia
Indonesia
     Foreign physicians   1443, 1850
     Need for women physicians   1850
     Practice patterns   2261
Indonesia, Kediri
     Clinic   1443
Indonesia, Semarang
     Physicians   2261
Industrial medicine see Occupational medicine
Industrialization of medicine   3003
Infirmary for Women and Children see New York City--New York
               Infirmary for Women and Children
Innsbruck, University of, Medical School (Austria)   1901, 2158
Inspector-General of British Army Hospitals see Armed services
               (Great Britain)--Inspector-general of army hospitals
Institute for Officers' Daughters see under Austria, Hernels
Institute of Pennsylvania, Strecker Award recipients   756
Insurance
     National health insurance   2201, 3239, 3284, 3327, 3983
Insurance companies
     Employment of women physicians   416, 2358, 2498, 2888
Insurance for women physicians   2341, 3921, 4074, 4075, 4087
Internal medicine, Work in   907, 2455
International Academy of Pathology   329, 342
International Association of Medical Museums   329, 342
International Association of Women Physicians see Medical Wo-
               men's International Association
International Conference of Women Physicians see Young Women's
               Christian Association Conference
International Council of Women Congress (1904)   3874
International Medical Woman's Association for the Promotion of
               Postgraduate Study   3354
Internships and residencies (See also Hospitals--Housing accommoda-
               tions for women interns)
     Association of Internes and Medical Students   1947
     Exclusion of women   300, 2046, 2060, 2068, 2071, 2072, 2109-
               2111, 3023, 3154, 3187
          Justification for   2059, 2106, 2107
          Specific physicians' experiences   1296
     Exclusion of women (1930-1940s)   2953, 3986, 4023
     First woman to intern with United States Army Medical Corps
               742
     Hospital administration attitude survey (1926)   2091, 2094, 2095
     Medical Women's Federation stand (1931)   2046
     Opportunities for women   2040, 2066, 2067, 2078-2080, 2084,
               2096, 2105
          Black interns   2093
          Catholic hospitals   2101
          Jewish hospitals   2092
          Temperance hospitals   3765
     Part-time training programs

      Psychiatry 2053, 2062-2065, 2073
      Surveys 2087, 2089
   Part-time training programs (specific) 2047, 2049, 2052, 2057,
      2076, 2102, 2103
   Preceptorship programs 2050
   Problems for women 2069, 2086, 3170, 3995
   Selection of hospital 2097
   Surveys 2054, 2061, 2075, 2081-2083, 2085, 2087, 2088
The Interpretator (Australia) 292
Inventions and innovations by physicians (See also Discoveries and
      descriptions (medical) by physicians)
   Chair for switchboard operators 1585
   Food storage techniques 1192
   Medical museum classification 348
   Medical record keeping 1585
   Return receipt for registered mail 868
   Subway seats 1749
   Surgeons' glove powder 4026
   Surgical needle 1253
Iowa
   Physicians (specific) 890, 1110, 1279, 1335, 1604
   Physicians (status) 2350, 3963
   State Society of Iowa Medical Women 954, 1406, 3488, 3557,
      3604, 3746
Iowa, Council Bluffs
   Physicians 827
Iowa, Des Moines
   Methodist Hospital 829
Iowa, Sioux City
   Florence Crittenden Home 1500
Iowa, University of (Iowa City) 784
Iran (See also Armenia)
   Physicians 1484, 3364
   Red Cross work in 270
Iran, Tabriz
   American missionaries 2521
Iran, Teheran
   Physicians 270
Iraq, Baghdad
   British physicians 519
Ireland
   History of women in medicine 114
   Medical education 1921, 1925, 2168, 2170
   Physicians (specific) 432, 435, 443, 444, 467, 2607
   Practice patterns 2168, 2170
Israel
   Physicians 273, 834, 2119, 2126, 3364, 3833, 3842
Israel, Haifa
   Hadassah Hospital 273
Israel, Jerusalem
   Museum of Pathology 273
Israel, Tel Aviv
   League of Equal Rights for Women 273

Israeli Women's Medical Association 3833
Italian Association of Women Physicians   465, 3877
Italy
    Deterrents to medical careers   59
    Healers   59, 60, 65, 76
    Medical education   60, 73
    Physicians (specific)   418, 457, 464-466, 476, 2383, 3892
    Physicians (status)   2156, 2173, 2874, 3364, 3877, 3878, 3892,
            3903, 3906
Italy, Rome
    First hospital   26
    Psychiatry clinic   418
Italy, Rome (ancient)
    Healers   46, 56, 67, 68, 132, 133, 159, 162
Italy, Salerno
    Healers   23

Jackson City, Michigan see Michigan, Jackson City
James Walker Memorial Hospital see under North Carolina, Wil-
            mington
Janet M. Glasgow Award (American Medical Women's Association)
            1345, 1549
Japan (See also American Women's Hospitals--Activities)
    American Women's Hospitals   3397
    History of women in medicine   280, 3198, 3199, 3856
    Medical education   286, 3195
    Missionaries   2656
    Physicians (specific)   277, 280, 281, 286, 696, 1772, 3844,
            3860
    Physicians (status)   3194, 3195, 3364, 3836, 3837, 3841, 3858,
            3859
Japan, Tokyo
    St. Luke's Hospital   3202
    Tokyo Medical Society for Women   3837
Japanese Medical Women's Society   3194, 3202, 3841
Jefferson Medical College (Philadelphia)   1274, 1305, 1917, 3622
Jerusalem, Israel see Israel, Jerusalem
Jessie Weston Fisher Laboratory see Connecticut, Middletown--
            Middlesex Hospital
Jewish physicians (See also Hebrew healers)   37, 70, 152, 155
Johannesburg, South Africa see South Africa, Johannesburg
John Ordonaux Prize (George Washington University Medical School)
            1515
Johns Hopkins University Hospital see under Maryland, Baltimore
Johns Hopkins University Medical School
    Admission of women   1977, 2034, 3091, 3383, 3434
    Alumnae survey (1960s)   2359
    Faculty   761
    Students (specific)   913, 1006, 1138
Journal of the American Medical Women's Association   3591, 3694,
            3761
Journal of the Association of Medical Women in India   2124

Journals, Medical women's see Journal of the American Medical
Women's Association; Medical Woman's Journal; and
Journal of the Association of Medical Women in India
Judson Health Center see under New York City
Jurors, Physicians as see Criminal law--Physicians as expert wit-
nesses and jurors
Juvenile court physicians 1289

Kalamazoo, Michigan see Michigan, Kalamazoo
Kansas
Physicians 1225, 1418, 3932
Kansas City, Missouri see Missouri, Kansas City
Karolinska Institute for Medicine and Surgery (Stockholm, Sweden)
1908, 1940, 2166
Kashmir, India see India, Kashmir
Kate Depew Strang Tumor Diagnostic and Treatment Clinic see
New York City--New York Infirmary for Women and
Children--Strang Cancer Clinic
Kate Hurd Mead Alumnae Award (Medical College of Pennsylvania)
1089
Kediri, Indonesia see Indonesia, Kediri
Kennedy, John F. , Physician to see White House physicians
Kentucky (See also American Women's Hospitals--Activities)
American Women's Hospitals 3584
Physicians 1662, 1809-1812
King Edward Hospital Medical School (Indore, India) 1876
King Edward Medical College (Lahore, India) 1876
King George's Medical College (Lucknow, India) 1876
Kings College (London, England) 1921
Kiukiang, China see China, Kiukiang
"Klumpke Palsy" 462
Kollontai, Alexandra 456
Korea
Missionaries 346, 351, 728, 1087, 1266, 1319, 2529, 2530,
2535
Physicians 3190, 3193, 3364, 3846, 3847
Korea, Seoul
East Gate Hospital 3193
Korea, Woman's Medical Institute of (Seoul) 1422, 1878, 3847
Korea, Yong Dong
Salvation Army Hospital 1649
Korean War
Physicians 1317
Krakow, University of, Medical School (Poland) 378
Kuwait
American missionaries 878, 1693
Kwangtung Medical College for Women see Hackett Medical Col-
lege for Women (Canton, China)
Kwashiorkor 533

Labrador

American physicians 1809
Ladies' Medical Missionary Society (Boston) 3540
Ladies' Physiological Institutes see under Massachusetts, Boston
Lady Chelmsford League (India) 2116
Lady Chichester Hospital for Women and Children see under England, Brighton
Lady Dufferin's Association see Dufferin Association
Lady Hardinge Medical College and Hospital (Delhi, India) 1366, 1876, 3341, 3852
Lady Willingdon Medical School for Women (Madras, India) 1876
Lafayette General Hospital see under New York, Buffalo
Lafayette, Louisiana see Louisiana, Lafayette
Lallemand Prize (Academy of Science, Paris) 466
Langley Porter Neuropsychiatric Institute see under California, San Francisco
Language
    Importance in denoting physicians' sex 3032
Lasker Awards (American Public Health Association) 1230
Latin America (See also specific countries)
    Missionary activity 2648
Laura Memorial Woman's Medical College (Ohio) 3549, 3965
        See also Cincinnati, University of, Medical School (Ohio)
Laval, University of (France) 2163
Lawyers
    Comparisons with physicians 3069, 3083, 3144
    Specific physicians as 911, 1628, 1793, 1820
League of Equal Rights for Women (Tel Aviv) 2090
League of Nations 710, 1437, 2260, 3282
Lebanon
    Missionaries 2526
Legal medicine see Forensic medicine
Legislation (See also under specific topics and specific countries)
    Anti-discrimination laws 1337, 2364, 2503, 3023, 3056, 3185, 3573
Leipzig, University of (Germany) 85
Leningrad Military Hospital see under USSR, Leningrad
Leningrad School of Medicine for Women see St. Petersburg School of Medicine for Women (USSR)
Leningrad, USSR see USSR, Leningrad
Lewis Maternity Hospital see under Illinois, Chicago
Libraries, Physicians' work in 810
Licensure (Great Britain) 2193, 2234
            See also Medical Register (Great Britain)
Licensure (Sweden) 63
Lincolnshire, England see England, Lincolnshire
Literature (See also Theater and films, Portrayal of women physicians)
    Dedications in books by women physicians 692
    Physicians and healers in 29, 43, 146, 149, 1251, 3227, 4017, 4052, 4057, 4058
Little Mothers' League see under New York City
Lockheed Aircraft Corporation, Plant physician 1831
Loma Linda University (California) 3816

London, England see England, London
London Homeopathic Hospital see under England, London
London Hospital see under England, London
London Hospital Medical School (England) 687
London School of Medicine for Women (England) (See also England,
          London--Royal Free Hospital)
     Effect of Goodenough Report on 1933
     Faculty and deans 655, 3302
     Founding 119, 679
     History 109, 496, 616, 666, 1926, 2193, 3244, 3310, 3926
London, University of (England) (See also specific colleges)
     Admission of women to medical degrees 3317
     Convocation, exclusion of women medical graduates 3289
     Exclusion of women medical students 1933, 2917, 2926, 2940,
          2941, 3259, 3275
     Regulations affecting women 3246, 3315, 3316
     Report on medical education of women 1916, 3243
     William Julius Mickle Fellowship 653
Long Beach, California see California, Long Beach
Long Island College of Medicine (New York) 2370
Longevity 2961, 3001
               See also Age distribution of physicians; and Character-
               istics of women physicians (specific)
Los Angeles, California see California, Los Angeles
Louisiana, Lafayette
     Physicians 876, 1387
Louisiana, New Orleans
     City Hospital of New Orleans 2101
     Orleans Parish Medical Society 819, 1404
     Physicians' activities 982, 3937
     Sara Mayo Hospital (formerly New Orleans Dispensary for Wo-
          men and Children) 1404, 1482
Loyalty among women physicians see Support among women physi-
          cians and medical students
Loyola University Medical School (Chicago, Illinois) 1532, 1550,
          1764, 2354e, 3069
Lubyanskie Course for Women (Moscow, USSR) 202
Lucretia Mott Dispensary and Infirmary see under New York,
          Brooklyn
Ludhiana, India see India, Ludhiana
Ludhiana Medical College (India) 1876, 3331, 3336
Ludhiana, Women's Christian Medical College of see Ludhiana
          Medical College (India)
Lund, University of (Sweden) 2166
Lutheran Hospital see under California, Pasadena
Luzancy, France see France, Luzancy
Lymphatic system 1576

MCAT see Medical College Admission Test
Macclesfield, England see England, Macclesfield
Macclesfield Infirmary see under England, Macclesfield
McGill University Medical School (Montreal, Quebec) 342, 350,

1611, 2260, 3211
McKinney Jr. High School see New York, Brooklyn--Dr. Susan
          Smith McKinney Junior High School
Macronisi
     Quarantine station (American Women's Hospitals) 1027, 1547
Madagascar
     Physicians 2126, 3364
Madera, California see California, Madera
Madras, India see India, Madras
Madras Medical College (India) 1876, 2616, 3330, 3335, 3832
Madura, India see India, Madura
Magistrates, Physicians as see under Politics
Maine
     Physicians 938, 1336
Malagasy Republic see Madagascar
Male attire and haircuts, Women physicians' and healers' use of
          137, 650, 667, 868, 1514, 1578, 1600
Male impersonators, Women physicians as 171, 528, 652, 661, 717
Malpractice insurance see Insurance for women physicians
Malpractice, Physician tried for 975
Management positions see Administrative positions for women
          physicians
Manchester, England see England, Manchester
Manchester Medical School (England) 578
Manchester University Medical School (England) 507, 2925
Manchuria, China see China, Manchuria
Mandar, India see India, Mandar
Manila, Philippine Islands see Philippine Islands, Manila
Manitoba, University of 318, 343
Manitoba, Whitemouth
     Physicians 314
Mankota, Minnesota see Minnesota, Mankota
Mao, Tse-tung 369
Margaret Williamson Hospital see under China, Shanghai
Marie Curie Hospital for Cancer and Allied Diseases see under
          England, London
Marie de Medicis, Queen, Consort of Henry IV, King of France
          692
Marihuana legalization, Attitudes towards 3983
Marire Hospital see under New Zealand, Stratford
Marital partners 2199, 3006, 3085, 4015
     Attitudes 2473, 3044, 3081
     Occupations 2189, 2286, 2297, 2336
Marital status (See also Divorce statistics)
     Statistics
          (1900-1930s) 2189, 2261, 2890
          (1950s) 2213, 2286, 2354, 2354h
          (1960s) 2146, 2175, 2199, 2211, 2224, 2236, 2332, 2342,
               2346, 2359, 4015
          (1970s) 2133, 2136, 2148, 2168, 2272, 3124
Marriage (See also Children--Marriage of; and Divorce statistics;
          and Single women physicians)
     Effects on and compatibility with medical activity 1759, 2180,

　　　　　2183, 2354b, 2845, 2919, 2925, 3150, 3156, 3160
　　　(1800s)　2284, 2876, 3053, 3131, 3168
　　　(1950s)　2226, 2354, 3149, 3162, 3167
　　　(1960s)　1862, 1867, 2197, 2209, 2216, 2217, 2240, 2336,
　　　　　2408, 2911, 2966, 2994, 3015, 3962, 3995
　　　(1970s)　2130, 2132, 2440, 2937, 2998, 3030, 3054, 3073,
　　　　　3119, 3127, 3144, 3163, 3182
　　Effects on and compatibility with psychiatric careers　2426,
　　　　2469
　　Effects on and compatibility with surgical careers　2446
　　Employment restrictions for women (Great Britain)　2194, 2195,
　　　　　2198, 2208, 2210, 2228, 2250, 2406, 2914, 2920, 2931
　　　Medical Women's Federation activities　2928, 3242, 3274,
　　　　　3277, 3282, 3325, 3327
　　Employment restrictions for women (Sweden)　2160, 2165
Martha Tracy Memorial Fund　3626
Mary J. Johnston Memorial Hospital　see under　Philippine Islands,
　　　Manila
Mary Putnam Jacobi Fellowship Fund　409, 1147, 1148, 1414, 1701,
　　　3485, 3999, 4000
Mary Taber Schell Memorial Hospital　see under　India, Vellore
Mary Thompson Hospital　see　Illinois, Chicago--Women and
　　　Children's Hospital of Chicago
Mary Thompson Statue　see　Art depicting women physicians
Maryland
　　Women's Medical Society of Maryland　1282, 3421, 3424
Maryland, Baltimore
　　Johns Hopkins University Hospital　2095
　　Medical education of women　1792
　　Physicians (specific)　1234, 1753, 1792, 3424
　　University of Maryland Hospital　744, 1310
Maryland College of Pharmacy (Baltimore)　1574
Maryland, University of, Medical School (College Park)　756
Massachusetts
　　Massachusetts Reformatory for Women　1624, 1716
　　Massachusetts State Medical Society　1783, 1809, 3070, 3387,
　　　　3422, 3431, 3732
Massachusetts, Boston
　　Boston State Hospital　1843
　　Eye and Ear Infirmary　1545
　　Female Medical Education Society　212, 3513, 3540
　　Gynecological Society of Boston　3736
　　History of women in medicine　248, 249, 1783
　　Homeopathic Medical Society　693
　　Ladies' Physiological Institutes　212
　　New England Hospital for Women and Children　247, 255, 1068,
　　　　1453, 1778, 3406, 3647, 3703
　　Peter Bent Brigham Hospital　2071
　　Physicians (specific)　1238, 1707, 1711, 1782, 1783, 2493
Massachusetts Eye and Ear Infirmary　see　Massachusetts, Boston--
　　　Eye and Ear Infirmary
Massachusetts Reformatory for Women　see under　Massachusetts
Maternal and child health care　see　Health care--Maternal and child

Maternité, La see under France, Paris
Maternity and Children's Hospital (Manila) see under Philippine
       Islands, Manila
Maternity Hospital (Mankota) see Minnesota, Mankota--St. Joseph's
       Hospital
Maternity Hospital (Minneapolis) see under Minnesota, Minneapolis
Mayo Clinic see under Minnesota, Rochester
Mayo Medical School (Rochester, Minnesota) 3803
          See also Minnesota, Rochester--Mayo Clinic
Medak, India see India, Medak
Medal of Honor recipients see Congressional Medal of Honor re-
       cipients
Medical Academy of Warsaw see Warsaw Medical Academy (Po-
       land)
Medical associations see Organizations, Medical
Medical College Admission Test (MCAT) 1855, 2007, 2008, 2031
          See also Medical schools--Admissions statistics; and
          Medical schools--Applicant statistics
Medical College for Women (Edinburgh, Scotland) 3934
Medical College of Georgia see Georgia, Medical College of
       (Augusta)
Medical College of Pennsylvania (Philadelphia)
    Activities (1930s-1950s) 3738, 3790, 3792, 3794-3797, 3799,
        3800, 3812
    Admission of males 3658, 3667, 3728, 3771
    Admissions criteria 3749
    Alumnae 265, 280, 370, 851, 866, 1687, 2284, 2649, 2653,
        3723
    American Medical Women's Association liaison 3611, 3822
    Building innovations 3653, 3715, 3791
    Centennial 3508, 3510, 3511, 3609, 3683, 3820
    Commencement addresses (1851-1891) 2284, 2967, 2986, 3020,
        3021, 3037, 3067, 3109-3111, 3131, 3133, 3163, 3708
    Commencement addresses (1893-1919) 2975, 3019, 3038, 3057,
        4037
    Commencements 3523, 3524, 3663, 3673, 3677
    Curriculum 2055, 3558, 3680
    Deans and presidents 243, 1507, 1734, 1789, 3389
    Faculty 629, 1407, 1448, 1784, 2354e, 3661, 3670, 3676, 3793
       Early years 212, 758, 3605, 3751, 3752, 3789
    Funding 3432, 3506, 3608, 3618, 3644, 3674, 3821
    History 932, 3389, 3509, 3572, 3624, 3635, 3718, 3719, 3734,
        3788, 3810
    Importance to women 253, 1993, 3389, 3428, 3607, 3620,
        3754, 3778, 3787
    Library 3559, 3638, 3640, 3747, 3781
    Opening addresses (1850-1923) 258, 1953, 2816, 2985, 2987,
        3107, 3970, 3994, 4014
    Proposed merger with Jefferson Medical College 3522, 3798
    Reminiscences 3552, 3753, 3777
    Retraining programs 2053, 2070, 2074, 2104, 3563
    Scholarships and awards 1089, 4006
    Special programs 1568, 2057, 3533

Specific departments   326, 952, 3605
Students   2016, 2984, 3492, 3529, 3671, 3679, 3739, 3786,
        3807, 3966, 4009
Medical consultants, Women as   2196, 2206
Medical Council of New Zealand   see   New Zealand Medical Council
Medical courses for women (Leningrad, USSR)   see   Nikolaev Mili-
        tary Hospital Medical Courses for Women
Medical education   see   Education--Medical
Medical Education for National Defense (MEND)   2429
Medical Evangelists   see   Loma Linda University
Medical historians   75, 333, 797, 947, 1371
        See also History of women in medicine
Medical Institute for Women (Leningrad, USSR)   203
        See also Nikolaev Military Hospital Medical Courses for
        Women (Leningrad, USSR)
Medical licensure   see   Licensure...
Medical Mission Sisters   see   Society of Catholic Medical Mission-
        aries
Medical museum classification   348
Medical organizations   see   Organizations, Medical
Medical practice   2147, 2175, 2230, 2369, 4028, 4036, 4071
        See also Practice patterns
    Earnings (pre-1950s)   2190, 2284, 2302, 2328, 2354b, 2357,
        2369, 2375, 2599, 3169
    Earnings (1950s-1970s)   2148, 2286, 2300, 2309, 2336, 2342,
        2346, 2374, 2452
    Socio-economic factors affecting   2138, 2226, 2290, 2373, 3928
Medical Practitioners' Union (United Kingdom)
    Surveys by   2216, 2220, 2227
Medical record keeping   1585
Medical Register (Great Britain)   1158, 3919
        See also Licensure (Great Britain)
Medical schools (See also Medical students; and Education, Medical;
        and Affirmative action; and specific schools)
    Admissions committees   1995, 3182
    Admissions criteria   1855, 1860, 1872, 1875, 1876, 1921, 2007,
        2028, 2971, 3958, 3973
    Admissions policies
        Legislation   1893, 1936, 1983, 3919
        Opinions on   1936, 3667, 4026
    Admissions quotas   1879, 1952, 2004, 2137, 3990
        Justification   2000, 2006, 2200, 2316, 2372
    Admissions statistics (1930s-1960s)   1915, 1933, 1959, 1992,
        1999, 2010, 2035, 2036
    Admissions statistics (1960s-1970s)   1924, 1946, 1966, 2013,
        4030
    Applicant statistics (1920s-1950s)   1959, 1992, 2020
    Applicant statistics (1960s)   1883, 1885, 1886, 1924, 1985,
        1986, 2017, 2023, 2024, 4030
    Applicant statistics (1970s)   1881, 1962, 1963, 1968-1971, 3122
    Attrition, Reasons for   1972, 1997, 1998, 2016
    Attrition statistics   1883-1885, 1924, 1959, 1972, 1987, 1988,
        2035, 3635

Backlash reaction to feminism   3039
Coeducational   1858, 1904
Coeducational question   1896, 1954, 1976, 1977, 2898
    Great Britain   1916, 1918, 1921, 2917, 2921, 2926
    United States   253, 1957, 1958, 1976, 2011, 2021, 2032,
        2034, 2983, 3386, 3995
Curriculum
    Need for revision   1608, 1990, 1994, 1997, 2001, 2007,
        3120, 3427, 3958
Deans' Delphi survey   1991
Debarment of women students   1920, 2193, 3487, 3699, 3908,
        4023
    Justification   1926, 2843, 2881, 2887, 2903
Discrimination studies   1955
Enrollment statistics (pre-1960)   1897, 1923, 1967, 2005, 2039,
        2868, 4008, 4045
Enrollment statistics (1960s-1970s)   1880, 1882-1884, 1960,
        1965, 3635
Examining boards   1925, 1928, 1929
Faculty
    Opportunities   2314, 2466
    Women as (specific)   356, 478, 1134
    Women as (status)   1991, 2174, 2204, 2256, 2284, 2305,
        2316, 2354e, 2364, 2425, 3986, 3995, 4042
Sectarianism as favorable for women   253
Sponsored by religious groups   1873, 1941, 2598
Support programs   1982, 2992, 3027, 3135
Medical schools, Women's   161, 164, 333, 1996, 3512, 3783
Need for   1984, 2100, 3031, 3454, 3496
Medical social service (See also Public health)
    Women in   627
Medical societies see Organizations, Medical
Medical students (See also Education, Medical; and Medical schools)
    Academic performance   1915, 2031, 3100, 3442
    Advice   1855, 1953, 2912, 3957, 3973
    Anxiety   2014, 2938, 3055
    Association of Internes and Medical Students   1947
    Attitudes of   2934, 2935, 2938, 2958, 3089, 3098, 3123, 3635
    Attitudes taught   1983, 2037
    Attitudes towards   249, 1903, 1905, 1955, 1983, 2037, 2868,
        2905, 3120
    Characteristics   1978, 2016, 2938, 2977, 2984, 3100, 3749
    Comparisons with law, nursing, and teaching students   3063
    Effects of studies   2893
    Finances   1860, 1862, 1947, 1956, 1974, 1975, 3958, 4028
    Geographical distribution   1883-1885, 1889
    Minority statistics   1946, 1965, 1966
    Parents of   1886, 1910, 3063
    Problems   1950, 1952, 1990, 3051, 3088, 3090
    "Rites of passage" (medical profession)   2016, 3092
    Role conflict   1982, 2001, 2007
    Sisterhood with non-physician health care workers   3064, 3089
    Specialty selection   1886, 1889, 2444, 2908

Undergraduate schools attended 1964
Medical Woman's Journal
    Editors 1423, 3632, 3633
    History 3531, 3534, 3556, 3560, 3591, 3722
    Purpose 1975, 3388, 3433, 3501, 3637, 3641, 3681, 3693,
        3730
    Stands 3093, 3562, 3630, 3631
Medical Women's Federation (Great Britain) (See also specific cities
        for branches. For campaigns and stands see under
        specific topics)
    Adjustment to wartime disruption 3276
    Cancer research committee 3915
    History 507, 512, 588, 3297, 3318
    Meetings, council (1920s) 3239, 3242, 3278-3282, 3328
    Meetings, council (1930s) 3277, 3283-3287, 3324-3327
    Meetings, general 3240, 3300
    Overseas reports 3241, 3288
    Purpose 3245, 3249, 3308
    Representation in British Medical Association 3262
    Surveys 2220, 2230, 2926
Medical Women's International Association
    Congresses 2259, 3352-3353, 3363-3365, 3376, 3935
    History 3355, 3358-3360, 3366, 3374
    Meetings 3348, 3356, 3361, 3362, 3370, 3377
    Purpose 3349, 3357, 3364, 3369, 3372
Medical Women's National Association see American Medical
        Women's Association
Medicine women see American Indian physicians and healers
Medico-Surgical Academy (USSR) 197
Melbourne, University of (Victoria) 7, 299, 2879, 3861
Melbourne, Victoria see Victoria, Melbourne
Memorial Hospital (Ludhiana) see under India, Ludhiana
Memorial Hospital (New York) see New York City--Memorial Hos-
        pital, Cancer Prevention Clinic
Memorial Hospital (Sialkot) see under India, Sialkot
Memorials to women physicians see Art depicting women physi-
        cians
MEND see Medical Education for National Defense
Meningitis research, Work in 1250
Menstruation, As deterrent to medical careers 2059, 2892, 3013
        See also Deterrents to medical careers--Biological
        makeup
Menstruation, Information on 3240, 3279, 3325
Mental hospitals see Psychiatric hospitals
Merida Medical College (Mexico) 716
Metabolic research, Work in 1447
Methodist Episcopal Church, Woman's Foreign Missionary Society
        2527
Methodist Episcopal Home see under New Jersey, Collingswood
Methodist Hospital see under Iowa, Des Moines
Metropolitan Asylums Board (England) see under Psychiatric hos-
        pitals
Mexican American women students, Statistics see Medical students--

Minority statistics
Mexico
    American missionaries 928, 1139
    Physicians (specific) 694, 707, 712, 716, 2947
    Physicians (status) 3364, 3945
Mexico, University of, Medical School 707
Miami Medical College see Cincinnati, University of, Medical
            School (Ohio)
Michael Reese Hospital see under Illinois, Chicago
Michigan
    Board of pharmacy 1447
    Physicians (specific) 916-920, 942, 951, 1655, 1664, 1670-
            1672, 1677-1686
    Physicians (status) 2327, 3075, 3725, 3939
Michigan, Ann Arbor
    Ann Arbor Private Hospital for the Mentally Disturbed 1557
    St. Joseph Mercy Hospital 1380
    University Hospital (University of Michigan) 3022
Michigan Asylum for the Insane see under Michigan, Kalamazoo
Michigan, Battle Creek
    Battle Creek Sanitarium 920, 1671, 1677, 1678
    Physicians 1420, 1673
Michigan, Detroit
    Blackwell Medical Women's Society 3521, 3725
    Grace Hospital 1447
    Woman's Hospital and Infants' Home 2095, 2096, 2367, 2368,
            3769
Michigan, Grand Rapids
    Physicians 1499
Michigan, Jackson City
    Children's Free Kindergarten 1401
    Home of the Friendless 1401
Michigan, Kalamazoo
    Michigan Asylum for the Insane 1679
Michigan, Muskegon
    Physicians 825
Michigan, Sturgis
    Physicians 1675
Michigan, University of (Ann Arbor) 1190
Michigan, University of, Medical School (Ann Arbor) 362, 372, 987,
            1498, 1670, 1671, 3157, 3442, 3805
Middle Ages (500-1500)
    Healers 15, 47, 53, 64, 69, 76, 149, 150, 159, 3923
    Jewish physicians 37, 70
    11th century healers 75, 150
    12th century healers 29, 59, 76, 89, 100, 152
    13th century healers 19, 59, 76, 152
    14th century healers 19, 22, 152
    15th century healers 152
Middle East (See also specific countries)
    Physicians 3843
Middlesex Hospital see under Connecticut, Middletown
Middlesex Hospital Medical School (London, England) 1915, 2217

Middletown, Connecticut see Connecticut, Middletown
Midwifery
     As forerunner to medical education   72, 252, 3216
     Attitudes towards 1382, 3012, 3239
     Education 197, 200, 1900
     History 27, 67, 144, 216
     Women in 32, 74, 248, 779, 1390, 2165
Military hospitals see Hospitals--Military
Milwaukee, Wisconsin see Wisconsin, Milwaukee
Mining company physicians 1061
Ministers, Physicians as see Clergy, Physicians as
Minneapolis, Minnesota see Minnesota, Minneapolis
Minnesota
     Minnesota State Medical Association 787
     Minnesota Suffrage Association 787
     Physicians 786, 787, 830, 1240
Minnesota, Mankota
     St. Joseph's Hospital (formerly Maternity Hospital) 786
Minnesota, Minneapolis
     Asbury Hospital 787
     City Hospital 787
     Maternity Hospital 786
     Northwestern Hospital for Women and Children 787
     St. Joseph Hospital 786
Minnesota, Rochester
     Crittenton General Hospital 1550
     Mayo Clinic 2077, 3407, 3803
               See also Mayo Medical School (Rochester, Minne-
               sota)
Mintsing, China see China, Mintsing
Mintsing Hospital see under China, Foochow
Misericordia Hospital see under Pennsylvania, Philadelphia
Missionaries
     Attitudes towards Dufferin Association 3340, 3342
     British physicians 530
     Canadian physicians 12
     Physicians (specific) 312, 313, 315, 351, 515, 657, 715, 1410,
               1592, 2945
     Recruitment 2515, 2596
     Training of 2510, 2657, 2663
Missionary activity 2254
               See also Society of Catholic Medical Missionaries; and
               Medical schools--Sponsored by religious groups; see
               also under specific countries
     History 2665
     In Africa 608, 685, 1042, 1201, 1468, 1521
     In Burma 1104, 1504
     In China 950, 1030, 1040, 1207, 1212, 1242, 1298, 1410, 1662
     In India 315, 435, 502, 546, 632, 634, 669, 1118, 1135, 1157,
               1235, 1277, 1581, 1641, 1805, 3338
     In Indonesia 1443
     In Korea 346, 1087, 1266, 1319
     In Kuwait 878, 1693

In Mexico 1139
In Middle East 3843
In Nepal 1135
In Philippine Islands 832
In Turkey 1565
In Zaire 514, 1351
Specific societies 1592, 2527, 2528, 2532, 3540
Mississippi
Mississippi State Medical Society 693, 847
Missouri
Physicians 815, 1703
Missouri, Kansas City
Children's Mercy Hospital 3759
Women's and Children's Hospital 1255
Missouri, St. Louis
Emmaus Home for Girls 1039
Monash University survey (Australia) 2133
Monopoly, Medicine as 2995
Montessori schools 418
Montevideo, University of (Uruguay) 701
Montpellier Medical School (France) 657
Montpellier, University of (France) 149
Montreal, Quebec see Quebec, Montreal
Mormons, Physicians as 1632
Morocco
French physicians 429, 440, 455
Morocco, Tangier
Missionaries 4060
Moscow, USSR see USSR, Moscow
Mothercraft 290, 298, 424, 533, 616, 1409, 2982
See also Health care--Maternal and child; and Ob-
stetrics and gynecology
Mothers and Babies Health Association (Australia) 298
Moulmein, Burma see Burma, Moulmein
Mount Holyoke College (South Hadley, Massachusetts) 1068
Mount Sinai Hospital see under New York City
Mount Sinai Medical School see New York, City University of,
Medical School
Movies, Portrayal of women physicians see Theater and films,
Portrayal of women physicians
Mrs. William Butler Memorial Hospital see under India, Baroda
Municipal Hospital and Polyclinic see under Czechoslovakia,
Bratislava
Municipal Tuberculosis Sanatorium see under Illinois, Chicago
Museums, Medical see Pathology--Museums
Museums, Medical--Classification system 348
Muskegon, Michigan see Michigan, Muskegon
Mymensingh, Bangladesh see Bangladesh, Mymensingh
Mythological healers 67, 137

Nanchang, China see China, Nanchang
Nasik, India see India, Nasik

Nathan Sites Memorial Good Shepherd Hospital see under China,
           Mintsing
National Academy of Sciences (U.S.) 1138, 1564
National American Woman Suffrage Association 967, 2790
National Association for Supplying Female Medical Aid to the Women
           of India see Dufferin Association
National Board examinations 2031
National Cancer Institute of Canada 356
National Congress of Dispensers (Hungary) 16
National Council on Health Careers (U.S.) 1866
           See also Vocational guidance
National Eclectic Medical Association (U.S.) 212
National health insurance see under Insurance
National Health Service (Great Britain) 2196, 2222
           See also Public health
     Women Doctors' Retainer Scheme 2048, 2203, 2235, 2249
     Women Doctors' Retraining Scheme 2048
National Institutes of Health (U.S.) 1713, 3808
National Medical and Dental University (Washington, D.C.) 3623
National Union of Women Workers (Great Britain) 616
National White Cross League (U.S.) 1591
National Woman's Party Convention (1942) 3678
National Working-Women's Association (U.S.) 1254
Navy (U.S.) see under Armed services (U.S.)--Physicians (spe-
           cific)
Nazism, Effects on women physicians 105, 2161, 2259, 3362, 3904
Near East (See also specific countries; and American Women's
           Hospitals--Activities)
     American Women's Hospitals 1106
Nebraska
     Nebraska State Medical Society 801, 1231
     Physicians 1078, 1113, 1365, 1592, 1720
Nebraska, Walthill
     Susan La Flesche Picotte Hospital 1592
Neemuch, India see India, Neemuch
Neilsville, Wisconsin see Wisconsin, Neilsville
Nepal
     American missionaries 1135
     Shanta Bhawan Hospital 1135
Netherlands
     Physicians (specific) 66, 417, 425, 445, 453, 461, 3901
     Physicians (status) 2167, 2261, 2380, 2387, 3364, 3884, 3901
Netherlands Company for the Promotion of Medical Sciences see
           Royal Netherlands Company for the Promotion of Med-
           ical Science
Netherlands East Indies see Indonesia
Netherlands Society of Women Physicians 3901
Neurasthenia, Physicians who have 895
Neurology (See also Pediatric neurology, Careers in)
     French Neurological Society 452
     Women in 452, 460a, 462, 466
Neuropathology, Women in 1155, 1843
           See also Pathology

Neuropsychiatry, Women in   1076
          See also Psychiatry
Neurosurgery, Careers in   2447
          See also Surgery
Nevada City, California see California, Nevada City
New Brunswick
     Physicians 355
New England (U.S.) (See also specific states)
     American Medical Women's Association 3568
     Physicians 1780
New England Female Medical College (Boston, Massachusetts) (See
          also Boston University Medical School (Massachusetts))
     Faculty 1585, 1781
     Founding 3034, 3526
     History 212, 223, 230, 3420, 3513, 3651, 3772, 3774, 4037
     Opening address (1852) 3065
New England Hospital for Women and Children see under Massa-
          chusetts, Boston
New England Journal of Medicine 2322
New England Women's Medical Society see New England--American
          Medical Women's Association
New Guinea
     American physicians 2514
New Guinea, Dewade
     Anglican Mission Dispensary 2514
New Hampshire
     Physicians 995, 1780
New Hampshire, Concord
     New Hampshire Memorial Hospital for Women and Children
          1558, 3780
New Hampshire Memorial Hospital for Women and Children see
          under New Hampshire, Concord
New Hospital for Women see England, London--Elizabeth Garrett
          Anderson Hospital
New Jersey
     Camden County Medical Society 1741
     Physicians' attitudes 3983
New Jersey, Bridgeton
     Bridgeton Hospital 1405
New Jersey, Collingswood
     Methodist Episcopal Home 1741
New Jersey Medical School (Newark) 2958
New Jersey, Newark
     Newark City Hospital 899
     Physicians 899
New Jersey, Nutley
     Hoffman-La Roche Plant physicians 1691
New Jersey, Somerville
     Somerset Hospital 1651
New Mexico
     Missionary activity 2660
New Mexico, Santa Fe
     Catholic Maternity Institute 2660

New Mexico, University of, Medical School (Albuquerque) 1731,
       3806
New Orleans Dispensary for Women and Children see Louisiana,
       New Orleans--Sara Mayo Hospital
New Orleans, Louisiana see Louisiana, New Orleans
New South Wales, Sydney
    Rachel Forster Hospital 289, 290, 3204, 3861
New Sussex Hospital see under England, Brighton
New Wilmington, Pennsylvania see Pennsylvania, New Wilmington
New York Academy of Medicine see under New York City
New York, Binghamton
    City physician 1447
    Well Baby Health Station 1409
New York, Brooklyn
    Dr. Susan Smith McKinney Junior High School 750
    First woman physician 1499
    Lucretia Mott Dispensary and Infirmary 964
    Williamsburgh Hospital 1412
New York, Buffalo
    Lafayette General Hospital (formerly Riverside Hospital) 1367
    Physicians (specific) 1018
    St. Rita's Home for Exceptional Children 1442
New York, Castile
    Greene Sanitarium 912, 1038, 1046, 1164, 1417
New York City
    Ambulance surgeons 785, 1108
    American Woman's Association Clubhouse 3701
    Babies' Hospital 1374
    Bellevue Hospital 2096
    Columbia Presbyterian Medical Center 1735
    Federal Reserve Bank of New York, medical division 1041,
           1412
    Federation of Children's Agencies 1601
    Galen Hall 1749
    Gotham Hospital 1564, 3530
    Gouverneur Hospital 785, 1077, 1462, 1535
    Judson Health Center 818
    Little Mothers' League 1601
    Memorial Hospital, Cancer Prevention Clinic 3657
    Mount Sinai Hospital 2092
    New York Academy of Medicine 1263, 1494
    New York Foundation, Population Council 2490
    New York Hospital Medical Center 3804
    New York Infirmary for Women and Children (formerly New
           York Dispensary for Poor Women and Children) (See
           also Women's Medical College of the New York In-
           firmary for Women and Children)
        Activities (1850s-1870s) 3445, 3447, 3450, 3451, 3453,
               3455, 3456, 3467
        Activities (1880s) 3473-3476, 3478-3483
        Building plans 3414, 3538, 3616, 3776
        Emily Blackwell Memorial 1456
        Founding 844, 1806, 3443, 3484

Funding 3811
History 3491
History by Annie Sturges Daniel 222, 932, 933, 3629
Importance of 3576
Male physicians 3448, 3449
Proposed merger with Columbia University-Presbyterian
    Hospital Medical Center 3437, 3724
Reopening (1924) 1111
Strang Cancer Clinic 896, 921, 1083, 1563, 1618
Survey by 4042
Trustees 3446, 3448, 3452
New York Posture League 1749
Out-patient services 817
Physicians (specific) 779, 1383
Public health administration 779, 822, 1031, 1601, 1836, 2358
St. Vincent's Hospital 2102
Settlement house work 1152
Town hall forum 1835
Women's Medical Association of New York City
    Femininity perception survey 3145, 3146
    History 3575, 3656
    Mary Putnam Jacobi Fellowship Fund 409, 1414, 3999,
        4000
    Meetings 3535, 3578, 3579
    Tributes to women physicians 537, 1264
    World's Fair activities (1939) 3697
New York, City University of, Medical School (New York) 2440
New York, Dryden Springs
    Physicians 897
New York, Geneva
    Physicians 694
New York Herald Tribune camp physicians 1447
New York Hospital Medical Center see under New York City
New York Hygeio-Therapeutic College (New York City) 212
New York Infirmary for Women and Children see under New York
    City
New York Medical College (New York City) 977, 1989, 1990
    Part-time residency program in psychiatry 2053, 2062, 2063,
        2065
New York Medical College and Hospital for Women (New York City)
        3514, 3717
New York Medical College of the Infirmary see Women's Medical
        College of the New York Infirmary for Women and
        Children (New York City)
New York, Oswego
    Physicians 1712
New York Post Graduate School (New York City) 2637, 3354
New York, Poughkeepsie
    Bowne Memorial Hospital 1167, 1837
    Physicians 393, 752
New York, Pulaski
    Physicians 701
New York, Rochester

Strong Memorial Hospital   2052
New York State
   Bronx County Medical Society   1383
   Columbia County Health Department   1062, 1344
   Dutchess County Medical Society   1496
   New York County Medical Society   1532, 3578
   New York State Medical Society   1447, 3698
   Physicians (specific)   750, 1018, 1133, 1836
   Physicians (status)   2317
   Tri County Medical Society of Buffalo, Trempealeau and Jackson counties   793
   Women's Medical Society of New York State
      History   1480, 3419, 3646
      Legislation activities   3486, 3544, 3642
      Meetings   2373, 3418, 3565, 3612, 3613, 3648, 3662, 3696, 3709-3711, 3720, 3726, 3744, 3815
      Purpose   3574, 3577
      Scholarship funds   1878, 3813, 3814
   Wyoming County Medical Society   1367
New York University Medical School (New York City)   3756
New York, Utica
   Physicians   1130
New Zealand
   American physicians   1532, 1767, 1768
   Native physicians   3364
New Zealand, Dunedin
   Society for the Protection of Women and Children   306
New Zealand Medical Council   2131, 2135
New Zealand, Stratford
   Marire Hospital   296
New Zealand, Wellington
   St. Helen's Maternity Hospital   301
   Women Students' Hostel   301
Newark City Hospital   see under   New Jersey, Newark
Newark, New Jersey   see   New Jersey, Newark
Newfoundland
   Physicians   316
Nigeria, Ibadan
   University College Hospital   3189
Nightingale, Florence   247, 617, 666, 844, 845, 2987
Nikolaev Military Hospital Medical Courses for Women (Leningrad, USSR)   197, 200, 202, 203, 207
      See also Medical Institute for Women (Leningrad, USSR)
Nineteenth century
   Social context   212, 225, 239, 1846, 3940
Nobel Prize recipients   1433, 3673
Noguchi Medal (Nebraska State Medical Society)   1231
Non medical activities (See also Vacations for women physicians)
   Bird watching   1589
   Bookstore operation   1633
   Carnival appearances   1085
   Collecting World War II mementos   1610

    Community participation 3701, 3968
    Congressional stenographer work 1721
    Cookery school management 1501
    Effects on medical activity 2852
    Figure skating 1646
    Mountain climbing 1083
    Playwriting 1706
    Poetry writing 424, 472, 1588, 1752
    Sculpting 867, 1743, 4082
    Short story writing 4084
    Weaving 1068
Norfolk, Virginia see Virginia, Norfolk
Norristown, Pennsylvania see Pennsylvania, Norristown
Norristown State Hospital see under Pennsylvania, Norristown
North Carolina (See also American Women's Hospitals--Activities)
    American Women's Hospitals 3584
    First woman to practice medicine in 1199
    North Carolina State Medical Society 221, 1199
    Physicians 254, 828, 1199, 1200-1208, 1210-1212, 1214, 1216,
        1217, 1219, 1220
North Carolina, Asheville
    Physicians 1213, 1447
North Carolina, Crossnore
    Crossnore School 828, 915, 1205, 1705
North Carolina Medical College 221, 1209, 1575
North Carolina, University of, Medical School (Chapel Hill) 1215,
        1982
North Carolina, Wilmington
    James Walker Memorial Hospital 1218
North Carolina, Winston-Salem
    City Hospital 744
    Physicians 744, 1310
North China Union Medical College for Women 4005
North Dakota
    Physicians 1193, 1315, 1613
Northern Ireland (See also Ireland)
    Physicians 421, 458
Northwestern Hospital for Women and Children see under Minne-
        sota, Minneapolis
Northwestern University Medical School (Chicago, Illinois)
    Arguments against readmitting women 3621
Northwestern University Woman's Medical College
    Closing (1902) 3048, 3669
    Commencement address 2973, 3496-3498, 3959
    Faculty and dean 3700
    History 1253, 1640, 1689, 3497, 3603, 3668, 3705
    Missionary alumnae 3498
    Survey of alumnae 3497, 3498
Norway
    Physicians (specific) 434, 442
    Physicians (status) 2167, 3364, 3888, 3893
Nottingham University School of Medicine (England) 2935
Nova Scotia

Physicians 332, 340, 345, 352, 357, 2148
Nu Sigma Phi fraternity 3495
Nunneries as hospitals see Hospitals--Nunneries as
Nuns as physicians 162
Nurses (See also Army Nurse Corps (U.S.))
    Cincinnati Visiting Nurse Association (Cincinnati, Ohio) 1258
    Physicians as 513
    Physicians' relationships with 247, 2191, 2726, 2747, 2946,
        3127
Nurses' education
    Role of physicians in 225, 451, 833, 869, 978, 2946, 3454,
        3883
Nursing service
    Physicians' work with 820
Nutley, New Jersey see New Jersey, Nutley
Nutrition, Women in 699, 713, 1026, 1370, 1691
        See also Rickets research, Women in
[Nyankunde] Medical School (Zaire) 514

Oberlin College (Oberlin, Ohio) 802
Obesity control, Physicians' work in 1609
Obstetrical Society of London (England) 3206, 3237, 3293, 3306
Obstetrical Society of Philadelphia 1435
Obstetrics and gynecology (See also Gynecologic endocrinology,
        Women in; and Mothercraft)
    American Academy of Obstetrics and Gynecology 811
    American Association of Obstetricians, Gynecologists and Ab-
        dominal Surgeons 2323
    Attitudes of women in 2490
    Boston Gynecological Society 3736
    Careers in 2463
    Education of women (19th century) 216
    History of women in 2
    Hysterectomy techniques 1097
    Obstetrical Society of London 3237, 3293, 3294, 3306
    Obstetrical Society of Philadelphia 1435
    Prenatal clinics 1150
    Proposed exclusion of male physicians 2472
    Royal College of Obstetricians 282
    Societies, Women members 3294, 3390
    Spanish Society of Gynecologists 422
    Suitability of women for 1858, 2032, 2202, 2384, 2405, 2472,
        2877, 3034, 3070, 3188, 3237
    Women in (specific)
        Canada 343, 354
        Hungary 387, 401
        Iraq 518
        New Zealand 295
        Philippine Islands 268
        U.S. 744, 1171, 1310, 1352, 1354, 1411, 1435, 1764,
           1774, 1804, 1844, 1845
        Western Europe 30, 36, 58, 80, 479, 483, 489, 619

Occupational medicine (See also specific companies)
    American Medical Women's Association activities 3695
    Careers in 2500
    Legislation affecting physicians 220
    Women in (specific) 722, 1091, 1177, 1447, 1524, 1691, 1831
Ohio
    Physicians (specific) 956, 997, 1227, 1494, 1554, 1726
    Physicians (statistics) 2317
Ohio, Cincinnati
    Christ Hospital 1258
    Cincinnati Medical Women's Club 1150
    Physicians (specific) 1150, 1168, 1258, 1606
Ohio, Cleveland
    Cleveland Academy of Medicine 1324, 1747
    Physicians 256, 775, 979
    Seaman Free Dispensary 775
    Woman's General Hospital (formerly Women's and Children's
        Free Medical and Surgical Dispensary) 3528, 3687
Ohio, Columbus
    Physicians 1084
Ohio, Toledo
    Ohio State Hospital for the Insane 2108
Olympic games, Exclusion of women 3699
Omsk Medical Institute (USSR) 723
Ontario
    College of Physicians and Surgeons 333
    Medical education 11
Ontario Medical College for Women (Toronto) 333, 2255
            See also Toronto, University of, Medical School (On-
            tario); and Ontario, Toronto--Woman's College Hos-
            pital
Ontario, Toronto
    Federation of Medical Women of Canada, Retraining programs
        2044
    Sunnybrook Medical Centre 2044
    Toronto General Hospital 693
    Woman's College Hospital 11, 354, 3208, 3212
            See also Ontario Medical College for Women (Toronto)
Ophthalmology
    Careers in 2435
    Women in (specific) 521, 717, 729, 1175, 1202, 1457, 1545,
        1721, 3218
Opium, Investigations of 1298
Opportunities for women physicians' employment see Employment
        opportunities and services for women physicians
Ordonaux Prize see John Ordonaux Prize
Oregon
    Oregon State Medical Society 1020, 1528
    Physicians 1080, 1088, 1119, 1325, 1561, 1638
Oregon, Portland
    Health department 794
    Physicians 1115, 1299
    Portland City Medical Society 759

Oregon, Salem
    Physicians 1523
Oregon, University of, Medical School (Portland) 1430
Organizations, Medical (See also specialty societies under their spe-
            cific specialty; and national associations under their
            specific names; and specific state and country societies
            under their geographic locations)
    Dues 2341
    Exclusion of women physicians 225, 4023, 4032
    Representation of women physicians 2284, 2354f, 2483, 3159,
        3504, 3768
    State societies 1399, 1528, 2318, 3431, 3684
    Suitability of women as members 3499
    Women's admission to 214, 2256
Organizations, Medical women's see national associations under
            their specific names
    Disinterest among younger women 3612
    Duties 2354f, 3818, 3953
    First in U.S. 1057
    Necessity for 3186, 3375, 3390, 3573, 3574, 3613, 3650,
        3689, 3713, 3757, 3758
    Need for women physicians to join 4076
Oriental medical students, Statistics see Medical students--
            Minority statistics
Orleans Parish Medical Society see under Louisiana, New Orleans
Orthopedics, Women in 699, 1234, 1348
Osmania Medical College (Hyderabad, India) 1876
Oswego, New York see New York, Oswego
Otago, University of, Medical School (Dunedin, New Zealand) 295,
        297, 304, 1879, 2136
Otolaryngology, Women in 699, 700, 740, 875, 1029, 1445, 2440
Overlook Sanitarium see under Pennsylvania, New Wilmington
Oxford Regional Hospital Board see under England
Oxford University Medical School (England) 642, 2232, 2236

Pacific Dispensary for Women and Children see under California,
            San Francisco
Pakistan (See also Bangladesh)
    American missionaries 2538, 2645
    Native physicians 2118
Pakistan, East see Bangladesh
Pakistan, Rawalpindi
    Holy Family Hospital for Women and Children 2516, 2628
    St. Catherine's Hospital for Women and Children 2605
Palestine see Israel
Palo Alto, California see California, Palo Alto
Palwal, India see India, Palwal
Pan American Medical Congresses 1382, 3378
Pan American Medical Women's Alliance
    Congresses 2947, 3350, 3351, 3381, 3382
    History 3368, 3380
    Purpose 3367, 3373, 3379

Paraguay
    Physicians 1944
Paramedical education see Education, Paramedical
Parasitology, Women in 1366
Parents of women medical students see Medical students--Parents
        of
Parents of women physicians, Attitudes see Attitudes towards
        women physicians--Family
Paris, Ecole de Medicine (France) 617, 1612
Paris, France see France, Paris
Paris, University of, Medical School (France) 33, 3228
Parole Board (U.S.), Physicians on 2339
Pasadena, California see California, Pasadena
Pathology (See also Neuropathology, Women in)
    American Society of Clinical Pathologists 1747
    Aviation pathology training programs 2429
    International Academy of Pathology 329, 342
    Museums 218, 273
    Obstacles for women in 2481, 2503, 2504
    Women in (specific) 309, 317, 342, 568, 723, 985, 1003, 1352,
        1444, 1520, 1692, 1808
    Women in (status) 2416, 2418, 2495
Patients (See also Psychiatry--Patients of women therapists)
    Attitudes towards women physicians 1867, 2007, 2465, 3008,
        3035, 3097, 3166, 3947
    Emotional involvement with 1984, 2996
Patients, Women
    Need for women physicians 3868
    Selection of women physicians 2186, 2295, 2358, 2853, 2888,
        2968, 3035, 3097, 3151, 3181
Patna, India see India, Patna
Pechey-Phipson Sanitarium see under India, Nasik
Pediatric allergy, Women in 773
            See also Allergy and immunology
Pediatric neurology, Careers in 2436
            See also Neurology
Pediatric surgery, Careers in 2438
            See also Surgery
Pediatrics (See also Health care--Maternal and child; and Adolescent
        girls, Work with)
    American Academy of Pediatrics 806
    American Pediatrics Society 1250
    British Paediatric Association 1051
    Paediatric Society (Hong Kong) 571
    Suitability of women for 1858, 2382, 2383, 2401
    Women in (specific)
        Australia 290
        Eastern Europe 410, 733, 2676
        Great Britain 533
        U.S. 743, 784, 806, 1239, 1511, 1586, 1611, 1744, 2496
    Women in (status) 2156, 2380, 2440, 2496
Peking, China see China, Peking
Peking Union Medical College for Women (China) 1771, 3192, 3853

Peking Union Medical College Hospital see China, Peking--Capital
        Hospital
Penicillin use 1448
Penn Medical College (Philadelphia, Pennsylvania) 3507
Penn Medical University (Philadelphia, Pennsylvania) 212, 3580,
        3773
Pennsylvania
    Allegheny County Medical Society 1849
    Attitudes of counselors towards women physicians 1870
    Congress of Women's Clubs of Western Pennsylvania 3548
    Montgomery County Medical Society 3438
    Pennsylvania Federation of Women's Clubs 1572, 3432
    Pennsylvania State Medical Society 3438, 3580
    Philadelphia County Medical Society 3108, 3131, 3173, 3438,
        3580, 3719, 3824
    Physicians 1174, 1427, 1616, 1654, 1695, 1754, 1817
    Public welfare department 904, 1103
    Women in Medicine Week (1967) 3980, 3981
Pennsylvania, Medical College of (Philadelphia) see Medical Col-
        lege of Pennsylvania (Philadelphia)
Pennsylvania, New Wilmington
    Overlook Sanitarium 1474
Pennsylvania, Norristown
    Norristown State Hospital 1823
Pennsylvania, Philadelphia
    Clinic of Notre-Dame des Malades 1873
    College of Physicians of Philadelphia 1435, 1733, 1789
    Department of health 1360
    Hospital of the Medical College of Pennsylvania 808, 1171,
        3389, 3688
        See also Medical College of Pennsylvania (Philadelphia)
    Misericordia Hospital 2101
    Obstetrical Society of Philadelphia 1435
    Petition against clinical instruction of women (1869) 2011
    Philadelphia General Hospital 923, 1790
    Philadelphia Heart Association 4009
    Physicians 807, 1696, 1733, 1784, 3073
    West Philadelphia Hospital for Women 3801
    Woman's Hospital of Philadelphia 1447, 3536, 3537, 3801
Pennsylvania, Pittsburgh
    Elizabeth Steel Magee Hospital 1447
Pennsylvania, University of, Medical School (Philadelphia) 2071,
        2342, 2956
People's Republic of China see China
Personality traits of medical students see Medical students--Char-
        acteristics
Personality traits of women physicians see Characteristics of wo-
        men physicians
Peru
    Physicians 3364
Peter Bent Brigham Hospital see under Massachusetts, Boston
Pharmacology, Women in 1752
Philadelphia College of Pharmacy and Science (Pennsylvania) 1249,
        1737

Philadelphia County Medical Society see under Pennsylvania
Philadelphia, Pennsylvania see Pennsylvania, Philadelphia
Philippine General Hospital see under Philippine Islands, Manila
Philippine Islands
    Foreign physicians 832, 1813, 2537
    Native physicians 266, 268, 2122, 3364, 3835, 3839
Philippine Islands, Manila
    Bethany Dispensary 832
    Mary J. Johnston Memorial Hospital 832, 3197
    Maternity and Children's Hospital 3191
    Philippine General Hospital 2040
Philippines, University of, Medical School (Manila) 2040
Physical rehabilitation, Women in 285, 2437, 2443, 2497
Physician shortage
    As determinant of medical career 2873, 2906
    Remedies 1869, 1951, 1993, 3872
    Women's role in 2022, 2247, 2292, 3056, 3928, 3978
Physiology, Women in 728, 864
Physostigmine, Discovery of 552
Pictorial Review Achievement Award recipients 1564
Pittsburgh, Pennsylvania see Pennsylvania, Pittsburgh
Pittsburgh, University of, Medical School (Pennsylvania) 3027,
    3548
Placement opportunities and services for women physicians see
        Employment opportunities and services for women
        physicians
Planned Parenthood Federation of America 877
Plantation health clinics 859
Plastic surgery, Women in 460, 485, 755, 867, 1610, 2471
Playground Association (U.S.) 694
Playwrights, Physicians as 1706
        (For other non-medical activities see under Non medical
        activities)
Poetry about women physicians and healers see Literature--Physi-
        cians and healers in
Poets as physicians 424
        (For other non medical activities see under Non medical
        activities)
Poland
    American physicians 1063
    American Red Cross 3555
    Medical education 1887, 1889
    Native physicians (specific) 14, 378, 381-385, 391-393, 396,
        397, 404, 411, 699
    Native physicians (status) 2151, 2855
    Youth organization physicians 407
Poland, Brzeziny
    Women's Hospital Camp 2153
Poland, Warsaw
    Emergency Hospital 1063
    Warsaw Medical Society 14, 381
Police physicians 431, 2385, 2396, 2400, 2412
Police women

British Medical Women's Federation stand   3242
Poliomyelitis, Work in   287, 1354
Politics
    Physicians as magistrates   549, 588
    Physicians as revolutionaries   3225
    Physicians in city government   496, 540, 617, 701, 904, 2323
    Physicians in national government   607, 686, 737, 756, 2159
    Physicians in state government   756, 1632
Population-physician ratio   2276, 3928
Pornography, Attitudes towards   3983
Portland, Oregon   see   Oregon, Portland
Portraits of women physicians (See also Art depicting women physicians)
    Inaccessibility   151
Portugal
    Physicians   424, 459, 3887, 3890
Postage stamps commemorating physicians   181, 190, 245
Postal innovations by physicians   868
Poughkeepsie, New York   see   New York, Poughkeepsie
Practice patterns (See also Specialties; and Geographical distribution of physicians; and Medical practice)
    Black women physicians (1970s)   2354a
    Comparisons between U.S. and USSR   2268
    Full-time
        Absenteeism   2270
        Attitudes of women in   2937
    Germany   2186
    Inactive
        Australia   2137, 2141
        Comparisons of Australia and U.S.   2264
        Comparisons with active practitioners   2297
        Myth of   2353
        Pakistan   2118
        Philadelphia   2074
        Reasons for   2195, 2216, 2935, 3005, 3073
        South Africa   2112
        Statistics (1970s)   2310
        Suggestions for activating   2050, 2145, 2149, 2200, 2207, 2242, 2288, 2356
    Part-time
        As relieving physician shortage   2292
        Attitudes of women in   2206, 2937
        Problems in   2271, 2341
        Suggestions   2307
        Suitability of married women for   2214
        Suitable areas of practice   2238
        Symposia and discussions   2226, 2393, 2409, 4044
    Review of surveys on   2209, 2227, 2246, 2251, 2336, 2363, 3068
    Statistics
        Misuse of   2285
    Statistics (1800s)   2284, 4017
    Statistics (1900-1920s)   2177, 2186, 2190, 2261, 2354b, 2772,

          2893, 2926, 3279
Statistics (1900-1970s) 3901
Statistics (1930s) 2185, 2218, 2925, 2974
Statistics (1940s) 2230, 2285, 4023
Statistics (1950s) 2213, 2282, 2286, 2335, 2344, 2354h, 2374,
          3875
Statistics (1960s)
      Australia 2138
      Canada 2144, 2146
      Germany 2179, 2908
      Great Britain 2211, 2216, 2219, 2220, 2224, 2236, 2240,
          2241, 2243, 2245
      Ireland 2170
      New Zealand 2139
      U.S. 2297, 2336, 2342, 2347, 2359, 3635, 4030
Statistics (1970s)
      Australia 2129, 2132, 2133
      Canada 2148, 2150
      Carnegie Commission Report correction 2287
      Comparing Australian and New Zealand physicians 2142
      Great Britain 2205, 2223, 2225
      New Zealand 2128, 2135, 2136
      USSR 2269, 2270, 2272
      U.S. 2308, 2309, 2327, 2333, 2334, 2338, 2351, 2356,
          3069, 3073
      Western Europe 2158, 2162, 2168
Pratt Hysterectomy see Obstetrics and gynecology--Hysterectomy
          techniques
Preceptorship programs 1980, 1981, 2050
Predictions regarding women physicians 1991
Pregnant therapists see under Psychiatry
Presbyterian Board of Missions 1592
Presidents' physicians see White House physicians
Preventive medicine, Women in 704, 795, 1032, 1404, 1534, 1592,
          2303, 2489
Princesses as physicians see Royalty as physicians
Prison (See also specific institutions under geographical location)
      Physicians incarcerated in 379, 632, 2587
Prison health care, Physicians in 448, 586, 620, 712, 988, 1083,
          1103, 1203, 1226, 1444, 1624, 1716, 2427
Prisons, Physicians as supervisors 550
Professional Corporation of Physicians and Surgeons of Quebec see
          under Quebec Province
Prostitution, Physicians' work with 274, 420, 445, 461
Protestant physicians as missionaries 2665
Prussia see Germany
Psychiatric hospitals
      Employment of women physicians 2108, 2258, 2289, 2304,
          2337
          Legislation 1480, 3438, 4031
          Medical Women's Federation activities 3281
          Statistics 2280, 2365, 3282
      Metropolitan Asylums Board (England) 2204

Physicians working in (specific) 2439
Psychiatry (See also Neuropsychiatry, Women in; and Psychiatric
       hospitals)
   American Psychiatric Association 2464, 3733
   Attitudes towards women therapists 2431
   Careers in 2423, 2426, 2427, 2434, 2478, 4013, 4049
   Characteristics of women in 2426, 2469
   Comparison of male and female therapists 2433, 2445, 3117
   Consciousness raising groups 2311
   Patients of women therapists 2445, 2474
   Practice patterns 2491
   Pregnant therapists 2420-2422, 2424, 2454, 2460, 2462, 2485
   Problems for women specializing in 2425, 2464, 2473
   Single women in 2461
   Students' performance in 2938
   Suicide of therapists 2981
   Suitability of women for 2456, 2465, 2469, 3078
   Therapists as role models 2425
   Training programs 1989, 2047, 2053, 2062-2065, 2421
   Women in (specific) 340, 814, 908, 1182, 1186, 1223, 1228,
          1476, 1599, 1609, 1727, 2434
   Women in (status) 2440, 2470
Psychiatry, Child
   Women in 699, 971, 1060, 1444
Psychosomatic medicine, Women in 1341
Public health (See also Social hygiene; and National Health Service
          (Great Britain); and Medical social service)
   American Public Health Association 795, 939, 1230, 1400
   Association of Women in Public Health 3569, 3570, 3660
   Careers in 2392, 2402, 2406, 2407, 2448, 2468, 2502, 3823
   Conferences in 2480
   Differential treatment of physicians in 2403
   Health Protection Clinic 886
   Medical Women's Federation activities 3239
   Public Health Bill (U.S. Senate Bill 2507) 2281
   Role of women in 2273, 2457, 2458, 2496
   Salary inequities 3280, 3285, 3325
   Suitability of women for 2397, 2921, 4022
   United States Public Health Service 1132
   Women in (specific) 451, 761, 779, 807, 821, 834, 856, 877,
          886, 1102, 1192, 1213, 1330, 1339, 1344, 1376, 1400,
          1404, 1503, 1576, 1597, 1601, 1626, 1647, 1725, 1836,
          1839, 2475
   Women in (status) 2199, 2270, 2391, 2410, 2452, 2483, 2494
   Women's acceptance of low-paying posts 2388, 3240, 3282
Public Law 38 see Armed services (U.S.)--Legislation
Public Law 252 see Armed services (U.S.)--Legislation
Public Law 408 see Armed services (U.S.)--Legislation
Publicity for women physicians 2354g, 3155, 3180
Puerto Rico
   Physicians 796, 910, 1089, 1436
Pulaski, New York see New York, Pulaski
Punjab, India see India, Punjab

Punjab Medical School for Indian Girls (Punjab, India)   2597
              See also Ludhiana Medical College (India)

Quack physicians   19, 28, 180
Quarterly Bulletin of the Medical Women's National Association   see
              Journal of the American Medical Women's Association
Quebec, Montreal
    Closed hospitals   310
Quebec Province
    Medical education   8
    Physicians   314, 609, 2150
    Professional Corporation of Physicians and Surgeons of Quebec
       2150
Quedlinburg, Germany   see   Germany, Quedlinburg
Queen Margaret College, University of Glasgow (Scotland)   3934
Queen Victoria Hospital for Women and Children (Melbourne)   see
              under   Victoria, Melbourne
Queens as physicians   see   Royalty as physicians
Queensland, University of   2129
Quincy, Illinois   see   Illinois, Quincy

Rachel Forster Hospital   see under   New South Wales, Sydney
Radcliffe College (Cambridge, Massachusetts)
    Alumnae physicians   4039
Radcliffe College Women's Archives   1445
Radiology, Women in   1101, 1257, 1615, 1707, 1849, 2381, 2477
Rajahmundry, India   see   India, Rajahmundry
Rajahmundry Mission Hospital   see under   India, Rajahmundry
Ramapatam, India   see   India, Ramapatam
Rawalpindi, Pakistan   see   Pakistan, Rawalpindi
Raymond, Henry Jarvis   3452
Record keeping, Medical   1585
Recruitment   1921, 1990, 2954, 3055, 3139, 3966, 3967, 3983, 4003
              See also under Missionaries
Red Army Medical Corps (USSR)   see   Armed services (USSR)
Red Cross work   2675, 2699, 2705, 2795, 2796, 2807, 2842, 3555
              See also under specific countries
Refugees, Physicians as   see   World War II--Physician refugees
Rehabilitation, Physical   see   Physical rehabilitation, Women in
Reims, France   see   France, Reims
Religion, Effects on physicians   see under   specific religions and
              sects
Reproductive system research   2472
Research (See also under specific topics)
    Careers in   2343, 2353, 2476, 2482
    Suitability of women for   2389, 2390, 2472, 2924
Residencies   see   Internships and residencies
Retarded children, Work with   743
Retirement Home for Aged Physicians   4085
Retraining programs
    Australia   2041-2043

Federation of Medical Women of Canada   2044
Medical College of Pennsylvania   2053, 2070, 2074, 2104, 3563
Necessity for   498, 1952, 2051, 2056, 2246, 2251, 2911
Physicians' experiences in   1571, 3015
Presbyterian Medical Center (San Francisco, California)   2051
Recommendations   2132, 3967
Surveys   2054, 2205
United States Public Health Service   2050
Women Doctors' Retraining Scheme (National Health Service,
       Great Britain)   2048
Retreat for women physicians   3393
Revolution (USSR)
Medical students during   208
Rhode Island
Physicians   772, 1161
Rickets research, Women in   653
       See also Nutrition, Women in
Riverside Hospital see   New York, Buffalo--Lafayette General
       Hospital
Robb-Smith, A. H. T.
Comments on Robb-Smith's Oxford medical women article   2232
Robertson Medical School (Nagpur, India)   1876
Rochester, Minnesota   see   Minnesota, Rochester
Rochester, New York   see   New York, Rochester
Rockefeller Foundation   3192, 3853
Rockefeller Institute for Medical Research   761, 850, 1138, 1564
Rockhill, Margaret H.   1386
Rohmatpur Hospital   see under   India, Palwal
Role conflict   3088
       See also Children of women physicians--Effects on med-
       ical activity; and Marriage--Effects on and compatibility
       with medical activity; and Deterrents to medical careers
Effects on specialty selection   2440, 2452
Suggestions for coping with   1855, 3967, 3973, 4013
Role models   1856, 2425, 2962, 2992, 3090
Romania
Physicians   402, 3867
Rome, Italy   see   Italy, Rome
Rome, University of (Italy)   476
Root Memorial Nursery of Stamford Hospital   see   Connecticut,
       Stamford--Stamford Hospital, Stella Quinby Root Memor-
       ial Nursery
Royal College of Obstetricians   see under   Obstetrics and gynecology
Royal College of Physicians   see under   England, London
Royal College of Physicians and Surgeons   see under   England, Lon-
       don
Royal College of Surgeons (England)   see under   England, London
Royal College of Surgeons (Scotland)   see under   Scotland, Edinburgh
Royal Free Hospital   see under   England, London
Royal Free Hospital School of Medicine (London, England)   1921,
       2211, 2935
Royal Infirmary   see   Scotland, Edinburgh--Edinburgh Royal In-
       firmary

Royal Medical College (Kingston, Ontario) 11
Royal Netherlands Company for the Promotion of Medical Science
        3884
Royal Victoria Hospital for Caste and Gosha Women   see under
        India, Madras
Royalty as physicians 406, 459
Royaumont, France see France, Royaumont
Royaumont Hospital see under France, Royaumont
Rumania
    Physicians 399
Runge, Max
    Comments on his book, Emancipation of Women 2886
Ruppertsberg Abbey see under Germany, Bingen
Rural practice, Women in 291, 304, 828, 903, 1816, 2345
Rush Medical College (Chicago, Illinois) 1627, 3409
Russell, Violet
    Comments on her public health letter 2406
Russia see USSR
Russian Women's Society 727
Russo-Turkish War, Physicians in 206, 2676
Rutgers University Medical School (New Brunswick, New Jersey)
        2958
Rydygiera, Ludwig
    Comments on his article on medical education 2850, 2851

St. Elizabeth's Hospital see under Washington, D.C.
St. George's Hospital Medical School (Great Britain) 1921, 1927
St. Helen's Maternity Hospital see under New Zealand, Welling-
        ton
St. Joseph Mercy Hospital see under Michigan, Ann Arbor
St. Joseph's Hospital see under Minnesota, Mankota
St. Louis, Missouri see Missouri, St. Louis
St. Luke's Hospital see under Japan, Tokyo
St. Mary's Dispensary for Women and Children see England,
        London--Elizabeth Garrett Anderson Hospital
St. Mary's Hospital Medical School (England) 2218
St. Petersburg Academy of Medicine (USSR) 3213
St. Petersburg School of Medicine for Women (USSR) 208, 1911,
        3214, 3216, 3217, 3937
St. Petersburg, USSR see USSR, Leningrad
St. Rita's Home for Exceptional Children see under New York,
        Buffalo
St. Stephen's Hospital see under India, Delhi
St. Vincent's Hospital see under Virginia, Norfolk
Saints as healers 180
Salaries see Medical practice--Earnings
Salem, Oregon see Oregon, Salem
Salerno, Italy see Italy, Salerno
Salerno Medical School (Italy) 22, 31, 47, 75, 132, 149, 152
Salt Lake City, Utah see Utah, Salt Lake City
Salvation Army Hospital see under Korea, Yong Dong
Salvation Army, Physicians in 1649, 3707

San Antonio, Texas see Texas, San Antonio
San Diego, California see California, San Diego
San Francisco, California see California, San Francisco
Sanitary Aid Commission see under Civil War (U.S.)
Santa Fe, New Mexico see New Mexico, Santa Fe
Sara Mayo Hospital see under Louisiana, New Orleans
Saskatchewan
    Physicians 312, 313, 318
Schelenz, H.
    Comments on Schelenz's Women in the Realm of Esculapius 35
School bussing, Attitudes towards 3983
School physicians 427, 448, 488, 1213, 1442, 2387, 2448, 2493,
        3908
Schroetter, Leopold Von 1905
Scientists, Relationships with physicians 2354c, 2482
Scotland
    Physicians 668, 686
Scotland, Edinburgh
    Edinburgh Hospital for Women and Children 679, 3313
    Edinburgh Royal Infirmary 3253, 3299
    Elsie Inglis Memorial Hospital 501, 3256, 3296, 3307, 3313
    Medical education 3267
    Royal College of Surgeons 282
Scottish Universities Commission (Ordinance 18) 1936
        See also Medical schools--Admissions policies--Legisla-
        tion
Scottish women's hospitals (See also under specific countries and re-
        gions)
    History 501, 612, 3272
    World War I activities 585, 2685, 2694, 2699, 2790
Sculptures of women physicians see Art depicting women physicians
Seaman Free Dispensary see under Ohio, Cleveland
Sectarianism in medical school see Medical schools--Sectarianism
    as favorable for women
Sedgwick, Theodore 3443
Semarang, Indonesia see Indonesia, Semarang
Seoul, Korea see Korea, Seoul
Serbia see Yugoslavia
Seventeenth century healers 36, 38, 77, 80, 152, 213, 227
Seventh Day Adventist physicians 1322, 2668, 3816, 3993
Seventh Day Adventist, Sanatorium at Iowa Circle see under Wash-
        ington, D.C.
Severance Medical College (Seoul, Korea) 3193
Sex education
    Sex Information and Education Council of the United States
        (SIECUS) 877
Sex education, Work in 420, 816, 955, 1097, 2349, 2982
        See also Social hygiene
Shanghai, China see China, Shanghai
Shanta Bhawan Hospital (Nepal) see under Nepal
Shantung Christian University see North China Union Medical Col-
       lege for Women
Shawmut Mining Company see under Illinois

Sheffield University, Medical School (England) 2224
Sheppard-Towner Act see under Health care--Maternal and child
Ships' physicians 455, 965, 3917
Sialkot, India see India, Sialkot
Siam see Thailand
Sierra Leone
    American missionaries 2508
Singapore
    British physicians 533
Single women physicians 1068, 2461, 3124, 3138, 3151, 3168
              See also Marital status; and Divorce statistics
Sioux City, Iowa see Iowa, Sioux City
Sixteenth century healers 32, 42, 54, 111, 152
Slaves
    Analogy of women physicians to freed slaves 2957
Smith College Medal recipients 1014
Social clubs for school girls 1126
Social hygiene (See also Sex education, Work in)
    Careers in 2450, 2501
    Physicians 419, 798, 837, 1066, 1570, 1774
    Social Hygiene Council of Chicago 1845
Social reform, Physicians in 1091
Socialism, Effects on physicians 369, 1287, 2671, 2672, 2908, 3225
Socialized medicine 3186, 3411, 3565, 3955
Society for the Propagation of the Gospel 2528
Society for the Protection of Women and Children see under New
              Zealand, Dunedin
Society of Catholic Medical Missionaries
    Activities 2605, 2628, 2647, 2648, 2660, 2664, 3430
    Founders 515, 2667
    History 1595, 2658, 2659, 2662, 2665, 2666
    Hospitals 2516, 2646
    Purpose 2661
Society of Friends 1180, 3453
Somerset Hospital see under New Jersey, Somerville
Somerville, New Jersey see New Jersey, Somerville
Soochow, China see China, Soochow
Soochow Woman's Medical School (China) 1030, 1124
              See also China, Soochow--Women's Hospital
Soroptimist Association 460
South Africa
    British physicians 596, 650, 680, 2113
    Missionaries 685, 2507
    Native physicians (specific) 261, 263, 264, 698
    Native physicians (status) 2167, 2843, 3364
South Africa, Cape Province
    Physicians 260
South Africa, Johannesburg
    Physicians 262, 633
South America (See also specific countries)
    Missionary activity 2665
South Carolina
    American Women's Hospitals 1698, 3584

                    See also American Women's Hospitals--Activities
          Physicians 798, 1214, 2317
South Dakota, Armour
     Physicians 1429
South Dakota, University of, Medical School 1280
South East Settlement House see under Washington, D.C.
South London Hospital for Women see under England, London
South Vietnam see Vietnam
Southern California, University of, Medical School (Los Angeles)
          1512, 1829, 2840, 3410
Southern Medical Association (U.S.) 798, 819, 1404
Southern Medical Women's Association (U.S.) 3714, 3731
Soviet Union see USSR
Spain
     Healers and physicians (specific) 18, 42, 422, 472
     Physicians (status) 2173, 2858, 3364, 3890, 3891 3897
Spanish-American War physicians 1307, 1539
Spanish Society of Gynecologists 422
Sparkman-Johnson Bill (U.S. Bill H.R. 1857) see under Armed
          services (U.S.)--Legislation
Specialties (See also Medical students--Specialty selection; and
          Practice patterns; and specific specialties)
     Factors governing selection 55, 2142, 2267, 3859, 3995, 4012,
          4015
     Relation to practice patterns 2214, 3073
     Statistics (1880s) 2284
     Statistics (1900-1930s) 2177, 2184, 2185, 2190, 2256, 2318,
          2354b
     Statistics (1940s) 2230, 2316, 2375, 3830
     Statistics (1950s) 2179, 2286, 2344
     Statistics (1960s)
          Canada 2144
          Great Britain 2211, 2224, 2236, 2240, 2241
          New Zealand 2139
          United States 2332, 2334, 2336, 2342, 2346, 4030
          Western Europe 2170, 2173
     Statistics (1970s)
          Australia 2129, 2132, 2264
          Eastern Europe 2152, 2266, 2270, 2271
          New Zealand 2131
          United States 2300, 2308, 2309, 2333, 2334, 2338, 2351
          Western Europe 2158, 2171, 2225
     Suggested for women 1855, 1858, 2156, 2329, 2376, 2895, 2919,
          2930, 3138, 3181, 3184, 3975
Spence Chapin Award recipients 741
Sri Lanka
     Missionaries 2517
     Physicians 3364
Stalin, Joseph 2671
Stalnaker and Dykman Survey see Dykman and Stalnaker
Stamford, Connecticut see Connecticut, Stamford
Stamford Hospital, Stella Quinby Root Memorial Nursery see under
          Connecticut, Stamford

Ständers, Rikets 2154
Stanford, California see California, Stanford
Stanford University Hospital see under California, Stanford
Stanford University Medical School (California) 1432, 1802, 3103,
          3427, 3494
State medical societies see under Organizations, medical. See
              specific societies under their geographic locations
Statues of women physicians see Art depicting women physicians
Stein, Gertrude 1692
Stella Quinby Root Memorial Nursery (Stamford Hospital) see
              Connecticut, Stamford--Stamford Hospital, Stella Quinby
              Root Memorial Nursery
Stenographers 1721
              (For other nonmedical activities, see under Non med-
              ical activities)
Stone, Lucy 1094, 1188
Strang Cancer Clinic see under New York City--New York In-
              firmary for Women and Children
Stratford, New Zealand see New Zealand, Stratford
Strecker Award (Institute of Pennsylvania) 756
Stritch Award recipients (Loyola University) 1532
Strong Memorial Hospital see under New York, Rochester
Student health see under Health care--Students
Sturgis, Michigan see Michigan, Sturgis
Suffrage see Woman suffrage
Suicide among women physicians 2981, 2993, 3125, 3140, 3147
Suitability of women for medical careers (See also Deterrents to
              medical careers)
     Historical justification 2899
Suitability of women for medical careers, Opinions on
     (Pre-1850) 2885, 2907
     (1850s) 2865, 2968, 2970, 2991, 3012, 3014, 3031, 3065, 3168
     (1860s) 2864, 2871, 2965, 2983, 3013, 3033, 3108, 3173, 3179
     (1870s) 1922, 2859, 2870, 2872, 2875, 2883, 2915, 2939, 3036,
              3070, 3490
     (1880s) 2033, 2973, 3045, 3163
     (1890s) 129, 2856, 2861, 2881, 2882, 2891, 2892, 2894, 2895,   -
              2900, 3099
     (1900-1920) 2862, 2930, 2999, 3057, 3176, 3181
     (1920s) 1901, 2893, 2929, 2978, 3022, 3157
     (1930s-1940s) 2944, 3028, 3080, 3151
     (1950s-1960s) 3060, 3074, 3077, 3174
     (1970s) 2959, 3078, 3172, 3975
Sunderland, England see England, Sunderland
Sunnybrook Medical Centre see under Ontario, Toronto
Support among women physicians and medical students 1955, 2124,
              2927, 2990, 3101, 3142, 3185, 3416, 3702, 4079
              See also Medical schools--Support programs; and Or-
              ganizations, Medical women's--Necessity for
Surgery (See also Pediatric surgery, Careers in; and Plastic sur-
              gery, Women in; and Neurosurgery, Careers in)
     American Association of Obstetricians, Gynecologists and Ab-
              dominal Surgeons 2323

Association of Military Surgeons   1539
Careers in   2446, 2488
Deterrents for women   1858, 2442, 2459
Suitability of women for   2376, 2419, 2987, 3016
Women in (specific)
    Austria   700
    Great Britain   534, 620, 655, 683
    United States   701, 849, 926, 930, 982, 1021, 1035, 1083,
        1086, 1166, 1259, 1301, 1397, 1455, 1459, 1485, 1488,
        1550, 1582, 1689, 1736, 1764, 2484, 3391
Women in (status)   2440, 2459
Susan La Flesche Picotte Hospital   see under   Nebraska, Walthill
Su-Tsierr-Ku, China   see   China, Su-Tsierr-Ku
Suva, Fiji   see   Fiji, Suva
Svensen, Carl John   1909
Sweden
    Debate over women's right to practice medicine   44, 63, 1909,
        2164-2166
    Medical education   1900, 1908, 1909, 1940
    Opportunities for women in government service   2159, 2160
    Physicians (specific)   44, 71, 419, 420, 426, 436, 441, 456,
        471, 473, 474, 2159
    Physicians (status)   2056, 2154, 2166, 2167, 3364, 3886, 3889,
        3895, 3898
    Practice patterns   2171, 2172
Sweden, Gothenburg
    Medical students   1910
Swedish medical societies   984, 2171
Switzerland
    History of women in medicine   24, 3875
    Medical education   72, 1912
    Physicians (status)   2173, 3364, 3905, 3941
    Physicians and healers (specific)   54, 446, 463, 468
    Practice patterns   2381, 3875
Switzerland, Zurich
    Swiss school for nurses and hospitals   463
Sydney, New South Wales   see   New South Wales, Sydney
Sydney, University of (New South Wales)   7, 300, 305, 2043,
        3861
Syphilis control   see   Venereal disease control
Syria
    American missionaries   2523, 2524

Tabriz, Iran   see   Iran, Tabriz
Taiwan
    Physicians   3364
Talbot, Israel Tisdale   3420
Tangier, Morocco   see   Morocco, Tangier
Taxes   2130, 2187, 2916, 3961, 4077, 4078
Teheran, Iran   see   Iran, Teheran
Tel Aviv, Israel   see   Israel, Tel Aviv
Tennessee

Physicians 1796
Tennov
    Comments on her paper, "Feminism, Psychotherapy, and Pro-
            fessionalism" 3117
Texas
    Physicians 803, 862, 949, 1133, 1477, 2371, 4047
Texas, San Antonio
    Academy of General Practice 1848
Thailand
    Missionaries 2537
    Physicians 274, 3364
Theater and films, Portrayal of women physicians 4053
            See also Literature
Theologians see Clergy, Physicians as
Thirteenth century healers see under Middle Ages (500-1500)
Thuruthipuram, India see India, Thuruthipuram
Tokyo, Japan see Japan, Tokyo
Tokyo Women's Medical College (Tokyo, Japan) 3195, 3198, 3199,
            3203, 3837, 3856, 3859, 3860
Toland Medical School (California) 863
Toledo, Ohio see Ohio, Toledo
Tombstone epitaphs of healers 46, 132
Toronto General Hospital see under Ontario, Toronto
Toronto, Ontario see Ontario, Toronto
Toronto School of Medicine see Toronto, University of, Medical
            School (Ontario)
Toronto, University of, Medical School (Ontario) 11, 333, 1881
Toulouse, Medical School of (France) 437
Transportation, High speed mass
    Attitudes towards 3983
Tropical medicine, Women in 490, 533, 2389
Tuberculosis control
    North Dakota Tuberculosis Association 1613
    Women in 420, 451, 512, 588, 749, 795, 995, 1205, 1747
Tufts University School of Medicine (Boston, Massachusetts) 2014,
            3055
Tulane University, Elizabeth Bass Collection on Women in Medicine
            see Bass Collection on Women in Medicine (Tulane
            University)
Tulane University School of Medicine (New Orleans, Louisiana)
            819, 3069
Turkey (See also Armenia; and American Women's Hospitals Ser-
            vice--Activities)
    American physicians 1082, 1106, 1167, 1304, 1565, 1837, 3590
    American Women's Hospitals 2677, 3599
    Missionary activity 2646
    Native physicians 3830
    Russian physicians 379
Twelfth century healers see under Middle Ages (500-1500)
Twilight sleep, Physicians' use of 1149, 1764
Tzechow, China see China, Tzechow

Union des Femmes (Geneva, Switzerland) 292
Union Medical College for Women (Peking) see Peking Union Med-
          ical College for Women (China)
Union Missionary Medical School for Women (Vellore, India) 2616,
          2630, 2634
USSR (See also American Women's Hospitals Service--Activities;
          and Armenia)
      American physicians 1177, 1567, 1575, 1596, 3873
      American Women's Hospitals Service 3392
      Art depicting women physicians 3871
      History of women in medicine 736, 1894, 3216, 3217, 3225
      Medical education 1888, 1891, 1892, 2671, 2856, 2857, 3940
      Native physicians (specific) 379, 723, 726, 729, 735, 736,
          2671, 2673, 2676, 2679, 2680, 3218, 3225
      Native physicians (status) 2056, 2672, 2853, 2869, 3407, 3866,
          3869, 3870
      Scottish physicians 585, 612
      Specialties 2379, 2381
USSR, Leningrad
      Clinics 199, 3215
      Day nursery for children of working women 727
      Leningrad Military Hospital 2678
USSR, Moscow
      International medical conference (1897) 3873
USSR, St. Petersburg see USSR, Leningrad
United Nations World Health Organization see World Health Or-
          ganization (United Nations)
United States
      Canadian physicians 345
      French physicians 454
      Hungarian physicians 409
      Medical education 3940
      Missionary activity 2648
      Native physicians 3929
      Physician comparisons with other countries 2671, 3950
      Scottish physicians 581
United States Children's Bureau see Children's Bureau (U.S.)
United States Department of Agriculture see Agriculture, United
          States Department of
United States Department of Labor, Women's Bureau Report on
          opportunities for women physicians see Women's
          Bureau (U.S.) report on opportunities for women
          physicians
United States Public Health Service see under Public health
United States Sanitary Aid Commission see under Civil War (U.S.)
Universidad Mayor de San Andres de la Paz (Bolivia) 708
University College Hospital see under Nigeria, Ibadan
University of Arkansas Medical School see Arkansas, University
          of, Medical School (Fayetteville)
University of Athens Medical School see Athens, University of,
          Medical School (Greece)
University of Bahia see Bahia, University of (Brazil)
University of Birmingham Medical School see Birmingham, Uni-

versity of, Medical School (England)
University of Bologna Medical School   see   Bologna, University of,
    Medical School (Italy)
University of Bombay Medical School   see   Bombay, University of,
    Medical School (India)
University of Bristol Medical School   see   Bristol, University of,
    Medical School (England)
University of California Medical School   see   California, University
    of, Medical School...
University of Cincinnati Medical School   see   Cincinnati, University
    of, Medical School (Ohio)
University of Copenhagen   see   Copenhagen, University of (Denmark)
University of Edinburgh   see   Edinburgh, University of (Scotland)
University of Freiburg   see   Freiburg, University of (Germany)
University of Giessen   see   Giessen, University of (Germany)
University of Glasgow Medical School   see   Glasgow, University of,
    Medical School (Scotland)
University of Glasgow, Queen Margaret College   see   Queen Marga-
    ret College, University of Glasgow (Scotland)
University of Graz Medical School   see   Graz, University of, Med-
    ical School (Austria)
University of Groningen   see   Groningen, University of (Netherlands)
University of Halle   see   Halle, University of (Germany)
University of Halle-Wittenberg   see   Halle-Wittenberg, University of
    (Germany)
University of Havana   see   Havana, University of (Cuba)
University of Hawaii Medical School   see   Hawaii, University of,
    Medical School (Honolulu)
University of Heidelberg Medical School   see   Heidelberg, University
    of, Medical School (Germany)
University of Helsingfors   see   Helsingfors, University of (Finland)
University of Helsinki   see   Helsinki, University of (Finland)
University of Hong Kong Medical School   see   Hong Kong, University
    of, Medical School
University of Illinois Medical School   see   Illinois, University of,
    Medical School (Urbana)
University of Innsbruck Medical School   see   Innsbruck, University
    of, Medical School (Austria)
University of Iowa   see   Iowa, University of (Iowa City)
University of Krakow Medical School   see   Krakow, University of,
    Medical School (Poland)
University of Laval   see   Laval, University of (France)
University of Leipzig   see   Leipzig, University of (Germany)
University of London   see   London, University of (England)
University of London School of Medicine for Women   see   London
    School of Medicine for Women (England)
University of Lund   see   Lund, University of (Sweden)
University of Manitoba   see   Manitoba, University of
University of Maryland Medical School   see   Maryland, University
    of, Medical School (College Park)
University of Melbourne   see   Melbourne, University of (Victoria)
University of Mexico Medical School   see   Mexico, University of,
    Medical School

University of Michigan Hospital   see   Michigan, Ann Arbor--University Hospital
University of Michigan Medical School   see   Michigan, University of, Medical School (Ann Arbor)
University of Montevideo   see   Montevideo, University of (Uruguay)
University of Montpellier   see   Montpellier, University of (France)
University of New Mexico Medical School   see   New Mexico, University of, Medical School (Albuquerque)
University of North Carolina Medical School   see   North Carolina, University of, Medical School (Chapel Hill)
University of Oregon Medical School   see   Oregon, University of, Medical School (Portland)
University of Otago Medical School   see   Otago, University of, Medical School (Dunedin, New Zealand)
University of Paris Medical School   see   Paris, University of, Medical School (France)
University of Pennsylvania Medical School   see   Pennsylvania, University of, Medical School (Philadelphia)
University of Pittsburgh Medical School   see   Pittsburgh, University of, Medical School (Pennsylvania)
University of Queensland   see   Queensland, University of
University of Rome   see   Rome, University of (Italy)
University of South Dakota Medical School   see   South Dakota, University of, Medical School
University of Southern California Medical School   see   Southern California, University of, Medical School (Los Angeles)
University of Sydney   see   Sydney, University of (New South Wales)
University of the Philippines, Medical School   see   Philippines, University of, Medical School (Manila)
University of Toronto Medical School   see   Toronto, University of, Medical School (Ontario)
University of Uppsala Medical School   see   Uppsala, University of, Medical School (Sweden)
University of Utrecht Medical School   see   Utrecht, University of, Medical School (Netherlands)
University of Vienna Medical School   see   Vienna, University of, Medical School (Austria)
University of Western Ontario, Medical School   see   Western Ontario, University of, Medical School
University of Wisconsin Medical School   see   Wisconsin, University of, Medical School
University of Zurich   see   Zurich, University of (Switzerland)
Uppsala, University of, Medical School (Sweden)   **2166**
Urology
    Exclusion of women   **2090, 2095**
    Women in (specific)   **1584, 1635**
Uruguay
    Physicians   **701, 710, 720, 721, 3944**
Utah
    Physicians   **791, 1533, 1632, 1760**
Utah, Salt Lake City
    Deseret Hospital   **1533**

Utica, New York see New York, Utica
Utrecht, University of, Medical School (Netherlands) 66

Vacations for women physicians 4070
Vallejo, California see California, Vallejo
Vandervall, Isabella
        Comments on her article about black women physicians 3023
Vellore, India see India, Vellore
Vellore Medical School (India) 1277, 1278, 3345
Venereal disease control
        French Society of Dermatology and Syphilology 1437, 1824
        Medical Women's Federation activities 3242, 3257, 3283, 3325,
            3326
        Women in (specific)
            Thailand 274
            United States 1289, 1327, 1448
            Western Europe 106, 415, 436, 446, 2386
Venezuela
        Physicians 195
Venezuelan Society of the History of Medicine 195
Vermont
        Vermont Medical Society 1305
        Vermont Women's Health Center 3964
Veteran's Administration Hospital, Lenwood Division see Georgia,
            Augusta--Lenwood Division of the Veteran's Administra-
            tion Hospital
Veteran's Administration Hospitals see Hospitals--Veteran's Ad-
            ministration
Victoria (Australia)
        Physicians 7, 3941
        Victorian Medical Women's Society 2138
Victoria, Melbourne
        Queen Victoria Hospital for Women and Children 2042, 3206,
            3861
Victoria University (Canada) 308
Vienna, Austria see Austria, Vienna
Vienna Medical Women's Association see under Austria, Vienna
Vienna, University of, Medical School (Austria) 1901, 2158, 3234
Vietnam
        Physicians 839, 1779, 3364
Viking healers 78
Virginia
        Physicians 1122, 1339, 4081
Virginia, Norfolk
        St. Vincent's Hospital 1215
Vocational guidance (See also National Council on Health Career
            (U.S.))
        Attitudes of counselors towards women physicians 1870, 2949
        Experiences in 1867
        Recommendations 1860, 1866, 1875, 2908, 3952
Volunteer activity statistics 2286
Volunteer medical service corps see under Armed services (U.S.)

Wages and Hours Bill (U.S., 1938)
    Effect on physicians 2357
Wai, India see India, Wai
Walker Dunbar Hospital see under England, Bristol
Walthill, Nebraska see Nebraska, Walthill
Warsaw Medical Academy (Poland) 1889
Warsaw, Poland see Poland, Warsaw
Washington, D.C.
    American Medical Women's Association 3567
    Children's Hospital Luetic Clinic 1448
    District of Columbia Medical Society 1447
    Ferdman Hospital 2093
    First gymnasium for women and children 994
    Garfield Memorial Hospital 1295
    Physicians 898, 1071, 2335, 2347
    St. Elizabeth's Hospital 1043, 1182, 1438, 2111, 3435, 4031
    Seventh-Day Adventist Sanatorium 1282
    South East Settlement House at Washington Circle 859
    Woman's Evening Clinic 2366
Washington state
    Physicians 865
Water cure 846
        See also New York, Castile--Greene Sanitarium
Waukesha County Medical Society see under Illinois
Wayne State University Medical School (Detroit, Michigan) 1033,
        4015
Wei Hien, China see China, Wei Hien
Welfare reform, Attitudes towards 3983
Well Baby Clinics 1613, 1748, 2851
Well Baby Health Station see under New York, Binghamton
Wellesley College (Wellesley, Massachusetts) 1599
Wellington, New Zealand see New Zealand, Wellington
Wesleyan University (Middletown, Connecticut) 1173
West China Union University (Chengtu) 2541
West London Hospital see under England, London
West Pakistan see Pakistan
West Philadelphia Hospital for Women see under Pennsylvania,
        Philadelphia
West Virginia University School of Medicine 2354h
Western Ontario, University of, Medical School 2144
Western Reserve College see Case Western Reserve University
        Medical School (Cleveland, Ohio)
White House physicians 1234, 1752, 3974
White slave market, Campaigns against 1298, 1591
Whitemouth, Manitoba see Manitoba, Whitemouth
Wiesbaden, Germany see Germany, Wiesbaden
Wilberforce University (Xenia, Ohio) 750
Willard, Frances 1164
Willard (Frances E.) National Temperance Hospital see Illinois,
        Chicago--Frances E. Willard National Temperance Hos-
        pital
William Butler Memorial Hospital see India, Baroda--Mrs. Wil-
        liam Butler Memorial Hospital

Williamsburgh Hospital see under New York, Brooklyn
Wills and testaments of women physicians 1420, 1421, 3674
Wilmington, North Carolina see North Carolina, Wilmington
Wilson, John Stainback 229
Winston-Salem, North Carolina see North Carolina, Winston-
          Salem
Wisconsin
     Physicians 903, 1292, 1574, 1579, 1803
     Racine County Medical Society 1747
Wisconsin, Milwaukee
     Milwaukee Medical Society 1579
Wisconsin, Neilsville
     Memorial Hospital 860
Wisconsin, University of, Medical School 3080
Witch doctors 236
Witches 144, 146, 175
Woman suffrage
     College Equal Suffrage League 779
     Dominion Women's Enfranchisement Association (Canada) 356
     Effects on physicians 1030
     Minnesota Suffrage Association 787
     National American Woman Suffrage Association 967, 2790
     Parade in support of 4080
     Physicians active in
          Canada 328
          Great Britain 515, 600, 602, 612, 615, 616
          Netherlands 445, 461
          Sweden 436
          USSR 737
          United States 787, 850, 1048, 1160, 1188, 1247, 1341,
               1579, 1601, 1612, 1694, 1712, 1792, 1847
Woman's British Temperance Society 1781
Woman's Christian Medical College (Shanghai, China) 3196
Woman's Christian Temperance Union 1298
          See also Hospitals--Temperance
     Physicians in 889, 922
Woman's College Hospital see under Ontario, Toronto
Woman's Evening Clinic see under Washington, D.C.
Woman's Foreign Missionary Society, Methodist Episcopal Church
          2532
Woman's Hospital and Infants' Home see under Michigan, Detroit
Woman's Hospital of Cleveland see Ohio, Cleveland--Woman's
          General Hospital
Woman's Hospital of Philadelphia see under Pennsylvania, Phila-
          delphia
Woman's Medical College (Toronto) see Ontario Medical College
          for Women (Toronto)
Woman's Medical College of Chicago see Northwestern University
          Woman's Medical College
Woman's Medical College of Cincinnati see Laura Memorial Wo-
          man's Medical College (Ohio)
Woman's Medical College of Pennsylvania see Medical College of
          Pennsylvania (Philadelphia)

Woman's Medical Institute see Korea, Woman's Medical Institute
    of (Seoul)
Woman's Medical Journal see Medical Woman's Journal
Woman's Medical School at Soochow see Soochow Woman's Med-
    ical School (China)
Women and Children's Hospital of Chicago see under Illinois,
    Chicago
Women Doctors' Retainer Scheme (Great Britain) see under Na-
    tional Health Service (Great Britain)
Women Physicians' Club of San Francisco see under California,
    San Francisco
Women's and Children's Free Medical and Surgical Dispensary see
    Ohio, Cleveland--Woman's General Hospital
Women's and Children's Hospital (Compton) see under California,
    Compton
Women's and Children's Hospital (Kansas City) see under Missouri,
    Kansas City
Women's and Children's Hospital (Nanchang) see under China,
    Nanchang
Women's and Children's Hospital (Punjab) see under India, Punjab
Women's Auxiliary Service Pilots (WASPs) 1317
Women's Bureau (U.S.) report on opportunities for women physicians
    (1945) 2375
Women's Christian Medical College see Ludhiana Medical College
    (India)
Women's Clinic of Helsinki see Finland, Helsinki--Helsinki Wo-
    men's Clinic
Women's Equity Action League 2364
Women's Hospital (Madura) see under India, Madura
Women's Hospital (Soochow) see under China, Soochow
Women's Hospital Camp see under Poland, Brzeziny
Women's Hospital Corps (Great Britain) see under World War I
Women's hospitals see Hospitals, Women's
Women's Labour League (Great Britain) 607
Women's League for Peace (USSR) 727
Women's Medical Association of New York City see under New
    York City
Women's Medical College (Ontario) see Ontario Medical College
    for Women (Toronto)
Women's Medical College of the New York Infirmary for Women and
        Children (New York City) (See also New York City--
        New York Infirmary for Women and Children)
    Activities
        (1850s-1860s) 3444, 3459
        (1870s) 3462-3464
        (1880s) 3477, 3482
    Catalogues and announcements 3460, 3471, 3472
    Closing 3785
    Commencements 2995, 3050, 3099, 3461, 3465, 3802
    Criticism of 2033
    Different from male and coeducational schools 3454
    Faculty reports (1880s) 3468, 3469
    Founders 212

History 3491
Incorporation 3457, 3484
Opening addresses 3051, 3413, 3458
Reminiscences 1374, 3617
Students 3447, 3461
Women's Medical Institute (Leningrad, USSR) 207, 739
Women's Medical School (Agra, India) see Agra, Women's Medical
        School of (India)
Women's Medical Society of New York State see under New York
        State
Women's Missionary Institute (London, England) 3322
Women's over-seas hospitals see under World War I
Women's Party (Yugoslavia) see Yugoslavia Women's Party
Women's rights movement (See also Equal rights; and Woman suf-
        frage)
    Attitudes towards 2952, 3042, 3072, 3141, 3983
    Physicians active in
        U.S. 802, 1238, 1601, 1806, 1834
        Western Europe 45, 415, 419, 456, 496
    Relation to women's education 212, 637, 2002, 2889, 3003
Women's War Service Auxiliary of New Zealand see under World
        War II
Woolston Memorial Hospital see under China, Foochow
Worcester Medical Institution (Massachusetts) 250, 1780
World Columbian Dental Congress 1448
World Health Organization (United Nations) 533, 939, 1822, 3369
World War I (See also Armed services)
    American physicians 1240, 1273, 1478, 1485, 1605, 1809, 1840,
        2318, 2681-2684, 2744, 2752, 2756, 2784, 2790, 2842
    Australian physicians 303
    British physicians 501, 585, 611, 686, 2193, 2694, 2696,
                2697, 2699, 2705, 2713, 2790, 3925
    Duties of women physicians 2751, 2759
    Effects on medical education 1927, 1939, 1961
    Opportunities for physicians 2711, 2712, 2716, 2718, 2772,
                2783, 2785, 2816, 2824, 2836, 4032
    Russian physicians 2672
    Serbian physicians 388
    Women's Hospital Corps (Great Britain) 560, 2193, 2705, 2714
    Women's Over-Seas Hospitals 974
World War II (See also Armed services)
    American physicians 831, 857, 883, 1610, 1827, 2701, 2709,
                2743, 2823
    Australian physicians 1505
    British physicians 2215, 2669, 2686, 2688, 2689, 2714
    Canadian physicians 2669
    Duties of women physicians 2740, 2768
    Effects on medical education 276, 2737
    Emergency Medical Service (Great Britain) 2698
    Finnish physicians 470
    Opportunities for physicians 2375, 2715, 2764, 2769, 2771,
                2776, 2791, 2805, 2806, 2828, 4046, 4049
    Physician refugees 3514

Polish physicians 699
Postwar predictions concerning physicians 4046, 4048
Russian physicians 2672, 2673, 2678-2680
Women's War Service Auxiliary of New Zealand 301
World's Fair (1939), Physicians' participation 3697
Writing, Medical
    Authorship and acknowledgements statistics 2322
    First article by a woman physician published in the U.S. 1650
    Opportunities for physicians 2301, 2358
    Women's contribution 160
Wuchang, China see China, Wuchang
Wuhu, China see China, Wuhu
Wyoming County Medical Society see under New York State

Yale University School of Medicine 3063
Yemen
    German physicians 487
Yong Dong, Korea see Korea, Yong Dong
Young, Brigham 1533
Young Women's Christian Association Conference 753, 2262, 3825
Yugoslavia (See also American Women's Hospitals Service--Activities)
    American physicians 1485
    American Women's Hospitals 3403, 3429, 3582, 3706, 3819
    British physicians 585, 612, 2674, 2675
    Hospitals run by women 2257
    Native physicians 13, 17, 377, 388, 388a, 389, 394, 398, 414
    Russian physicians 379
Yugoslavia, Bosnia and Herzegovina
    Physicians 34, 413, 439, 3868
Yugoslavia, Herzegovina see Yugoslavia, Bosnia and Herzegovina
Yugoslavia Women's Party 388

Zaire see Congo
Zenana Medical College (London, England) 2651
Zeta Phi fraternity 3495
Zurich, Switzerland see Switzerland, Zurich
Zurich, University of (Switzerland)
    Women medical students 1895, 1896, 3219, 3221, 3226, 3232,
        3233
        Russian 376, 380, 739, 3225

Abbott, Eulalie M. (20th C)
1206
Abbott, Julia Holmes see
Smith, Julia Holmes
Abbott, Maude Elizabeth Sey-
mour (1869-1940) 307, 311,
320, 324, 329, 331, 347, 350,
353, 671, 705, 952, 1439
Biographies 161, 309, 342,
348
Career sketches 12, 317,
326, 349
Personality traits 321, 358
Abella (Middle Ages) 31, 70,
134
Abercrombie, Anna S. (MD
1908) 3421
Abouchdid, Edma (20th C) 3843
Abt, Theresa Knauf (b1866)
1193, 1315
Acosta-Sison, Honoria Herminia
(b1890) 268, 1537, 3835,
3839
Acres, Louise (b1858) 884
Adair, Bethenia see Owens-
Adair, Bethenia Angelina
Adams, Fae M. (b1918) 1573
Adams, Letitia Douglas (b1878)
1301
Adams, Myrta Mae Wilson
(b1897) 1726
Adams, Sarah E. (1779-1846)
802, 803
Adams-DeWitt, Lydia (1859-
1928) 917
Adamson, R. H. B. (20th C)
2694
Adamson, Sarah Read see
Dolley, Sarah Read Adam-
son
Addams, Mary see Leslie-
Smith, Mary Addams

Afable, Trinidad (b1908) 266
Agnodice (c300 BC) 25, 62,
132, 137, 153, 171, 3913
Aguirra, Maria Luisa (20th C)
703
Ahlem, Judith Emelia (b1895)
1461
Ai, Hee Kim (20th C) 3786
Aigner-Rollett, Oktavia (1877-
1959) 416
Airmedh (8th C) 156
Akers, L. Stella (d1929) 2656
Akin, Mabel M. (b1879) 826,
1080, 1357
Albrecht, Margarete (b1894?)
2178
Albright, Tenley Emma (b1935)
1646
Aldegunde de Nolde, Helena
(18th C) 135
Aldrich-Blake, Louisa Brandreth
Euclid (1865-1925) 534, 655
Aleixandre y Ballestar, Maria
Concepcion (19th C) 18
Alexander, Annie Lowrie (1860-
1917) 1199
Alexander, Christina McCulloch
see Blaikie, Christina Mc-
Culloch Alexander
Alexander, Harriet C. Beringer
(1858-1938) 1197, 1228
Alexander, Hattie Elizabeth
(1901-1968) 1250
Alexander, Ida Mary F. (b1877)
749
Alexander, Lilian Helen (1861-
1934) 299
Alexander, Virginia Margaret
(b1899) 1180
Algee, Madeline Johnston (b1897)
1832
Ali, Safieh (Safiye) (20th C)

3830, 3843

Allen, Florence see Inch, Florence Allen

Allen, Maud (19th C) 2594

Allen, Mira (Miranda) May (b1870) 1678

Alley, Reuben Gertrude (b1897) 1219

Allison, Mary Bruins (20th C) 878, 1518

Alsop, Gulielma Fell (b1881) 757, 4051

Alvarez, Virginia Pereira (MD 1920) 195

Amable (fictional) 149

Amelie, Queen of Portugal (20th C) 459

Andersen, Judith Cooper (b1944) 1713

Anderson, Belle see Gemmell, Belle Anderson

Anderson, Camilla (MD 1929) 1080

Anderson, Eleanor see Campbell, Eleanor Milbank Anderson

Anderson, Elizabeth Garrett see Garrett-Anderson, Elizabeth

Anderson, Kathryn D. (b1939) 3046, 3072

Anderson, Susan M. (b1870) 1738

Anderson-McIntyre, Justina (d1938) 796

Anderson-Riffle, Kathleen (b1879) 796, 3893, 3894

Andersson, Hedda (1861-1950) 44, 2159

Andreen-Svedberg, Andrea (19/20th C) 2154

Andrews, Mabel L. V. (20th C) 498

Angell, Harriet see Gerry, Harriet Angell

Angelucci, Helen Marguerite (b1896) 1541

Angwin, Maria (MD 1892) 12, 352

Anthony, Catherine Wilson (b1921) 882

Anyte (of Epidaurus) (3d C BC) 20

Apgar, Virginia (1909-1974) 1064

Archangelskaya, A. G. (19th C) 205, 207

Ardery, Mary Dugan (b1842) 1406

Armstrong, Frances see Rutherford, Frances Armstrong

Armstrong, Sarah B. (b1857) 1680

Arnine, Queen (literary) 149

Arnold, Anna Whelan (b1897) 2956

Arnold, Jean (20th C) 3127

Arnold, Jeannie Oliver (b1860) 772

Aronson, Emma Selkin see Selkin-Aronson, Emma

Artemisia II (3d C BC) 20

Arthurs, Ann Catherine (b1889) 875

Ashby, Winifred Mayer (b1879) 1122

Ashkenazi (Middle Ages) 70

Ashton, Dorothy Laing (b1888) 3605

Aspasia (2d C) 62, 134, 153

Aspinall, Jessie Strahorn (20th C) 300

Atkins, Louise (19th C) 3232

Atkinson, Dorothy Wells (b1893) 1072

Atkinson, Kate see King May-Atkinson, Kate

Attkins, Evelyn Jeffrey Forgan (1911-1963) 495

Austin, Ella see Enlows, Ella Morgan Austin

Auten, Alcinda see Pine, Alcinda Auten

Avery, Caroline Louise (1865-1949) 1421

Avery, Mary Alice (1849-1904) 1336

Babel (19th C?) 2869

Bacon, Mary (b1893) 1405

Baer, Mary (b1863) 3338

Bain, Katherine (b1897) 2496

Baker, Charlotte Le Breton Johnson (b1855) 2323

Baker, Mary (b1897) 3780

Baker, May Davis (b1866)
1311, 4023
Baker, Mercy N. (1840-1918)
931
Baker, Minnie Dell Sprague
(1858-1934) 1682
Baker, Sara Josephine (1873-
1945) 861, 1055, 1437,
1601, 1636, 2090, 2260, 3576,
3656, 3666, 3701
Biographies 779, 1056, 1121,
1553
Memorials 1645, 1836,
3672
Baker-McLaglan, Eleanor
Southey (1879-1969) 288,
293
Bakhireva, E. V. (20th C)
2673
Bakwin, Ruth Morris (b1898)
1510
Baldwin, Evelyn (d1917) 1800
Baldwin, Helen (1865-1946)
1006, 1252, 3576
Baldwin, Janet Sterling (1908-
1958) 1444
Bale, Rosa (d1941) 658
Balfour, Margaret I. (20th C)
2116, 3840
Ball, Elizabeth Browning
(b1882) 780
Ballard, Cora Marie (b1865)
3354
Ballard, Edith Loeber (b1875)
982
Ballard, L. Anna (b1848)
1679
Bamford, Rachel Ethel (1889-
1958) 458
Bancroft, Mabel Harvey Falk
(MD 1903) 2682
Bang, Dagny (MD 1896) 442
Banks, Sarah Gertrude (MD
1873) 1685
Barahona, Ernestina Perez
(MD c1890) 3948
Barbara (of Frankfurt) (Middle
Ages) 70
Barker, Anna E. (1861-1929)
1305
Barker-Ellsworth, Alice
(1875-1947) 955, 1425
Barlow, Agnes see Harrison,

Agnes Barlow
Barlow-Brown, Alice (b1869)
2682, 3582
Barnard, Margaret Witter
(b1896) 1031
Barrett, Clara Binns (b1894)
1444
Barrett, Florence Willey (d1945)
597, 3359
Barrett, Kate Waller (d1925)
972
Barringer, Emily Dunning (1877-
1961) 167, 785, 998, 1077,
1108, 1109, 1121, 1134,
1462, 1535, 2484, 3656
Barrows, Isabel (1845-1913)
1721
Barry, James (Miranda Stewart)
(1795-1865) 8, 12, 138, 167,
356, 528, 596, 609, 625,
650, 652, 661, 662, 667,
2706, 2714, 2717, 4064
Barry, Miranda see Barry,
James (Miranda Stewart)
Barsness, Nellie O. (b1875?)
830, 1240, 1447
Bartlett, Esther E. (b1902)
1381
Bartlett-Tyson, Frances (b1874)
1312, 1442
Bartsch-Dunne, Anna (b1876)
898
Bartuska, Doris Gorka (b1929)
1860
Bass, Mary Elizabeth (1876-
1956) 240, 819, 1404, 1482
Bassi, Laura Maria Catarina
(1711-1778) 36, 53, 108,
135, 137
Bateman, Jeanne Cecile (b1903)
823
Bateman, M. Mitchell (MD
1946) 756
Bates, Mary Elizabeth (1861-
1954) 161, 700, 805, 1036,
1347, 1471, 2099, 3705
Batzer, F. Marian Williams
see Williams, F. Marian
Bauer, Lydia see Hauck,
Lydia Roselle Bauer
Bauer, Marjorie L. Frantz
(b1916) 1829
Baumann, Frieda (b1887) 923,

1790

Baumgartner, Leona (b1902)
1019, 1134, 1330, 1331,
1446, 2972, 3177

Bayer, Anna (19th C)   34, 439

Bayerova, Anna see Bayer,
Anna

Baylis, Katherine see MacInnis, Katherine Baylis

Beals, Rose Fairbank (b1874)
2652, 3829

Beamis, Louise W. (b1878)
3565

Bean, Achsa Mabel (b1900)
857, 1827, 2701, 2709,
2714

Beatty, Elizabeth (MD 1884)
12, 344

Beatty, Geneva (b1911)   1444

Beauperthy de Benedetti, Rosaria (20th C)   195

Bebinn (pre-19th C)   156

Beckett, Elizabeth see
Matheson, Elizabeth Beckett
(Scott)

Bedell, Leila Gertrude (d1914)
1198

Bednyakova, V. (19th C)   736

Beecher, Mabel see King,
Mabel Beecher

Beglarion, [Dr.] (b1870?)
406

Beilby, [Dr.] (19th C)   3329

Belkind, Alexandria (20th C)
273

Bell, Jane L. Heartz (b1870)
317, 352, 357

Bell, Muriel (20th C)   297,
304

Bellhouse, Helen Wynyard
(b1910)   1597

Ben-Ami-Soloder, Sara (20th
C)   273

Bendahan, Chocron (MD 1939)
195

Bender, Lauretta (b1897)   699,
887, 1444

Benedetti, Rosaria see Beauperthy de Benedetti, Rosaria

Benedict, Sr. M. (20th C)
2511-2513, 3550

Benetar, Judith (pseud). (20th

C)   814

Bengtson, Ida (20th C)   3808

Benham, Alice Marion (d1939)
580

Bennett, Agnes (b1872)   301

Bennett, Alice G. (19/20th C)
2963

Bennett, Doris R. Rubin (b1924)
2972

Bennett, Emma (medical student)
(20th C)   2963

Bennett, Marjorie (b1909)   335

Bennett, (Mary) Alice (1852-
1925)   3609

Bennette, Marie Antoinette
(b1857)   1162

Benoit (19th C)   2869

Benson, Annette (19/20th C)
3330

Bentham, Ethel (d1931?)   607

Beregoff-Gillow, Pauline (b1901)
310, 704, 705

Bergere, Violette (MD 1917)
1063

Beringer, Harriet C. see
Alexander, Harriet C. Beringer

Bernard, Betty (b1933)   1829

Bernard, Marcelle (b1920)
1383

Berne, Georgina Dagmar (1866-
1900)   300, 305

Berry, Alice see Graham,
Alice Berry

Berry, Katherine see Richardson, Katherine Berry

Berry, [Lady] F. M. Dickenson
see Dickenson-Berry,
[Lady] F. M.

Bertine, Eleanor (1887-1968)
753

Bestuzheva, Sofia Ivanovna
(1840-1912)   2676

Betlheim, Vanda (19th C)   13

Betty, [Dr.] (fictional)   4067

Beucker, Andreae see Dorp-
Beucker, Andreae van

Beverly, Julia A. (1814-1876)
1161

Bickel, Beatrix Adelaide (b1875)
810, 2945

Bielby, Elizabeth (d1929)   502,
2116, 2604

Bien, Gertrude (19/20th C)
    3234
Bienenfeld, Bianca (MD 1916)
    3234
Biffin, Harriet (20th C) 289,
    300, 3204
Bigland, Phoebe Mildred Powell
    (d1930) 587
Billett, Helen Louise (d1926) 631
Billings, Cora see Lattin,
    Cora Billings
Bingen, Hildegard von (1098-
    1179) 100, 101
Binn see Bebinn
Binney, Nancy Elizabeth see
    Clark-Binney, Nancy Eliza-
    beth Talbot
Birch, Carroll La Fleur (1896-
    1969) 1366, 3550
Bissell, Helen M. (19th C)
    1679
Bissell, Heleń W. (20th C)
    1206
Bisyakina, V. P. (20th C)
    723
Bitting-Kennedy, Miriam
    (d1933) 1208
Black, Dora (20th C) 2196
Black, Elinor Francis Eliza-
    beth (b1905) 318, 343
Black, Louisa Teresa (b1866)
    1615
Blackman, Julia Cole (b1849)
    1197, 1640
Blackwell, Edith B. (MD 1891)
    1203
Blackwell, Elizabeth (1821-
    1910) 158, 219, 1158, 1464
    Biographical sketches 161,
    167, 174, 177, 180, 212,
    497, 697, 702, 777, 841,
    1105, 1329, 1338, 1342,
    1493, 1555, 1622, 1718,
    1841, 3923, 4034
    Biographies (complete) 566,
    778, 844, 888, 1188, 1303,
    1364, 1489-1492, 1637, 1648,
    1801, 1806
    Career sketches 991, 1095,
    1763
    Early life 989, 1483, 1776
    Education 221, 1286, 1709,
    3940

Graduation to 1853 927, 990,
    1067, 1755
Letters and writings 239,
    1094, 1636, 1650
Memorials 181, 1454, 1676
New York Infirmary for Wo-
    men and Children 932, 1778,
    2755, 3444, 3446, 3447, 3451,
    3454, 3459, 3576
Nonmedical concerns 799,
    1340
Nursing experiences 513
Observations by others 624,
    843, 929, 1263, 1302, 1393,
    1715
Relationship with Florence
    Nightingale 247, 845
Blackwell, Emily (1826-1910)
    219, 799, 1094
    Biographies 161, 174, 177,
    842, 925, 1188, 1493, 4034
    Memorials 1263, 1454,
    1569, 1676
    New York Infirmary for Wo-
    men and Children 3444,
    3446, 3450, 3576
    Relationships with other phy-
    sicians 926, 934, 1264
    Reminiscences by others
    210, 1374
    Western Reserve Medical
    School 3809
    Work with Elizabeth Black-
    well 844, 888, 1364, 1806
Blaikie, Christina McCulloch
    Alexander (1866-1945) 659
Blair, Lovisa I. (1878-1944)
    1616
Blake, Charlotte see Brown,
    Charlotte Amanda Blake
Blake, Sophia Jex see Jex-
    Blake, Sophia
Blampin, Winifred (b1896) 4006
Blanchard, Frances S. Carothers
    (b1856) 1481
Blandy, Marjorie (1887-1937?)
    622
Blanton, Libby (medical student)
    (20th C) 3098
Blatchford, Ellen Henrietta
    Comisky (b1900) 354
Blink-Rolder, J. W. van den
    (MD 1925) 3884

Bliss, Barbara E. (b1924)
2427
Bliss, Clara see Hinds, Clara
Bliss
Blount, Anna Ellsworth (1872-
1953) 766, 816, 2100
Bluestone, Naomi Ruth (b1936)
2428
Bluhm, Agnes (19th C) 101,
2869, 2884
Bocchi, Dorothea (1390-1436)
180, 3227
Bodley, Rachel L. (1831-1888)
243, 265, 758, 1496, 1687,
2055, 3389, 3537
Bogan, Isabel Katherine (b1889)
1615
Bogle, Kate Breckinridge see
Karpeles, Kate Breckinridge
Bogle
Bogolepova, Lyudmila Sergeevna
(1889-1969) 722
Boivin-Gillain, Marie-Anne-
Victoire (1773-1841) 87,
132, 141, 159, 182
Bokova-Sechenova, M. A. (MD
1871) 197, 205, 376, 380,
734, 3225, 3232
Bolibot, Sofia Ivanovna (1850-
1918) 2676
Bolton, Elizabeth (1878-1961)
500
Bolton, Ruth (fictional) 4058
Bolza, Anna (19th C) 16
Bond, Roberta see Nichols,
Roberta Bond
Bone, Honor (20th C) 663
Bono, Silvia Maria (20th C)
3875
Bonomi, Ester (20th C)
3892
Bonser, Georgiana M. (20th
C) 647
Boose, Emma see Tucker,
Emma Boose
Borden, Sallie see Hutton,
Sallie Borden
Borrino, Angela (20th C)
3892, 3906
Bostwick, Sara Howard see
Hoffman, Sara Howard Bost-
wick
Boteford, Mary E. (19/20th C)

863
Boulding, Dorothy see Fere-
bee, Dorothy Boulding
Bourdeau-Sisco, Patience S.
(b1869) 1282, 3421
Bourgeois-Boursier, Louyse
(1563-1636) 32, 36, 38, 69,
74, 138, 141, 153, 154, 159
Boursier, Louise see Bourgeois-
Boursier, Louyse
Bower, Emma Eliza (b1849)
1672
Bowerman, Mary see Purvine,
Mary Bowerman
Bowles, Katharina (17th C) 36,
135, 180
Bowman, Mary M. (19/20th C)
2537
Bowser, Hilda Crichton (1892-
1941) 567
Boyd, Lois see Gaw, Lois
Boyd
Boyle, Helen (19th C) 687,
2193
Boylen, Alice Lois McCollough
(b1937) 1829
Brabb, Alice Amelia (1856-1917)
1681
Brackett, Elizabeth Rock (b1892)
1532
Bradford, Mary Elizabeth (b1858)
2521
Bradley Bystrom, Elizabeth
(1852-1906) 871
Branham, Sara Elizabeth (b1888)
1445
Brant, Cornelia Chase (MD
1903) 902
Braunwarth, Anna M. (b1857)
796
Braunwarth, Emma W. (1859-
1940) 796
Braunwarth, Jannette Sarah
(1853-1927) 796
Breed, Mary E. (19th C) 3447
Breen, Grace (fictional) 4056,
4058
Breeze, Gabrielle (19th C)
2505
Brekke, Viola G. (b1904) 1448
Brent, Helen (fictional) 4058
Brenton, Helen see Pryor,
Helen Brenton

Brês, Madeleine (MD 1875)
    33, 72, 3940
Breymann, Margaretha (19/
    20th C) 99
Brinck, Julia (19th C) 2390
Brindley, Clare Evalyn (b1920)
    2430
Brison, Eliza P. (1881-1974)
    340
Brodie, Jessie Laird (b1898)
    760, 858, 885, 1080, 1119,
    3379
Broido (20th C) 455
Broman, Anna (d1962) 499
Brookins, Jennie see Clark,
    Jennie Brookins
Brooks, Rachel see Gleason,
    Rachel Brooks
Broomall, Anna E. (1847-
    1931) 1171, 1248, 1368,
    1688, 1845, 3536, 3537,
    3605
Brown, Adelaide (1868-1940)
    953
Brown, Alice (US) see Bar-
    low-Brown, Alice
Brown, Alice (Great Britain)
    (d1941) 574
Brown, Amy Garrison see
    Kimball, Amy Garrison
    Brown
Brown, Charlotte Amanda
    Blake (b1846) 236, 863,
    978, 1432, 1495, 1621, 3742
Brown, Dorothy L. (b1916)
    756, 1559
Brown, [Dame] Edith (MD
    1891) 3336
Brown, Edith Petrie (b1900)
    1580
Brown, Fanny Hurd (b1867)
    1266
Brown, Lucy see Hughes-
    Brown, Lucy
Brown, Madelaine Ray (b1898)
    1442
Brown, Mary (19th C) 2540
Brown, Vera Scantlebury
    (d1946) 3861
Brownell, Emily A. see Var-
    ney-Brownell, Emily A.
Bruce, Maybel (b1924) 2649
Bruch, Hilde (b1904) 1609

Brucke-Teleky, Dora (20th C)
    427, 700
Brueckner, [Dr.] (18th C) 135
Brul, Marcella Du see Du
    Brul, M. Marcella
Brun, Thyra Sloth see Sloth-
    Brun, Thyra
Brunander, Siri see Wikander-
    Brunander, Siri
Brunyate, Annie Tombleson
    (d1937) 613
Bryant, Alice Gertrude (b1862)
    700
Bryant, Ruth Ophelia Leake
    (1856-1914) 1208, 1677
Bryce, Lucy (20th C) 3861
Buček, Augusta (MD 1903) 13
Buchanan, Mary (1870?-1946)
    4079
Buckel, Chloe Annette (1843-
    1912) 236, 863, 1432, 1501,
    1621, 3447
Buckley, Emma (MD 1902)
    3204
Buckley, Olive B. (20th C)
    2514
Buckley, Sara Craig (1856-
    1922) 796, 1125
Buckley, Winifred (20th C)
    2705
Budzinska-Tylicka, Justyna
    (1867-1936) 404
Bugbee, Marion Louise (b1871)
    3780
Bullard, Rose Talbot (b1864)
    236
Burnett, Mary Weeks (MD
    1879) 3765
Burr, Carrie see Simpson-
    Coleman-Burr, Carrie
Burr, Elizabeth see Thelberg,
    Elizabeth Burr
Bushnell, Katharine C. (b1855)
    873, 1298, 2527, 2534
Butin, Mary see Ryerson,
    Mary Butin
Butler, Alice (1863-1929) 956
Butler, Fanny Jane (1850-1889)
    546, 2604, 2632
Butler, Josephine (1828-1906)
    874, 1187, 3188
Butler, Margaret F. (d1931)
    1029, 1833

Butler, Miriam (b1898) 1472

Button, Helen Louise (b1900)
  3174

Byett, Hilda (d1942) 590

Byington, Mary Kate (1869-
  1935) 1678

Bystrom, Elizabeth see Bradley Bystrom, Elizabeth

Calderone, Mary S. (b1904)
  877

Caldwell, Margaret (1845-1938)
  905, 1579

Calenda, Costanza (Middle
  Ages) 31, 59, 70, 134

Call, Emma Louisa (b1847)
  3732

Callendar, Emma Huddah
  (1839-1878) 1305

Calopathaki (17th C) 62

Calverley, Eleanor Jane Taylor (b1886) 878, 1693

Campbell, Eleanor Milbank
  Anderson (b1878) 818

Campbell, Elizabeth (b1862)
  1258

Campbell, Grace (MD 1899)
  3341

Campbell, Mabel R. (d1939)
  689

Campbell, Susan (d1930) 634,
  2608

Campbell-Mackie, Mary (20th
  C) 518, 519

Candia, Beatrice di (19th C)
  180

Cannon, Martha Hughes Paul
  (1857-1932) 1533-1632

Carcupino-Ferrari, Myra (20th
  C) 465

Cardwell, Mae H. Whitney
  (b1864) 759

Cargill, Winifred Drummond
  (1901?-1930) 672

Carleton Jessica Royce (b1862)
  2618

Carleton, Mary Eline (MD
  1886) 1194

Carleton, May (d1927) 2535

Carothers, Frances see
  Blanchard, Frances S.
  Carothers

Carpenter, Julia W. (b1840)
  1606

Carr, Catherine Creighton
  (b1893) 1195

Carr, Lucinda (d1914) 1198

Carrasco, Maria Luz Donoso de
  (b1916) 708

Carroll, Delia Dixon (1872-
  1934) 1203

Carswell, Harriet see Mc-
  Intosh, Harriet Carswell

Carter, Mary (20th C) 2994

Carvajal y del Camino, Laura
  see Martinez de Carvajal y
  del Camino, Laura

Carvill, Lizzie Maud (b1873)
  1545

Cashatt, Effie Faye see Lewis,
  Effie Faye Cashatt

Castaneda, Martina (MD 1882)
  3897

Castells, Martina (d1884) 18,
  3890

Castex-Sturgis, Margaret
  see Sturgis, Margaret Castex

Castro-Carro, Carmencita (19th
  C) 796

Castro-Carro, Celeste (19th C)
  796

Castro-Carro, Marisa (19th C)
  796

Castro-Carro, Providencia (19th
  C) 796

Castro-Carro, Teresita (19th
  C) 796

Castro Ischiae, Thomasia de
  Matteo (Middle Ages) 59,
  70, 180

Catani, Guiseppina (19th C)
  158

Catlin, Marion Woolston (b1931)
  1294, 1466

Catz, Charlotte (b1925) 1379

Caven, Evangeline R. (b1876)
  3582

Cavov, Miliea Sviglin see
  Sviglin-Čavov, Milica

Cesar, Antonieta see Dias,
  Antonieta Cesar

Chabanow, Anna N. see
  Shabanoff, Anna N.

Chadburn, Maud Mary (19/20th

C) 3303

Chadwick, Sarah (19th C) 3809

Chadwick, Sarah Ann see Clapp, Sarah Ann Chadwick

Chalmers, Alexandra (Mona) Mary see Watson, Alexandra (Mona) Mary Chalmers

Chambers, Helen (20th C) 2705, 3295

Chaplin, Matilda (student?) (19th C) 119

Chappell, Amey (b1900) 1146

Chard, Marie Louise (b1868) 934, 1785, 2484

Chase, Cornelia see Brant, Cornelia Chase

Chase, Lillian Alice (b1894) 341

Chase-Willson, Sara Thomasina (b1865) 918

Cheney, Lucilla Green (19th C) 2527, 2655

Chenoweth, Alice Drew (b1903) 1153, 1586

Chess, Stella (b1914) 1060

Chestnut, Eleanor (19/20th C) 2532

Chestwick, Marie (fictional) 4066

Chiao-chih, Lin see Lin, Chiao-chih

Childs, Mary E. see MacGregor, Mary E. Childs

Chilia, Elvira Rey (b1915) 711

Chisholm, Catherine (MD 1904) 507

Chopin (19th C) 2869

Chou, Rosalie see Han, Suyin

Chow, Anna M. Y. (20th C) 373

Christiancy, Mary (MD 1883) 2535

Christine (of Pisa) (1363-1431) 154

Christine, Barbara D. Weed (b1922) 3962

Chubb, Elsie M. (d1958) 260

Chun Wai Chan, Daphne (20th C) 275, 276, 282, 283

Ch'un Yü-yen (Han dynasty) 4

Chung, Ho Kei Ma see Ma, Chung Ho Kei

Chung, Margaret Jessie (b1889) 1610, 1665, 1765

Church, Ruth E. (b1905) 2748

Cilento, Phyllis (20th C) 1321

Cisinato, Venturela (Middle Ages) 70

Ciszkiewicz, Teresa (d1920) 404

Clapp, Sarah Ann Chadwick (d1908) 1196

Clarice of Rouen (14th C) 19, 28

Clarisse, Jehanne (14th C) 19

Clark, Annabel see Gale, Annabel Burdock

Clark, Daisy see Gale, Annabel Burdock

Clark, Esther Bridgman (b1900) 806

Clark, Jennie Brookins (1862-1946) 1617

Clark, Katherine Jane Stark (1866-1958) 660

Clark, Margaret Vaupel see Vaupel-Clark, Margaret

Clark, Mary Grover (19th C) 1686

Clark, Murdoch (19/20th C) 2229

Clark, Nancy (MD 1852) 3809

Clark-Binney, Nancy Elizabeth Talbot (1825-1901) 255, 1666, 1783

Cleaves, Margaret A. (19/20th C) 895

Clemmer, Virginia B. (b1944) 1236

Clendon, Clara Kate (b1868) 3687

Cleopatra (69-30 BC) 62, 132, 153

Cleveland, Emeline Horton (1829-1878) 851, 1171, 1494, 1687, 2755, 3509, 3536, 3537, 3605

Cleveland, Martha see Dibble, Martha Cleveland

Clisby, Harriet (b1830) 292, 573, 636, 691

Clow, Alice Sanderson (1876-1959) 591

Clower, Virginia Lawson (b1920) 2434

Clowes, Gertrude see Seabolt,
   Gertrude Clowes
Cobb, Isabel (b1858) 1011
Cochran, Gloria Grimes (20th
   C) 882
Cochrane, Margaret see
   Cooper, Margaret Cochrane
Cochrane, Martha see Strong,
   Martha Cochrane
Cogan, Sarah Edith Ives (b1873)
   1545
Coghlan, Isa F. (20th C) 300
Cohen, Elizabeth (1820-1921?)
   803
Cohen, Raquel Eidelman (b1922)
   2972, 3046
Cohen Stuart, N. see Stokvis-
   Cohen Stuart, N.
Colby, Margaret Ewart (b1855)
   890
Colby, Sarah A. (b1824) 1178
Cole, Carol Skinner (b1888)
   4070
Cole, Julia see Blackman,
   Julia Cole
Cole, Rebecca (1846-1922)
   866, 1052
Coleman, Carrie see Simp-
   son-Coleman-Burr, Carrie
Colinet, Marie (15th C) 180,
   489
Collins, A. Dorothy (20th C) 2198
Combs, Lucinda (MD 1873)
   2527, 2593, 2655
Combs-Strittmatter, Lucinda
   (19th C) 2527, 2649
Commena, Anna (1083-1148)
   154, 2717
Comstock, Elizabeth (b1875)
   793
Condat, M. (20th C) 437
Condict, Alice Bryan (MD 1883)
   2600
Cone, Claribel (MD 1890)
   1081, 1692
Conley, Frances K. (b1940)
   1802
Connor, [Dame] Jean see
   MacNamara, Annie Jean
Converse, Jehanne (Jeanne) of
   Salins (14th C) 19, 28
Cook, Clara Gathright (b1882)
   1442

Cook, Dana G. see Warner-
   Cook, Dana G.
Cook, Mary Anna see Thomp-
   son, Mary Anna Cook
Coolidge, Marie Belle (b1876)
   2744
Cooper, Elsie Thomson Douglas
   (d1958) 563
Cooper, Lillian (19th C) 6
Cooper, Margaret Cochrane
   (d1907) 1685
Copple, Peggy Jean (b1934)
   2436
Corbett, Catherine (d1960) 578
Cords, Elisabeth (19/20th C)
   99
Corey, Katherine Anne (d1936)
   2656
Cori, Gerty T. (1896-1957)
   887, 1092, 1433, 1710, 3673
Corpening, Cora Zetta (b1892)
   1215
Cory, Harriet Stevens (b1883)
   837
Coryllos, Elizabeth Vasiliki
   Despina (b1929) 2438
Cosa, Garcia de (20th C)
   3897
Cote, Marie M. (19th C) 914,
   1640, 2518
Coudray, Angelique see Du
   Coudray, Angelique
Craggs, Joyce E. see Roffey,
   Joyce E.
Craig, Anna B. G. (b1928)
   1125
Craig, Barbara (medical stu-
   dent) (20th C) 1349
Craig, Marion see Potter,
   Marion Craig
Craig, Sara see Buckley,
   Sara Craig
Craighill, Margaret D. (b1898)
   900, 1028, 1129, 1214, 1710,
   2771, 2774, 2838, 3389, 3509,
   3795, 3798
Cramer, Marjorie S. (b1941)
   2952
Craven, Judith (medical student)
   (b1945) 1140
Crawford, Mary M. (b1884)
   1041, 1412, 1527, 3701
Creighton, Catherine see

Carr, Catherine Creighton

Crescentius, Stephania (Pre-20th C) 132

Cringan-McIntyre, Lillias (b1890) 343

Croasdale, Hannah T. (MD 1880) 3552, 3605

Crocker, Diane H. Winston (b1926) 1829

Crockett, E. Ethelene J. (b1914) 3075

Crosby, Elizabeth C. (PhD, MD hon) (20th C) 992, 1690, 3805

Crosse, Victoria Mary (MD 1930) 645

Cross-Gray, Catherine see Gray, Catherine Cross

Crowder, Grace L. Meigs see Meigs, Grace Lynde

Cruickshank, Margaret (MD 1897) 297

Crump, Jean (b1892) 773

Culbertson, Emma V. P. B. (b1854) 1501

Cummings, Emma J. (19th C) 2601, 2602, 2619

Cunningham, Gladys Story (b1895) 2541

Curtis, Margaret see Roberts, Margaret Curtis Shipp

Cushier, Elizabeth M. (1837-1932) 224, 799, 861, 926, 1264

Cushman, Beulah (1890-1964) 1175, 1457, 2099

Cushman, Mary Floyd (b1870) 2506

Cusina, Donna (Middle Ages) 60

Cuthbert, Grace (20th C) 3861

Cutler (20th C) 3847

Czarnecki, Nancy Sonia Szwec (b1939) 1274

Daily, Ray Karchmer (b1891) 1445

Dakin, Marion Janet (b1912) 1831

Dale, Esther H. (b1897) 1446

Dale, Katherine Neel (1872-1941) 928, 1139

Dalyell, Elsie (19th C) 300

Danforth, Josephine see Gilette, Josephine Danforth

Danforth, Mary S. (b1882) 3780

Daniel, Annie Sturges (1858-1944) 767, 776, 779, 1246, 1479, 3576, 3629

Daniello, Maestra Antonia del Maestro (Middle Ages) 70, 132

Daniels, Anna Kleegman (1894-1970) 1702

Dann, Margaret (b1902) 1180

d'Arcy, Constance Elizabeth (20th C) 300, 3204, 3861

Darling, Dorothy Ruth (b1914) 882

Darrow, Anna Albertina Lindstedt (1876-1959) 1221, 1530, 1546

Darrow, Ruth Renter (1895-1956) 1699

Da Silva, Yamei Kin see Kin, Yamei

Daum, Susan Carol Moss (b1941) 3177

Davenport, Mary R. Myers (1858-1887) 1042, 2509

Davidson, Gisela Kaufer (b1908) 938

Davidson, Virginia Mayo (b1940) 1117

Davies, Veronica Catherine Jessica see McPherson, Veronica Catherine Jessica

Davies, Virginia Meriwether (d1949) 804

Davies-Colley, Eleanor (1874-1934) 524

Davis, Amanda (fictional) 4069

Davis, Elizabeth Bishop (b1920) 756

Davis, Katharine Bennent (20th C) 3188

Davis, May see Baker, May Davis

Davison, Rachel J. (d1912) 1679

Dawson, Emma see Parsons, Emma Dawson

Day, Isabel I. Thomas (b1891)
    334
Day, Mary see Gage-Day,
    Mary
Deacon, Ariel R. S. see Mc-
    Elney, Ariel R. S. Deacon
Deal, Louise Bacon (d1931)
    1022
de Allende, Ines L. C. (MD
    1934) 706
Dean, Jennie A. (20th C) 2682
Deane, Gertrude see Seabolt,
    Gertrude Clowes
de Carvalho, Domitila (20th C)
    424
Decker-Holcomb, Amy Amanda
    (1865-1936) 1683
De Garis, Mary C. (20th C)
    291
Dejerine-Klumpke, Augusta
    (1859-1927) 159, 447, 449,
    452, 460a, 462, 469
de la Marche, Marguerite
    (Margarethe) (17th C) 36,
    77
de Lange, Cornelia Catharine
    (20th C) 461, 2261, 3901
Delano, Barbara Gustin (b1940)
    2952
Delanöe, Eugenia (MD 1910)
    429
Delgado de Solis Quiroga, Mar-
    garita (20th C) 707, 712
DeLiee-Burke, Elvira (b1911)
    1107
Delle Donne, Maria (c1777-
    1842) 159, 180, 457, 3227
Dempsey, Lillian Elizabeth
    (b1873) 945
Dengel, Anna (b1892) 515, 693,
    1595, 2516, 2605, 2648,
    2659, 2662, 2665-2667,
    3564
Denko, J. Joanne Decker (b1927)
    2998
Denman, Charlotte see
    Lozier, Charlotte Denman
Dennis, Mary E. (1870-1938)
    1037, 1458
de Olloqui, Maria Juanita (d1957)
    355
de Procel, Matilda Hidalgo see
    Hidalgo de Procel, Matilda

Děrerová, Elena (20th C) 384a
de Rodriguez, Maria Luisa
    Saldún see Saldún de
    Rodriguez, Maria Luisa
de Solis, Margarita Delgado
    see Delgado de Solis
    Quiroga, Margarita
De Vilbiss, Lydia Allen (b1883)
    1647
DeVore, Louise (20th C) 981,
    2743
De Vriese, Bertha (MD 1900)
    423
DeWitt, Lydia see Adams-
    DeWitt, Lydia
Dexter, Martha Edith MacBride
    (b1887) 3609
Dias, Antonieta Cesar (1869-
    1920) 721
Diaz, Eloisa see Inzunza
    Eloiza Diaz
Dibble, Martha Cleveland
    (d1944) 1255
di Candia, Beatrica Gherardo
    (Pre-20th C) 132
Dickens, Helen Octavia (b1909)
    756, 1532
Dickenson-Berry, [Lady] F. M.
    (19/20th C) 508, 2928
Dickinson, Frances (b1856)
    1169
Didriksen, Sarah see Rose-
    krans, Sarah Hoff Didriksen
Diest, Isala see Van Diest,
    Anne Catherine Albertine
    Isala
Diez, Mary Luise (1879-1942)
    1411
Dikanskaya, Evgenia Elizarovna
    (19/20th C) 729, 3218
Di Lotti, Vlasta Kalalova (20th
    C) 390, 403, 3843
Dimock, Susan T. (1847-1875)
    803, 1178, 1199, 1271, 1453,
    1495, 1778, 1977, 3232,
    3647, 3662, 3732
Disosway, Lula Marjorie (b1897)
    1218
Dixon, Delia see Carroll,
    Delia Dixon
Dmitrienko, Lidia Stepanovna
    (20th C) 2679
Dmitrieva, Vera Michailovna

(d1901) 2676

Doane, Harriet M. (1872-1940)
    701, 946, 1005

Dobrska, Anna see Tomasze-
    wicz-Dobrska, Anna

Dodd, Katharine (b1892) 1445

Dodge, Eva Francette (b1896)
    744, 1310

Doherty, Kate C. (20th C)
    2804

Dole, Mary Phylinda (b1862)
    1068

Dolley, Sarah Read Adamson
    (1829-1909) 174, 1057-
    1059, 1178, 1480, 1494,
    1666, 1781, 2999, 3419,
    4034

Dombrowiecki, Alexandra
    (b1924) 2952

Dominga, Luisa (19th C) 18

Donahue, Julia Maud (1892-
    1942) 1069, 2536

Donald, Mary E. May (b1931)
    3127

Donaldson, Nettie see Grier,
    Nettie Donaldson

Donhaiser-Sikorska, Helena
    (1873-1945) 378

Donovan, Mabel (d1942) 576

Dorp-Beucker, Andreae van
    (20th C) 2261

Douglas, Letitia see Adams,
    Letitia Douglas

Douglas, Margaret Ellen (1878-
    1950) 317, 323, 355

Douglas, Maria Collins (1833-
    1899) 1504

Dove, Lillian E. Singleton
    (b1895) 756

Dowling, Emma see Kyhos,
    Emma Dowling Brindley

Down, Monica (d1927) 577

Downarowicz, Elzbieta (19/
    20th C) 404

Doyle, Helen MacKnight (b1873)
    1074

Doyle, Janet (fictional) 4058

Dranga, Amelia A. (20th C)
    3548

Drips, Della Gay (b1884) 1708

Drooz, Irma H. Gross (b1913)
    1076

Dryden, Mary Victoria (1868-

1946) 1419

Du Breel, Louise (20th C) 1726

Du Brul, M. Marcella (20th C)
    893

Duckering, Florence West
    (b1870) 3406

Du Coudray, Angelique (b1713)
    30

Du Fay, Thecle Felicita (18th
    C) 135

Duff-Good, Ella Ishbel (b1896)
    355

Dugan, Mary see Ardery,
    Mary Dugan

Dugès, Marie Jonet (18th C)
    3222

du Lee, Joan see Joan du Lee

Dundas, Grace see Giffen
    Dundas, Grace

Dunham, Ethel Collins (b1883)
    939, 3666

Dunn, Fannie see Quain,
    Fannie Dunn

Dunn, Thelma Brumfield (b1900)
    1444

Dunning, Emily see Barringer,
    Emily Dunning

Durgin, Bernice Elise (b1917)
    1543

du Saar, Marie (19/20th C)
    461

Duthie, Georgiana see Bonser,
    Georgiana M.

Eaba (2000 BC) 156

Earle, Elizabeth C. (1856-1940)
    1672

Easby, Mary Hoskins (b1898)
    4009

Easton, Anna see Lake, Anna
    Easton

Eby, Lauretta see Kress,
    Lauretta Eby

Ecklund, Effie Matilda (b1901)
    1657

Eddy, Mary Pierson (19th C)
    177, 1082, 2523, 2524,
    2653, 3843

Edelstein, Merle (b1941) 908

Eder, Stefanie (19/20th C)
    3234

Edmonds, Florence (MD 1921)

687

Edward, Mary Lee (b1885) 12

Edwards, Addie M. (b1872)
1208

Edwards, Anna Spencer see
Rankin, Anna Spencer

Edwards, Lena Frances (b1900)
699, 1559

Edwards, Mme. see Pilliet,
Mme. Edwards

Eggleston, Suzanne (medical student) (20th C) 1281

Ehrenthal, Gabriele Possaner
von (19/20th C) 34, 51, 55,
416, 2869, 3234, 3936

Ehrlich, Marta (20th C) 404

Eichelberger, Agnes (1863-1923)
954, 1500

Eisenhardt, Louise (1891-1967)
1155

Elders, M. Joycelyn Jones
(b1933) 756

Eleonore, Dutchess of Tropan
(17th C) 135

Elgood, Mrs. Sheldon Amos
(MD 1900) 628

Elias, Dorothy Armstrong
(b1910) 2748

Eliot, Martha May (b1891)
887, 939, 1092, 1376, 1400,
1710, 1822, 3666

Elisabeth, Queen of the Bel-
gians (MD 1900) 181

Elise, Sr. M. see Wyne, Sr.
M. Elise

Elizabeth of Hungary (b1207)
47

Elizabeth of Kent (17th C) 135

Elliott, Lucy MacMillan (20th
C) 3682

Elliott, Mabel Evelyn (1881-
1968) 696, 1027, 1106,
1509, 2677, 3202, 3502,
3582, 3596, 3649, 3682

Elliott, Mary Hughes (b1880)
2842

Elliott, Minnie Agnes Howard
(d1902) 1681

Ellis, Effie O'Neal (b1913)
756

Ellis, Elizabeth Hunter Lange
(b1902) 1220

Ellis, Ruth M. (b1927) 3503

Ellison, Lois Taylor (b1923)
1269, 2360

Ellsworth, Alice see Barker-
Ellsworth, Alice

Ellsworth, Anna see Blount,
Anna Ellsworth

Elsom, Katharine O'Shea (b1903)
699

Eltsina, A. A. (20th C) 730

Emans, Jean (20th C) 1294,
1466

Emanuel, Vera (b1906) 262

Emery, Allen Daisy (19/20th C)
1133

Empiria (1st C) 21

Eng, Hu-King see Hu, King
Eng

Eng Yu, Poe see Hu, King
Eng

Engbring, Gertrude Mary (b1897)
1532

Engert, Rosa E. (MD 1873)
1640

England, Grace Ritchie see
Ritchie-England, Octavia
Grace

Engström, Sigrid see Nolander-
Engström, Sigrid

Enlows, Ella Mortan Austin
(b1889) 1445

Epler, Blanch Nettleton (b1866)
1217, 4005

Epps, Roselyn Payne (b1930)
882, 1053

Erko, Matrena (20th C) 2680

Erlanger, Viola Janet (b1891)
1328

Ernest, Elvenor A. (b1872)
3695

Ernst, Alice Lucretia (b1861)
2525

Ernull, Clara see Jones,
Clara Ernull

Erxleben, Dorothea Christiana
Leporin (1715-1762) 69, 79,
82, 90, 91, 93-96, 98,
101-103, 105, 108, 132, 159,
162, 180, 479, 2906, 3934

Esaa, Dolores Maria see
Pianese de Esaa, Dolores
Maria

Eshelman, Lillian see Magan,
Lillian Eshelman

Eskelin, Karolina Sidonia (1867-1936) 3909

Eskridge, Belle Constance (1859-1941) 1477

Espino-Cabatit, Belen (20th C) 3835

Esterly, Nancy Burton (b1935) 2441

Estrela, Maria Augusta Generoso (b1861) 721

Ettinger, Alice (b1899) 1707

Evans, Alice (MD 1898) 3808

Evans, Amanda J. (1844-1909) 1670

Evans, Florence L. A. (b1872) 1208

Evans, Helen Glover (b1913) 119

Everaert, Clemence (MD 1893) 423

Everitt, Ella B. (1866-1922) 1251, 1598, 3605

Exley, Maud Conyers (1876-1924) 1427

Faber, Henrietta (aka Henry) (b1791) 132, 171, 717

Fabiola (d399) 26, 137, 162

Fairbank(s), Charlotte (19/20th C) 3402

Fairfield, Letitia (20th C) 2694, 2714

Fairlie, Margaret (d1963) 649

Fajans, Olga (19th C) 99

Fannon, Margaret Ann see Osborn, Margaret Ann Fannon

Farrand, Elizabeth M. (MD 1887) 1680

Farrar, Emma (19th C) 1754

Farrar, Lillian Keturah Pond (MD 1900) 1021, 2484

Fauquet (17th C) 135

Fawcett, Millicent Garrett (d1929) 684

Fay, Marion Spencer (PhD) (b1896) 243, 941, 1290, 1450, 1572, 3366, 3389, 4011

Fearn, Anne Walter (1870-1939) 969, 1121, 1124, 1821

Feder, Ellen W. Posnjak (b1917) 1661

Feilberg, Johanna Hvallmann see Hvallmann-Feilberg, Johanna

Feinberg, Olga J. Pickman (b1886) 273

Félicie, Jacobe(a) (14th C) 19, 28, 146, 149, 175, 180

Fenlon, Roberta F. (b1911) 1446, 3177

Ferebee, Dorothy Boulding (b1898) 756, 859, 1070, 1639

Feretti, Zaffira (d1817) 117, 157

Ferguson, Agnes Burns (b1885) 2100

Ferguson, Angella D. (b1925) 756

Ferguson, Ellen B. (1844-1920) 1632

Ferguson, Wilhelmina (19th C) 7, 300

Ferguson, Winifred (19th C) 6

Ferrari, Myra Carcupino see Carcupino-Ferrari, Myra

Ferretti, Maria Madalena see Pettraccini-Ferretti, Maria Madalena

Ferris, Phoebe A. (1869-1945) 1581

Fetterman, Julia Faith Skinner (b1887) 3605, 3789

Feyler, Marie (20th C) 3355

Fiedler, Dolores E. (b1926) 839

Field, Constance Elaine (20th C) 571

Field, Edna Ricker (b1848) 863

Filzherbert, Selina see Fox, Selina Filzherbert

Fimpel, Lena see Schreier, Lena Fimpel

Finch, Sarah Elizabeth (1881-1921) 1538

Findlay, Jessica White (MD 1889) 1164

Fink, Emma Sloop (MD 1906) 1705

Finkler, Rita Sapiro (b1888) 699, 1448, 1620

Finley, Caroline Sandford

(1875-1936) 974

Fischer-Pap, Lucia T. (b1933)
    3015

Fish, Barbara (b1920) 971

Fisher, Jessie Weston (b1872)
    3675

Fitfield, Emily Walworth (18/
    19th C) 3634

Fitzjames (fictional) see Bar-
    ry, James (Miranda Stewart)

Flanagan, Katharene Wave Allee
    (1869-1946) 1674

Fleming, Bethel G. Harris
    (b1901) 1135

Fleming, Lula C. (1862-1899)
    1201, 1351

Fleming, Mary Randolph (b1877)
    3338

Flesche, Susan La see Pi-
    cotte, Susan La Flesche

Flood, Mabel E. (20th C)
    3582

Flood, Regina see Keyes,
    Regina Flood

Florence, Loree (b1896) 1746

Flounder, Fanny (20th C) 233

Folger, Lydia see Fowler,
    Lydia Folger

Folkeson, Maria (19/20th C)
    2159

Folkmar, Eleanor (19/20th C)
    2366

Follansbee, Elizabeth A. (MD
    1884) 236, 863

Föllinger, Elis (20th C) 99

Fontaine, Therese Bertrand
    (20th C) 887, 1092, 1710

Foote, Lois Brooke see
    Stanford, Lois Brooke Foote

Forbes, Audrey Elaine (b1934)
    756

Forcee, Margaret (19th C)
    1754

Ford, Estella see Warner,
    Estella Ford

Ford, Harriet Rosa Delo
    (1873-1960) 521

Forgan, Evelyn see Attkins,
    Evelyn Jeffrey Forgan

Formad, Marie K. (b1863)
    1614

Forrester, Deborah P. M.
    (b1937) 1829

Fosness, Edith (b1853) 786

Foulks, Sara E. (b1881) 1141

Fowler, Laura (19th C) 3916

Fowler, Lydia Folger (1822-
    1879) 161, 216, 224, 255,
    1666, 1781

Fox, Elsie (MD 1911) 1257

Fox, Selina Filzherbert (d1958)
    627

Foye, Amelia Frances (b1871)
    1308, 4080

Fraenkel, Friederike (19/20th
    C) 3234

Frame, Mary see Thomas,
    Mary Frame Myers

Francis, Irene Susanne Pierre
    (b1908) 1526

Francis, Sr. M. (20th C)
    2609

Frank, Lou (medical student)
    (20th C) 3098

Frank, Thelma Edna (b1910)
    1446

Frankowski, Clementine Eliza-
    beth (b1906) 1445

Fraser, Catherine (d1926) 631

Fraser, Margaret Ethel Vic-
    toria (b1871) 2684, 2804

Frazer, Mary Margaret (b1891)
    1442

Frederic, Sr. M. (20th C)
    2610, 2611

Freese, Annie Elizabeth (b1874)
    1615

Frei, Theresa Hueter (19th C)
    99, 157

Freitag, Julia L. (b1927) 3177

Freitas Pereira, Maria Joana
    de (20th C) 3887

French, M. Isabella (19th C)
    3937

Frenkel, B. Barbara (19th C)
    99

Frenkel, Raisa Samoilovna see
    Svyatlovskaya, Raisa Samoi-
    lovna

Friedland, Else (19/20th C)
    3234

Friedmann, Amalie (19/20th C)
    3234

Frost, Mary Elizabeth (aka Ag-
    nes Stewart) (medical student)
    (19th C) 3580

Fulton, Annie Maxwell see
   Maxwell-Fulton, Annie
Fulton, Mary (d1929) 4, 950,
   2532, 2656, 3853
Funamura, Janwyn (medical
   student) (20th C) 1350
Furtos, Norma Catherine
   (b1905) 2749

Gage, Shirley Elliott (b1918)
   1180
Gage-Day, Mary (b1857) 1145
Galbraith, Katherine C. see
   Manion, Katherine C.
Gale, Annabel Burdock (d1931)
   525, 531
Gale, Rhoda (fictional) 4058,
   4063
Galt, Eleanor see Simmons,
   Eleanor Galt
Gambrell, Winton Elizabeth
   (b1903) 1732
Gantt, L. Rosa Hirschmann
   (b1875) 798, 1214, 1577,
   1602, 1603, 3714
Gardner, Emily (1899-1956)
   1147, 1148, 1339
Gardner, Mabel E. (b1883)
   701, 1168, 1363, 1447,
   2978
Gardner, Penney E. A.
   (b1943) 1151
Garfield, Brian (20th C) 696
Garis, Mary De see De
   Garis, Mary C.
Garrett, Mary (20th C) 3964
Garrett-Anderson, Elizabeth
   (1836-1917) 50, 158, 513,
   551, 665, 666, 679, 844,
   1806, 2411, 3290, 3294,
   3310, 3926
   Biographies (complete) 496,
   566, 617
   Biographies (sketches) 161,
   167, 174, 177, 497, 540,
   560, 584, 697, 702, 2864,
   3923
   Fight for recognition of women physicians' struggle 125,
   1931, 2193, 3940
Garrett Anderson, Louisa (b1873)
   496, 560, 611, 2705

Garrison, Harriet E. (b1848)
   1184
Garrison, Penelope Knapp
   (b1943) 3046, 3072
Gaskill, Cornelia Jane (b1912)
   2837
Gaston, Mary (b1855) 1651
Gates, Irene (b1900) 1152
Gauzon, Marie Paz Mendoza
   see Mendoza-Gauzon, Marie
   Paz
Gavrančič-Novak, Milana (19th
   C) 13
Gaw, Lois Boyd (b1878) 1206
Gay, Claudine Moss (b1915)
   882
Geib, M. Eugenia (b1918) 1788
Geisel, Carolyn E. (1862-1932)
   1677
Gelber, Anita (b1895) 763
Gelderblom, C. Auguste 99
Gemmell, Belle Anderson
   (b1863?) 791, 796, 813,
   1440
Gemwold, E. (20th C) 3893
Gering, Franziska Maria Char-
   lotte (18th C) 106, 2386
Gerish, Nettie Luella (b1884)
   694, 1511
Gerry, Harriet Angell (d1889)
   1672
Getty, Mary (b1859) 2804
Getzowa, Sophie (20th C) 273
Giannini, Margaret J. (b1921)
   743, 3177
Gibson, Freda (20th C) 294
Gibson, Julia Roberts (b1877)
   1157
Giddings, Aurora (19th C)
   1240
Giffen Dundas, Grace (d1934)
   529
Gilbert, Elsie Martinson (b1875)
   920
Gilchrist, Ella (d1884) 2656
Gilette, Josephine Danforth
   (19/20th C) 3687
Giliani, Alessandra (d1326?)
   15, 60, 76, 149, 1943
Gillain-Boivin, Marie-Anne-
   Victoire see Boivin-Gillain,
   Marie-Anne-Victoire
Gillette, Harriet E. (b1914)

1447, 2443

Gillie, K. Annis (20th C) 575

Gillmore, Emma Wheat (b1867)
2752

Gilmore, Marguerite (20th C)
3962

Ginko, Ogino (MD 1890) 3837,
3844, 3860

Ginsberg-Shimkin (20th C)
273

Giorgi, Elsie A. (b1911) 3177

Giz, Suat (20th C) 3830

Gjorgjevic, Vladana (19/20th
C) 394

Glascock, Joy Harris (1863-
1945) 1202, 1465

Glasgow, Maude (d1955) 906,
1159, 1160, 1404, 1607,
3176

Glassen, Mary see Townsend-
Glassen, Mary

Gleason, Margaretta B. (19/
20th C) 1781

Gleason, Rachel Brooks (1820-
1905) 1666, 1781

Gleiss, M. Wilhelmine (19/
20th C) 99

Gloeckner, Mary Louise Carpenter (b1904) 3177, 3385

Gloss, Anna D. (20th C)
2535, 3192

Glover, Mary Elizabeth (b1881)
1745

Glud, Margrete (20th C) 441

Glueck, Helen Iglauer (b1907)
1168

Goldsmith, Luba Robin (b1879)
3548

Golovina, A. 405

Golubeva, Nadezhda see Suslova, Nadya Prokofievna

Good, Ella Ishbel see Duff-
Good, Ella Ishbel

Goodman, Harriet see Mc-
Graw, Harriet Goodman

Gordon, Doris Jolly (20th C)
295, 296

Gordon, J. Mary Louisa (b1941)
550, 586, 690

Gorinevskaya, Valentina V.
(20th C) 2672, 2679

Goudsmit, Helene (20th C) 417

Gould, Mary see Hood,
Mary Gould

Gould, Sue Hurst Thompson
(b1899) 1062, 1133, 1344

Gove, Anna M. (1868-1948)
1200

Gowanlock, Jennie see Trout,
Jennie Gowanlock

Grace, Sr. M. (20th C)
2526

Grad, Marjorie Ann (b1921)
1168

Graff, Elfie Richards (b1876)
3598

Graham, Alice Berry (d1913)
3759

Gray, Catherine Cross (b1900)
1217

Gray, Etta G. (b1880) 3546,
3582, 3586, 3706, 3819

Gray, Sarah (19/20th C) 569,
3290

Grayson, Ellin (fictional) 4068

Green, Lucilla see Cheney,
Lucilla Green

Green, Mary E. (19th C) 1685

Greene, Cordelia Agnes (1831-
1905) 912, 1046, 1164,
1497, 1666, 3809

Greene, Marjorie Pearl Christine (1897-1964) 682

Greene, Mary Theresa (b1866)
701, 1038, 1046, 1164, 1367,
1417

Greenfield, Rose (19th C?)
2604

Gregory, Gertrude Betty (b1933)
951

Gregory, Mildred Geraldine
(b1894) 854, 1446

Greisheimer, Esther M. (b1891)
864

Grey, Anna Barbara (b1895)
2519

Grier, Nettie Donaldson (b1869)
1207

Grierson, Cecilia (MD 1889)
3946

Griffin, Edna L. (b1905) 855

Grigsby, Margaret Elizabeth
(b1923) 756

Grim, Ella Williams (b1877)
1044, 4079

Griscom, Mary W. (b1866)

220, 1172, 1368, 3192

Griselle, Elizabeth (19th C)
3809

Grogan, Gertrude (d1930) 538

Grover, Mary see Clark,
Mary Grover

Gstettner, Mathilde (19th C)
3234

Guarna, Rebecca (Middle Ages)
31, 59, 70, 132, 134, 155

Gueldenapfel, Anna Elisabet
see Horenburg, Anna Elisabet

Guest, Edith Mary (20th C)
572

Guierson, Cecilia (MD 1889)
721

Guion, Connie Myers (b1882)
879, 880, 887, 907, 980,
1134, 1213, 1436, 2484,
3656

Gullattee, Alyce McLendon
Chenault (b1928) 1173

Gullen, Augusta Stowe see
Stowe-Gullen, Augusta Ann

Gullett, Lucy (20th C) 289,
300, 3204

Gurd, Adeline Emma (1856-
1941) 1680

Guryan, A. S. (19th C?)
205

Guthrie, Mamie see Pallesen,
Mamie Guthrie

Guthrie, Sylvia Kema (MD
1926) 648

Hadden, Winifred Eileen (d1960)
505

Haffner, Vortha M. Baliman
(b1899) 1174

Haines, Blanche Moore (1865-
1944) 1680, 3666

Haines, Frances Edith (b1882)
2756

Halkett, Anne Murray (1622-
1699?) 154, 159, 180,
2717

Hall, D. Winifred (d1958) 556

Hall, Lucinda Susannah Capen
(1815-1890) 250, 1780

Hall, Rosetta Sherwood (b1865)
1422, 2529, 2535, 3193,

3847

Hall, Winifred S. (20th C)
2396

Halpir, Salomee see Rusiecki-
Halpir-Pilstein, Salomee

Ham, Goldie Suttle (b1896) 862

Hamann, Anna (1894-1970) 1615

Hamilton, Alice H. (1869-1970)
167, 697, 957, 1091, 1134,
1177, 1287, 1318, 1567,
1636, 1643, 1710, 1714,
4022

Hamilton, Annie Lee (b1864)
352

Hamilton, Lillias (d1925?) 547,
664

Hamilton, Norah (d1961) 630

Hamilton-Muncie, Elizabeth
(b1866) 1097

Hampton, Victoria (19/20th C)
1080

Han, So Jeai (20th C) 3190

Han, Suyin (aka Rosalie Chou)
(20th C) 363-365

Hanchelt, Juliet (1856-1921)
1498

Hannington, Mabel Louise
(d1966) 355

Hansen, Karen Marie (MD
1923) 441

Hansen, Mary Larney (b1921)
4023

Hansen-Hein, Estrid (b1873)
441

Hanson, Helen Beatrice de Rastricke (1874-1926) 493, 595,
2674, 2675

Harbou-Hoff, Alvida (b1862)
45, 441

Harding, Eva (19th C) 1574

Harding, Frances June Keller
(b1906) 148, 245, 1445

Hardy, Harriet Louise (b1906)
1447, 1643

Harlin, Vivian Krause (b1924)
882

Harper, Margaret (1879-1964)
290, 300, 3204

Harper, Mary McKibbin see
McKibbin-Harper, Mary

Harris, Alice (19th C) 2508

Harris, Jean Louise (b1931)
756

Harris, Joy see Glascock,
Joy Harris

Harris, Lillian N. (1863-1902)
2537, 3193

Harris, Thelissa (medical student) (20th C) 1140

Harrison, Agnes Barlow (b1860)
865

Hartgraves, Ruth (b1901) 1532

Hartig, Hermina Hermansen
(b1889) 1181

Hartley, Harriet Louise (b1874)
3609

Hartman, Mary Ellen (b1924)
1407

Haslinger, Hildegard (20th C)
2178

Hastings, Alicia E. (b1934)
756

Hatch, Edith Rebecca (b1876)
1445

Hauck, Lydia Roselle Bauer
(b1886) 1444

Havens, Mary P. (1839-1908)
1686

Haverfield, Addie R. (b1858)
786

Havliček, Zlata (MD 1911) 13

Haycock, Christine E. (b1924)
882, 2446

Hayden, Catharine Phoebe
(1858-1939) 1204

Hayden, Eleanor (b1907) 1656

Hayes, Marie Elizabeth (1875?-
1908) 435

Hayhurst, Susan (1820-1909)
1737, 3537

Haynes, Bessie Park (19th C)
786

Hayward, Carrie M. (d1906)
884

Hayward, Martha (1868-1942?)
1211

Heafitz, Lesley Bunim (b1940)
1294, 1466

Healy, Mildred M. (20th C)
1660

Hearst, Bella R. (b1920)
3174

Heath, Lillian (1865-1962)
1470

Hedger, Caroline (b1868) 3666

Heer, Anna (1863-1918) 463

Heerden, Petronella van see
van Heerden, Petronella

Heidenreich-von Siebold, Charlotte Heiland (1788-1859)
36, 83, 101, 157, 479, 481,
483, 486, 489

Heikel, Rosina (19th C) 3907

Heiland, Charlotte see Heidenreich-von Siebold, Charlotte
Heiland

Heim-Vögtlin, Marie see
Vögtlin, Marie Heim

Hein, Estrid Hansen see
Hansen-Hein, Estrid

Heinemann, Käthe (1899-1972)
477

Heins, Marilyn (b1930) 3075

Held, Antonia Elisabeth de
(18th C) 2386

Helfand, Toby Scheintaub (b1931)
3962

Hemenway, Ruth V. (b1894)
1641, 2544-2579

Hendershott, Lizzie Amanda
(b1859) 1681

Henderson, Orra Miller Baxter
(1895-1931) 1216

Hendrick, Rhoda Grace (b1874)
917

Hendrickson, Anna Rose Mc-
Nalley (b1892) 1615

Heney, Alice Kirk Roehrig Ryan
(b1867) 1682

Henning, Josepha see Siebold,
Regina Josepha von

Henry, Annie see McClung,
Annie Mae Henry

Henry, Frances J. (b1873)
1703

Henry, Mary Azalea Mitchell
(b1900) 1448, 1848

Hersend, [Mistress] (13th C)
19

Herwerden, Marianne van (19/
20th C) 461, 2261

Herz, Flora see Levy, Flora
Herz

Herzfeld, Gertrude (20th C)
581

Herzig, Emma Maria (19/20th
C?) 416

Herzog, Sophie (d1927) 803,
949

Hewell, Barbara Ann (b1903)
1726
Hewitt, Dorothy (b1902) 811
Heyes, Elizabeth (20th C)
1061
Hickey, Eileen Mary (d1960)
421
Hickey, Rachel (19/20th C)
2099
Hicks, Ernestine Julia (1859-
1938) 1681
Hidalgo de Procel, Matilda
(MD c1922) 2948, 3949
Hielscher, Helen Hughes (1863-
1935) 786
Higgins, Alice E. Kelly (b1883)
863
Hight, Gertrude (b1916) 1797
Hilborn, Carolina Lunetta
(1876-1948) 1216
Hildebrand, Jennie (19th C)
1723
Hildegard of Bingen, Saint
(1098-1178?) 26, 47, 69,
76, 89, 101, 104, 137, 138,
149, 150, 153, 158, 159,
162
Hilden, Marie Colinet de (16th
C) 132, 135, 159
Hill, Armina Sears (b1895) 771
Hill, Emily A. (d1902) 997
Hill, Emma Linton (1858-1943)
1225, 1757
Hill, Ethel see Sharp, Ethel
Hill
Hill, Isabel (d1933) 599
Hill, Lillie Rosa Minoka (d1952)
824, 1525, 1634
Hill, Xa Cadenne Averyllis
(b1909) 756
Hilliard, Marion (1902-1958)
319, 354
Hillyer, Frances Van Vechten
(1846-1924) 1679
Hinds, Clara Bliss (20th C)
2335
Hinterbuchner, Catherine
Nicolaides (b1926) 977
Hirschmann, L. Rosa see
Gantt, L. Rosa Hirschmann
Hirszfeld, Hanna (20th C) 699
Hishikawa, Yasu (19th C) 281,
1640, 2535

Hissong, Cecelia Ferne (b1939)
3075
Hoag, Lucy (19/20th C) 2656
Hoashoo (20th C) 271
Hobart, Mary Forrester (b1851)
1068
Hocker, Elizabeth M. Van Cort-
landt (MD 1897) 1262, 2758
Hodgman, Joan Elizabeth (b1923)
1829
Hodgson, Amy (d1930) 651
Hoebeke, Eli Ann (20th C) 450
Hoenigsberg-Hilferding, Marga-
rete (MD 1903) 34, 3234
Hoff, Alvida Harbou see Har-
bou-Hoff, Alvida
Hoffman, Sara Howard Bostwick
(1860-1926) 1682
Hofma, Elizabeth (1859-1938)
1682
Hogle, Kate A. see Mason-
Hogle, Kate A.
Holbrook, Mary Ann (19th C)
2656
Holcomb, Amy Amanda see
Decker-Holcomb, Amy Aman-
da
Holland, Margaret Ellen (1840-
1921) 949
Hollister, Mary C. (MD 1882)
1640
Holm, Sigrid (20th C) 417
Holmes, Elizabeth Jardine
(b1928) 2458
Holmes, Julia see Smith,
Julia Holmes
Holmgren, Sofia (19/20th C)
2159
Holst, Marie (MD 1893) 3893
Holth, Helga Spangborg (19th
C) 442
Holth, Marie Spaangberg (1865-
1942) 3888
Holtz, Anne (19th C?) 423
Holtzmueller, Ann see Schutt,
Ann
Hood, Mary Gould (b1850) 786,
787
Hoogh, Esperanza Oteo de
(b1904) 719
Hoon, Pierra Vejjabul see
Pierra Hoon Vejjabul
Horenburg, Anna Elisabet (16th

C) 36

Horilleno, Fe (20th C) 3835

Horn, Paula Marie (b1908) 1354

Horney, Karen (b1885) 1134

Horton-Underwood, Lillias (19th C) 1087, 2520, 2528

Hosmer, Harriett Goodhue (medical student) (19th C) 1743, 4082

Hostetter, Peggy (medical student) (20th C) 4026

Houston-Patterson, Anne (b1867) 1237

Howard, Lenora see King, Lenora Howard

Howard, Meta (b1862) 1680, 2528, 2530, 2535

Howe, Martha Elizabeth (b1902) 1658

Howe, Suzanne Adele L. (b1914) 740

Howe, Willella see Waffle, Willella Howe

Howell, Mary C. (b1932) 2037, 2972

Hu, King Eng (b1865?) 4, 366, 368, 2745, 3853

Hubert, Anna (1879-1956) 887, 966, 1083

Hubert, Elinor (20th C) 2178

Hughes, Helen see Hielscher, Helen Hughes

Hughes, Martha see Cannon, Martha Hughes Paul

Hughes-Brown, Lucy (1863-1911) 1200

Hugonni-Wartha, Vilma (1847-1922) 16, 386, 395, 400, 408, 412

Humphrey, Amy Rawson (b1876) 1208

Humphreys, Eleanor Mary (1892-1971) 1444, 1808

Hunt, Barbara (b1884) 1441, 2804, 3402

Hunt, Harriot Kezia (1805-1875) 212, 216, 239, 248, 249, 802, 1105, 1178, 1185, 1238, 1782, 3011, 3082, 3183

Hunter, Gertrude T. (20th C) 1239

Hunter-Newlove, Mary Myrtle Pennington (1865-1931) 1678

Hunt-Peters, Lulu see Peters, Lulu Hunt

Hurd, Annah (b1871) 786

Hurd, Ethel Edgerton (b1845) 786, 1240

Hurd, Fanny see Brown, Fanny Hurd

Hurd-Mead, Kate Campbell (1867-1941) 163, 797, 1297, 1346, 1371, 1403, 3552, 4055

Hurdon, Elizabeth (d1941) 541, 542, 561, 621, 3247

Hurrell, M. Louise (b1871) 2681, 3553, 3554

Hurst, Sue Thompson see Gould, Sue Hurst Thompson

Huson, Florence (d1915) 1680

Hutchins, Fannie Collins (d1944) 1123

Hutchinson, Adelle Stewart (d1909) 786, 1240

Hutchinson, Alice (20th C) 3272

Hutton, Isabel Emslie (d1960) 585, 654, 1241, 2694

Hutton, Sallie Borden (20th C) 1202

Hvallmann-Feilberg, Johanna (MD 1895) 442

Hyde, Laura (19th C) 2656

Hygeia (mythology) 150, 181, 185

Iglauer, Helen see Glueck, Helen Iglauer

Imison, Isabel Elizabeth (d1928) 633

Inberg, Lya (MD 1936) 195

Incarnata, Maria (Middle Ages) 70, 180

Inch, Florence Allen (b1875) 917

Ingelman-Sundberg, Maria (19/20th C?) 44

Ingersoll, Louise Mason (1877-1962) 1212

Ingham, Loy McAfee see McAfee, Loy

Ingleby, Helen (1887-1973)

568, 629

Inglis, Elsie Maud (1864-1917)
159, 501, 543-545, 611,
612, 2193, 2714, 3272, 3923

Inouye, Tomo (20th C) 3202,
3355, 3397

Inunzo, Eloisia Dias see Inzunza, Eloiza Diaz

Inzunza, Eloiza Diaz (MD 1877)
721, 1945, 3948

Irby, Edith Mae (20th C) 1559

Isabel (Elizabeth), Queen of
Portugal (15th C) 19

Isachsen, Louis (d1932) 442

Isolt, Queen of Ireland (literary) 149

Israeli, Clara (20th C) 792

Izquierdo, Eleanor R. (20th C)
1089

Jackson, Edith Banfield (b1895)
1794

Jackson, Josephine Agnes
(1865-1945) 805, 1016,
1424, 1627

Jackson, Mercy B. (b1802)
1178

Jacobi, Mary Corinna Putnam
(1842-1906) 158, 178, 210,
234, 785, 799, 933, 1264,
1494, 1778, 3656
Biographies 167, 697, 948,
1134, 1270, 1285, 1341,
1415, 1669, 1756, 1835, 3485
Letters and other writings
935, 940, 1612, 1623

Jacobina (14th C) 132

Jacob-Peller, Anna (20th C)
273, 3833

Jacobs, Aletta Henrietta (1854-
1929) 66, 158, 425, 445,
453, 461, 2261, 3884, 3901

Jaeger, Dorothy Steinle (b1917)
1071

Jaganadhan, Anni (19th C)
2123

Jakoby, Ruth Kerr (b1929)
2447

Jakshicj-Radulaski, Katitsa
(b1884) 389

Jalas, Rakel (20th C) 3907

James, Mary Latimer (b1883)

1410, 1519, 2581

Janeway, Margaret M. (b1896)
1128, 1378

Jankowska, Helina (20th C?)
384

Jauregui, Pilar (Pre-20th C)
158

Jefferson, Mildred F. (b1927)
2972

Jeffery, M. Pauline (b1898)
1278

Jennings, Mary Louise (b1868)
694

Jewell, Catherine Underwood
(19th C) 1178

Jex-Blake, Sophia (1840-1912)
624, 679, 799, 844, 1158,
1806
Biographical sketches 125,
161, 187, 496, 497, 697,
3461, 3923
Edinburgh struggle 116, 117,
119, 614, 1925, 2193, 3310,
3940

Joan du Lee (15th C) 175

Johns, Juanita Pearl (b1888)
1545

Johnson, Alice Elizabeth (1873-
1945) 1204

Johnson, L. Carrie (19th C)
975

Johnson, L. M. (19th C) 1574

Johnson, Nora see Ross, Nora
Johnson

Johnson, Sophia Eliza (19th C)
2535, 2613, 2614, 2633

Johnson-Marsh, Lucille (d1965)
1170

Johnston, Frances (20th C)
3256, 3307

Johnston, Helen (20th C) 1448

Johnston, Zoe Allison (1889-
1961) 1615, 1849

Johnstone, Mabel see Thorburn-Johnstone, Mabel

Jokl, Helene (20th C) 431

Jolly, Doris see Gordon,
Doris Jolly

Jones, Beatrice O. (19th C)
1747

Jones, Bess Violet Puett (d1938)
1206

Jones, Clara Ernull (b1847)

1200

Jones, Edith Irby (b1927) 756
Jones, Jane C. see Wright,
    Jane Cooke
Jones, Kathleen Carmen
    (b1922) 1443
Jones, Louise Taylor see
    Taylor-Jones, Louise
Jones, Lucy C. (MD 1898)
    1203
Jones, May Farinholt (b1866)
    693, 847
Jones, Mrs. Edward see
    Taylor-Jones, Louise
Jones, Vera Heinly (b1897)
    2448
Jordon, Sara Murray (b1884)
    1134
Jorgensen, Anna M. (20th C)
    417
Jorgensen-Krogh, Marie
    (b1874) 441
Joshee, Anandabai (1865-
    1887) 158, 265, 267, 279,
    2604, 3683
Joteyko, Josephine (1866-1929)
    159
Jull, Roberta Stewart (MD
    1895) 6
Junovitz, Rina (20th C) 273

Kagan, Helen (20th C) 273
Kahane, Regine (19/20th C)
    3234
Kahler, Elizabeth Sartor
    (b1911) 1594
Kahn, Ida (1873-1931) 4, 359,
    362, 372, 2592, 3853
Kaijser, Anna (19/20th C?)
    44
Kalalova, Vlasta see Di Lotti,
    Vlasta Kalalova
Kalopothakes, Mary (19th C)
    451
Kalyan, Valentina see
    Gorinevskaya, Valentina V.
Kanof, Naomi M. (20th C)
    2449
Kaplow, Gwen Harriet Katz
    (b1941) 944
Kappes, Johanna (19th C) 99
Karpeles, Kate Breckinridge

Bogle (b1887) 1295, 1296
Kascherwarowna-Rudnewa,
    B. K. see Kashevarova-
    Rudneva, Varvara Alexandra
    Nafanova
Kashevarova-Rudneva, Varvara
    Alexandra Nafanova (1844?-
    1889) 180, 197, 205, 724,
    734, 738
Katona, Ibolya (19th C?) 408
Katsigra, Anna (19/20th C?)
    448
Katysheva, L. (20th C) 2673
Kâzim, Müfide see Külley,
    Müfide
Kazmierczak, Mary J. (b1893)
    1018, 1442
Kearney, Elizabeth Frances
    (1858-1923) 1500
Kearsley, Mary Jeannette
    (b1867) 1830
Keatinge, Harriette (1837-1909)
    1528
Keck, Bohuslava (19th C)
    413, 2869, 3868
Kectova, Bohmuila (19th C)
    439
Keen, Agnes (d1932) 675
Keith, Maria (19th C) 3937
Keller, Elizabeth C. Rex (b1837)
    1178
Keller, Florence Nettie Arm-
    strong (b1875) 1532
Kellogg, Helen R. (d1917)
    1787
Kellogg, Lena see Sadler,
    Lena Kellogg
Kellogg, Margaret M. McCauley
    (b1853) 1680
Kelly, Gertrude B. (b1862)
    779, 3576
Kelly, Jane see Sabine, Jane
    Downes Kelly
Kelynack, Violet McLaren
    (d1940) 554
Kemp, Minta Proctor (1874-
    1934) 919
Kennedy, Miriam Bitting see
    Bitting-Kennedy, Miriam
Kent, Leslie Swigart (1882?-
    1953) 1020, 1080, 1119,
    1332, 1528
Kerr, Charlotte Herman

(b1920) 882, 3962

Kerschbaumer, Rosa (19th C)
34

Ketcham, Jane Merrill (b1880)
1795

Ketring, Mary (b1865) 1040

Kettle, Marguerite H. (d1939)
517

Keyes, Regina Flood (20th C)
2682, 3582

Khati Lim see Lin, Chiao-
chih

Kilham, Eleanor B. (b1858)
983, 2683

Killain, Maud (19th C) 2580

Kimball, Amy Garrison Brown
(1847-1911) 1401

Kimball, Grace Niebuhr (1855-
1942) 958, 1004, 1167,
1265, 1304, 1837, 3591

Kimball, Julia see Qua, Julia
Kimball

Kin, Yamei (Jamei? Dschamei?)
(b1864) 4, 177, 360,
361, 367, 368, 693, 2535,
3853

Kinberg, Julia (1874-1945)
44

King, Lenora Howard (19th C)
2527, 2534

King, Mabel Beecher (1838-
1920) 1670

King, Violet Redman (d1941)
681

King, Y. May (You-me May)
see Kin, Yamei

King-eng, Hu see Hu, King
Eng

King May-Atkinson, Kate (d1934)
526

King-Salmon, Frances (MD
1921) 1306

Kipiani, Varvara Nikolaevna
(b1879) 728

Kirby, Millie see Upjohn,
Millie Kirby

Kirkland, Helen Maria Upjohn
see Upjohn, Helen Maria

Kittredge, Elizabeth Amanda
(b1889) 1098

Klajewska (pre-20th C) 2869

Klausner, Irma (19th C) 99,
484

Kleiman, Anna (19th C) 380

Kleinert, Margaret Louise
Noyes (b1879) 1445

Kleinman, Elizabeth Zelda
(b1892) 3582

Klenerman, Pauline (20th C)
263

Klumpke, Augusta see Dejerine-
Klumpke, Augusta

Knauf, Helena see Wink, Helena Knauf

Knauf, Mary see McCoy,
Mary Knauf

Knauf, Theresa see Abt,
Theresa Knauf

Knight, Elizabeth (d1933) 600

Knott, Harriet Ann (1867-1947)
1683

Knowles, Frances Ivens (20th
C) 2694

Knudsen, Helen L. (b1911)
1448

Kobayashi, Aya (b1928) 277

Koch, Margaret (b1864) 786

Kochurova, S. A. (pre-20th C)
205

Koenigsberger, Lea (MD 1897)
16

Komyo, Empress (1st C) 3844

Kornegay, Cora Zetta Corpening
see Corpening, Cora Zetta

Kornreich, Helen Kass (b1931)
1829

Kosnowska, [Mme] see Kra-
jewska, Theodora

Kovrigina, Maria Dmirievna
(b1910) 725

Kraft, Ruth M. (b1905) 1447

Krajewska, Theodora (19th C)
158, 3868

Kraker, Florence Elizabeth
(b1877) 1306

Krasuskaya, A. A. (20th C)
207, 730

Kratz, Esther Clarice Cumberland (b1887) 2741

Krayevska (19th C) 413

Kress, Lauretta Eby (b1863)
1322, 1678

Krey, Phoebe see Lanzoni,
Phoebe Krey

Krishnabai (20th C) 192

Kroeger, Hilda H. (b1903) 1447

Krogh, Marie Jorgensen see
  Jorgensen-Krogh, Marie
Krug, Else see Weyman,
  Else M. Krug
Kugler, Anna S. (1856-1930)
  2616, 2629, 2656, 3338
Kuhnow, Anna (19th C) 2869
Kuji, Naotaro (20th C) 3195
Küley, Müfide (20th C) 3830
Kusumoto, Ine (1827-1893)
  3844
Kvyatkovskaya, Julia Alex-
  androvna (19th C) 729
Kyhos, Emma Dowling Brindley
  (b1892) 1691
Kying, Yuo Me see Kin,
  Yamei
Kynett-Parmele, Lydia Estelle
  (1865-1935) 920

Lachapelle, Marie Louise
  Dugès (1769-1861?) 87,
  141, 159, 182, 3222
Ladds, Winifred (1905?-1930)
  1625
La Flesche, Susan see Picotte,
  Susan La Flesche
Laird, Emma see Perrine-
  Laird, Emma
Laird, Jessie see Brodie,
  Jessie Laird
Lais (of Athens) (3d C BC)
  20
Lake, Anna Easton (1849-1899)
  1234
Lakeman, Mary Ropes (MD
  1895) 3571
Lalinsky, Helen (MD 1935)
  1595, 2628, 3430
Lalinsky, Sr. M. Alma see
  Lalinsky, Helen
Lamb, Gail (medical student)
  (20th C) 3098
Lamont, Margaret Traill
  Christie (d1931) 506,
  2648, 2665
Lamson, Phoebe (d1883) 1671
Lancaster, Dorothy (d1961)
  656
Land, Gerda van't (19/20th C)
  3901
Lane, Bessie Evans (1891-

1968) 1219
Lane-Claypon, Janet (20th C)
  2390
Lange, Amelia (1825-1897?)
  3937
Lange, Linda Bartels (d1947)
  1537
Langford, Jane (fictional) 4061
Lanzoni, Phoebe Krey (20th C)
  3061
Lapham, Mary E. (1860-1936)
  1205, 3714
Lappits, M. Eleanor (20th C)
  3430
La Roe, Else K. (20th C) 485,
  1434
Larsson, Elisabeth (b1895)
  984, 1222, 1728
Laszlo, Ingrid M. L. (b1940)
  1568
Latham, Vida Annette (b1866)
  1441, 1448, 1640
Lattin, Cora Billings (MD 1894)
  2182
Laurence (wife of Jehan de Gail-
  lon) (14th C) 19
Lautzenheiser, Alma see
  Rowe, Alma Matilda Laut-
  zenheiser
Lavinder, Mary (1776-1845)
  802, 803
Lawney, Josephine Carrier
  (b1881) 3196
Lawrence, Harriet J. (b1893)
  1080
Lawrence, Margaret Morgan
  (b1914) 756
Lazarevitch, Radmila Milio-
  vitch (20th C) 398,
  3355
Lazarus, Hilda (19/20th C?)
  2652
Lazíc, Emilia (19th C) 13
Lea, Juanita Isabella (b1872)
  1211
Leake, Ruth Ophelia see
  Bryant, Ruth Ophelia
  Leake
Leavitt-Goff, Sarah (1854-1917)
  1679
Lee, Joan du see Joan du
  Lee
Lee, Rebecca (b1905) 1052,

1559

Lee, Yeu-Tsu Nee (b1936)
1829

Lefort, Marie Louise (b1875)
3235

Legey, Francoise Entz (d1935)
440, 455

Lehmus, Emilie (19th C)   83,
101, 108, 480, 482, 491,
492, 2869, 3232

Leidenius, Laimi (1877-1938)
3907, 3909

Le Marquis, Antoinette (b1907)
881, 1127

Lemcke, I. Dorothea (b1898)
1524

Leonard, Eliza E. (20th C)
3192

Leonard, Ethel (1871-1944)
1717

Leporin, Dorothea Christiana
see Erxleben, Dorothea
Christiana Leporin

Lesher, Mabel Grier (20th C)
1356

Leslie-Smith, Mary Addams
(d1961)   688

L'Esperance, Elise Strang
(d1959)   887, 896, 921,
985, 1092, 1618, 1710,
3656, 3657, 4023

LeVasseur, Irma (MD 1900)
12

Levy, Flora Herz (b1895)
640

Lewis, Effie Faye Cashatt
(b1896)   1280, 1335

Lewis, Margaret Cummings
(b1890)   1384

Lewis, Mary R. H. (1879-
1968)   1044, 2467

Leyen, Else von der (19th C)
99, 484

Li, Katherine (20th C)   699

Li, Yuin T'sao see T'Sao,
Li Yuin

Lin, Chiao-chih (aka Khati
Lim) (20th C)   369

Lin, Lan Ying (20th C)   3192

Lindenfield, Matilda May
(b1875)   918

Lindforss, Bengt (19/20th? C)
44

Lindforss, Gerda (19/20th? C)
44

Lindsay, Catherine (b1842)
1671

Lindsay-Wynekoop, Alice Lois
see Wynekoop, Alice Lois
Lindsay

Lindstedt, Anna Albertina see
Darrow, Anna Albertina Lindstedt

Lines, Amelia Wilkes (1823-
1909?)   1499

Linton, Emma see Hill, Emma
Linton

Linton, Laura (1834-1915)   786

Lippert, Frieda (1867-1946)
1574

Lippits, Marie Eleanor (b1907)
3430

Little, Elaine Marjory (1884-
1974?)   303

Liu, Felicia Hsin (medical student) (b1947)   3064

Ljocic-Milosevic, Draga (1855?-
1926)   13, 17, 388, 394

Lleonart y Casanovas, Dolores
(19th C)   18

Lloyd, Hilda (20th C)   118

Lobato, Rita (19/20th C)   718

Locatelli, Piera (b1900)   466

Locke, Eva May (b1874)   1218

Lockwood, Myrtle Spencer (MD
1900)   920

Loeber, Edith see Ballard,
Edith Loeber

Loizeaux, Marion Cotton (b1904)
883

Lollini, Clelia (20th C)   3355,
3892

Longo, Margaret Fay (b1936)
1387

Longshore, Hannah Elizabeth
Myers (1819-1902)   212,
796, 1105, 1179, 1668, 1784,
3752

Longshore-Potts, Anna M.
(b1829)   1686, 1723

Lopes, Rita Lobato Velho
(b1886)   196, 721

Lopez, Carmen (20th C)   3835

Lord, Margery Juline (b1891)
1213, 1267, 1327, 1447

Lore, Julia (19th C)   2527, 2655

Lorska, Dorota 396
Lotti, Vlasta Di see Di Lotti, Vlasta Kalalova
Lovejoy, Esther Clayson Pohl (1869-1967) 794, 848, 872, 999, 1116, 1284, 1449, 1475, 1742, 3358, 3589
    Biographies 1115, 1325, 1430, 1593, 1619, 1761, 3229, 3355, 3366
Lowell, Mary C. (19/20th C) 1820
Lowrie, Annie see Alexander, Annie Lowrie
Lozier, Charlotte Denman (1844-1870) 1254
Lozier, Clemence Sophia (1812?-1888) 242, 902, 943, 1105, 1247, 3717
Lubchenko, Portia Mary McKnight see McKnight-Lubchenko, Portia Mary
Lubinger, Friederike (19/20th C?) 3234
Luden, Georgine (20th C) 1438
Luisi, Paulina (19th C) 701, 710, 721
Lukacs, Elizabeth (20th C) 3177
Lukanin, Adelheid (MD 1876) 380
Luke, Jaya (19th C) 1747
Lundberg, Mathilda (19/20th C) 44, 2154
Lyle, Edna see Thomas, Edna Lyle
Lyndon, Mary see Nichols, Mary Sargent (Neal) Gove
Lynn, Ethel Grace (b1881) 1353
Lynn, Kathleen (19/20th C) 444
Lyon, Ellen M. (19th C) 1640
Lyons, Joanna (b1892) 515, 2665

Ma, Chung Ho Kei (20th C) 278
Mabie, Catharine Louise Roe (b1872) 2652

McAfee, Loy (d1941) 911
McAndrew, Helen Walker (1826-1906) 1664, 1684
McAvoy, Eileen B. (MD 1952) 742
MacBride, Edith see Dexter, Martha Edith MacBride
McBroom, F. Pearl (20th C?) 756
McCall, Annie (19th C) 2193
McCalmont-Stone, Harriette Osborn (1837-1931) 1683
McCann, Gertrude F. (b1889) 909
McCarroll, Ernest Mae (b1898) 899
McCarthy, Marguerite Patricia (b1901) 1388
McClung, Annie Mae Henry (b1878) 1703
McCombs, A. Parks (b1902) 745, 2455
McCormick, Ruth Anne (b1929) 1829
McCowen, Jennie (b1846) 1279, 1382
McCoy, Bernice (b1896) 1142, 1337
McCoy, Mary Knauf (MD 1890) 1193, 1315
McCulloch, Christina see Blaikie, Christina McCulloch Alexander
McDaniels, Oreanna (19/20th C) 786, 1240
McDonald, Belle J. (MD 1886) 2458
MacDonald, Carolyn Nicholas (1887-1942) 1320, 1358
McDowell, Kate (19th C) 2535
McEachen, Esther Isabella (b1892) 1113
McElney, Ariel R. S. Deacon (1904-1933) 593
Macfarlane, Catharine (1877-1969) 976, 1230, 1314, 1435, 1436, 1733, 2298, 3355, 3670, 3678, 4023
McGeachy, Jessie Ann Evelyn (1903-1966) 330
McGee, Anita Newcomb (1864-1940) 764, 769, 869, 1307, 1539, 2717, 2794

McGeorge, Mary (d1893) 2607, 2620

McGillwray, Alice Skimmen (20th C) 12

McGraw, Harriet Goodman (b1881) 1078, 1365

Macgregor, Daisy Annabelle Bennett (19/20th C) 532

McGregor, Dora Ann Sweezey (MD 1864) 1697

MacGregor, Mary E. Childs (1896-1955) 1584

McGrew, Elizabeth A. (b1916) 1446, 3611, 3962

McHardy, Caroline Gordon Lennox (d1929) 520

McIlroy, Louise (19/20th C) 585

MacInnis, Katherine Baylis (b1902) 1216

McIntosh, Harriet Carswell (1888-1971) 1183, 1615

Mackay, Helen Marion Mac-Pherson (MD 1917) 653, 887, 1092, 1710, 4035a

Mackay, Mary (d1935) 352

McKee, Mary H. (1865-1947) 1723

McKeeler, Margaret (19/20th C) 2606

Mackenzie, Mary Smith (1867?-1955) 318

McKenzie, Myra (19/20th C) 585

Mackerras, Josephine (20th C) 3861

McKibbin-Harper, Mary (b1873) 800, 1368, 1369, 1372, 1373, 1560, 3341

Mackie, Janet (20th C) 3550

McKinney, Susan Maria Smith (1847-1918) 750, 756, 1052

Mackinnon, Emily H. see Siedeberg-Mackinnon, Emily Hancock

MacKnight, Helen see Doyle, Helen MacKnight

McKnight-Lubchenko, Portia Mary (MD 1912) 1209, 1575

McKune, Joanne (b1938) 3075

McKusick, Marjorie J. K. (1923-1975) 3046, 3072

McLaglan, Eleanor see Baker-McLaglan, Eleanor Southey

McLaren, Agnes (1837-1913) 142, 162, 515, 530, 657, 1595, 2648, 2659, 2662, 2665, 2667

McLaren, Alice (19/20th C) 531

McLaren, Jennette (b1857) 786

McLaren, Violet see Kelynack, Violet McLaren

McLaughry, Elizabeth (b1865) 1474

McLean, Helen Vincent (b1894) 887, 1092, 1710

McLean, Mary Hancock (b1861) 1039, 1764

MacLeod, Jessie McGeachy see McGeachy, Jessie Ann Evelyn

MacLeod, Mary Elizabeth (d1936) 355

McLorinan, Margaret Harkness (b1887) 302

MacMillan, Ada J. (20th C) 589

MacMillan, Kate (19/20th C) 351

MacMurchy, Helen (1862-1953) 12, 322, 336, 353a, 693, 887, 1092, 1710

McNair, Dorothy (20th C) 646

MacNamara, Annie Jean (d1968) 287

Macnaughton, Mona (d1964) 509

McNeal, Alice (b1897) 2746

MacNeil, Phyllis (b1923) 1582

McNeill, Mary Lauchline (1874-1928) 608

McNicholas, Kathleen (b1948) 1735

McNutt, Julia G. (b1844) 1374

McNutt, Sarah J. (b1877) 1374, 3617

McPherson, Veronica Catherine Jessica (1895-1975) 680

Macrina (pre-Middle Ages) 162

McSherry, Elizabeth (20th C) 1099

Magan, Lillian Eshelman (b1870) 919

Magier, Nina G. (b1910) 3619

Maher, Irene Eleanor (b1910)
    1542
Maiden, Joanna Cranston (b1929)
    2649
Malahlele, Mary Susan (19/
    20th C) 2652
Malecove, Ida (19/20th C) 195
Mallison, Elizabeth Carr
    (1865?-1942) 1305
Maltraversa, Adelmota (15th
    C) 134, 180
Malyarskaya, Ekaterina Chris-
    tofovna (1852-1904) 2676
Mamontova, I. G. (20th C)
    723
Mandelevy, Y. A. (20th C)
    2671
Manion, Katherine C. (b1867)
    1299
Mansell, Nancie Monelle (19/
    20th C?) 2527, 2652, 2655
Manzolini, Anna see Morandi-
    Manzolini, Anna
Marble, Ella Marie Smith
    (b1850) 994
Marchand, Dolores Perez (20th
    C) 1436
Marchant, Juliet E. (1844-
    1929) 949
Marguerite of Naples (15th C)
    134
Mark, Nellie V. (b1867) 1672
Marmorston, Jessie (b1898)
    1829
Marquis, Antoinette see Le
    Marquis, Antoinette
Marrat, Muriel (19/20th C)
    644
Marsh, Lucille see Johnson-
    Marsh, Lucille
Marshall, Clara (1848-1931)
    242, 243, 1249, 3389, 3719
Martin, Helen Eastman (b1906)
    1829
Martin, Martina Mockaitis
    (b1939) 1695
Martin, Mary see Sloop,
    Mary T. Martin
Martindale, Louisa (20th C)
    548, 616, 619, 620, 1438,
    2193, 3324, 3359
Martinez de Carvajal y del
    Camino, Laura (1869-1941)

717
Marting, Ann D. (MD 1927)
    796
Marting, Esther Clare (b1908)
    796, 1448, 1750
Marting, Miriam Ruth (b1905)
    796
Martinson, Elsie see Gilbert,
    Elsie Martinson
Mashkovtseva, Olga Arkadevna
    (1851-1933) 729
Mason, Letitia (19th C) 2527
Mason-Hogle, Kate A. (b1859)
    937, 1604
Mason-Hohl, Elizabeth Pearl
    (b1890) 49, 993, 1100, 1447,
    1828
Mastellari, Maria (pre-20th C)
    157
Matheson, Elizabeth Beckett
    (Scott) (MD 1898) 12, 312,
    313
Mathis, Lane (medical student)
    (20th C) 3098
Matlack, Ann see Shearman,
    Ann Matlack
Matthews, Caroline (d1927)
    632
Matveena, Vera Petrovna
    (1851-1916) 205, 2676
Maxwell-Fulton, Annie (1848-
    1889) 345, 352
May-Atkinson, Kate see King
    May-Atkinson, Kate
Mayo, Helen Mary (b1878) 298
Mazzola, Linda (b1911) 2952
Me, Kying Yuo see Kin,
    Yamei
Mead, Ella Avery (b1874) 820,
    1444, 1522
Mead, Kate Campbell Hurd see
    Hurd-Mead, Kate Campbell
Meade, Euthanasia Sherman
    (19th C) 1432, 1621
Meader, Isabel M. (1857-1932)
    1244
Mears, Isabella (d1936) 623
Mechthilde of Magdeberg (13th
    C) 101
Mecredy, Emily M. Spencer
    (d1958) 564
Medford, Effie (b1937) 1731
Meigs, Grace Lynde (b1881)

3666

Meine, Berta M. (1886-1973) 1447

Meitner, Gisela (19/20th? C) 3234

Meiyie, Shie see Stone, Mary

Mei-yu, Shih see Stone, Mary

Melior (fictional) 149

Mendenhall, Dorothy Reed (b1874) 913

Mendenhall, Jean Clements (b1886) 1273

Mendoza-Gauzon, Marie Paz (b1884) 3839

Mercuriade (15th C) 22, 31, 132, 134

Mergler, Marie Josepha (d1901) 930, 1397, 1496, 1629, 1640, 3438, 3700, 3705, 3764

Mermod, Camille (b1900) 1154, 1445, 3962

Merrick, Myra K. (1825-1899) 1666, 3687, 3716

Merrill, Julia Dyer (1861-1914) 1243

Merrimon, Louise see Perry, Louise A. Merrimon

Merritt, Doris M. Honig (b1923) 3079

Merritt, Emma Sutro (b1856) 863

Metcalf, Chris (fictional) 4065

Meyer, Blanche Montgomery (MD 1939) 2456

Meyers, Marjorie see Peebles-Meyers, Marjorie

Miall-Smith, Gladys (20th C) 2914

Michel, Auguste Marie (19/20th C) 454

Middelhoven, Ada (20th C) 417

Miles, May S. (b1870) 1204

Miliovitch, Radmila see Lazarevitch, Radmila Milovitch

Miliovitch, Rosalie (19th C) 398

Miller, Adaline Nancy (20th C) 3917

Miller, Elizabeth (20th C) 1135

Miller, Emma (b1864) 3843

Miller, Florence Fenwick (medical student in 1869) 624

Miller, Janet (20th C) 1468

Miller, Leona Vivien (b1928) 1829

Milobar, Karola (19/20th C) 13

Milosevic, Draga Ljocic see Ljocic-Milosevic, Draga

Miner, Thelma Sylvia (b1920) 318

Minoka, Lillie Rosa see Hill, Lillie Rosa Minoka

Minyailo, E. K. (20th C) 723

Mishimura, Eiko 3199

Mitchell, Ellen E. (b1829) 1104

Mitchell, Elsie Reed (b1871) 3338

Mitchell, Isabel (18/19th C) 637

Mitchell, Mary see Henry, Mary Azalea Mitchell

Mix, Josephine B. Dexter (b1837) 1178

Moeller, Eli (b1863) 45, 441

Moffett, Elisabeth Jane (1866-1960) 562

Moller, Eli see Moeller, Eli

Monelle, Nancie see Mansell, Nancie Monelle

Montague, Mary Wortley (1689-1762) 159

Montessori, Maria (1870-1952) 418, 464, 476

Montoya, Matilde P. (19th C) 2947, 3942

Montreuil-Straus, Germaine (20th C) 428

Moralt, Marie (d1931) 676

Morandi-Manzolini, Anna (1716-1774) 73, 137, 159, 180, 3227, 3906

Morani, Alma Dea (b1907) 754, 755, 867, 959, 3688

Morawitz, Lucia (19/20th C?) 3234

Morgan, Frances Elizabeth (1843-1927) 1943, 3232

Morgan le Fay, Queen (literary) 149

Morgan the Wise see Morgan
le Fay, Queen
Morgans, Dollie (b1907) 2799
Morizaki, Hoyu 3199
Morris, Sarah I. (b1879) 1540,
1583, 3080
Morrow, Laura Ehrlich (b1913)
1775
Morse, Eliza Roxana (MD
1888) 1642
Morse, Marian Shaffner (1894-
1973) 3671
Morton, Helen (MD 1862)
1007, 1495, 3662
Morton, Rosalie Slaughter
(b1876) 782, 861, 1121,
1439, 1484, 1485, 1636,
1819, 2784, 2794, 4081
Moschek, Lydia (1887-1954)
416
Mosher, Clelia Duel (b1863)
1486, 1487
Mosher, Eliza Maria (1846-
1928) 241, 781, 783, 987,
988, 1190, 1191, 1226, 1423,
1493, 1556, 1624, 1716,
1749, 1826, 2323, 3159,
3256, 3662, 3938
Mosleva, Maria (20th C) 2671
Moss, Emma Sadler (b1898)
1747
Mowry, Martha H. (1818-
1899) 1161
Mueller, Merna (20th C) 294
Muellerin, Antonia Elisabeth
de Held see Held, Antonia
Elisabeth de
Mühl, Anita May (1886-1952)
1505, 1506, 1727
Muir, Kathleen (1899-1962)
601
Munch, Kristine (19/20th C)
3355
Mundo, Fe del (20th C) 472,
3835, 3839
Munson, Arley (19/20th C)
2622
Murav'eva, E. F. (20th C)
2673
Murdoch, Agnes Gordon (b1880)
2652
Murdoch, Charlotte Soutter
see Young, Charlotte Sout-

ter Murdoch
Murdoch, Mary (1864-1915)
616, 620
Murdock, Virginia C. (19th C)
2543, 2584
Murray, Anne see Halkett,
Anne Murray
Murray, Doris Audrey (b1893)
355
Murray, Flora (20th C) 560,
611, 2705
Murray, Florence Jessie (1894-
1975) 346, 351
Murray, Virginia (20th C) 3555
Murrell, Christine (1874-1933)
138, 539, 598, 663, 3262,
3277, 4072
Myers, Hannah E. see Long-
shore, Hannah Elizabeth
Myers
Myers, Jane Viola (1831-1918)
796, 1784
Myers, Lonny (b1922) 3177
Myers, Mary Frame see
Thomas, Mary Frame Myers
Myers, Mary R. see Daven-
port, Mary R. Myers

Nakling, Ida (20th C) 434
Nasmyth, Dorothea (1879-1959)
642
Navas, Mariana (17th C) 717
Nayar, Sushila (20th C) 4004
Neal, Josephine Bicknell (b1880)
1017, 3656
Neel, Katherine see Dale,
Katherine Neel
Neild, Edith (d1927) 559
Nekrasova, V. S. (19th C)
202
Nelson, Ida Shively (1868-1947)
1260
Nelson, Mrs. Lou J. see
Heath, Lillian
Nelson, Olivia M. (20th C) 1200
Nemir, Rosa Lee (b1905) 1838,
3962
Nerbone, Giletta di (pre-20th
C) 180
Nesbitt, Irene Thornton (b1880)
1206
Newcomb, Anita see McGee,

Anita Newcomb

Newcomb, Kate Pelham (b1885) 903

Newcomer, Elizabeth Horneman (b1880) 1101

Nichols, Mary Sargent (Neal) Gove (19th C) 212, 846, 1531

Nichols, Roberta Bond (1901-1966) 332

Nichols, Victoria Raye (b1944) 1777

Nicholson, Marianna Parker (1888-1924) 1210

Nicolette (fictional) 149

Nielsen, Nielsine Mathilde (1850-1916) 45, 63, 71, 415

Niles, Gussie Annice (1896-1948) 1523

Niles, Mary Frost (1854-1932) 2656

Niles, Mary W. (19th C) 2585, 2586

Nilsson, Ada (19/20th C) 456, 2154

Nilsson, Betty Augustina (b1878) 3338

Nilsson, Hanna Christer (19/20th C) 2159

Nivison, Samantha S. (1820-1915) 897

Noble, Mary Riggs (b1872) 1416

Noble, Nelle S. (b1878) 829, 1446

Noël, Suzanne Blanche Marguerite Gros Pertet (1878-1954) 460

Nofach, Miriam (20th C) 273

Nolander-Engström, Sigrid (19/20th C) 44, 2159

Nonaka, Enko (19/20th C) 3199, 3844

Nordhoff-Jung, Sofie Amalia (b1867) 2869

Norgan, Anne Fisher (b1920) 951

Norris, Amanda Taylor (b1849) 803, 853

Norris, Frances M. Sochor (b1932) 3177

Norris, Grace M. (b1875) 1130

Norris, Maria Whittelsey (1856-1938) 1682

Norris, Sarah (19th C) 2604

Norstrand, Iris Fletcher (b1915) 2952

Norton, Annie (b1846) 2537

Norton, Blanche (19/20th C) 1807

Novak, Milana Gavrancic see Gavrančič-Novak, Milana

Noyes, Margaret see Kleinert, Margaret Louise Noyes

Nusbaumer, Pauline S. (1858-1927) 1590

Oakley, Geraldine (b1891) 343

Odecrantz, Elin (19/20th C) 2154

Odell, Anna (1874-1929) 919

Oetiker (19/20th C) 2863

Offenbach, Bertha (b1908) 1545

Ogino, Ginko see Ginko, Ogino

Ogorek, Flora (19/20th C) 3234

O'Grady, Lois Frances (b1936) 774

O'Hara, Margaret (b1855) 2623

Okami, Keiko (1859-1941) 280

Okunkova-Goldinger, Z. N. (19/20th C) 205

Oliver, Belle Chone (1875-1947?) 315

Olloqui, Maria Juanita de see de Olloqui, Maria Juanita

Olney, Mary Belle (b1908) 1447

Olsen, Frances Adams (b1916) 1730

O'Malley, Mary (b1867) 1043, 1182, 1438, 3435

Oppenheimer, Ella (b1892) 1532

Orchard, Ethel (20th C) 638

O'Reilly, Susie (20th C) 300, 3204

Orosa, Severina Luna (b1890) 3835

Ortmayer, Marie (b1894) 1447

Orzeszkowa, Eliza (19th C?) 397

Osborn, Harriette see Mc-

Calmont-Stone, Harriette
    Osborn
Osborn, Margaret Ann Fannon
    (MD c1897) 1554
Osborn, Mary E. (1856-1896)
    1606
O'Sullivan, Gertrude (b1866)
    916
Oteo de Hoogh, Esperanza
    see Hoogh, Esperanza
    Oteo de
Otis, Clara Lee Beckner
    (b1875) 919
Outwater, Eva Shedd (1856-1906)
    1672
Ouzts, Katharyn Butts (b1946)
    3098
Owen, May R. (b1896) 1447,
    3634
Owens, May Rodgers (MD
    1883) 4026
Owens-Adair, Bethenia Angelina
    (1840-1928?) 1080, 1088,
    1119, 1467, 1561, 1562,
    1638

Painter, Hetty K. (19th C)
    1009
Pak, Esther Kim (MD 1900)
    3193, 3846, 3847
Pallesen, Mamie Guthrie
    (b1896) 1343
Palmer, Alice Freeman (20th
    C) 174
Palmer, Mary Simpson Mc-
    Carty (b1861) 1680
Palmer, Sarah Ellen (1856-
    1946) 1259
Panacea (mythology) 185
Panagiotatu see Panayotatou,
    Angélique G.
Panayotatou, Angélique G.
    (20th C) 62, 448, 3843
Papara, Dora (20th C) 433
Papgeorgion, Vessalide (20th
    C) 448
Paraclita, Sr. M. (20th C)
    1758
Pardee, Emily (19th C) 4017
Park, Bessie see Haynes,
    Bessie Park
Park, Maybelle M. (b1871)

1579
Parker, Harriet H. (20th C)
    1799
Parker, Madeline Phyllis (19th
    C) 557
Parker, Marianna see Nichol-
    son, Marianna Parker
Parks, Margaret (d1955) 355
Parmele, Lydia Estelle see
    Kynett-Parmele, Lydia Es-
    telle
Parmelee, Ruth A. (b1885)
    833, 1565, 3397, 3398, 3597
Parrish, Rebecca (b1869) 832,
    1566
Parry, Angenette (1857-1939)
    962, 1437, 3597, 3598
Parsons, Emma Dawson (b1859)
    1110
Parsons, Kate (19/20th C)
    3687
Parsons, Mary Almera (b1850)
    3714
Paschalis, Michalina (19th C)
    404
Paso, [Senorita] (19th C)
    3946
Pasquale, Virdimuna (Middle
    Ages) 59
Pastino, Cusina di Filippo de
    (Middle Ages) 70
Paterson, Elizabeth Park Young
    (d1928) 633
Patterson, Ellen James (b1873)
    1572
Pattison, Jean Harwood (b1896)
    2684
Paul, Martha Hughes see
    Cannon, Martha Hughes Paul
Paull, Amanda (fictional) 4059
Paulson-Neall, Mary Wild
    (b1872) 1678
Pavlekovic, Ema (MD 1903)
    13
Paykull, Lilly (19/20th C)
    2154
Payne, Helen Nora (d1958)
    511
Payne, Helen V. (b1917) 756
Payne, Roselyn see Epps,
    Roselyn Payne
Pearce, Louise (1885-1959)
    809, 1023, 1134, 1507

Pearce-Dickinson, Beatrice
(1866-1948) 1261
Pechey-Phipson, Mary Edith
(1845-1908) 119, 602-606,
624, 678, 679, 2116, 2531
Peck, Eleanor Kellogg (b1908)
1051
Peck, Elizabeth L. (b1854)
3537
Peckham, Adelaide Ward
(b1848) 747
Peebles-Meyers, Marjorie
(20th C) 951, 1033
Pelzel, Jane M. Barksdale
(b1924) 1571
Pennington, Mary Engle (20th
C) 1192
Penrose, Romania Bunnell
Pratt (1839-1932) 1533,
1632
Pereira (Middle Ages) 70
Pereira, Maria Joana de Freitas
see Freitas Pereira, Maria
Joana de
Pereira, Virginia see Al-
varez, Virginia Pereira
Perelokina, M. I. (20th C)
723
Perez, Ernestina (MD 1887)
1945
Perkins, Anna (b1899) 1816
Perla (Middle Ages) 70
Perretti, Zaffira (pre-20th C)
180
Perrill, Wilma E. Conger
(b1914) 2643
Perrine-Laird, Emma (b1868)
919
Perry, Isabella Hester (b1892)
3672
Perry, Louise A. Merrimon
(b1878) 1202
Pertelote (fictional) 149
Pertet, Suzanne Blanche Mar-
guerite Gros see Noel,
Suzanne Blanche Marguerite
Gros Pertet
Peters, Lulu Hunt (1873-1930)
1026, 1370
Petrardini, Maria (19/20th C)
157
Petrie, Edith see Brown,
Edith Petrie

Pettraccini-Ferretti, Maria
Madalena (19th C) 53, 132,
1943
Pfeifer, Elizer see Stone,
Elizer Pfeifer
Phelps, Cecily (d1936) 510
Phelps, Dale Lee King (b1945)
1165
Phillips, Frances J. (b1904)
768
Phillips, M. Alice (b1894)
1740
Phillips, Mildred E. (b1925)
756
Pianese de Esaa, Dolores
Maria (MD 1912) 195
Pickett, Frances E. (b1886)
1445
Picotte, Susan La Flesche
(1865-1915) 693, 1131, 1592
Pierce, Priscilla Adella (20th
C) 1681
Pierra Hoon Vejjabul (MD 1932)
161, 274
Pierson-Eddy, Mary see Eddy,
Mary Pierson
Pigott, May (d1930) 634
Pike, Ann Hollingsworth (b1920)
1696
Pilliet, Mme. Edwards (19th C)
33
Pilstein, Salomee see Rusiecki-
Halpir-Pilstein, Salomee
Pincock, Carolyn Hannah Sny-
der (b1910) 1448
Pine, Alcinda Auten (b1858)
786
Piñero, Dolores Mercedes
(b1892) 910
Pires, Carmen Escobar (20th
C) 196
Pirret, Mary J. (19/20th C)
674
Pischinger, Olga (20th C) 438
Plantz, Laura Marion (1829-
1923) 1798
Platt, Kate (20th C) 3341, 3840
Platter, Mary Ann (b1851)
2633
Poe-Eng Yu see Hu, King
Eng
Poelz, Anna (19/20th C) 3234
Pohl, Esther see Lovejoy,

Esther Clayson Pohl

Polk, Margaret Harrison (MD 1893) 1030, 1596

Polk-Peters, Ethel (1883-1961) 1596, 2587

Polydaemona (Antiquity) 62

Ponce-Vargas, Tegualda (20th C) 709, 714

Pope, Emily Frances (MD 1870) 4017

Poplawska, Stanislawa (20th C) 404

Popova, A. P. (20th C) 732

Popovici, Antoinette F. (b1908) 402

Possaner von Ehrenthal, Gabriele see Ehrenthal, Gabriele Possaner von

Potter, Ellen Culver (1871-1958) 701, 808, 904, 996, 1102, 1103, 1503, 1529, 1570, 3786, 3795

Potter, Marion Craig (1864-1943) 796, 1032, 1125, 1440, 1516

Potts, Anna M. see Longshore-Potts, Anna M.

Pouzin, Yvonne (20th C) 3355

Powell, Janet Travell (MD 1929) 1446, 1599, 1752, 3974

Powers, Isadora Sharring (1860-1940) 1683

Powers, Lunette I. (b1875) 825, 916, 1525

Pratt, Emily Adelaide (b1890) 3555

Pratt, Romania Bunnell see Penrose, Romania Bunnell Pratt

Pray, Susan R. (19th C) 1839

Presley, Sophia (1834-1909) 1741

Pressly, Maude Stoovall (1898-1962) 1220

Preston, Ann (1813-1872) 224, 239, 765, 1291, 1494, 4055
    Biographies 212, 963, 1105, 1171, 1398, 1663, 3734
    Woman's Medical College of Pennsylvania affiliation 243,
306, 1734, 1781, 2055, 3509, 3536, 3537, 3751, 3754, 3777

Preston, Frances I. (MD 1922) 304

Price, Dorothy Stopford (20th C) 443

Price, Mary A. Moss (b1917) 1429

Priestly, Mary see Rupert, Mary Priestly Sheriff

Pringle, Isabella Ferrier (d1963) 673

Pringle, Julia (d1960) 594

Procel, Matilda Hidalgo de see Hidalgo de Procel, Matilda

Prokofeva, M. S. (20th C) 730

Pryce, Ethel (d1937) 536

Pryor, Carol Graham (b1918) 1446

Pryor, Helen Brenton (1898-1972) 1744

Puckey, Mary (20th C) 289

Puett, Bess Violet see Jones, Bess Violet Puett

Purdy, Ann (b1888) 1611, 1653

Purnell, Caroline M. (1860-1923) 973, 1488, 3231, 3402

Purvine, Mary Bowerman (b1881) 1080

Puscariu, Elena (1875-1965) 399

Putnam, Catherine (b1851) 786

Putnam, Helen Cordelia (b1857) 1814

Putnam, Mary Corinna see Jacobi, Mary Corinna Putnam

Putyata-Kershbaumer, P. V. (19th C) 376

Qua, Julia Kimball (1862-1936) 918

Quain, Fannie Dunn (b1874) 1613

Queen, Oceola C. (b1864) 1559

Quiroga, Margarita Delgado de Solis see Delgado de Solis Quiroga, Margarita

Rabinoff, Sophie (b1889)
  699, 834, 1517
Rabinowitsch, Lydia (19th C)
  4016
Radcliff, Sue (1894-1924)
  1502, 1552, 3396, 3595
Radcliffe, Jean see Vernier,
  Jean
Ragland, Wilhelmina Afton
  (b1883) 1065
Ralli, Elaine Pandia (b1894)
  817, 1447
Ramabai, Pundita (19th C)
  2603
Ramey, Estelle (PhD) (20th
  C) 3113
Ramsey, Florence Muriel
  (b1902) 1120
Ramsey, Mabel L. (20th C)
  2694
Ranes, Annie R. (b1870) 970
Rankin, Anna Spencer (b1821)
  1679
Rankin, Hattie Love (1884-
  1960) 2587
Ratterman, Helena Teresa
  (b1882) 1150, 1168, 1363,
  1444
Ratynska, Maria (d1920) 404,
  411
Raven, Clara (b1907) 2794,
  3999
Raymond, Aimee (MD 1889)
  3452
Read, Jessie D. (b1903)
  2826
Rebecca of Salerno see
  Guarna, Rebecca
Redding, Lucia see Thomp-
  son, Lucia Redding
Redmond, Sophie (19/20th C)
  3901
Reed, Dorothy see Menden-
  hall, Dorothy Reed
Reese, Clare N. (b1905) 894
Reid, Ada Chree (1895-1974)
  887, 1245, 1532, 3359
Reid, Eva Charlotte (MD
  1907) 4084
Reifsnyder, Elizabeth (1858-
  1922) 1654, 2656, 3196
Renshaw, Josephine (b1910)
  1447, 3177

Renter, Ruth see Darrow,
  Ruth Renter
Renthe, Barbara von (20th C)
  105
Reynolds, Ellis see Shipp,
  Ellis Reynolds
Reynolds, Helen E. see Ryan,
  Helen E. Reynolds
Reynolds, Mary Ann V. (b1934)
  1803
Rezhabek, Olga Yaroslavovna
  (b1897) 731
Rice, Grace Elizabeth Bernard
  (b1879) 352
Rice, Roberta (b1917) 1319
Richards, Esther Loring (b1885)
  1114
Richards, Florence Harvey
  (1877-1944) 4079
Richards, Kathryn E. (b1934)
  1380
Richards, Mabel see Tarbell,
  Mabel Richards
Richardson, Katherine Berry
  (b1887) 3759
Richardson, Mary McDaniel
  (b1893) 1649, 1732
Ricker, Marcena Sherman (MD
  1888) 698
Ridout, Lilla (b1882) 3582
Ripley, Martha G. (1843-1912)
  786, 787, 1240
Ritchie-England, Octavia Grace
  (20th C) 12, 3355
Ritter, Mary Bennett (b1859)
  863, 1432, 1621
Robbins, Felicia Autenried
  (1869-1950) 870
Robbins, Jane E. (MD 1890)
  1126, 3597
Roberts, Lois M. (b1922) 2649
Roberts, Margaret Curtis Shipp
  (d1926) 1533
Roberts, Regina Flood Keyes
  (20th C) 1840
Robinson, Daisy Maude Orleman
  (1869-1942) 1232, 1437,
  1478, 1824
Robinson, Doreen M. Stranger
  (1896-1935) 527
Robinson, Florence M. (d1931)
  668
Robinson, Grace T. (MD 1895)

300

Robson, Elsie Thomson Douglas
see Cooper, Elsie Thomson
Douglas

Rochford, Grace Elizabeth
(b1882) 1166

Rodriguez, Maria Luisa see
Saldún de Rodriguez, Maria
Luisa

Roffey, Joyce E. (d1958) 639

Rogers, Dorothy M. (20th C)
1446

Rogers, Vesta Marie (b1909)
699

Rohde, Alice (b1883) 1414

Rolder, J. W. van den Blink
see Blink-Rolder, J. W.
van den

Roll, Barbara Von see Von
Roll, Barbara

Rollett, Oktavia Aigner see
Aigner-Rollett, Oktavia

Roma, Francesca de see
Romana, Francesca

Romaine, Adelaide (b1896)
1532, 3578

Romana, Francesca (Middle
Ages) 22, 31, 59, 60, 70

Root, Eliza H. D. (1846-1926)
986, 1382, 1589, 1629,
1640

Root, Stella Quinby (1872-
1941) 3493

Rose, Frances Eastman (b1872)
700, 766, 1002, 1316

Rosekrans, Sarah Hoff Didriksen (b1901) 860

Rosencrantz, Esther (b1876)
947

Rosenthal-Thompson, Augusta
Louise (b1859) 1672

Roseveare, Helen (b1925?)
514

Ross, Charlotte Whitehead
(1843-1916) 314

Ross, Mary J. (MD 1907)
1409, 1447

Ross, Nora Johnson (1876-
1916) 1049

Ross-Wolcott, Laura J. (19th
C) 1579

Roth, Linda Gage (1873-1944)
1673

Rothchild, Alice (medical student) (b1948) 3064

Rowe, Alma Matilda Lautzenheiser (19th C) 789

Rowe, Anna Forest (d1920) 964

Rowley, Ethel (19/20th C) 579,
2652

Roys, Elmina M. see Roys-
Gavitt, Elmina M.

Roys-Gavitt, Elmina M. (1828-
1898) 3591, 3632

Rozelle, Charlotte (20th C)
1209

Ruddock, Agnes Julia Scholl
(b1889) 2742

Rude, Anna Elizabeth (b1876)
3666

Rudneva, V. A. Kashevarova
see Kashevarova-Rudneva,
Varvara Alexandra Nafanova

Rukhmabai (b1864) 192, 269,
603, 2123

Rule, Amy J. (1870-1946) 1309

Rundell, Annie Margaret Stevens
(b1867) 916

Rupert, Mary Priestly Sheriff
(1880-1939) 1413

Rusiecki-Halpir-Pilstein, Salomee (b1718) 132, 158, 159

Russell, Elizabeth Dill (d1928?)
261

Russell, Gladys J. C. (19/20th
C) 592

Russell, Jane Anderson (b1931)
3127

Russell, Julia Eastman Wallace
see Wallace-Russell, Julia
Eastman

Russell, Marie Oliviera (b1945)
1355

Rutherford, Frances Armstrong
(1842-1922) 942, 1499, 1686

Ruthven, Jane Henderson (d1928)
633

Ruud, Helga Mariane (b1860)
1640, 1652

Ruys, A. Charlotte (20th C)
3359

Ryan, Helen E. Reynolds (1860-
1947) 337

Ryder, Claire F. (20th C) 886

Ryerson, Mary Butin (d1944)
801

Sabin, Florence Rena (1871-1953) 219, 761, 795, 852, 901, 1137, 1323, 1377, 1452, 1473, 1513, 3701
Biographies 697, 838, 850, 1001, 1523, 1564, 1576
Honors and awards 1136, 1138, 1710
Sabine, Jane Downes Kelly (1894-1950) 1326
Sabuco, Oliva (b1562) 42, 158, 159
Sachs, Bernice Cohen (b1918) 1073
Sadler, Lena Kellogg (b1875) 1441, 1534
Safford, Mary (19th C) 1721
Saint Gilles, Sara di (Middle Ages) 70
Saint Hildegarde see Hildegarde of Bingen, Saint
Saint Jutta (13th C) 19
Saint Nicerata (5th C) 26, 134
Saint Philomela (pre-6th C) 26
Saint Theodosia (pre-6th C) 26
Saint Zenais (pre-6th C) 26
Salamanca, Olivia (MD 1910) 3839
Saldún de Rodriguez, Maria Luisa (20th C) 720
Salerno, Rebecca of see Guarna, Rebecca
Salerno, Trotula of see Trotula de Ruggiero Platerius
Salpis (BC) 62
Sanapia (1895-1968) 1288
Sandelin, Ellen (19/20th C) 2159
Sandeman, Laura Stewart (d1929) 686
Sanderson, Alice see Clow, Alice Sanderson
Sanderson, Harriet Phoebe (1861-1921) 1677
Sanderson, Susanne Munro (b1879) 1441
Sandes, Gladys M. (1897-1968) 432
Sanford, Amanda (d1890) 1498, 1685

Sanford, Mary Blanche Waterman (b1876) 3707
Sapoznikova, Elena (20th C) 2671
Sarah (la Mirgesse) (Middle Ages) 70
Sarah (of Paris) (13th C) 155
Sarah (of Würzburg) (15th C) 70, 155
Sarah (wife of Abraham) (14th C) 19
Sartor, Elizabeth see Kahler, Elizabeth Sartor
Satthianadham, S. (d1894) 2535
Saunders, Sabine (b1520) 111
Savage, Anne (20th C) 2238
Saville, Lily (20th C) 3192
Sawin, Martha A. Hayden (1815-1859) 216, 1782
Sawyer, Annie Laurie (1865-1933) 1402
Sawyer, Grace M. (b1889) 1442
Scarlett, M. J. (19th C) 1697
Schaeffer, Charlotte (1874-1927) 949
Scharlieb, Mary Bird (d1930) 109, 504, 535, 549, 551, 553, 666, 683, 2116, 2193
Scharlieb, Mary Ethel Sim (d1926) 631
Scharnagel, Isabel Mona (b1906) 1268, 1563
Schetky, Martha G. K. (1870-1951) 1551
Schilder, Lauretta Bender see Bender, Lauretta
Schloezer, Dorothea von (18th C) 79
Schmidt-Schütt, Margarete (20th C) 490
Scholl, Agnes see Ruddock, Agnes Julia Scholl
Schorr, Matild (MD 1897) 16
Schraders, Catharine-Gertrude (pre-20th C) 159
Schreier, Lena Fimpel (b1884) 1760
Schroeder, Mary G. (b1868) 1186
Schugens, M. Elizabeth (d1907?) 1144
Schuhmeister, Maria (19/20th C) 416

Schulze, Margaret (b1893) 1352

Schutt, Ann (b1932) 3803

Schwartz, Fannie Adele (1882-
1946) 748

Schwendener, Hattie A. Galen-
tin (1858-1942) 1655, 1667,
1679

Scoresby-Jackson, Margaret
(20th C) 522

Scott, Eleanor (b1908) 1090

Scott, Emma (19/20th C) 2537

Scott, Kate Frances (b1890)
1293

Scudder, Ida Belle (b1900)
2626, 2649

Scudder, Ida Sophia (b1870)
285, 699, 812, 1010, 1275-
1278, 1313, 1805, 1877, 2626,
2630, 2634, 2649, 2652,
3834, 4023

Scully, A. Lois (b1922) 882

Seabolt, Gertrude Clowes
(b1881) 1156

Seaman, Cleora Augusta (1814-
1869) 775, 979, 1498, 3716,
4010

Sears, Armina see Hill, Armina Sears

Sebesta, Vilma (20th C) 409

Sebire, Irene (20th C) 3861

Sechenova, M. A. see Bo-
kova-Sechenova, M. A.

Secord, Elizabeth C. (1841-
1916) 355

Seevers, Ruth (b1883) 815

Selekeid (of Frankfurt) (Middle Ages) 70

Selig, Hedwig (19/20th C) 99

Selkin-Aronson, Emma (20th
C) 1111

Selmon, Bertha Eugenia Loveland (1877-1949) 835, 836,
1189, 1420, 2589

Sercombe, Harriet Frances
(b1848) 924

Serebrennaya, A. (19th C)
380

Sermour, Mary A. (19/20th
C) 786

Sewall, Lucy Ellen (d1890)
614, 624, 679, 1025,
1495, 1778, 3662

Seward, Sarah C. (19th C)
2604, 2627, 2655

Sexton, Lucinda see Wilcox,
Lucinda Sexton

Shabanoff, Anna N. (1848-1932)
207, 441, 727, 730

Shabanova, A. N. see Sha-
banoff, Anna N.

Shafer, Bertha Meserve (b1890)
837

Shafer, June Carol (b1913) 1446

Shaibany, Homa (20th C) 270

Shamer, Bertha Tapman (b1886)
1289, 3421

Shanamova, A. N. (19th C)
205

Shane, Jessie F. (b1859) 2345

Sharkhovaya, S. (19/20th C)
736

Sharp, Ethel Hill (1876-1952)
922

Sharp, Helen Carmeleta (b1905)
2538

Sharring, Isadora see Powers,
Isadora Sharring

Shattuck, Elizabeth (19/20th C?)
2531, 3447, 3754

Shaw, Anna Howard (1847-1919)
967, 1164, 1694, 1825, 3644

Shearman, Ann Matlack (b1905)
3177

Shemonsky, Natalie Kaplin
(b1934) 1797

Shepard, Louisa (19th C) 803

Sheppard, Alice Elizabeth
(b1898) 1817

Sheppard, Amy (20th C) 2705

Sherbon, Florence Brown (b1869)
1000, 1440, 1748

Sheriff, Hilla (b1903) 1698

Sherman, Jeanette Hurd (b1875)
4079

Sherwood, Mary (b1856) 1792

Sherwood, Rosetta see Hall,
Rosetta Sherwood

Shih Mei-Yu see Stone, Mary

Shipp, Ellis Reynolds (1847-
1939) 1533, 1632

Shively-Nelson, Ida May (1868-
1947) 1678

Shlikova, V. (19th C) 376

Shmits (19th C) 729

Shoemaker, Rosemary (b1909)
1635

Short, Libby (MD 1968) 1802

Shortt, Elizabeth Smith (d1949)
12, 327

Shuey, Sarah I. (19th C) 1432,
1621

Shumova-Simanovskaya, E. O.
(19th C) 376

Shutt, Margaret Taylor (1868-
1903) 1628

Siebold, Charlotte von see
Heidenreich-von Siebold,
Charlotte Heiland

Siebold, Marie (19th C) 379,
2869

Siebold, Regina Josepha von
(1771-1849) 36, 83, 101,
479, 481, 486, 489

Siedeberg-Mackinnon, Emily
Hancock (19/20th C) 297,
306

Siegemundin, Justine (1648-
1705) 36, 69, 72, 77, 80,
101, 489

Siewers, Sarah M. (MD 1891)
1588

Simecek, Angeline Frances
(b1903) 762, 1701

Simmons, Eleanor Galt (1854-
1909) 1729

Simonovich, Rosalinda (19th
C) 380

Simpson, Abbie see Winegar,
Abbie

Simpson, Joan (medical student) (b1936) 1431

Simpson-Coleman-Burr, Carrie (1867-1944) 916

Sinclair, Julie (19th C) 3232

Sison, Honoria Herminia
Acosta see Acosta-Sison,
Honoria Herminia

Sizemova, G. A. (20th C)
723

Skimmen, Alice see Mc-
Gillwray, Alice Skimmen

Skinner-Fetterman, Faith see
Fetterman, Julia Faith Skinner

Skolfield, Jane Wilkie Manning
(b1866) 1533

Slade, Mary I. (b1850) 1164

Slater, Catherine Brown
(b1844) 1640

Slater, Iris (b1935) 2952

Slaughter, Rosalie see Morton,
Rosalie Slaughter

Slava, Draga (14th C) 13

Slobodinsky, Rachelle see Yarros, Rachelle Slobodinsky

Sloop, Emma see Fink, Emma
Sloop

Sloop, Mary T. Martin (1873-
1962) 254, 828, 915, 1205,
1705

Sloth-Brun, Thyra (20th C) 441

Smart, Isabelle Thompson
(b1869) 1375

Smith, Alice Maude (b1867)
1706

Smith, Almira Mary (1850-1923)
3232

Smith, Annie Thompson (b1895)
1215

Smith, Elizabeth C. see Secord, Elizabeth C.

Smith, Elizabeth Helen (1861-
1938) 610

Smith, Ella Marie see Marble,
Ella Marie Smith

Smith, Ethel Stackhouse (b1936)
876

Smith, Julia Holmes (1838-1930)
803, 1226, 2100

Smith, Margaret H. D. (b1915)
2496

Smith, Mary Alma (1850-1923)
1035, 1501

Smith, Mary Joyce (b1934)
1484, 3843

Smith, Mary Mackenzie see
Mackenzie, Mary Smith

Smith, Nora (b1935) 2952

Smith, Pat (20th C) 1779

Smith, Pearl (b1883) 1163

Smith, Susan Maria see Mc-
Kinney, Susan Maria Smith

Smith-Shortt, Elizabeth see
Shortt, Elizabeth Smith

Snoddy, Mary Jane see Whetstone, Mary Jane Snoddy

Snow, Edith (20th C) 1774

Snyder, Carolyn Hannah see
Pincock, Carolyn Hannah
Snyder

Snyder, Elizabeth Ryland (1857?-
1945) 1723

Sokolova-Ponomareva, O. D.
    (20th C)   723
Solera   62
Solis, Jeanne Cady (1867-1947)
    1557, 1682
Solis, Manuela (b1862)   422
Somerville, Margaret Ewart
    see Colby, Margaret Ewart
Sorenson, Mary (19/20th C)
    1045
Soriano, Elise (20th C) 3890,
    3897
Sorrentini, Emilia (20th C)
    3363
South, Lillian Herald (b1878)
    1439
Southey, Eleanor see Baker-
    McLaglan, Eleanor Southey
Soyster, Eliza Shumaker
    (b1923) 1515
Spaangberg, Marie see Holth,
    Marie Spaangberg
Spackman, Mary Dora (20th C)
    2335
Span, Julia (19th C) 2527
Spangborg, Helga see Holth,
    Helga Spangborg
Speetjens, Anna see Paraclita,
    Sr. M.
Spencer, Myrtle see Lockwood,
    Myrtle Spencer
Sperry, Mary A. (MD 1890)
    1068
Spiegel, Else (d1960)   626
Spiegelman, Anna (b1903)
    2952
Spitaleri, Joan Florence (b1935)
    2952
Spivack, Elizabeth F. Cole
    (b1930) 3127   ·
Sprague, Minnie Dell see
    Baker, Minnie Dell Sprague
Spurlock, M. Jeanne (b1921)
    756
Stacey-Cleminson, Florence
    (d1935)   494
Stacy, Ethel Maud (1876-1938)
    516
Staley, Mildred (20th C)   3201
Stanford, Lois Brooke Foote
    (b1896) 1218
Stang, Regina (20th C) 442,
    3355

Stannard, Amy Nivison (b1894)
    2339
Stanojevicj, Nadezda S. (b1887)
    388a
Starbuck, Amber Angelia (b1878)
    1075
Starkowskie, Wandzie (19/20th
    C) 391
Starr, Lillis Adora see Wood,
    Lillis Adora
Stasova, Nadezhda Vasilyevna
    see Suslova, Nadya Proko-
    fievna
Stastny, Olga Frances (b1878)
    831, 1050, 1231, 1547, 1548,
    1605, 1719, 1720, 3407
Stebbins, Margaret (b1914) 1661
Stecksén, Anna (1870-1904) 473,
    474, 2159
Stein, Helen Dym (b1931) 2952
Steinbiss, Viktoria (20th C?)
    2178
Steiner-Wourlisch, Aida (1896-
    1931) 446
Stenhouse, Evangeline (b1893)
    1791
Stephens, J. (18th C) 135
Stephens, Nannie A. (MD 1878) 2
Stephenson, Bette (20th C) 356
Stephenson, Catherine (20th C)
    2471
Stephenson, Violet Elma (b1924)
    3177
Steppanen, Anni (20th C) 470
Stern, Lena (20th C) 2671
Stetler, Pearl Mae (b1884)
    1804
Stevens, Annie Margaret see
    Rundell, Annie Margaret
    Stevens
Stevens, Caroline North (b1874)
    1164
Stevens, J. 135
Stevens, Marion C. (19/20th C)
    2682
Stevenson, Milda Ida (19th C) 2536
Stevenson, Sarah Hackett (1841-
    1929) 1178, 1196, 1382,
    1497, 1631, 1640, 2021,
    2100, 2354f, 3516, 4032
Steward, Susan Maria Smith
    McKinney see McKinney,
    Susan Maria Smith

Stewart, Adelle see Hutchin-
son, Adelle Stewart
Stewart, Agnes see Frost,
Mary Elizabeth
Stewart, Eleanor Bittinger
Wolf (b1886) 3338
Stewart, Mary R. (b1875)
1725
Stewart, Wendy (b1906)
1793
Stewart, Zella White (1878-
1943) 1436, 1724, 1847
Stimson, Barbara Bartlett
(b1898) 1536, 1827, 2709,
2714, 2746
Stinson, Mary H. (19/20th C)
2531
Stockham, Alice Bunker (d1913)
1196, 4017
Stokvis-Cohen Stuart, N. (20th
C) 1850, 2261
Stoltz, Elise (MD 1894) 442
Stone, Alice see Woolley,
Alice Stone
Stone, Clara (b1883) 7, 796
Stone, Constance (20th C) 6,
7, 796, 3861
Stone, Elizer Pfeifer (20th C)
236
Stone, Harriette see Mc-
Calmont-Stone, Harriette Os-
born
Stone, Mary (aka Mei-yu Shih)
(b1873) 4, 362, 368, 371,
372, 374, 2592, 3853
Stone, Mary Page (19th C)
796
Stoney, Edith (20th C) 3272
Stoney, Florence Ada (d1932)
467, 611
Stowe, Emily Howard (1832-
1903) 12, 328, 333, 356
Stowe, Emily Jennings (19th C)
161
Stowe-Gullen, Augusta Ann
(1857-1935) 12, 308, 339,
356
Stranger, Doreen M. see
Robinson, Doreen M. Stran-
ger
Strong, Martha Cochrane
(b1843) 1670
Struthers, Jacqueline (b1935)

2952
Stuart, Anabel McG. (19/20th
C) 863
Stuart, N. see Stokvis-Cohen
Stuart, N.
Sturges, Annie see Daniel,
Annie Sturges
Sturgis, Katharine R. (b1903)
1797
Sturgis, Margaret Castex (1885-
1962) 1211, 1362, 1385,
3605
Suat, Rasim Kizi (19/20th C)
3830
Subbotina, E. (19th C) 376
Sullivan, Margaret P. (b1922)
4026
Summerskill, Edith (19/20th C)
699
Sundberg, Maria see Ingelman-Sundberg, Maria
Sundquist, Alma (1872-1940)
426, 436, 441, 2159, 3355,
3359, 3895
Suslova, Nadya Prokofievna
(d1895) 64, 139, 157, 158,
197, 205, 209, 376, 380,
734, 739, 2869, 2881, 3225,
3232, 3905
Sutherland, Annie Christina
(1869-1933) 570
Sutton, Lucy Porter (b1891)
1024
Svartz, Nanna (20th C) 44,
471, 3898
Šviglin-Čavov, Milica (MD 1893)
13
Svyatlovskaya, Raisa Samoilovna
(1853-1914) 2676
Swain, Clara A. (1834-1910)
220, 1134, 1164, 1235, 1497,
2116, 2527, 2532, 2604,
2643, 2649, 2652, 2655,
3142, 3507, 3509, 3570,
3702
Swain, Mary Lizzie (MD 1877)
786
Swigart, Leslie see Kent,
Leslie Swigart
Sykes, Elisabeth (20th C) 558
Szagunn, Ilse Tesch (b1887)
488
Szczawinska, Wanda (1866-

1955)   404

Szendeffy, Ida (MD 1897)   16

Szentpeterr, Ilonka (19th C)
16

Taggart, M. Barbara (20th C)
3857

Talbot, Nancy see Clark-
Binney, Nancy Elizabeth Talbot

Talbot, Rose see Bullard,
Rose Talbot

Talyzina, N. K. (20th C)   723

Tamm, Afhild (19/20th C)   44

Tapman, Bertha see Shamer,
Bertha Tapman

Tarbell, Mabel Richards
(b1886)   1532

Tarrash, Hertha (b1900)   1223

Taussig, Helen B. (b1898)
697, 887, 1008, 1092,
1582, 1710

Taverna, Raimonda Di (Middle
Ages)   60

Taylor, Ann Gray (b1893)
1445

Taylor, Eleanor Jane see
Calverley, Eleanor Jane
Taylor

Taylor, Lois see Ellison,
Lois Taylor

Taylor-Jones, Louise (b1871)
790, 1644, 3740

Teleky, Dora (MD 1904)   3234

Temple, Ruth Janetta (b1892)
856

Tertre, Marguerite de la
Marche see de la Marche,
Marguerite (Margarethe)

Tesch, Ilse see Szagunn,
Ilse Tesch

Thackrah, Margaret (d1937)
643

Theano   62

Thelander, Hulda Evelyn
(b1896)   1532, 1608, 1744

Thelberg, Elizabeth Burr
(b1860)   958, 1096, 1439,
3576, 3597

Thomas, Edna Lyle (20th C)
694

Thomas, Isabel I. see Day,

Isabel I. Thomas

Thomas, Julia Carlile (MD
1891)   300

Thomas, Mary Alice Howe
(b1922)   1871

Thomas, Mary Frame Myers
(1816-1888)   796, 1714,
1784

Thompson, Augusta Louise see
Rosenthal-Thompson, Augusta
Louise

Thompson, Lucia Redding (MD
1891)   1199

Thompson, Mary (19/20th C)
3755

Thompson, Mary Anna Cooke
(1825-1919)   1080, 1119

Thompson, Mary Harris (1829-
1895)   1198, 1253, 1408,
1455, 1496, 1689, 3566,
3659, 3705, 3721, 3764,
3823

Thompson, Sue Hurst see
Gould, Sue Hurst Thompson

Thompson-Stevens, Mary Ella
(b1864)   1680

Thomson, Bertha Virginia
(b1861)   1574, 1579

Thorbecke, Geertruida Jeanette
(b1929)   1003

Thorburn-Johnstone, Mabel
(20th C)   677

Thorne, Isabel (medical student)
(b1853?)   109, 119, 124,
678, 3310

Thorne, May (19/20th C)   624

Thornton, Irene see Nesbitt,
Irene Thornton

Thorpe, Juliet M. (19th C)   1606

Thuillier-Landry, L. (20th C)
3355

Tiburtius, Franziska (1843-
1927)   101, 108, 180, 480,
482, 491, 492, 632, 2869,
3232, 3908, 3940

Tichauer, Ruth Wresinski (20th
C)   713

Tillman, Mary Anne Tuggle
(b1935)   756

Timms, Edna D. (1869-1910)
1080

Tingvald-Hannikainen, Gota
(20th C)   3907

Tinley, Mary Louise (1869-
1953) 827
Tissheim, Catharine (17th C)
135
Tkatcheff, Alexandrine (20th
C) 3940
Toland, Gertrude M. B. (20th
C) 2710
Tomaszewicz-Dobrska, Anna
(1854-1918) 381-383, 385,
392, 393, 404, 3232
Toral, Petra Bonilla (b1866)
715
Towers, Elizabeth A. (20th
C) 1751
Towles, Caroline Benson
Shamer (b1872) 3421
Townsend-Glassen, Mary
(1902-1972) 1418, 1786
Tracy, Martha (1876-1942)
243, 701, 1360, 1361,
1626, 1789, 3389, 3509,
3522, 3626, 3753, 4007
Trapp, Ethlyn (1891-1972)
356, 2669
Trask, Sigourney (19th C)
2527, 2655
Travell, Janet see Powell,
Janet Travell
Travis, Elma Allen (1860-
1917) 1199
Trento, Brunetta di (Middle
Ages) 70
Tretjakova, Eugeniia Niko-
laevna (20th C) 733
Trotula de Ruggiero Platerius
(d1097) 22, 23, 26, 31, 43,
48, 49, 58-62, 64, 69, 70,
75, 76, 132, 138, 149,
150, 152, 162, 175, 178
Trotula of Salerno see Trotula
de Ruggiero Platerius
Trout, Emily (19/20th C) 12
Trout, Jennie Gowanlock
(d1921) 333, 356
Trowell, Amy Becky (medical
student) (b1946) 3098
T'Sao, Li Yuin (MD 1911) 370
Tse-Tse, Rosie see Young,
Rosie Tse-Tse
Tucker, Emma Boose (b1870)
1525, 1662, 1769
Tucker, Margaret Emmeline

(b1907) 1662
Turnbull, Jane H. (1871-1958)
582
Turner-Watts, [Dr.] (20th C)
3840
Turpin, Mollie (20th C) 1176
Tussenbroek, Catherine van
(1852-1925) 66, 461, 2261,
3901
Tydeman, Emily F. (1870-1945)
1208
Tylicka, Justyra see Budzin-
ska-Tylicka, Justyna
Tyson, Frances Bartlett see
Bartlett-Tyson, Frances

Ulezro-Stroganova, K. A. (19/
20th C) 207
Ulrich, Mabel S[imus] (b1876)
1633, 1759
Underwood, Lillias Horton see
Horton-Underwood, Lillias
Upjohn, Helen Maria (1839-1901)
1685
Upjohn, Millie Kirby (19th C)
1670

Vachovskaya, V. (19th C) 376
Vadillo Gutiérrez, Consuelo
(20th C) 694, 716
Van Cortlandt, Elizabeth see
Hocker, Elizabeth M. Van
Cortlandt
Van den Blink-Rolder, J. W.
see Blink-Rolder, J. W. van
den
Vandervall, Isabella (19/20th C)
3154
Van Diest, Anne Catherine Al-
bertine Isala (1842-1916) 423
Van Dorp-Beucker, Andreae van
see Dorp-Beucker, Andreae
van
Van Gasken, Frances C. (1860-
1939) 1143
van Heerden, Petronella (20th
C) 264
Van Herwerden, Marianne see
Herwerden, Marianne van
Van Hoosen, Bertha (1863-1952)
1438, 2095, 3638, 3705, 3805

Biographies 1149, 1459,
1681, 1764, 3559
Honors and awards 746,
1229, 1233
Surgical skills 1736, 2312,
3157
Travels 1765-1773, 3376,
3378
Tributes, memorials 1460,
1550, 3782
Van Loon, Emily Lois (b1898)
699
Vann, Elizabeth Rogers (b1897)
1220
Van Schoonhoven, Mary Emma
(MD 1891) 1533
Van't Land, Gerda see Land,
Gerda van't
Van Tusschenbroek, Catherine
see Tussenbroek, Catherine
van
Vargas, Tegualda Ponce see
Ponce-Vargas, Tegualda
Varman, E. G. (20th C) 723
Varney-Brownell, Emily A.
(d1906) 1305
Vasconcelos, Ermelinda Lopes
de (d1952) 196, 721
Vasseur, Irma see LeVas-
seur, Irma
Vassilaidon, Anthe (20th C)
448
Vaughan, Kate Marion (d1926)
631
Vaughan-Sawyer (19/20th C)
2193
Vaupel-Clark, Margaret (1853-
1932) 784
Vedin, Alma (MD 1899) 960
Vejjabul, Pierra Hoon see
Pierra Hoon Vejjabul
Veres, Palne (19/20th C)
16
Veretennikova, A. I. (19/20th
C) 207, 735
Verghese, Mary (b1926) 285
Vernier, Jean (1874-1942)
919
Vickery, Alice (19/20th C)
635
Vilar, Lola (20th C) 472
Vincent, Jane (19th C) 1754
Vines, Charlotte S. (19/20th C)

2635
Virdimura (Middle Ages) 70
Vitale, Frederica (1059-1080)
15, 59, 70
Vögtlin, Marie Heim (1845-
1916) 72, 463, 468, 3905
Volna, Grażyna (1919-1974)
410
Von Bose, Edda (b1887) 1444
von Poswick, Gisela (1875-1940)
1615
Von Roll, Barbara (1502-1571)
54
Von Roth, Georgine (19/20th C)
475
Voorhis, Anna H. (b1866) 965
Votaw, May (b1931) 1428
Vucetic-Prita, Marija (1866-
1954) 388
Vuckovich, Nancy Jean (b1947)
1508

Wadleigh, Lydia (1817-1888)
3482
Waffle, Willella Howe (b1854)
236
Wagner, Mathilde (19/20th C)
99
Wagner, Ruth Evangeline (b1892)
1444
Waite, Lucy (19th C) 2100,
3764
Waite, Netta May (1868-1925?)
1209
Wakefield, Emma (19/20th C)
3936
Walker, Ada Francis Harris
(b1889) 1520
Walker, Eliza (19th C) 3232
Walker, Emma Elizabeth (b1864)
2358
Walker, Helen see McAndrew,
Helen Walker
Walker, Jane Harriett (d1938)
512, 537, 588, 4072
Walker, Maggie Laura (b1918)
756
Walker, Mary (20th C) 552
Walker, Mary Edwards (1832-
1919) 132, 218, 247, 788,
868, 961, 1047, 1048, 1084,
1085, 1234, 1451, 1514,

1578, 1600, 1712, 1834,
2794, 2864, 3795, 4054
Wallace, Ada Isabella Wilson
(b1896) 318
Wallace, Ellen Alfleda (b1853)
995, 1558, 1747
Wallace, Helen Margaret
(b1913) 822
Wallace, Joyce Irene (b1940)
2102
Wallace-Russell, Julia Eastman
(19th C) 1558, 3780
Wallin, Mathilda Kristina
(b1858) 1348, 1426
Walrath, Belle (1849-1910)
786
Walter, Josephine (MD 1882)
1224
Walter, Regina Rosa (19/20th
C) 3234
Walters, Bernice R. ("Burma")
(b1912) 1317
Walters, Mary Jane (b1894)
1079
Wang, Hsiao-Chen (fictional)
4060
Wang, Pao Chun (20th C)
3192
Wanstrom, Ruth Cecilia (b1893)
1219, 3805
Wanzer, Lucy Maria Field
(b1841) 138, 236, 863,
1463
Ward, Mildred Elsie (b1913)
3177
Warfield, Mary Cabell (b1894)
1220
Warner, Estella Ford (1891-
1974) 180, 821, 1112,
1132, 3550
Warner, Helen Frances (1843-
1905) 1685
Warner, Nancy Elizabeth
(b1923) 1512
Warner-Cook, Dana G. (1855-
1932) 917
Warren, Marjory Winsome
(d1960) 618
Wartha, Vilma see Hugonni-
Wartha, Vilma
Watarai, Sono (pre-20th C)
3199
Waterston, Jane (d1932) 685,

698
Watney, Lilian Enid (d1933)
503
Watson, Alexandra (Mona) Mary
Chalmers (d1936) 615
Watson, Anna Boggs (b1867)
1521
Watters, Ethel M. (b1888)
1815
Watters, Hyla S. (b1893) 1242
Wauchope, Gladys Mary (20th C)
687
Waugh, Elizabeth Sides (b1904)
1359
Way, Edith Waldie (b1882)
1208
Weaver, Ruth Hartley (1893-
1973) 807, 1448
Weber, Laura E. (b1914) 1659
Webster, Gladys M. R. (d1925?)
632
Webster, Helen Baker Worthing-
ton (1837-1904) 1496
Webster, Sr. Frances (20th C)
2625
Weinberg, Ethel Schwartz
(b1936) 2074
Weintrauben, Barbara (pre-18th
C) 135, 1943
Weiseger, Ethel M. Sutton
(b1905) 756
Weitz, Hanna (20th C) 273
Weizenblatt, Sprinza (b1898)
1218
Wells, Beulah (b1886) 1762
Welpton, Martha (b1884) 3355
Welsh, Lilian (1858-1938) 1753,
1792
Wengberg, Hilma (19/20th C)
44
Wensel, Louise Oftedal (b1918)
1599
Werne, Joellen (b1944) 1802
West, Emma Jane (1859-1927)
918
Westgate, Letitia (b1866) 1334
Wetmore, Mary Rhoda (1870-
1944) 917
Weyman, Else M. Krug (b1915)
2492
Wharton, May Cravath (b1873)
1796
Wheelock, Zilpha Rosannah Baily

(1854-1919) 1680

Wherry, Marie Nast (20th C)
1168

Whetstone, Mary Jane Snoddy
(1849-1929) 786, 787

Whipper, Ionia Rollin (b1875)
3666

Whipple, Electa B. (1848-1907)
1144

White, Frances Emily (d1903)
1630, 3552

White, Jean G. (b1927) 3205

White, Julia A. (b1875) 920

White, Margaret Ellen (b1927)
3861

White, Marguerite (19/20th C)
2713

White, Maria (19th C) 2633,
2636-2642

White, Priscilla (b1900) 887,
1092, 1532, 1710

White, Zella see Stewart,
Zella White

Whitehead, Charlotte see
Ross, Charlotte Whitehead

Whiteside, Margaret (b1880)
1210

Whitmore, Clara Beatrice
(b1873) 3200

Whitney-Morse, Jean Calista
Harris (1872-1940) 1678

Whittaker, Mary Achsah (1853-
1928) 1681

Whitten, Kathryn Marion (b1882)
189, 1300

Widerström, Karolina Olivia
(1856-1941?) 44, 63, 71,
419, 420, 441, 2154, 2159,
3895, 3898

Wiedmann, Barbara (17/18th
C) 36

Wijnen, M. Elise (20th C) 3430

Wikander-Brunander, Siri
(19/20th C) 44

Wilberforce, Octavia Margaret
(1888-1963) 583

Wilcox, Lucinda Sexton (b1820)
1686

Wildenow (19th C) 1943

Wilkerson, Nina Copeland (1890-
1946) 1675

Wilkes, Addie (d1958) 641

Wilkins, Jeanette (b1936) 1829

Willard, Luvia Margaret (b1882)
3404, 3601, 3712

Willets, May (19th C?) 3509

Willey, Florence see Barrett,
Florence Willey

Williams, Anna Wessels (b1863)
968, 2494

Williams, Cicely Delphin (b1893)
533

Williams, Clara (b1870) 3582

Williams, Ethel Lauretta Hennes-
sy (b1893) 2411

Williams, F. Marian (b1903)
1544, 4023

Williams, Mary Achsah see
Whittaker, Mary Achsah

Williams, Mary Edith (1883-
1956) 1722

Williamson, Cecilia F. (1884-
1964) 523

Willits, Emma K. (b1869) 1086

Wills, Lucy (d1964) 565, 653

Willson, Sara Thomasina see
Chase-Willson, Sara Thomasina

Wilson, Ida M. (b1866) 1201

Wilson, Kathleen (b1886) 670

Wilson, May Georgiana (b1890)
887

Wilson, Miriam (b1922) 1829

Windsor, Sarah Sweet (MD 1885)
693

Winegar, Abbie (20th C) 1678

Wink, Helena Knauf (b1854)
1193, 1315

Winsome, Marjory see War-
ren, Marjory Winsome

Winterhalter, Elise (19th C?)
2869

Wistein, Rosina (1867-1937)
936, 1054

Withington, Alfreda Bosworth
(b1860) 1121, 1809-1812

Witthoff, Evelyn (b1912) 1118,
1813

Wittner, Asta J. (b1902) 2952

Woerner, Lydia (b1860) 3338

Wojcik, Ladislas D. (b1918)
2496

Wolcott, Laura J. see Ross-
Wolcott, Laura J.

Wolf, Eleanor B. see Stewart,
Eleanor Bittinger Wolf

Wolf, Helena   407
Wolfe, Mary Moore (b1874)
     1823
Wolley, Anna (17th C)   135
Wollstein, Martha (b1868)   3576
Wong, Helena (20th C)   375
Wong, Louise May (b1949)
     1345
Wong, Rose Victoria Goong
     (b1896)   892
Woo, Theresa Ting (b1911)
     2748
Wood, Jane E. (d1931?)   555
Wood, Lillis Adora (1865-1938)
     1677
Wood-Allen, Mary (1841-1909)
     889, 1144
Woodhull, Kate C. (10th C)   2583
Woodman, Marjorie (b1897)
     3703
Woodroffe, Helen L. Hill
     (b1878)   2684
Woodward-Marshall, Louie
     Frances (MD 1945)   1034
Woodworth, Elizabeth A.
     (b1864)   1240
Woodzicka, Julia L. (b1865)
     1292
Wooley, Mary E. (20th C)
     770
Woolley, Alice Stone (1882-
     1946)   751, 752, 840, 958,
     1333, 1739, 3419
Woolston, Henrietta B. (19th
     C)   2527, 2534
Wortley, Mary see Montague,
     Mary Wortley
Wright, Jane Cooke (b1919)
     741, 756, 1012-1015,
     1272, 1559
Wright, Katharine Wright
     (b1892)   1476
Wyne, Sr. M. Elise (20th C)
     2645
Wynekoop, Alice Lois Lindsay
     (MD 1895)   1764, 3823
Wynen, Elizabeth (19/20th C)
     2649

Yamei Kin see Kin, Yamei
Yaroslavovna, Olga see Rezha-
     bek, Olga Yaroslavovna

Yarros, Rachelle Slobodinsky
     (MD 1894)   1066, 1438,
     1774, 1844, 1845, 2323,
     3188, 4022
Yavein, Schischkina (20th C)
     737
Yeomans, Amelia (MD 1883)
     338
Yeomans, Lilian B. (MD 1882)
     12
Yoh, Helen (MD 1930)   2541
Yonis, Bathsheba (Bat-Sheva)
     (20th C)   273, 3842
Yoshioka, Arata   3199
Yoshioka, Yayoi (1871-1959)
     286, 3195, 3199, 3203, 3837,
     3844, 3856, 3860
You-me May King see Kin,
     Yamei
Young, Anna M. (b1898)   1324,
     1747
Young, Charlotte Soutter Mur-
     doch (d1947)   1469
Young, Edith Louisa (d1930?)
     669
Young, Evangeline Wilson (b1874)
     3548
Young, Lois A. (b1934)   756
Young, Nellie Louise (b1907)
     756
Young, Rosie Tse-Tse (MD
     1959)   284
Young, Ruth (19/20th C)   2116
Ytting, Helene (20th C)   417
Yu, Poe-Eng see Hu, King
     Eng

Zachariasz, Janina   407
Zakrzewska, Marie Elizabeth
     (1829-1902)
     158, 219, 239, 249, 799,
     1390, 1394, 3809
     Biographies   161, 212, 891,
     1134, 1389, 1493, 1585,
     1711, 1778, 4034
     New England Infirmary for
     Women and Children   247,
     1391, 1392, 3444, 3446,
     3447, 3576, 3647, 3703
     Reminiscences by others
     844, 929, 1238, 1395, 1396,
     1814

Work with other physicians
888, 1164, 1364, 1393

Zalivako, M. T. (20th C) 730

Zandowa, Natalia see Zilberlast-Zandowa, Natalia

Zawisch-Ossenitz, Carla (MD
1923) 55

Zay, Dr. (fictional) 4058,
4062

Zeller, Fredericka C. (d1944)
1256

Zerlin (of Frankfurt) (15th C)
70, 155, 1943

Zeterberg, Marie Therese
(b1928) 2952

Ziber-Shumova, N. O. (19th
C) 376

Zibold, Maria Alexandrovna
(19th C) 2676

Ziegler, Amelia (b1861) 1080

Zilberlast-Zandowa, Natalia
(20th C) 404

Zimmerman, Jean Turner
(d1927) 1591

Zotova, O. D. (20th C) 723

15